AF327314

OPERATIVE CHALLENGES IN
OTOLARYNGOLOGY–HEAD AND
NECK SURGERY

Operative Challenges in Otolaryngology–Head and Neck Surgery

Harold C. Pillsbury III, M.D., F.A.C.S.
Professor and Chief
Division of Otolaryngology–Head and Neck Surgery
University of North Carolina School of Medicine
Chapel Hill, North Carolina

Manning M. Goldsmith III, M.D.
Clinical Assistant Professor
Division of Otolaryngology–Head and Neck Surgery
University of North Carolina School of Medicine
Chapel Hill, North Carolina

YEAR BOOK MEDICAL PUBLISHERS, INC.
CHICAGO • LONDON • BOCA RATON • LITTLETON, MASS.

1 2 3 4 5 6 7 8 9 0 P R 94 93 92 91 90

Library of Congress Cataloging-in-Publication Data
Operative challenges in otolaryngology : head and neck surgery /
 [edited by] Harold C. Pillsbury III, Manning M. Goldsmith III.
   p.   cm.
   Includes bibliographical references.
   ISBN 0-8151-6708-3
   1. Head—Surgery. 2. Neck—Surgery. 3. Surgery, Plastic.
 I. Pillsbury, Harold C. II. Goldsmith, Manning M.
   [DNLM: 1. Head—surgery. 2. Neck—surgery. 3. Surgery,
   Plastic.
 WE 705 061]
 RF51.06 1990   89-25050
 617.5'1—dc20   CIP
 DNLM/DLC
 for Library of Congress

Sponsoring Editor: David K. Marshall
Assistant Managing Editor, Text and Reference: Jan Gardner
Production Project Coordinator: Gayle Paprocki
Proofroom Supervisor: Barbara M. Kelly

*To my wife, Sally; my parents, Harold C. Jr.
and Athena; and my children, Matt, Ben, and
Tom, who supported me, nurtured me, and
provided me the positive outlook it took to
produce this volume.*

H. C. P.

*To the residents who asked these questions; to
Ruth, Miles, David, and Ben, who patiently
awaited these answers; and to my parents and
Mrs. Beulah Harper, who taught me to
communicate both.*

M. M. G.

CONTRIBUTORS

I. KAUFMAN ARENBERG, M.D., F.A.C.S.
Clinical Associate Professor of Otolaryngology
University of Colorado Health Science Center
Director Audio Vestibular Lab
Swedish Medical Center
Engelwood, Colorado

THOMAS BALKANY, M.D., F.A.C.S., F.A.A.P.
Adjunct Professor
University of Northern Colorado
Director of Research
Colorado Otologic Research Center
Attending Surgeon
Porter Memorial Hospital
Denver, Colorado

W. PAUL BIGGERS, M.D., F.A.C.S.
Professor, Division of Otolaryngology–Head and
  Neck Surgery
University of North Carolina School of Medicine
Attending Physician
North Carolina Memorial Hospital
Chapel Hill, North Carolina

ROGER BOLES, M.D.
Professor and Chairman
Department of Otolaryngology
University of California at San Francisco
San Francisco, California

EUGENE M. BOZYMSKI, M.D.
Professor of Medicine
University of North Carolina School of Medicine
Chief, Division of Digestive Diseases and Nutrition
Diagnostic and Treatment Center
North Carolina University Hospital
Chapel Hill, North Carolina

DERALD E. BRACKMAN, M.D.
Clinical Professor of Otolaryngology
University of Southern California
Chief of Otology
St. Vincent Medical Center
Los Angeles, California

NICHOLAS J. CASSISI, D.D.S., M.D.
Professor and Chief
Division of Otolaryngology
Department of Surgery
University of Florida
Shands Hospital
Gainesville, Florida

J. RICHARD CASUCCIO, M.D.
Attending Physician
Plastic and Reconstructive Surgery and Loudoun Hospital
  Center
Attending Physician
Otolaryngology–Head and Neck Surgery
Reston Hospital Center
Reston, Virginia

MACK L. CHENEY, M.D.
Department of Otolaryngology
Harvard Medical School
Boston, Massachusetts

NEWTON J. COKER, M.D.
Associate Professor
Baylor College of Medicine
The Methodist Hospital
Houston, Texas

ROBIN T. COTTON, M.D.
Professor, Otolaryngology and Maxillofacial Surgery
University of Cincinnati
Director, Otolaryngology and Maxillofacial Surgery
Children's Hospital Medical Center
Cincinnati, Ohio

SADY S. daCOSTA
International Hearing Foundation
Sao Paulo, Brazil

DOUGLAS D. DEDO, M.D.
Clinical Assistant Professor
Otolaryngology–Head and Neck Surgery
University of Miami Medical School
Active Staff
Good Samaritan Hospital
Miami, Florida

LAWRENCE W. DeSANTO, M.D.
Professor and Chairman
Department of Otorhinolaryngology–Head and Neck Surgery
Mayo School of Medicine
Mayo Clinic—Scottsdale
Scottsdale, Arizona

AMELIA F. DRAKE, M.D.
Assistant Professor
Division of Otolaryngology–Head and Neck Surgery
University of North Carolina School of Medicine
Attending Physician
North Carolina Memorial Hospital
Chapel Hill, North Carolina

EDWARD H. FARRIOR, M.D.
Associate Clinical Professor
University of South Florida
Tampa General Hospital
Tampa, Florida

RICHARD T. FARRIOR, M.D.
Clinical Professor
University of Florida
Gainesville, Florida
University of South Florida
Tampa General Hospital
Tampa, Florida

SIDNEY S. FEUERSTEIN, M.D., F.A.C.S.
Clinical Professor
Otolaryngology–Head and Neck Surgery
Mount Sinai School of Medicine
Attending Otolaryngology
Mount Sinai Hospital
New York, New York

NEWTON D. FISCHER, M.D., F.A.C.S.
Professor
Division of Otolaryngology–Head and Neck Surgery
University of North Carolina School of Medicine
Attending Physician
North Carolina Memorial Hospital
Chapel Hill, North Carolina

M. SEAN FREEMAN, M.D.
Resident Physician
Department of Otolaryngology
Washington University
St. Louis, Missouri

TERRY L. FRY, M.D., F.A.C.S.
Associate Professor
Division of Otolaryngology–Head and Neck Surgery
University of North Carolina School of Medicine
Attending Physician
North Carolina Memorial Hospital
Chapel Hill, North Carolina

W. P. R. GIBSON, M.D., F.R.C.S., F.R.A.C.S.
Sydney, Australia

MICHAEL E. GLASSCOCK III, M.D., F.A.C.S.
Clinical Professor of Surgery (Otology and Neurotology)
Clinical Associate Professor, Neurosurgery
Vanderbilt University School of Medicine
Nashville, Tennessee

JACK L. GLUCKMAN, M.D., F.A.C.S.
Professor of Otolaryngology
Associate Dean for Clinical Affairs
University of Cincinnati
Cincinnati, Ohio

MANNING M. GOLDSMITH III, M.D.
Clinical Assistant Professor
Division of Otolaryngology–Head and Neck Surgery
University of North Carolina School of Medicine
Chapel Hill, North Carolina

JEROME C. GOLDSTEIN, M.D., F.A.C.S.
Visiting Professor
Otolaryngology–Head and Neck Surgery
The Johns Hopkins Medical Center
Baltimore, Maryland
Adjunct Professor, Otolaryngology
Albany Medical Center
Albany, New York

KENNETH M. GRUNDFAST, M.D., F.A.C.S., F.A.A.P.
Associate Professor
Division of Otolaryngology
George Washington University School of Medicine
Chairman, Department of Otolaryngology
Children's National Medical Center
Washington, D.C.

PATRICK J. GULLANE, M.D., F.R.C.S.(C)
Associate Professor
Department of Otolaryngology
University of Toronto
Deputy Otolaryngologist-in-Chief
Toronto General Hospital
Toronto, Canada

STEVEN D. HANDLER, M.D.
Associate Professor of Otolaryngology and Human
* Communication*
University of Pennsylvania School of Medicine
Associate Director of Pediatric Otolaryngology
The Children's Hospital of Philadelphia
Philadelphia, Pennsylvania

MICHAEL J. HOLLIDAY, M.D.
Associate Professor
Department of Otolaryngology–Head and Neck Surgery
The Johns Hopkins Hospital
Baltimore, Maryland

JACK VAN DOREN HOUGH, M.D.
Clinical Professor
Otolaryngology–Head and Neck Surgery
University of Oklahoma Health Sciences Center
Chairman, Department of Otolaryngology–Head and
* Neck Surgery*
Baptist Medical Center of Oklahoma
Oklahoma City, Oklahoma

WILLIAM F. HOUSE, M.D.
Clinical Professor of Otolaryngology
University of Southern California School of Medicine
Active Staff—Otology
St. Vincent Medical Center
Los Angeles, California

C. GARY JACKSON, M.D., F.A.C.S.
Associate Clinical Professor
Otology and Neurotology
Vanderbilt University School of Medicine
Nashville, Tennessee

FEDERICK JANCZVK, D.O.
Fellow—Cosmetic Surgery
The Graduate Hospital
Philadelphia, Pennsylvania

HERMAN A. JENKINS, M.D.
Professor and Vice Chairman
Department of Otorhinolaryngology and Communicative
Sciences
Baylor College of Medicine
Houston, Texas

MICHAEL E. JOHNS, M.D.
Andelot Professor and Chairman
Department of Otolaryngology–Head and Neck Surgery
Dean
The Johns Hopkins University School of Medicine
Baltimore, Maryland

GLENN D. JOHNSON, M.D.
Assistant Professor of Clinical Surgery (Otology and
Neurotology)
Dartmouth-Hitchcock Medical Center
Clinical Staff
Mary Hitchcock Memorial Hospital
Hanover, New Hampshire

JONAS T. JOHNSON, M.D., F.A.C.S.
Professor and Vice Chairman of Otolaryngology
University of Pittsburgh
Eye and Ear Hospital
Pittsburgh, Pennsylvania

RALEIGH O. JONES, JR., M.D
Chief, Division of Otolaryngology–Head and Neck Surgery
University of Kentucky College of Medicine
A. B. Chandler Medical Center
Lexington, Kentucky

ALFRED D. KATZ, M.D.
Chief of Head and Neck Clinic
Attending Surgeon
Cedars-Sinai Medical Center
Los Angeles, California

ROBERT M. KELLMAN, M.D.
Director, Maxillofacial Trauma Surgery
Assistant Professor
Department of Otolaryngology and Pediatrics
State University of New York
Health Sciences Center at Syracuse
Syracuse, New York

JOHN L. KEMINK, M.D.
Associate Professor
University of Michigan Medical Center
Department of Otolaryngology–Head and Neck Surgery
Director, Division of Otology, Neurotology and Skull Base
Surgery
University of Michigan Hospitals
Ann Arbor, Michigan

MARGARET A. KENNA, M.D.
Associate Professor
Surgery (Otolaryngology) and Pediatrics
Yale University School of Medicine
Attending Physician
Yale-New Haven Hospital
New Haven, Connecticut

DAVID W. KENNEDY, M.D.
Associate Professor
Otolaryngology–Head and Neck Surgery and Neurosurgery
The John Hopkins Medical Institutions
Attending Physician
The Johns Hopkins Hospital
Baltimore, Maryland

EUGENE B. KERN, M.D., M.S.
Professor of Otorhinolaryngology
Mayo Medical School
Rochester, Minnesota

YOSEF P. KRESPI, M.D.
Professor and Chairman
Department of Otolaryngology
State University of New York
Health Sciences Center at Brooklyn
Chief, Department of Otolaryngology
Long Island College Hospital
Brooklyn, New York

PAUL A. LEVINE, M.D.
Professor and Vice-Chairman
Department of Otolaryngology–Head and Neck Surgery
Director, Division of Head and Neck Surgical Oncology
University of Virginia Health Sciences Center
Charlottesville, Virginia

RICHARD J. LIPTON, M.D.
Instructor in Otolaryngology
Mayo Medical School
Chief Resident Associate
Department of Otolaryngology
Mayo Clinic
Rochester, Minnesota

WILLIAM F. LUXFORD, M.D.
Clinical Assistant Professor of Otolaryngology
University of Southern California School of Medicine
Associate, House Ear Institute
Los Angeles, California

ANTHONY E. MAGIT, M.D.
Division of Otolaryngology
Duke University Medical Center
Durham, North Carolina

LEONARD I. MALIS, M.D.
Professor and Chairman
Department of Neurosurgery
Mount Sinai School of Medicine
Neurosurgeon in Chief and Director
Mount Sinai Hospital
New York, New York

BERNARD R. MARSH, M.D.
Associate Professor
The Johns Hopkins University School of Medicine
Active Staff
The Johns Hopkins Medical Institutions
Baltimore, Maryland

ROBERT H. MATHOG, M.D.
Professor and Chairman
Wayne State University
Chairman, Department of Otolaryngology
Harper Hospital
Detroit, Michigan

DOUGLAS E. MATTOX, M.D.
Associate Professor
The Johns Hopkins Hospital
Baltimore, Maryland

JOHN T. MCELVEEN, JR., M.D.
Assistant Professor
Duke University Medical Center
Durham, North Carolina

KATHRYN E. MCGOLDRICK, M.D.
Associate Professor of Anesthesiology
Yale University School of Medicine
Attending Anesthesiologist
Yale-New Haven Hospital
New Haven, Connecticut

W. FREDERICK MCGUIRT, M.D.
Professor of Surgery (Otolaryngology)
The Bowman Gray School of Medicine
Wake Forest University
Winston-Salem, North Carolina

ROBERT H. MILLER, M.D., F.A.C.S.
Professor and Chairman
Department of Otolaryngology–Head and Neck Surgery
Tulane University School of Medicine
New Orleans, Louisiana

WILLIAM W. MONTGOMERY, A.B., M.D., F.A.C.S.
Professor of Otolaryngology
Harvard Medical School
Surgeon, Massachusetts Eye and Ear Infirmary
Boston, Massachusetts

MICHAEL R. MORRIS, M.D.
Department of Otolaryngology–Head and Neck Surgery
Madigan Army Medical Center
Tacoma, Washington

MICHAEL S. MORRIS, M.D.
Assistant Professor
Department of Otolaryngology–Head and Neck Surgery
Georgetown University Medical Center
Washington, D.C.

MANI NAMBIAR, M.D.
Kenosha Hospital and Medical Center
Kenosha, Wisconsin

J. GAIL NEELY, M.D., F.A.C.S.
Professor and Chairman
Department of Otorhinolaryngology
University of Oklahoma College of Medicine
Health Sciences Center
Oklahoma City, Oklahoma

JULIUS NEWMAN, M.D.
Chairman, Department of Cosmetic Surgery
Graduate Hospital
Chairman, Department of Cosmetic and
   Reconstructive Surgery
The Mount Sinai Hospital
Philadelphia, Pennsylvania

EDWARD A. NORFLEET, M.D.
Professor of Anesthesiology
University of North Carolina School of Medicine
Vice Chairman
Department of Anesthesiology
North Carolina Memorial Hospital
Chapel Hill, North Carolina

TIMOTHY P. O'DWYER, M.B., B.C.R., F.R.C.S.(L), F.R.C.S.
Clinical Fellow
Department of Otolaryngology
University of Toronto
Toronto General Hospital
Toronto, Ontario

JOHN DAVID OSGUTHORPE, M.D.
Professor of Otolaryngology
Medical University of South Carolina
Charleston, South Carolina

WILLIAM R. PANJE, B.S., M.S., M.D., M.S.(OTOL)
Professor and Chairman
University of Chicago Pritzker School of Medicine
Mitchell Hospital
Chicago, Illinois

MICHAEL M. PAPARELLA, M.D.
Clinical Professor and Chairman Emeritus
University of Minnesota
Department of Otolaryngology
Minnesota Ear, Head and Neck Clinic
Minneapolis, Minnesota

IRA D. PAPEL, M.D.
Director, Facial Plastic and Reconstructive Surgery
Department of Otolaryngology–Head and Neck Surgery
The Johns Hopkins Hospital
The Johns Hopkins Medical Institutions
Baltimore, Maryland

NIGEL R. T. PASHLEY, M.B., B.S., F.R.C.S.(C), F.A.A.P.
Clinical Associate Professor
University of Colorado School of Medicine
Chairman, Pediatric Otolaryngology–Head and Neck Surgery
The Children's Hospital
Denver, Colorado

N. CLIF PATTERSON, M.D., F.A.C.S.
Clinical Assistant Professor
University of North Carolina School of Medicine
Chapel Hill, North Carolina

BRUCE W. PEARSON, M.D., F.R.C.S.(C)
Serene M. and Francis C. Durling Professor of
   Otolaryngology
Mayo Medical School
Mayo Clinic—Jacksonville
Consultant in Otorhinolaryngology
St. Lukes Hospital
Jacksonville, Florida

MYLES L. PENSAK, M.D.
Associate Professor
Department of Otolaryngology
University of Cincinnati College of Medicine
Active Medical Staff
University Hospital
Cincinnati, Ohio

LOUIS G. PETCU, M.S., M.D.
Instructor, Otolaryngology
Department of Surgery
Yale University School of Medicine
Chief Resident, Otolaryngology–Head and Neck Surgery
Yale-New Haven, Hospital
New Haven, Connecticut

HAROLD C. PILLSBURY III, M.D., F.A.C.S.
Professor and Chief
Division of Otolaryngology–Head and Neck Surgery
University of North Carolina School of Medicine
Attending Physician

DENNIS S. POE, M.D.
Clinical Assistant Professor
Tufts University Medical School
Lahey Clinic Medical Center
Burlington, Massachusetts

DUNCAN S. POSTMA, M.D., F.A.C.S.
Assistant Clinical Professor
Department of Surgery
University of North Carolina School of Medicine
Chapel Hill, North Carolina

JOHN C. PRICE, M.D.
Clinical Assistant Professor
The Johns Hopkins School of Medicine
Baltimore, Maryland

DALE H. RICE, M.D.
Professor and Chairman
Department of Otolaryngology–Head and Neck Surgery
University of Southern California
Los Angeles, California

FRANK N. RITTER, M.D.
Clinical Professor of Otolaryngology
University of Michigan Medical Center
Active Staff
St. Joseph Mercy Hospital
Ann Arbor, Michigan

CLARENCE T. SASAKI, M.D.
Ohse Professor and Chief
Section of Otolaryngology
Yale School of Medicine
Chief, Otolaryngology
Yale-New Haven Hospital
New Haven, Connecticut

HAROLD F. SCHUKNECHT, M.D.
Walter Augustus LeCompte Professor Emeritus
Harvard Medical School
Emeritus Chief of Otolaryngology
Massachusetts Eye and Ear Infirmary
Boston, Massachusetts

DAVID E. SCHULLER, M.D.
Professor and Chairman
Department of Otolaryngology
Ohio State University
Director, Comprehensive Cancer Center and
  Arthur G. James Cancer Hospital and
  Research Institute
Ohio State University Hospitals
Columbus, Ohio

STANLEY M. SHAPSHAY, M.D.
Clinical Associate Professor of Otolaryngology
Boston University School of Medicine
Chairman, Department of Otolaryngology–Head and
  Neck Surgery
Director, Eleanor Naylor Dana Laser Research Laboratory
Lahey Clinic Medical Center
Boston, Massachusetts

JOHN J. SHEA, JR., M.D.
Clinical Professor
Otologic Consultant
University of Tennessee
Consulting Physician
St. Joseph Hospital
Memphis, Tennessee

WILLIAM W. SHOCKLEY, M.D., F.A.C.S.
Associate Professor
Department of Otolaryngology–Head and Neck Surgery
Louisiana State University Medical Center
Shreveport, Louisiana

SALLY R. SHOTT, M.D.
Assistant Professor
University of Cincinnati
Assistant Professor
Children's Hospital Medical Center
University Hospital
Cincinnati, Ohio

CARL E. SILVER, M.D.
Professor of Surgery and Otolaryngology
Albert Einstein College of Medicine
Chief, Head and Neck Surgery
Montefiore Medical Center
Bronx, New York

HERBERT SILVERSTEIN, M.D., F.A.C.S.
President, Ear Research Foundation
Clinical Professor of Surgery
Division of Otolaryngology
University of South Florida
Tampa, Flordia

HOWARD W. SMITH, M.D., D.M.D., F.A.C.S.
Clinical Professor, Surgery (Otolaryngology)
Columbia University School of Medicine
Attending Physician
Columbia/Presbyterian Medical Center
New York, New York

FRED J. STUCKER, JR., M.D., F.A.C.S.
Professor and Chairman
Department of Otolaryngology–Head and Neck Surgery
Louisiana State University School of Medicine
Shreveport, Louisiana

ELLEN K. TABOR, M.D.
Assistant Professor of Radiology
University of Pittsburgh
Staff Radiologist
Eye and Ear Hospital
Pittsburgh, Pennsylvania

M. EUGENE TARDY, JR., M.D., F.A.C.S.
Professor of Clinical Otolaryngology–Head and Neck Surgery
Director, Division of Facial Plastic Surgery
University of Illinois at Chicago
Chicago, Illinois

J. REGAN THOMAS, M.D., F.A.C.S.
*Director, Division of Facial Plastic and
    Reconstructive Surgery*
Department of Otolaryngology
Washington University School of Medicine
St. Louis, Missouri

JAMES N. THOMPSON, M.D., F.A.C.S.
Associate Dean
Professor of Surgery (Otolaryngology)
The Bowman Gray School of Medicine
Wake Forest University
Winston-Salem, North Carolina

HARVEY, M. TUCKER, M.D., F.A.C.S.
*Chairman, Department of Otolaryngology and
    Communicative Disorders*
Cleveland Clinic
Cleveland, Ohio

PAMELA A. TURNER, B.A.
Harvard Medical School
Boston, Massachusetts

PAUL H. WARD, M.D., F.A.C.S.
Professor of Surgery and Chief
Division of Head and Neck Surgery
UCLA School of Medicine
Los Angeles, California

MARK C. WEISSLER, M.D., F.A.C.S.
Assistant Professor
Division of Otolaryngology–Head and Neck Surgery
University of North Carolina School of Medicine
Attending Physician
North Carolina Memorial Hospital
Chapel Hill, North Carolina

FOREWORD

On Parents' Day our children would sometimes lay down the rules by which I might come to meet their schoolteachers and classmates: "You may come provided you do not say anything." Now I have been invited to say something in a foreword to this modern volume. I am caught between saying, on the one hand, too little and, on the other hand, crowing as the clarion cock. I hope I will be excused if I tend toward the latter.

I am very proud of the energy and enthusiasm of these two young men, their distant vision of the explorer, and their endurance to reach land after all. It was not easy.

Now the record of their adventures and safe return lies before you. They tell you of their experiences and those of their best friends. The written word is often not enough to tell the story. Illustrations are helpful, but they are no substitute for good seats at a live performance.

I believe you will find the material to be presented in a clear and lively manner. The topics are of enduring interest. Contrasting points of view are presented in an open forum. Indications for specific therapy are clearly identified. These are based, of course, on intuitive interpretation of the patient's history as well as expert examination. With agreement for classification and description of the disease as a foundation, we can proceed with a comparison of therapeutic results—even prospective and double-blind studies. The authors are collegial, stimulating, and experienced. They speak with confidence that they are offering the patient the best chance for improvement.

Not all of us would agree with the steps they take in diagnosis and management, but that is the reason the book is called *Challenges in Otolaryngology–Head and Neck Surgery.*

NEWTON D. FISHER, M.D.
Thomas J. Dark Distinguished Professor of
Otolaryngology
Division of Otolaryngology–Head and Neck Surgery
Department of Surgery
University of North Carolina School of Medicine
Chapel Hill, North Carolina

PREFACE

As a teacher of otolaryngology–head and neck surgery for the past 12 years, I constantly ask my colleagues and quiz my residents on how they would extricate themselves from difficult surgical situations. I have been fascinated to learn and observe the various techniques other surgeons have developed to deal with surgical dilemmas. It is clear that the thought process that goes into developing one's own style determines much of what will make a surgeon more or less successful in the operating room. One of my favorite exercises with house officers is to develop a surgical scenario in which a combination of complex issues requires thoughtful intervention by the resident in the operating room. After hearing their plan, we discuss it; then I present my approach to the problem. They constantly ask what the experts would do with the proposed scenario. The inspiration for this book was to develop two approaches to a variety of head and neck surgical challenges. We hope readers find this information useful. As I have found, one is seldom a prophet in one's own hometown.

Harold C. Pillsbury III, M.D.

PREFACE

Whereas the *science* of clinical medicine is predicated on the principles of scientific method and the prospective randomized clinical trial, the *art* is derived from an intangible assortment of clinical adages and anecdotes to which we attribute the term "clinical experience." As a resident in otolaryngology, I was impressed with the many different approaches and opinions regarding surgical issues within our specialty. Although there are many ways to skin a cat, it was often difficult to decide whose way was best, and thus the opinions of the experts became important in the formulation of my surgical judgment. However, I found that this information was difficult to access in print, because most textbooks and journal articles presented more traditional, well-referenced discussions of the accepted pathophysiology, diagnosis, and treatment of diseases. The personal approach to challenging surgical issues was conspicuously absent.

This book is a conglomeration of expert opinion regarding operative challenges within the specialty of otolaryngology–head and neck surgery. The challenges discussed include surgical indications, operative technique, anatomic anomalies, postoperative management, and complications. In short, it is a book of clinical pearls and "how I do its" in otolaryngologic surgery. Because of the inherent anecdotal nature of this book, two experts were chosen to comment on their personal approaches to the challenges in their respective chapters. At the risk of occasional redundancy, this format underscores areas of controversy and most thoroughly accesses a wealth of experience from its 94 contributors.

We are most grateful to the contributors for their time and effort in sharing their surgical judgment and experience with us. We are confident that all levels within our specialty will learn and profit from *Operative Challenges in Otolaryngology–Head and Neck Surgery*.

Manning M. Goldsmith III, M.D.

ACKNOWLEDGMENT

We would like to acknowledge the prodigious work done by Edith Calhoun in the editorial preparation of this text. We believe that without her constant vigilance this book would not have become a reality.

Harold C. Pillsbury III, M.D.
Manning M. Goldsmith III, M.D.

CONTENTS

CHAPTER 1

Tympanostomy Tubes

Approach of

Kenneth M. Grundfast, M.D.

INDICATIONS

The indications for insertion of tympanostomy tubes are controversial.[1–4] In fact, some pediatricians believe that tympanostomy tubes are more harmful than helpful, and one well-known pediatrician has even called for a moratorium on the insertion of tympanostomy tubes in the ears of children.[5] Despite the controversy regarding indications, tympanostomy tubes are frequently inserted in the ears of children in the United States. Though methods for reporting surgical procedure statistics do not yield dependable information about the exact number of children having insertion of tubes in the ears, estimates suggest that approximately 2 million children in the United States have tubes inserted in the ears each year.[1] Though all parties involved in this controversy about the indications for tympanostomy tubes might like to believe that the dispute is centered entirely on interpretation of scientific data without the influence of pecuniary factors, such is probably not the case.[6] After all, for the primary care physician who has been following a patient with persistent otitis media or recurring episodes of acute otitis media, myringotomy with insertion of a tympanostomy tube may demarcate the point at which care is transferred from the primary care physician to a surgical subspecialist. In this modern era of medicine with increasing competition among physicians for patients and economic pressures of all sorts, primary care physicians may be less willing than ever before to relinquish care of patients. Conversely, even though all surgeons like to believe they never recommend surgical intervention when other modes of therapy might achieve a desired outcome, nowadays the surgeon must be on guard to avoid letting economic pressures and attempts to maximize income per unit of time expended influence the choice for surgical vs. nonsurgical intervention. Though all physicians involved with management of patients with otitis media might prefer to ignore these po-

lemics, the controversy about the indications for insertion of tympanostomy tubes has become a public debate. Magazines, newspapers, and radio and television commentaries have focused public attention on the lack of agreement among physicians regarding indications for tympanostomy tubes.[7, 8]

In the midst of all this controversy, how is the otolaryngologist to arrive at a rational decision regarding indications for insertion of tympanostomy tubes? A reasonable approach is to carefully collate data on each patient and then group patients into categories according to the abnormal middle ear conditions that are manifest and according to the severity of the disorder in each patient. When this logical approach is taken, some general guidelines can be applied in deciding which patients are likely to benefit from insertion of tympanostomy tubes and which patients might be better managed with continued medical or other therapy. Table 1–1 provides a summary with definitions of commonly encountered clinical disorders, and the indications for insertion of tubes related to each of the conditions are described.

Even though Table 1–1 provides a helpful summary of indications for insertion of tympanostomy tubes, the otolaryngologist must remember that many factors influence decision making. Table 1–2 summarizes the many factors that need to be considered when one is attempting to decide whether benefits outweigh risks for any given patient who is being considered for insertion of tubes. Perhaps, the very controversy about overuse or misuse of tympanostomy tubes is a result of an attempt to oversimplify the process of decision making regarding indications for insertion of tubes.

In working with children, the otolaryngologist is advised to carefully describe to the parent all alternatives available and to make sure that the parent understands and is comfortable with the decision to insert tubes before attempting to schedule a child for the surgical procedure. Keeping in mind the

TABLE 1–1. Indications for Insertion of Tubes

Descriptive Term (Condition)	Definition	Symptoms	Signs	Advisable Prior Management	Indications for Insertion of Tympanostomy Tubes
Acute otitis media	Rapid onset of middle ear infection	Ear pain, fever, conductive hearing loss	Red, yellow, pink bulging eardrum	1. Antimicrobial, administered orally for 10 days 2. Analgesic, antiypyretic	1. Usually not indicated 2. Indicated if there is manifest or incipient complication (e.g., facial paralysis, labyrinthitis)
Frequently recurrent acute otitis media	More than four episodes of acute otitis media occurring within 3 mo.	Same as above, but otalgia and fever subside within 48 hr after starting antimicrobial treatment	Same as above, but appearance of eardrum returns to normal between each episode	1. Same as above given for each episode 2. Antimicrobial prophylaxis to reduce frequency of infections	Three or more episodes of acute otitis media occurring in each of two consecutive seasons
Persistent otitis media with effusion	Middle ear effusion present for 10 wk or longer	Minimal ear discomfort, conductive hearing loss, usually no fever	Dull, opaque, pink or amber eardrum with sluggish or no mobility on pneumatic otoscopy; flat tympanogram	1. Antimicrobial given for 10 days if not administered within 3 wk prior to diagnosis 2. Trial with prolonged low-dose antimicrobial administered for 1 to 2 mo 3. In some cases, trial of anti-inflammatory agent (steroid) may be attempted 4. Tympanocentesis, or myringotomy in infants or in cooperative children, usually most beneficial in spring and summer	One ear involved, normal hearing opposite ear, minimal associated symptom wait until effusion has been present approximately 3 mo. Both ears involved, hearing impaired significantly, or associated speech language abnormality or learning disability, consider inserting tubes when effusion persists longer than 10 wks; recurs within 3 wk after tympanocentesis
Middle ear ventilation disorder	Frequently recurring or persistent negative middle ear pressure with observable findings and confirmation by tympanometry; eustachain tube dysfunction; may be a subacute, underlying condition with recurrent acute otitis media	Ear discomfort, constant or intermittent; mild conductive hearing loss	Retracted eardrum, prominent lateral process and appearance of foreshortened manubrium of malleus; tympanometry demonstrates normal eardrum compliance with peak at or exceeding negative pressure of 250 mm H_2O	1. Attempts at control with autoinflation techniques 2. Politzerization 3. Adenoidectomy (?) 4. Antihistamine, decongestants, if indicated, for control of perennial or allergic rhinitis	Signs and symptoms present longer than 3 mo Diagnosis confirmed with pneumatic otoscopy and tympanometry
Structural changes in the eardrum	Changes in the integrity of the eardrum that would be evident on histopathologic examination (e.g., monomeric, atrophic area, adhesion of medial surface of eardrum to lenticular process of incus or to mucosa over promontory of the middle ear; granulation tissue or cholesteatoma)	Ear discomfort, hearing loss, otorrhea	Retracted, hypermobile portions of the eardrum; inability to lift eardrum off middle ear structures when negative pressure is applied with pneumatic otoscope; mild to moderate conductive hearing loss; excessive eardrum compliance or significant reduced compliance on tympanogram; Radiographic changes may be apparent on CT scan	1. Antimicrobial therapy 2. Politzerization 3. (Tympanostomy tube)	Insertion of a tympanostomy tube, alone, usually is not the definitive therapy where structural changes have occurred; tympanoplasty, sometimes combined with mastoidectomy, usually is necessary; a tympanostomy tube may be inserted at the time of tympanoplasy to provide aeration during a healing phase postoperatively

TABLE 1–2.
Factors to be Considered in Deciding
When to Insert Tubes

Past medical history
  Frequency of prior infections
  Duration of middle ear effusion
  Allergy: foods, inhalants, medications
Physical findings
  Palate abnormalities
  Craniofacial anomaly
  Appearance of eardrum
Audiometric data
  Pure tone thresholds
  Speech reception thresholds
Impedance data
  Compliance
  Pressure
Communication skills
  Speech development
  Articulation
Psychosocial
  Patient/parent compliance, anxiety level
  Personal hygiene
  Affinity for, frequency of water sports
Legal
  Litigiousness
Other
  Season
  Risks for anesthesia
  Attention deficit disorder
  Learning disability
  Intelligence

CHOOSING THE PROPER VENTILATION TUBE

Table 1–5 provides a description of the technical design components of a tympanostomy tube along with examples of some commonly used types of tubes. I have summarized the factors to be considered in choosing one particular type of tympanostomy tube.

Ease of Insertion

Although insertion of a tympanostomy tube is not a difficult procedure to perform in the technical sense, anatomic variation in the size of the external auditory canal or tortuosity of an ear canal can make the insertion of one type of tube difficult, whereas another type of tube can easily be inserted given the anatomic limitations. In general, I find the Armstrong Teflon beveled edge tympanostomy tube one of the easiest types of tubes to insert in most ear canals.

Tube Composition

Currently, materials used for the manufacture of tympanostomy tubes include fluorocarbon (Teflon) silicone, gold, titanium, and stainless steel. All of these materials are biologically inert. However, in soft tissue pockets, silicone rubber potentiates infections more often than does fluorocarbon.[9] I have found Teflon tubes to be most reliable in terms of lack of problems with infection and tendency for the tube lumen to become occluded. Sometimes, when Silastic tubes remain in an ear for more than 1 or 2 years, I have seen the development of granulation tissue at the junction between the eardrum and the shaft of the tympanostomy tube. Also, I have noticed a slightly

outcome that is expected from insertion of a tympanostomy tube may assist the otolaryngologist in decision making. Table 1–3 summarizes the desired outcomes divided into categories corresponding to the arbitrarily defined disorders listed in Table 1–1. Insertion of a tympanostomy tube can help to achieve a desired outcome; however, before recommending insertion of tubes for a given patient, the otolaryngologist should explore the possibility that nonsurgical modes of therapy might also achieve the desired outcome. The time to recommend insertion of tubes is when alternative methods of therapy have proved ineffective in achieving the desired outcome or when a patient or parent chooses the insertion of a tympanostomy tube as preferable to an alternative mode of therapy that might be equally effective. That is, we must remember that parents and patients do have choices. Although antimicrobial prophylaxis and tympanostomy tubes might offer an equal chance for diminishing the frequency of acute otitis media, one parent may choose the medical therapy, and another might prefer the surgical approach. Table 1–4 provides a summary of questions frequently asked by parents about tympanostomy tubes. The answers provided in Table 1–4 are my own, and they are not meant to be definitive; each surgeon may have a different opinion or way of answering the questions.

TABLE 1–3.
Expected Outcome From Insertion of Tympanostomy Tube

Condition	Outcome
Acute otitis media	Resolution of infection without complication or sequela
Frequently recurring acute otitis media	Significant diminution in frequency of acute otitis media; arbitrarily, <3 episodes of acute otitis media in 4 mo
Persistent otitis media with effusion	Evacuation of fluid from middle ear, prevention of reaccumulation of middle ear effusion, improvement in hearing; arbitrarily, sustained normal hearing for >6 mo
Middle ear ventilation disorder	Return of eardrum to neutral position, no ear discomfort, normal hearing; signs and symptoms may recur after tube becomes extruded
Structural changes in the eardrum	Aeration of the middle ear during the healing phase after definitive surgery undertaken to correct the eardrum abnormality or to remove cholesteatoma

TABLE 1–4.
Frequently Asked Questions

	Questions	Answers
Indications	Why does the primary care physician say that tubes are unnecessary and possibly harmful?	Some physicians take a dogmatic approach. The insertion of tympanostomy tubes is one of many methods for managing otitis media. Like any medical or surgical treatment, the use of tympanostomy tubes has advantages and disadvantages.
	Why does one otolaryngologist suggest tubes, another otolaryngologist suggest adenoidectomy alone, and a third otolaryngologist say that both tubes and adenoidectomy are indicated?	There is no single best method for treating otitis media. Many methods are available, and many are effective. Each parent, patient, and physician must select the treatment method with which he or she is most comfortable. The best that anyone can do is to make a rational decision based on available data.
Duration in situ	How do you know when the tube has come out of the eardrum?	The physician who inserted the tube will check the ears at least every 6 mo. In most cases, the tube will work its way out of the eardrum and into the ear canal within 18 mo. after the tube was inserted. When the tube is seen lying in the ear canal, the physician can use a small instrument to grasp and remove the tube from the ear.
	How long are the tubes supposed to stay in the eardrum?	The length of time that a tube stays in the eardrum depends on the size and design of the tube, the site within the eardrum at which the tube is inserted, and the structural integrity of the eardrum. Some tubes are designed to stay in the eardrum until they are removed by the surgeon.
	What happens if the tubes come out too soon?	Depending on the appearance of the eardrum, the frequency of infection, and the hearing, tubes may or may not need to be reinserted. Certainly, in most cases, there will not be a need to immediately reinsert a tube that has come out.
	What happens if the tubes do not come out when they are supposed to come out?	If a tube has not come out 2 yr after having been inserted, the tube may have to be removed. Usually, removal of the tube can be done as an office procedure without requiring general anesthesia.
Curative or pallative	Will my child be completely free of ear infections while the tubes are in the ears?	Not necessarily. The tubes should diminish the frequency of ear infections, but infections can still occur.
	Will another set of tubes be needed after the first set comes out?	Not necessarily. In most cases children have outgrown or are beginning to outgrow the problems of frequent ear infections and persistent middle ear fluid by the time the tubes come out.
Care	Is swimming permissable after tubes are inserted?	Yes. Some physicians recommend use of ear plugs when swimming; others do not. Some tubes are specifically designed to allow the patient to swim without a need for ear plugs.
	How is an ear infection diagnosed and treated when there are tubes in the ears?	Usually, yellowish sticky liquid will be seen draining from the ear. Sometimes, if the tube becomes blocked, there may be an infection without fluid draining. If your child is acting as if he or she has an ear infection, examination by a physician is a good idea.
Complications	Can anything go wrong at the time of surgery?	Little can go wrong when the tube is being inserted. Sometimes there can be bleeding, and dried blood can clot inside the lumen of the tube. The ossicles should not be damaged if the tubes are being inserted by an experienced ear surgeon. Patients in good health should be able to tolerate the brief anesthesia without a problem.
	Can the tube cause scarring of the eardrum or damage to the eardrum?	There can be some thickening or thinning of the eardrum at the site where a tube has been inserted, but these blemishes on the eardrum rarely cause any future problems. A permanent hole can remain in the eardrum at the site where a tube was inserted. If this happens, an operation may be necessary to surgically repair the persistent eardrum perforation.
	What happens if the opening in the tube gets plugged up?	The tube will not function properly if the lumen of the tube becomes blocked. Sometimes instillation of antibiotic or anti-inflammatory eardrops can reopen the tube. In other situations, the physician may be able to reopen the tube by using small instruments under a microscope in the office.

TABLE 1–5.
Design of Tympanostomy Tubes

Biosurgical material
　Hydrofluorocarbon (Teflon)
　Polyethylene
　Silicone rubber (Silastic)
　Titanium
　Gold
　Stainless steel
Outer flange
　Same size and shape as inner flange—grommet, collar button
　　(Sheehy, Reuter bobbin, Soileau, Pappas, Donaldson)
　Differs in size and/or shape from inner flange
　　Wire attached (Shepard tube)
　　Extension for grasping (Moretz, collar button with tail)
Inner flange
　Same size and shape as outer flange (grommet)
　Differs in size and/or shape from outer flange
　　T shape (T tube, butterfly tube, Touma T type)
　　Wide circumference (Per Lee tube, spoon bobbin)
Shaft
　short grommet
　long T tube, Armstrong type V
Air permeable/liquid barrier—designed to prevent water from en-
　tering middle ear when one is swimming or bathing
　Castelli tube (no longer availabe)
　Narrow lumen tube (Teflon vent tube 0.89 mm inner diameter
　　and 7 mm long); Schreiber tube (in clinical trials)
Shaft/flange angle
　Perpendicular
　Angled (Armstrong bevel, Pope)

higher rate of persistent perforation with use of stainless steel and Silastic tubes than with the Teflon tubes.

Shape and Design of Tube

The myriad shapes and types of tympanostomy tubes and the seemingly never ending introduction of new and improved types of tubes may be more a reflection of the degree of egocentricity among otolaryngologists rather than true evidence of a continuing evolution toward an optimally developed biosurgical implant device. That is, newly developed tympanostomy tubes seem to come and go, and no single tube seems to be optimal for all cases.[10] The array of tubes available allows the surgeon to select a size and shape tube that best meets the needs of the clinical situation encountered. Quite obviously, the tiny grommet tubes are well designed for insertion through stenotic ear canals, typically encountered in children with Down syndrome. In general, the larger the inner flange compared with the size of the shaft, the longer the tube will remain in the eardrum. Therefore, the T-shaped tubes tend to be best for long-term use. However, T tubes with long shafts tend to get plugged with debris, and even though the tube remains in the ear for several years, the tube may become dysfunctional because of an occluded tube lumen. In contrast, the Paperella no. 2 tube has a relatively wide inner flange and a wide-bore lumen that is not long. Thus, the Paparella no. 2 tube remains in the eardrum for a long time, and there is little tendency for the lumen to become occluded. However, the Paperella no. 2 tube is a bit difficult to insert and often requires a surgical procedure with anesthesia for removal of the tube. Also, there seems to be a relatively high rate of perforation associated with the use of the Paperella no. 2 tube.

Duration In Situ

Perhaps one of the most important factors to be considered when one is choosing a tympanostomy tube is the length of time that the surgeon desires the tube to remain in the eardrum. All other factors being equal, the smaller the tube's size, and the smaller the inner flange diameter, the sooner the tube will become extruded spontaneously. Therefore, tiny grommet tubes may remain in the eardrum for less than 6 months, whereas the larger tubes can remain between 9 and 18 months. I would consider the average length of time for a tube to remain in the eardrum to be approximately 18 months. If you want to choose a tube that will remain in the eardrum for approximately 2 years or more, it is probably best to choose a T tube or a butterfly-type tube. Patients who are likely to require a long-term tympanostomy tube include children with craniofacial anomalies, children with overt or submucous cleft palate, adults who have had extirpative surgery and who have impaired eustachian tube function, and patients who have begun to manifest structural changes in the eardrum such as retraction pocket or adhesive changes.

The recent report of a randomized study comparing four types of commonly used tympanostomy tubes yielded results as follows[11]:

> In respective order of listing, the Shepard grommet, the Armstrong grommet, the Armstrong tube, the Reuterbobbin tube, and the Goode T tube had extrusion rates at 24 months of 94%, 80%, 66%, and 31%; obstruction rates of 11%, 25%, 74%, and 36%; associated otorrhea rates of 0%, 17%, 42%, and 50%; and residual perforation rates (without all tubes yet being extruded) of 0%, 0%, 0%, and 5%. No other complications were noted. The authors concluded that the Shepard- and Armstrong-type tubes were preferable in the majority of first-intubation pediatric patients and that the Goode T tube, with its longterm retention rate and higher perforation rate, should be reserved for patients requiring more prolonged intubation or for patients in whom perforation might even be useful, such as those with tumor or cleft palate.

ADHESIVE OTITIS MEDIA

There is some controversy about the value of tympanostomy tubes in the management of adhesive otitis media. The central question in this controversy is, if structural changes in the eardrum and middle ear have progressed to a point that adhesive otitis media has developed, can insertion of a tympanostomy tube provide aeration of the middle ear sufficient to prevent further deterioration, and can the insertion of a tube reverse the process that has already developed? Probably, there is no simple answer to this question. When the question is considered, the most useful approach is to view the development of adhesive otitis media as one aspect of a continuum in the development of structural changes that occur in the eardrum and middle ear as a result of inadequate aeration of the middle ear (Table 1–6). The continuum begins with the mildest forms of eardrum retraction, then continues through such manifest disorders as localized retraction pockets, pars flaccida retraction, myringostapediopexy, erosion of the lenticular process of the incus, erosion of the stapes superstructure, adherence of the eardrum to the promontory, and then, in the most severe forms, retraction of the eardrum into the sinus tympani and facial recess with extension into the aditus ad antrum. Insertion of a tympanostomy tube may truncate a process of progressive eardrum retraction, leading to adhesive changes. Tos et al. have shown that 4% of children less than 5 years of age with "secretory otitis" go on to develop atrophic changes in the eardrum compared with 10% of ears in children with similar conditions who are 6 to 10 years of age.[12] In a more recent report on the "dynamics of eardrum changes following secretory otitis," Tos et al. affirm that the combination of poor eustachian tube function and an atrophic and retracted eardrum represents potential risk for further progression of the retraction.[13] I think that there is a point within the continuum of progressive structural eardrum changes after which insertion of a tympanostomy tube is probably not very helpful and certainly would not be the definitive method for management of the otologic problem (see Table 1–6). In my opinion, that point is when the eardrum has actually become adherent to a middle ear structure such as an ossicle (lenticular process of incus) or the mucosa overlying the promontory of the middle ear. In situations where there is anatomic adherence between the medial surface of the eardrum and another structure, insertion of a tympanostomy tube alone

would not be sufficient to cure the abnormal condition. If the eardrum is elevated with tympanoplasty surgery and absorbable gelatin film (Gelfilm) or Silastic sheeting is inserted in the middle ear and a tympanostomy tube is inserted in the anteroinferior quadrant of the eardrum, the tube may provide aeration for the middle ear, and the Gelfilm or Silastic sheeting prevents recurrence of the adhesion. Table 1–6 provides a guideline for determining when insertion of a tympanostomy tube alone can be sufficient in curing the abnormal condition compared with those situations in which the insertion of the tympanostomy tube can be considered adjunctive to another procedure that is necessary for curing the abnormal condition.

ADENOIDECTOMY

Despite recent reports suggesting the usefulness of adenoidectomy in the management of otitis media with effusion in children,[14, 15] I remain hesitant to routinely recommend this procedure. In children who are less than 2 years of age and who do not manifest signs or symptoms of nasal obstruction or adenoid hypertrophy, I usually recommend insertion of tympanostomy tubes and do not recommend adenoidectomy. For children 2 years of age and older who manifest signs and symptoms of nasal obstruction and who have radiographic evidence of adenoid hypertrophy or evidence of partial or complete obstruction of the choanae with adenoid tissue observed on posterior rhinoscopy (flexible fiberoptic nasopharyngoscope or rod lens telescope), I do recommend adenoidectomy. In children between the ages of 2 and 8 years who have previously had insertion of tympanostomy tubes and then develop symptoms of frequent ear infections or persistent middle ear effusion, I will recommend adenoidectomy regardless of whether or not

TABLE 1–6.
Stages in Development of Sequelae From Inadequate Middle Ear Ventilation

	Early*	Progressive*	Late†
Observed findings	Subtle, detectable	Manifest; confined to eardrum	Obvious, unequivocal
	Retracted tympanic membrane; foreshortened manubrium of malleus	Retraction pocket, tympanic membrane on incudostapedial joint	Deep retraction pocket, flaky white debris (cholesteatoma), granulation tissue, tympanic membrane adherent to ossicles or promontory
Symptoms	Minimal or none	Mild ear discomfort, mild conductive hearing loss	Ear discomfort, ear drainage, hearing loss
Audiogram	Normal	Normal or 5–10 dB air-bone gap	15–30 dB air-bone gap
Impedance	Normal compliance	Normal compliance	Reduced compliance
	Peak from -200 to -300 mm H_2O	Peak from -300 to -400 mm H_2O, may have atypical, biphasic peaks	No peak or flattened peak
Ossicles	Not eroded	Partial erosion, normal continuity and conduction	Impaired mobility, significant erosion
Management	Politzerization	Politzerization	Tympanoplasty (with mastoidectomy?)
	Autoinflation	Autoinflation	Tympanostomy tube (?)
	Decongestant	Decongestant	
	Hyposensitization	Hyposensitization	
	Tympanostomy tube	Tympanostomy tube	
	Adenoidectomy(?)	Adenoidectomy (?)	

*Tube alone may be helpful.
†Tube alone is not curative.

there are signs and symptoms of nasal obstruction. That is, I believe that the adenoidectomy may be helpful in alleviating the problem with otitis media if the problem has persisted after one set of tympanostomy tubes has been inserted previously, and I am not as stringent about basing a recommendation for adenoidectomy on symptoms of nasal obstruction in the child who is having repeat insertion of tympanostomy tubes.

Even though several studies have investigated the advisability of recommending adenoidectomy in the management of otitis media, the results still appear to be inconclusive. Several studies seem to demonstrate the effectiveness of adenoidectomy as an adjunct to insertion of tympanostomy tubes, other studies suggest that adenoidectomy alone is preferable to insertion of tympanostomy tubes, and still others seem to suggest that adenoidectomy has little effectiveness in the management of otitis media. The more recent studies seem to suggest that adenoidectomy is valuable in the management of otitis media and I think that best results can be achieved by selecting carefully the patients for adenoidectomy. Even though the study by Gates et al. suggest that the size of the adenoid on lateral neck radiograph does not correlate well with the outcome to be achieved after adenoidectomy,[16] I continue to believe that the best results can be achieved by recommending adenoidectomy only for those children who have demonstrable evidence of significant adenoid enlargement on a lateral neck film or for children who are manifesting signs of nasal obstruction that is attributed to obstruction in the choanae or nasopharynx from adenoid tissue.

OTORRHEA FOLLOWING INSERTION OF TUBES

Otorrhea can and does occur in a proportion of any group of patients who have had insertion of tubes.[17, 18] A review of relevant reports in the medical literature suggests an incidence of postoperative otorrhea between 14% and 41%, with an average rate of 26%.[19] One prospective study investigating the causes and methods for preventing otorrhea following tube insertion drew three conclusions[20]:

1. The incidence of postoperative tympanostomy and tube infection is in the range of that previously reported—up to 15%.
2. The rate of infection was reduced by the use of prophylactic antibiotic/steroid drops and to a lesser extent by the use of prophylactic oral ampicillin.
3. Posttympanostomy tube infections were statistically related to the middle ear findings prior to insertion of the tube; the more evidence of middle ear infection preoperatively, the more likely the development of otorrhea postoperatively.

In my practice, approximately 25% to 30% of the patients have otorrhea at some time while the tube remains in the eardrum. I view the problem with otorrhea in several ways. First, before inserting tympanostomy tubes in any child, I discuss with the parent the likelihood that otorrhea may occur when the child has an upper respiratory tract infection with purulent rhinorrhea and nasal obstruction. I explain that the middle ear is connected by the eustachian tube to the "back of the nose and mouth" and that it will be reasonable to expect that "mucus" that is discharging from the nose will also be seen coming out of one or both ears for a few days when a child has a severe upper respiratory tract infection characterized by nasal obstruction and nasal discharge. Second, I am aware that surgical technique at the time of insertion of tympanostomy tubes may be a factor in causing postoperative otorrhea. Although some otolaryngologists do not use sterile technique for insertion of tympanostomy tubes, quite obviously, sterility in technique can help to avoid the postoperative otorrhea caused by bacterial infection. One report suggests that postoperative otorrhea can be avoided by sterilizing the ear canal with providone iodine.[21] I like to cleanse the ear canal with instillation of 70% alcohol, which is removed by suction after remaining in the ear canal for 60 seconds. Also, I instill antibiotic–steroid otic suspension in the ear canal after the tube has been inserted. One prospective study demonstrated a reduction from 16% to 4% in the incidence of postoperative otorrhea when the middle ear was irrigated with saline through the tympanostomy tube at the time of insertion.[22] Another recent report suggests that postoperative otorrhea can be prevented with instillation of gentamicin ophthalmic solution immediately following insertion of a tube in the ear.[23]

The matter of otorrhea related to swimming in children with tympanostomy tubes remains controversial. Although some physicians believe that there is no need to prevent water from entering the ear canals in patients with tympanostomy tubes,[24–26] I have noticed a correlation between swimming and the development of otorrhea, and, therefore, I prefer that ear plugs be used when swimming.

A fourth situation associated with otorrhea seems to be atopy. I have found that children between the ages of 3 and 6 years who have marked hypersensitivity, especially inhalant allergies, seem to have more problems with otorrhea than do other children who have had insertion of tubes. I suspect that the problem may be one of chronic weeping from mucous membranes. I know of no specific way to prevent this type of otorrhea associated with allergies; however, I like to caution parents of allergic children that there is a higher chance of otorrhea because of the allergies, and I also mention to the parents my impression that the tendency for a child to develop otorrhea is correlated with the adequacy of allergy management. The better the allergies are controlled with management, the less likely otorrhea is to develop. Recently, some otolaryngologists have perceived a correlation between otorrhea in children with tympanostomy tubes and measurable deficiencies in some of the subclasses of immunoglobulins. When such correlations are detected, the children are often given prophylactic doses of antimicrobial agents to prevent otorrhea. Since otorrhea itself is relatively common, and since the clinical significance of measurably lower than normal levels of subclasses of immunoglobulins is not yet clear, I am skeptical of this seemingly plausible explanation of the cause of otorrhea. Until further scientific data are available, I would not recommend testing for deficiency of subclasses of immunoglobulins in most children with intermittent otorrhea. Perhaps in unusual cases, when the otorrhea is unremitting, immunologic evaluation may be warranted.

Finally, there is a sixth situation in which otorrhea can be expected, and that is the situation characterized by poor personal hygiene. The child who is seen to be unkempt on office visits and preoperative examination is likely to be a child who will develop otorrhea with more frequency than a child who is cared for meticulously and who is always clean and neat when examined in the office. The rule here is: The child who has a soiled shirt and dirt around the pinna on preoperative examination is likely to be the child who will return at the first postoperative visit with otorrhea.

My method for managing otorrhea in a child with tympanostomy tubes is as follows:

1. Inform parents during preoperative counseling that yellowish discharge is likely to occur whenever the child has purulent rhinorrhea, as with an upper respiratory tract infection. When otorrhea does occur, parent wipes away sticky mucoid discharge with cotton-tipped applicator and instills antibiotic–steroid otic suspension three times daily for 3 days.

2. If otorrhea persists after the third day, the parent calls for an office appointment.

3. In the office, suction mucoid discharge from the ear canal so that the tube lumen is visible, then insert a dry compressed expandable ear canal wick (Pope earwick Merocel fiber sponge). Instill 4 drops of antibiotic-steroid suspension into the ear canal so that the otic suspension soaks into and expands the wick. Show the parent the location of the wick in the ear canal, and instruct the parent in the method of removing the wick with "tweezers" at home. Give the parent an additional sterile wrapped dry compressed wick to keep in the medicine cabinet at home. The parent instills 4 to 5 drops of otic suspension three times daily for 3 days, then removes the wick at home, and continues the drops three times daily for 2 more days after the wick is removed (total of 5 days for instillation of drops).

4. Wait 2 days after the 5-day regimen of instillation of otic suspension is completed. If otorrhea persists, the parent inserts a sterile wrapped wick in the child's ear at home in the same manner as the wick had been inserted by the physician in the office. The parent calls the office to inform the physician that otorrhea is persisting and requests that a prescription for a systemic antibiotic be called to a local pharmacy. The parent again instills otic suspension three times daily for 3 days, removes the wick at the end of the third day, continues instillation of the otic suspension 2 more days, and administers an oral antibiotic such as amoxicillin or cephalosporin in appropriate dose for 10 days.

5. If otorrhea persists, a repeat office examination is necessary. For recalcitrant otorrhea, frequent ear suction and debridement may be necessary. In general, culture of the mucopurulent discharge is not helpful. Cultures will frequently grow *Pseudomonas aeruginosa.* Nonetheless, almost all cases of otorrhea can be treated without administering either topical or systemic aminoglycoside antibiotics.

When these enumerated measures fail to alleviate the problem or the problem of otorrhea recurs frequently, suspect undetected middle ear cholesteatoma, allergy, immunodeficiency, or poor hygiene as etiologic factors.

TUBE OBSTRUCTION

Obstruction of a tympanostomy tube can occur when fluid produced in the middle ear enters the medial end of the tube lumen and becomes inspissated or when cerumen produced in the ear canal enters or overlies the outer orifice of the tube lumen. Every attempt should be made at the time of insertion of the tube to prevent blood from filling the middle ear and entering the medial orifice of the tympanostomy tube. Prevention begins with careful technique. Usually, if the middle ear mucosa is not accidentally incised at the time that the eardrum is being incised, there will be minimal bleeding from the middle ear. When bleeding does occur, it is worthwhile to continually suction the blood from the tube by applying the suction tip to the outer lumen of the tube until the bleeding slows and ceases. If the bleeding is troublesome and persistent, a solution containing 1:1,000 epinepherine can be instilled in the middle ear by taking a 3 mL syringe and injecting through the tympanostomy tube lumen using an Argyle Medicut tip with the 22-gauge metal needle removed. If this does not stop the bleeding, an antibiotic-steroid such as Cortisporin ointment can be instilled into the tube to keep the lumen patent until the middle ear bleeding stops. Then the ointment can be suctioned from the tube lumen at the time of the first postoperative visit. If the skin of the ear canal is abraded or accidentally incised at the time that a tympanostomy tube is inserted, blood can fill the medial portion of the external ear canal and become clotted on the surface of the outer orifice of the tube lumen. This can be avoided by using meticulously careful techniques so that the tympanostomy tube and instrument do not come in contact with the ear canal skin during the insertion of the tympanostomy tube. When bleeding from the skin of the external ear canal does occur, a small piece of cotton soaked in the epinepherine 1:1,000 can be placed in the ear canal over the tympanostomy tube until the bleeding has stopped. Again, if the bleeding is troublesome and continues, the antibiotic-steroid ointment can be instilled in the medial portion of the ear canal and then suctioned later at the postoperative visit.

In patients who are known to produce large amounts of cerumen, frequent office visits are helpful in removing the cerumen and preventing the cerumen from occluding the outer lumen of the tympanostomy tube.

When a patent tympanostomy tube has been observed at the time of the first postoperative visit but a patient returns at some time later with evidence of occlusion of the lumen of the tympanostomy tube, several procedures can be helpful in restoring patency of the tube lumen. I used to advise use of antibiotic–steroid otic suspension in an attempt to dissolve the plug in a tube lumen. Now, after a recent report showing the efficacy of hydrogen peroxide,[27] I usually suggest instillation of 6 drops of hydrogen peroxide in the ear canal twice daily, with massage of the tragus to pump the instilled solution that is filling the ear canal into the tympanostomy tube. In many cases, after this has been done for 5 days, the patient will return, and the tube lumen is seen to be patent. When this fails to restore patency of the tube lumen and the patient is sufficiently co-operative, I am usually able to open the tube lumen by inserting the stilette from an 18-gauge spinal needle into the tube under direct vision using the microscope.

RESIDUAL PERFORATION FOLLOWING TUBE EXTRUSION

Residual perforation after extrusion of tympanostomy tubes can and does occur. Therefore, all patients who are having insertion of tubes and the parents of children who are having insertion of tympanostomy tubes should know about the possibility of a perforation developing. In fact, misunderstandings and potential litigation can be avoided by including on the operative permit a statement about the possibility of a perforation in the eardrum remaining at the site where a tympanostomy tube has been inserted and then becomes extruded. The reported incidence of persistent perforation varies from 0.5% to 3.0%, with a mean of 1.4%.[19] However, when parents ask me about my own rate of persistent perforations, I usually answer by saying that the occurrence of a persistent perforation is not as common as 1 in 100 cases but not as rare as 1 in 1,000 cases. Parents seem to be satisfied by this rather broad range given for the likelihood of the occurrence of a persistent perforation. When I am recommending insertion of a long-term tympanostomy tube such as a T tube or a Paparella-type no. 2 tube, I usually stress that the rate of persistent perforation is higher than would be expected with use of a short-term ventilation tube. When I am providing this explanation, I am always quick to add that a persistent perforation is really not necessarily a "complication" in children who are having insertion of one of the tympanostomy tubes designed for long-term ventilation of the middle ear. After all, the goal in using one of the long-term types of tympanostomy tubes is prolonged aeration of the middle ear through the eardrum. In such cases, the decision to depend on a tube for aeration of the middle ear is based on the assumption that eustachian tube function is poor and the additional assumption that eustachian tube function will not be improving within a short amount of time. Therefore, a persistent perforation in a patient with chronically poor eustachian tube function may be considered to be advantageous. This being the case, I think it is a good idea to spend some extra time with patients or parents of patients who are having insertion of a tympanostomy tube designed for long-term use so that the advantages and disadvantages of a persistent perforation are put in proper perspective.

The two factors that are correlated with persistent perforation are length of time that the tube has remained in the eardrum and location that the tube has been placed within the eardrum. Tubes placed in the anterosuperior quadrant of the eardrum seem to have a higher rate of residual perforation compared with tubes placed in the anteroinferior quadrant of the eardrum. I do not insert tubes in the posterior portion of the eardrum. Also, as mentioned earlier, the longer that a tube remains in the eardrum, the more likely that a persistent perforation will remain after the tube extrudes spontaneously or is surgically removed.

When a persistent perforation develops after spontaneous extrusion of a tympanostomy tube that was intended for short-term use, I usually wait between 1 and 2 years for the perforation to close before even considering myringoplasty surgery. The younger the child, the less likely I would be to recommend surgical repair of the perforation at the site where a tympanostomy tube had been inserted. When children reach approximately 10 years of age and still have a small perforation at the site where a tympanostomy tube had been placed in the eardrum, I will recommend myringoplasty or tympanoplasty surgery for closure of the eardrum perforation.

FAILURE OF TUBE TO EXTRUDE SPONTANEOUSLY

When a child who has had insertion of a tympanostomy tube designed for short-term use still has the tympanostomy tube in situ beyond 2 years from the time of insertion, I begin to consider the possibility of removing the tube from the eardrum. Removal of a tube from the eardrum can be done as an office procedure or under general anesthesia. Depending on the age of the child, the degree to which the child is cooperative for ear examinations, and the child's tolerance for insertion of instruments in the external ear canal, removal of a nonextruded tube as an office procedure may be feasible. When I have a cooperative child, I instill 4 drops of a solution containing benzocaine (Auralgan) in the ear canal approximately 15 minutes before removing the tube. Then I make a tiny incision in the eardrum next to the shaft of the tympanostomy tube. The tube is grasped with alligator forceps, rotated, and gently removed. The benzocaine eardrops do not necessarily always provide complete anesthesia of the eardrum, and sometimes this procedure is slightly uncomfortable for patients. However, I am usually able to remove the tube, and the child may whimper or cry for a moment or two; the procedure is brief, however, and both parent and child appreciate having had the tube removed as an office procedure rather than requiring a trip to the operating room for use of general anesthesia. When there are nonextruded tympanostomy tubes in both ears, or when the nonextruded tube is in one ear but the patient is uncooperative, I will recommend the use of general anesthesia for removal of the tube. However, when I use general anesthesia for removal of a tympanostomy tube, I apply 10% trichlorocetic acid to the edges of the eardrum perforation and then apply a cigarette paper patch to the eardrum. The rationale for combining the paper patch with removal of the tube under general anesthesia is based on my concern about the likelihood of a persistent perforation after failure of a tympanostomy tube to spontaneously extrude. If a child requires general anesthesia for removal of a nonextruded tympanostomy tube, that means the tube must have been in the ear for more than 2 years, and based on my experience, the likelihood of a residual perforation is higher in such cases than when a tube extrudes spontaneously within the first 2 years after insertion. Thus, I like to use the acid technique to debride the edges of the eardrum perforation and the paper patch to facilitate healing of the eardrum so that a child who has had to have general anesthesia for removal of the tympanostomy tube has every chance of having the eardrum perforation close without having to return to the operating room at some later time for myringoplasty surgery.

SECONDARY ACQUIRED CHOLESTEATOMA

Does insertion of a tympanostomy tube prevent development of secondary acquired cholesteatoma? Can insertion of a tympanostomy tube be an etiologic factor in the development of secondary acquired cholesteatoma? Logic would tell us that the answer to both of these questions cannot be affirmative. Nonetheless, although many otologists believe that insertion of a tympanostomy tube can play a role in preventing the development of secondary acquired cholesteatoma,[28] other physicians have published reports suggesting that insertion of a tympanostomy tube may play a role in the development of cholesteatoma.[29, 30] Actually, I believe that part of this confusion is related to a semantic issue. Those who believe that the insertion of a tympanostomy tube may be related in some way to the development of cholesteatoma are probably using the term "cholesteatoma" to describe an eardrum inclusion cyst that can develop at the site where a tympanostomy tube had been inserted. Or there may be some cases in which a tympanostomy tube had been inserted in an eardrum because of eardrum retraction, poor eardrum mobility on pneumatic otoscopy, and conductive hearing loss. In some of these situations, a small congenital middle ear cholesteatoma may have gone undetected at the time that the tympanostomy tube was inserted, and then, with time, the cholesteatoma grows and becomes detectable. In such cases, even though the tympanostomy tube can be implicated, I think it is not really causally related to the development of the cholesteatoma.

I do think that insertion of a tympanostomy tube can be helpful in attenuating a process of progressive eardrum retraction that can eventually lead to the development of secondary acquired cholesteatoma. When I see persistent retraction of the posterosuperior quadrant of the eardrum, and when I see the eardrum resting on the incudostapedial joint, I describe the situation as an "incipient cholesteatoma." Tos et al. have reported an incidence of 0.8% for the development of cholesteatoma in a group of 278 children followed and observed for "secretory otitis."[13] Of course, even though all ears manifesting findings of deep posterosuperior retraction pocket with contact between the medial surface of the eardrum and the ossicles will not go on to develop cholesteatoma, I believe that it is extremely important to frequently examine and monitor the hearing of patients who are showing signs of developing progressively deepening posterosuperior retractions of the eardrum. The problem in managing a patient with a progressively deepening posterosuperior eardrum retraction pocket is the timing of intervention. As soon as progression and further deep-

ening of the eardrum retraction pocket is noted, I recommend insertion of a tympanostomy tube. In many cases, the eardrum retraction disappears, the ear becomes stable, and hearing improves as soon as the tympanostomy tube has been inserted. However, there is a significant likelihood that the process of progressive posterior retraction with potential for development of cholesteatoma will recur as soon as the tympanostomy tube has become extruded. When it becomes evident to me that a patient is developing progressive retraction of the posterosuperior portion of the eardrum and it is clear that insertion of a tympanostomy tube has not attenuated or prevented this process from occurring, I recommend a tympanoplasty procedure to prevent further structural changes from occurring and also to prevent the development of cholesteatoma. Depending on the patient's prior otologic history, the audiogram, and findings on CT scan of the temporal bone, I may recommend mastoidectomy along with the tympanoplasty. The mastoidectomy is recommended when the CT scan demonstrates poor pneumatization of the mastoid air cell system, when there is clouding in the epitympanum, when the scutum is partially eroded, or when there are other radiologic findings suggestive of extension of disease into the aditus or antrum. On the other hand, if radiographic findings suggest normal mastoid pneumatization and the problem seems to be localized to the eardrum itself, I recommend tympanoplasty surgery alone. Whether or not mastoidectomy is combined with the tympanoplasty, I usually will insert a grommet type of tympanostomy tube in the anteroinferior quadrant of the eardrum when I am doing a tympanoplasty procedure to strengthen the posterosuperior portion of the eardrum. I like to use a tragal perichondrium and cartilage graft placed medial to the posterosuperior quadrant of the eardrum, which usually is atrophic. Most of the time, the atrophic eardrum can be carefully dissected and removed intact from the facial recess area. However, in some cases, the eardrum has become adherant to the mucous membranes in the region of the sinus tympani and the facial recess. When this has occurred, surgical repair is extremely difficult, a facial recess (posterior tympanotomy) may be required, and the chance for development of cholesteatoma in the mesotympanum is reasonably high. A second look procedure may be required if the surgeon has the impression that epithelium has been left within the sinus tympani of the middle ear.

One of the greatest dilemmas in otologic management is the matter of deciding when to recommend tympanoplasty surgery for the patient who is showing signs of deep posterosuperior retraction pocket and "incipient cholesteatoma." The dilemma can be described as follows: How can the otologic surgeon recommend a surgical procedure for a patient who has minimal or no ear discomfort, normal hearing, and no otorrhea when the risks of the surgical procedure might include perforation of the eardrum, worsening of hearing, and intermittent otorrhea? Stated in this way, it would seem that the risks outweigh the benefits of surgical intervention. However, as the years have passed and I have had an opportunity to follow many patients over the course of time, I have been impressed that there definitely is an optimal time to surgically intervene to prevent hearing loss and irreversible structural changes of the eardrum and ossicles. The optimal time to intervene is when insertion of a tympanostomy tube has proved not to be the definitive therapy in preventing progressive deepening of a posterosuperior retraction pocket. When I have observed the progression of structural changes in the posterosuperior quadrant of the eardrum and I have not operated, I have sometimes seen the development of polypoid granulation in a deep posterosuperior retraction pocket. I also have seen erosion of the ossicles, otorrhea, and hearing loss. Now, my goal is to intervene before these irreversible changes occur. The only problem with taking this somewhat aggressive approach is that there may be cases in which the indication for surgery was "incipient cholesteatoma" in a patient with normal hearing and a dry ear, and then the result of surgery may be mild conductive hearing loss, an eardrum perforation, and temporary otorrhea. Certainly, when these are the postoperative findings, the result is discouraging. Nonetheless, failure to intervene at the proper time can lead to worse hearing and less chance for achieving the desired ultimate outcome of normal hearing, dry ear, and intact eardrum.

OSSICULAR INJURY FROM INSERTION OF TYMPANOSTOMY TUBE

The chance of injuring an ossicle from inserting a tympanostomy tube is extremely low. When an otolaryngologist uses an operating microscope and ear speculum to insert a tympanostomy tube in a patient under general anesthesia, the tube can be carefully placed in portions of the eardrum that are not near the ossicles. Specifically, the tube usually can be placed in the anteroinferior quadrant of the eardrum, and the tube should not come in contact with the ossicles. Unless a mishap such as sudden head movement occurs in an awake patient or the surgeon's hand is bumped or jarred, damage to the ossicles should not occur.

INJURY TO A DEHISCENT JUGULAR BULB

Injury to a dehiscent jugular bulb can be avoided by carefully examining the eardrum prior to making an incision for insertion of a tympanostomy tube. The dehiscent jugular bulb will appear as a bluish structure medial to the inferior aspect of the eardrum. Despite admonitions that appear in textbooks, the dehiscent jugular bulb actually is quite easily discernible on careful examination of the eardrum, and injury should be avoided by not incising the eardrum near any bluish structure that appears to be medial to inferior portions of the eardrum. When I encounter an eardrum with the obvious or questionable appearance of a dehiscent jugular bulb, I do not make an incision and insert a tympanostomy tube. Usually, alternative modes of therapy are acceptable if the potential risk outweighs the benefit of inserting a tympanostomy tube. Then I order a CT scan of the temporal bone to determine the presence or absence of a dehiscent jugular bulb or to detect any other abnormality that could account for the bluish structure that had been previously observed on examination of the ear in the operating room.

REFERENCES

1. Paradise JL: On tympanostomy tubes: rationale, results, reservations, and recommendations. *Pediatrics* 1977; 60:86–90.
2. Black N: Surgery for glue ear—a modern epidemic. *Lancet* 1984; 11:835–837.
3. Gonzalez C, Arnold JE, Woody EA, et al: Prevention of recurrent acute otitis media: Chemoprophylaxis versus tympanostomy tubes. *Laryngoscope* 1986; 96:1330–1334.
4. Maw AR: Is your grommet really necessary [letter]? *Arch Dis Child* 1987; 62:656–658.
5. Stickler GB: The attack on the tympanic membrane. *Pediatrics* 1984; 74:291–292.
6. Grundfast KM, Carney C, in *Ear Infections in Your Child*. New York, Warner Books, 1989, pp 10–16.
7. Gates GA, Paradise JL: Do ear tubes help chronic ear infection? *Physician's Weekly* and *Washington Post* May 3, 1988.
8. Brody J: Personal health. *The New York Times,* April 23, 1986.
9. Karlan MS, Mufson RA, Grizzard MB, et al: Potentiation of infections by biomaterials: A comparison of three materials. *Otolaryngol Head Neck Surg* 1981; 89:528–534.
10. Crysdale WS: Comparative study of various ventilating tubes. *Ann Otol Rhinol Laryngol* 1976; 85(suppl 25):268–269.
11. McGuirt WF: Medical news report on "A prospective randomized study of four commonly used tympanostomy tubes" by Weigel MT, et al. *Arch Otolaryngol Head Neck Surg* 1988; 114:612–613.
12. Tos M, Stangerup SE, Holm-Jensen S, et al: Spontaneous course of secretory otitis and changes of the eardrum. *Arch Otolaryngol Head Neck Surg* 1984; 110:281–289.
13. Tos M, Stangerup SE, Larse P: Dynamics of eardrum changes following secretory otitis—a prospective study. *Arch Otolaryngol Head Neck Surg* 1987; 113:380–385.
14. Brenman AK, Milner RM, Weller CR: Use of hydrogen peroxide to clear blocked ventilation tubes. *Am J Otol* 1986; 7:47–50.
15. Gates GA, Avery CA, Prihoda TJ, et al: Effectiveness of adenoidectomy and tympanostomy tubes in the treatment of chronic otitis media with effusion. *N Engl J Med* 1987; 317:1444–1451.
16. Gates GA, Avery CA, Prihoda TJ: Effect of adenoidectomy upon children with chronic otitis media with effusion. *Laryngoscope* 1988; 98:58–63.
17. Slack RW, Gardner JM, Chatfield C: Otorrhea in children with middle ear ventilation tubes: A comparison of different types of tubes. *Clin Otolaryngol* 1987; 12:357–360.
18. Gates GA, Avery C, Prihoda TJ, et al: Delayed onset post-tympanostomy otorrhea. *Otolaryngol Head Neck Surg* 1988; 98:111–115.
19. Goldofsky E: Tympanostomy tubes for chronic serous otitis media: A literature review. *Mt Sinai J Med* 1987; 54:355–358.
20. Balkany TJ, Barkin RM, Suzuki BH, et al: A prospective study of infection following tympanostomy and tube insertion. *Am J Otol* 1983; 4:288–291.
21. Gates GA, Avery C, Prihoda TJ, et al: Post tympanostomy otorrhea. *Laryngoscope* 1986; 96:630–634.
22. Balkany TJ, Arenberg IK, Steenerson RL: Ventilation tube surgery and middle ear irrigation. *Laryngoscope* 1986; 96:529–532.

23. Baker RS, Chole RA: A randomized clinical trial of topical gentamicin after tympanostomy tube placement. *Arch Otolaryngol Head Neck Surg* 1988; 114:755–757.
24. Wight RG, Jones AS, Connell JA, et al: Three year follow-up (1983–1986) of children undergoing bilateral grommet insertion in Sheffield. *Clin Otolaryngol* 1987; 12:371–375.
25. Becker GD, Eckberg TJ, Goldware RR: Swimming and tympanostomy tubes: A prospective study. *Laryngoscope* 1987; 97:740–741.
26. el Silimy O, Bradley PJ: Bacteriological aspects of swimming with grommets. *Clin Otolaryngol* 1986; 11:323–327.
27. Tos M, Poulsen G: Secretory otitis media: Late results of treatment with grommets. *Arch Otolaryngol* 1976; 102:672.
28. Gunderson T, Tonning FM, Dveberg KH: Ventilating tubes in the middle ear. Longterm observations. *Arch Otolaryngol* 1984; 110:783–784.
29. Stangerup SE, Tos M: Treatment of secretory otitis media and pneumatization. *Laryngoscope* 1986; 96:680–684.
30. Slack RWT, Maw AR, Capper JWR, et al: Prospective study of tympanosclerosis developing after grommet insertion. *J Laryngol Otol* 1984; 98:771–774.

Tympanostomy Tubes

Approach of

Steven D. Handler, M.D.

The use of tympanostomy tubes in the management of middle ear disorders has increased dramatically in the past years. Since Armstrong reintroduced the concept of an indwelling tympanostomy tube in 1954, the procedure to place tympanostomy tubes has become the most common operation in the United States today. The purpose of this chapter is to acquaint the reader with indications for and the management of tympanostomy tubes in the treatment of middle ear disorders.

INDICATIONS

Tympanostomy tubes are indicated in the management of the following conditions:

1. Recurrent acute otitis media that has not responded to medical management with chemoprophylaxis for at least 4 to 6 weeks. Since this disease is most often bilateral, tympanostomy tubes are placed in both ears.
2. Persistent serous otitis media that has not responded to medical management with chemoprophylaxis for at least 4 to 6 weeks. Since the fluid is most often bilateral, tympanostomy tubes are placed in both ears. If middle ear effusion is present in one ear only, the use of tympanostomy tubes depends on other criteria. If the child is of normal intelligence, has language skills appropriate for his or her age, normal hearing in the contralateral ear, and we are into the spring or summer months (less infections), I usually do not recommend tympanostomy tubes in these patients. However, if the child is developmentally delayed, has other handicaps such as visual or auditory processing problems, and we are approaching the fall and winter months (more infections), I would strongly recommend bilateral tympanostomy tube placement.

3. Severe atelectasis and tympanic membrane retraction. The unilateral or bilateral placement of tympanostomy tube in this condition depends on the presence of pathology. If only one ear is affected, the contralateral ear would not be a candidate for a tympanostomy tube.

4. High negative middle ear pressure with resultant conductive hearing loss that is affecting speech and language development.

5. The presence of a complication of acute otitis media, such as acute coalescent mastoiditis, facial nerve paralysis, or meningitis. (Although the acute episode can certainly be treated

with myringotomy alone, the placement of tubes allows for chronic ventilation and permits complete resolution of the process while giving some protection from recurrence in the next 6 to 12 months.) Although a complication of middle ear disease is usually unilateral, these occur most often in otitis-prone children. For this reason, tympanostomy tubes are usually placed bilaterally.

PROCEDURE

When the decision to place tympanostomy tubes has been reached, arrangements are made to have this performed under a general anesthesia. I do not perform these procedures in children under local anesthesia or without anesthesia as some surgeons suggest for very young children. Local injections to the ear are often quite painful, and I have found that iontophoresis is often undependable in its ability to obtain anesthesia for the external auditory canal and tympanic membrane. To perform the procedure without any anesthesia is cruel and barbaric. In addition, the extremely loud noise created by suctioning the middle ear fluid adds to the discomfort and fear of the child. The preferred anesthestic is an inhalation agent administered by mask. Intubation is usually not required.

A sterile clear plastic drape with a center hole (eye drape, Microtek 4914) is placed over the first ear as the head is rotated to the opposite side by the anesthesiologist. The ear is examined using the operating microscope, and wax and debris cleared from the external auditory canal. No attempt is made to sterilize the external canal by use of any antiseptic preparation solution. A circumferential incision is made in the anterosuperior or anteroinferior quadrant using a pediatric myringotomy blade (Beaver 7121). The middle ear is suctioned clear of all fluid that is found after the myringotomy. If the mucus is too thick to be evacuated with a no. 5 French suction tube, a no. 7 French suction tube is used to evacuate the middle ear contents. A second hole (beer can effect) is rarely needed to aid in mucus removal. I do not flush or irrigate the middle ear contents since I find this to be unnecessary to remove the fluid, and its efficacy in cleansing the middle ear is questionable. A myringotomy tube is placed in the incision site, and any blood and secretions are suctioned to clear the tube lumen. Antibiotic-containing otic drops (Cortisporin otic suspension) are placed in the external canal, and the procedure is repeated in the other ear. The procedure is terminated, and the child taken to the recovery room.

I routinely have the parents administer otic drops (Cortisporin otic suspension or Garamycin ophthalmic solution) to the ears twice daily for 2 days to make sure the tube lumen stays patent. In the case of excessive bleeding during tympanostomy tube placement, Afrin solution may be placed in the ear to slow down the bleeding prior to terminating the procedure. In those instances of significant bleeding, otic drops are continued for 7 to 10 days postoperatively to ensure patency of the tube lumen. In addition, if purulent fluid is found at the time of myringotomy, oral antibiotics are prescribed for 7 to 10 days.

The tympanostomy tube that I use for the majority of my patients is a silicone Paparella tube with an internal diameter of 1.0 mm (Microtek 2445). I have these tubes customized for my practice without tabs on the lateral flange. I have found these tabs to be more of a nuisance in that they often will scrape against the medial external auditory canal during insertion. This can cause a laceration and resultant meddlesome bleeding during tube insertion. I find the flexibility of the silicone tube allows the tube to be popped into a small myringotomy incision without tearing the tympanic membrane. The silicone appears to have little tendency to occlude with cerumen or secretions when compared with other tube materials. In fact, I have had the opportunity to compare several other materials to the silicone tube, and I have found the silicone tube to be as good as, if not better than, Biolite, titanium, and gold ventilating tubes of similar design.

I do not use long ventilating tubes (Armstrong I or Goode T tube) because these long thin tubes tend to lie up against the external canal and become easily encrusted with wax and skin debris. In addition, it is difficult to treat otorrhea from these tubes with topical drops alone, since the drops have to traverse such a long distance. The T tubes have two other disadvantages: (1) a general anesthetic is usually necessary to remove the tube from the tympanic membrane, and (2) they have a high incidence of postoperative permanent perforation. The long ventilating tube does have its use, however, in the very thickened tympanic membrane that will not allow placement of a standard double-flanged Paparella tube. If a T tube is placed in such an ear, the medial flanges are trimmed so that they do not extend so far beneath the tympanic membrane, and the lateral end of the tube is trimmed so that it does not lie against the external auditory canal.

In the case of the child who has required multiple insertions of tubes (at least three) or the child in whom the standard Paparella tube extrudes within 2 or 3 months, a Paparella tube with a larger internal and external diameter is used. The Paparella II tube has an internal diameter of 1.27 mm (Microtek 2446) and tends to remain in the tympanic membrane for 12 to 24 months. Although the majority of Paparella II tubes spontaneously extrude at the end of this time, a small number will remain in place and have to be removed, usually under a general anesthetic. The incidence of postoperative perforation after spontaneous extrusion is only slightly higher than that of the standard Paparella tube.

In the case of severe tympanic membrane atelectasis or adhesive otitis, a tympanostomy tube should be considered as the first line of treatment. I will often have the anesthesiologist maintain as much positive pressure as possible to attempt to inflate the middle ear with nitrous oxide. Often the tympanic membrane will lift off of the promontory and present an adequate site for tympanostomy tube placement. If the tympanic membrane does not lift off the promontory with this maneuver or after an incision in the tympanic membrane, consideration must be given to a formal tympanoplasty. In the case of a severe tympanic membrane retraction, I find it is very important to make sure there is no squamous debris or wax within the retraction pocket that might prevent its return to a normal position with ventilation from the tympanostomy tube. Often, a plug of wax and skin debris can line the sides and fill the retraction pocket. If this plug is not removed, the retraction pocket cannot evert sufficiently. In all cases, attempt is made to evert the retraction pocket with a small (18- or 20-gauge) suction tube prior to termination of the procedure.

Although placement of the tympanostomy tube in the anterior quadrants may be technically more difficult, studies show that tubes placed in these quadrants tend to remain in place for longer periods of time compared with those placed in the posterior quadrants. Since the anterior quadrants are not so readily visible during routine office otoscopy, I may have to tell the family that the tubes are far anterior so that the pediatrician or family practitioner can locate the tube during office examinations.

ADENOIDECTOMY

Adenoidectomy as a primary therapy for management of middle ear disorders is still quite controversial. At the present time, I believe that adenoidectomy is indicated in cases of recurrent adenoiditis or upper airway obstruction secondary to adenoid hypertrophy. I do not believe that adenoidectomy alone for management of middle ear disease is indicated unless at least some of these symptoms are present. However, in the case of recurrent or persistent middle ear disease that requires multiple insertions of tubes, consideration should be given to performing an adenoidectomy with the next set of tympanostomy tubes even if there is not clear-cut evidence of recurrent adenoiditis or adenoid hypertrophy. I do not believe that tonsillectomy plays a role in the management of middle ear disease. Consequently, unless there are specific indications for tonsillectomy, adenoidectomy alone would be performed.

INTRAOPERATIVE COMPLICATIONS

Although ossicular injury secondary to myringotomy and tympanostomy tube placement is a possible complication of the procedure, it is a very rare occurrence and should be prevented by staying away from the posterosuperior quadrant. In addition, excessive manipulation of the malleus should be avoided during the procedure.

Often, the operating room personnel wince at the loud noise generated by suctioning middle ear contents. We wondered if this noise could conceivably cause a sensorineural hearing loss. We have never demonstrated any postoperative hearing losses that could be attributed to high noise levels. However, our measurements of the suctioning noise at the level of the patient's ear indicate that the decibel level is probably high enough to induce a temporary threshold shift in some of these patients. This may be the reason that some children do not notice or demonstrate an improvement in their hearing immediately after myringotomy.

The incidence of entry into a dehiscent jugular bulb during tympanostomy tube placement is extremely rare if myringotomy is confined to the anterior quadrants. In addition, care should be taken not to allow the myringotomy blade to extend deep to the tympanic membrane and touch the promontory where the jugular bulb might be located. However, if profuse bleeding should occur during myringotomy from a dehiscent jugular bulb, the procedure should be terminated and the external canal packed with cotton packing. If this is successful in stopping the hemorrhage, CT scan of the temporal bone should be performed to determine the source of the bleeding. Rarely, surgical intervention with exploratory tympanostomy is required to control the bleeding.

An ectopic carotid in the middle ear space is a very uncommon anomaly. Since it may appear in the anteroinferior quadrant, it may be injured by myringotomy in that position. An ectopic carotid is usually visible through an intact tympanic membrane and appears as a dull hypotympanic mass. However, serous otitis fluid behind the tympanic membrane may obscure the aberrant vessel. Damage to this vascular structure should be managed in a manner similar to that described for the dehiscent jugular bulb.

POSTOPERATIVE CONSIDERATIONS

The incidence of posttympanostomy tube otorrhea in my practice runs approximately 10% to 20% over the duration of tube placement. The majority of these bouts of otorrhea are associated with upper respiratory tract infections. I am able to clear the majority of these cases of otorrhea with drops for 10 days. I use either Cortisporin otic suspension or Garamycin ophthalmic solution should the child not tolerate the Cortisporin. Occasionally, the child is brought into the office so that the ear canal and tube lumen can be suctioned clear of secretions prior to institution of topical drop therapy. This is especially important in cases of profuse otorrhea where the drops cannot enter the ear canal. If the external auditory canal is so swollen that drops will not enter, a wick must be placed for 2 to 3 days to allow drops to come into contact with the tube and tympanic membrane. Some of the children do not respond to this regimen of topical drops, and these will require a course of oral antibiotics. The choice of antibiotics is the same as that for the treatment of a bout of acute otitis media, with amoxicillin being the primary drug of choice.

A few children have frequent bouts of otorrhea with every upper respiratory tract infection. These may occur at 2- to 3-week intervals and clear completely between episodes. These children are placed on a course of antibiotic prophylaxis for 8 to 12 weeks. This regimen is often very successful in preventing these recurrent bouts of otorrhea.

In the case of persistent otorrhea that does not clear with topical or oral antibiotics (or both), the child is admitted to the hospital for intravenous antibiotics and daily suctioning of the external canal secretions. Antibiotic choice is based on culture and sensitivity of the secretions. The most common organisms responsible for these infections are *Staphylococcus* and *Pseudomonas*. If the course of intravenous antibiotics does not clear the otorrhea, or if the otorrhea recurs soon after the treatment is stopped, the myringotomy tubes are removed (either in the office or in the operating room, depending on the patient). In this way, the foreign body is removed, and the chronically infected ear is allowed to "cool down." The discharge usually decreases dramatically as the tympanic membrane heals. Serous (noninfected) fluid will often reappear behind the intact tympanic membrane. The child is then kept on antibiotic prophylaxis to keep the ear clear before reinsertion of tympanosotomy tubes is considered.

Residual perforation of the tympanic membrane after tympanostomy tube placement is a bothersome problem. I have found an incidence of approximately 1% of my patients sustaining permanent perforation after spontaneous extrusion of the Paparella 1.0 mm tympanostomy tube. The incidence of persistent perforation after the use of the Paparella 1.27 mm tube or the T tube is about 5% to 10%. Placing a tympanostomy tube in an atrophic portion of the tympanic membrane may increase the incidence of postoperative permanent perforation. If a ventilating tube remains in place for more than 3 years, I usually remove the tube to see if the child has outgrown the eustachian tube problem and subsequent middle ear disease. This procedure is usually performed under a general anesthetic in the operating room. After the tube is removed, the perforation is cauterized with trichloroacetic acid, or the edge is surgically rimmed with a straight pick to freshen up the edges. A patch of cigarette paper is then placed over the perforation to help guide squamous epithelial healing. If the perforation does not heal after 6 months, a formal tympanoplasty can be performed to close the perforation. A small perforation that occurs after spontaneous extrusion of a tympanostomy tube may be treated in the same way. A paper patch myringoplasty may be attempted before a formal tympanoplasty is considered.

Obstruction of the lumen of the tympanostomy tube can be a difficult problem to treat. Occlusion of the tube lumen with blood can occur in the immediate postoperative period or as a result of hemorrhagic otorrhea at a later date. If the clot is fresh, it can be suctioned out in the office under the operating microscope and the patency of the tube lumen assured. Otic drops can also be used to loosen and dissolve the fresh clot. If the clot is already hardened, I have been successful in using hydrogen peroxide to dissolve the clot or hardened wax. I prescribe 4 drops three times daily until the child complains of discomfort from the peroxide solution entering the middle ear. At that time, I know that the tube lumen has been opened, and the peroxide drops are discontinued. Antibiotic-containing otic drops are now prescribed for 3 days to prevent or treat the inflammatory response that might occur as a result of the per-

oxide entering the middle ear cavity. Occasionally, the lumen of the tube becomes plugged with dried middle ear secretions. This appears as an amber plug within the tube lumen. This may be successfully treated in the office under the operating microscope. The plug of dried secretions is manipulated with a straight pick and either removed or pushed into the middle ear space. Any fluid in the middle ear is then suctioned out, and otic drops are used for 5 to 7 days to keep the tube lumen open.

Secondary acquired cholesteatoma from tympanostomy tube placement is very uncommon. I do not believe that any particular tube has an increased incidence of this problem. The main consideration would be anything that causes inward migration of squamous epithelium. Certainly, care should be taken not to push squamous epithelium medial to the tympanic membrane during tympanostomy tube placement. An indwelling tympanostomy tube and any residual perforation after spontaneous extrusion of the tube should be examined at 3- to 6-month intervals to detect any inward migration of squamous epithelium. If it does occur, surgical intervention with tympanoplasty and excision of the cholesteatoma should be performed. Occasionally a small squamous pearl will form on the lateral surface of the tympanic membrane at the site of the previous myringotomy. Since this pearl is usually small, localized, and on the lateral surface of the tympanic membrane, I will observe it for some time before considering surgical excision. Often, this pearl will spontaneously separate from the tympanic membrane and require no further treatment. If it does persist on the surface of the tympanic membrane, removal may require a brief general anesthetic.

A granuloma of the external canal may form as a result of the body's attempt to reject the ventilating tube. I attempt to gently suction the secretions and the granuloma free from the ventilating tube if possible. A no. 5 suction tube is often successful in removing the granuloma from the underlying ventilating tube. Grabbing the granuloma with cup or alligator forceps usually results in fragmentation of the tissue and meddlesome bleeding. Any granuloma that is not easily removed is cauterized with a silver nitrate stick, and the patient is treated with antibiotic and steroid-containing otic drops and an oral antibiotic effective against *Staphylococcus* species. If the granuloma does not resolve with this treatment, the ventilating tube and granuloma must be removed in the operating room under a general anesthetic.

CHAPTER 2

Tympanoplasty

Approach of

John T. McElveen, Jr., M.D.

PREOPERATIVE EVALUATION

Successful reconstruction of the tympanic membrane and ossicular chain requires an accurate preoperative assessment and attention to surgical technique. In addition to a complete otologic history and routine audiometric studies, the preoperative evaluation should include careful microscopic inspection of the ear. Particular attention should be paid to the type of perforation (marginal or central), the condition of the middle ear mucosa, the presence of purulent discharge, and the status of the ossicular chain.

Tympanic membrane perforations can be divided into central or marginal perforations. The central perforations may vary in size but always have a margin of drum remnant surrounding them (Fig 2–1). Marginal perforations extend to the tympanic sulcus and fail to have a surrounding drum remnant. Meticulous care is needed in evaluation of marginal perforations, particularly those involving the attic or the posterosuperior aspect of the tympanic membrane. The apparent marginal perforation may actually be the opening to a cholesteatoma sac (Fig 2–2).

Whereas normal middle ear mucosa is a positive prognostic finding, diseased or absent mucosa may indicate the need for intraoperative placement of silicone rubber (Silastic) sheeting. Mucosal disease in association with ossicular defects may indicate the need to "stage" the operation.

Although reports in the literature indicate comparable results in discharging and nondischarging ears, it is preferable to resolve the drainage before the surgical procedure is performed. Topical application of CSF powder—a mixture of chloramphenicol (50 mg), sulfanilimide (50 mg), and amphotericin B (Fungizone; 5 mg)—is particularly effective in resolving the drainage.

Preoperative evaluation of eustachian tube function is generally not necessary since the presence of poor eustachian tube function is not a contraindication for surgery. However, cleft palate patients may be poor surgical candidates. I evaluate the contralateral ear; if it is normal, the prognosis is much improved. During the surgical procedure, all patients have eustachian tube patency confirmed using a lacrimal probe. If the eustachian tube orifice is obstructed by redundant mucosa or granulation tissue, the tissue is removed and a sliver of 0.005-in. Silastic sheeting is placed.

Tympanic membrane repair is not contraindicated in young children. If the contralateral ear has been free of recurrent serous otitis and the child is a good surgical risk, the drum can be reconstructed. I tend to favor the postauricular approach in children.

Flaccid Drum

The management of the flaccid tympanic membrane remains controversial. The presence of an abnormal flaccid tympanic membrane is not an indication to replace it. However, if the patient perceives a hearing loss and there is a conductive loss greater than 10 dB, or if the flaccid drum is adherent to the promontory or ossicles (unable to lift off with pneumotoscopy or politzerization), a tympanoplasty is appropriate. An asymptomatic flaccid drum, retracted, yet not attached to the promontory, can be managed conservatively. The patient should be instructed to do the Valsalva maneuver at regular intervals to aerate the middle ear space and relieve the retraction.

Vascular Masses

In addition to assessing the status of the tympanic membrane and ossicular chain, the surgeon should note the presence of any vascular masses. Glomus tumors, an aberrant internal carotid, or a dehiscent jugular bulb may occasionally be seen

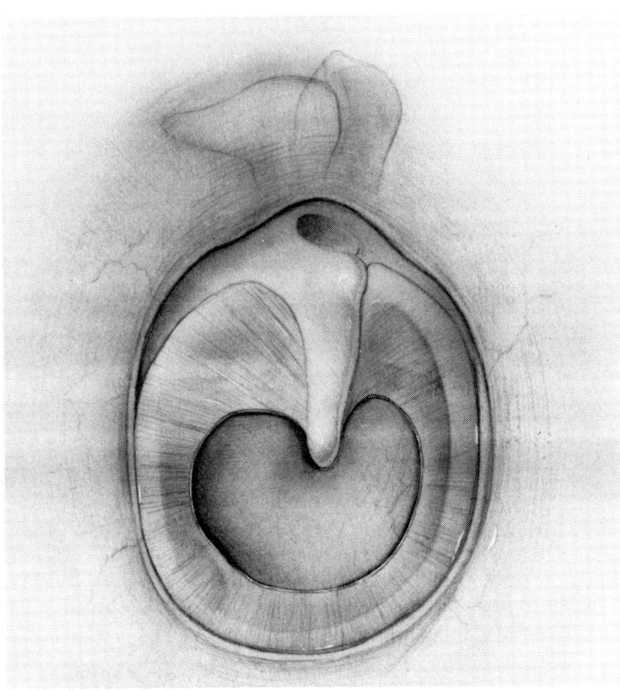

FIG 2–1.
Central perforation.

through the tympanic membrane defect. Although I do not routinely obtain preoperative radiographs for tympanoplastic procedures, the presence of a vascular mass extending beyond the annulus requires radiographic evaluation.[1]

SURGICAL TECHNIQUE

The techniques involved in tympanic membrane grafting fall into one of two categories: lateral or medial. The terms lateral graft and medial graft refer to the location of the graft relative to the annular ligament. The graft is placed medial to the handle of the malleus in both techniques. The decision as to which technique I use is based on the location and size of the perforation, the presence of extensive tympanosclerosis, and whether the patient has previously undergone an unsuccessful tympanoplasty in the involved ear.

The lateral graft technique is used in patients with perforations involving the anterior quadrant of the tympanic membrane, patients who have failed a previous tympanoplastic procedure, and patients with posterior quadrant perforations and extensive tympanosclerosis. (It is important to remove the tympanosclerosis surrounding the perforation; however, removal of the tympanosclerosis may convert a small posterior perforation into a subtotal perforation, thus requiring a lateral graft technique.)

The lateral graft technique is well described.[2] Briefly, it consists of the following steps: (1) creation of a vascular strip, (2) elevation and anterior retraction of the vascular strip through a postauricular incision, (3) temporary removal of the anterior

canal wall skin, (4) removal of the tympanic membrane's squamous layer (Fig 2–3), (5) placement of the temporalis fascia graft medial to the handle of the malleus and lateral to the annular ligament (Figs 2–4 to 2–6), and (6) replacement of the anterior canal skin and vascular strip.

Removal of the anterior canal skin and thinning of the anterior bony overhang afford excellent exposure of the tympanic membrane's anterior sulcus. However, blunting of the anterior sulcus may occur if the fascia overlaps the anterior canal wall skin or if an inadequate sulcus exists for the fascia graft. Occasionally the malleus handle is not present due to chronic ear disease or prior surgery (Fig 2–7). In such cases the lateral graft technique needs to be altered to prevent lateralization of the graft. The graft is anchored by placing a flap of fascia from the graft into the posterior aspect of the epitympanum, preventing lateralization (Fig 2–8).

With any postauricular approach, it is important to accurately reapproximate the skin and subcutaneous tissue to ensure that the auricle is returned to its preoperative position. The mastoid dressing is removed on the first postoperative day, and the patient is discharged from the hospital with a 7-day course of a first-generation cephalosporin. The postauricular incision is inspected on the seventh postoperative day. The patient is instructed to begin using antibiotic eardrops (3 drops three times daily) for 2 weeks beginning on the twenty-first postoperative day. The drops dissolve the absorbable gelatin sponge (Gelfoam) packing in the external canal and prevent infection. The patient is then seen 3 months following surgery, and any residual packing is removed from the external canal. The graft should be completely healed at this point, and, thus, no further water precautions are necessary.

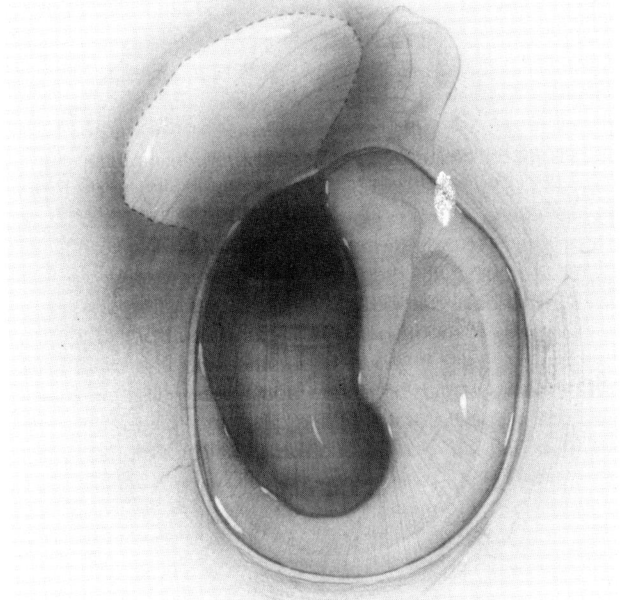

FIG 2–2.
Cholesteatoma mimicking a marginal perforation.

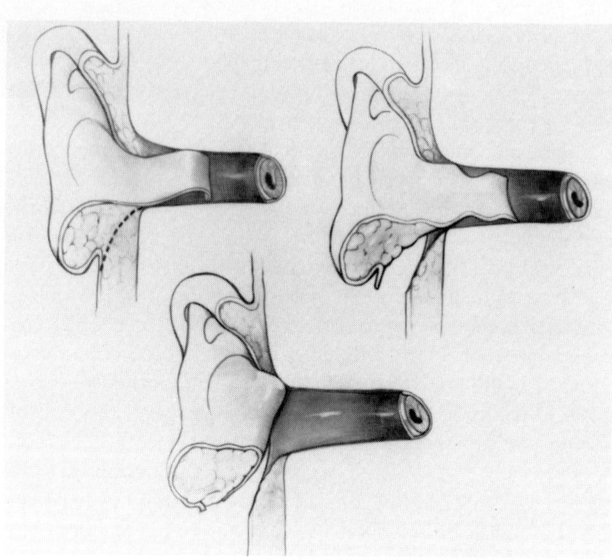

FIG 2–3.
Lateral graft technique.

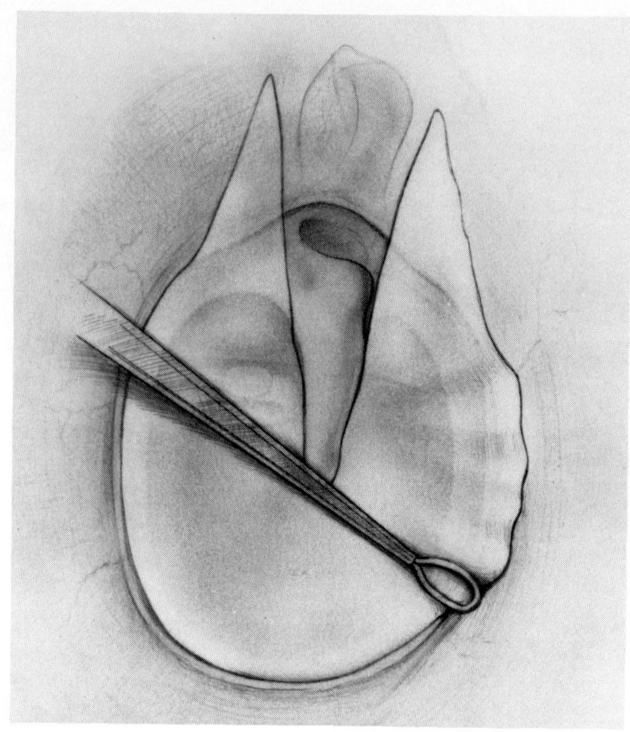

FIG 2–5.
Lateral graft technique. Fascia placed lateral to annular ligament.

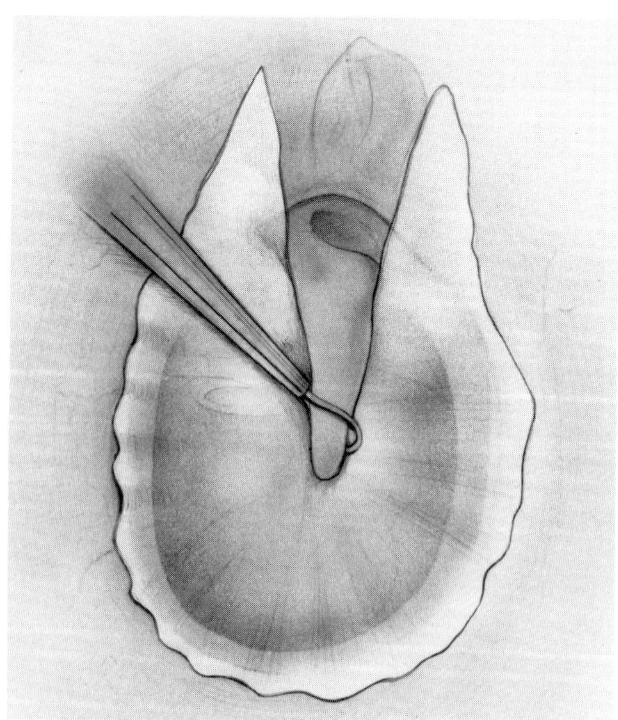

FIG 2–4.
Lateral graft technique. Fascia placed medial to malleus handle.

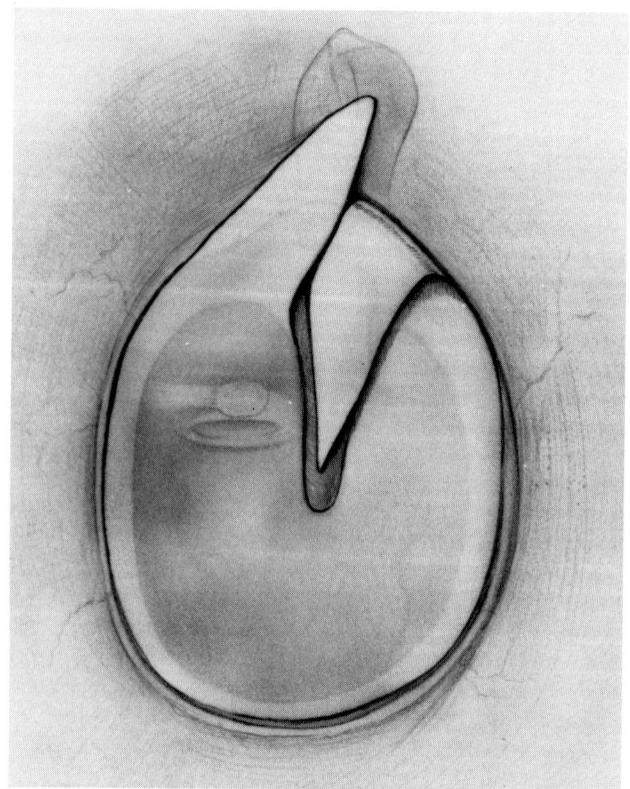

FIG 2–6.
Lateral graft technique. Strip of fascia covering handle of malleus.

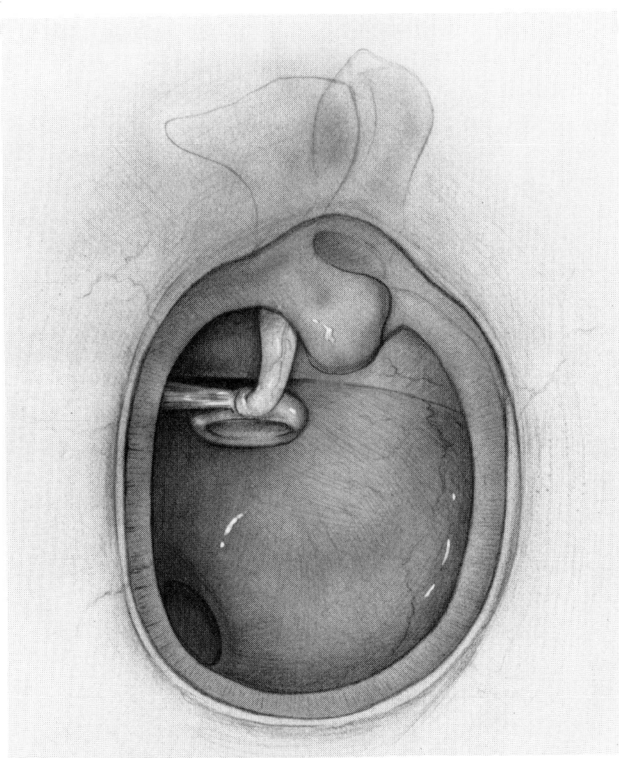

FIG 2–7.
Tympanic membrane perforation with absent malleus handle.

Medial Graft

Suitable candidates for the medial graft technique are patients with uncomplicated tympanic membrane perforations limited to the posterior quadrant of the drum.

There are many variations of the medial graft procedure; however, my personal preference is the technique advocated by Dr. Jack Hough.[3] It consists of the following steps: (1) rimming the perforation of squamous tissue, (2) elevating a tympanomeatal flap and removing squamous remnants from the membrane's medial surface, (3) placing the fascia medial to the handle of the malleus and the annular ligament, and (4) returning the tympanomeatal flap. The procedure is usually performed transcanal, but in cases of canal stenosis, the tympanomeatal flap can be elevated using a postauricular approach.

Unless a postauricular incision is performed, patients are not seen in follow-up until their sixth postoperative week. As with the lateral graft procedure, the mastoid dressing is removed on the first postoperative day, and patients are discharged on first-generation cephalosporin therapy; however, the antibiotic eardrops are not started until the fourth postoperative week. During the postoperative visit, any residual Gelfoam is removed from the external canal, and the graft is inspected. Barring complications, no further water precautions are necessary.

Combined Membrane and Ossicular Defects

The management of combined membrane and ossicular defects is based on the condition of the middle ear mucosa, the presence of residual squamous tissue in the middle ear space, and the status of the remaining ossicles (particularly the stapes). If the middle ear mucosa is absent, or if residual squamous epithelium is present, staging is required. During the first stage, reinforced Silastic sheeting (Supramid 0.02) is placed in the middle ear space, preventing the formation of adhesions between the tympanic membrane and the promontory. If the stapes footplate is fixed, the tympanic membrane is repaired and a stapedectomy deferred to a later time.

The interval between the initial operative procedure and the second stage procedure is, in part, a matter of personal preference. I generally delay the second procedure for 1 year. By this time the mucosa has healed, and the majority of the middle ear adhesions have resolved spontaneously. In children with residual squamous tissue in the middle ear space, the interval between the first and second stage is decreased to 6 months.

In ears where no staging is required, the management of the concomitant ossicular problem depends on the preference of the surgeon. Whereas there is general consensus regarding the materials used to reconstruct the tympanic membrane, there is no general consensus with respect to the materials used in ossicular chain reconstruction. Alloplasts in the forms of Plasti-Pore partial ossicular replacement prostheses (PORPs) and Plasti-

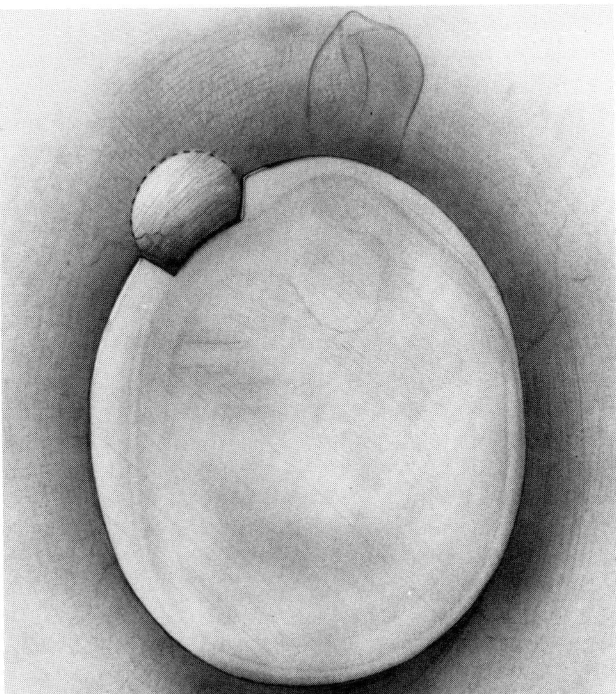

FIG 2–8.
Modified lateral graft technique to prevent lateralization.

Pore total ossicular replacement prostheses (TORPs) are routinely used by some, whereas others exclusively use nonalloplastic materials such as homografts and autografts.

Regardless of the surgeon's preference for alloplasts or nonalloplasts, the ossicular problems that confront the surgeon are similar and can be grouped into one of the following three categories: (1) an absent or fixed incus with a normal stapes, (2) an absent or fixed incus with an absent stapes suprastructure (mobile footplate), and (3) an absent or fixed incus with a fixed stapes.

Absent or Fixed Incus With Normal Stapes (Figure 2–9)

The alloplastic surgeon uses a PORP interposed between the tympanic membrane and the capitulum of the stapes. A piece of cartilage is interposed between the prosthesis and the tympanic membrane. The edges of the cartilage should be beveled, and the composite prosthesis should create only a slight bulge in the tympanic membrane. If too much tension is placed, one risks the problems of extrusion and stapes subluxation. (Determining the exact amount of tension needed is the most difficult assessment for the inexperienced otologist.)

The nonalloplastic surgeon uses the patient's incus or a homograft ossicle to bridge the gap between the handle of the malleus and the capitulum of the stapes. (It is preferable to have the handle of the malleus overlying the stapes capitulum. This is not always the case and may make the placement of the ossicle more difficult and compromise the hearing result.)

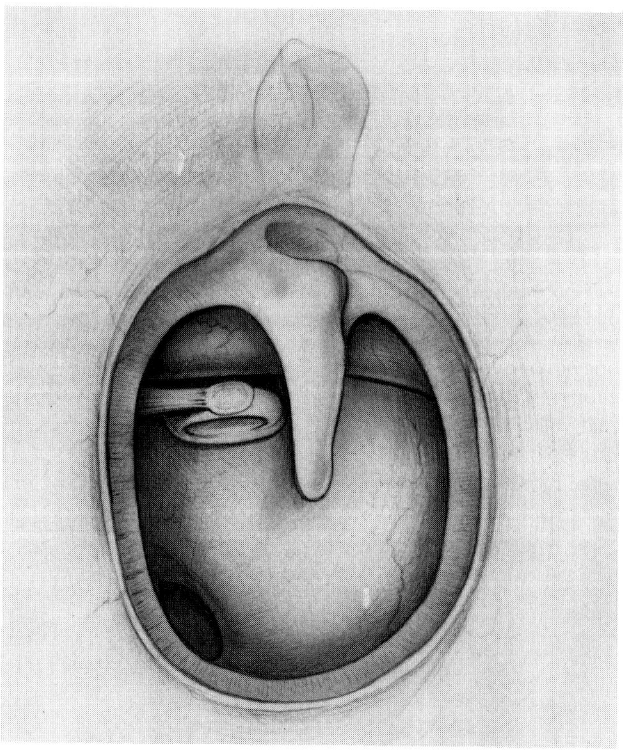

FIG 2–9.
Absent incus and mobile stapes.

Absent or Fixed Incus With an Absent Stapes Suprastructure, or Mobile Footplate (Figure 2–10)

The alloplastic surgeon uses a TORP in such cases. As with the partial replacement prosthesis, cartilage is interposed between the prosthesis and the tympanic membrane. The prosthesis extends from the tympanic membrane to the mobile footplate. Some of the alloplastic prostheses have a small protruding wire to prevent slippage off the footplate.

The nonalloplastic surgeon uses an incus crutch without the acetabulum. It extends from the handle of the malleus to the footplate.

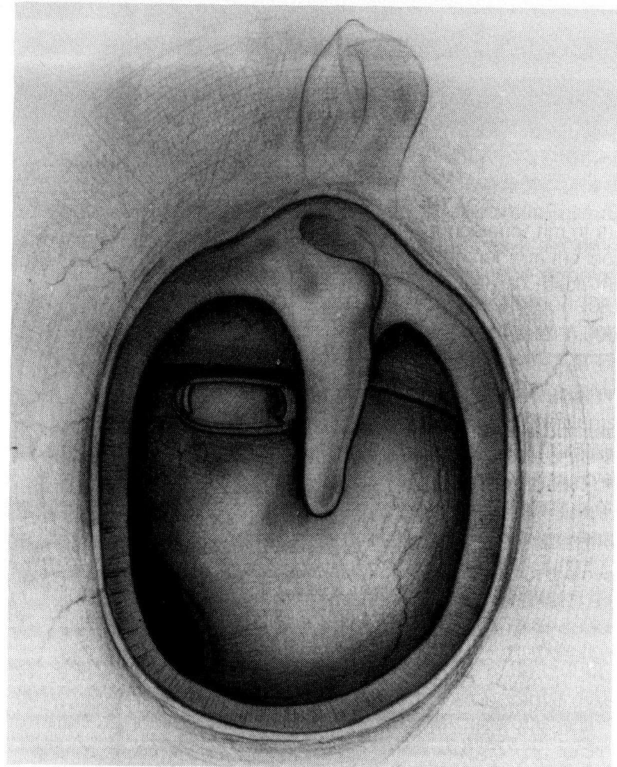

FIG 2–10.
Absent incus and missing stapes suprastructure (mobile footplate).

Absent or Fixed Incus With a Fixed Stapes

This is the most challenging reconstruction problem for both alloplastic and nonalloplastic surgeons. The alloplastic surgeon may use either an incus replacement prosthesis (IRP) that loops around the handle of the malleus and extends to the (tissue-covered) oval window or a TORP. Although the IRP is technically more difficult to place, it is firmly attached to the malleus and is less likely to be displaced into the vestibule.

The nonalloplastic surgeon uses a longer version of the incus crutch without the acetabulum. It extends from the malleus handle to the (tissue-covered) oval window.

Although similarities between alloplastic and nonalloplastic techniques exist, the role of the malleus in nonalloplastic procedures is much more critical. If the malleus is malpositioned or absent, staging may be required. A malleus is incorporated into the tympanic membrane during the first stage, and in the second stage the ossicular reconstruction is completed. With most alloplastic procedures, the presence or absence of the malleus is superfluous to the reconstruction.

After the ossicular reconstruction is completed, the canal is packed with antibiotic-soaked Gelfoam, and the patient is discharged on first-generation cephalosporin therapy. The patient is instructed to place antibiotic drops in the canal during the fourth postoperative week. The ear is evaluated on the sixth postoperative week, and any residual packing is removed. The hearing is evaluated 3 months after surgery and then annually. Long-term follow-up is essential in all patients undergoing ossicular reconstruction.

COMPLICATIONS: PREVENTION AND MANAGEMENT

Complications can occur with any operative procedure, and tympanic membrane repair is no exception. The complications more likely to be encountered in type 1 tympanoplasties include the following: (1) graft failure, (2) blunting of the anterior sulcus, (3) graft lateralization, and (4) graft medialization.

Graft failure should be limited to less than 10% and preferably less than 5%. The most common cause of failure is postoperative infection. To minimize this possibility, perioperative antibiotics should be administered and the middle ear and external canal Gelfoam packing impregnated with an antibiotic solution. (I generally use Colymycin Otic Solution.) If the patient develops purulent drainage prior to the third postoperative week, the antibiotic drops are instilled in the ear before the normally scheduled time.

Graft failures, not related to infection, may occur as a result of improper placement of the Silastic sheeting. The chance of extrusion is minimized if the edges of the Silastic sheeting are beveled and the Silastic is not under tension.

Blunting of the anterior sulcus is a complication generally associated with the lateral graft technique. In removing the anterior canal skin and the squamous layer of the tympanic membrane, one potentially loses the sharp angle created at the anterior sulcus. This blunting is minimized by creating a "neosulcus" just lateral to the annular ligament. The graft abuts the anterior canal skin at 90 degrees and does not extend onto the anterior canal wall. A small piece of Gelfoam is placed in the anterior sulcus to keep the fascia and anterior canal skin in this position. If severe blunting occurs, one should regraft the ear approximately 1 year following the previous procedure and adhere to the previously mentioned techniques. In patients with a foreshortened or absent manubrium, one may have difficulty seating the graft, resulting in graft lateralization. To minimize the likelihood of graft lateralization, hemostasis should be obtained, the nitrous oxide should be discontinued 20 to 30 minutes before the graft is placed, and a portion of the graft should be tucked into the epitympanum. As with the previous complications, lateralization of the graft requires regrafting approximately 1 year after the previous surgery.

Graft medialization may result in obliteration of the middle ear space and compromise the hearing result. This usually occurs as a result of fibrous tissue developing between the denuded promontory and the graft. It may also occur in medial grafting if the fascia is not adequately supported by the Gelfoam packing. Proper use of the Silastic sheeting will prevent this complication. If the complication does occur, the ear may need to be regrafted or the graft reflected off the promontory and a piece of reinforced Silastic interposed between the drum and the promontory.

CONCLUSION

Careful preoperative evaluation, meticulous surgical technique, and appropriate postoperative care will minimize postoperative complications and maximize the chances for successful otologic surgery.

REFERENCES

1. McElveen JT Jr, Lo WWM, El Gabri TH, et al: Aberrant internal carotid artery: Classic findings on computed tomography. *Otolaryngol Head Neck Surg* 1986; 94:616–621.
2. Sheehy JL: Surgery of chronic otitis media, in English GM (ed): *Otolaryngology*. New York, Harper & Row, Publishers, 1977, vol 1, pp 1–86.
3. Hough JD: Tympanoplasty with the interior fascial graft technique and ossicular reconstruction. *Laryngoscope* 1970; 80:1385.

Tympanoplasty

Approach of

J. Gail Neely, M.D.

Any discussion of technique tends to immediately imply that other techniques are inferior or that basic surgical principles tend to apply only to the ascribed technique. I disagree. Certainly in tympanoplasty there are many ways to accomplish a successful result. Basic surgical principles apply to each of these techniques; variance from those surgical principles creates suboptimal results. Each technique has its own special set of advantages, disadvantages, and special approaches to obviate the disadvantages. Repetitive experience with a given technique is probably the most important component to success, because try as we might, we cannot describe or illustrate every one of the important subtle details that makes one effort at the procedure fail and another effort at the procedure succeed.

Despite these inherent limitations of procedural description, I will attempt to convey, in as much detail as possible, my approach to tympanoplasty.

TECHNIQUE

Approach

A postauricular approach using a medial grafting technique with autogenous temporalis fascia is my procedure of choice.

Injections

One percent lidocaine with epinephrine 1:100,000 is injected into the canal and the postauricular area; approximately 3 to 4 mL is used in the canal, and approximately 3 mL postauricularly. If the patient is hypertensive, only 2 mL is used in the canal injunction, and no injection is made in the postauricular area.

The canal injection is begun by inserting the needle through the skin at the lateral margin of the vibrissae and impinging on the bone of the lateral osseous canal. The injection (1 mL) is first delivered to the thicker skin overlying the squamous bone contribution to the external auditory canal (i.e., that skin that is posterior to the tympanosquamous suture line and anterior to the tympanomastoid suture line). A posteroinferior injection of 1 mL into the densely adherent thinner skin overlying the

tympanic bone contribution to the external auditory canal is made, followed by an anterior injection of 1 mL. At the completion of these injections, the external auditory canal skin appears blanched, and no blebs are present. An additional 1 mL injection may be used in any area needed.

The postauricular injection is made approximately in the dermis along the line of incision; about 2.5 mL is used. The needle is then positioned medial to the superior aspect of the concha and lateral to the temporalis fascia, and 0.5 mL of solution is injected.

Smaller amounts of solution are used in fragile adults and children. In children, extra care must be taken not to position the needle external to the auditory canal, particularly inferiorly or anteriorly, in an effort to avoid facial paralysis from the injected anesthetic.

Incisions

Using the operating microscope, I make a longitudinal incision along the tympanosquamous suture line with a sickle knife. This incision extends from the anterior aspect of the notch of Rivinus to the lateral most extent of the osseous canal.

A horizontal incision is made approximately 2 mm lateral to the notch of Rivinus extending from the tympanosquamous suture line incision to the tympanomastoid suture line. This is made with a round knife, or "weapon." This incision can rarely be made by sliding the instrument along this course because of the thick, loosely attached skin. It is best done by pressing the instrument against the bone, cleanly severing that component of tissue, and then lifting the instrument to impinge another aspect of the proposed incision line and again pressing the instrument against the bone. When the horizontal incision reaches the tympanomastoid suture line, the character of the skin changes markedly to thin skin, tightly adherent to the tympanic bone. The knife is held tightly against the tympanic bone and slid posteroinferiorly along the tympanomastoid suture line, creating the second longitudinal incision ending at the lateral edge of the osseous canal.

Following this, the postauricular incision is made without the use of the microscope. This incision is a curvilinear line connecting three points. The first point is the anterior most extent of the postauricular sulcus. The second point is 1 cm posterior to the postauricular sulcus on a line tangent to the superior wall of the external auditory canal. The third point is at the very center of the inferior extent of the mastoid process. The postauricular incision is carried medially through layers to ultimately incise the periosteum over the mastoid and the areolar tissue and vestigial postauricular musculature over the temporalis fascia.

The lateral surface of the temporalis fascia is widely exposed and dissected inferiorly to the inferior margin of the temporalis muscle, taking care not to transect the skin of the external auditory meatus. A periosteal incision is made from the center of the mastoid process superiorly to the inferior margin of the temporalis muscle attachment. A second incision is made from the root of the zygoma along the inferior margin of the temporalis muscle to connect with the first periosteal incision; in making this incision, one should remember that the mastoid cortex is, at that point, curvilinear and extending into the external auditory meatus as the squamous bone contribution to the osseous canal. It is necessary to rotate the transverse axis of the knife inferiorly approximately 45 degrees, so as to make the periosteal incision perpendicular to the plane of the bone and avoid severing the external auditory canal skin.

The completion of these two periosteal incisions creates a triangular, anteriorly based soft tissue and periosteal flap, which is then elevated anteriorly to the posterosuperior margin of the osseous external auditory canal.

One failure to achieve adequate exposure is in not elevating the periosteum attached to the temporalis muscle slightly superiorly and the periosteum attached to the canal skin slightly inferiorly to expose the origin of the zygomatic process. This exposure is a necessary step to allow ultimate visualization of the anterior canal wall.

Temporalis fascia may be taken at this point and spread on a Teflon block and allowed to dry. Temporalis fascia, devoid of extraneous connective tissue, muscle, and fat, is my grafting tissue of choice.

A 6 $^1/_4$ in. Weitlander retractor is placed anteroposteriorly to hold the ear forward. The periosteum of the mastoid at the lateral margin of the posterosuperior osseous canal and the periosteum of the canal are elevated to the previous canal incisions. When the canal skin incision along the tympanomastoid suture line is first encountered, it should be extended laterally with a no. 15 blade to allow the pinna to be moved forward. If the canal skin incision along the tympanosquamous suture line is not severed far enough laterally to allow the rest of the pinna to move forward, that incision may be extended laterally as well with a no. 15 blade; this allows the canal skin between the incisions to fall free as a laterally based, conchal or vascular strip flap. Properly done, this flap and the attached pinna will move forward with retraction to allow complete visualization of the external auditory canal, including the anterior canal wall and its attendant skin. No additional ties or retractors are needed for this. If the pinna does not move easily forward, usually the canal incisions along the tympanosquamous and tympanomastoid suture lines have not been extended far enough laterally.

The periosteum remaining over the mastoid posteriorly and superiorly is elevated, and the second 6 $^1/_4$ in. Weitlander retractor is positioned to hold the wound open in a superoinferior direction.

Flaps

Before the tympanomeatal flaps are created, the margin of the perforation or the mouth of the cholesteatoma is incised so as to separate any abnormal skin bearing tissue from the drum remnant.

Some care is necessary in excising and removing the margin of the perforation. A small no. 3 Baron suction, a sickle knife, and small cup forceps are used to incise into the drum remnant, adjacent to the perforation, through the squamous layer and the fibrous layer of the drum, making every attempt not to incise the medial mucosal layer. The mucosal layer is separated from the medial aspect of the fibrous layer and is inspected for evidence of skin extending medially beyond the perforation. If skin is noticed to extend medially, the mucosal layer is dissected until the dissection is beyond the migrating skin. At that point the mucosal layer is severed, and the perforation margin, with the underlying mucosal layer and invading skin, is removed with cup forceps. In grasping the tissue with the cup forceps, one should shear the tissue along the plane of the fibrous layer rather than simply pulling the tissue at right angles from the wound. This shearing maneuver will assist in the complete removal of the perforation margin in one contiguous piece. Fragmented removal of this tissue increases the possibility of leaving skin behind in the middle ear.

The small amount of canal skin remaining between the tympanosquamous incision and the tympanomastoid incision and superior to the notch of Rivinus is elevated and discarded.

The remaining skin in the external auditory meatus is thin, tightly adherent skin attached to the tympanic bone. A portion of this skin is elevated into two tympanomeatal flaps: a posterior flap and an anterior flap. The posterior tympanomeatal flap is developed by elevating the canal skin from its lateral extent to the fibrous annulus and elevating the fibrous annulus, with attendant drum remnant, from the posterior edge of the notch of Rivinus to just short of the 6 o'clock position. The anterior tympanomeatal flap is accomplished by elevating the complete length of the canal skin from the lateral osseous canal to the fibrous annulus in continuity with the fibrous annulus and the anterior drum remnant. This elevates the anterosuperior flap one-fourth the circumference of the canal skin and tympanic membrane. The majority of the anterior canal skin and fibrous annulus remains tightly adherent to bone. Care is taken not to elevate this skin so as to avoid anterior canal skin blunting (discussed later).

The posterior tympanomeatal flap is carried anteriorly to the periosteum attaching the drum remnant to the posterior aspect of the manubrium. This is elevated from the manubrium and incised with Bellucci scissors along the posterior edge of the manubrium from the superior edge of the incision to the perforation. The anterior tympanomeatal flap is dissected through the periosteum attached to the manubrium and reflected down to, but not completely through, the attachment of the pars tensa to the umbo. Every effort is made to leave the pars tensa attached to the umbo if it is originally attached. In a total tympanic membrane perforation or large tympanic membrane perforation in which the pars tensa is not attached to the umbo, the anterior tympanomeatal flap is severed with Bellucci scissors along the anterior aspect of the manubrium into the perforation. The anterior tympanomeatal flap is reflected inferiorly, and the posterior tympanomeatal flap anteroinferiorly, allowing good visualization of the middle ear.

A special problem complicating exposure is an unusual posteriorly bulging anterior and anteroinferior osseous canal wall. The problem can be dealt with in several ways. One way is to divert to a lateral graft technique. Another way is to elevate the anterior canal skin down to, but not beyond, the fibrous annulus via a lateral circumferential incision at the lateral edge of the bulging canal. This anterior canal skin can be elevated around the bulging bone and that bone removed carefully with either mastoid curettes or a small fine cutting or diamond drill. Care must be taken not to catch the canal skin with the drill. A variant of this technique is to create an anterior canal wall skin, inferiorly based, flap by incising circumferentially along the lateral edge of the osseous canal and then just lateral to the fibrous annulus and elevating the canal skin posteroinferiorly to allow exposure of the obstructing bone.

Resection of Disease

A basic principle of disease resection, whether squamous epithelium from adhesions between the perforation and the promontory or cholesteatoma or granulation tissue, is to resect the disease in broad sheets, precisely constructed and excised, as opposed to fragmented and piecemeal removal.

Dissection of disease proceeds in the following order. First, Prussak's space is dissected to the neck of the malleus. If a primary acquired cholesteatoma is present, the dissection is done to separate the cholesteatoma matrix from the notch of Rivinus and the neck of the malleus, being careful not to break the continuity of the matrix. If no primary acquired cholesteatoma is present, the tissue is dissected from the notch of Rivinus and the neck of the malleus and discarded. The dissection is then directed toward the middle ear. If granulation tissue, or cholesteatoma, exists in the middle ear, the dissection begins along the superoanterior mesotympanum by exposing the hemicanal of the tensor tympani muscle and cochleariform process. The dissection is carried along the promontory and toward the protympanum in a sheetlike fashion, dissecting toward the hypotympanum and into the hypotympanum, ultimately ending at the posterior tympanum and the superior mesotympanum in the area of the stapes. At that point, contiguous disease is incised and removed, leaving disease only in the area of the posterior tympanum and about the stapes.

If the disease is limited to the mesotympanum and can clearly be seen and evaluated through the canal, completion of the middle ear disease removal is done through the canal before mastoidectomy. If, however, the disease extends out of view in the posterior tympanum or superior mesotympanum into the epitympanum, a mastoidectomy with resection of the canal wall or a mastoidectomy with the use of a facial recess approach is done prior to the final mesotympanic disease removal.

Mastoidectomy will be considered in detail in another section of this book. However, I would emphasize that the first step toward adequate visualization and disease removal is the posteriorly positioned postauricular incision, which affords wide exposure of the mastoid cortex. Extensive beveling of that cortex allows a near tangential view through the mastoid toward the middle ear, either in the removal of the posterior external auditory canal or in the facial recess approach to the middle ear.

Disease in the mastoid is dissected from lateral to medial and posterior to anterior. All disease is dissected, again in sheets, to the level of the horizontal semicircular canal, facial nerve, and stapes. This region is approached when exposure is maximal. Special considerations for handling labyrinthine fistulae will be discussed elsewhere in this book.

Grafting

Temporalis fascia devoid of extraneous muscle, fat, and connective tissue is used. This tissue is allowed to dry before cutting and fashioning just prior to closure.

It is advantageous for the surgeon to study the external auditory canal and tympanic membrane dimensions and equate some of the critical dimensions to their own body parts, such as how does the area of the tympanic membrane compare to their own thumbnail. Alternatives to this are the prior construction of templates that can be sterilized and placed in the operative set or actual measurements being made of the amount of tissue required for reconstruction. In any event, it is important to structure the graft so that it is not too small, which would result in reperforation, and not too large, which would result in difficulty of graft placement or reduced hearing result.

The dried temporalis fascia is cut to fit medial to the drum remnant, the manubrium, and the anterior and posterior tympanomeatal flaps. To accomplish this, I make a vertical slit in the superior part of the graft. The concept is to place the graft completely medial to the plane of the pars tensa and then up on the superior canal wall, anterior to the malleus, and the other portion posteriorly onto the posterosuperior canal wall from approximately 12 to 6 o'clock. Some modification in the total extent of this coverage can, of course, be made with smaller perforations.

When this single fascial graft is cut, it is useful to think of its construction as two parts: a circle and a rectangle. The circle is that portion of the graft that will fit over the mesotympanum with enough margin to extend onto the posterior canal wall medial to the posterior tympanomeatal flap and medial to the bony annulus anteriorly and inferiorly. The rectangular portion is that which ultimately extends onto the superior canal wall, posterior to the manubrium, and onto the superior and anterosuperior canal wall, anterior to the manubrium. The vertical slit separates the rectangular portion into an anterior one third and a posterior two thirds. The slit extends to but not beyond the imaginary superior margin of the circle. The anterior and posterior edges of the rectangle are tangents to the anterior and posterior margins of the circle. Structuring the graft in this way creates a single graft that is rectangular on its superior half and curvilinear, or circular, on its inferior half with a slit in the superior half. It is important to imagine the structure of a circle and rectangle rather than one single piece that is oval since cutting the fascia in an oval fashion frequently results in a piece of fascia that is too small in an anteroposterior direction.

Placement of the graft requires an absolutely dry field. This can be accomplished by placing Gelfoam or cotton pledgets that have been soaked in epinephrine (Adrenalin) in the middle ear and point coagulation to canal bleeding sites with very low coagulating current delivered through a fine drum elevator by touching the cautery tip to the handle of the drum elevator.

Gelfoam soaked in saline solution is placed sparingly at the mouth of the eustachian tube to temporarily occlude the tube and to offer support for the graft anteriorly.

The graft is grasped posteriorly with fine alligator forceps and rehydrated briefly with saline solution and placed in the middle ear, first positioning it medial to the bony annulus inferiorly and anteriorly, and onto the anterosuperior osseous canal wall. The anterior tympanomeatal flap is replaced lateral to the graft anteriorly. The graft is then placed medial to the manubrium by placing the apex of the slit at the umbo and carrying the graft medial and superiorly to the manubrium with a 1 mm right-angle pick. Ultimately the apex of the slit is approximately at the level of the tensor tendon. The graft is then secured in its position medial to the inferior bony annulus and remnant and then brought onto the posterosuperior canal posterior to the manubrium. The graft position is inspected, and a few small pieces of Gelfoam soaked with saline are placed in the middle ear, placing them from posterior to anterior, to secure the graft against anteroinferior drum remnant and bony annulus. The posterior tympanomeatal flap is then positioned lateral to the graft. The graft should assume somewhat of a conical shape.

Anterior canal skin blunting and lateralization of the drum are not expected with this technique. The primary complication that can occur with this technique is retraction of the drum anteromedially, away from the drum remnant, resulting in an early (usually discovered within the first 6 to 8 weeks) perforation. This complication is obviated by constructing the anterior tympanomeatal flap, placing the graft onto the superior and anterosuperior canal wall, and securing the graft medial to the bony annulus anteriorly with Gelfoam soaked with saline.

Late graft perforation is poorly understood. It is assumed to occur from avascular necrosis of the graft material and is not specific to any grafting technique.

Closure

The graft is supported in its position by placing pledgets of Gelfoam, soaked with Coly-Mycin otic suspension or equivalent antibiotic solution over its lateral surface and by completely filling the external auditory canal with this material. These pledgets are placed carefully to adhere to the surfaces of the graft, drum remnant, and external auditory canal. No medially directed pressure is applied. These pledgets hold by surface tension and mass. Medially directed force simply serves to displace graft elements or the ossicular reconstruction.

During the placement of the Gelfoam pledgets, the space on the posterosuperior canal wall is left unpacked for the even-

tual placement of the conchal flap (vascular strip). After the pledgets have been placed adjacent to the lateral surface of the drum but prior to the complete filling of the external auditory canal with the pledgets, the postauricular wound is closed. The conchal flap is straightened with forceps so that it is not contracted and not rolled on itself, and then it is carefully placed adjacent to the canal wall bone posterosuperiorly. Gelfoam pledgets soaked with antibiotic suspension are placed adjacent to it, and the external canal is completely filled with these pledgets.

The postauricular wound is closed by a loose approximation of the periosteal flap with several 3-O interrupted sutures of absorbable material such as Dexon or Vicryl. Subcutaneous closure is with 3-O interrupted sutures. The skin is approximated with a running 4-O Dexon or Vicryl running subcuticular closure. Half-inch Steri-Strips are positioned longitudinally along the incision. A mastoid dressing is applied.

Postoperative Care

With very few exceptions, tympanoplasty is performed in adults and children in an ambulatory surgery setting in which the patient is discharged the afternoon of surgery. The dressing is removed on discharge from the hospital or allowed to remain until the next morning. If extensive muscle pedicles have been used to obliterate a mastoid cavity, the dressing may be changed daily but kept on the patient for 5 days. This is an unusual situation.

The patient is seen in the office 1 week later. The Steri-Strips are removed, and one or two pieces of the Gelfoam in the external auditory meatus are removed. The patient is started on a regimen of 1 dropper of Cortisporin otic suspension or its equivalent three times daily. One month later the ear canal is evacuated by suction of all remaining Gelfoam unless a particularly adherent piece is adjacent to the drum; in that case, it is allowed to remain. Drops are continued twice daily, and the patient is seen again 1 month later. Usually at that time the ear is healed.

In cases in which the superoposterior osseous external auditory canal has been removed and a cavity constructed, the postoperative course is the same except the patient is followed at 2-month intervals until the cavity is completely epithelialized. Any excessive granulation tissue is removed with suction, cup forceps, and/or a wire loop. In areas far lateral to the facial nerve, limited cautery with silver nitrate on a stick is done.

In cavities that are slow to epithelialize (longer than 3 or 4 months), Cortisporin drops are discontinued, and a regimen of filling the cavity with 3% hydrogen peroxide for 5 minutes, evacuating the cavity by gravity, and filling the cavity with Domeboro otic suspension for 5 minutes, repeated three times daily, usually speeds cavity healing.

Rarely is it necessary to skin graft the cavity. In those cases that have had several operations and are known to have abundant granulation tissue formation, skin grafting may be necessary. This is usually done 10 days after the initial surgery when a fine granulation bed has developed. It is done in the operating room, and a split thickness skin graft 12/1,000 in. thick is taken with a Brown or Padgett dermatome. The epithelialized surface of the skin is laid on rayon that has been spread with bacitracin ointment. The rayon-ointment-skin composite is cut into small squares, and these are individually laid in the cavity and the rayon removed. This allows precise placement of the skin graft and complete coverage of all surfaces. The cavity is filled with Gelfoam soaked with antibiotic drops, and the postoperative visits begin 1 week later, as mentioned earlier. The graft site is covered with a sterile wound dressing (Op Site) in the operative room; it is allowed to remain on the wound until it spontaneously separates from it in approximately 6 weeks.

TOTAL PERFORATIONS

Total (100%) tympanic membrane perforations are managed exactly as described above.

TYMPANOSCLEROSIS

Tympanosclerosis involving the tympanic membrane is left attached to the drum remnant. It has not been necessary to remove this material unless it fixes the malleus. In that case, it is important to remove all or a portion of the offending plaque.

Tympanosclerosis of the middle ear mucosa fixing the head of the malleus laterally, anteriorly, or superiorly may be easily removed by removing adjacent bone and the tympanosclerosis. If it is necessary to remove the scutum to free the malleus, the scutum is reconstructed with a piece of postauricularly obtained conchal cartilage. Tympanosclerosis of the middle ear mucosa fixing the incus is handled in the same way.

Tympanosclerosis on the promontory about the oval window fixing the stapes should not be manipulated in a case of perforated drum. This may be approached later after the drum is healed; a stapes replacement prosthesis may be placed if manipulating the tympanosclerotic plaque does not free the stapes. Tympanosclerosis is hyaline degeneration in an area of avascular necrosis, predominantly of the lamina propria of the mucous membrane of the drum, middle ear, or both. The noxious events that thus cause tympanosclerosis may have involved the otic capsule to an extent that removal of the tympanosclerotic plaque can possibly open the perilymph space. This is a very rare situation but should be kept in mind when one is approaching tympanosclerosis over the otic capsule.

SECONDARY ACQUIRED CHOLESTEATOMA

Negative middle ear pressure and infection certainly play major roles in the development of secondary acquired cholesteatoma. Potential prevention of secondary acquired cholesteatomas incorporate middle ear ventilation with tympanostomy tubes and the use of systemic antibiotics. However, the frequent observation of quiescent posterosuperior pars tensa retraction pockets that never develop into cholesteatomas on one hand, and the already established secondary acquired cholesteatoma on the other hand, clearly suggest that other factors are involved. At this time, the other causal factors are not clearly

identified, and, therefore, prevention is limited. This is an area of rapidly developing new knowledge that hopefully will yield better methods of prevention in the future.

Therapeutically, the secondary acquired cholesteatoma is managed by resection. The secondary acquired cholesteatoma, in contradistinction to the primary acquired cholesteatoma, extends immediately on to the stapes and expands medial to the ossicular chain. It is usually associated with very poor eustachian tube function and infection. Thus, with few exceptions, the resection of the cholesteatoma requires removal of the incus and, frequently, the head of the malleus for exposure and total resection. Because poor eustachian tube function increases the risk of development of recurrent cholesteatoma and because the unusually aggressive nature of this type of cholesteatoma (e.g., migration along haversian canals and crevices) increases the risk of residual cholesteatoma, I prefer to construct a modified radical cavity with drum and ossicular reconstruction. In these cases, pneumatized spaces of the temporal bone are less well developed, and the size of the resultant cavity is rarely so large as to create a problem postoperatively.

Primary acquired cholesteatomas and congenital cholesteatomas tend to have better eustachian tube function and more extensively developed pneumatized spaces, and occasionally they may remain lateral to the ossicular chain. In some of these cases, intact canal wall techniques are used if the patient or the family understand that reexploration within 1 year, looking for evidence of hidden residual cholesteatoma, is preferred.

There are three principles of surgical resection of cholesteatoma, regardless of the technique employed. These are (1) direct visualization of the cholesteatoma, (2) resection of the cholesteatoma matrix and attendant granulation tissue in continuity avoiding shredding or uncontrolled piecemeal removal, and (3) resection of margins whenever possible. Bone adjacent to cholesteatoma that can easily be removed should be removed. In areas such as the otic capsule, fallopian canal, or stapes, in which removal of bone is not possible, careful dissection of all granulation tissue and soft tissue overlying the bone should be done by using the technique of elevating sheets and layers of tissue rather than piecemeal removal and shredding of tissue. The concept of removing margins about the cholesteatoma whenever possible relate to the propensity of cholesteatomas to send squamous epithelial excrescences that may be invisible even under the operating microscope into granulation tissue, haversian canals, and bony crevices. This kind of aggressive behavior is much more prominent in children than in adults.

DEHISCENT JUGULAR BULB

Dehiscence in the osseous jugular foramen may be occult or apparent. The occult variety is most common. In these cases the superolateral osseous jugular foramen is dehiscent immediately adjacent to the fibrous annulus, and the fibrous annulus is adherent to the dura of the foramen. This occult variety remains occult only until the surgeon elevates the tympanic membrane, at which time a copious amount of venous blood fills the operative field. This can rarely, if ever, be preoperatively or even intraoperatively identified prior to this spectacular event.

The second type of dehiscent osseous jugular foramen is fairly obvious. In this event not only is the osseous foramen dehiscent, but it is positioned much more superiorly than ordinarily. The jugular bulb may be visible in the mesotympanum and may extend superiorly even to the level of the stapes and facial nerve. It may extend far anteriorly to the protympanum and be indented by the manubrium.

The treatment of the suddenly lacerated jugular bulb in the occult variety is to gently and immediately replace the annulus in its original position and hold it in place with the drum elevator to tamponade the flow of blood. Small pieces of oxidized cellulose (Surgicel) and quarter-inch cottonoid squares with attached sutures are used to secure the area before the surgery is continued. The small cottonoid is gently slipped under the annulus to extraluminally tamponade the lacerated foramen. It is held in place with a suction tip, and the drum is elevated to a level necessary to complete the surgery. Then a small piece of Surgicel is placed under the cottonoid and the cottonoid placed back on the Surgicel to hold it in place. Several other pieces of Surgicel are placed over the lacerated foramen, and a fresh cottonoid is held in place to control the bleeding. The cottonoid and the Surgicel are allowed to remain, and the procedure is completed. At the end of the case, the cottonoid is removed, the Surgicel is allowed to remain, a fresh piece of Surgicel is placed over that area to reinforce it, and a small piece of fascia is placed on top of that and held in place with Gelfoam pledgets soaked with saline solution. The tympanoplasty is completed in the usual manner, and the packing of the external auditory meatus or cavity is done in the usual fashion. In this instance, it may be prudent to keep the patient in the hospital overnight for observation.

An obviously high lying jugular bulb extending through a dehiscent jugular foramen is occasionally obscured by serous or mucinous middle ear effusion, though with some care and cautious awareness of this problem, it can be identified by a discretely demarcated bluish area. It is necessary to think of this high-lying exposed bulb in all cases of idiopathic hemotympanum in which the complete middle ear looks bluish. In these instances, a very carefully done myringotomy anterosuperiorly should avoid the dehiscent bulb. This situation can usually be determined by microscopic observation through the drum prior to myringotomy. If it cannot be clearly identified as to what the situation is, a limited carefully done tympanomeatal flap can be raised to inspect the middle ear before any incisions are made.

An ear that requires surgical intervention for cholesteatoma or other disease and that has a high-lying exposed bulb can be operated by taking care not to rupture the bulb during the standard procedure. At the close of the procedure, a piece of conchal cartilage should be placed lateral to the exposed bulb to protect the bulb in the future from some inadvertent injury. It is also very important to explain to the patient and the family what the condition is and what has been done.

If manubrium is indenting the jugular bulb, it might be feared that ultimate erosion of the bulb might occur. In that instance, surgery to place a piece of cartilage between the manubrium and bulb appears to be an appropriate course. Otherwise, a completely asymptomatic high-lying jugular bulb requires no surgery but does require informing the patient or legal guardian of the anatomic variant.

ABERRANT CAROTID ARTERY

I have no personal experience with an aberrant carotid artery, although personal discussions with those who have the experience and literature review suggest that an aberrant carotid artery can look exactly like a glomus tympanicum, or glomus jugulare tumor. This entity should be ever present in the mind of an otologic surgeon.

Injuries to the tympanic portion of a normal internal carotid artery are usually fatal before the otolaryngologist sees the patient. If an injury occurs in a time frame and a condition in which intervention may be rendered, the first step is to tamponade the site directly, preferably without compressing and occluding the lumen of the artery. The patient's hemodynamic state should then be brought to normal with transfusion and time; occlusion of the internal carotid artery in a compromised hemodynamic state frequently results in cerebral infarction. When the patient is in satisfactory condition, an attempt to graft or repair the lesion can be done. It is possible to approach the internal carotid artery and the temporal bone by displacing the mandibular condyle anteriorly and approaching the protympanicum through radical mastoidectomy. The carotid canal can be opened with a diamond burr and the internal carotid artery isolated circumferentially. Surgical repair is difficult in that area, however, even when exposure is achieved. Occlusion of the internal carotid artery in the tympanic segment can be done with circumferential ligature, proximally and distally, to the injured segment or can be accomplished by angiographically placing a detachable balloon through the cervical carotid to the temporal bone segment. We have successfully used these techniques in trauma, carcinoma, and osteoradionecrosis.

MIDDLE EAR MUCOSAL DISEASE

Normal middle ear mucosa is exceedingly thin and, when viewed en face, is almost invisible except for a slight glistening surface on the slightly cream-colored bone of the otic capsule. Diseased middle ear mucosa is relatively easily classified into three types by gross observation under the operating microscope. The first is an obvious layer of mucosa that is pink and slightly edematous appearing, which unlike the normal mucosa, obscures the cream color of the underlying bone and is obviously present as a layer, as opposed to the normal mucosa, which is almost invisible. Histologically this tissue still maintains most of the characteristic anatomy of mucosa, with considerable changes in the epithelium and edema in the lamina propria. The second category appears grossly like markedly thickened mucosa, which is still flat but 1 mL or more thick. Histologically this material rarely looks like mucosa and generally has the appearance of thin granulation tissue. The third category is obvious, thick, somewhat polypoid granulation tissue, both grossly and histologically.

Normal-appearing middle ear mucosa, except when there is a coexistent cholesteatoma, rarely, if ever, indicates the need for a mastoidectomy at the time of tympanoplasty.

Diseased middle ear mucosa of any variety is a satisfactory indicator for mastoidectomy to explore the other pneumatized spaces for irreversible disease; however, very often in the first category of disease described, the mastoid is normal or with similar edematous mucosa, particularly at the proximal antrum. The second category bears approximately a 50:50 chance of discovery of similar or worse mucosal disease in the mastoid. The third type of mucosal disease seen through a tympanic membrane perforation in the middle ear is almost always associated with similar disease in the mastoid. This type of disease is irreversible and should be removed when found. The decision to do a mastoidectomy at the same time as tympanoplasty is a liberal one. Certainly if there is cholesteatoma, a mastoidectomy is done. If middle ear mucosa is diseased, a mastoidectomy is done in most instances and is certainly performed in the second and third category of middle ear disease. Mastoidectomy might not be done in cases in which only the first category of mucosal disease is seen in the middle ear and in which the ear has never spontaneously discharged but discharged only transiently when induced to do so by water contamination or an upper respiratory tract infection.

Every attempt is made to leave as much mucosa in the middle ear as possible in an effort to avoid adhesions between the promontory and the graft. Of course, normal middle ear mucosa is allowed to remain. The first classification of mucosal disease is allowed to remain in the middle ear. The second type is removed in areas where this disease may be obstructive, as in the protympanum and mouth of the eustachian tube. This type of diseased mucosa is usually attempted to be left over the promontory when possible. The third type of disease is removed whenever and wherever encountered, since its propensity for inciting recurrent infections is considerable.

Mucosal disease rarely contraindicates ossicular reconstruction. An occasional exception to this is when the middle ear is abundantly filled with granulation tissue polyps, there is little or no normal mucosa in the middle ear, and the stapes superstructure is absent. In this case, ossicular reconstruction might be delayed for a second stage, following an attempt to achieve a mucosal-lined, aerated middle ear space with the placement of thick Silastic sheeting.

Severe mucosal disease and poor eustachian tube function predispose to adhesive otitis media. Methods to avoid adhesive otitis media include the placement of a thick Silastic sheet into the middle ear and extending it into the mastoid, either lateral to the stapes footplate or stapes capitulum, if present, or about the stapes when an ossicular reconstruction is done. Thick Silastic sheeting, without ossicular reconstruction, when mucosal disease is severe and no stapes superstructure exists is perhaps the best tact to take initially. If the stapes superstructure is present, thick Silastic sheeting laying on the stapes capitulum and extending into the mastoid may actually serve as an ossicular reconstruction in and of itself, as well as serve to maintain the middle ear space.

If mucosal disease is less severe and some mucosa has been removed from the promontory, a thin piece of Silastic sheeting laid over the exposed bone is usually satisfactory to avoid adhesions. Small tympanostomy tubes do improve the aeration of the middle ear while it is in the processs of healing; however, they will not prevent adhesions between the graft and exposed bone. Both Silastic sheeting and small tympanostomy tubes can be used in concert.

Completely satisfactory mechanisms to ensure an aerated middle ear space in severely diseased ears still awaits development.

CANAL WALL BLUNTING

Canal wall blunting refers to blunting or obliteration of the acute angle between the anterior canal wall and the plane of the drum. This is a significant problem because anterior angle blunting reduces the vibratory surface of the drum and creates a significant conductive hearing loss. The second problem with blunting is that it is difficult to treat once it has occurred. This complication is almost never encountered in medial graft techniques. The problem is reasonably frequently encountered in lateral graft techniques in the hands of individuals who are not experienced in that grafting technique. Experienced individuals do get some blunting or slightly more blunting than in the medial graft technique, but it is usually minimal and does not have an adverse effect.

If anterior canal wall blunting does occur and proves to be significant, the canal is allowed to heal for approximately 6 months or longer, and then reoperation is done using the lateral graft technique. The scar formation, which composes the blunted area, is resected, and the canal skin is repositioned adjacent to the bone, the fibrous annulus, and the drum.

If a lateral graft technique is employed an impeccably dry grafting area should be secured; the fascia must be placed to the anterior canal wall but not on it, and the skin must be placed around the angle of the anterior sulcus and tightly approximated to the osseous anterior canal wall.

GRAFT LATERALIZATION

Graft lateralization is distinctly different from anterior canal wall blunting and from canal stenosis, described later in this section. Lateralization of the graft is defined as the new tympanic membrane pulling laterally from the manubrium. It results when the lateral grafting technique is used and the fascia is not placed medial to the manubrium. If the fascia is placed just laterally onto the manubrium, the conical shape of the drum cannot be maintained as the wound heals, because wounds tend to heal across curvilinear surfaces in a straight line. Healing tissue tends to create a cord across an arc rather than maintaining the arc configuration.

When lateralization of the drum occurs, a maximum conductive hearing loss to a 50- to 55-dB hearing level usually ensues. Management of this complication is to reoperate and completely redo the graft as though a total tympanic membrane perforation existed.

Canal stenosis is sometimes erroneously called lateralization of the graft; this is a distinctly different entity. Canal stenosis is defined as the occlusion of the canal lateral to the plane of the drum. It can be fairly far laterally and can result in the trapping of squamous epithelium medial to the stenotic area, thus creating a canal cholesteatoma. Canal stenosis can be more medial, closer to the drum surface, and the complete region medial to the stenotic area can be filled with thick fibrous tissue.

Medial canal stenosis occurs when ulcerations and lack of viable squamous epithelium are at and just lateral to the graft. If they exist, the area will obliterate with fibrous tissue.

A lateral stenotic area occurs when there is a circumferential break in the squamous epithelium. This phenomenon can occur when the anterior canal skin is removed and replaced further medially than ordinary, thus allowing an anterior non-epithelialized area of the canal to be adjacent to the posterior conchal flap incisions. This, in effect, creates a circumferential deepithelialized area that granulates and ultimately obliterates that segment of the canal with fibrous tissue. Another way lateral canal stenosis can occur is with poor positioning of the conchal flap, or vascular strip. If this flap is not carefully positioned against the posterior canal wall during closure, it can adhere to the anterior canal wall and thus create a lateral canal stenosis.

Management of canal stenoses requires removal of canal stenotic areas with the attendant scar, saving as much skin of the canal as possible. Strips of thin, full-thickness, postauricular skin can be used to augment the lack of available canal skin. This full-thickness skin can be in the form of free grafts or pedicled grafts into the canal. Special care must be taken to avoid adjacent nonepithelialized areas.

OSSICULAR RECONSTRUCTION

Stiffness seems to be much more important to a satisfactory hearing result than is mass. Thus, the smaller the reconstructive components and the more tightly their approximation, the better. It is more advantageous to create a tight osseous strut from the manubrium to the stapes capitulum than to place a moderately large piece of cartilage or bone lateral to the stapes capitulum.

With this concept in mind, the following ossicular reconstructive strategies are employed:

1. If the ossicular chain is intact and mobile, every attempt is used to maintain that configuration. Occasionally, cholesteatomas can be totally removed from the ossicular chain without disarticulating the chain.

2. If the ossicular chain is intact but not mobile, the ossicular chain is left intact and the ankylosing area removed with the otologic drill, preferably the diamond drill, and the scutum is rebuilt with cartilage. The ossicular chain can be left intact, even in a cavity situation. If the stapes is fixed, a stapedectomy obviously is not done in an unsterile, open environment. Stapedectomy may be done at a later date if the middle ear is aerated and remains normal for a considerable period of time.

3. If the incus is partially eroded and the stapes is present, a cortical bone fragment is constructed to wedge between the manubrium, the incus, and the stapes capitulum. This maneuver

is capable of creating a very stable, stiff, vibratory mechanism that seems to work well. An alternative is to remove the incus and create a strut between the medial surface of the manubrium and the capitulum by creating a notch in articulating surface of the incus and a facet in the short process of the incus to fit on the stapes capitulum.

4. If the stapes superstructure is not present, the oval window nitch is widely open, and the patient is an adult, a bone strut of the incus is made. A portion of the incus strut is placed medial to the manubrium. A larger portion is placed posterior to the manubrium to bulge the drum slightly laterally, and a fine blunt point of the incus strut is placed squarely in the center of the stapes footplate. If the patient is a child or the oval window is narrow, such a bony strut tends to fuse to the promontory or the fallopian canal. In this case, a cartilage wedge made out of postauricular or tragal cartilage is placed posterior to the manubrium and down on the stapes footplate.

These ossicular reconstruction methods are employed initially, and alloplastic materials are not used in the contaminated ear. Alloplastic materials can be used in second stage operations.

POSTOPERATIVE INFECTION

Postoperative infection in otologic surgery is unusual. However, an occasional postauricular incision abscess can occur. If it does occur, it is opened, irrigated, and packed with a small piece of gauze, which is changed daily. Oral antibiotics for gram-positive organisms are given for 7 to 10 days, and the wound is daily swabbed with hydrogen peroxide and bacitracin ointment.

Another unusual complication is an acute canal infection. It is easily treated by evacuating the Gelfoam with suction and instilling Cortisporin otic suspension into the canal. Oral systemic antibiotics for gram-positive organisms can be added to this regimen, particularly if there is a component of surrounding cellulitis.

Short-duration perioperative antibiotics may very well be worthwhile in these contaminated cases. Clear evidence to support the efficacy and cost effectiveness of such treatment is not readily available, but extrapolation from experiences with other contaminated operative sites suggests it may be an appropriate approach.

FLACCID TYMPANIC MEMBRANE

A flaccid tympanic membrane that is not adherent to the promontory but sufficient to create significant middle ear atelectasis occasionally will contract and tighten when the middle ear is ventilated with an anteriorly placed tympanostomy tube.

A flaccid tympanic membrane that is adherent to the ossicular chain and promontory may contract and tighten when the middle ear is ventilated and the adhesion between the tympanic membrane and the promontory and ossicles is incised. In both of these cases, however, the hearing may be quite good, and the role of surgical intervention is questionable.

When hearing is significantly reduced as the result of a flaccid tympanic membrane adherent to the promontory and ossicular chain, a step-wise approach can be used, pending the patient's agreement to a serial approach. It can begin with careful elevation of the adhered membrane and placement of an anteriorly positioned tympanostomy tube. If satisfactory results are not achieved, resection of the atelectatic adherent drum with performance of tympanoplasty and the addition of a tympanostomy tube intraoperatively may improve the hearing.

In a number of these cases, the ossicular chain may be obviously or less obviously restricted, and the repair of the drum may not result in the hearing improvement expected.

This particular problem of the flaccid not adhered or flaccid adhered drum with hearing loss is poorly understood and less than satisfactorily treated. Therefore, a very conservative approach is warranted, and the patient should be informed of the limits to hearing improvement in this situation.

CHAPTER 3

Ossicular Reconstruction: Stapedectomy and Incus Replacement

Approach of

J.V.D. Hough, M.D.

STAPEDECTOMY

Perilymph Gusher

Etiology and Incidence

An abnormally large or open cochlear aqueduct, allowing free unrestrained flow of cerebrospinal fluid (CSF) into the perilymph of the labyrinthine chambers, may be present in a rare congenitally maldeveloped inner ear. From my experience, I would estimate its occurrence to be 1 in 1,000 ears. This may be with or without other more obvious malformations. It may also be due to other cavity-forming lesions, such as a syphilitic gumma of the labyrinth.

Recognition

This malformation may be detected, or at least suspected, with well-done roentgenograms prior to surgery. However, routine preoperative roentgenograms in stapedectomy would seldom change the surgical indications and would increase the costs inordinately. Congenitally malformed ears suspected of having this should have preoperative computed tomography (CT) scans.

The principal suggestion indicating the presence of this condition is the observation of other congenital otic malformations. Lack of proper development of the oval window and its stapedial footplate may first be suspected by the history of conductive deafness in early childhood. Otosclerosis superimposed on this condition is very rare but may be present if there is childhood impairment with additional progressive hearing loss in adulthood.

The presence of a Mondini deformity places this complication in a much higher risk category. Indeed, the finding of a congenitally malformed pinna, external ear canal, or tympanic membrane should also cause a surgical alert.

The true recognition of the perilymphatic gusher occurs the moment an opening is made through the footplate into the labyrinth. The CSF may spout like a gusher or may weld up to fill the oval window niche. Whether or not the cochlear aqueduct is open enough to cause significant postoperative complications cannot, in most cases, be determined before the footplate is opened. I have not seen evidence that the malformed cochlear aqueduct was the cause of the hearing loss. Also, in most ears with this problem, the final hearing results have been quite satisfactory.

Surgical Management

Because of the possibility of a CSF perilymphatic fistula in any ear, the footplate should always be opened precisely in the thinnest portion with a very fine sharp pick. Once one has determined that a CSF perilymphatic fistula does indeed exist, one must determine (1) whether the operation should continue with the hope of improving hearing and (2) how the fluid leak, caused by the fistula, can be controlled.

The decision as to continuing the restorative procedure depends primarily on the severity of the fistula, the pathology causing the loss, the amount and type of hearing loss in the opposite ear as related to the surgical ear, the age of the patient, the possibility of hearing aid utilization, and the ease of the surgical technique.

Once the gusher occurs, it should be observed for several minutes. It may spurt like a geyser or may pulsate. Both indicate a more open system of the CSF. The fluid may only gradually fill the oval window niche. One should, with a footpedaled controlled suction, gradually reduce the level of the fluid down to the footplate, repeatedly clearing the area.

To reduce the fluid flow volume, one can initiate several measures in the operating room. The head of the patient can be raised significantly. Usually this, plus patiently waiting, allows the flow to subside enough to continue the surgical procedure. I have not had to resort to any other more complicated or radical techniques. A cerebrospinal tap with an indwelling catheter and brain shrinking and dehydrating agents (e.g., mannitol) may be instituted if needed and should be in the surgeon's armamentarium.

Normally, removal of the footplate sufficiently to perform the stapedectomy neither hinders healing nor apparently compromises the final functional result. Unfortunately, the flow of CSF may obstruct proper visualization, making the procedure more difficult. If one determines to proceed with the stapedectomy, one should definitely not use a technique that fails to include a total, very firm, connective tissue seal over the open area of the oval window. I consider perichondrium best suited for this. I also consider a piston procedure to be contraindicated unless it calls for vein or perichondrium medial to the prosthesis. A small hole with a piston protruding through it with a small amount of soft tissue tucked around it is not adequate.

In those cases in which I can preserve the posterior crus (80%), I cut the anterior crus high, cut the tendon, cut the posterior crus at the footplate, and lift the arch out of the oval window, resting it on the promontory. A perichondrial graft is then taken from the tragus and custom trimmed to seal the oval window. The footplate is removed, and the perichondrial graft, which is shaped like a little boat, is then placed firmly over the oval window so as to totally seal the opening. The posterior crus is rotated back into the niche so that its medial end is in the center of the oval window, resting on the perichondrial graft. This technique uses the natural forces of the ossicular chain to hold the graft firmly against the oval window and provides the preservation of the natural tissue for rapid healing over the oval window.

It is important that the graft be held down in place over the opening; otherwise, it will simply float away postoperatively. To hold it in place, I use either the posterior crus, as mentioned earlier, or a nonossicle sculptured homograft in the shape of a piston. It is placed between the lenticular process of the incus and the perichondrium, which has sealed the oval window. If it is not available, I use a well-measured, prefabricated House or Robinson prosthesis between the incus and the footplate.

Postoperative Management

Frequently, there continues to be a slight ooze around the graft for several minutes to hours after the termination of the operation. Postoperatively, the patient's head should be wrapped

in a very large mastoid dressing. The head of the bed should be elevated at least 60 degrees. The patient should have absolute bed rest until the drainage has stopped. A laxative is ordered to prevent straining. Physical activity, such as leaning or blowing the nose should not be permitted. The temperature should be monitored for at least 2 weeks following the operation, and the patient should be instructed to observe any dripping from the nose when the head is bent over.

If CSF drainage has not been stopped within 24 hours or is excessively profuse after 12 hours, a spinal tap for removal of CSF should be done and repeated daily as needed.

This regime has been successful in all of my patients thus far. Fortunately, I have not had a patient suffer a total sensorineural loss following a perilymphatic gusher.

If drainage is profuse without showing signs of abatement after 3 days, I would suggest (1) the use of a CSF or cisternal catheter for continuous reduction in CSF pressure and (2) medications to reduce fluids.

If the flow is not controlled, surgical closure of the cochlear aqueduct will need to be considered.

None of my patients, to date, has required surgical ablation of the cochlear acqueduct or the internal auditory canal. Fortunately, none has had persistent vertigo, and none has had a continued CSF leak past 3 days.

Floating Footplate

When the annular ligament or the bony bridges of the otosclerosis between the margins of the oval window and the footplate break prematurely during manipulation of the stapes, a floating footplate may occur. This important complication may occur during any stapedectomy procedure.

Cause and Prevention

The axiom that should always be remembered is that the only safe footplate is one with a hole in it large enough to get an instrument through the opening and under the footplate. The surgical complication of a floating footplate may occur even in the hands of the most skillful and experienced otologist.

In the United States, otosclerosis is confined to the anterior portion of the footplate in approximately 80% of patients affected. In this group of patients, the major portion of the footplate is thin. This is in contrast to some other parts of the world, such as Australia and India. If the bridge of the otosclerotic bone is small or fragile, it may be fractured easily by pressure or manipulation. When fracture occurs, the remainder of the annular ligament tears easily and results in a floating footplate.

A biscuit-type footplate always presents the threat of becoming a floating footplate. In this instance, otosclerosis growth spreads across the annular ligament in a limited area, then proceeds to cover the entire footplate. Otosclerosis seems hesitant to invade the fibrous connective tissue of the annular ligament and, therefore, does not involve the fibrous annular ligament. It builds up on the edges of the footplate into a thick biscuit-like mass, moving completely to the edge, without involving the ligament itself. This produces a discrete or circumscribed biscuit-type footplate. Obviously, making an opening through a thick footplate of this type will require increased instrumentation, possibly causing premature breaking up of the annular ligament so that the entire thick footplate becomes floating.

In addition to the use of instruments directly on the footplate, external manipulation of the ossicular chain lateral to the footplate may also cause this premature dislodgment. Because of this possibility, a major error in technique is the use of any instrumentation on the stapes prior to making an opening in the footplate. This is a cardinal rule.

To prevent a floating footplate:

1. Always use a very sharp pick to penetrate the footplate, using as little pressure as possible. Penetration should be in the thinnest area of the footplate.

2. Use a pick that is slightly curved on the shaft near the end, so that one can see the tip engage the footplate.

3. Firmly press the shaft of the pick against the arch of the stapes so that the stapes is "wedged" as the tip of the sharp pick makes the first hole through the footplate if there is any footplate mobility felt or visualized. All of the structures—the incudostapedial joint, the promontory, the tendon, and the remaining annular ligament—are used in this maneuver to keep the stapes frozen while the opening of the footplate is being made.

4. Do not remove the arch before the oval window has been opened unless absolutely necessary. Removal of the arch will frequently cause the footplate to become dislodged. The stapedial superstructure is the handle of safety if the footplate begins to float.

5. Begin with the initial examination of the patient. A person with evidence of very early involvement with otosclerosis has a greater possibility of a premature floating footplate. If the SRT is less than 40 dB and there is a narrow air-bone gap, the ear poses a greater chance of presenting this problem. If the problem has occurred in one ear, the opposite side is likewise more predisposed to the same condition. If a previously successful simple stapes mobilization has been done in the ear, one would consider the possibility of a floating footplate to be greater during a revision stapedectomy. Likewise, if during previous stapedectomies the opposite ear was observed to have a biscuit-type circumscribed pathologic involvement of the footplate, one should be aware of a greater chance of causing a floating footplate.

6. Observe the footplate during surgery. Frequently, a small area of the footplate is thin and requires little effort in its penetration. Therefore, choose this area to open. If the footplate is extremely thick, it may be approachable with a microdrill, which requires only slight pressure against the footplate. This need is rare, but when necessary, I prefer to make a troughlike cut across the center of the footplate with as little downward pressure as possible. An opening can often be made large enough to admit an excavator hoe or pick to begin the routine footplate removal. Fortunately, those footplates with circumscribed otosclerosis are frequently removed in large segments because of the presence of a normal annular ligament around most of its circumference.

Management

In spite of all precautions, a floating footplate is a surgical problem in stapedial surgery that any otologic surgeon must be prepared to face. If it occurs, the dilemma now is that one cannot provide or enlarge an opening in the footplate enough to allow proper extraction. Every attempt to enlarge the opening for further instrumentation causes the footplate to become more freely floating and to be in more danger of sinking into the labyrinthine fluids. When a floating footplate occurs, one must then make the decision to either (1) stop the procedure altogether and consider it to be a simple stapes mobilization or to (2) continue toward the goal of stapedectomy with its attendant higher risk of inner ear trauma. The mobilization choice is certainly the most conservative and may be the most prudent, especially in the hands of those surgeons who either are early in their experience or do only occasional stapedectomies. The initial hearing result with mobilization may be good but has an 80% chance of gradual regression due to refixation. The refixation is frequently not firm; therefore, at revision, one usually encounters, and must be prepared for, the same situation to occur again.

Use of a Laser in the Floating Footplate

Use of a laser in the floating footplate is perhaps one of the most practical applications of the laser in the middle ear surgery. An opening can usually be made without major disturbance to the fluids of the labyrinth or risk of pushing the floating footplate into the labyrinth. The laser can definitely vaporize any portion of footplate desired if it can be visualized properly. A routine stapedectomy or stapedotomy may then be carried out.

Major stumbling blocks in the use of the laser is its limited availability, the increase in procedural cost, and the surgical awkwardness produced when this rather massive piece of equipment is attached to the microscope.

I do not use a laser in doing a routine stapedectomy. I have the laserscope available specifically in readiness for this particular complication.

When the footplate is quite thick and floating, I still do not use a laser. Because of the amount of laser energy required and the manipulation required to remove the char from the massive floating footplate, I use the standard "pothole" technique.

Pothole Technique

In the pothole technique the labyrinth is entered by making a small hole through the promontory bone immediately inferior to the footplate. Avoiding touching the footplate, shave the promontory using sharp fenestration excavators or by carefully using a slow-speed microdrill. The opening is made large enough to admit a right-angle excavator hoe. This instrument is dull and therefore not as dangerous to the membranous labyrinth. It is placed immediately below the footplate and turned at right angles to the footplate, whereupon it is lifted laterally with the precise force necessary to remove the footplate or to break it in half. The various footplate portions are then removed.

Thick Floating Footplate

The thick footplate is frequently trapped in a bottleneck restriction due to the bony overhang along the promontory side. Entrapment is especially common at the posteroinferior aspect of the oval window. It is important to remove this projecting bone before any attempt is made to remove the footplate. If this is not done, lifting the footplate may cause it to wedge, flip over, and fall into the depths of the labyrinth.

If the fragment of the footplate, or even the entire footplate, falls free into the depths of the labyrinth, the surgeon should not attempt to go deep into the labyrinth to retrieve it. The fragment, even if large, will usually fall into the deeper posterior aspects of the vestibule and adhere to the membrane lining of the walls. If no deep instrumentation within the vestibule is done, the presence of this fragment usually does not cause difficulty.

If bone fragments or small portions of the footplate still remain attached to the oval window edge, an excavator hoe can be used. With only shallow entry into the labyrinth, the portions of the footplate can then be lifted out. Frequently, not only that portion of the footplate will come safely out of the labyrinth but other fragments as well due to the "blanket-holding effect" of the mucous membrane and endosteum attached to the fragments of the footplate, allowing the fragments to hold together in unity.

Persistent Stapedial Artery

There is usually a blood vessel that is more distinct than the others crossing the footplate near its center, extending from the promontory down into the oval window niche, then across the footplate, and disappearing into the facial ridge. This most prominent blood vessel crossing the footplate is usually seen near its center or slightly anteriorly. It is usually lying in the mucous membrane against the stapedial footplate but may be free standing in a mucosal web through the obturator foramen. Occasionally, the vessel is quite large and, in some instances, may almost fill the obturator foramen. I believe even small blood vessels such as these represent remnants of the original stapedial artery. Furthermore, these small blood vessels are seen in most ears. Large ones, which interfere with techniques in and around the oval window, are rare (Figs 3–1 and 3–2).

It is my practice to look for this vessel, or this artery-vein complex, when I first examine the oval window niche. If the blood vessel is relatively small, I immediately cut it with a sharp pick or hook so as to give time for proper vasoconstriction and cessation of bleeding prior to footplate removal. Usually, bleeding subsides rather quickly without further intervention. However, in some instances, the small artery may bleed rather briskly. Gelfoam applied directly to the obturator foramen usually suffices; however, pressure with a blunt chisel directly over the vessel for a few minutes may be necessary. I rarely use epinephrine 1:10,000 on absorbable gelatin sponge (Gelfoam) since

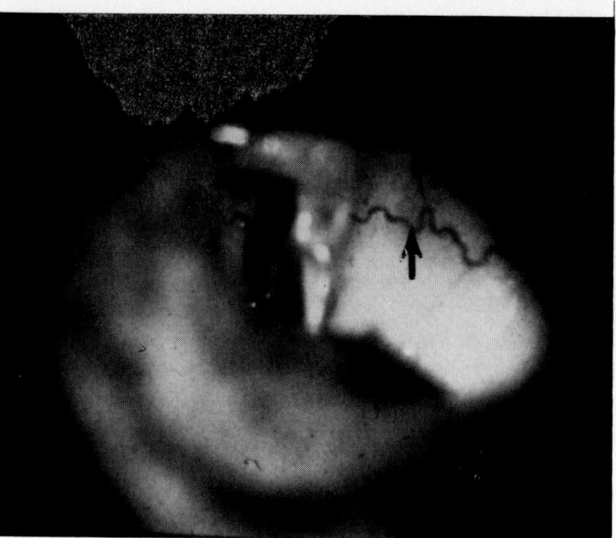

FIG 3–1.
Arrow points to persistent stapedial artery passing freely through obturator foramen.

the rebound vasodilatation may cause further hemorrhage later in the midst of the footplate removal.

I have seen a number of quite large, persistent stapedial arteries that require change in the surgical technique. If these vessles are opened or severed, there will be profuse hemorrhage that may make it impossible to carry out a successful stapedectomy.

In the presence of a large vessel, the surgeon has two choices. First, the artery can usually be bypassed and left undisturbed. The arterial blood vessel wall is frequently well formed and can occasionally be safely mobilized and moved with its mucosal attachments anteriorly to give a more generous working area. If a sufficient area of the footplate can be seen and removed posteriorly or from beneath the vessel, an effective conductive mechanism can usually be established. This is certainly the most preferable choice. The alternative approach to the problem of a large stapedial artery is its coagulation with a bipolar cautery. The use of a unipolar cautery is contraindicated, but bipolar coagulation with long fine-tipped bipolar forceps can sometimes be accomplished. The risks of cauterizing this large vessel might be that retrograde thrombosis could cause swelling, which could conceivably affect the facial nerve. Also, the nearby Jacobson plexus could be damaged.

Incudal Subluxation or Dislocation

Cause and Avoidance

Collision of the curette on the body, or long process of the incus while removing the bone of the posterior superior bony canal wall, is the most common cause of this complication.

Improper visualization of the actual point of contact of the curette with the bone, improper application of the instrument on the bone, improper direction of the force applied, and improper instrumental design may cause this unnecessary complication. Also of great importance is the position and stability of the surgeon's hands.

To obtain proper visualization of the oval window, one must curette for bone removal of the bony posterior superior canal wall in the majority of the cases requiring stapedectomy. To properly accomplish this, grasp the curette between the thumb, index finger, and forefinger, with the ring and little finger resting on and in solid contact with the speculum and the head. This should prevent the instrument from slipping medially when irregular pressure requirements suddenly occur. The instrument should be slightly cupped with prominent, very sharp edges. The face of the curette should be made so that it is tilted slightly toward the handle. I use curettes that have a number of small serrations on the sharp edges of the cup, which allows for good purchase of the instrument against the bone and discourages slippage as the curette moves along and bites into the edge of the bone.

The curette should first be placed so as to engage the bone at the notch of Rivinus with the face of the curette directed posteriorly and slightly superiorly, dipping into the bone but directed so as to stay lateral and superior to the chorda tympani nerve. When thinned, the bone is then curetted away from the chorda tympani nerve by twisting motions of the curette, chipping the bone inferiorly and posteriorly. This, plus proper securing of the hand position, prevents the instrument from drifting medially. It is very important that this instrument remain quite lateral to the long process of the incus.

A second cause for producing subluxation or dislocation of the incus is instrumentation in and around the oval window. This can occur when the stapes footplate is frozen solidly by otosclerosis, making it hard to remove. A right angle excavator hoe or pick may slip off the edge of the firmly fixed footplate, causing a sudden jerk. One may be lifting, with considerable energy, in an attempt to dislodge the fixed footplate. If the hands are not properly prepared for this, as the tip is suddenly released, the incus may be dislodged. Also, moving picks and right-angled instruments in and out of the ear, if done too rapidly, may cause the sharp right angle ends of the instruments to impale against the long process of the incus and pull it outwardly, causing it to dislodge.

Treatment

Most frequently, the incus is not entirely dislodged. The ligaments of the malleus-incus articulation may be only partially severed. With gentle manipulation, the incus may be returned to its normal position. Usually, this heals with no serious untoward effects. In some instances, the incus may be torn completely free from both the fossa-incudus attachment and the malleus-incus articulation. This may allow the body of the incus to dislocate medially and superiorly into the attic, or it may be pulled almost completely into the middle ear. This total displacement is very difficult to reduce to an effective reapproximation. In this event, the ossicular chain should be reconstructed using either an autograft or homograft transplant. Techniques to accomplish reconstruction of the malleus to the stapes are quite effective and will be discussed in the following section on malleus fixation.

Malleus Fixation

Upper ossicular chain fixation may occur either with or without simultaneous stapedial fixation. The reconstruction of the conductive mechanism would obviously be different in the two circumstances.

Any time we otologists raise the tympanomeatal flap in surgery, both mental and physical preparation is important. The axiom for the whole surgical team should be: When the tympanomeatal flap is elevated, expect anything and be prepared for everything.

Other than otosclerosis, malleus fixation is the most common noninflammatory progressive conductive hearing loss in adulthood. One may be tipped off by the otoscopic examination or the tympanogram. One should also remember that it is commonly a unilateral problem. Progressive hearing impairment is found in otosclerosis, osteogenesis imperfecta, "congenital" cholesteatoma, and upper ossicular chain fixation. Nonprogressive hearing loss may be the result of traumatic ossicular chain injury, congenital malformations, incus necrosis, lightning injury, and soft tissue impairments. Conditions other than otosclerosis are more apt to be unilateral.

As to pathology, the head, neck, or even the long process of the malleus may be fixed. Congenital fixation of the incudostapedial joint or bony fusion with the upper tympanic walls may occur. Massive congenital bony fusion may occur. Other causes of attic osteogenesis are those stimulated by head trauma, inflammatory disease, or surgical manipulation. In many instances, one may be unable to discover the etiology. On rare occasions, congenital bony bridges from the long process of the incus to the malleus or from the malleus to the promontory may occur. In most instances, malleus fixation, discovered at the time of stapedectomy, is due to bony fixation of the anterior ligament of the malleus. Although I do not have an accurate

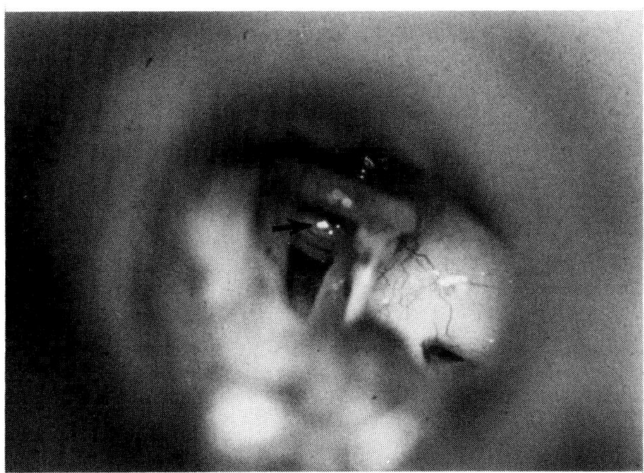

FIG 3–2.
Arrow points to huge persistent stapedial artery.

count, it is my impression that this would occur in 2% to 3% of ears undergoing middle ear surgery.

Management

When a stapedectomy is being performed, one must consider the earlier part of the operation to be a continuation of the clinical examination. After the tympanomeatal flap has been reflected forward and sufficient bony canal wall has been removed to examine the oval window, one should first examine the mobility of the ossicular chain. Its mobility is observed by moving the malleus and observing the incus, stapes, the tendon of the stapedial muscle, and the round window for motion. To omit this step and begin the process of the stapedectomy may lead to a major error.

If the malleus is fixed, it is my present choice to bypass the attic. I do this by using a sculptured ossicle, fitted between the head of the stapes and the handle of the malleus, as will be discussed later. I first cut the incudostapedial joint, releasing the long process of the incus from the head of the stapes. The incus is then disarticulated by moving the long process forward. The stapedial tendon acts as an anchor to the stapes. With the cup forceps, the incus is removed from the attic. The neck of the malleus is then cut with the House-Deiter malleus nipper. If the head is frozen in the attic, by fixation of either the anterior ligament or the superior ligament, break it free by downward-forward push using a Derlacki mobilizer. The head of the malleus is then removed from the attic with cup forceps. Quite often it is necessary to free the head of the malleus before the incus can be removed. The incus is then sculptured and used as an autograft. The head of the malleus may also be used if the distance between the head of the stapes and the handle of the malleus is not too great. The bone is delicately sculptured and precisely fitted over the head of the stapes and clamped to the handle of the malleus, as will be discussed later. The results should be in the realm of 85% air-bone gap closure to within 10 dB of the preoperative bone conduction.

On rare occasions, the stapes is also fixed with otosclerosis. In this event, a stapedectomy should be done, and the oval window must be covered with a substantial soft tissue seal (perichondrium). A homograft ossicle, sculptured to extend from the handle of the malleus to the center of the oval window graft, is then placed in position.

One should always remember that many cases of primary or secondary causes of conductive hearing impairment are completely diagnosed only after microscopic examination of the tympanic cavity. One should consider every operation as a reasonable continuation of a good examination. It is no dishonor for an otologist to make the final diagnosis at the time of tympanotomy.

Dehiscent Facial Nerve Overlying Oval Window

Embryology and Anatomy

The horizontal fallopian canal traverses the upper tympanic cavity from the geniculate ganglion anteriorly to the second genu of the facial nerve posteriorly. This nerve runs through its bony canal in the labyrinthine capsule just above the oval window. Very frequently (in at least 60% of ears), there is, in some portions of the fallopian canal, an opening or lack of bony covering of the facial nerve and its soft tissue sheath. Because this is so common, it is considered to be a normal variation. The location of this dehiscence in the bony canal, whether large or small, is almost always immediately superior to the stapedial footplate on the inferior circumference of the facial canal. It is usually quite small and is of no consequence, save that it should be known to the surgeon, so that injudicious movements of sharp right angle picks should not be made in that direction while working in the oval window niche.

Frequently, however, the lack of bony covering of the facial nerve may be quite extreme, even to the point of the entire nerve from the cochleariform process to the pyramidal eminence being unprotected by a bony covering. This still is not a deterrent to careful instrumentation of the oval window. Unfortunately, this variation from normal may be much more extensive. The facial nerve may herniate through the bony dehiscence and encroach over a portion of the footplate or even bulge inferiorly, so that a soft tissue mass may fill the obturator foramen of the stapes and may almost completely obstruct one's view of the entire stapedial footplate. One must presume this soft tissue mass to contain the fibers of the seventh cranial nerve, although it may simply be soft tissue accompanying the sheath. Finally, on rare occasions, one may find major developmental malpositioning of the facial nerve in the temporal bone. These have been described extensively in the scientific literature and should be in the memory bank of every otologic surgeon doing stapedial surgery. One may find the nerve running over the promontory inferior to the oval window. In this position, it may or may not have a bony covering. One must not make the mistake of thinking that the nerve across the promontory is the ponticulus, Jacobson's plexus, an unimportant adhesion, or a residual rope of mesenchymal tissue. When one is looking above the oval window, the absence of the characteristic large facial ridge above the oval window niche should give guidance suggesting that it may be inferior to the oval window niche on the promontory side. The nerve may be found also running directly across the stapedial footplate completely covering it. In these instances, other crude distortions of surrounding anatomical features, including the ossicles, are usually present.

In very rare conditions, the nerve may be bifid, that is, the nerve may split into two branches—one going above the oval window and one going below. Because of the developmental events of mesenchymal tissue of the first branchial arch incorporating the stapedial arch and the facial nerve, there is, perhaps, a strong predisposition for this malplacement to specifically occur at the oval window area. In all cases in which this has been reported, there have been other major ossicular malformations or anomalies observed.

A very important tipoff of an anomalous facial nerve may come from first observing the chorda tympani nerve as the tympanotomy begins. It may be malpositioned. Also, if it is definitely larger than normal, one should be alert. I have found this correlation to be present frequently (Fig 3–3).

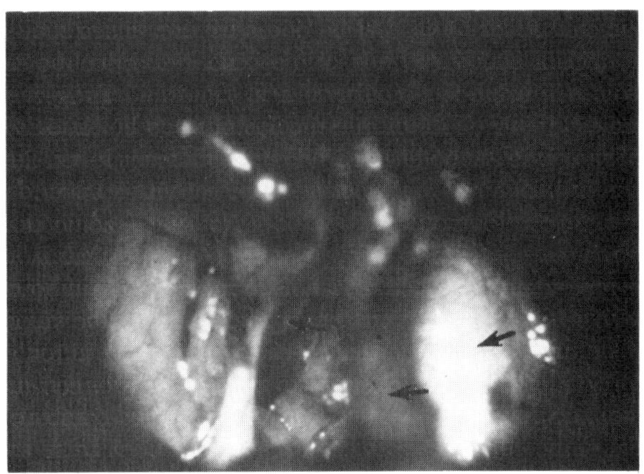

FIG 3–3.
Arrows point to misplaced facial nerve on promontory. Note very large chordi tympani nerve and, consequently, malformed unicrurate stapes with absence of oval window.

Surgical Management

A simple dehiscence of the bony covering of the facial nerve is not a contraindication to stapedectomy and only warns the surgeon to be careful and respectful of its presence. However, a nerve sheath that bulges down, obscuring a large portion of the footplate, may cause difficulty in the manipulative process. The soft tissue of the nerve and its sheath may need to be retracted gently to visualize enough of the footplate to allow its removal. Adjustment of the prosthesis (if one is used) on the long process of the incus or bending the prosthesis so as to go around the bulging nerve may be necessary. If the nerve is grossly bulging into the obturator foramen, one may see that it is being deeply indented by the crural arch. This is not a physiologic deterrent to its normal function. Therefore, it is permissible for the prosthesis to, at least slightly, indent the sheath of the nerve without causing long-term damage. Likewise, in the stapedectomy procedure in which the posterior crus is preserved and used, this indentation is obviously permissible.

Many major anomalies of the facial nerve are recognizable preoperatively by the presence of other accompanying branchial anomalies and may be seen in roentgenologic findings.

If the nerve is bifid, one is now in the midst of a major anomaly. There will probably be complete agenesis of the oval window with improper development of the stapedial arch and its footplate. If the area of the oval window is thin, and the two branches of the facial nerve are separated widely enough to permit access to the vestibule through the area of the footplate, an opening can be made and a prosthetic conductive mechanism established, providing, of course, there is a functional malleus and incus. This was the dilemma faced by John Shea (personal communication) in the early 1960s. His solution was the use of a very heavy large-diameter wire attached to the incus with its shaft extending slightly through the hole into the labyrinth. His ingenuity gave birth to the piston concept now so commonly used in stapedectomy.

If the nerve is misplaced on the promontory side of the oval window, this is, again, a major anomaly usually accompanied by massive agenesis of the oval window, the stapes, and its footplate. As far as the nerve itself is concerned, the issue is identification. The nerve should not be disturbed. The labyrinth should be opened, the oval window created, and the conductive mechanism established as seems prudent, taking into consideration all other factors such as the age of the patient, and the condition of the opposite ear.

I have had only two ears in which the facial nerve was completely filling the oval window niche, causing total coverage of the area where the oval window should be. There was, in those instances, a total agenesis of the oval window. In both of these, there was also an anomalous stapedial structure with an incomplete development of the crural arch. I was able to displace the nerve inferiorly enough to open the labyrinth above it.

In general then, seventh nerve malformations in the region of the oval window are quite common, occasionally very disturbing, and sometimes awesome. Usually, they do not prevent the surgeon from performing a successful stapedectomy; however, the principles of handling the facial nerve begin with the proper recognition and honoring its integrity.

Tympanic Membrane Perforation Related to Stapedectomy and Otosclerosis

Perforation Resulting From Disease in the Presence of Otosclerosis

A basic rule is that the labyrinth should not be opened in the presence of a tympanic membrane perforation caused by disease (past or present). Therefore, the disease in the tympanic cavity, mastoid, and nasopharynx that caused the perforation must be brought under control if still present and the perforation closed with tympanoplasty. Stapedectomy may be done several months later as a secondary procedure but only after elimination of disease and restoration of the tympanic membrane.

The reader is doubtless aware that the tympanic membrane closure may be done by a variety of techniques, including chemical cautery in the office, onlay-patch techniques, stuff-through techniques, and so forth. I prefer to use the underlay fascial graft technique as the most practical and the most successful procedure in my hands. The stapes should not be disturbed during this procedure. Six months after, the stapedectomy may be performed.

Primary and Secondary Perforations Caused by Stapedectomy

The tympanic membrane may be torn while the stapedectomy is done. It usually occurs in the posterior margin of the tympanic membrane at the superior end of the fibrous annulus. To prevent perforation, the surgeon should be very careful in lifting the tympanomeatal flap. The incision should be made with a sharp knife completely through the periosteum. The periosteum and skin should be elevated with the sharp elevating instrument, scraping hard against the bone so that the periosteum remains intact. Care should be made that tears do not occur at the tympanomastoid suture line where the tympanomeatal flap is quite vulnerable. When the sulcus of the annular ligament of the tympanic membrane is approached, even more care should be given so that the dissecting instrument stays against the bone and does not push against the soft tissue. Prepackaged, long stable dental cotton balls (no. 3) will help considerably in both providing a dry field and protecting the tympanomeatal flap. When the sulcus is reached at the edge of the tympanic membrane, the elevating instrument is moved more in a linear fashion parallel to the sulcus rather than pushing straight forward at right angles to the sulcus. The annular ligament is clearly visible, and if one dissects under it by lifting it out of its sulcus, a perforation will not occur. If this is ignored and the dissection is attempted over the annular ligament between the squamous epithelium and the fibrous annular ligament, a perforation is quite likely to occur.

In some ears, very heavy bands or sheets of scar tissue occur from the incus and stapes to the tympanic membrane. Removal of these, especially in ears that have had previous perforations, may cause a perforation. Perforation may be anticipated preoperatively by observing thin areas of monomeric membranes in which the middle fibrous layer of the drum has been destroyed.

Treatment of Intraoperative Perforation

During the procedure of stapedectomy, I almost always use a perichondrial graft from the tragus to cover the oval window. There is always plenty of perichondrial material from this site to provide graft tissue for any intraoperative perforation that may occur. The perichondrium is custom trimmed and placed under the tympanic membrane in a position so that it will close the perforation with ample extension under the surrounding tympanic membrane and flap. It is supported and held laterally against the drum with blood-soaked Gelfoam.

If the perforation is small and only a linear slit occurs, wet Gelfoam can be positioned under the drum and the edges of the membrane tear teased back together with picks and a foot pedal–controlled suction tip. The outer surface of the drum is then covered with a cast of wet blood-soaked Gelfoam.

If these techniques are used, a postoperative perforation from an otherwise uncomplicated case usually provides excellent results.

Secondary Poststapedectomy Perforations

Very rarely, an acute otitis media occurs during the first week after a stapedectomy. Obviously, the threat of labyrinthitis is a major concern. For this reason and others, I believe that a solid connective tissue graft that provides a seal over the oval window is important in stapedectomy. The oval window seals quickly with perichondrium, fascia, or vein. This and the administration of specific antibiotics are usually successful in preventing serious secondary complications, even in the presence of postoperative otitis media.

After the otitis media subsides, the resultant tympanic membrane perforation usually heals. If it persists beyond 4 to 6 months, it may then be successfully closed with an underlay fascialgraft tympanoplasty.

Obliterative Otosclerosis

The definition of obliterative otosclerosis is important. From a surgical standpoint, the pathology of diffuse obliterative otosclerosis is considerably different from the thick, biscuit-type circumscribed otosclerosis.

Circumscribed (biscuit-type) otosclerosis occurs in approximately 15% of the footplates involved with otosclerosis in the United States. It is reported to be more frequent in Australia and India. In this pathologic involvement, the otosclerosis crosses the annular ligament, usually anteriorly in a relatively small area, and builds up into a large, thick mass occupying the entire footplate before it attempts to invade or cross any of the remaining annular ligament onto the surrounding oval window. This apparent ligamentous deterrent to otosclerosis is helpful to the surgeon inasmuch as these otosclerotic footplate masses often shell out, leaving a healthy, well-defined window margin.

In contrast, diffuse obliterative otosclerosis occurs in approximately 2% of ears affected with otosclerosis in the United States and is relentlessly aggressive in its diffuse invasion of the temporal bone. It crosses all areas of the annular ligament, obliterating it, and invades the entire oval window, the promontory, and the surrounding labyrinthine bone. It produces a solid mass of thick, hard bone over the entire valley of the oval window, obliterating all of the landmarks of the annular ligament. This, indeed, is its identifying characteristic. One cannot see the location of the former annular ligament, and one cannot know the definite position of the original oval window margin.

Management

This pathologic problem of diffuse obliterative otosclerosis, to me, is the absolute indication for the use of the piston technique. Since one cannot safely recreate an oval window, or even identify its margins, the recreation of an opening into the labyrinth is all one should do. After removing the stapedial superstructure, I simply drill a shaft like a well through the bone into the vestibule. After careful measurement, a piston is placed into the opening and attached at the opposite end to the incus. It is measured so that it extends approximately 0.25 mL into the labyrinth. Soft tissue is then placed around the opening. I make the shaft barely large enough to admit the piston (which is usually 0.6 mm in diameter).

In the late 1950s and the early 1960s, the prevailing surgical philosophy was to drill out the bone in the oval window, saucerizing it widely, hopefully to prevent as much regrowth of bone as possible, and to gradually thin the bone down over the proposed oval window so as to finally remove it to create a new oval window. Unfortunately, creating such a large oval window caused excessive labyrinthine trauma. The bone dust and the bone removal also seemed to promote postoperative osteogenesis and labyrinthine reaction. As a result, we were most dissatisfied with the high percentage of postoperative sensorineural losses, vertigo, and so forth. My response has been a total reversal of my former surgical approach from aggressively drilling out the entire oval window to that of opening only a small hole into the labyrinth, with as little drilling as possible.

This newer procedure is much easier and provides a better long-term hearing result with much less risk of inner ear damage.

Revision

Unfortunately, because of the pathologic characteristics of diffuse obliterative otosclerosis, the prognosis for both the initial as well as long-term hearing improvement is not nearly as good as in the remaining 98% of the patients with otosclerosis. When regression occurs, one is then faced with a decision of choosing whether or not to (1) reenter the ear for possible revision, (2) use a hearing aid, or (3) implant the electromagnetic conduction device, the Xomed Audiant Bone Conductor. These alternatives are available, of course, only if there has been no sensorineural drop postoperatively that might preclude surgical intervention.

In trying to visualize what might have occurred to cause a recurrence of a conductive loss, one must think of the possibility of (1) massive regrowth of bone around and under the prosthesis, which fixes it again; (2) dislodgement of the prosthesis from the incus due to poor application or pathologic processes that may have pushed it off of the incus; and (3) the prosthesis being too short and resting on the edge of the stapedotomy opening.

I would consider reexploration of an ear only if there is a strong possibility of a repair such as (1) loose wire on the incus or (2) prosthesis too short to reach the oval window. Other important factors would be that the ear in question be the poorest ear, that there be no evidence of high-frequency loss following previous surgery, and that the patient has a good chance of restoration of hearing to a socially adequate level. Age considerations would also be taken into account with these factors. I would be extremely conservative in the younger age group.

Revision Stapedectomy of All Ears

One must realize that the results following revision stapedectomy, overall, are considerably poorer than with the original operation. For this reason, one must be much more conservative in both the decision to operate and expectation for success. Points to consider in making the decision include:

1. Condition of the opposite ear. One should follow the axiom of always operating on the poorest ear.

2. History as to the type of procedure previously done and the pathology encountered at that time.

3. History and progress of the improvement following the original surgery. For example, if the previous surgery was done 20 years ago with maintenance of good hearing until recent sudden loss, one might think of a displaced prosthesis or an erosion of the incus.

4. Ability to wear a hearing aid satisfactorily.

5. History of vertigo. If the events during the previous surgery, especially if done by someone else, is unknown and the patient remembers significant intraoperative or postoperative vertigo, this might be an important deterrent. The inner ear may be fragile.

6. History of previous surgery, the immediate postoperative course, and any long-term sequela are extremely important, especially if done by another surgeon and if the records are unreliable or absent. The length of the operation, the intraoperative happenings (e.g., vertigo), and the immediate postoperative severity of vertigo may give good indication as to the mechanical difficulty the previous surgeon found in doing the procedure. Labyrinthine trauma occurring at that time may cause the ear to be very fragile.

7. Pathology seen at the time of the original surgery and anatomic difficulty in doing the previous surgery. The pathology would be very important in determining the disease progress and the prognosis for the future. For example, if diffuse obliterative otosclerosis was seen in a young adult and the hearing remained good for only 3 months postoperatively, then slowly deteriorated after a well-done piston technique, revision surgery would be contraindicated. The alternative of using a hearing aid or using the implantable electromagnetic bone conductor (Xomed Audiant Bone Conductor) should be offered. The anatomic difficulty in doing the previous surgery must also be considered. These restrictions can reduce the chances for success for even the most skillful surgeon.

8. Health, age, and psychologic commitment of the patient. Any one of these can play a major role toward vetoing the surgical reentry into the ear and must be added into the formula for reaching the final decision.

Cause of Stapedectomy Failure During or Soon After Stapedectomy

Some of the common causes of immediate failure at the time of surgery and regression in the early postoperative period (within 2 weeks) are:

1. Severe labyrinthine reaction. Severe reaction may be due to instrumental trauma, biochemical reaction, fluid pressure changes, serous labyrinthitis, acute labyrinthitis, and so forth. Any of these, if significant, can produce a sensorineural loss of hearing. Revision surgery is contraindicated. It is my belief that one is rarely justified in reopening the labyrinth within the first 2 weeks following surgery.

2. Ossicular chain discontinuity. A prosthesis poorly attached to the incus or a prosthesis that has not been properly placed in the oval window will cause an immediate failure. This ear may have an excellent chance for success with revision surgery. This condition should be rare if the initial surgery has been well planned and well executed. One of the problems commonly causing difficulty for the inexperienced surgeon is proper measurement of the prosthesis. If the prosthesis is too short, poor hearing results will occur. If it is too long, labyrinthine trauma with long-term postoperative vertigo may result.

3. Occurrence of postoperative oval window fistula. Again, this will be extremely rare if the oval window is well covered with a viable connective tissue graft.

4. Regrowth of bone causing recurrent ankylosis. This, too, is almost nonexistent during the first few weeks after surgery.

5. Marked adhesive otitis media. This may occur, especially if there is postoperative otitis media or granuloma formation (see later discussion of reparative granuloma).

6. Cochlear block. It is widely recognized that conductive hearing impairment may still present itself in the presence of a normally mobile ossicular chain and without any apparent conductive lesion. The etiology and pathology of this are unknown, but one must, of course, be very sure that proper diagnostic testing has been accomplished.

7. Upper ossicular chain fixation with or without stapedial ankylosis. If one does not observe the mobility of the malleus and the incus, one may fail to recognize upper ossicular chain fixation even though a complete stapedectomy has been done. Upper chain fixation may also occur concomitantly with stapedial ankylosis due to otosclerosis. It is also possible that the malleus-incus articulation may slowly ankylose in the early postoperative period secondary to surgical trauma.

8. Misdiagnosis of a conductive hearing impairment in a patient with a unilateral sensorineural loss. This may be due to the lack of proper masking during the preoperative audiologic examination and the improper use of tuning forks.

Common Causes of Long-Term Failure With Recurrence of Conductive Loss After Initial Successful Results

Common causes of failure months to years postoperatively with recurrence of conductive loss after initial successful results include:

1. Erosion of the long process of the incus due to necrosis caused by the prosthesis
2. Migration of the prosthesis from the oval window to its edge, causing secondary ankylosis
3. Narrowing of the oval window with bony fixation
4. Regrowth of otosclerosis
5. Perilymphatic fistula
6. New pathology occurring elsewhere in the conductive mechanisms causing ankylosis (i.e., upper ossicular chain fixation)

Intraoperative Vertigo

The most common causes for intraoperative vertigo are some of the following:

1. Change in fluid levels in the labyrinth
2. Hyperactive labyrinth (patients who have motion sickness, excessive anxiety, etc.)
3. Instrumental trauma to the labyrinth
4. Prolonged surgical exposure causing drying out of the labyrinth due to long exposure to the intense heat from the microscope light
5. Chemical imbalance in the labyrinthine fluids
6. Prosthesis too long
7. Labyrinthine otosclerosis
8. Organic brain stem disorders
9. Preoperative medication
10. Labyrinthine hydrops

Management

The severity of intraoperative vertigo is not necessarily related to surgical technique. For instance, a patient may have stimulation of the vestibular labyrinth because of fluid motion during the stapedectomy from which one might expect a very mild vertiginous response, but in patients with a hypersensitive labyrinth such as those subject to motion sickness, the intraoperative vertigo may be quite severe.

Unusual labyrinthine sensitivity may also be present if the patient gives a preoperative history of previous episodes of spontaneous vertiginous attacks. It becomes important that one differentiates preoperatively between true Meniere's type of hydrops and vertigo caused by labyrinthine otosclerosis. In my patients, I have found that 35% of the patients with otosclerosis have a preoperative history of episodes of typical labyrinthine vertigo at some time in the past. These episodes, and accompanying symptoms, are usually distinguishable from typical Meniere's type of vertigo. However, both of these entities do cause the labyrinth to be more predisposed to operative disturbance. Of great importance, also, is the instruction and psychologic preparation of the patient. Although the patient should be informed of every fact related to the operation and to the events they are to experience, this should, in no way, be done in a frightening manner. Calm reassurance by the surgeon and the surgical nurses may prevent, or reduce, the perceived severity of any labyrinthine reaction or systemic shock.

Proper attention to the preoperative history may also allow one to omit certain sedatives and so forth that have caused trouble in the past. I do not use meperidine (Demerol) because I have found adverse reaction in many patients who become violently nauseated, even before the operation starts. I believe it is important not to use a large number of medications at the same time.

On the other hand, certain medications may be needed to suppress certain responses. For cardiovascular protection, I give atropine as a preoperative medication. In addition, I have available a few other carefully chosen drugs for specific pharmacologic actions. If a patient is extremely tense in spite of preoperative medication or has a history of suggesting the possibility of labyrinthine hyperirritability, 5 to 10 mg of diazepam may be given intravenously at the beginning of the surgical procedure. Diazepam works directly on the vestibular nucleus in the brain stem and is quite effective as a vestibular suppressant. Midazolam (Versed R) may be given intravenously. It is very similar to diazepam and is faster acting.

If vertigo occurs during the surgical procedure, I find oxygen to be of great benefit.

Two of the most important factors in intraoperative vertigo are the length of the procedure and the exposure of the labyrinth to the heat generated by the microscope light. The labyrinth should be left open only a very short period of time. Everything should be in perfect preparation before the procedures on the footplate are to be accomplished so that there is no delay in moving through this critical stage of the operation.

It is always important to guard against the sudden inordinate removal of perilymph with the suction. For this reason, I consider a foot pedal suction a must, so that removal of perilymph does not occur suddenly and uncontrollably.

The labyrinth should not be entered with sharp instruments. A very fine 0.3-mm right-angle pick may be used to remove the first tiny portion of the footplate. Immediately, the dull right-angle footplate excavator (the Hough hoe) should be used to remove the remaining portions of the footplate. Properly used, this instrument is not likely to damage the membranous labyrinth. Once the labyrinth is open, no other fluids should enter the ear. Irrigation of the ear is definitely contraindicated. The delicate chemical balance of the perilymph and the endolymph cannot be matched with any physiologic solution available.

Intraoperative vertigo most frequently is the response to the surgeon's activities and techniques. Therefore, prevention is more personal than pharmacologic.

Postoperative Vertigo

Several factors need consideration when there is postoperative vertigo. First, mild postoperative vertigo is common for the simple reason that the labyrinthine fluids have been entered. Therefore, it seems best to require several hours of bed rest with the head elevated and very little motion postoperatively. No routine medication is given to control or prevent vertigo, and normally, recovery is quite rapid.

Second, if a patient has a known hypersensitive labyrinth (motion sickness, etc.), it may be wise to use mild postoperative labyrinthine sedation with diazepam (Valium), dimenhydrinate (Dramamine), or promethazine (Phenergan), etc. We should expect all postoperative vertigo to gradually diminish.

The third type of postoperative vertigo is serous labyrinthitis, which is characterized by normal recovery, but 2 to 3 days later, the patient experiences an onset of moderate to even severe vertigo, often with accompanying nausea and vomiting. Cochlear suppression with roaring tinnitus may also be experienced. The etiology is speculative but is probably an altered aseptic histochemical response to healing. I always start the patient on steroid therapy immediately unless there is a medical contraindication. The results are usually good, with the patient slowly recovering to a completely normal state. Some patients, unfortunately, suffer severe sensorineural loss. Two things are important. First, these patients should not have immediate revision surgery. The ear is undergoing healing at a very critical stage and is already fragile. If one reenters the ear, resolving blood clots, fibrous tissue, and thickened mucous membrane will be encountered. In attempting to remove this, perhaps thinking it is a granuloma, one may well convert the fragile ear into one with a permanent functional loss.

Another factor is that in the very early onset of delayed postoperative vertigo, it is impossible to distinguish serous labyrinthitis from acute septic labyrinthitis. For this reason, I not only start the patient on steroid therapy but also use heavy doses of a broad-spectrum antibiotic, such as amoxicillin.

Acute septic labyrinthitis is another cause of postoperative vertigo. Fortunately, it is extremely rare. It is usually secondary to postoperative acute otitis media, and early surgical reentry is contraindicated.

I will give little attention to the fifth cause of postoperative vertigo, that is, a stapedial prosthesis that is too long. It is the result of improper measurement during the surgical technique. Revision in this instance is the only answer.

Finally, a postoperative perilymphatic fistula may be the cause of vertigo. This is rare and is more likely to occur if the oval window has not been properly sealed with a strong tissue graft such as perichondrium, vein, or fascia. In my experience, certain piston techniques, which do not use a complete connective tissue oval window seal, are more prone to develop this complication. Diagnosis is difficult without direct visualization, and early reentry in an already fragile ear is dangerous.

Reparative Granuloma

So-called reparative granuloma is the overabundance of granulation tissue in the healing area of the oval window and the tympanomeatal flap. When viewed otoscopically, the tympanic cavity, especially the superior posterior region, seems to be filled with a beefy red mass. This condition is extremely rare and is probably caused by foreign body contaminates such as glove powder, lint, fibers, or hair. Resolving blood clots in the tympanic cavity, hematomas under the tympanomeatal flap, and hyperreactive mucous membranes can be diagnosed improperly as a reparative granuloma. This appearance, to some extent is seen in every ear recovering from stapedectomy. Thus, differential diagnosis between these normal healing responses and a reparative granuloma is a matter of degree.

In my opinion, few, if any, of these conditions are improved by early revision surgery. In most cases, the already fragile ear is functionally destroyed by the surgical reinvasion. My choice for therapy is the use of steroids and broad-spectrum antibiotics.

Tympanosclerotic Footplate Fixation

Tympanosclerosis is not an epithelial disease but, rather, arises in the connective tissue elements. It is probably secondary to an altered healing response. Once established, it is thought to be nonprogressive. Being connective tissue, the fibrous annular ligament, bridging the space between the stapedial footplate and the oval window, is prone to involvement. Likewise, the stapedius muscle, tendon, and the connective tissue of the submucosal layer in the oval window may be involved, causing fixation. When the oval window is diffusely involved with tympanosclerosis, it is understandably very difficult to remove the plaque and recreate a smooth oval window. Frequently, small pieces of tympanosclerosis remain, restricting the mobility of the footplate. Furthermore, if the surgical removal is too aggressive, one may enter the labyrinth.

If a concomitant tympanic membrane perforation exists, one must consider the ear as being possibly contaminated, and, therefore, aggressive removal of plaques on the footplate should not be done. In this situation, the stapedectomy should be done as a secondary procedure 6 months after repair of the tympanic membrane.

Although one may occasionally improve hearing to a somewhat adequate level by removing tympanosclerosis over the footplate without doing a stapedectomy, the results are usually poor, especially if there is minute annular ligament infiltration. The decision as to the removal of tympanosclerosis in the oval window and over the footplate must be made on an individual basis after all of the factors are weighed.

In clean ears with an intact tympanic membrane, total stapedectomy can often be performed as in otosclerosis with good results. However, the remainder of the conductive mechanism (tympanic membrane and upper ossicular chain) may also be involved to some degree with tympanosclerotic pathology. Therefore, results are usually not as good as with stapedial surgery for otosclerosis. Furthermore, because of other complicating factors caused by more generalized pathology and perhaps a more fragile ear, the risk of sensorineural loss is somewhat greater with stapedectomy for tympanosclerosis (2%–5%) compared with stapedectomy for otosclerosis (<1%).

Lenticular Process Erosion

Erosion of the long process of the incus has created one of the major objections to the use of some types of artificial stapedial prostheses. The original polyethylene prosthesis (Shea) very frequently caused a severance of the long process. Fortunately, erosion of the long process of the incus is rare with most of the modern artificial prostheses; however, an even better choice is the technique of maintaining the posterior crus, as in a stapedectomy with preservation of the posterior crus. One may also use a homograft strut from a lenticular process to the oval window. If one of these more physiologic techniques is used, the problem of incus erosion is eliminated.

Wire loops, crimped around the long process of the incus over a long period of time, usually produce some erosion of the bone. This erosion may be due to anemic necrosis, vibratory action, or both. If left long enough, it may produce not only indentation in the bone but also complete division of the long process. Fortunately, it usually requires many years to occur, and the vast majority of ears have continued to function well even 25 years later.

One must consider that the long process of the incus is further away from soft tissue blood supply than any other part of the ossicular chain. If one removes the stapedial superstructure, cuts tendon of the stapedius muscle, and uses a prosthesis of any kind, the entire soft tissue blood supply, except the mucous membrane along the long process of the incus, has been swept away, leaving the incus extremely vulnerable to necrosis. For these reasons, in doing a stapedectomy, I have continued to preserve the incudostapedial joint and the posterior crus of the stapes as often as possible (in 80% of stapedectomies). When accomplished, this eliminates the concern of incus necrosis.

When a prosthesis is applied, one should attempt a firm connection. Normally, if one uses a wire loop, it should be near the end of the long process just superior to the lenticular process. Occasionally, the long process overhangs the oval window far inferiorly. In this instance, the loop should be tightened so that it will be in good functional alignment with the center of the oval window graft. If the facial nerve overhang is great and the incus is short, it may be necessary to provide a bend in the wire to accommodate for the facial nerve.

If a part or most of the long process of the incus has been eroded away by a previous prosthesis, reapplication more proximally may be possible. In many instances, to attempt a revision with another incus attachment is unreasonable. The better choice is to connect the oval window directly to the handle of the malleus with a sculptured homograft ossicle (see later discussion).

Chorda Tympani Nerve

If the tympanic membrane is elevated in any surgical procedure, every patient should be warned that disturbance of taste or some dryness of the mouth may occur, either temporarily or permanently, after the operation. My experience is that approximately 5% of the patients notice dryness of the mouth. Most of these recover, but some very slowly, over a period of 3 to 8 months. For a rare few, however, it becomes a very annoying problem. Strangely enough, cutting the nerve may or may not cause symptoms.

If the ear has had long-lasting inflammatory disease and undergoes tympanoplastic surgery, the patient is much less likely to notice postoperative disturbance and seldom notices it if the nerve requires sacrificing.

I believe great care should be taken to preserve the chorda tympani. It should not be stretched or dried out. The method I use for removal of the bony overhang of the posterior superior bony canal wall has been described previously.

In revision surgery, the problem is identification and separation of the nerve from the scar tissue fibers at the tympanic membrane margin. I find it useful to first lift the tympanic membrane anteriorly and superiorly in the region of the malleus, entering the middle ear superiorly rather than posteriorly and inferiorly. This allows one to first identify the chorda tympani as it runs under the malleus and between the incus and the malleus. In this location, it is usually free from scar tissue and easily identified. It can then be carefully dissected free from the tympanic membrane posteriorly to the iter chorda posticus, where final sharp dissection of the scar tissue is used to free it from the tympanic membrane.

INCUS REPLACEMENT

Conditions For Ossicular Reconstruction

The most ideal condition for ossicular reconstruction is one in which the tympanic membrane is intact, the eustachian tube functions normally, the mucosa of the tympanic cavity is healthy, the malleus is normal, the stapes is normal and mobile, but the bridge provided by the incus is missing or nonfunctional. Such a situation, as in a longitudinal basilar skull fracture, upper ossicular chain fixation, or erosion of the long process of the incus due to previous but inactive middle ear disease, is frequently found. In all cases, strive to obtain:

1. A permanently functioning and efficient connective bridge from the tympanic membrane to the inner ear

2. An aerated tympanic cavity
3. A tympanic membrane that is in normal position and well attached to the handle of the malleus
4. A healthy middle ear mucosa
5. A tympanic cavity of sufficient depth to support an ossicular bridge
6. A healthy external canal and mastoid environment

Some of these may be obtained only partially, yet this lack may not deter a surgical attempt toward reconstruction. Tympanomastoid surgery is done primarily to eliminate disease and prepare the foundations for reconstruction. Ossicular reconstruction is the placement of the capstone with tympanoplasty. Surgeons vary in what they consider as to conditions necessary for ossicular chain repair. Thus, some may more frequently plan a two-stage procedure than others. I seldom plan a two-stage procedure because I find that mucosal healing and control of inflammatory disease provided through surgical procedures, combined with effective medical therapy, frequently, and often surprisingly, allow excellent healing. The grafts usually remain in place and function well postoperatively. This, then, eliminates the need for a second surgical procedure. I see no need in denying the patient this opportunity of success with the first operation by withholding ossicular chain reconstruction until a later date.

The one exception, in which a planned second procedure is necessary, is when the stapedial footplate is fixed, and there is also a tympanic membrane perforation or inflammatory disease of the middle ear mucosa. In this event, a second-stage stapedectomy can be done after complete healing of the tympanic cavity.

Tympanoplasty with ossicular reconstruction is often contraindicated in several conditions, such as:

1. When it is the only hearing ear and it is functional with a hearing aid.
2. When the tympanic cavity is atelectatic and it is impossible to restore the eustachian tube to proper function.
3. When the sensorineural loss is so great that restoration of hearing cannot be obtained so that the ear becomes useful to the patient (one must always consider the possibility of hearing-aid utilization and consider the function of the opposite ear).
4. When the age and general condition of the patient causes the planned procedure to be unreasonable.
5. When chronic inflammatory disease of the tympanomastoid complex is locally uncontrollable.

Materials for Ossicular Reconstruction

In the late 1950s and the early 1960s, a number of artificial prosthetic materials were used. At the same time, I, as well as others, discovered that autograft human bone, and even homograft bone, could be used to bridge gaps in the ossicular chain. Even in air-containing cavities, the graft would almost always take, bone would be revitalized, and resorption was rare. On the other hand, the first plastic and metal prostheses we used were very often rejected and dislodged, cutting through their bony attachments. Fortunately, materials that are more biocompatible have been introduced in later years, and the success rate has been greatly improved. Nevertheless, it makes sense to me that an artificial prosthesis can never integrate with human tissue and will continue to be somewhat less physiologic for long-term use. Since autograft ossicular bone is usually not usable, it was a great boon to our efforts when it was found that homograft bone, particularly ossicles, could be used. Furthermore, many of us found that with sculpturing techniques, we could design units that would custom fit almost any need, thus, giving a higher degree of good function.

Technique of Malleus to Footplate Reconstruction

For malleus to footplate reconstruction, I usually use a portion of a homograft malleus (Fig 3–4). The handle of the homograft malleus from the lateral process to the tip is almost always the right length to fit between the footplate of the stapes and the medial aspect of the handle of the malleus. In some cases, the promontory may be high, overhanging the footplate. It may be best to use the homograft from the right ear for the patient's left side. The reason is that the malleus makes a slight curve anteriorly as it nears the umbo. This curve is helpful when it is applied to the footplate, allowing it to arch around an overhanging promontory.

This sculptured homograft can be applied by maneuvering the saddle end of the bone graft in place under the handle of the malleus using foot pedal–controlled suction and forceps to guide it into place against the malleus. Once it is engaged, the

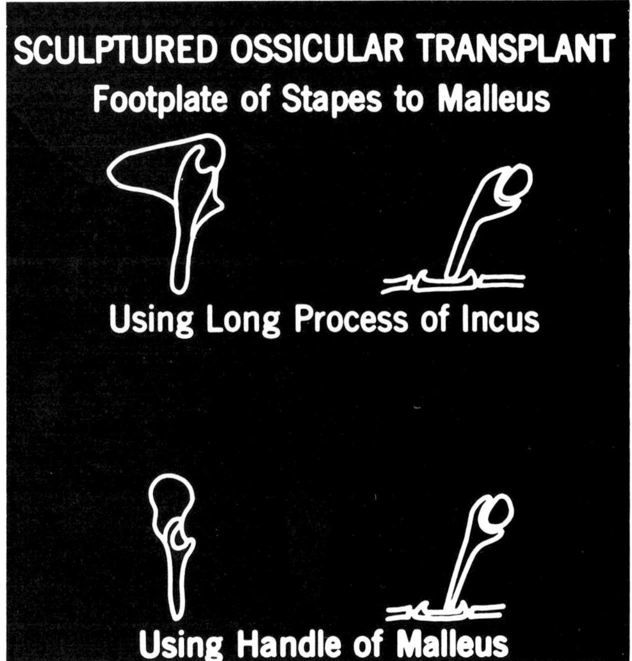

FIG 3–4.
Incus and malleus sculptured to reconstruct ossicular chain from footplate of stapes to handle of malleus.

malleus is raised and pushed slightly forward, and at the same time, the shaft of the homograft is rotated into the oval window niche, allowing it to finally rest in the center of the oval window either directly on the footplate or in the center of a perichondrial graft over the oval window. After it is in place, I use a stabilizing cast of wet Gelfoam pledgets around the homograft.

Occasionally, the distance from the malleus to the footplate is excessive. In these instances, I use a homograft incus that is sculptured to fit (see Fig 3–4).

Frequently, the tip of the handle of the malleus is displaced medially so that it is almost in direct contact with the promontory. Also, occasionally, the head of the malleus is fixed with bony union at its anterior or superior ligament. In these conditions, the neck of the malleus can be cut with the House-Dieter malleus nipper, releasing the handle of the malleus for better positioning and mobility. When this is done, it is usually best to either remove the head of the malleus with cup forceps or dislodge it into the attic area so that it will not cause further ankylosis.

When there is no handle of the malleus, one may use a homograft shaft of bone approximately the same size of the handle of the malleus. It can be placed on the medial surface of the new tympanic membrane in the desired position. It retains its position quite well, especially when a fascial graft has been used for tympanic membrane reconstruction.

Technique For Malleus To Head of Stapes Reconstruction

Malleus to head of stapes reconstruction is the most common ossicular chain reconstruction and, fortunately, the most easily accomplished, and it provides the best results. Thirty years ago, some of us began rotating ossicular remnants to bridge the gaps in the conductive mechanism. We proved that bone would revitalize and retain its mass. Soon afterward, House[1] used the body of the incus on the stapedial head. Although some excellent results were obtained, the application was crude, and more consistent stability was desired. For instance, the massive body of the incus frequently attached to the tympanic membrane, and as it tensed during healing, it lifted the bone graft laterally away from the stapedial head. In some instances, it migrated and became ankylosed to the promontory or the posterior wall of the tympanic cavity, thus preventing good sound transmission.

Soon after, it was found that more definite sculpturing techniques of these bone grafts suggested by Pennington[2] and later by others, eliminated some of the problems. This sculpturing provided a custom fit within the ossicular chain, giving needed stability, with better and more uniform long-term results.

For reconstruction of the ossicular chain, from the head of the stapes to the handle of the malleus, I use an autograft or homograft incus sculptured to fit (Fig 3–5). If the autograft incus is not diseased, after disarticulating it from the head of the malleus, I grasp it with cup forceps and rotate it out of the attic. Holding the incus at its short process with a Sheehy or Derlacki bone holder, I sculpture it with a 1-mm diamond burr. The long process is cut off at the body of the incus. At this surface, a cup is made with the 1-mm diamond burr for the head of the

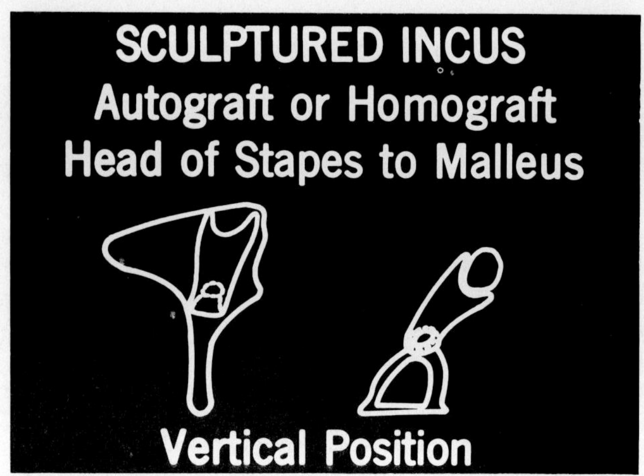

FIG 3–5.
Incus sculptured to reconstruct ossicular chain from head of stapes to handle of malleus.

stapes. A saddle indentation is then made on the superior surface of the body of the incus graft to receive the handle of the malleus. The bone is sculptured with the burr so as to create a more delicate shaft between these two new articulating surfaces (see Fig 3–5).

The sculptured bone is now introduced into the ear so that the saddle end is secured to the undersurface of the malleus. With firm but gentle lateral pressure, the bone graft and malleus are lifted and the opposite cupped end of the graft brought into position and rested over the head of the stapes. This remains quite stable even without a Gelfoam support and usually provides an excellent restoration of hearing.

Prosthesis Extrusion

Prevention and Management

The most effective prevention is not to use artificial prostheses in reconstructing the ossicular chain. If one uses either autograft or homograft ossicles, the chances of extrusion are very limited. Other cortical bone may also be used effectively.

Because I have not used artificial prostheses for a number of years, I am not an authority and will not discuss the value or describe other well-known methods of prevention of prosthetic extrusion such as the use of a cartilage interface. Since the introduction of the use of artificial prosthetic materials (polyethylene tubes etc.) in the tympanic cavity about 30 years ago, there has been a never-ending stream of new materials advocated. The biocompatible materials now used in these prosthetic devices have been improved. Some have also found that tissue reinforcement, such as the use of a cartilaginous interface between the tympanic membrane and the prosthesis, may diminish the rate of rejection. Their convenience and the improved reliability of these materials have become a great boon. Nevertheless, we must await long-term results for the final assessment.

Even presently, results are still no better, and perhaps not as good, as those results seen when human bone has been used. Historically, long-term breakdown and extrusion have caused the advocates of prosthetic materials to repeatedly devise newer techniques and use different materials through the years.

The question of transmission of the acquired immune deficiency syndrome (AIDS) virus through the use of homograft transplants is answered and made inconsequential by (1) the proper screening of donors; and (2) the fact that this virus is easily destroyed by the commonly used methods of sterilization with alcohol or formaldehyde, sterilization by autoclaving, or sterilization by irradiation. These methods may be used singly or in combination to provide proper preparation of the bone bank ossicle for transplantation.

Management of Failed Ossicular Reconstruction

How does the patient and physician face and assess a failure to obtain a good hearing result after ossicular reconstruction? The answer must begin in the original examination and discussion with the patient. The patient must be prepared for failure. The reasons for the procedure, the percentage chance of success and failure, and the prognosis for disease elimination and hearing recovery must be openly discussed. The alternatives must also be described to the patient and well understood. For instance, many procedures, such as tympanomastoidectomy, are done primarily for disease elimination and prevention and only secondarily for hearing restoration. Due to various factors, such as eustachian tube function, these procedures may have a very poor prognosis for hearing restoration. Even so, one may, in some instances, attempt functional restoration during the first procedure. If the patient has been well instructed preoperatively, they will have reasonable expectations and an understanding when failure to regain hearing occurs. Patients are usually pleased when they have a healthy, safe ear for the future. Even in those cases in which improved function is the primary objective, if patients know that their chances are quite limited in obtaining this, they can reasonably accept the failure and their future alternatives.

The presence of failure requires a thorough analysis of all the factors and uses all of the acumen of a good otologist. Many questions concerning the reason for the failure arise. Can the cause be corrected so that another operation might be successful? What is the status of the bone conduction? What is the status of the opposite ear and the patient's general health, age, and attitude toward another procedure? What are other alternatives for better function?

If at the time of the original procedure there was extensive disease in the tympanic cavity and mastoid, the chances of success and hearing restoration are obviously reduced due to the massive amount of healing required in the tympanic cavity. Therefore, once the tympanic cavity is healed, even if the original attempt of ossicular reconstruction failed, one may have a better chance of a more stable reconstruction with a secondary revision tympanoplasty. This possibility should be explained to the patient beforehand.

One factor cannot be overemphasized: the presence of a functional eustachian tube is the essential cornerstone for successful hearing restoration. If it is not present or cannot be obtained, then repeated surgical attempts are futile. To overlook this factor leads to repeated disappointments.

The presence of the handle of the malleus is important. Although success may be obtained by double grafting of bone or by a prosthesis to the tympanic membrane, both are more unstable without the normally attached malleus and have less chance of success.

Finally, one must be very pragmatic, and even somewhat pessimistic, in considering revision surgery. Despite the patient's desire and willingness to participate, there is a time to advise against low-yield, high-cost surgery and to encourage other alternatives. These other alternatives should be outlined before the first procedure and should be represented when surgical failure occurs. Depending on the function of the opposite ear, the cochlear function of the ear in question, and the status of the ear canal (and possibly the mastoid bowl), a conventional air-conduction hearing aid may be a reasonable alternative.

Again, depending on all of these factors, the new implantable electromagnetic bone conduction hearing device (Xomed Audiant Bone Conductor) is an excellent solution to middle ear mastoid malformation and disease. Since an ear canal mold is not needed with this device, it may be used when there is intermittant or chronic otorrhea. Likewise, dermatitis, caused by canal molds, is not a factor.

With this implantable electromagnetic device, hearing can be obtained not only in the lower frequencies, as with conventional hearing aids, but in the important high frequencies as well. Furthermore, hearing will be very predictable because the postoperative threshold will be at or near the audiometric bone conduction threshold.

If after the initial surgical procedure or procedures have failed there is still (1) a good cochlear reserve, (2) an air-containing, disease-free middle ear, and (3) an intact tympanic membrane, and if the patient is still socially inadequate due to a hearing deficit and strongly desires to have another surgical try attempted, the surgeon may be again inclined toward trying to restore hearing with tympanoplastic reconstruction. In the face of these diminishing odds for success, if I attempted further middle ear revision, I would consider making, at the same time, a separate incision postauricular and implanting the magnet of the Xomed Audiant Bone Conductor in the temporal bone. This, then, will provide a safety net in case the tympanoplasty fails again or there is, in the future, periodic eustachian tube dysfunction, disabling the conductive mechanism.

REFERENCES

1. House WF, Patterson ME, Linthicum FH: Incus homografts in chronic ear surgery. *Arch Otolaryngology* 1966; 84:148–153.
2. Pennington CL: Incus interposition techniques. *Ann Otol Rhinol Laryngol* 1973; 82:518–531.

Ossicular Reconstruction

Approach of

John J. Shea, M.D.

Stapedectomy, with reconstruction of the sound-conducting mechanism of the middle ear with an artificial prosthesis, which I introduced in 1956, was the first successful use of an artificial plastic prosthesis to replace the stapes bone. After the success of this operation was established by many years of use by surgeons all over the world, prostheses have been developed to replace the arch of the stapes, incus, and malleus. All of these prostheses will be explained, with the indications for their use and technique of insertion.

STAPEDECTOMY

The usual indication for stapedectomy is otosclerosis, although in ears with congenital and other defects of the stapes with good eustachian tube function, stapedectomy is also the operation of choice.

In tympanoplasty, in those ears with poor eustachian tube function, stapedectomy is not indicated because of the danger of getting material from the middle into the inner ear through the oval window because of the negative pressure that can and most often does develop in the middle ear after closure of the perforation of the drum. After the drum perforation is closed and the infection controlled, in these ears with good eustachian tube function, no negative pressure will develop in the middle ear. Stapedectomy may be performed to reconstruct the sound-conducting mechanism of the middle ear.

In ears with nonobliterative otosclerosis, the lining membrane of the middle ear is removed from the footplate and around the oval window for a distance of 1 mm, and any bleeding is controlled. The posterior half of the footplate is removed, and the oval window opening is sealed with a large (4 by 6 mm) vein from the back of the hand, previously pressed, to thin the vein and eliminate its tendency to curl, with the adventitia down.

Any type of piston prosthesis with a cup in its head can be used. I prefer the Shea platinum Teflon cup piston prosthesis (Richards Medical; Fig 3–6), because with the platinum wires you can make a firm attachment of the prosthesis to the lower incus to hold it in the cup, which you cannot always do with the cup piston prosthesis with a bale handle wire at its lower

end. In about 5% of ears, the lenticular process extends beyond the oval window, so that a cup piston prosthesis cannot be used. In this situation, the old-style Teflon piston with a loop in its upper end is slipped around the lower incus (Fig 3–7). The distance from the undersurface of the lower incus to the center of the vein over the oval window is measured, and the correct length prosthesis is used. The tip of the prosthesis should extend about 0.25 mm beyond the inner rim of the oval window opening into the vestibule. After the prosthesis is inserted, Gelfoam is packed around the lower end of the prosthesis to hold it in the center of the opening in the oval window and to hold the vein down onto the denuded bone.

In ears with obliterative otosclerosis, now very rare, a small opening is made in the center of the oval window in the thinnest portion of the bone with the Shea microdrill using a 0.65-mm diameter diamond burr. This opening is covered with an inferiorly based flap of lining membrane of the middle ear, elevated from the promontory, and a 0.6-mm diameter platinum Teflon cup prosthesis or Teflon piston with a loop in its end is inserted, depending on the position of the lenticular process with reference to the oval window opening. Once again the tip of the prosthesis should extend about 0.25 mm beyond the inner rim of the oval window opening into the vestibule. Gelfoam is packed around the Teflon piston to hold it in the oval window opening and to hold the lining membrane of the middle ear down on the oval window opening (Fig 3–8).

In those ears with otosclerosis in which the incus is not suitable to use, for any reason, one half of the stapes footplate is removed, the oval window is covered with a vein graft, and a malleus attachment Teflon piston prosthesis is inserted between the handle of the malleus and the oval window opening covered with vein. This prosthesis has a larger loop in the upper end, which is at an angle of 30 degrees with the shaft of the prosthesis to accommodate the angle of malleus with reference to the plane of oval window opening. Results with this malleus attachment Teflon piston prosthesis are good, better than with any other way to reconstruct the sound-conducting mechanism of the middle ear when the incus is not usable, but they are not as good or dependable as when the prosthesis can be attached to the incus. A small piece of loose connective tissue is inserted between the loop at the end of the large-headed malleus Teflon piston as it fits around the malleus and the overlying drum to prevent erosion of the drum (Fig 3–9).

Results with this technique of stapedectomy using Teflon piston prostheses have been good, with 90% closure of the air-bone gap and less than 1% made worse. Over time, about 30% of those operated, especially those ears with widespread, invasive otosclerosis, particularly those beginning early in life, develop enough sensorineural hearing loss and must return to the use of a hearing aid.

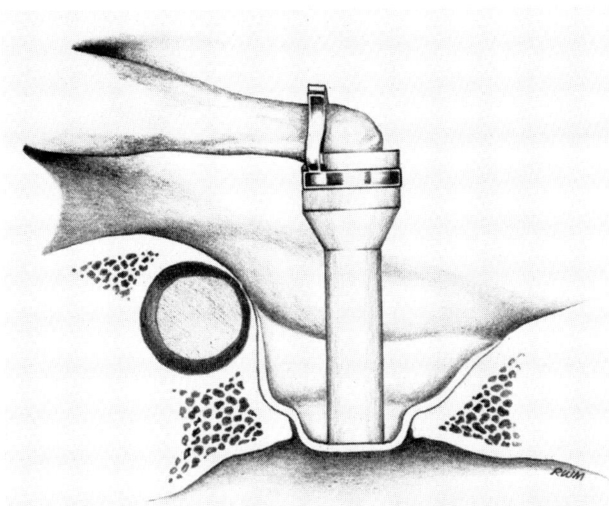

FIG 3–6.
Shea platinum Teflon cup piston prosthesis.

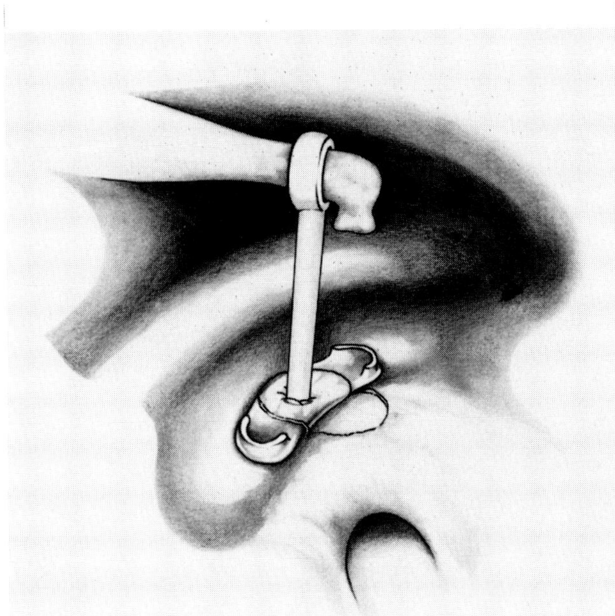

FIG 3–7.
Teflon piston prosthesis attached to incus.

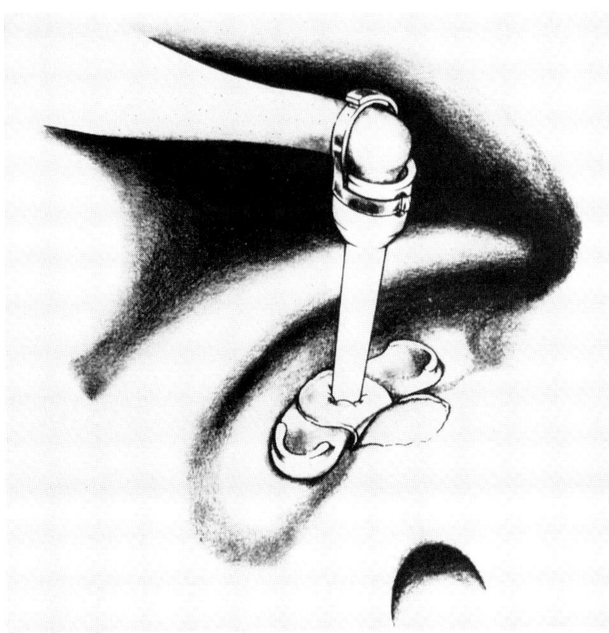

FIG 3–8.
Prosthesis is placed into the small opening in the thinnest portion of the footplate after it is covered with flap of lining membrane of the middle ear.

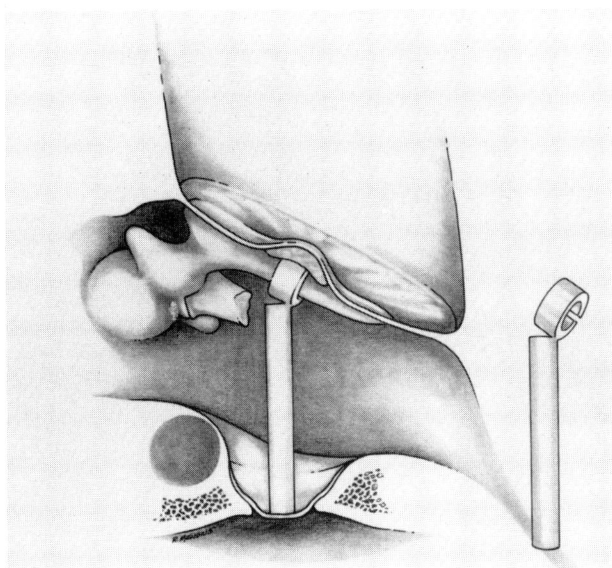

FIG 3–9.
Malleus attachment prosthesis in place.

INCUS REPLACEMENT

In ears with a poor connection of the incus to the stapes head, which is a large and difficult group to treat successfully, a simple "incus necrosis" prosthesis (Richards Medical) has been developed. This prosthesis is a hollow tube of high-density polyethylene sponge, with a slit in its underside to press down

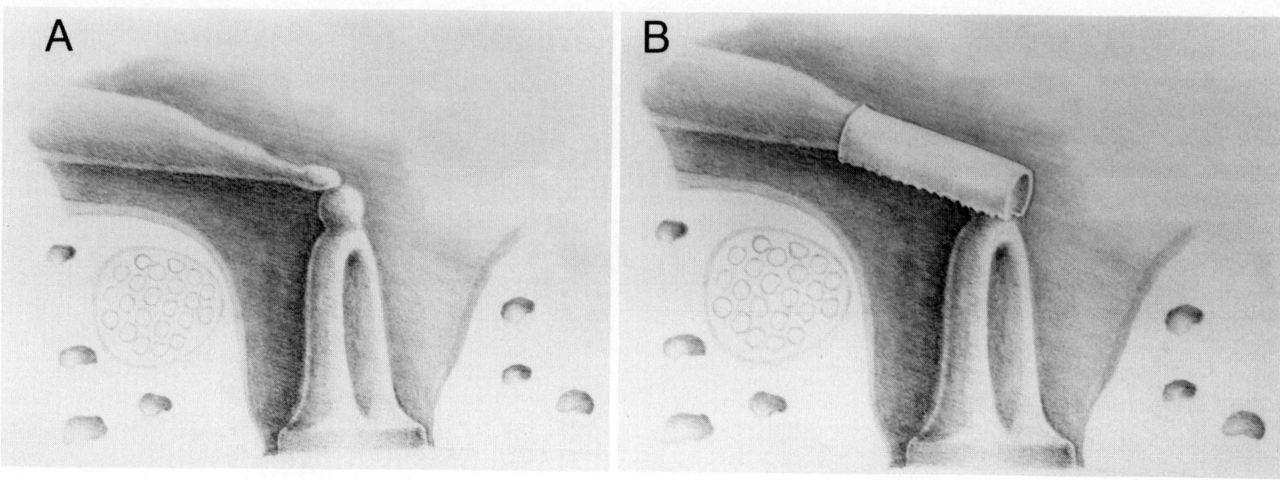

FIG 3–10.
Incus necrosis prosthesis. **A**, incus necrosis. **B**, prosthesis in place.

onto the lower incus and a hole in its lower end to fit down onto the head, neck, and arch of the stapes (Fig 3–10). Results with this prosthesis have been good, even in ears when the tip of the incus was gone, and I am confident they will continue to stand the test of time.

Many of these ears with incus necrosis have poor eustachian tube function, and the drum is often plastered down onto the lower incus and stapes head. In such ears, it is necessary to insert an underlay graft of perichondrium, fascia, or vein beneath the atrophic drum and insert a small ventilation tube in the anterior superior quadrant of the drum, away from the underlay graft during the healing process, and permanently if the eustachian tube function is not good. I prefer titanium tubes because they stay in longer and become blocked less.

If more of the lower end of the incus is missing and is far from contact with the stapes so that the incus necrosis prosthesis cannot be used, the best way to reconstruct the sound-conducting mechanism of the middle ear is to put a tack-shaped prosthesis made of high-density polyethylene (HDPE) sponge, known as a partial ossicular replacement prosthesis (PORP), with a hollow shaft down onto the head, neck, and arch of the stapes, with the flat head under the malleus handle or drum. A small piece of cartilage is interposed between the undersurface of the drum and the head of the PORP to prevent extrusion of the prosthesis if the drum collapses (Fig 3–11). If the eustachian tube function is not good, it is necessary to insert a small ventilation tube in the anterior superior quadrant of the drum to prevent collapse during the healing process. Results with this PORP prosthesis have been good, especially in those ears with adequate eustachian tube function.

In ears with absent arch of the stapes and incus, with mobile footplate and adequate eustachian tube function, the prosthesis of choice is another tack-shaped prosthesis, the total ossicular replacement prosthesis (TORP), also made of HDPE sponge. This prosthesis has a solid narrow shaft that fits onto the mobile footplate and a flat head that fits under the malleus handle or drum. Thin slices of Proplast (Vitek Corporation) are packed around the shaft of the TORP to hold it on the footplate. A small piece of cartilage is interposed between the head of the TORP and the undersurface of the drum to prevent extrusion if the drum collapses (Fig 3–12). If the eustachian tube function is not good, a small ventilation tube should be inserted in the anterosuperior quadrant of the drum to ventilate the middle ear during the healing process. Results with the TORP have been good, better than those with autograft or homograft ossicles and various solid prostheses, but not as good as with the PORP prosthesis.

MALLEUS REPLACEMENT

In ears with an absent or unusable malleus, the incus is never usable. If the stapes is in place and freely movable, a PORP can be inserted between the stapes head and arch and the undersurface of the drum. It is necessary to interpose a small piece of cartilage onto the head of the PORP beneath the drum to prevent extrusion. A small titanium ventilation tube is inserted in the anterosuperior quadrant of the drum if the eustachian tube function is not good. Results are good most of the time.

If the arch of the stapes is missing but the footplate is in place and freely movable, a TORP can be inserted with the flat head beneath the undersurface of the drum, with cartilage interposed, and the shaft on the center of the movable footplate, being held there by thin slices of Proplast. A small ventilation tube should be inserted in the anterosuperior quadrant of the drum if the eustachian tube function is not good to prevent collapse of the drum on the prosthesis.

Results with this type of reconstruction with the TORP have been good but not as good as those with the PORP onto the head and arch of the stapes because of the poor connection of the lower end of the TORP to the movable footplate.

SUMMARY AND CONCLUSION

The simple design of the prostheses described is the secret of their success, because they are easy to insert, are well tolerated by the body, and do reconstruct the sound-conducting mechanism of the middle ear. The success of the solid Teflon or metallic stapes replacement prostheses in stapedectomy is well established. Despite the initial opposition, most otologists worldwide have come to accept and use the porous plastic implant prostheses in preference to autograft and homograft ossicles and solid plastic or metallic prostheses. The one big drawback with these porous plastic implants was rejection, but with cartilage interposed between the head of the prosthesis and the undersurface of the drum and a ventilation tube inserted, this problem has been reduced to insignificance.[1]

There are several important principles in the use of these prostheses:

1. Proper length. The prosthesis must be cut to the proper length so that when cartilage is interposed it does not protrude beyond the normal position of the drum.

2. Free from attachment. The prosthesis must be away from the bone of the canal wall or promontory so that if it moves a little, which it will, it will not come in contact with the bone of the canal wall or promontory.

3. Supported during healing. The prosthesis must be held into the desired position by Gelfoam in the middle ear plus

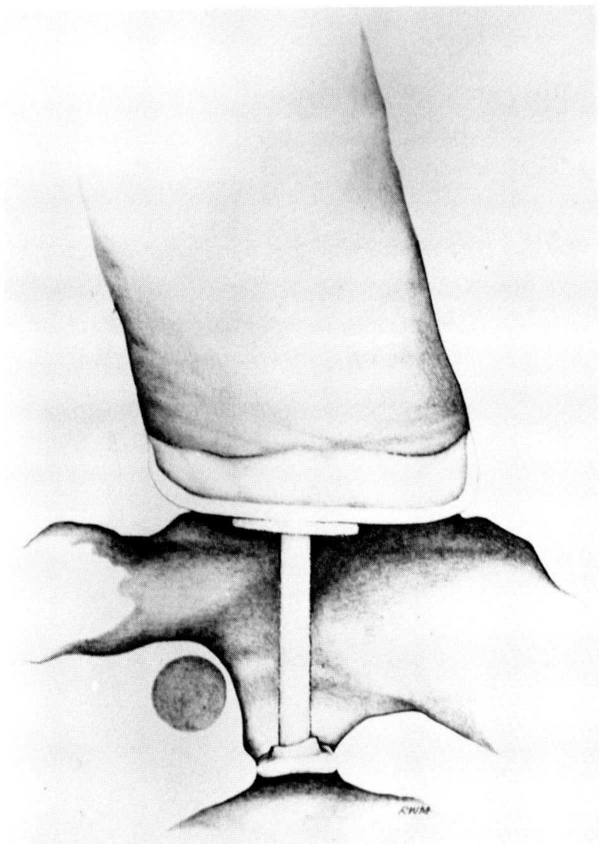

FIG 3–12.
Total ossicular replacement prosthesis in place.

Proplast around the shaft of a TORP as it rests on a mobile footplate, so that it does not move until it becomes encapsulated by tissue above and below.

4. Insertion of a small ventilation tube in the anterosuperior quadrant of the drum if the eustachian tube function is not good.

These porous plastic prostheses are easy to alter at operation in contrast to the solid plastic or metallic prosthesis. These prostheses are sterile and free of AIDS and other diseases in contrast to the homograft cartilage and bony implants about which there is always some doubt about the sterility.

Ossicular reconstruction either by stapedectomy with a Teflon or stainless steel cup piston prosthesis or by tympanoplasty using the various porous plastic prostheses has stood the test of time and now, after 30 years of use, can be said to be the solid foundation of modern otologic surgery.

REFERENCE

1. Emmett JR: Biocompatible implants in tympanoplasty. *Am J Otol* 1989; 10:215–219.

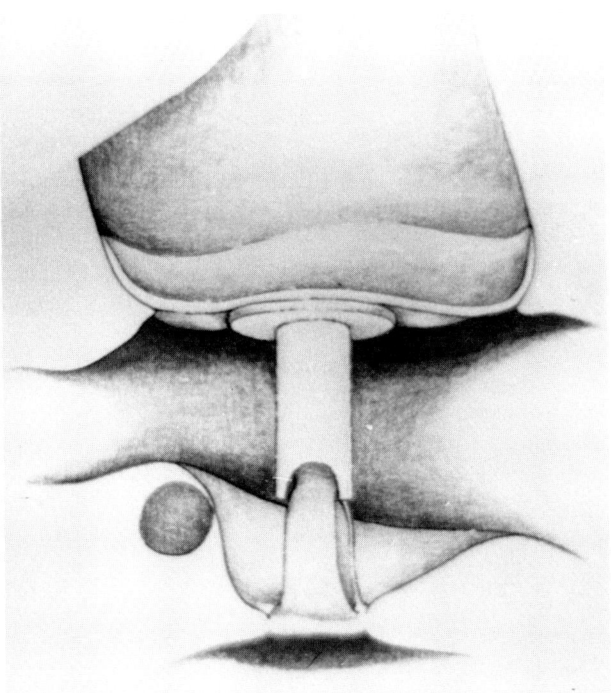

FIG 3–11.
Partial ossicular replacement prosthesis in place.

CHAPTER 4

Mastoidectomy

Approach of

Manning M. Goldsmith III, M.D.

FACIAL NERVE INJURY

Injury to the facial nerve is the most common serious complication of mastoidectomy. The incidence of this complication is approximately 1 in 1,000 cases as reported by ten experienced otologists at one facility.[1] Prevention of this complication is contingent on a thorough knowledge of the anatomy of the facial nerve as well as the principles of proper operative technique. The incidence of iatrogenic injury is highest when tissue planes and landmarks are distorted by previous surgery, trauma, tumor, or congenital anomalies. Therefore, even the most careful otologist must be prepared for iatrogenic facial nerve injury, and the patient and family must be fully informed regarding the risk and consequences of this complication.

An important philosophical point regarding intraoperative identification of the facial nerve in mastoid surgery should be underscored at this time. My policy is to always identify (not expose) the facial nerve for the following reasons: (1) it facilitates complete exenteration of all mastoid air cells, particularly those contiguous to the facial nerve and in the mastoid tip region; and (2) one never has to worry about the integrity of the nerve should postoperative paralysis occur. The experienced otologist will use the facial nerve as a landmark and useful guide for surgical dissection of the temporal bone. Fear and avoidance of the facial nerve, particularly in the settings of tissue plane and landmark distortion mentioned earlier, may lead to iatrogenic injury.

Several considerations are paramount to the prevention, evaluation, and management of facial nerve injury in mastoidectomy. Two commonly encountered settings occur and warrant separate discussion: (1) intraoperative recognition and (2) postoperative recognition of facial nerve injury.

Intraoperative Recognition

Normal and Abnormal Anatomy

The most common site of injury to the facial nerve in mastoid surgery is the second genu at the junction of the tympanic and mastoid segments. Knowledge of the normal anatomy of the facial nerve in the tympanic and mastoid segments is imperative for the avoidance of injury. In the attic, the nerve lies medial to the head of the malleus. It then courses superior to the oval window, where overlying bone is dehiscent approximately 50% of the time. Approaching the mastoid segment, it courses inferior to the horizontal semicircular canal and superior to the oval window. The second or external genu, which marks the beginning of the mastoid segment, is lateral and posterior to the pyramidal process. The facial nerve is usually found at a level just medial to the short process of the incus in a line between the short process of the incus and the anterior extent of the digastric ridge. The nerve courses from the medial point at the horizontal canal laterally toward the stylomastoid foramen at a 15-degree angle. The periosteal fibers of the digastric muscle blend with sheath of the facial nerve at the stylomastoid foramen, providing a landmark for its identification. Approximately 50% of the time, the vertical part of the facial nerve crosses the plane of the annular sulcus, and in another 50% it is medial to this plane in its descent to the stylomastoid foramen.[2] Because of the variability of the facial nerve in this area, it is best to identify the nerve at a more constant location, either inferiorly at the digastric ridge or at the second genu, and follow its course toward the annulus.

Numerous anatomic variations of the facial nerve are reported. They vary from total absence or poor development to abnormalities in the course of the nerve. The former anomalies are most commonly seen in the presence of other congenital anomalies, thalidomide toxicity, and the Möbius syndrome.[3] Almost every possible aberrant course of the vertical segment of the mastoid has been described,[4] but the most common in my experience is posterolateral displacement such that the nerve is encountered posterior to the lateral canal in the dissection, which is also where it is most frequently injured.

Mastoid anatomy may also predispose to facial nerve injury, particularly in individuals in whom there is a low middle fossa dural plate or a poorly pneumatized mastoid. If the antrum is not easily encountered and the dura of the middle cranial fossa is low, the surgeon may be tempted to drill medially in a perpendicular plane instead of finding the tegmen and then hugging the tegmen as the dissection is carried medially toward the attic. If the tegmen is pursued in the latter way and the surgeon continues the exposure superiorly and anteriorly, the antrum is encountered, and the attic is exposed, as is the incus, which is the first landmark for determining the depth of the facial nerve. The short process of the incus usually points to the pyramidal turn of the facial nerve just inferior to the horizontal canal. If the mastoid is poorly pneumatized and the incus is not well demonstrated early in the case, the depth of the facial nerve is very difficult to ascertain. Most commonly, facial nerve injuries that I have encountered have occurred where the surgeon has not found the antrum and has drilled medially well inferior to the antrum. Two complications can occur in this scenario. Most commonly, the horizontal canal is opened, and next most commonly, the facial nerve is injured. It is possible that injury would occur more often were not the endochondral bone of the labyrinth so distinct from mastoid bone. Where there is infection and especially if there is tympanosclerosis extending into the mastoid, this delineation can be difficult.

Operative Technique

A proper technique for identifying the facial nerve is to begin the dissection along the linea temporalis of the mastoid and identify the tegmen early. The dissection must be carried medially with dissection anteriorly into the antrum and posteriorly to the sinodural angle. A triangular dissection incorporating the sigmoid sinus posteriomedially and the digastric ridge inferiorly is then developed. My particular preference in doing a mastoidectomy is to find the tegmen first, the sigmoid sinus second, and the digastric ridge third. I then thin the posterior canal wall and follow the dissection into the antrum, finding the incus and exposing its head and the short process. Next, I dissect the digastric ridge and establish a line using the digastric ridge as the depth inferiorly and the incus superiorly so that the Körner septum and petrosal cells medial to it but lateral to the facial nerve are removed. In the process, there is usually a somewhat vascular area lateral to the facial nerve supplied by the stylomastoid artery commonly referred to as the *sentinel row of bleeders*. It is the first landmark in encountering the facial nerve and allows the surgeon to know when the nerve is near.

Once the short process of the incus is well exposed or the digastric ridge has been found, I generally employ a medium polishing burr with generous irrigation in pursuing the dissection. By thinning down the posterior external canal wall in doing

the mastoidectomy, the surgeon will generally find the chorda tympani nerve anterior and lateral to the facial nerve. It should not be routinely exposed and can generally be identified through a thin layer of bone.

In dissecting more posteriorly and medially, the surgeon will generally encounter the branches of the stylomastoid artery that supplied the mastoid in this area. These branches ultimately can be followed to the fallopian canal. It is important to grasp the drill firmly in doing this part of the dissection so that the drill does not jump or run, with the possibility of flukes catching and digging into thin ridges of bone overlying the facial nerve.

When the vessels overlying the nerve in the mastoid are encountered, it is advisable to switch to a large diamond burr. Smooth, slow strokes in the superior to inferior direction are generally recommended in drilling the mastoid adjacent to the nerve. The surgeon must allow the drill to progress more laterally as the strokes are continued inferiorly or the nerve may be encountered inferiorly in a more unexpected way than is desirable. When a diamond burr is used, copious irrigation is required to avoid thermal trauma from frictional heating of the nerve. Occasionally, granulation tissue will confuse the surgeon by obscuring the nerve. When encountering this situation, one should drill both proximal and distal to the area of granulation tissue, identifying the nerve, and working from known to unknown anatomy.

Injury

If the sheath is exposed but is not injured, no further dissection need be performed. If, however, the nerve sheath has been injured to any extent, the nerve sheath should be exposed 2 to 3 mm proximal and distal to the site of suspected injury. I do this by thinning the bone with a diamond burr to the point where the fine vessels of the sheath are easily visible. I then use a small endaural knife to lift the bony fragments off the nerve. One should not use the facial nerve or the fallopian canal itself as a fulcrum on which to rock the base of the endaural knife because doing so will only create a greater injury to the nerve than one is trying to prevent by doing the additional exposure. The theory behind exposing the facial nerve on two sides of a suspected nerve sheath injury is to prevent nerve ischemia resulting from swelling of the nerve within the fallopian canal in the postoperative period. If the nerve sheath has not been injured, there is no point in incising it, and this should be actively discouraged. If the surgeon encounters an abnormally positioned facial nerve or if it is exposed in the course of the dissection, it should be well documented in the operative report since many individuals undergo repeated mastoid surgery, and this is important information for the second surgeon.

If a partial transection of the nerve is observed, management depends on the degree of injury. Animal studies have shown that nerve loss of 80% is required before weakness is observed. This means that 80% of the random axons can be injured without loss of facial function. An 80% segmental section, however, is obviously a disaster. In my experience, if there is more than a 30% transection of the nerve, the nerve should be exposed well above and below the injury, and an attempt

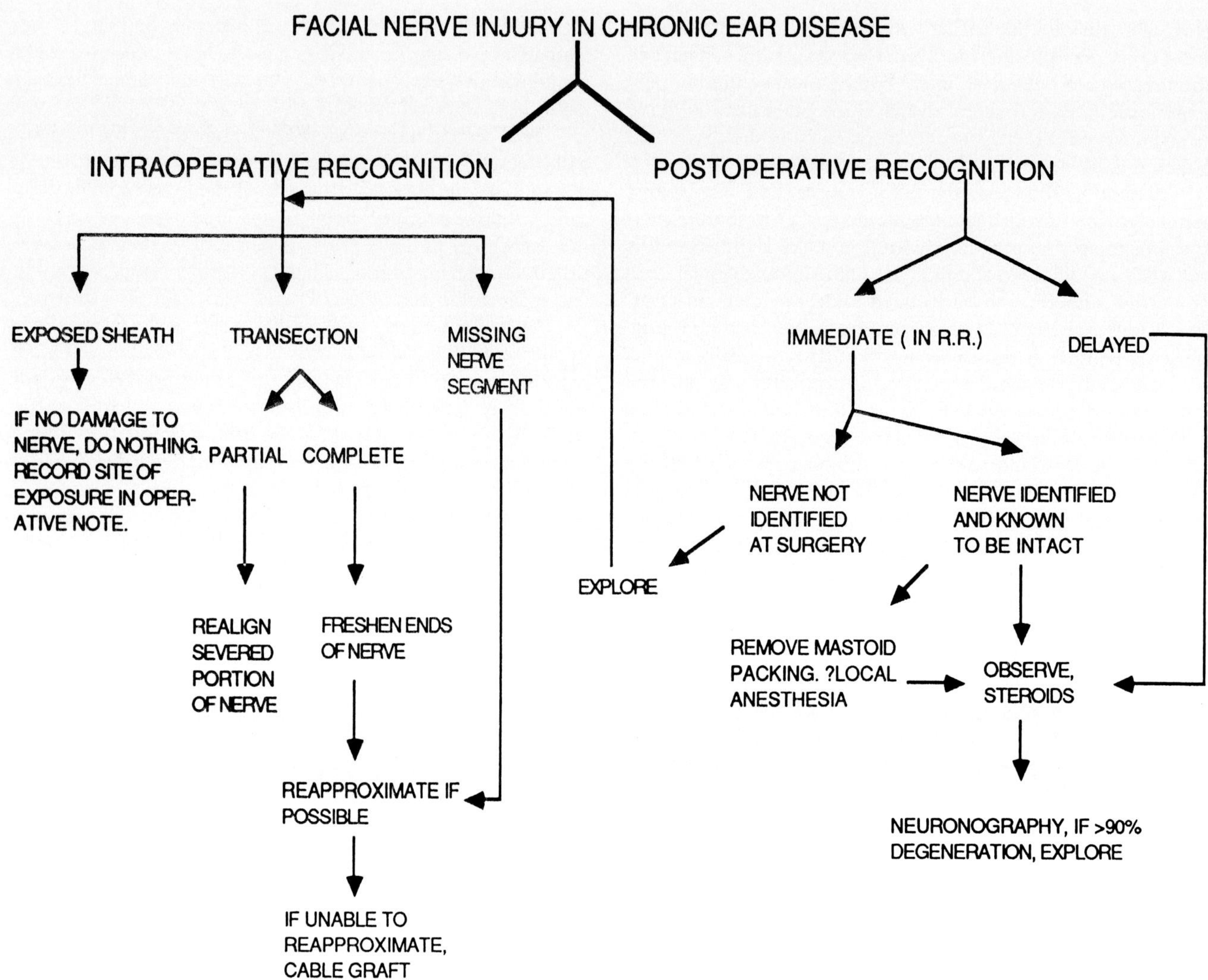

FIG 4–1.
Facial nerve injury in chronic ear disease.

should be made to reapproximate the severed ends (Fig 4–1). If mobilization of the nerve is insufficient for reapproximation without undue tension, I prefer to complete the transection and perform a cable graft. The greater auricular nerve is readily available within the surgical field and is most commonly harvested in this setting. The greater auricular nerve is noted as it extends from the posterior border of the sternomastoid to its anterior border, bisecting the midpoint of a line drawn from the mastoid tip to the angle of the mandible. I have found that by going more inferiorly, one tends to encounter fewer branches of the nerve. If the greater auricular nerve is unavailable, the sural nerve can be used as an alternative cable graft. The two ends to be approximated should be cleanly and sharply incised so that any fraying of the neurons will be minimized, which inhibits the formation of a neuroma at the anastomotic site. I recommend an epineural repair with placement of three or four 7.0 monofilament permanent sutures, depending on how the nerve comes together. If the nerve seems to come together

well with three well-placed sutures, I do not place a fourth one.

Postoperative Recognition

When facial nerve paralysis is noted postoperatively, several important considerations direct the treatment approach. The first and foremost consideration is whether or not the nerve was identified and noted to be intact at the time of surgery. The second important factor is whether the paralysis is of immediate or delayed onset. Facial nerve function should always be assessed as the patient is arising from anesthesia. I generally do this by observing flaring of the ala nasi following brief pinching of the nose or gentle manipulation of the endotracheal tube if it is still in place.

I have often noted facial nerve paralysis postoperatively after middle ear or mastoid surgery where local anesthetic has infiltrated into the middle ear dissecting beneath the middle ear mucosa and into a dehiscent facial nerve at the oval window niche. It generally resolves within 2 hours if lidocaine (Xylocaine) is the anesthetic and 4 hours if bupivocaine is used. The second cause of facial nerve paralysis in the recovery room not requiring reexploration is the presence of excessive packing in the mastoid. I prevent this by using absorbable gelatin sponge (Gelfoam) within the mastoid and only a light packing in the cavity when a canal wall down procedure is performed. I might add that I try to avoid exposing the facial nerve in the mastoid as much as possible under these circumstances. In doing a canal wall-up procedure, I commonly use a rigid tubular mastoid drain that is left in place for approximately 5 days to allow for prevention of a hematoma, which theoretically could cause facial nerve paresis but which, in fact, I have never seen.

If the paralysis does not recover within 4 to 6 hours after the above-mentioned etiologies have been ruled out, the management depends on whether the surgeon is convinced that the nerve was identified in the dissection and noted to be intact. If paralysis is immediate and the nerve was not identified in the operation, I recommend immediate exploration since the probability of iatrogenic damage is high, the medicolegal consequences of this complication are substantial, and early exploration obviates obscuration of the surgical field by granulation tissue, inflammation, and scar tissue.

Delayed postoperative paralysis may occur up to 14 days after surgery. If the paresis is incomplete, the prognosis for total recovery is excellent, and no treatment is necessary. If there is total paralysis, the nerve should be evaluated by evoked electromyography (EEMG) daily for 2 weeks. If the response to EEMG drops to less than 10% of normal, indicating severe degeneration, the nerve should be reexplored. Repair of injury is as described earlier. The prognosis for delayed paralysis is satisfactory for the majority of patients.

Recovery

After injury to and repair of the facial nerve, one should allow at least 4 to 8 months for any kind of recovery to occur. My knowledge about this is based on two episodes of facial nerve paralysis following Gelfoam embolization of the external carotid artery in which the stylomastoid artery was, in fact, thrombosed. In both of these instances, it took 4 months for the nerve to recover when, in fact, it was known to be intact. With this as a baseline, facial nerve recovery after grafting or anastomosis should be expected within 1 year of the repair. If recovery does not occur, the nerve should be reexplored. If any problem with the nerve anastomoses or the graft has occurred, a new graft should be placed. There are occasions when we as otolaryngologists and head and neck surgeons are confronted with the tragedy of a patient who has had a long-standing facial paralysis with no effort at diagnosis or repair. In these instances, I generally believe that once 2 years has elapsed, the chance of meaningful nerve anastomosis is very low. I generally use 2 years as my cutoff after the injury for enthusiastic perusal of nerve exploration and potential nerve grafting. There is literature to support the premise that 18 months is the outside limit of motor end-plate survival following loss of proximal innervation, but this should always be determined on an individual basis by EEMG.

VASCULAR INJURY

Major vascular injury is a rare complication of mastoidectomy. A thorough knowledge of temporal bone anatomy and meticulous surgical technique are the keys to avoiding this complication. Minor vascular injury is quite common and, if not controlled, can lead to further complications as a result of obscuration of the surgical field.

Dural Bleeders

Dural bleeders are most often a result of exposed dura while drilling in the vicinity of the tegmen tympani. There are a number of ways to control these bleeders. Bipolar cautery is a safe method of coagulating these vessels. Monopolar cautery is to be discouraged because resultant greater tissue damage may on occasion lead to cerebrospinal fluid (CSF) leakage postoperatively.

A very small dural dehiscence and vascular injury may be controlled with application of bone wax. In addition, tightly packed microfibrillar collagen (Avitene) balls may be applied to the area of bleeding, followed by the application of wet cottonoid balls. The cottonoid is pressed against the Avitene with a Frazier tip sucker and subsequently removed in 30 to 45 seconds, which leaves a deposit of Avitene over the dural dehiscence and injured vessel with quite effective coagulation.

Facial Nerve Epineural Bleeders

One often encounters a row of bleeders while exposing the facial nerve during mastoidectomy. It occurs as a result of damage to the epineurial vasa nervora from contact by the mastoid drill. One must not use heating techniques from reversing the polarity of the drill to stop these bleeders, because damage to the facial nerve will result. If bleeding is troublesome and obscures the surgical field, I use the previously mentioned Avitene and wet cottonoid technique to stop the bleeding. I discourage the use of bipolar cautery, but I am aware of otologists who use bipolar cautery at the lowest setting to control these bleeders.

Sigmoid Sinus Injury

Injury to the sigmoid sinus can be quite impressive. It usually occurs in a setting of a contracted mastoid cavity with an anteriorly located sigmoid sinus. Damage occurs as one tries to drill anteromedial to the sigmoid sinus in the constricted area between the facial nerve, posterior semicircular canal, and endolymphatic sac–posterior fossa dura. In this setting, one must create a bony island (Bill's island) and carefully deflect the sigmoid sinus posteriorly to obtain greater exposure in this area.

When drilling over the sigmoid sinus, one is forewarned of its presence by a change in the frequency of the sound made by the drill (a higher frequency sound is elicited from contact of a cutting burr against compact bone overlying this sigmoid sinus). In addition, the blue color from the vein is readily discernable as bone is thinned around the sinus.

Minor injury to the sigmoid sinus can usually be controlled by application of bone wax or the previously mentioned Avitene and cottonoid technique. Gelfoam should not be used to pack off the injured sinus, unless the jugular vein has been tied off in the neck, because it may readily embolize systemically. Pulmonary embolism has been documented by the Otologic Medical Group.[5] More significant injury to the sigmoid sinus is rare, but almost any degree of injury can be controlled by the Avitene-cottonoid application. It is conceivable that a fascial graft could be necessary to repair larger defects in the sigmoid sinus following control by the Avitene-cottonoid application. The temporalis fascia is most useful and could be harvested from within the surgical field. The fascial graft should be tucked within the bony margins surrounding the injury to the sigmoid sinus and stabilized by external Gelfoam packing.

Carotid Artery Injury

Carotid artery injury should be extremely rare, if not impossible, during routine mastoidectomy. It is a more significant potential problem during procedures that require exposure of the jugular bulb, as is the case for removal of glomus jugulare tumors. In the latter circumstance, the carotid artery is routinely exposed in the neck and controlled with vessel loops prior to exposing the "crotch" (between the jugular vein and carotid artery) via the mastoidectomy approach. Should carotid artery injury occur during removal of a glomus tumor, the immediate response is of course application of pressure to the injured vessel, followed by constriction of the proximal vessel by the vessel loop. The vessel should then be repaired, if possible, by a running 7-0 Prolene suture in a transverse fashion so as not to constrict the vessel diameter.

LABYRINTHINE FISTULA

It can be quite disheartening for the inexperienced otologic surgeon to see "snake eyes," indicating fenestration of a semicircular canal by the mastoid drill. If recognized early, it does not always mean that the patient will suffer profound hearing loss and severe postoperative vertigo. When it is recognized, one should stop drilling immediately and apply no suction to the area. A temporalis fascia graft should be rapidly harvested and applied to the area of fenestration with external stabilization by Gelfoam packing. It is the opinion of some otologists that the prognosis for long-term hearing is poor regardless of immediate postoperative results. It is also widely held that traumatic fenestration of semicircular canals in the setting of endolymphatic hydrops is nearly always followed by profound hearing loss.

One frequently worries about labyrinthine fistula when cholesteatoma matrix is found directly overlying the lateral semicircular canal. There are two approaches to this problem. In either approach, one should first open the cholesteatoma and suction the keratinaceous debris from within the cholesteatoma, initially leaving the matrix intact overlying the semicircular canal. One could then perform a modified radical mastoidectomy,

taking down the posterior canal wall, and exteriorizing the cholesteatoma into the mastoid cavity. It is quite important to have an adequate meatoplasty in this setting to facilitate hygiene and cleansing of the mastoid cavity. I take this latter approach when there is a small contracted mastoid cavity and when gentle palpation of the matrix overlying the semicircular canal reveals soft areas suggestive of bony dehiscence that might make an attempt at matrix elevation precarious. If one does not feel these soft areas, careful matrix elevation may be feasible, allowing one to remove the cholesteatoma and still maintain an intact posterior canal wall. This is an acceptable approach to cholesteatoma overlying the lateral semicircular canal for experienced otologists. Should a labyrinthine fistula become evident on elevation, the cholesteatoma matrix should be immediately replaced, and an additional temporalis fascia graft should be applied to this area and stabilized by Gelfoam. In addition, the posterior canal wall should be taken down, allowing exteriorization of the cholesteatomatous process.

OSSICULAR INJURY

Stapes Subluxation and Dislocation

Stapes subluxation can conceivably occur during elevation of the tympanomeatal flap for repair of a tympanic membrane perforation associated with chronic ear disease. It usually occurs when inexperienced otologists make a less than delicate movement with the canal wall elevating instrument, making contact with the incudostapedial joint and subluxing the stapes from its oval window nitch. Mild subluxation should be treated with returning the stapes to its proper position within the oval window. Should perilymph leakage be visualized, fat may be harvested and placed within the oval window to seal the leakage. Stapes dislocation should be extremely rare. It should be treated with completion stapedectomy, followed by a perichondrial graft to the oval window nitch and an appropriate stapes prosthesis. I prefer the Robinson-Well prosthesis in this setting.

CEREBROSPINAL FLUID OTORRHEA

Cerebrospinal fluid otorrhea implies damage to the dura, which can be avoided by adhering to the operative concepts of mastoid drilling technique discussed earlier in this chapter. When one approaches the dura, a higher frequency will be noted as the mastoid drill contacts more compact bone overlying dura. In addition, there is frequently more bleeding in the vicinity of the dura. Should the drill, nevertheless, gouge into the dura with a resultant significant injury allowing CSF leakage, repair of the injured dura should be undertaken. Generally, lacerations can be repaired with 6-0 Prolene sutures in a watertight fashion. Avulsion defects in the dura require fascial repair. Most commonly, temporalis fascia is employed because it is readily accessible within the operative field. Quite large bony dehiscences of the tegmen with resultant dural injury require not only fascial repair but support from an additional cartilage graft, which is usually harvested from the conchal area of the pinna.

Delayed recognition of CSF otorrhea is unlikely unless it occurs from dural damage from monopolar cautery of an extensive area. Once it is recognized, I would perform immediate exploration of the area. Contrary to management of CSF otorrhea in temporal bone trauma, delayed and profuse CSF otorrhea in this setting indicates a significant dural defect that usually will not heal with conservative therapy. The technique of repair should follow the principles outlined earlier for the CSF leak that is recognized intraoperatively.

BRAIN HERNIA

Herniation of the temporal lobe into the mastoid cavity is most frequently seen when there is a bony dehiscence of the tegmen tympani created by either iatrogenic drill trauma or the presence of a cholesteatoma. Small herniations with viable brain tissue can be elevated from below using a mastoidectomy approach. The bony defect can be repaired with a composite temporalis fascia and conchal cartilage graft, which is tucked beneath the bony margins of the hernia circumferentially. More significant herniations with nonviable brain tissue require amputation of the brain herniation with subsequent repair of the dura and bony defect. More commonly these require a middle cranial fossa approach via a temporal bone flap. The bony defect can then be successfully repaired with a pericranial fascial graft.

INCUDAL DRILL TRAUMA

Incudal drill trauma usually occurs while rounding the corner after having entered the mastoid antrum during mastoidectomy. It is particularly common in the setting of a contracted mastoid cavity with a low-lying middle cranial fossa dural plate. One approaches this situation by staying high and anterior along the tegmen tympani and carefully thinning the posterior canal wall as one approaches the fossa incudis. When the midpoint of the lateral semicircular canal is sited, one can apply clear water to the area, and the differential refractive index allows visualization of the short process of the incus through the operating microscope. In addition, a right-angle pick can be used to gently palpate the mobile ossicle. Overlying bone is then thinned and curretted, exposing the incus. If drill trauma should occur, it is readily recognized intraoperatively by flattening of the contour of the ossicle. Postoperatively, minor drill trauma usually results in profound high-frequency sensorineural hearing loss beginning at 4,000 Hz. Frequently it is not readily noticed by the patient because the high-frequency hearing loss is out of the speech frequency range and because it is

well compensated for by a normal hearing contralateral ear.

In settings where there is a contracted mastoid cavity and I know that I will perform a modified radical mastoidectomy, I separate the incudostapedial joint prior to drilling in the vicinity of the incus to prevent the transfer of energy from the mastoid drill through the ossicular chain to the membranous labyrinth. If a type 3 myringostapediopexy is not subsequently performed, the reapproximation of the incudostapedial joint and ossicular complex is performed with subsequent healing of the incudostapedial joint in most instances.

SCLEROTIC MASTOID WITH NO ANTRUM

The key to avoiding injury to all of the aforementioned structures in this setting is staying high and anterior during drilling. In this way one will avoid the lateral canal and second genu of the facial nerve inferomedially as one finally exposes the aerated epitympanum. This is the most common setting, nevertheless, for injury of the lateral semicircular canal to occur because there is no mastoid air cell architecture from which to differentiate the endochondral bone overlying the semicircular canals. One must proceed cautiously and slowly when performing these mastoidectomies. Injury to the lateral semicircular canal, facial nerve, dura, or ossicular complex in this setting should be managed as outlined earlier.

SUMMARY

Proper knowledge of temporal bone anatomy and precise and controlled operative technique is essential for avoiding complications of mastoidectomy. It is certainly one operation in which haste can make waste. The occasional otologist should be advised to undertake this operation only after practice in a properly equipped temporal bone laboratory.

REFERENCES

1. May M, Klein SR: Facial nerve decompression complications. *Laryngoscope* 1983; 93:299–305.
2. Litton WB, Krause CJ, Anson BA, et al: The relationship of the facial canal to the annular sulsus. *Laryngoscope* 1969; 79:1584–1664.
3. Sando I, English GM, Hemenway WG: Congenital anomalies of the facial nerve and stapes. A human temporal bone report. *Laryngoscope* 1968; 78:316–23.
4. May M: *The Facial Nerve.* New York, Thieme, 1986.
5. McElveen J: Personal communication, 1984.

Mastoidectomy

Approach of

Michael J. Holliday, M.D.

FACIAL NERVE INJURY

Intraoperative Recognition

Exposed Sheath

During the performance of mastoid surgery, it may be desirable to demonstrate the facial nerve in its vertical mastoid segment or its genu blending into the middle ear portion. Less frequently, complete removal of disease also requires uncovering the bone overlying nerve in the horizontal tympanic portion. During nerve exposure, the epineurium can be inadvertently abraded with the drill, cauterized with the electrocautery, or lacerated with sharp instruments. If blunt trauma to the perineurium and the endoneurial tubules results, the degree of this injury is frequently inapparent in the operating room. Prevention of harm to the facial nerve requires both the mental recognition of those conditions that can predispose to inadvertent trauma and the avoidance of these pitfalls. Knowledge of normal anatomy of the facial nerve and the use of guiding landmarks is imperative for anticipation of nerve exposure. If the surgeon is lacking recent experience in mastoid surgery, it is to his or her benefit to review otosurgical technique and anatomy in the temporal bone laboratory prior to the performance of surgery. When one is drilling during exposure of the facial nerve, continuous water irrigation with a suction irrigator is mandatory. Bone dust or bone paste obscures recognition of the nerve position until bleeding from epineural injury or the appearance of soft tissue shreds herald the insult that has occurred. Before epineural exposure, the nerve should be identified through a thin bony layer, appearing as a white cord running from the stylomastoid foramen on the anterior edge of the digastric ridge to the anteroinferior border of the lateral semicircular canal. Progressively smaller diamond burrs and ample suction irrigation should be used until final light brushing strokes create the eggshell thin bone that protects the nerve. Only if nerve manipulation is required in dealing with the particular disease state is this shell very carefully removed with the use of fine instruments. Any bleeding from the epineural vessels should be controlled before proceeding, or damage to the nerve can result. A fine-tipped microbipolar cautery, used very briefly with a low current setting and in combination with continuous saline irrigation, or alternatively, a hemostatic agent such as oxidized cellulose (Surgicel), Gelfoam, Avitene, or topical thrombin, is effective. In these latter instances, excess hemostatic material and clot may need to be irrigated away before proceeding.

Once trauma to the epineural sheath has occurred and bleeding is controlled, no further repair is necessary if no fascicular transection has occurred. However, if blunt trauma to the nerve is suspected, the patient should be considered a candidate for intraoperative intravenous steroids and ranitidine in an attempt to decrease nerve edema. The dosage should be generous, such as 4 to 10 mg of dexamethasone intravenously and continued postoperatively, with tapering over 3 to 7 days, depending on the clinical situation. Coexistent conditions such as diabetes mellitus, duodenal ulcer, and positive tuberculous skin test history must be simultaneously managed.

Partial Transection

When there has been a partial transection of the nerve, normally little in the way of repair is indicated. If the partial transection is sharp, transected axons are stabilized and endings opposed. If a portion of the axons is missing, as would occur if they were bitten away by cup forceps, the surgeon has several options. If the missing segment is less than 50% of the circumference of the nerve, nothing need be done because only 10% to 50% of intact fibers need to remain to have eventual satisfactory facial strength. If however, greater than 50% of the thickness of the nerve is interrupted, with a gap greater than 2 mm, repair would be in order. The options in this case include:

1. If the missing segment is 90% of the nerve thickness or greater, the transection is completed and the nerve endings coapted by either epineural or perineural suture repair. The approximation should be achievable without tension. If extra length should be necessary, it is best achieved by nerve mobilization whenever possible.

2. When the gap is 50% to 80% of the nerve diameter, an onlay free nerve graft may be placed to bridge the gap. It can be stabilized with suture or coaptation alone. This maneuver should avoid the kinking compression of the remaining intact axons that might occur with an end-to-end anastomosis, possibly

sparing the patient a total nerve degeneration with its attendant temporary, but significant, period of total facial paralysis and ultimate synkinetic facial function.

3. When very few axons remain, or when obvious blunt trauma to remaining axons has already occurred, suture approximation of the transected epineurium and fascicles may be performed. This, of course, can cause a kinking compression of remaining intact tubules and often requires some degree of nerve mobilization to have a tension-free anastomosis. One obvious advantage is that the epineurium is stabilized in a setting where nerve degeneration is already imminent.

Complete Transection

Once complete transection has occurred, sharply freshening ragged or oblique edges and approximation of the nerve endings is advisable. End-to-end anastomosis of the facial nerve is always preferable to interposition nerve grafting. Interfascicular repair, when it is feasible, may achieve superior results to epineural repair but is technically more challenging and may be impractical in many situations. It generally requires personal familiarity with the technique as well as negligible loss of nerve tissue in the intervening damaged segment. Because the nerve fascicles repeatedly separate and rejoin throughout its course through the temporal bone, the surgeon may find unequal fascicles at the two ends of the transected nerve if even a small segment is missing. One obviously loses the advantage of fascicular repair if dissimilar fascicles are wedded in reanastamosis. Proper orientation of the individual fascicles is dependent also on identical positioning of the ends of the individual fascicles in addition to assurance of reunification with its prospective partner unit if synkinetic regeneration is to be minimized.

Postoperative Recognition

Facial function should be checked as soon as possible postoperatively to be sure that inadvertent trauma has not occurred. The time-honored dictum that immediate paralysis requires exploration and that delayed or partial palsy demands only loose packing and watchful waiting does not always apply in modern surgery. Blunt trauma, pressure from tight mastoid packing, diffusion of injected local anesthetic, or, in rare instances, systemic medication (e.g., phenothiazines) all may be etiologic in the development of a facial palsy and would not be indicative of a need for exploration. Packing loosening, steroids, and head elevation all may be helpful in reversal of palsy progression. Watchful waiting is indicated if the surgeon can be reasonably certain that disruption of nerve continuity has not occurred and that no compressive force such as sutures, clips, bone fragments, or packing remains. Final visualization of the integrity of the nerve at the end of the operation using high-power magnification is the best assurance that surgical exploration and repair will be unnecessary should a facial nerve deficit become apparent in the recovery room. Marked inflammatory disease with granulations, polypoid disease, and bleeding obscures clear identification of the nerve. With modern microsurgical techniques, this situation is less frequent than in the past. Often the facial nerve is well identified in the mastoid and middle ear

segments, and the chief risk to the facial nerve is in its blind side labyrinthine segment during skeletonization of the anterior aspect of the superior semicircular canal. When a canal wall down mastoidectomy results in facial malfunction, usually the facial nerve has been well identified to safely lower the facial ridge, and the integrity of the facial nerve is not in question. If this is not the case, the mastoid and middle ear cavities may be directly examined microscopically under sterile conditions in the clinic and, therefore, resolve the question of reoperation. If a question of nerve separation or compression still exists, EMG may exhibit voluntary potentials, eliminating the possibility of a complete anatomic interruption. If these physiologically conducted action potentials cannot be demonstrated, and the surgeon believes that destructive insult to the nerve was not delivered, the patient can be serially followed with electroneuronography for evidence of degeneration beginning at 48 hours following surgery. This presumes that nerve transection, not nerve compression, is at question. If no nerve degeneration is demonstrated by electroneuronography in 7 days, it is highly probable that spontaneous recovery of nerve function will occur. If nerve degeneration is demonstrated, and any possibility of neural compression has been dismissed, I have found that the surgeon's initial impression of the possibility of transection is usually accurate in predicting the status of nerve integrity. If the surgeon identified what he or she believed was an intact nerve at the completion of surgery, even if epineural trauma occurred, the nerve will usually spontaneously recover. Watchful waiting in many cases will spare the patient an extra surgical procedure. The surgeon has to weigh the patient's and surgeon's own anxiety during the waiting period against the morbidity of the additional surgery while simultaneously attempting to predict the anticipated final functional cosmetic result. If the surgeon is very uncertain about nerve interruption, having never identified what he or she believed was nerve tissue, the probability of nerve interruption is magnified. Although much has been written about the ideal time for nerve exploration and anastomosis, it has been our experience that neurorrhaphy performed anytime within the first year following disruption has similar ultimate results. The grade of facial nerve spontaneous recovery following a nerve degeneration may be difficult to differentiate from the appearance of a surgically anastomosed nerve. There is little question that ultimate results deteriorate if repair is undertaken after 1 year, and the resultant function obtained from neurorrhaphy performed after 2 years is essentially always doomed to a poor result.

VASCULAR INJURY

Dural Bleeders

When the tegmental or posterior fossa bony plates are thinned, it is desirable to switch from a cutting to a diamond or polishing burr to avoid abrasion trauma to the dura. The inner cortex of bone in either of these areas is commonly uneven, producing dips of dura that otherwise may be exposed and lacerated, even though the bone immediately adjacent may still have considerable thickness. Usually small dural bleeders are easily controlled with a fine-point microbipolar cautery set at a moderate current level. If the current is set too high, one runs the risk of opening the dura. Once the dura has been opened, two primary dangers are possible: (1) the potential for bleeding into the subarachnoid space arises, (2) chronic expulsion of intracranial contents (i.e., CSF and brain) can occur.

Therefore the dural defect must be repaired, but only after being absolutely certain that all dural bleeding is permanently controlled. The details of management are discussed later. Suctioning on a cotton ball that has been placed next to the bleeding site and irrigating away any accumulated blood allow good visualization of the dural vessels, pinpointing any locations that must be coagulated. This technique can also be effective with medium-sized vessels coursing intradurally. Sometimes these vessels are troublesome, because they tend to retract within the dura. If the surgeon is planning on opening the dura eventually, as during the performance of a complete mastoidectomy, preparatory to translabyrinthine removal of a cerebellopontine angle tumor, it is best to control bleeding temporarily with coagulation or a hemostatic agent and later suture ligate the vessel after the dura has been opened and the vessel can be isolated. When dural opening is not planned, a retracted vessel can sometimes be controlled with hemostatic agents. Some examples of hemostatic agents that can be effectively used include Gelfoam, Avitene, thrombin, and Surgicel.

Sigmoid Sinus Injury

The lateral sinus is probably most frequently violated during the purposeful creation of Bill's island. The area of entry is often at the exiting mastoid emissary vein, which joins the upper third of the sinus posteriorly. Peeling tumor or cholesteatoma off of the vein after bone has been eroded by a disease process can end up with the same result. During extended mastoid surgery for removal of glomus jugulare tumor, the lateral sinus and jugular bulb are intentionally entered to accomplish removal of both the invading tumor and the lateral half of the vein. Packing the vein with Gelfoam or Avitene facilitates bloodless accomplishment of this task.

I have found that placing a tightly balled Avitene wad over a bleeding defect of the lateral sinus, jugular bulb, or emissary vein and maintaining its position by covering it with a larger wad of wet cotton, held steady by a suction for several minutes, and periodically flushing the cotton with saline solution from the irrigator until it is clear of blood will eventually achieve hemostasis. The compressed Avitene pad is allowed to remain in place, flushing away the excess amount later. At the end of the procedure, when surrounding visualization is no longer necessary, additional Avitene may be placed over the area as extra insurance.

Any of the techniques that occlude the vein, namely, ligation of the lateral sinus, packing of the sinus with hemostatic agents, or compression collapse of the sinus, as with the use of bone wax, should be used with caution unless the patient has been studied preoperatively regarding venous drainage from the opposite side. Although unusual, an occasional patient has a rudimentary, stringlike venous drainage, or even none at all, serving the opposite side. Stopping venous outflow can result in marked facial and cerebral edema in the postoperative period with catastrophic results.

Whenever the sinus is ligated or occluded, the blockage is ideally below the level of the mastoid emissary vein, so that at least this collateral route may be able to provide some venous drainage.

Carotid Artery Injury

In most cases of injury to the internal carotid artery in its petrous segment, arterial exposure is intentional, because disease is extending directly onto the artery or into bony pericarotid air cells. Therefore, some anticipation of potential hemorrhage exists prior to arterial encounter, and advance preparation for immediate management of hemorrhage is possible. As with the sigmoid sinus, a set of various sized Avitene balls are prepared and readied on a tray, available for immediate application. A pair of bayonet forceps lies beside them. Adjacent to this setup are soppy wet cotton wads varying from several millimeters to several inches in greatest dimension. If arterial bleeding occurs, a large-bore suction (e.g., no. 8 Frasier tip) is placed next to the bleeding to identify the arterial laceration. The bleeding site is immediately covered by an appropriately sized, tightly packed, Avitene ball, held in place with suction until the larger wet cotton wad is placed over the ball. The suction is then immediately transferred to the cotton. If bleeding is not controlled, the cotton is wetted and removed and a larger ball placed, repeating the later steps of the process. Only if the bleeding is so voluminous that this technique is ineffective is the artery temporarily compressed by finger or tamponade packing. Then a large wet cotton ball with a generous Avitene ball applied to its front surface can be immediately applied and compressed on removal of the tamponade. In this circumstance, additional Avitene is applied shortly after and wetted down well to relieve any compressive effect that could completely occlude the artery. When an arterial laceration occurs in a radical mastoid cavity, the artery should be covered also by a fascial graft, dermal graft, or a temporalis muscle flap if at all possible. It may have to be placed in an overlapping fashion, covering both the artery and the Avitene.

LABYRINTHINE FISTULA

Traumatic Fenestration of Semicircular Canals

The opening of a semicircular canal can result in an immediate partial or complete sensorineural hearing loss. We also know from fenestration surgery literature that if membranous labyrinth exposure is very carefully performed, little or no long-term hearing loss may result. Since in most cases today we are not intentionally skeletonizing the lateral semicircular canal membranous labyrinth, this area, when opened, is most often accidentally traumatically performed with drilling. In the cases of which I am aware, the patient initially retained some hearing in the damaged ear for a while but eventually serially progressed to a profound hearing loss or total anacusis. The surgeon has little to lose by repairing the fistula with autologous tissue coverage (e.g., fascial graft muscle flap, areolar tissue). The surgeon may, in fact, stabilize the inner ear damage if it has been minimal or if there is none. More important, the inner ear structures are protected from potential contamination. The benefits of protecting against a purulent labyrinthitis with its secondary bacterial meningitis and labyrinthitis ossificans as well as diminishing the ongoing problems of vertigo and fluctuant hearing that exists with a persistent perilymphatic fistula are obvious. Avoidance of labyrinthine entry is preferable to repair. After entering the antral air cell, the surgeon should refrain from drilling on the floor of the antrum unless the lateral semicircular canal has been clearly identified or unless an experienced surgeon is blue-lining the canal for definitive identification.

Cholesteatoma Overlying Semicircular Canals

When cholesteatoma overlies the semicircular canals, it is best to begin dissection of the cholesteatoma and its matrix from the periphery, advancing toward the centralized semicircular canals. Because bulky-sized cholesteatomas are more likely to have accompanying bony labyrinth erosion, with the lateral semicircular canal at greatest risk, a gentle debulking of the major portion of the cholesteatoma while leaving the medial matrix in situ allows visualization of the interface between the cholesteatoma and the semicircular canals prior to matrix removal. Some authors believe that if the bony lateral canal has been eroded, it is best to leave the cholesteatoma matrix in place and to create a radical cavity, lest the inner ear inadvertently be opened. It is one acceptable solution. However, when an intact canal wall procedure has been planned, and if the surgeon is comfortable with the task, the remaining matrix may be successfully dissected off of bone or even the membranous labyrinth by using high-power magnification in a bloodless field. The removal requires very careful dissection with small sharp instruments such as needle picks, microknives, and microdissectors. All matrix must be removed if the canal is to be covered with tissue. When the matrix has been completely removed, the exposed membrane should be covered with a small fascial graft in the case of a radical cavity. There is no need for coverage in a simple mastoid cavity, but a second look mastoidotomy is required between 6 and 12 months later.

Stapes Subluxation and Dislocation

When inadvertent subluxation of the stapes footplate occurs during mastoidectomy, it is best to gently replace the stapes into its original position so that the annular ligament is reunited. Small strips of autologous tissue are then placed to overlie the ligament defect. Gelfoam may be carefully placed over the area to help hold the grafts in place. If the stapes has been totally dislocated, the oval window should be covered with a tissue graft of fascia, fat, vein, or perichondrium. The stapes may be replaced on top of the graft. Alternatively, ossicular reconstruction can be delayed until a second-stage operation. The staged procedure is somewhat safer, because there is less chance of the graft being moved or subluxed into the vestibule by the weight of the stapes. If audiometric follow-up shows poor cochlear reserve, the second-stage reconstruction is unnecessary.

Sometimes, when the middle ear of a patient who has had chronic inflammatory disease or who has had prior surgery is examined, the stapes will be found to be partially subluxed into the vestibule. This most commonly would be medially displaced in the region of the anterior footplate but also occurs in the inferior oval window region. Medial displacement is often associated with trauma to the ossicular chain. It appears that inward pull of a chronically retracted drum and attached ossicles is responsible for the second condition. It is best to accept this abnormal partial subluxation if no perilymph fistula is present. Manipulation to a normal position can cause tearing of adherent neuroreceptors of the saccule or utricle. Sensorineural hearing loss or chronic vertigo may result.

CEREBROSPINAL FLUID OTORRHEA

Intraoperative Recognition

During the performance of a mastoidectomy, a CSF leak would not normally be anticipated. Should a leak occur, it would most often be located in the tegmental dura either adjacent to the mastoid antrum or in the region of the epitympanum. The next most frequent location for a leak to be encountered is the posterior fossa dura, anterior to the lateral sinus and posterior and inferior to the posterior semicircular canal. The dura in this area is usually not exposed unless extensive disease is present. Most commonly, dural misadventure occurs while one is using a cutting burr, with poor direct visualization of the burr and bone contact point. This may result in failure of recognition that dura is dipping down into bony valleys created by concavities of the inner cortex. Saucerization of the outer bony cortex and progressive medialward observation of the bone being skeletonized while the microscope or the patient's head is moved as necessary to allow a right-angle view of the drilling may prevent inadvertent dural trauma. As the bone is about to be leveled, it is safest to switch from a cutting to a diamond burr. To efficiently work on the posterior fossa bone plate between the facial nerve and lateral sinus, the surgeon must create Bill's island and depress the lateral sinus medially to allow full visualization while drilling. It is especially helpful when one is dealing with a small, constricted mastoid with a very anterior sinus. Once a leak is discovered, its source should be identified. If the dural defect is small, it may be repaired primarily with a fine suture. The operating microscope should be used during the repair, lessening risks of intracranial or dural vessel impalement. The dural repair is covered with a soft tissue graft, preferably fascia, tucked beneath the edges of the bony defect, whenever possible. The free graft can be incorporated into the dural repair sutures, ensuring its fixed centering over the repair. Layered Gelfoam supports the fascial graft. With an intact canal wall mastoidectomy, the anterior antrum and the epitympanum may be sealed off from the rest of the mastoid system by covering the entrance to the epitympanum with temporalis muscle fascia and then packing the entire mastoid with free abdominal fat. If however, significant mucosal remnants remain, the patient can develop pockets of cholesterol granuloma or retention cysts that might become symptomatic of postauricular pain and can be destructive of bone and neural structures over time. A drain assists epitympanic graft healing, effectively halting mastoid CSF drainage from flowing around the graft, which otherwise is its natural egress toward the nasopharynx. A postincisional drain of sterile intravenous tubing attached to a butterfly needle and draining into a standard Vacutainer allows ambulation and regulated lowering of CSF pressures. An alternative repair of a medium-sized or larger meningeal defect is the use of a local pedicled flap such as a temporalis muscle flap or postauricular flap composed of muscle with its attached fascia and periosteum. The former flap is bulky, has tendencies to retract readily, and can be difficult to stabilize in position. Tight packing presents the risk of flap strangulation and aditus blockage.

A CSF leak during radical mastoidectomy may require double-layer blind sack closure of the external auditory canal, along with eustachian tube obliteration, and mastoid fat packing. Repair from above or behind by neurosurgical craniotomy is an alternative if the leak persists despite initial attempts at correction of the problem.

Postoperative Recognition

It is imperative whenever a CSF leak is suspected postoperatively that its presence or absence is confirmed. Establishing the diagnosis can be as simple as sitting the patient at the bedside and asking the patient to lean forward for several minutes, with periodic coughing. A unilateral watery rhinorrhea, seen as gross dripping from the nose, is unlikely to be from another cause. It is more accurate in establishing a presumptive diagnosis than testing nasal mucus for glucose and protein content. Both of these latter tests commonly lead to false conclusions. Absence of rhinorrhea does not, of course, rule out the diagnosis.

Following the performance of intact canal wall mastoid surgery, microscopic examination of the tympanic membrane may reveal a clear pulsatile fluid. Tympanic membrane inspection while the patient coughs may reveal drum bulging, which is more prominent with the person assuming the supine position. Because of middle ear swelling and persistent clot, this examination, unfortunately, is not very helpful for the first 10 postoperative days.

Following radical mastoidectomy, the diagnosis is strongly suspected if persistent watery soaking of the mastoid dressing occurs. The diagnosis may be established through computed tomography (CT) scanning following intrathecal injection of metrizamide, but a small or intermittent leak may be missed with this technique. Radionucleotide scanning with intrathecally injected indium or radioactive iodinated serum albumin is quite accurate, but even with this investigation, false results are possible. It is important to place pledgets at another anatomic area where moist mucosal membranes exist, so that a background comparison count can be established. Intrathecal dyes aid in visual development of a diagnosis of leak but generally are not much advantage over the observation of gross clear fluid and do have some inherent risks. Fluorescein can cause seizures, especially if in a concentrated solution, and can introduce infection when not absolutely sterile. Indigo carmine red dye and methylene blue are less toxic but may be sufficiently dilute that their diagnostic colors may be inapparent.

Once the diagnosis of CSF leak is established, a definitive plan for handling the problem must be carried out. The patient is ordered to refrain from nose blowing. Autoinflation of the ears with the Valsalva maneuver can produce pneumocephalus and subsequent seizures, as well as forcefully introduce bacteria, with resultant meningitis. Antibiotic prophylaxis during active CSF otorhinorrhea continues to be controversial. A multitude of broad-spectrum antibacterial drugs are available today, and their potential protective benefits far outweigh the small risks of development of drug-resistant bacterial strains and of drug allergy. The exception might be the rare patient with allergies to most known antibacterial medications. In such a case, choosing to hold the drug in reserve is reasonable. A modified form of protective isolation must then be instituted.

A decision between watchful waiting or more aggressive treatment measures is based on the amount and frequency of drainage and on a reasonable prediction of the natural course of the leak, gained from intraoperative knowledge of the meningeal defect and the details of its primary operative repair. Ultimately the patient is informed of the indications for each possible treatment alternative for the problem. The advantages and disadvantages of each respective treatment, with its attendant risks, as well as all reasonable alternatives, are stated, and the patient is then invited to participate in the decision making of the final choice of management, after recommendations are made. Since no method of dealing with CSF leaks is foolproof, the patient must fully understand that a repeat of the procedure or an alternate treatment method may become necessary.

When the drainage is fairly profuse, repeat lumbar punctures performed two to three times daily, withdrawing 30 to 50 mL of CSF with each tap will slow down the drainage sufficiently that it may cease. An alternative choice would be to place an indwelling lumbar drain that has been attached to a sterile water seal bottle or to a dependent sterile collection container. Either of these techniques runs the risk of diminishing CSF pressures sufficiently that a negative pressure can result, especially when the patient is in the upright position. The net danger is the potential for inward vacuuming of upper respiratory tract secretions, which can result in meningitis. There is also an increased hazard of tearing bridging arachnoidal veins with resultant subdural bleeding once the supportive effect of the protective fluid is absent. If significant drainage is ongoing, with resultant low pressure, the patient should be lying in a horizontal position or with the head elevated no more than 10 to 15 degrees. This diminishes both the aforementioned risks and headaches. If, on the other hand, there is minimal leakage even though no indwelling drain has been placed and no reason exists to suspect low pressures in the CSF circulation, it is reasonable to maintain head elevation of 30 to 45 degrees, which will lower CSF pressures and encourage spontaneous healing of the fistula. Ambulation is allowed, but bending, straining, and heavy lifting are prohibited until the leak is stopped. Regular nursing neurochecks for evidence of evolving meningitis should be performed, with emphasis on level of consciousness, mental status, and increasing headache.

When these nonoperative measures fail, surgical intervention is necessary. If approached extracranially, blind sack closure of the external auditory canal, along with cavity obliteration, allows sterility. With a simple mastoidectomy, other options are possible (see the discussion of intraoperative recognition). In certain cases, intracranial repair from above or behind, performed by our neurosurgical colleagues, may be more prudent.

BRAIN HERNIA

Brain herniation in mastoid surgery is more often a result of radical mastoid cavity surgery than arising from intact canal wall procedures. Exposure of large areas of dura during intact canal wall surgery does not appear to be a long-term problem in most cases as long as rents have not been made in the dural surface. Chronic exposure of dura in the presence of continuous infection, as in the wet radical mastoid cavity, appears to weaken the dural lining. The weight and persistent pulsations of the brain seem to have a compromising effect on fine dural vessels, adding to the eventual thinning of the meninges. The herniation may be sufficiently large to fill the entire cavity and, on occasion, to protrude through the meatus. The meninges may be intact, adherent, and tightly thinned over the dehiscent brain or may have ruptured with resultant CSF otorrhea. The bony defect can be slowly enlarged by the developing meningoencephalocele. When the bony opening is small, the pouching meningoencephalocele can be dumbbell shaped, with a portion of the brain being strangulated and ischemic or necrotic. This damaged cerebral cortex can be an epileptogenic focus. Amputation of abnormal ischemic or infarcted brain, followed by postoperative antiseizure medication, may therefore be in order.

Repair of the skull defect should be multilayered, simulating the original layers of tissue. Involved dura should be reinforced with free tissue graft or pericranial flap. The skull defect can be replaced with a bone graft of temporal squama or cartilage. Care must be taken not to bury any squamous epithelium from cholesteatoma matrix or radical mastoidectomy bowl lining. Long-term annual magnetic resonance imaging (MRI) scans are ordered to safeguard against recurrent silent cholesteatoma or encephalocele.

INCUDAL DRILL TRAUMA

Drilling on an intact ossicular chain can transmit vibratory trauma to the inner ear, resulting in sensorineural hearing loss, or worse, can create an avulsion injury of ossicles with resultant anacusis. Avoidance of such cochlear trauma should be emphasized in technique. Careful curetting or drilling of the bone of the anterior antrum and aditus, attaining early identification of the incudal short process, helps avoid ossicular trauma. During drilling in the aditus area, if clear saline is allowed periodically to pool in the antrum, the bending of light created by the air-water interphase permits the operator to visualize the incudal short process while it still remains protected under the scutum. Disarticulation of the incudostapedial joint before drilling in the mesotympanum decreases risk of direct high-energy trauma transmission along the ossicular chain into the inner ear. Maintaining the superior bridge of bone, lying posterior to the incudal fossa, during the performance of a facial recess approach assists incus shielding. Once direct drilling on the

ossicular chain has occurred, audiometric follow-up and avoidance of further trauma are usually all that is possible. If significant disruption to the ossicles has been inflicted, ossicular reconstruction and oval window tissue coverage are often necessary.

POSTERIOR CANAL WALL FENESTRATION

The creation of defects of the posterior canal wall is easier to avoid than to repair. Defects of the posterior or superior bony wall take place while thinning bone from the mastoid side in intact canal wall mastoidectomy or from inside the canal during canalplasty. Failure to repair this bony defect eventually results in a canal skin retraction pocket and a canal cholesteatoma that extends into the mastoid. If the defect is repaired primarily, it can be handled satisfactorily by bone or cartilage graft placement over the defect between the canal wall and the canal skin. If it can be wedged into position in a dovetail fashion, it is more secure and less apt to migrate during healing. An intermediate fascial layer helps prevent canal skin breakdown.

Anterior canal defects, on the other hand, may be more difficult to deal with. The capsule of the temporomandibular joint is immediately anterior to the midportion of the anterior canal wall. Creation of a bony dehiscence in the area usually results in a herniation of the soft tissues of the joint, which is aggravated by the constant pressure exerted by the strong sliding movements of the mandibular condyle. The bulging tissue can obstruct the view of the anterior tympanic membrane or, if marked, may fuse with the drum, causing blunting of its anterior angle, dampening drum mobility, and creating a conductive hearing loss. In the extreme, the entire external canal can be stenotic or obstructed. Although small defects may be repaired from the canal side with bone or cartilage free grafts wedged into the bone defect, larger openings require a preauricular repair with a more generous exposure of the joint space.

SCLEROTIC MASTOID WITH NO ANTRUM

The poorly developed air cell system can be difficult to deal with if the surgeon is to perform an intact canal wall mastoidectomy. The lack of an identifying antral air cell, the usual first distinct landmark, means that the semicircular canals must be definitively identified by a blue-lining technique. The denser endosteal bone of the otic capsule appears slightly more cream colored, but it is not a reliable sign.

This frustrating experience can be avoided through preoperative radiographic evaluation, preferably with CT scanning, using bone window settings, which allows the luxury of identifying important structures such as the facial nerve, ossicles, vestibule, and epitympanum from the middle ear side first. With poor pneumatization of the temporal bone and limited disease extension, the surgeon is justified in proceeding directly to a modified radical or radical mastoidectomy technique. This is true with chronic inflammatory processes and cholesteatoma. If the surgeon is dealing with tumor in the hypotympanum, jugular fossa, and petrous apex areas, canal wall preservation is most likely inhibitory to disease eradication anyway. The fortunate aspect of performing a canal wall down or a Bondy type of modified radical mastoidectomy in the face of a sclerotic mastoid is the small resultant cavity, not much bigger than the normal canal, as the usual end result. With moderate or generous pneumatization, the surgeon must reconsider the ramifications of long-term care of the large cavity created. Canal wall up surgery, under these conditions, is undertaken with much less attendant risk than in the severely sclerotic temporal bone.

CONGENITAL ATRESIA

No Tympanic Ring

When no tympanic ring is present and the canal has a medial bony atresia plate, the main problem in most cases is the resultant conductive hearing loss present. Since most cases are unilateral, surgery is elective. The child can have preferential seating in school and will function quite normally in the educational process. In the much less common bilateral situation, hearing aid amplification is an option that is feasible, particularly if the cartilaginous external canal is well formed. Surgery is dictated by the presence of cholesteatoma. It is quite often located in a position lateral to the bony atresia plate. Surgery in this instance may be approached from an anterior or a posterior position but should be initiated superiorly, identifying tegmental plate, zygomatic root, ossicular structures, and then facial nerve. Preoperative reconstructed CT scans will inform the surgeon of the course of the facial nerve, which is often more superior and posterior than would be anticipated. The surgeon who is about to operate on a congenitally malformed ear would do well to review the classic articles of other surgeons' experiences. The writings of Dr. Robert Jahrsdoerfer, who in recent years has obtained superior results in this special field of ear surgery, is especially recommended.

Poor or Absent Pneumatization

The less sculpting of the temporal bone that nature provides with the pneumatization process, the more work that is required of the surgeon if the surgeon is to carve out critical structures without injury to them. This also presents greater risks to the patient that has congenital ear malformations. Therefore, the surgeon should perform the amount of bony dissection necessary to reverse the progressing disease process but not continue with drilling if it adds nothing to the patient's safety or to the ultimate functional result.

Facial Nerve Overlying the Oval Window

An overlying facial nerve is not a major problem if the stapes superstructure is intact and the footplate remains mobile. When ossicular reconstruction using a total ossicular replacement prosthesis or a malleus-stapes footplate assembly is required, or when stapedotomy or stapedectomy is indicated, the risk of injury to the overhanging facial nerve comes into play. We know that the horizontal segment of the nerve within the mesotympanum has bony dehiscenses in 60% of temporal bones.

A rigid or sharp object, such as a prothesis, resting on the exposed overlying nerve can cause a facial nerve compression and clinical palsy. The degree of coverage of the footplate by the nerve can be variable. In the more severe anomaly, where the nerve hides the stapes footplate, the surgeon would be prudent to reconnoiter and consider hearing aid amplification as a viable alternative. Aggressive approaches to such a situation can be the classical fenestration operation or a careful exposure of the membranous mucoperiosteum of the basal turn of the cochlea just below the oval window. The problems with either of these techniques are the risk of traumatic membranous entry and the significant incidence of eventual bony reclosure.

When cholesteatoma encases the nerve, conversion to a radical cavity or at least total removal of the tympanic membrane is required if the cholesteatoma matrix cannot be totally removed safely. If the matrix is believed to be totally eradicated, a second look operation is necessary when an intact drum has been maintained.

Sequence of Pinna Versus External Auditory Canal Reconstruction

If pinna reconstruction is to be coordinated with canal reconstruction, a joint decision must be made between the otologic and reconstructive surgeon involved as to what is the most reasonable sequence. The ability to use adjacent skin for canal relining in the case of mild deformity would speak for the otologic surgeon initiating the order. In the more severe deformity, the need for as much available contiguous skin as possible favors the reconstructive surgeon in deciding on the position of the initial skin incisions. The otologist may then, by necessity, be forced to use full thickness skin grafts for canal skin reconstruction. In some cases, previous surgery limits possibilities for incisional lines. It is even more critical for cooperative discourse between the surgeons in this instance if skin loss and unfavorable scar formation are to be avoided.

CHOLESTEROL GRANULOMA OF THE PETROUS APEX

We used to think of cholesterol granuloma of the petrous apex as a relatively rare problem. With the advent of CT and MRI scans, this diagnosis is becoming more common. Earlier and more frequent usage of antibiotics in the treatment of otitis media of childhood has probably played some etiologic role in increasing the incidence of this disorder. It is only in a well-developed air cell system of the petrous apex that this entity can occur. The developmental arrest of pneumatization occurring with severe and chronic inflammatory ear disease in the young child may be protective of later development of these cysts. Prior to CT and MRI scans, patients usually presented with multiple cranial nerve palsies, often of many years' duration. Now we find them incidentally or because minimal symptoms led to performance of a scan. This allows the possibility of preservation of cranial nerve function. It, therefore, also increases the possible methods of surgical treatment. Whereas the surgeon previously could easily justify a transcochlear or translabyrinthine drainage operation in the anacusic patient, to halt progressive cranial nerve destruction, he or she now must attempt to preserve hearing and yet provide good long-term cyst drainage. Cyst marsupialization into the posterior fossa via a retrosigmoid approach was reasonably straightforward when the large cysts had eroded the medial petrous pyramid and the posterior fossa dura was bulging well into the cerebellopontine fossa. With the early cases now seen radiographically, quite often thick sclerotic bone persists in the medial wall of the pyramid, requiring drilling before posterior fossa drainage is possible. This bone drilling is hampered by the intervening seventh and eighth nerve complex exiting the internal auditory meatus and coursing through the angle on its way to the pons. Ironically, these patients usually have normal eustachian tube function, so that if the cyst can be drained into the middle ear space, it will be well cleared into the nasopharynx. I am currently using this approach as advocated by Dr. Derald Brackmann for drainage. A complete mastoidectomy with facial recess approach and extended hypotympanotomy with placement of Silastic sheeting drain provides marsupialization if the cyst extends posteriorly to the jugular bulb. Unfortunately, in the early cysts, such posterior extension does not exist, and therefore pericarotid cellular exteriorization of the internal carotid artery through an extended facial recess approach may be the only transmastoid access to the cyst. The problems in this situation are possible damage to the bony eustachian tube during drilling and the tendency of this route to seal off. The pulsations of the carotid artery encourage extrusion of the Silastic drain. Constant contact of the artery to the adjacent bony structures leads to fibrous adherence. I have tried many different surgical approaches in treatment of this disorder, including retrosigmoid craniotomy, lateral transtemporosphenoid approach, radical transcochlear-

translabyrinthine exteriorization, transseptal transsphenoid marsupialization, and complete mastoidectomy with extended facial recess and extended hypotympanotomy approach, and pericarotid apicotomy. Each of these approaches has its own peculiar problems, risks, and difficulties with long-term drainage. The decision on the proper approach should be based on the patient's hearing, age, and extent of disease found on high-definition CT scans with bone window cuts. Magnetic resonance imaging can give similar information. Since this entity gives a high-intensity signal on both T_1- and T_2-weighted images, it is able to differentiate this diagnosis from many others. One problem I have found is distinguishing the early cyst from retained marrow of the petrous apex. Both CT and MRI have a similar appearance with both entities. The final chapter on diagnosis and treatment of this disorder has not yet been written.

BIBLIOGRAPHY

Gherine SG, Brachmann DE, Lo WWM, et al: Cholesterol granuloma of the petrous apex. *Laryngoscope* 1985; 95:659–664.

Jahrsdoerfer R: Congenital malformation of the ears: Analysis of 94 operations. *Ann Otol Rhinol Laryngol* 1980; 89:348–352.

Jahrsdoerfer RA: Congenital atresia of the ear. *Laryngoscope* 1978; 88(suppl 13):1–48.

Jahrsdoerfer RA: Congenital absence of the oval window. *Trans Am Acad Otolarngol* 1977; 84:904–914.

Jahrsdoerfer RA, Yeahly JW, Hall JW, et al: High resolution CT scanning and auditory brain stem response in congenital aural atresia: Patient selection and surgical correction. *Otolaryngol Head Neck Surg* 1985; 93:292–298.

CHAPTER 5

Temporal Bone Trauma

Approach of

Myles L. Pensak, M.D.

Despite the fact that the structures of the middle ear and temporal bone are harbored and relatively protected from many traumatic events, they are not immune to the traumatic insults perpetrated by high-speed motor vehicle accidents or sharp missle injury or the blunt trauma resultant from blows to the skull. Moreover, because of the irregular and complex osteology of the bony skull base, the concomitant potential for injury to vital neural and vascular structures is ever present. Therefore, to understand the evaluation and management of traumatic injuries to the temporal bone, the physician must be intimately familiar with the regional anatomy and the physiologic functioning of both the seventh and eighth cranial nerves.

ANATOMIC CONSIDERATIONS

The temporal bone, made of four constituent parts, including the mastoid process, the squamosa, tympanic ring, and petrous portion, occupies a pyramidal position forming a portion of the skull base interposed between the middle and posterior cranial fossae. Three sides are described: the inferior, anterior, and posterior surfaces.

The auricle opens into the external auditory canal, which is formed by both cartilagenous and osseous segments ending at the tympanic membrane. The middle ear space houses the ossicular chain, with the malleus firmly attached at several crucial points, including the tympanic membrane, incudomalleolar joint, anterior, lateral, and superior malleolar ligaments, and at the cochleariform process by the tendon of the tensor tympani. The incus, supported by the superior and posterior incudal ligaments, occupies the least stable position of the ossicles juxtaposed between the malleus and the capitulum of the stapes.

The stapes suprastructure is held posteriorly by the stapedial tendon fixed at the pyramidal eminence and medially by the footplate that sits in the vestibular fenestra held by the annular ligament.

The cochleovestibular end organ is housed within the otic capsule with the cochlea directed anteromedially from the more posteriorly directed vestibular labyrinth.

Along the roof of the petrous ridge, the superior petrosal sinus runs posteriorly to join the sigmoid sinus proximal to the jugular bulb. The posterior face of the petrous bone opens to the internal auditory canal through which passes the seventh and eighth cranial nerves. The eighth nerve, subserving both the cochlear and vestibular functions, divides distal to the root entry zone. Within the internal auditory canal, the divisions of the eighth nerve are well defined. The facial nerve is located in the canal anterosuperior to the cochlear nerve, and the posterior compartment houses the superior and inferior vestibular nerves. The transverse crest separates the inferior compartments from the superior, and a vertical ridge of bone referred to as Bill's bar separates the facial nerve from the superior vestibular nerve.

At the end of the internal auditory canal, the facial nerve passes through its narrowest channel as it traverses the labyrinthine segment. Laterally, the geniculate ganglion is situated giving off at a sharp angle the greater superficial petrosal nerve, which supplies preganglionic parasympathetic fibers for lacrimation. Turning abruptly in a posterior direction, the facial nerve passes through its tympanic segment just above the cochleariform process and the oval window niche.

At the level of the horizontal canal, the facial nerve turns inferiorly at the region of the second genu and passes toward the stylomastoid foramen in its vertical segment. Along its distal course, the facial nerve gives off two branches that may be of diagnostic importance; these are the nerve to the stapedius muscle and the chordae tympani nerve. Hyperacusis or loss of taste function suggests dysfunction in the aforementioned region of the seventh nerve.

TRAUMATIC EVALUATION

In general, the otolaryngologist may be involved in the initial evaluation and management of the injured patient regarding airway management; however, evaluation of the temporal bone is often delayed until life-threatening injuries are addressed and the patient is stabilized.

Many traumatic injuries to the temporal bone result from more severe basilar skull fractures. Consultation with the otolaryngologist is usually made after the patient has undergone an initial battery of diagnostic tests obtained by the general surgeon or the neurosurgeon. Unfortunately, these examinations often will not address pathology limited to the temporal bone.

Physical examination is of utmost importance, as is obtaining information regarding the patient's antecedent history of otologic or neurotologic pathology. The neurotologic examination centers around the detailed evaluation of the cranial nerves. In the comatose patient, facial grimacing may be noted with sternal pressure or looking for nasal flaring. In patients with significant facial skeletal and soft tissue trauma, this may be particularly difficult.

The auricle should be examined after gentle cleansing. Traumatic soft tissue injuries should be noted and treated promptly, with exposed cartilage debrided and covered as needed. The external auditory canal should be optimally examined under clean otomicroscopic conditions. Manipulation of debris, foreign bodies, or clot should be discouraged in the emergency room but reserved for treatment under sterile bedside or operating room conditions. When cleaning the ear, the physician need be cognizant of bone fragments, soft tissue disruptions, the relative position of the temporomandibular joint, and the integrity of the tympanic membrane. Uncommonly, significant trauma may result in the displacement of an ossicle through a tympanic membrane perforation, and the injudicious extirpation of a soft tissue mass from the external auditory canal may result in further disability, especially if the stapes is dislocated from the oval window niche.

Examination should be made for the presence of cerebrospinal fluid (CSF) otorrhea, recognizing that CSF, when present, is frequently mixed with blood. Therefore, the ear should not be packed unless there is life-threatening hemorrhage, because packing may serve only as a nidus for bacterial growth, and though it may retard CSF leakage, it will not result in its cessation.

In situations wherein the external auditory canal has been torn or contaminated as a result of a traumatic event, topical otic drops may be employed; however, in cases of tympanic membrane perforations that are clean and dry, all agents are discouraged, and the ear is maintained in a dry state.

Following initial evaluation, diagnostic acoustic and neural electrophysiologic tests, as well as radiographs, may be obtained when the patient is stable.

In summary, the physical examination may reveal several findings that will provide insight into the nature of the injury sustained. Questions that should be answered include:

1. Is the patient awake and responsive to sounds?

2. Is the ear canal torn, is there otorrhea, and what is its nature?
3. Is there a hemotympanum?
4. Does the patient complain of vertigo, and is there nystagmus present?
5. Does the facial nerve work? Is there weakness?

NATURE OF TEMPORAL BONE TRAUMA

When viewed in the broad perspective, temporal bone trauma may result from direct lancinating injury as caused by a Q-tip, slag projectile, or bullet, or it may result from the blunt trauma incurred when the skull is thrown against a firm resistant surface as frequently occurs in motor vehicle accidents or from an industrial blast injury.

Lancinating trauma frequently results in significant soft tissue destruction to the ear canal and tympanic membrane. Fortunately, traumatic tympanic membrane perforations are most commonly found in an inferior location and do not require emergency treatment. However, a traumatic perforation that is located in the posterosuperior quadrant associated with vertigo or facial nerve dysfunction frequently requires surgical intervention. In the case of missile injuries, the caliber of the bullet, its direction, velocity, and mass all will be factors that determine the nature and extent of resultant injury. Certainly in this latter case, bone destruction is not an uncommon concomitant to the soft tissue destruction.

Blunt trauma to the temporal bone may result in several types of fractures. Classically, these lesions have been described as transverse or longitudinal in nature. Frequently, however, we observe a mixture of the two.

A longitudinal fracture is one that is characterized by a break in the bone beginning at the squamosa and directed through the external auditory canal, tympanic membrane, and middle ear, sparing the otic capsule and ending at the level of the foramen lacerum or foramen spinosum. Bloody otorrhea with hearing loss are the cardinal findings associated with this type of fracture.

Transverse fractures are seen less commonly, perhaps because the mortality is higher in accidents that result in this type of fracture. The fracture line at the base of the skull begins at the level of the foramen magnum and passes transversely across the long axis of the petrous ridge, disrupting the otic capsule or structures within the lateral portion of the internal auditory canal. The fracture line ends at the level of the foramen lacerum in the floor of the middle cranial fossa (Fig 5–1).

Although hemotympanum and profound sensorineural hearing loss are the salient clinical features of this injury, CSF otorhinorrhea, vertigo, and facial paralysis are frequently observed in patients with this type of fracture.

Mixed lesions may manifest with a myriad of associated deficits. Moreover, complex fractures of the skull base frequently raise some difficult managerial questions for the physician. Four areas that require evaluation and management are (1) facial paralysis, (2) vertigo, (3) CSF leak, and (4) hearing loss.

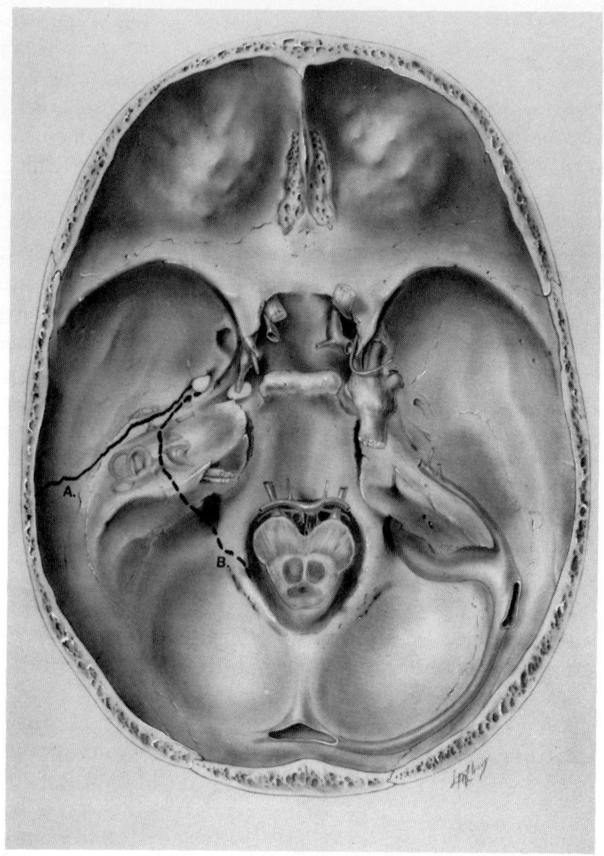

FIG 5–1.
A, pathway of a longitudinal fracture. **B**, fracture pattern of the transverse temporal bone fracture.

Facial Nerve Paralysis

It is highly desirable to establish whether or not the patient had any antecedent history of facial nerve dysfunction if the victim presents for evaluation with either facial paresis or paralysis. For the clinician, the salient question that must be answered is: Was the paralysis of immediate onset, or was it delayed? From a pragmatic point, the latter is often difficult to determine. Delays in arrival to a hospital setting, prolonged diagnosis, especially if the patient has had concomitant facial injuries, or more commonly, situations wherein the patient is too ill to be thoroughly evaluated often occur.

Several testing modalities, including diagnostic imaging and electrophysiologic tests, are employed when a patient with facial nerve paralysis is being evaluated.

Historically, from a diagnostic perspective, polytomography offered an optimal view of the facial nerve. Currently, high-resolution computed tomography (CT) scanning is employed. It is of utmost importance that the radiologist be informed of the nature of the injury prior to performing a study of the thin section cuts (1.5 mm) that will allow for optimal visualization of the seventh nerve. Both axial and coronal views are required to optimize visualization of the complete course of the seventh nerve. Presently, we have not found mastoid films or plain skull radiography to be of value.

Initial electrical testing is first performed 72 hours after paralysis with a bedside Hilger nerve stimulator when the functioning side is compared with the paralyzed side. Remember that this test as well as that employing electroneurography (ENoG) or evoked electromyography (EEMG) depends on the fact that the nonparalyzed side is functioning in a normal fashion. The principle on which the aforementioned electrically evoked action potential test is predicated results from the ability of the nerve to conduct a stimulus impulse. In cases of conduction block resultant from neural compression or disruption while stimulation may be conducted distal to the lesion, proximal stimulation will result in no response. It is important, however, to be cognizant of the fact that once complete wallerian degeneration has occurred, evoked potentials will not be obtained with stimulation at any point along the nerve.

Electroneurography thresholds for nerve stimulation are obtained and recorded in the patient's bedside chart. It is important to note that in the patient with traumatic facial nerve injury, localization of the site of injury is of utmost importance. Although we continue to employ Schirmer's test to establish proximal conduction block, the work by Gantz et al.[1] is considered significant because these authors demonstrated the inconsistency of Schirmer's test when compared to the identification of a neural conduction block by employing intraoperative EEMG.

Audiometry is routinely employed, and tympanometry is performed to establish the presence of an acoustic reflex where possible. I do not specifically test taste function for localization purposes of facial nerve deficit but do make note of aguesia or hypoguesia if the patient reports this.

In patients in whom we demonstrate no facial mimetic function, the history is good or highly suggestive for immediate onset facial paralysis, and the patient is stable, we will recommend facial nerve exploration. If the eye is tearing without problem, exploration is planned to begin through a transmastoid route with the patient prepared for a possible middle fossa approach. In cases involving a dry eye, combined middle fossa–transmastoid exploration is required. The aforementioned surgical approaches are determined by the presence or absence of hearing. In the patient who is able to cooperate for audiometrics, an anacusic ear indicates a tympanomastoid translabyrinthine exploration of the nerve. If the patient is not alert enough for reliable audiometrics and despite an auditory brain stem evoked response that shows no response, we will perform a middle fossa–transmastoid nerve exploration because the hearing threshold may be greater than 65 dB but the ear may still be serviceable with amplification.

The approach is begun with a cortical mastoidectomy. The facial nerve is identified at the level of the digastric ridge and followed cephalically, opening the facial recess. The incus is removed, if it is not already disarticulated, and the nerve is followed to the level of the cochlearform process. Because of our experience with finding facial nerve tears along the medial wall of the fallopian canal, we now mobilize the nerve for full visualization during exploration if fracture lines involve the canal.

Bone spicules and fracture fragments are removed. If the nerve is partially transected, the edges are coapted. Complete transection requires that the freshened nerve endings be juxtaposed without tension. If an irregular tear has occurred, the facial nerve is mobilized and sutured together. Loss of nerve length requires a graft interposition, and because of its location, the greater auricular nerve is an excellent choice.

In cases requiring a middle fossa approach, the technique described by Fisch and Esslen is employed.[2]

The management of a delayed paralysis is more difficult. At the University of Cincinnati, our current protocol requires that the patient be followed with serial ENeGs. In cases in which greater than 90% to 95% wallerian degeneration is demonstrated, exploration surgery is offered.

In cases of delayed onset paralysis, we are dealing with a presumed compressive phenomenon resultant from edema within the narrow confines of the bony fallopian canal. On several occasions, however, it will be found that depressed bone spicules are lying on the facial nerve. Our experience has been that the most common site for this is at the level of the geniculate ganglion, and, therefore, we have routinely prepared the patient for a middle fossa exploration. This route is followed in cases of delayed paralysis following temporal bone trauma with hearing preservation to allow for optimal exposure with the smallest chance for injury to the facial nerve by traction or the inadvertant moving of the depressed bone spicule onto the facial nerve. This is especially true in cases where the geniculate ganglion is naturally exposed. Removal of all bone spicules is performed.

The aforementioned paragraphs address decisions regarding the surgical management of patients with facial nerve paralysis. Nevertheless, protocols for the management of those individuals with a weakened face or those who refuse surgery should be established.

In principal, management goals must aim to minimize damage to the eye that may result from poor lubrication or from an inability to close the eye as part of a protection (blink) response. Although a tarsorrhaphy may be done early on for an anticipated period of seventh nerve dysfunction, a spring or weight may be placed by a surgeon experienced in oculoplastic techniques.

On a more limited basis, the use of Lacri-Lube and natural tears should be employed. In addition, taping the eye closed at night will help to maintain moisture within the eye chamber. Presently, we recommend that patients employ an eye bubble (Pro-Optics) during the day so that vision is not restricted to one eye.

The employment of steroids is controversial. Because of the concussive effect of a temporal bone fracture, if the paralysis is of a delayed nature, we will recommend 80 mg of prednisone to be employed and tapered over a 10- to 14-day period. The aim of the prednisone is to minimize the amount of swelling and edema associated with the neural trauma. In addition to recommended surgical intervention, the employment of steroids in cases of immediate onset facial paralysis is routine.

Posttraumatic Vertigo

Vertigo, lightheadedness, dizzy feelings, or manifestions with equilibrium and gait imbalance following significant head injury are not uncommon. Nevertheless, it is of paramount importance that early on the clinician establish whether or not the labyrinth has been directly involved. Initial evaluation is done again by close questioning of the patient. Duration and frequency of the vertigo spells are important. What provokes the attack? What will lessen its severity or cause the abatement of symptoms? Patients with whiplash injuries can be particularly difficult to evaluate, because often there is lightheadedness but no true vertigo. The latter symptoms may last for years after a head injury and often result in physician skepticism.

Objective evaluation begins with the otoneurologic examination. Cerebellar testing is done looking for signs of loss of fine motor coordination skills. Dix-Hallpike maneuvers are performed in an attempt to reproduce the vertigo by defining a position that may provoke the symptoms and demonstrate nystagmus. In some patients, the physician may be required to perform bedside caloric tests; however, they are generally reserved for patients unable to complete a formal caloric examination as part of an electronystagmography (ENG) battery.

Physiologic testing that may be employed includes ENG, platform posturography, and rotational chair evaluation. Although the methodology and testing parameters established by these tests are beyond the scope of this review, the physician should be aware of the limitations of these diagnostic tests. Moreover, as with any testing technique, the information gleaned is most often reflected by the experience of the tester and the individual interpreting the obtained results.

The differential diagnosis of posttraumatic vertigo or balance dysfunction includes those injuries that are directed toward the middle ear (stapes), the oval and round window regions, the labyrinth, seventh nerve, brain stem, cerebellum, and craniocervical junction. Generally, immediate surgical intervention is rarely required, because most patients will be satisfactorily cared for with the recommendation of rest and vestibular suppressants.

Perilymphatic fistulae may be suggested by a positive fistula test; however, the test is not pathognomonic, and a high degree of suspicion needs to be considered. Significant concomitant sensorineural hearing loss, fluctuant hearing loss, or a progressive sensorineural hearing loss is suggestive. Initial treatment if hearing is stable is to place the patient at bedrest with the head elevated and to employ a nonconstipating diet and stool softeners. If symptoms do not abate over several days and hearing is unstable, middle ear exploration is recommended. Whether or not an active fistula is noted, the round and oval windows should be packed with autogenous tissue. Presently we use fascia or perichondrium.

In cases of ossicular disruption and concomitant subluxation of the stapes, a stapedectomy will need to be performed with the oval window niche covered by a tissue graft. Reconstruction may be done with a homograft or autograft incus or any number of middle ear prostheses presently available. On occasion a small anterior subluxation and associated perilymph leak may be treated by soft tissue packing, leaving the footplate undisturbed.

Cupulolithiasis as described by Schuknecht[3] results from the displacement of the otoconia from the saccular or utricular maculae into a gravity-dependent positioning on the cupula of a dependent semicircular canal, with the posterior canal being the most commonly effected. A conservative approach is recommended, with limited vestibular suppressive medications to allow for early and rapid compensatory mechanisms to begin to take effect. Cawthorne head exercises have been employed with success in some cases. Surgery (singular neurectomy or selective vestibular neurectomy) is reserved for those with intractible symptoms that do not improve over a 1-year period.

Labyrinthine concussion is treated with vestibular suppressant medications, as are cases of vestibular neuronitis. Delayed posttraumatic endolymphatic hydrops patients are managed in the same fashion as the idiopathic Meniere patient, that is, with a low-salt diet, diuretic therapy, and mild vestibular suppressants. Surgery is reserved for refractory cases. If symptoms persist, an endolymphatic mastoid shunt or vestibular nerve section or labyrinthectomy may be performed, depending on auditory thresholds and degree of symptomatology.

Cerebrospinal Fluid Otorrhea

The general approach to CSF otorrhea is conservative. In many cases of transverse temporal bone fracture, the leakage of CSF may manifest as rhinorrhea, and only if the tympanic membrane or roof of the external auditory canal is lacerated will a fluid flow be noted through the ear.

In most cases, CSF otorrhea is not difficult to identify. Fluid that comes out of the ear canal, especially in a dependent position, is unmistakable. However, in many cases there is an admixture of blood and spinal fluid, and here the diagnosis is not clear. The classic "double ring" sign may not be positive. Nevertheless, since life-threatening hemorrhage is the only indication for packing of the ear canal, it is only infrequently that a CSF leak will go undeclared.

Diagnosis is made on clinical grounds most times. Computed tomography imaging that demonstrates a significant fracture line lends credible support. Diagnostic studies may be performed with radioactive isotope imaging techniques.

The treatment consists of bed rest and head elevation. Like the perilymph fistula, stool softeners and a nonconstipating diet are recommended. This approach is done for 10 days to 2 weeks if the volume of fluid flow is noted to be decreasing and resolves. If at that point leakage persists, I will explore the ear.*

Placement of a lumbar catheter or the performance of serial lumbar punctures to lower the volume of CSF fluid flow often has a dramatic effect. In some cases the placement of a ventriculoperitoneal shunt by the neurosurgeons will have a dramatic effect on the CSF otorrhea.

We do not routinely employ antibiotics for CSF otorrhea; however, aural and nasopharyngeal cultures are obtained as a baseline. Should a patient with recognized CSF otorrhea develop signs of meningeal irritation or intracranial infection, appropriate antibiotic therapy will be instituted.

In cases that do not respond to conservative management, the patient is prepared for both a transmastoid and middle fossa exposure. I have found it difficult to close tegmental deficits from the mastoid and, therefore, prefer the latter approach. Following retraction of the temporal lobe, both bone and fascia are used to cover the tegmental defect. Dural defects are closed primarily or a graft of lyophilized dura may be used.

*In cases of brisk CSF leak early in the course, I routinely place a lumbar drain prior to considering surgery.

Hearing Loss

The hearing loss associated with temporal bone trauma is highly variable, covering the range from mild conductive losses due to debris in the ear canal to profound sensorineural hearing loss or a mixture of the two.

The assessment of audiometric thresholds is performed once a patient is stabilized and before surgical intervention is undertaken. For the alert patient, a routine audiogram is performed. For those who are unconscious, an auditory brain stem evoked potential is done; however, in the face of significant debris in the canal or blood in the middle ear or a hearing loss at or above the 65- to 75-dB region, the auditory brain stem response will not give a definitive level of auditory threshold. This latter point is important if a procedure that may violate the otic capsule, resulting in further hearing loss, is planned.

Physical examination may reveal the presence of a tympanic membrane perforation, hemotympanum, or sometimes visualization of a disrupted ossicular chain.

Radiographics (CT images) will help establish whether a transverse or longitudinal temporal bone fracture has occurred. In case of the former, sensorineural hearing loss is anticipated, and the patient and patient's family are so informed.

In cases of longitudinal fracture, most commonly the incudostapedial joint is disrupted. The second most common source of an ossicular disruption is fracture of the suprastructure of the stapes, resulting in a conductive hearing loss.

The management of hearing loss should also take into account the possibility of nonorganic hearing loss because of the compensation that may be obtained due to claims resultant from accidents. The physician and audiologist should be cognizant of this fact and be prepared to recognize the occasional fraudulent patient.

Except in cases of suspected perilymphatic fistula, hearing loss associated with trauma does not constitute an emergency.

In the former case, however, it is imperative that the leak be sealed as soon as possible, because even under the best of circumstances, hearing loss is only occasionally reversed or brought back to pretrauma levels. Associated with the group of patients who are noted to have sensorineural hearing loss with vertigo is a small group who will be found to have subluxation of the stapes footplate. In this uncommon condition, stapedectomy is performed and the oval window sealed with a tissue graft as described previously.

I allow 1 month to pass before a traumatic tympanic membrane perforation is closed. If the ear is clean and dry, no topical otic preparations are employed, and the patient is instructed to keep the ear dry. In an ear that has developed a secondary infection, I will treat with both topical drops and systemic antibiotics. Following resolution and nonspontaneous closure of the tympanic membrane, a tympanoplasty will be performed.

In cases of conductive loss wherein the ossicular chain has been disrupted, a sculptured incus will be engaged between the malleus and stapes. In cases where the stapes suprastructure is fractured a fitted incus will be placed from the malleus to the footplate.

Patients who have sustained sensorineural losses will be fitted with a hearing aid if indicated.

CONCLUSION

Trauma to the temporal bone may lead to significant functional debility. Fortunately, life-threatening injuries are uncommon. Close attention should be directed to the function of the facial nerve and the presence of CSF leak. Conservative treatment is reserved for the vertiginous patient, and for those with auditory deficits, appropriate surgical intervention is undertaken. For individuals who are not surgical candidates, aural rehabilitation with amplification is recommended.

REFERENCES

1. Gantz B, Gmur A, Fisch U: Intraoperative electromyography in Bell's palsy. *Am J Otolaryngol* 1982; 3:273.
2. Fisch U, Esslen C: Total intratemporal exposure of the facial nerve. *Arch Otolaryngol* 1972; 95:335.
3. Schuknecht HF: *Pathology of the Ear.* Cambridge, Mass, Harvard University Press, 1974.

RECOMMENDED READING

Cannon CR, Jahrsdoerfer RA: Temporal bone fractures: Review of 90 cases. *Arch Otolaryngol* 1983; 109:285.
Emmett JR, Shea JJ: *Traumatic perilymph fistulae. Laryngoscope* 1980; 90:1513.
Goodhill V: Leaking labyrinthine lesions, deafness, tinnitus and dizziness. *Ann Otol Rhinol Laryngol* 1981; 90:96.
Hicks GW, Wright JW Jr, Wright JW III: Cerebrospinal fluid otorrhea. *Laryngoscope* 1980; 90(suppl 25):1–25.
Hough JVD: Fractures of the temporal bone and associated middle and inner ear trauma. *Proc R Soc Med* 1970; 63:245.

Temporal Bone Trauma

Approach of

Douglas E. Mattox, M.D.

FACIAL PARALYSIS

Site of Injury

Fractures can take a number of paths through the temporal bone, and the prognosis for recovery of the facial nerve and other injuries depends on the site and severity of the temporal bone fracture. Fractures of the temporal bone are classified as transverse and longitudinal with respect to the long axis of the temporal bone. Temporal bone fractures usually are caused by occipital or temporal trauma; frontal trauma rarely causes a fracture of the temporal bone. Signs of temporal bone fracture include ecchymosis of the postauricular skin (Battle's sign), bleeding from the ear or hemotympanum, CSF otorrhea, hearing loss (conductive or sensorineural), and facial paralysis.

Transverse fractures, which run anteroposteriorly through the skull across the long axis of the temporal bone, are associated with severe injuries and a high mortality rate. In the temporal bone the fracture may cross the internal auditory canal or pass through the vestibule and inner ear. Since the tympanic membrane remains intact, blood accumulation will cause a hemotympanum, and a CSF leak may be unrecognized because it drains through the eustachian tube. The facial nerve is injured in one half of transverse temporal bone fractures. Ninety percent of the injuries of the facial nerves in transverse fractures are in the labyrinthine segment of the nerve, and 10% are within the posterior fossa or internal auditory canal. There is also a high incidence of sensorineural hearing loss from the fracture of the cochlea.

Longitudinal fractures of the temporal bone follow the long axis of the temporal bone starting in the temporal squama and follow the external auditory canal to the petrous apex. Eighty percent of temporal bone fractures are longitudinal.[1] They are frequently bilateral. There is usually conductive hearing loss from laceration of the tympanic membrane or disruption of the ossicles. Facial paralysis occurs in about 20% of longitudinal fractures of the temporal bone. The part of the facial nerve most commonly injured by longitudinal fractures is the geniculate ganglion. The fracture usually passes anterior to the otic capsule and curves over the cochlea through the thin cortical bone over the geniculum of the facial nerve.

Damage of the facial nerve in the mastoid and distal tympanic segments of the facial nerve can also occur, especially in ballistic injuries, which can shatter the temporal bone.

Mechanism of Injury

The facial nerve can be damaged in several ways by temporal bone fractures, including transection (30%), compression (20%), and stretch injury with intraneural hematoma (50%).[2] Transection of the nerve is caused by movement of the bone fragments during the injury. Compression of the nerve can occur from a shift of the bony fallopian canal at the fracture site or from a fragment of bone impinging on the nerve.

Stretch injury at the geniculate ganglion is the most common facial nerve injury in longitudinal fractures of the temporal bone. It is caused by traction on the ganglion by the greater petrosal nerve. The greater petrosal nerve is firmly attached to the dura of the middle cranial fossa. When the fracture occurs, the temporary displacement of the anterior bone fragment and the attached dural segment stretch the petrosal nerve away from the geniculum. The stretch injury can damage nerve fibers directly or can cause rupture of small capillaries within the nerve, causing an intraneural hematoma. This intraneural hematoma will organize, and the resulting fibrosis can inhibit axon regeneration through the damaged segment.

Indications for Exploration

The indications for exploration of the facial nerve in temporal bone fractures are not as simple as the old dictum that immediate-onset paralysis should be explored and delayed paralysis should not be. Many paralyses in both categories will recover spontaneously without surgical intervention.[3] Electrophysiologic criteria can now be applied to determine if the nerve needs exploration (Fig 5–2).[4]

The criteria for exploration of facial nerves after temporal bone fracture are similar to those used for acute idiopathic paralysis (Bell's palsy).[5] Patients who do develop a complete paralysis, regardless of whether it occurs immediately after the trauma or after some delay, should be followed with ENeG. If patients develop more than 95% degeneration (as measured by comparison of the peak-to-peak muscle compound action potential between the injured and the normal side) within 21 days of the onset of the paralysis (not the trauma), they are candidates for surgical exploration. Patients who do not reach more than 95% degeneration have an excellent prognosis and are treated conservatively with steroids. Patients allowed to go on to 100% degeneration before exploration and patients who develop

greater than 95% degeneration more than 21 days after the onset of paralysis have poorer prognoses and are unlikely to benefit from surgery.

Unfortunately, many patients are not seen early after their trauma or other injuries prevent them from being accurately followed, and decisions about management of the facial nerve must be made in the absence of serial electrophysiologic recordings. Patients seen in the first month after injury in whom there is no demonstrable response on neuronography and in whom there is CT evidence of displacement of the fallopian canal should be explored. Patients seen at longer intervals and those in whom displacement of the fallopian canal cannot be demonstrated should be given 6 to 9 months for spontaneous recovery and explored only if they have no return of function.

In those cases that meet the ENoG criteria for exploration, Fisch and Mattox have suggested immediate facial palsies are best explored weeks after the injury and that delayed paralysis should be explored immediately after they occur.[2] The rationale of the delayed exploration of acute paralysis is that the nerve is probably severely crushed or transected and that an accurate diagnosis and management of the problem of the nerve is easier after the hematoma and edema within the temporal bone have resolved. The delayed paralysis, however, is a more moderate injury where decompression of the nerve is likely to have the greatest impact on facial function and therefore should be done immediately after 90% to 95% degeneration has occurred.

Management of Longitudinal Fractures

The method of exploration and management of the facial nerve are dictated by the location and severity of the injury.

Longitudinal fractures of the temporal bone are explored through the middle cranial fossa approach. Although the tympanic and mastoid segments of the facial nerve can be exposed through the mastoid and facial recess (with or without removal of the incus), the geniculate ganglion and labyrinthine segments of the facial nerve can be adequately exposed only through the middle cranial fossa.

The middle cranial fossa has few reliable landmarks. The transtemporosupralabyrinthine approach described by Fisch relies on a positive identification of the blue line of the superior semicircular canal to identify the internal auditory canal for exact orientation of the surgeon.[6] This landmark will allow wide opening of the internal auditory canal and decompression of the labyrinthine course of the facial nerve without additional damage of this delicate portion of the nerve.

The procedure is performed through a preauricular and temporal incision extending from the root of the zygomatic arch to 7 cm above the pinna. The temporalis muscle is exposed and divided. A 3 by 4 cm craniotomy in the temporal skull is made with diamond and cutting burrs. The craniotomy should have its center over the anterior edge of the external auditory canal. The rectangular bone flap is removed, and additional bone is removed inferiorly until the craniotomy is flush with the floor of the middle cranial fossa.

The dura is carefully elevated over the middle cranial fossa until the arcuate eminence and the meatal plane (flat bone anterior and medial to the arcuate eminence that covers the

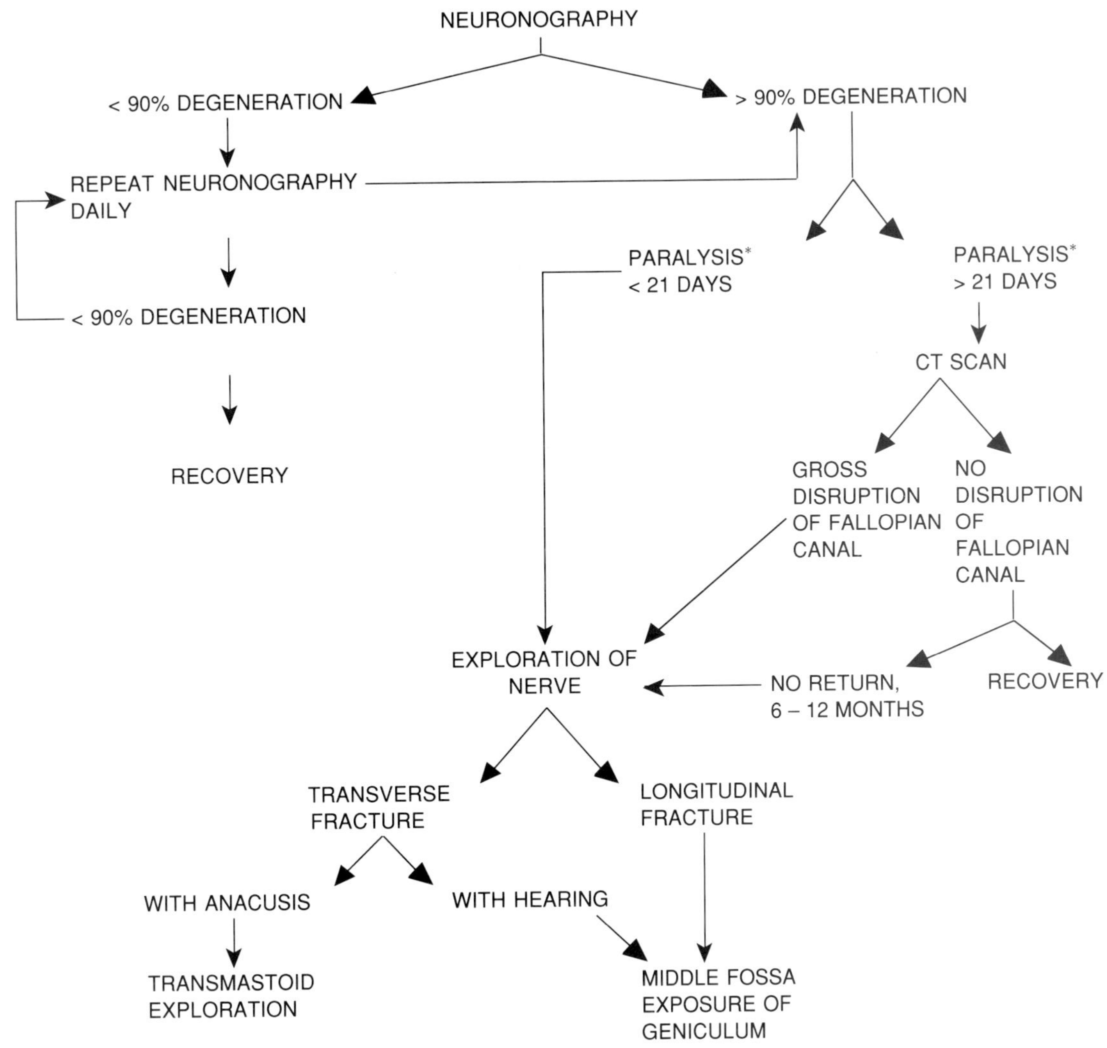

FIG 5–2.
Facial nerve injury in temporal bone trauma. The underlying concept in this algorithm is that surgical intervention in temporal bone fractures depends on the electrical integrity of the nerve rather than on the old division between immediate and delayed paralyses. Many immediate paralyses do not achieve the criteria of 90% degeneration on ENoG and have a high probability of satisfactory recovery. On the other hand, some delayed paralyses progress to total degeneration and therefore would benefit from exploration. If the patient is not seen early after the fracture (within 21 days) and there is already total degeneration of the nerve, the decision to explore the nerve is based on the integrity of the fallopian canal on high-resolution CT scan. If the canal is not grossly disrupted, time should be allowed for spontaneous recovery. If there is gross disruption of the canal, the nerve should be explored. The most common site of injury of the facial nerve in longitudinal fractures of the temporal bone is at the geniculate ganglion. This area can be satisfactorily exposed and repaired, while preserving middle and inner ear function, by using the middle cranial fossa approach. If hearing is destroyed by the fracture, it is less technically demanding to explore the nerve through a transmastoid-translabyrinthine approach.

internal auditory canal) are identified. A middle cranial fossa retractor is used to maintain the retraction of the dura. Extensive exposure of the floor of the middle fossa, including the middle meningeal artery and petrosal sinus, is not required if the following landmarks are used.

The arcuate eminence itself is a poor landmark for the superior semicircular canal because the otic capsule and membranous canal have a variable relationship to the arcuate eminence depending on the pneumatization of the temporal bone. There may be only thin bone over the membranous labyrinth, or the bone may be a few millimeters thick. Identification of the superior canal is facilitated by penetrating the mastoid tegmen and approaching the superior canal through the pneumatic bone lateral and posterior to it. Once the bony superior semicircular canal is identified, the bone is taken down on its superolateral surface with a diamond burr until the blue line is identified. The blue line is followed anteriorly until the area of the superior ampulla is identified to prevent it from being inadvertently opened as the nerve is exposed.

After the superior semicircular canal is blue lined, the internal auditory canal is identified along a 60-degree angle anterior to the superior semicircular canal. The bone of the meatal plane is drilled away until the internal auditory meatus is blue lined and eventually exposed along its entire superior surface. Exposure of the labyrinthine segment of the facial nerve is obtained by extending the dissection lateral and anterior to the fundus of the internal auditory canal to the geniculate ganglion. The tympanic segment of the facial nerve also can be exposed through this approach by removing additional bone over the tegmen tympani.

Once the nerve is fully exposed, the extent of injury can be accessed. If it is simply a matter of a bony fragment impinging on the nerve, the fragment can be removed. The epineurium of the facial nerve should be incised to allow decompression.

If the nerve is transected close to geniculate ganglion, it is possible to excise the ganglion and obtain an end-to-end reanastomosis by rerouting the labyrinthine and tympanic segments directly from the fundus of the internal auditory canal to the tympanic segment.

If an intraneural hematoma is noted, the epineurium should be incised and the hematoma evacuated. The rationale for this is that an organized hematoma within the nerve may block axons attempting to regenerate through the nerve sheath.

The wound is closed by placing a muscle graft over the internal auditory canal, and a piece of bone from the craniotomy is used to reconstruct the tegmen to prevent a postoperative encephalocele in the middle ear. The dura is sutured to the overlying muscle to prevent a postoperative epidural fluid accumulation. The bone flap is replaced, and the temporalis muscle and skin are closed.

Management of Transverse Fractures

Facial nerve injuries associated with transverse fractures of the petrous bone should be approached through a transmastoid approach, since cochlear and vestibular function are usually destroyed by the fracture. The internal auditory canal and labyrinthine and tympanic segments of the facial nerve all are readily identifiable after a complete mastoidectomy and labyrinthectomy are performed. If the injury is confined to the portion of the nerve adjacent to the geniculate ganglion, a direct rerouting from the internal meatus to the mastoid or tympanic segment of the nerve can be performed. If the injury is in the internal auditory canal, a cable graft is usually required.

Extensive injuries of the temporal bone from ballistic trauma or crush injuries of the skull can injure the facial nerve in many areas, and the surgical approach should be guided by high-resolution CT scanning and preoperative evaluation of hearing and vestibular function. If sensory function is not impaired, the entire intratemporal course of the facial nerve can be exposed without loss of vestibular or cochlear function by combination of the transmastoid and transtemporal approaches. If the ear is anacusic, a translabyrinthine approach to the facial nerve and internal auditory canal can be used.

POSTTRAUMATIC HEARING LOSS

Posttraumatic hearing loss can be either conductive or sensorineural.

Conductive Hearing Loss

Longitudinal fractures of the temporal bone pass through the external auditory canal, tympanic membrane, and middle ear. There is usually a tympanic membrane laceration. Not infrequently a fragment of the scutum impinges on the body of the incus, causing a conductive hearing loss. In addition, many injuries of the ossicular chain can occur; separation of the incudostapedial joint, fracture of the long process of the incus, and fracture of the crura of the stapes are the most common.[7] On occasion the incus can be totally dislocated into the external auditory canal or the hypotympanum. All of these injuries should be repaired using standard tympanoplastic and ossiculoplastic techniques.

Sensorineural Hearing Loss

Sensorineural hearing loss is commonly seen with a transverse temporal bone fracture when the fracture goes through the vestibule or cochlea. These losses are usually profound and are irreparable. Sensorineural hearing loss from perilymphatic fistula and posttraumatic Meniere's disease are discussed under posttraumatic vertigo.

A concussive injury of the inner ear has also been described.[8] The exact pathophysiology of inner concussion is unknown, although it is thought to be related to high-energy traveling waves, reflex hyperemia, or hemorrhage. The severity of the symptoms does not necessarily correspond to the apparent severity of the injury. The hearing loss may be bilateral and symmetric, although asymmetric and unilateral cases also occur.

Experimental animals subjected to head concussion with the head fixed showed a loss of inner and outer hair cells in the basilar turn and corresponding hearing loss without evidence of fracture of the otic capsule.[9] However, other studies in which the head was not fixed at the time of impact have shown little cochlear and vestibular damage.[10]

POSTTRAUMATIC VERTIGO

Posttraumatic vertigo can occur from destruction of the peripheral labyrinth by the fracture, perilymph fistula, posttraumatic hydrops, posttraumatic benign positional vertigo (cupulolithiasis), and brainstem injury.

Labyrinthine Fracture

A transverse temporal bone fracture through the vestibule

produces an immediate destruction of the end organ and loss of vestibular function. The patient is readily identified, having a total sensorineural hearing loss as well as total absence of caloric response. There is an acute severe dizziness lasting 5 to 10 days, followed by a progressively decreasing degree of disequilibrium. After full central nervous system compensation, the patient with a unilateral vestibular loss will be indistinguishable from normal except in the most complex physical activity and testing procedure. The patient's rehabilitation can be facilitated by appropriate vestibular exercises.[11]

Perilymph Fistula

A great deal of attention has been focused recently on fistulae between the perilymphatic space and the middle ear. In addition to rupture of the membranes of the oval and round windows, it is theoretically possible to have membrane ruptures of Reisner's membrane or the basilar membrane of the scala media.[12,13] These membrane ruptures could cause a sensorineural hearing loss without external leak of fluid. Patients with perilymph fistula generally have both a sensorineural hearing loss and disequilibrium, although either symptom can occur alone. The disequilibrium is most commonly described as a chronic disorientation, often associated with positional dizziness in addition.[14] The diagnosis is easy when the injury results from an abrupt pressure change within the middle ear space, for instance, from changes in atmospheric pressure, scuba diving accidents, and slap injuries to the external auditory canal. However, perilymph fistulas can also occur with much less severe trauma or may occur spontaneously, making the diagnosis much more difficult to establish.

Unfortunately, there is no diagnostic test pathognomonic for perilymph fistula short of exploratory tympanotomy, and even this may not be totally reliable because some fistulas can leak intermittently. Therefore, absolute criteria for exploration of the middle ear do not exist. The issue is further clouded by the fact that it is likely that a substantial number of perilymph fistulas heal spontaneously. To foster spontaneous healing, any patient with an acute injury causing cochlear and vestibular loss should be restricted to bed rest.

Exploration of the middle ear is indicated in patients who have a progressive sensorineural loss or in whom the hearing loss is stable but vestibular symptoms continue despite conservative therapy. Some patients with chronic disequilibrium combined with positional vertigo also may have perilymph fistulas.

The middle ear is explored through a standard endaural or transcanal tympanotomy. Absolute hemostasis of the canal incisions should be obtained before the tympanic annulus is elevated because any blood staining of the middle ear will obscure the fistula. The scutum should be curetted until there is a clear view of the oval and round windows. Having the patient in the Trendelenburg position performing the Valsalva maneuver may facilitate the identification of a fistula. If a fistula is identified, the mucosa around it is scarified and the area is packed with small pieces of connective tissue taken from the canal incision (it has been suggested that recurrence rates are higher when the grafting material is fat).[15,16] The graft may be further stabilized with small pieces of absorbable gelatin sponge (Gelfoam). Since perilymph leaks may be intermittent, most surgeons pack both the round and oval windows if no perilymph leak is identified.

The results of fistula closure had been very encouraging in terms of control of vertigo and preservation of residual hearing. Hearing improvement can occur but is seen in less than one third of patients.

Posttraumatic Hydrops

Episodic vertigo reminiscent of Meniere's disease can be seen in patients with previous head injury, often many years after the acute injury. Temporal bone histopathology has documented hydrops of the endolymph system in these patients. Usually the symptoms can be controlled with antihistamines or benzodiazephines. Labyrinthectomy can be considered in patients with severe symptoms and nonserviceable hearing. Patients with residual hearing can be considered for middle fossa or retrosigmoid vestibular nerve section, although the results of these patients are not as good in those with idiopathic Meniere's syndrome.

Benign Paroxysmal Positional Vertigo

Schuknecht coined the term cupulolithiasis to describe the presence of an amorphic basophilic calcium deposit on the ampulla of the posterior semicircular canal.[17] He proposed that these deposits are the result of degeneration of otoconia that become loosened from the otolith membranes during head trauma. The additional mass on the ampulla of the posterior semicircular canal leads to symptoms of benign paroxysmal positional vertigo (BPPV). It is a brief, intense vertigo and nystagmus that occurs when the patient is rapidly rotated to a head back position with the affected ear down. The nystagmus typically has a latency of 10 to 20 seconds, has a crescendo-decrescendo pattern, and extinguishes after 20 to 30 seconds. Repeated positioning of the patient causes habituation of the symptoms. Rehabilitative physical therapy has been extremely successful in the management of BPPV.[18]

Surgical Management

Although most patients can be managed with a combination of appropriate physical therapy and pharmacotherapy, destructive labyrinthine procedures are effective in the remaining patients. These procedures include transcanal or transmastoid labyrinthectomy when hearing loss is severe and vestibular nerve section when hearing should be preserved.

Middle fossa vestibular nerve section is performed similar to facial nerve decompression described earlier. The procedure is modified in that the dura of the internal meatus is incised over the vestibular nerve. The vestibular nerve is cut distal to Scarpa's ganglion and ganglionectomy is performed.[2,5]

CEREBROSPINAL FLUID LEAK

The dura is tightly adherent to the middle and posterior fossa aspects of the temporal bone and is frequently torn by both transverse and longitudinal fractures. The initial evaluation may be confounded by active bleeding or blood clot within the external auditory canal. Any patient with head trauma and bleeding from the canal should be examined only with sterile instruments and speculum to prevent contamination of a potential CSF leak. The examination is often best delayed 2 to 3 days until after the acute edema and active bleeding have subsided. If the tympanic membrane is intact (transverse fractures), a CSF leak may present as a middle ear effusion or as CSF rhinorrhea. Small leaks may be asymptomatic and not detected until the patient develops meningitis, often years after the initial trauma.

The initial management of CSF otorrhea should always be conservative because there is a high spontaneous healing rate. Closure of the CSF leak can be assisted by reducing CSF pressure with serial lumbar punctures or a lumbar drain.

Patients with persistent CSF leaks should have the site of bony defect documented with high-resolution CT. Active CSF leaks should be closed surgically if they do not clear in 14 days. The most difficult cases are those in which the leak is intermittent or of low volume, making localization of the site of leak difficult. In these cases the only sign of persistent CSF leak through the eustachian tube may be recurrent meningitis.

A radioactive iodine serum albumin (RISA) scan may be useful in localizing the site of the CSF leak. Autologous albumin tagged with iodine 131 is injected into the subarachnoid space by a lumbar puncture. Cotton pledgets are placed in the nasopharynx adjacent to the eustachian tube, sphenoid ostium, and superior meatus of the nose. The pledgets are extracted 6 hours later and assayed on a scintillation counter. An increase of 1.3 over the simultaneous serum level is indicative of a CSF leak.

The most common site for CSF otorrhea is from the middle fossa through the tegmen tympani or tegmen mastoideum. If the patient has no history of meningitis and the hearing function is intact, this may be repaired through a small middle fossa craniotomy or from below through the mastoid. In either case a strong fascial support such as fascia lata or temporalis fascia is placed between the temporal bone and the dura.

In cases where there is severe hearing loss or recurrent episodes of meningitis, the middle ear should be sacrificed and a subtotal petrosectomy performed.[19] In this procedure the external auditory canal and eustachian tube are closed, and all pneumatic spaces of the bone are exenterated. The cavity is obliterated with abdominal fat and temporalis muscle. This obliteration gives the most secure and reliable closure of the CSF leak and prevents retrograde infection from the eustachian tube.

LATE COMPLICATIONS

The most significant late complication of temporal bone fractures is encephalocele formation. Constant pressure of the brain and dura on a tegmen tympani dehiscence will cause resorption of bone and an expanding herniation of temporal lobe into the middle ear and mastoid.

On CT evaluation there will be an identifiable dehiscence in the bone of the tegmen, and the mass is in continuity with the temporal lobe. On magnetic resonance imaging scan, the brain tissue will have the same intensity signal as brain tissue unless it has undergone necrosis or cystic degeneration.

Encephaloceles can be repaired from the mastoid or from a small temporal craniotomy. A small herniation can be reduced and reinforced from below with fascia and cartilage and bone graft. A large encephalocele with necrotic brain must be amputated and the dura repaired.

REFERENCES

1. Fredrickson JM, Griffity AW, Lindsay JR: Transverse fracture of the temporal bone. A clinical and histopathologic study. *Arch Otolaryngol* 1963; 78:770–784.
2. Fisch U, Mattox DE: *Microsurgery of the Skull Base.* New York, Thieme Medical, 1988.
3. Maiman DJ, Cusick JF, Anderson AJ, et al: Nonoperative management of traumatic facial nerve palsy. *J Trauma* 1985; 25:644–648.
4. Holliday M, Mattox DE, Price JC, et al: Decision making in facial nerve surgery. Exhibit presented at the American Academy of Otolaryngology–Head and Neck Surgery. Washington, DC, Sept 25–29, 1988.
5. Fisch U: Surgery for Bell's palsy. *Arch Otolaryngol* 1981; 107:1–11.
6. Fisch U: Surgery of the internal acoustic meatus, in Naumann HH (ed): *Head and Neck Surgery.* New York, Thieme Medical, 1982, vol 3, pp 465–551.
7. Hough JVD, Stuart WD: Middle ear injuries in skull trauma. *Laryngoscope* 1968; 78:899–937.
8. Snow JB: Management and therapy of trauma to the external ear and auditory and vestibular systems, in Alberti PW, Ruben RJ (eds): *Otologic Medicine and Surgery.* New York, Churchill Livingstone, 1988, pp 1561–1576.
9. Schuknecht HF, Neff WO, Pearlman HB: Experimental study of auditory damage following blows to the head. *Ann Otol* 1951; 60:273–289.
10. Makishima K, Sobel SS, Snow JB: Histologic correlates of oto-neurologic manifestations following head trauma. *Laryngoscope* 1976; 86:1306–1314.
11. Zee DS: The management of patients with vestibular disorders, in Barber HO, Sharpe JA (eds): *Vestibular Disorders.* Chicago, Year Book Medical Publishers, 1988, pp 254–274.
12. Simmons FB, Mongeon CJ: Endolymphatic duct pressure produces cochlear damage. *Arch Otolaryngol* 1967; 88:143–150.
13. Simmons FB: Theory of membrane breaks in sudden hearing loss. *Arch Otolaryngol* 1968; 88:41–48.
14. Kohut RI: Perilymph fistulas, in Cumming CW, Fredrickson JM, Harker LA, et al (eds): *Otolaryngology—Head and Neck Surgery: Update I.* St Louis, CV Mosby Co, 1989, pp 370–379.
15. Singleton GT, Karlan MS, Post KN, et al: Perilymph fistulas: Diagnostic criteria and therapy. *Ann Otol Rhinol Laryngol* 1978; 87:797–803.
16. Love JT Jr, Waguespack RW: Perilymphatic fistulas. *Laryngoscope* 1981; 91:1118–1128.
17. Schuknecht HF: Cupulolithiasis. *Arch Otolaryngol* 1969; 90:765–778.
18. Brandt T, Daroff RB: Physical therapy for benign paroxysmal positional vertigo. *Arch Otolaryngol* 1980; 106:484–485.
19. Coker NJ, Jenkins HA, Fisch U: Obliteration of the middle ear and mastoid cleft in subtotal petrosectomy: Indications, technique and results. *Ann Otol Rhinol Laryngol* 1986; 95:5–11.

CHAPTER 6

ACOUSTIC TUMOR*

Approach of

William M. Luxford, M.D.

and

William F. House, M.D.

In the early 1900s, Dr. Harvey Cushing delineated the characteristic symptoms of large acoustic tumors through careful questioning of the patient. However, it was not until the 1920s that Dr. Walter Dandy[1] reported the first total removal of an acoustic tumor in a patient who survived. Dandy used the suboccipital approach. This technique was the standard approach for the next 30 years. Morbidity and mortality were high. Forty percent of patients died from surgery. Of the survivors, one half were totally disabled by ataxia, cranial nerve involvement, and in some cases, hemiparesis. In the late 1950s, the transtemporal approach, using the operating microscope, dramatically altered the mortality and morbidity associated with acoustic tumor surgery.

Since the late 1950s, surgeons at the Otologic Medical Group have removed more than 2,000 acoustic tumors. In the majority of these cases the translabyrinthine approach was used. However, in patients with good hearing, small intracanicular tumors were removed by a middle fossa approach in an attempt to preserve hearing. Recently, a retrosigmoid approach has been used for patients with serviceable hearing who have less than 1.5-cm tumor extension into the cerebellopontine angle in an attempt to preserve hearing. We believe that the translabyrinthine approach is the preferred route for removal of the majority of acoustic tumors.

*Sponsored by a grant from the House Ear Institute, an affiliate of the University of Southern California School of Medicine, Los Angeles.

TRANSLABYRINTHINE APPROACH

At the Otologic Medical Group, we use the translabyrinthine approach to remove the majority of acoustic tumors because it has many advantages.[1a] It is the most direct route to the cerebellopontine angle and requires minimum cerebellar retraction that is extradural, decreasing the incidence of postoperative ataxia. Dissection of the lateral end of the internal auditory canal ensures complete tumor removal from that area and allows definitive identification of the facial nerve with less risk of injury to it.

If the facial nerve is lost during acoustic tumor removal, the translabyrinthine approach offers the best opportunity for immediate repair by end-to-end anastomosis or interposition of a nerve graft.[2] Finally, and most important, this approach carries the lowest morbidity and mortality rates. The mortality rate for a recent series of 500 cases operated at the Otologic Medical Group was 0.4% (2/500).

The obvious disadvantage of the translabyrinthine approach is the sacrifice of any residual hearing in the operated ear. We believe that the loss of hearing is a small price to pay for the other advantages of the approach, particularly for cases in which the chance of saving hearing with other approaches is slight.

Surgical Technique

The patient is placed in the supine position on the opeating

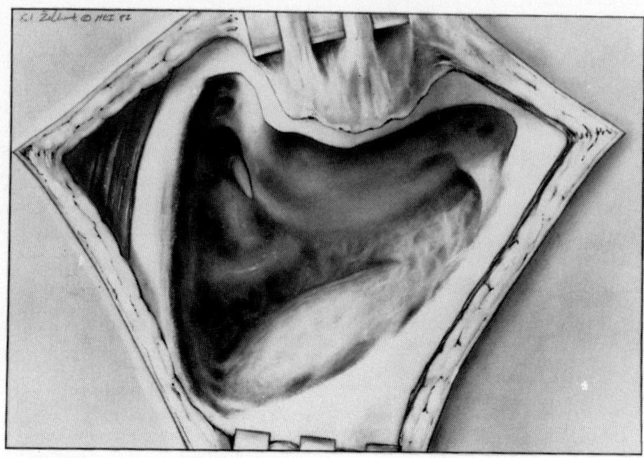

FIG 6–1.
Mastoidectomy is completed, and the lateral and posterior semicircular canals are identified.

room table with the ear to be operated on facing up. An extended mastoid shave is performed, facial nerve monitoring electrodes placed, the skin prepared with povidone-iodine (Betadine) solution, and plastic drapes applied.

A postauricular incision is made approximately 2.5 cm behind the postauricular crease. A complete simple mastoidectomy is carried out. Posteriorly, bone is removed over the sigmoid sinus to the posterior fossa dura. Final bone removal over the sigmoid sinus is undertaken with a large diamond burr. The lateral semicircular canal and fossa incudis are identified.

The labyrinthectomy is begun by removal of bone in the sinodural angle along the superior petrosal sinus (Fig 6–1). As the dissection is carried medially, hard labyrinthine bone is encountered and the posterior semicircular canal opened. Dissection is carried forward to the lateral semicircular canal, which is removed from postero superiorly toward the facial nerve. As the dissection is carried medially, the common crus is identified, and the superior semicircular canal is opened and removed. The vestibule is then opened, and the facial nerve is skeletonized from the mastoid genu to near the stylomastoid foramen. After the labyrinthectomy and the medial skeletonization of the facial nerve are completed, dissection of the internal canal is started. The posterior fossa dura behind the internal auditory canal is identified and the vestibular aqueduct identified and removed. The dissection is carried inferiorly to the jugular bulb and forward to the cochlear aqueduct. The cochlear aqueduct is not always readily identifiable. In large tumors it will be occluded at its medial oriface, and cerebrospinal fluid (CSF) is not likely to escape. It is an important landmark because it identifies the location of the 9th, 10th, and 11th cranial nerves in the neural compartment of the jugular foramen anterior to the jugular bulb. If the dissection is confined to the area superior and the posterior to the cochlear aqueduct, these nerves will not be injured. After the cochlear aqueduct is identified, the removal is carried medially around the internal auditory canal to the porus acusticus until the entire inferior lip of the internal auditory canal is removed. Dissection is then carried superiorly and anteriorly around the internal auditory canal. Removal of

the superior lip of the porus acusticus is tedious, but it is one of the most important parts of the dissection. If this is not entirely removed, the facial nerve will underlie the ridge of bone at the porus and will make identification and removal of the tumor from the nerve in the area very difficult. The dissection of the lateral end of the internal auditory canal is begun inferiorly with identification of the singular nerve, which is followed to the inferior vestibular nerve. The transverse crest and the superior vestibular nerve are identified above the inferior vestibular nerve. The superior aspect of the internal auditory canal is then dissected and the facial nerve identified as it exits the internal auditory canal and begins in the labyrinthine segment. Finally, Bill's bar, or island, which separates the vestibular nerve from the facial nerve, is identified. Bone is removed from two thirds of the circumference of the internal auditory canal. The wound is irrigated profusely with bacitracin solution to remove all bone chips and loose debris.

The dura is opened along the superior petrosal sinus, around the porus acusticus, and inferiorly along the jugular bulb. When opening the dura, be careful not to injure the petrosal vein along the superior petrosal sinus and the antero inferior cerebellar artery, which can loop up to the dura inferiorly. This dural flap is designed to protect the cerebellum and the petrosal vein and is placed between the cerebellum and the posterior tumor mass.

With a long fine hook passing inferiorly to Bill's bar, the superior vestibular nerve can be separated from the facial nerve (Fig 6–2). Removal of the superior vestibular nerve laterally from its canal allows identification of the facial nerve anteriorly and the plane between the facial nerve and tumor.

When an acoustic tumor is 2 cm or less, it may be separated from the facial nerve without first reducing its size, but when

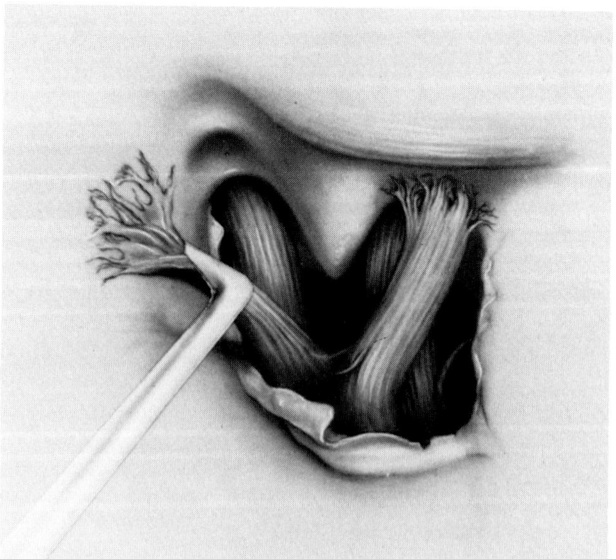

FIG 6–2.
A long fine hook passing inferiorly to Bill's bar separates the superior vestibular nerve from the facial nerve.

the tumor is larger, it usually must be reduced first before it can be mobilized off of the facial nerve.

The capsule of the tumor is incised over an avascular area. The main bulk of the tumor is removed with small dissectors and forceps. In large tumors the Urban dissector is used to gut the tumor prior to capsule removal. The posterior portion is removed initially, and attention is turned to separation of the tumor from the facial nerve.

The dura of the internal auditory canal is divided along margins of the bony dissection to allow release of the tumor within the internal auditory canal posteriorly. The superior and inferior edges of the facial nerve are then identified, and the arachnoid sheath that binds the nerve to the surface of the tumor is carefully divided by sharp dissection. Small hooks are used to separate the facial nerve from the tumor by gently retracting the tumor posteriorly and laterally. It is important not to push the tumor medially into the cerebellopontine angle, because it stretches the nerve where it exits the internal auditory canal and may lead to facial paralysis.

The facial nerve usually separates readily from the tumor in the internal canal, but the tumor is usually quite adherent to the nerve at the porus acusticus, and often the plane between the nerve and tumor is indistinct in this area. Rather than continue the dissection at this point, it is best to roll the tumor posteriorly while gently retracting it laterally to identify the facial nerve near the brain stem; the facial nerve originates medially and slightly caudad to the eighth cranial nerve and appears very wide at this point. After the facial nerve has been identified near the brain stem, dissection should be continued from medial to lateral toward the point of adherence of the facial nerve at the porus acusticus. The plane between the nerve and tumor usually becomes apparent at the porus acusticus as its dissection is carried out. In most cases, the facial nerve will lie anteriorly to an acoustic tumor. Occasionally when the tumor originates on the inferior vestibular nerve, the facial nerve may course over the tumor. In these occasional cases, the tumor should be rotated gently anteriorly.

Following tumor removal the wound is profusely irrigated with Ringer's solution to remove blood clots. Hemostasis is accomplished with bipolar cautery or clips. The dural defect and the mastoidectomy are obliterated with strips of abdominal fat. The skin is closed in three layers. A bulky mastoid dressing is applied.

MIDDLE FOSSA APPROACH

Most acoustic tumors arise from the vestibular nerves, and if diagnosed while still intracanicular, these tumors may be removed through the middle fossa approach in an attempt to preserve hearing.[3] The advantages of this approach are several. First, most of the dissection is extra dural, thereby lowering morbidity. Second, the lateral end of the internal auditory canal is exposed, which ensures removal of all the tumor. Third, positive identification of the facial nerve is possible at the lateral end of the internal auditory canal. This facilitates tumor dissection from the facial nerve (Fig 6–3).

The first disadvantage of this approach is that the surgeon

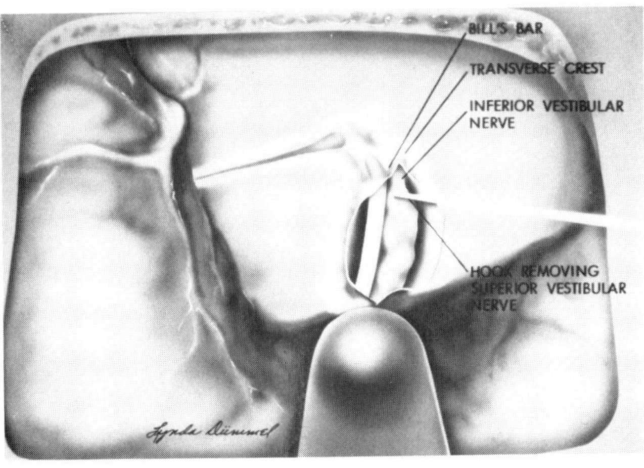

FIG 6–3.
Middle cranial fossa approach for acoustic tumor removal. Hearing preservation depends not only on maintaining integrity of cochlear nerve but, more important, on maintaining the blood supply to the cochlea.

must work past the facial nerve to remove the tumor. This subjects the facial nerve to more manipulation that does the translabyrinthine approach. A second problem sometimes encountered with the middle fossa approach is postoperative unsteadiness resulting from a partial preservation of vestibular function. This problem also occurs with the retrosigmoid approach, but it rarely occurs after total vestibular denervation with the translabyrinthine approach. Careful section of the remaining nerve fibres reduces the incidence of postoperative unsteadiness but also increases the risk of hearing loss. The final problem of the middle fossa approach is limited access to the posterior fossa in the event of bleeding either at surgery or after surgery. Despite these disadvantages, we recommend the middle fossa approach for small intracanicular acoustic tumors.

LARGE ACOUSTIC TUMOR REMOVAL

Tumor size, measured on cranial computed tomography (CT) or magnetic resonance imaging (MRI), has been reported as extension into the cerebellopontine angle. Small tumors are those that extend less than 0.5 cm into the cerebellopontine angle; medium tumors are those that extend 0.5 to 2.0 cm into the cerebellopontine angle; large tumors are those extending from 2 to 4 cm into the cerebellopontine angle; and tumors that extend more than 4 cm into the cerebellopontine angle are considered giant tumors.

We prefer the translabyrinthine approach for the large and giant tumors.[1] Because it is highly unlikely due to the almost inevitable damage to inner ear blood supply that hearing can be preserved in patients with tumors larger than 2 cm, we do not believe that the increased risk associated with the other approaches warrants the attempt to save hearing in such patients.

Removal of a larger tumor requires intracapsular decompression of the tumor to reduce its size before the superior and inferior planes are developed. The posterior surface of the tumor is carefully inspected for nerve bundles. On rare occasions, the facial nerve may lie on the posterior surface of the tumor. Beginning the dissection at Bill's bar establishes the location and direction of the facial nerve. If, on careful inspection, no nerve bundles are present, the capsule of the posterior tumor surface is incised, and intracapsular removal of the tumor is begun with the House-Urban dissector. During intracapsular removal of the tumor, it is important to avoid excessive movement and pressure on the tumor because they may stretch and injure the facial nerve. We believe facial nerve monitoring has been very helpful in decreasing injury to the facial nerve. Once the interior of the tumor has been extensively gutted, development of the tumor plane is carried out further inferiorly and superiorly. Since the tumor has been extensively gutted, the capsule is displaced into the interior of the tumor. The surface of the capsule is then followed to the brain stem. Inferiorly, an attempt is made to localize the ninth cranial nerve, which can be best identified near its exit medial to the jugular bulb. In larger tumors, the ninth cranial nerve may be stretched over the surface of the tumor. This plane is carefully developed, and the ninth cranial nerve is isolated from the field with cottonoids. During manipulation of the ninth and tenth cranial nerves, there are often changes in the pulse rate. If these occur, we stop manipulation of the nerves and allow the vital signs to stabilize.

Often large vessels, particularly the anteroinferior cerebellar artery, are located around the inferior aspect of the tumor, and these must be carefully separated from the tumor capsule and preserved. After the inferior aspect of the tumor has been developed down to the brain stem, additional debulking of the tumor and removal of a portion of the capsule can be completed. The superior aspect of the tumor capsule is next developed. The petrosal vein will be encountered in this location and must be carefully separated from the tumor. The facial nerve usually lies more anteriorly, but it is not unusual for it to come over the top of the tumor. The fifth cranial nerve is identified at the medial superior aspect of the tumor. In most cases the plane between the fifth nerve and the tumor is easily developed, and trauma to the fifth nerve is uncommon. Preservation of corneal sensation is important in avoiding corneal damage, especially in patients with facial paralysis.

Once the facial nerve has been separated from the tumor to the brain stem, the bulk of the tumor is removed with the House-Urban dissector, leaving only a small portion of the tumor attached to the brainstem. Removing the bulk of the tumor allows greater visibility of the tumor-brain stem plane.

Large acoustic tumors may cause considerable displacement of the brain stem. Fortunately, adhesions between the tumor and the brain stem are not usually dense and can be easily lysed. Bleeding in this area is controlled with bipolar cautery. Only those vessels that actually enter the tumor capsule are coagulated. Removal of the tumor from the brain stem may cause changes in the vital signs. It has been shown that cardiac changes precede respiratory changes by several minutes. When changes in vital signs are noted by the anesthesiologist, manipulation is stopped, and any cottonoids packing the tumor are removed to eliminate pressure on surrounding vessels outside the tumor capsule. Several minutes are allowed to lapse before dissection is started again. Usually attention is turned to an area where cardiac changes are not produced and where the size of the tumor can be reduced. If changes in the vital signs persist in the previous dissection area, tumor manipulation is stopped after the tumor has been debulked as much as possible. Surgery is terminated, and the wound closed in the usual manner. A second-stage procedure is carried out in 6 to 12 months. At this time, decreased tumor size allows increased brain stem circulation, and residual tumor removal is usually possible without further vital sign changes.

Complications

Venous Bleeding

Bleeding may be encountered from several sources, including mastoid emissary veins, sigmoid sinus, jugular bulb, superior petrosal sinus, and petrosal vein. Fortunately, the use of the supine position prevents air embolism. The most efficient method to control the mastoid emissary veins is to cauterize using bipolar cautery and divide the vessels prior to their entry into the sigmoid sinus. If an emissary vein is torn at its junction with the sigmoid sinus, bleeding usually can be controlled with bipolar cautery. If this is not successful, the lumen may be packed with a strip of oxidized cellulose (Surgicel); small pieces are not used, because embolization may occur if the Surgicel inadvertently slips into the lumen of the sinus. If further bone removal in the area is necessary, bone wax is placed over the Surgicel to prevent displacement during drilling. Small tears in the sigmoid sinus may be controlled with Surgicel packing or with microfibrillar collagen (Avitene). In cases where bleeding cannot be controlled, the incision may be extended into the neck and the internal jugular vein ligated. Following ligation, the sinus may be packed intraluminally as well as extraluminally without fear of embolization.

The level of the jugular bulb is variable and may actually reach the level of the internal auditory canal. In these cases, it is necessary to skeletonize the jugular bulb and to work behind it to remove the interior aspect of the internal auditory canal. It is difficult to compress the jugular bulb as one can the sigmoid sinus. If the bulb is inadvertently injured, a large piece of Surgicel packed around the margins of the bony defect will control bleeding. This packing is done carefully to avoid undue pressure on cranial nerves IX, X, and XI in the pars nervosa of the jugular foramen. If packing does not control bleeding, the internal jugular vein is ligated and the lumen of the jugular bulb packed.

If bleeding occurs from the superior petrosal sinus, it is best to totally occlude it. Distal control near the sigmoid sinus is best accomplished with neurosurgical clips passed on either side of the sinus. Proximal control may be obtained by using Surgicel to occlude the lumen of the sinus after distal ligation or by packing Surgicel between the sinus and the petrous ridge at the most anterior aspect of the dissection above the internal auditory canal. This compresses the sinus and prevents proximal bleeding.

The petrosal vein is large and drains the cerebellar hemisphere. It enters the superior petrosal sinus above the internal auditory canal. In most cases it is possible to keep the dura flat over the vein, compressing it against the cerebellum and protecting it from surgical trauma. If the petrosal vein is damaged, it may be clipped or bipolarally coagulated.

Anteroinferior Cerebellar Artery

The lateral branch of the anteroinferior cerebellar artery is intimately associated with the internal auditory canal. The branch may loop into the internal auditory canal and is usually on the anterior surface of the cochlear nerve close to the tumor. If one stays in the plane between the surrounding arachnoid sheath and the tumor capsule, only small tumor-feeding vessels are divided. These may be separated from the tumor surface and clipped or cauterized with bipolar cautery without causing retrograde thrombosis to the main lateral branch of the anteroinferior cerebellar artery.

Removal of tumor from the brain stem may cause changes in the vital signs. These changes are related to ischemia of the brain stem in the distribution of the anteroinferior cerebellar artery. Manipulation of the tumor may cause compression of the anteroinferior cerebellar artery with changes in pulse and blood pressure. Complete interruption of the blood vessel may cause infarction of the lateral tegmental pons with resultant death (Atkinson's syndrome). Continuous monitoring of the vital signs to prevent this problem is discussed under surgery for large acoustic tumors.

Cerebrospinal Fluid Leaks

Closure of the wound begins with partially reapproximating the edges of the dural flap. Abdominal fat is then used to obliterate the remaining dural and bony defect.[4] The fat is cut into thin strips approximately 1 cm in width and 5 cm in length. These adipose strips are packed into the defect in layers, working from the posterior to the anterior aspect. Small pieces are placed into the vestibule of the inner ear and the fossa incudis. The skin is closed in three layers, taking special care not to push the adipose packing around the partially closed dural flap into the cerebellopontine angle, which could place pressure on the facial nerve. A compression mastoid dressing is left in place for 72 hours. If any CSF is noted at this time, the dressing is replaced for an additional 72 hours. Persistent leakage after this time almost always requires wound revision. Additional abdominal fat saved from the original procedure is placed in the area of leakage, and a mastoid dressing is reapplied for 72 hours. Only rarely has a lumbar subarachnoid catheter for CSF decompression been necessary in persistent leaks.

Less than 10% of patients will develop a CSF leak. Most of these leaks will respond to a compression dressing. In a recent series of 230 acoustic tumor surgery patients, only 1 had a postoperative leak that required surgical closure.[4]

Facial Nerve

One of the great advantages of the translabyrinthine approach for acoustic tumor removal is that consistent identification of the facial nerve at the lateral end of the internal auditory canal can be made. The lateral end of the internal auditory canal is dissected, and the plane of the facial nerve is skeletonized in its labyrinthine portion. It allows identification of Bill's bar, which separates the facial nerve from the superior vestibular nerve.

Smaller tumors usually separate easily from the facial nerve. However, in some cases when the tumor is large, the facial nerve fibers are completely splayed widely over the surface of the tumor like a thin ribbon. A difficult decision must be made in managing the facial nerve during acoustic tumor removal when the nerve is obviously greatly thinned and damaged but appears to be uninterrupted and free of tumor. Hopefully with advances in facial nerve monitoring interoperatively, we will develop prognostic indicators for facial nerve function that will improve our facial nerve results.[5]

By use of the techniques described, facial nerve continuity can be maintained in 97% of all cases. Most of those patients will have normal facial function 1 year after surgery. If the facial nerve is thought to be intact at the completion of the operation but the patient awakes with a total facial nerve paralysis, the prognosis for complete return of facial function is poor.

The first concern in the early postoperative period is protection of the eye, particularly if there is an associated corneal hypesthesia from fifth cranial nerve involvement. In these cases, an opthalmologist is consulted early, and the appropriate measures are instituted.

The patient is observed for at least 1 year for return of facial function before a nerve substitution procedure is considered. Fortunately, the majority of patients in whom facial nerve continuity was preserved will recover facial function. Patients who begin to notice return of function within several weeks postoperatively should expect a satisfactory recovery. However, patients who do not notice any return of function until 3 to 6 months postoperatively usually have an imcomplete return of function. Hypoglossal-facial anastomosis is reserved for those patients who do not have return of facial movement in 12 to 18 months despite an apparently intact nerve at the completion of surgery.[6]

If the facial nerve is severed during the course of acoustic tumor removal, it is best to repair it immediately.[2] Repair is accomplished by either end-to-end anastomosis of the nerve following rerouting of the distal segment or by the insertion of a great auricular nerve graft (Fig 6–4).

BILATERAL ACOUSTIC TUMORS

In cases of bilateral acoustic tumor or a tumor present in the only hearing ear, alternatives are considered in an attempt to save residual hearing. An alternative to be considered in some cases of bilateral acoustic tumor is middle fossa decompression of the internal auditory canal with opening of the dura. Several patients who have undergone this procedure have maintained their hearing while the tumor has grown slowly. This method stalls the inevitable loss of hearing.

In many cases of bilateral tumors, the cochlear nerve courses directly through the tumor, and so even partial tumor removal will result in loss of hearing; in other cases, the cochlear nerve

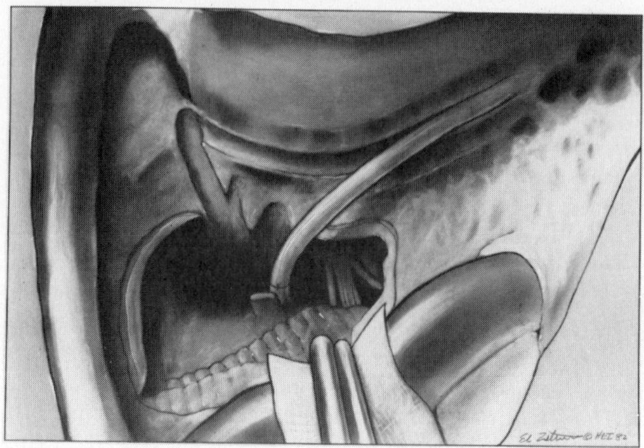

FIG 6–4.
Facial nerve repair in the cerebellopontine angle. Rerouted fascia allows for tension-free anastomosis.

apparently lies at the periphery of the tumor, as in unilateral cases. We evaluated a young teenager without any symptoms but with a strong family history of von Recklinghausen's disease. She had bilateral very small intracanicular tumors. She underwent successful middle fossa removal of the acoustic tumors with hearing preservation.[7] In most cases of bilateral tumor, preservation of hearing is impossible because the nerve either courses through the tumor or has been invaded by tumor. In bilateral tumor cases or in cases where the tumor involves the only hearing ear, an attempt at hearing preservation is probably warranted, even though a small scrap of tumor may remain on the cochlear nerve.

Another alternative is use of the stereotactic gamma knife radiation in lieu of surgery for bilateral acoustic tumors or cases of tumor involving the only hearing ear.[8] Unfortunately, not all of the patients who have been treated with gamma knife radiation have maintained their hearing.[9]

HEARING PRESERVATION

Early diagnosis with accurate imaging techniques has modified the philosophy that all acoustic tumors should be removed immediately after discovery. We still remove tumors on detection in people 20 to 50 years old, the most common age range for development. Older patients who thoroughly understand the slight risk of allowing a small tumor to grow may elect follow-up only with imaging every 6 months. If the tumor appears to enlarge, surgical removal is indicated. For most patients, acoustic tumors, like all tumors, are best treated when they are small. The larger the tumor, the greater the incidence of mortality and morbidity.

Today the most frequent deficit after acoustic tumor surgery is unilateral deafness. With tumors confined to the internal auditory canal, or with small tumors that extend less than 1.5 cm into the cerebellopontine angle, we may attempt preser-

vation of hearing through the middle fossa approach or the retrosigmoid approach.

Shelton has recently reviewed the middle fossa series of the Otologic Medical Group.[10] The middle fossa approach has been used in approximately 5% (106/2,157) of the cases. Good preoperative and postoperative audiometric data are available on 97 patients. Although the cochlear nerve was preserved anatomically in 89% of the cases, measurable postoperative hearing was preserved in only 59% of the cases. Hearing was preserved to within 10 dB of the preoperative speech reception threshold and within 15% of the preoperative speech discrimination score in 35% of the cases.

Although 59% of the cases had any degree of measurable hearing postoperatively, 43% had speech reception threshold (SRT) less than or equal to 50 dB and speech discrimination score greater than or equal to 50%; only 31% had a postoperative SRT less than or equal to 30 dB and speech discrimination score greater than 70%.

It is important to understand that not only must the cochlear nerve be preserved but also the blood supply to the inner ear maintained. Maintaining circulation is the more difficult task because the cochlear blood supply is often involved by tumor.

We have recently begun using the retrosigmoid approach in selected cases attempting to preserve hearing. We believe the best candidate for a retrosigmoid approach is the patient with a 1.5 cm or smaller tumor in the cerebellopontine angle, especially if there is little or no extension from the angle into the internal auditory canal. Visualization of the lateralmost portion of the internal auditory canal is more difficult with the retrosigmoid than the middle fossa approach; therefore, we prefer the middle fossa approach removal of intracanicular tumors that have less than 1-cm extension into the cerebellopontine angle.

There is a wide range of audiometric criteria for hearing preservation surgery. We believe the best candidate for hearing preservation has a speech reception threshold of 30 dB and a speech discrimination score equal to or greater than 70%. The chances for hearing preservation would appear to be improved in those patients who have hypoactive calorics on electronystagmography (ENG) testing and an auditory brain stem response intraaural wave V latency difference of less than 0.4 ms.

The focus of acoustic tumor surgery has changed from being concerned about a high mortality rate to being concerned about decreasing morbidity, especially the incidence of facial nerve paralysis, to finally being concerned about hearing preservation. Improvements in surgical technique, instruments, and the use of the operating microscope have markedly decreased both mortality and morbidity. Increased physician awareness of symptoms, improvements in diagnostic screening procedures (audiometric brain stem response), and newer imaging techniques (CT scan and MRI) have allowed the physician to make an accurate diagnosis of an acoustic tumor earlier than in the past decade. As a result, more patients will have smaller tumors and less hearing loss at the time of diagnosis. The development of interoperative monitoring of eighth nerve function has heightened the interest in hearing preservation in acoustic tumor surgery.[11, 12]

SUMMARY

Advances in surgical techniques and the use of the operating microscope have markedly decreased the mortality and morbidity of acoustic tumor surgery. Advances in diagnostic and imaging techniques have allowed the accurate diagnosis of tumors when they are smaller and produce fewer symptoms. Therefore, the major focus in acoustic tumor surgery now is on hearing preservation. We prefer the middle fossa approach for removal of intracanicular tumors and the retrosigmoid approach for removal of tumors that have a 1 to 1.5 cm extension into the cerebellopontine angle in an attempt to preserve hearing in patients with good preoperative hearing levels. For patients with nonserviceable hearing or in patients with unilateral tumors that extend more than 1.5 cm into the cerebellopontine angle, we prefer the translabyrinthine approach because it has the lowest mortality and morbidity. At the present time, the majority of our patients undergo a translabyrinthine removal of their acoustic tumor. For patients with bilateral acoustic tumors or tumors present in the only hearing ear, alternative techniques are considered in a desperate attempt to preserve the hearing.

REFERENCES

1. House WF: History of acoustic tumor surgery, in House WF, Luetje CM (eds): *Acoustic Tumors,* vol 1: *Diagnosis.* Baltimore, University Park Press, 1979, pp 1–75.
1a. House WF: Translabyrinthine approach, in House WF, Luetje CM (eds): *Acoustic Tumors,* vol II: *Management.* Baltimore, University Park Press, 1979, pp 43–87.
2. Barrs DM, Brackmann DE, Hitselberger WE: Facial nerve anastomosis in the cerebellopontine angle: A review of 24 cases. *Am J Otol* 1985; 5:269–272.
3. Brackmann DE: Middle cranial fossa approach, in House WF, Luetje CM (eds): *Acoustic Tumors,* vol II: *Management.* Baltimore, University Park Press, 1979, p 15.
4. House JL, Hitselberger WE, House WF: Wound closure and cerebrospinal fluid leak after translabyrinthine surgery. *Am J Otol* 1982; 4:126–128.
5. Harner SG, Daube JR, Beatty CW, et al: Intraoperative monitoring of the facial nerve. *Laryngoscope* 1988; 98:209–212.
6. Luxford WM, Brackmann DE: Facial nerve substitution: A review of 66 cases. *Am J Otol* Nov 1985; Suppl: 55–57.
7. Dutcher PO Jr, House, WF, Hitselberger WE: Early detection of small bilateral acoustic tumors. *Am J Otol* 1987; 8:35–38.
8. Kamerer DB, Lunsford LD, Møller M: Gamma knife: An alternative treatment for acoustic neurinomas. *Ann Otol Rhinol Laryngol* 1988; 97:631–635.
9. Brackmann DE: Personal communication, 1988.
10. Shelton C, Brackmann DE, House WF, et al: Middle fossa acoustic tumor surgery: Results in 106 cases. *Laryngoscope* 1989; 99:405–408.
11. Silverstein H, McDaniels A, Norrell H, et al: Hearing preservation after acoustic neuroma surgery with intraoperative direct eighth cranial nerve monitoring: II. A classification of results. *Otolaryngol Head Neck Surg* 1986; 95:285–291.
12. Hammerschlag PE, Berg HM, Prichep LS, et al: Real-time monitoring of brainstem auditory evoked response (BAER) during cerebellopontine angle (CPA) surgery. 1986; 95:538–542.

Acoustic Tumor

Approach of

Leonard I. Malis, M.D.

Twenty-five years ago neurosurgical removal of acoustic neuromas carried a high mortality and a poor end result for a strikingly high number of patients. William House and the Los Angeles Otological Group demonstrated that the use of the microscope with a translabyrinthine approach could produce a major improvement in the results. The neurosurgical community was forced, protesting bitterly, into the microsurgical era. It is my contention that neurosurgeons, using all of the advantages of microsurgical procedure, have now equaled even further the improvements of the otologic approaches, with the added advantages of preservation of hearing as well as a higher percentage of total removal, particularly in the larger tumors.

DIAGNOSIS

Auditory brain stem evoked response testing is the least expensive method of ruling out an acoustic neuroma. If the evoked response suggests a retrocochlear lesion, the best study for present-day demonstration of the lesion is the gadolinium-enhanced MRI examination, which will demonstrate even the smallest acoustic neuroma quite readily. Nevertheless, at the present time the high-resolution contrast-enhanced thin-section CT scan provides information regarding the distance that can be drilled to spare the vestibule as well as the size and position of the acoustic neuroma in a fashion that gives the operative information required most accurately. If one is reasonably certain an acoustic neuroma is present, the use of the CT scan is, at present, more cost effective. If the diagnosis is doubtful, the gadolinium-enhanced MRI is the answer but may still have to be followed by the high-resolution CT scan to get the bony structural information for more adequate surgery. We no longer use air or dye cisternography.

Pure tone audiometry and speech discrimination testing are carried out to provide comparison for postoperative preservation. The sophisticated audiologic studies formerly used are not now required. Vestibular testing with or without ENG has been abandoned in the interest of cost-effective simplification. Angiography, once almost routine, is now reserved for glomus tumors and large meningiomas.

Decision on the need for surgery is age related. In patients less than 40 years of age with an acoustic neuroma, I believe the tumor should be removed at the earliest reasonable moment, no matter how small the tumor. For older patients, 70 years or so, the duration of the history and the size of the tumor, as well as the physical condition of the patient, require additional evaluation. A patient who has had decreased hearing for 20 years in whom a 1 cm tumor is demonstrated at the age of 70 years will be most unlikely to have an increase in size of that tumor during his or her expected lifetime. It is reasonable, therefore, to do yearly MRI or CT, assuming there is no further change in anything else to require earlier evaluation. One of my patients now with 10 years of CT follow-up has actually decreased his tumor size from 1.6 cm down to 1.4 cm over the long interval. On the other hand, a college student who had a 1.4 cm tumor at the beginning of the school year in September had been advised to wait so as not to interfere with his schooling. He had a 1.8 cm tumor at Christmas and was still advised to delay. He had a 3 cm tumor and virtually complete hearing loss in that ear when he was referred in June.

At the opposite extreme, I have had only one 70-year-old who had a doubling in size of his tumor in 1 year between CT scans before referral. I am currently following 24 unoperated tumors, all in older people, all with long histories, none of whom has shown measurable change on CT or MRI over more than 1 year and, in some cases, more than 10 years of follow-

up. Some of these patients may, indeed, come to surgery if growth rate begins, but at the present their growth rate has been so slow as to suggest that they will never require surgery. Again, I would like to emphasize that if these patients had good hearing with modest tumors, I would not delay but would operate quite early in the course.

SURGICAL TECHNIQUE

In an earlier era, neurosurgeons used either a straight up sitting position or a prone position for their approach to the tumor. Both have been almost completely abandoned. My own preference is for a semisitting position with the back up only 30 degrees, with the knees above heart level and the patient supported in a pressure suit. The fear of air embolism from the sitting position has been minimized by this low position and the pressure suit. One can monitor it with the Doppler unit, listening over the right atrium to detect the least amount of entering air, and with the end expiratory carbon dioxide monitor to determine if the amount of air might be serious. Air embolization has, accordingly, not been a significant problem in thousands of operations in this position in our department.

Other neurosurgeons have adopted a position sometimes called the park bench position, essentially supine oblique, with the head rotated so that the mastoid of the affected side is almost upright. This position has the advantage of relatively little possibility of air embolization, though I find it more awkward for large tumors that may go through the tentorial notch, and therefore have preferred the semisitting position.

Preoperative and perioperative considerations are important to the end result. The banning of aspirin or aspirin-containing compounds for 1 week or more preoperatively as well as the stopping of the use of heparin flushes for keeping arterial or venous lines open intraoperatively has greatly decreased the threat of postoperative hemorrhage. The use of an intraoperative antibiotic regime with no preoperative or postoperative antibiotics has, in my series, essentially eliminated the threat of operative infections. Anesthesia is essentially fentanyl and nitrous oxide with total curarization and completely controlled respiration, permitting maintenance of blood gasses at optimal levels. The absence of brain stem damage or brain stem changes long ago eliminated the need for respiratory monitoring for protection of brain stem function. Intraoperative auditory evoked potential monitoring, sometimes mentioned as useful for recognition of brain stem involvement, has not been necessary.

The use of auditory evoked potentials to monitor the preservation of hearing seemed completely logical; however, a trial of 100 consecutive cases monitored for auditory responses did not demonstrate any difference in the percentage of hearing preservation between the monitored cases and those not monitored, probably because the surgical technique was identical and in all cases based on the technical surgical considerations most likely to preserve hearing.

I use a 7- to 8-cm straight line incision just medial to the mastoid posteriorly. The mastoid process and the adjacent suboccipital bone are exposed and a 4 cm craniectomy, including resection of the mastoid process, is made, exposing the sigmoid sinus completely. Dural separation as the craniectomy is carried out permits preservation of the unopened dura without injury to the sigmoid sinus. The rather constant emmisary vein can be sealed with the bipolar coagulator as the bone removal is carried out. Dural incision is semicircular with its base medially, with two relaxing incisions carried lateralward toward the sigmoid sinus. The mastoid cells are waxed with bone wax, and then traction sutures are used to sew the lateral tab of dura to the adjacent muscles, drawing the lateral sinus over the cut surface of the mastoid and providing exposure in a direct line along the petrous pyramid without the need for significant cerebellar retraction.

In an earlier era, bone removal went quite medial and included the foramen magnum rim. Resection of the lateral third of cerebellum was recommended by the premicrosurgical authors in neurosurgery, who also recommended that the bony resection be carried only to the medial margin of the lateral sinus. The resulting curve of the posterior fossa required either marked cerebellar retraction or cerebellar resection. With the present purely lateral opening and with much less need for wide exposure with microtechnique, neither cerebellar resection nor cerebellar retraction is required.

The arachnoid is now opened above the 9th nerve if the tumor is small or further down toward the foramen magnum if the tumor is quite large and obscures the 9th, 10th, and 11th nerves. Drainage of CSF from the open arachnoid provides all the additional room required. Spinal drainage, ventricular puncture, or shunt are not required.

The arachnoid dissection is carried upward along the margin of the tumor at the cerebellum and permits the cerebellum to be supported in the plane of the petrous pyramid by a self-retaining (never hand-held) retractor, which is used for support and to keep the cerebellum protected rather than for retraction. The space available between the petrous pyramid and the cerebellum is usually about 1.5 cm, which is all that is necessary for even the large 5 to 6 cm tumors.

In this posterior arachnoid, there are generally two fine arteries only 200 μm or so in diameter: (1) the arcuate arteries, residual anastomoses between the external circulation; and (2) the posteroinferior cerebellar artery (Fig 6–5).* They carry no significant supply and are in no way related to the anteroinferior cerebellar artery loop. They are coagulated and divided since they are part of the exposure pathway.

The petrosal vein, joined by the vein of the lateral recess, enters the superior petrosal sinus most frequently just a bit posterior to the opening of Meckel's cave. If the tumor is fairly large, the vein has usually been lengthened to the point that there is adequate room and it can be preserved. With a very small tumor, however, the petrosal vein may hold the cerebellum within a few millimeters of the petrous. Coagulation and division of the petrosal vein has not produced any deficit, because there is always a very adequate collateral. Most often it is preserved on the basis that no anatomic structure should be sacrificed unless absolutely necessary.

*For Figs 6–5 to 6–16, the right cerebellopontine angle is shown. The vertex is up, and the self-retaining cerebellar retractor is in the upper left-hand corner. Unless otherwise stated, the horizontal diameter viewed in the photographs is 2.0 cm.

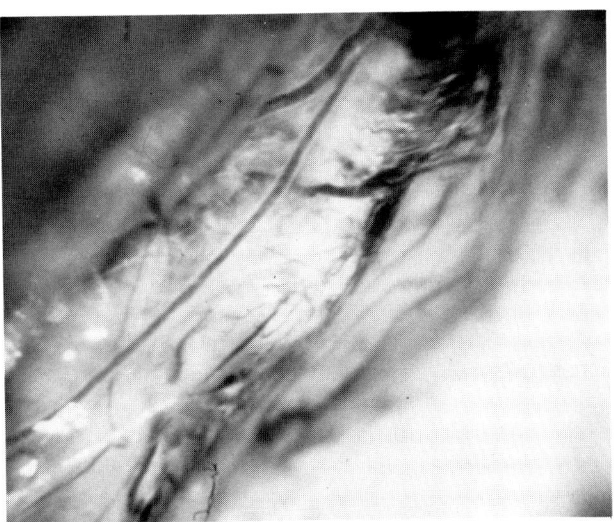

FIG 6–5.
A leash of small vessels attaches the tumor to the petrous pyramid on the right. The arcuate arteries run in the arachnoid, which has not yet been opened over the tumor and flocculus.

The anteroinferior cerebellar artery is in close relationship with virtually all acoustic neuromas. The artery is a direct branch of the basilar, usually arising about midway between the junction of the two vertebral arteries and the basilar apex. Its course is variable, but most frequently it curves laterally in the normal individual to reach almost to the internal auditory meatus and then to return medially between the eighth and ninth nerves to reach the brain stem and cerebellum anterior to the flocculus. With an acoustic neuroma it most frequently forms a loop curving laterally inferior to the neuroma (Fig 6–6), but its course is variable enough so that the lateral curve of the loop may be within the internal auditory canal, or it may perforate the dura

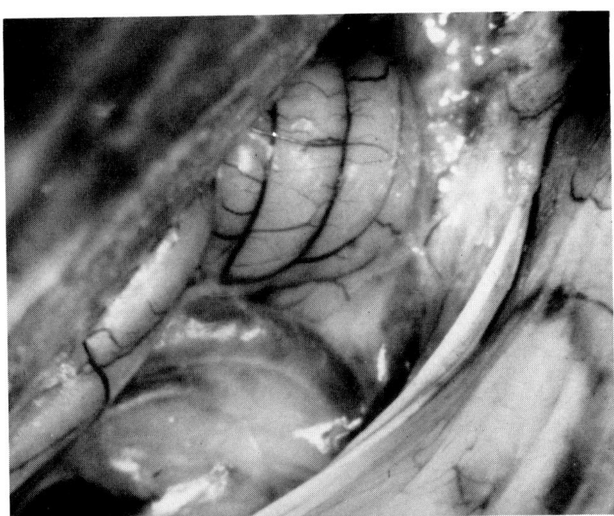

FIG 6–6.
The anteroinferior cerebellar artery can be seen through the arachnoid above the ninth nerve and below the cerebellum, with the tumor coming into view just superiorly and anteriorly.

and bone of the posterior wall of the canal before turning backward to the brain stem (Fig 6–7). The probability of severe brain stem damage if the anteroinferior cerebellar artery is occluded is quite high. There is an anastomotic network in the lateral cerebellar hemisphere between the superior cerebellar, the anteroinferior cerebellar, and the posteroinferior cerebellar arteries that may be able to carry the supply retrograde if the anterointerior cerebellar is damaged. Again, in an older era, when lateral resection of the cerebellum was carried out, this anastomotic network was destroyed and the risk much increased. Nevertheless, preservation of the anteroinferior cerebellar artery is a requisite, regardless of the approach.

Sharp dissection of the arachnoid attachments frees the usual anteroinferior cerebellar artery variations. If the artery perforates the internal auditory canal wall, a bit of bone is cut from the canal and turned medially with the arterial loop (Fig 6–8).

Finally, branches of the anteroinferior cerebellar artery supply the medial part of the tumor. Later in the dissection, under high magnification, the branches are sealed with the bipolar coagulator under saline irrigation and divided, protecting the main trunk.

The 9th, 10th, and 11th nerves enter the jugular foramen lateral to and just superior to the hypoglossal foramen. The hypoglossal nerve tends to cross the vertebral artery at the origin of the posteroinferior cerebellar artery, whereas the posteroinferior cerebellar artery curves upward on the brain stem inferior to the medullary attachment of the 11th nerve. Unless the tumor is more than 2.5 cm in diameter intracranially, these inferior

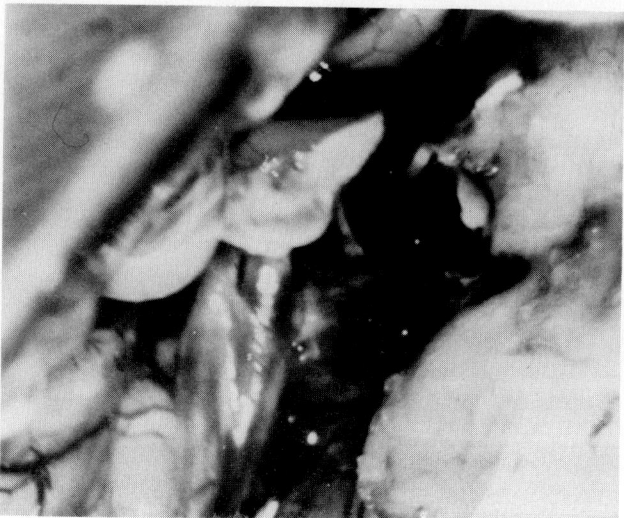

FIG 6–8.
This is the same patient as in Figure 6–7. The posterior rim of the internal auditory canal has been carved away together with the loop of the anterior cerebral artery and reflected medially to reach the retractor.

nerves and the posteroinferior cerebellar artery are not involved by the tumor. After dissection of the arachnoid, these nerves may simply be protected during the rest of the dissection by covering them with a strip of glove rubber, which keeps them moist and does not adhere or traumatize.

In my series, when it has been possible to determine the nerve of origin, more than 90% arose from the superior vestibular nerve in the lateral part of the canal. They tend to displace a sheath of arachnoid from within the canal, invaginating it into the arachnoid layer of the angle. In so doing, a double layer of arachnoid is formed over the tumor; the inner layer is densely adherent to the tumor, and the outer layer may be separable and can, indeed, protect the facial nerve and the auditory nerve during the dissection. When the tumor is quite large, these layers may fuse together and the protection may be lost, but if it is present, it makes the dissection significantly easier.

In the smaller tumors (Fig 6–9), I generally prefer to open the meatus and internal auditory canal early on in the dissection. A segment of dura is resected between the internal auditory canal and the sigmoid sinus, and then with a 4 or 5 mm high-speed turbine-driven diamond burr, the posterior wall of the internal auditory canal is carved away to reach the dura along the posterior limit of the canal. The opening is then widened around the curve of the dura with a 1 or 2 mm burr (Fig 6–10). The dura is opened sharply, and the arachnoidal dissection is carried around the rounded end of the intracranial extension of the medial end of the tumor. The nerve of origin is identified, nearly always the superior vestibular nerve, which can then be divided medial to the tumor and the tumor reflected laterally using round canal knives in various configurations. The drilling

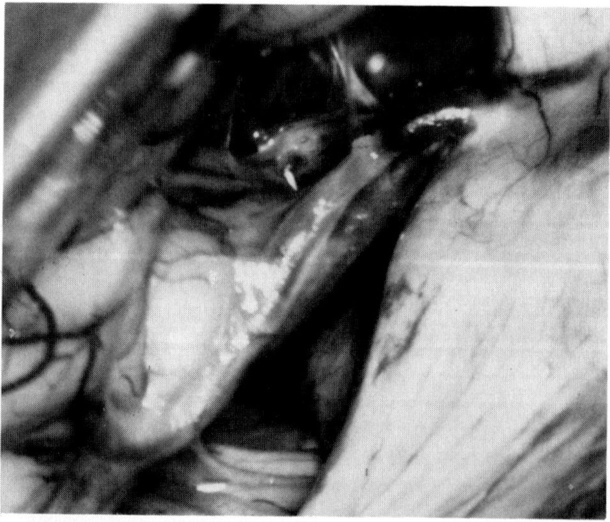

FIG 6–7.
In this case the anterior cerebellar artery runs upward from the basilar artery to enter the internal auditory canal and then penetrates the posterior wall of the canal and returns as a loop back to the flocculus. Inferiorly the ninth and tenth nerves are visible. The tumor extends anteriorly.

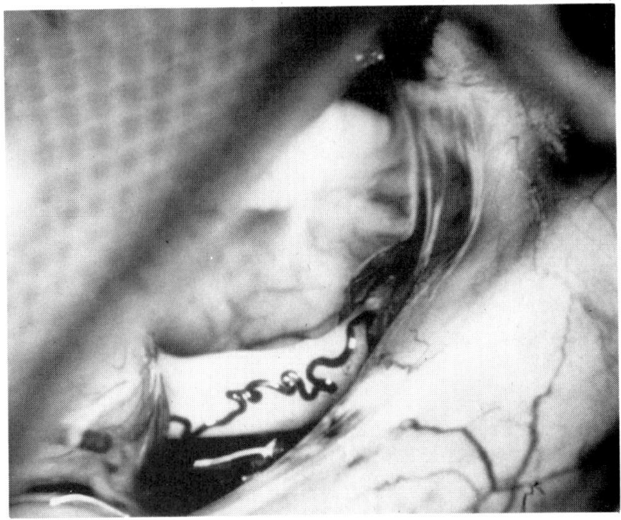

FIG 6–9.
A largely intracanalicular tumor bulges from the canal only a few millimeters. The vestibular nerves are seen crossing to enter the canal with the tumor. The facial and auditory nerves are concealed by the vestibular nerves.

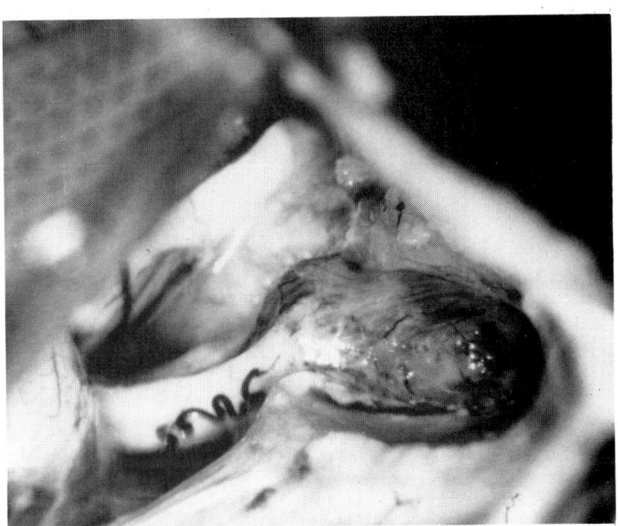

FIG 6–10.
This is the same patient as in Figure 6–9. The posterior wall of the internal auditory canal has been drilled away for 10 mm horizontally, which, as measured on the CT scan, was 1 mm from reaching the vestibule. Vertically the drilling has been carried for 6 mm, the actual height of the canal. The tumor is seen arising from the superior vestibular nerve.

of the canal has been carried laterally either to the extent of the tumor if it does not reach the crista or as far as possible without entering the vestibule. High-resolution CT scan with 1.5 mm cuts with the bone algorithm permits precise measurement preoperatively of the permissible opening. Nearly always this opening is between 10 and 13 mm from the meatus

and usually permits full exposure of the crista without entering the vestibule. In any case, dissection in the internal auditory canal should be carried from medial to lateral to avoid tension on the neural vestibular or cochlear attachments by lateral to medial dissection, which will readily destroy hearing. There are sufficient space and slack at the auditory nerve attachment to the brain stem to permit medial to lateral dissection to be atraumatic (Fig 6–11). The artery that supplies the cochlea is either a branch of the arteroinferior cerebellar artery or a direct branch of the basilar artery. It most often lies on the upper surface of the auditory nerve and may be adherent to the tumor capsule. Preservation of this auditory artery is requisite for hearing. The artery is followed from mediad to laterad at high magnification, usually with sharp dissection. Again there may be small branches to the tumor, which are sealed using the bipolar coagulator at a setting of 15 or 20, with saline solution wash, then divided.

The facial nerve in these small tumors is almost invariably anterior and just a bit superior to the auditory nerve, with the two vestibular nerves superiorly and inferiorly placed along the posterior surface of the canal. Because of this arrangement, the tumor virtually always fills the posterior surface of the canal; therefore, it protects the facial and auditory nerves during the drilling. Clearing of the tumor within the internal auditory canal will be accomplished using round canal knives of different angles. They include the usual 45 degrees from the line of the handle, a 90-degree knife, and one that is bent 135 degrees toward the handle, which is particularly useful for removing the last small segment of tumor between the superior vestibular canal and the posterior wall of the internal auditory meatus when drilling cannot safely be carried another 1 or 2 mm laterally. This last millimeter and the appearance of the crista can be checked with the dental mirror, though it is unusual to have the vestibule so medially placed.

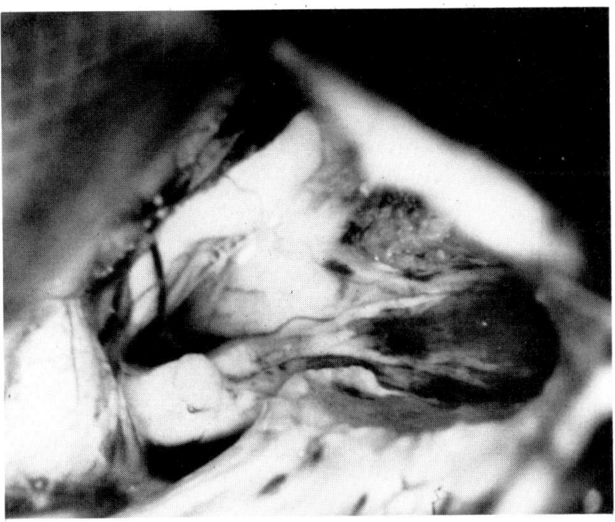

FIG 6–11.
This is the same patient as in Figures 6–9 and 6–10. The superior vestibular nerve has been divided and the tumor reflected from the facial, auditory, and inferior vestibular nerves, which are intact.

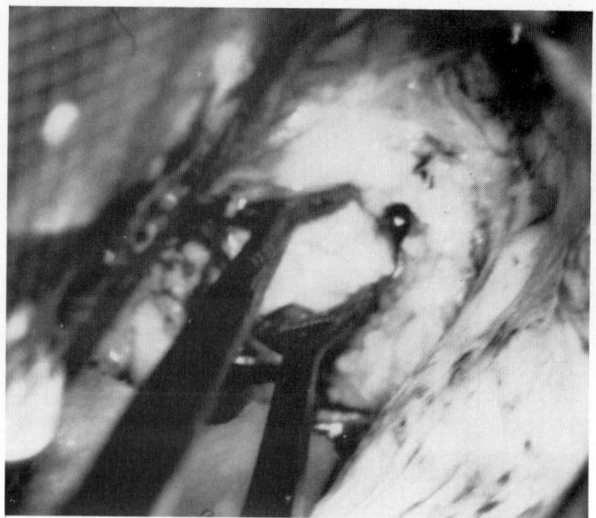

FIG 6–12.
A segment of tumor is removed bloodlessly with the cutting loop.

With the larger tumors, coring of the tumor permits the appropriate medial dissection. I prefer to incise the tumor with the bipolar coagulator along the lateral margin close to the petrosal surface. Through this incision segments of the tumor can be removed. Coring of the tumor may be carried out in a number of ways. Cup forceps or curettes or hard suction are commonly used, none of which I consider reasonable because of the lack of counterpressure or countertraction to protect the adjacent structures. More frequently the ultrasonic aspirator has been used to fragment and remove tissue progressively. The only disadvantage of this technique is its lack of hemostasis, though this can be achieved by using the bipolar coagulator as cottonoids are moved around within the cavity. In recent years I have preferred to core the tumors with the bipolar cutting current under continuous saline irrigation. This technique is rapid and almost completely bloodless. It can be done using sharp fine bayonet forceps to carve out segments, resecting blocks of tumor with several cuts. Still more recently, I have used mainly ring bipolar cutting forceps that remove segments of tumor on each application (Fig 6–12). Because of the bipolar configuration, there is no current spread. When they are used appropriately under continuous irrigation, there is no significant adjacent tissue heating as well, and yet the procedure is virtually bloodless. The devascularized portions of tumor can readily be lifted out with bayonet cup forceps.

The use of a laser in acoustic neuroma surgery presents a special question. I have used only the CO_2 laser and have not worked with the sapphire or the Nd-YAG laser. Using the CO_2 laser on a number of acoustic neuroma patients, I have found no situation where I cannot do so much better without the laser than I can with it. The laser is part of the operating room armamentarium, but over the years since its introduction has been used less and less as we decided that its limitations as an aid are greater than its advantages. Although I still use it for other types of lesions, I no longer use the laser appreciably in acoustic neuroma surgery.

Coring along the plane of the petrous interrupts most of the lateral blood supply to the tumor, coming from the external supply, the ascending pharyngeal and preauricular arteries, and makes the more medial tumor significantly less vascular. When a portion of the tumor has been cored laterally, it is possible to displace the tumor from medial to lateral to fill the cavity and then to repeat the process. Since this is done several times, even the largest tumor can be progressively displaced so that all that is needed for the medial dissection is the original 1.5 cm of available space. The coring of the tumor should be carried out until the medial wall is as thin as possible, and then dissection up along the medial surface from the posteroinferior aspect can be performed.

Anterior to and just superior to the lateral recess the facial nerve can be visualized. In any tumor large enough to reach this area of the brain stem, the facial nerve will have, at least at the beginning, an anterior course attached to the stem. The facial nerve is readily recognized since it is tan compared to the white stem or the 9th or 10th nerves (Fig 6–13). The nerve can be identified by bipolar stimulation, permitting recording of the potential with a recording electrode applied to the face 1 or 2 cm lateral to the nostril. Facial movement will not be apparent in the well-curarized patient, so that an evoked potential technique is required to demonstrate the effect of stimulus. I have personally not found the need for facial nerve stimulation, relying on visual recognition at high magnification.

Tumors that are between 3.5 and 4.5 cm in intracranial diameter tend to push the fifth and fourth nerves upward slightly through the tentorial notch. They deeply cup the brain stem, but when the coring has been adequate, bringing this medial layer over and down from above to the 1.5-cm lateral exposure

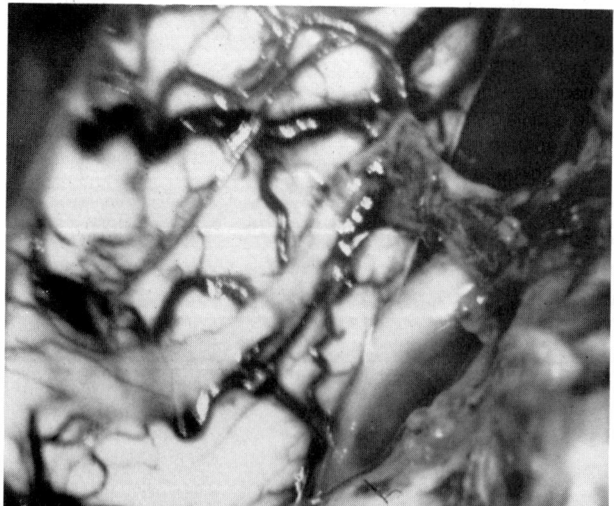

FIG 6–13.
After the removal of a 4.5-cm tumor, the facial nerve can be seen as a somewhat darker structure running along the well-preserved brain stem and then turning sharply laterally to enter the drilled out canal. The sixth nerve can be seen inferiorly, taking an upward course between the brain stem and the dural floor, then disappearing beneath the facial nerve as it heads toward the cavernous dura.

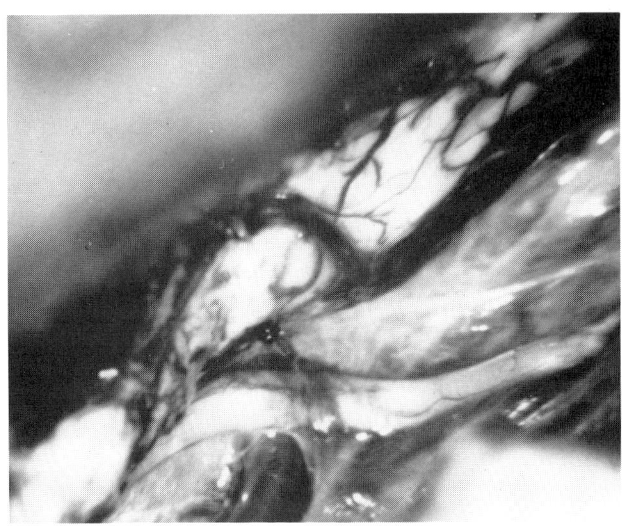

FIG 6–14.
A 6-cm tumor has been removed, exposing the basilar artery. The brain stem has been pushed to the left side, drawing the sixth nerve over the basilar artery, which it crosses at the point where the anteroinferior cerebellar artery branches from the basilar. The anteroinferior cerebellar artery can be seen at about the midpoint of the lower edge of the photograph, coursing downward.

is readily accomplished. Tumors more than 5 cm in diameter may extend between the fifth nerve and the tentorium, pushing the fifth nerve forward and downward instead of upward through the notch, and these tumors may extend along the basilar artery apex up past the posterior clinoids to reach the posterior cerebral artery, third nerve, and posterior communicating artery after passing the superior cerebellar artery. Occasionally in the largest tumors, they will get all the way to the carotid artery along the posterior communicating arteries. This area is easier to bring down because the membrane of Lilliequist virtually always has a separate plane from the tumor and permits, after coring, the displacement of this portion of the tumor downward and lateralward. These very large tumors displace the brainstem past the midline and across the basilar artery, with the sixth nerve then having to cross the basilar artery on its way to the cavernous sinus (Fig 6–14). This crossing characteristically is at the origin of the anteroinferior cerebellar artery from the basilar artery. At this point the sixth nerve is often deeply grooved over the anteroinferior cerebellar artery.

Some of these very large tumors also extend posteriorly down the foramen magnum and lie on the vertebral artery at the point where the 12th nerve crosses the vertebral artery. Here too, there is a characteristic neural crossing with the three fascicles of the 12th nerve pressed against the origin of the posteroinferior cerebellar artery as they cross its origin from the vertebral artery. The facial nerve in most of the patients proceeds anteriorly along the brain stem and then curves around the anteroinferior surface of the tumor (Fig 6–15). This is by no means invariable, and the facial nerve may be pushed downward to lie on the 12th nerve and the vertebral artery and then along the 9th nerve, which it passes to curve up to the internal

auditory meatus. In other cases the facial nerve may be displaced upward along the fifth nerve, even lying superior to the fifth nerve, first crossing the fifth nerve medially as it passes upward toward the middle fossa, turning laterally, and then again crossing the fifth nerve near the entrance to Meckel's cave as it returns toward the internal auditory meatus.

One of the most dangerous areas for dissection of the facial nerve occurs in a large tumor where the facial nerve, coming from an anterior displaced position around the front of the tumor, lies against the petrous dura running posteriorly and then makes a sharp right-angle bend to enter the anterior rim of the internal auditory canal. Dissection of this sharp bend must be done most precisely, usually with razor blade or microscissors, since at this point the nerve is very vulnerable to any stretch or trauma.

On only 4 occasions in more than 500 acoustic neuroma operative removals, was the facial nerve on the posterior surface of the tumor. Anatomically, the nerve would not have been identified unless by electrical stimulation. Since I have considered it necessary to attempt to save either vestibular nerve if it was not involved, the coring has been carried out both above and below the nerve to preserve it. Despite the delay in recognition, the facial function was preserved by the "preserve everything" approach.

The position of the auditory nerve has been far less variable

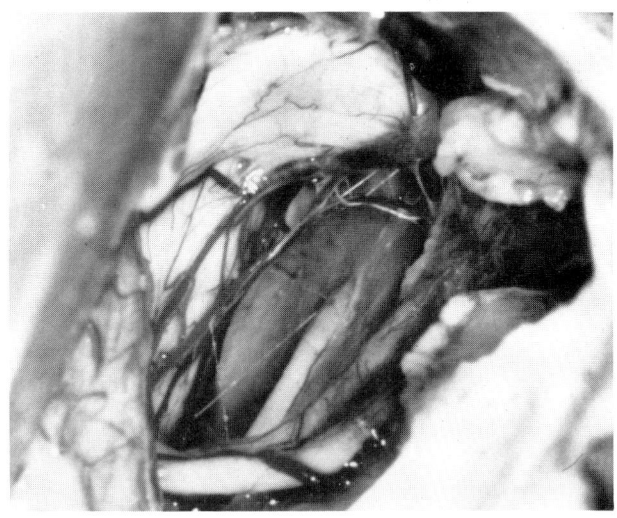

FIG 6–15.
A 3.5-cm acoustic neuroma has been removed. The fifth nerve can be seen curving along the upper margin of the center of the photograph. The facial and auditory nerves curve downward from the brain stem and then upward at the drilled out internal auditory canal. The sixth nerve goes diagonally upward from medial to lateral anterior to the seventh nerve. The anteroinferior cerebellar artery can be seen just at the lower edge of the photograph just beneath the eighth nerve. The flocculus is visible below the retractor in the lower left-hand corner, whereas in the upper right-hand corner, by the tentorium, the petrosal vein can be seen joined by the vein of the lateral recess, which crosses the fifth nerve at this point. Horizontal diameter of view is 3 cm.

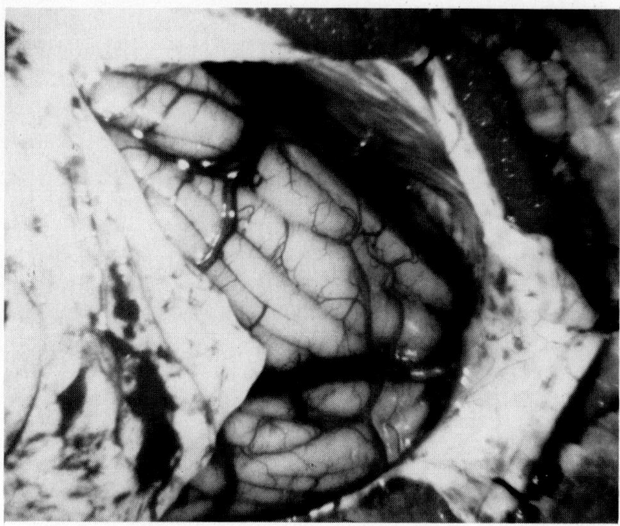

FIG 6–16.
Tumor removal has been completed, and the self-retaining cerebellar retractor has been removed. The cerebellum has dropped back into the angle, visualizing the tentorium. Laterally, the tab of dura with the stay sutures that draws the sigmoid sinus over the cut mastoid surface remains attached. These sutures will be cut and the dura closed. Horizontal diameter of view is 3 cm.

than that of the facial nerve. It has almost routinely been displaced inferiorly along the lower pole of the tumor anterior to the ninth nerve and has curved along the dural floor to come up to the internal auditory meatus just anterior to the ninth nerve. The inferior vestibular nerve has usually been just posterior to the auditory nerve. In the large tumors, these nerves may no longer be distinguishable in the capsular structure unless the double arachnoid layer has been preserved.

Mastoid cells opened during the drilling of the posterior wall of the meatus are filled by packing with little nodules of fat from the subcutaneous layer at the lower end of the skin incision. A segment of fat about 1.5 cm in diameter cut from the same area is then used to fill the drilled-out canal. In Europe and most of the rest of the world, fibrin glue is used to attach this fat pad, but since this is not available in the United States, I suture the fat pad to the adjacent dural margins with a 6-0 monofilament suture.

After the completeness of hemostasis is tested with bilateral jugular compression to distend the venous structures both before and after the retractor is removed (Fig 6–16), the posterior fossa dura is closed essentially watertight. Bone wax is able to seal the external portion of the mastoid cells, since they are not in contact with CSF.

A number of patients have complained of postoperative aching in the area above the incision after vigorous activity. I believe that this was probably due to adherence of the muscle layers to the dura and pulling of the muscles on the sensitive dura. After reoperating in a few such patients and placing a cranioplasty across the defect, I have demonstrated that this procedure had been effective in relieving the pain. In previous cases of vigorous young athletes where I had put in cranio-

plasties for protection at the time of surgery, postoperative pain had not been seen. Accordingly, for the past year I have been placing a titanium mesh and acrylic cranioplasty as part of the procedure. It takes little extra time and is carried out by carving a diploic groove with a high-speed cutting burr around the upper and medial margin of the bony opening and then bowing a sheet of titanium mesh into the groove across the dura, which has been covered with a sheet of absorbable gelatin sponge (Gelfoam). A thin layer of acrylic is then spread through the mesh and its heat of polymerization controlled by continuous saline irrigation. The polymerized acrylic surrounds the mesh and secures it into position. The titanium and acrylic cranioplasty has been used in more than 100 procedures in our department other than acoustic neuromas, and its lack of complications and total tolerance have been demonstrated. The titanium is virtually radiolucent, is nonmagnetic, and is the most biocompatible metal known. It does not interfere with CT scanning or with MRI.

Patients are awakened in the operating room at the end of the procedure when the anesthesia and curarization are reversed and are returned to the intensive care unit (ICU), alert and conversing, for 1 day of postoperative observation before return to their regular rooms. During that first night in the ICU, they are kept relatively dry with a serum osmolarity of about 310 and blood pressure maintained at less than 90 mean to avoid any threat of postoperative bleeding. They are allowed out of bed the next day and are returned to their regular rooms. Patients with small tumors are able to leave the hospital on the fifth day; others with larger tumors may require 7 days.

POSTOPERATIVE RESULTS

In the past 20 years, I have personally operated on 504 patients with acoustic neuromas. In the first 252 cases, there were 6 deaths, for a mortality of 2.4%. In the last 252 cases, there was 1 death, for a mortality of 0.4%. Major disability not present preoperatively has occurred in two patients, both as a result of postoperative hemorrhages.

Facial nerve function was rarely preserved with complete removals prior to the microsurgical era. Now it is routinely expected. Table 6–1 depicts the postoperative facial function results in 200 consecutive tumors measured by CT.

TABLE 6–1.
200 Consecutive Primary Acoustic Neuromas May 1977 to May 1984, All Totally Removed

Size (cm)	No. of Cases	No. of Facial Nerve Paralyses	Outcome Functional (%)
<2	48	1	98
2–3	30	1	97
3–4	55	7	87
>4	67	17	75
Total	200	26	87

*Size is CT measurement of intracranial diameter.

These are intracranial measurements only, not counting the size of the segment of the tumor in the internal auditory canal. If they were to be counted with that additional space, one would have to add another centimeter or so to each measurement. Clearly the major need is for earlier detection and operation on the growing acoustic neuroma before it is 2 cm in diameter. In addition to the correlation with tumor size and facial nerve preservation, the patient who has a preoperative palsy on the tumor side has a significantly worse prognosis than the patient with normal facial movement, regardless of the size of the tumor. There is a correlation, however, in that the patients with significant preoperative facial weakness generally have a fairly large tumor as well. The combination of a 4 to 5 cm tumor and a rather marked facial weakness indicates the high probability of infiltrated facial nerve fascicles, most likely at the anterior margin of the internal auditory meatus, and a very poor prognosis for facial nerve preservation.

Almost 50% of those patients with good function had mild, moderate, or even severe dysfunction for a few weeks to a few months postoperatively. Patients whose facial nerve was anatomically intact have recovered their function even though immediately markedly impaired. If the palsy is minimal, a Guibor bubble is used to protect the cornea until full eye closure and tearing have returned. If the palsy is severe, a lateral tarsorrhaphy is used until recovery is complete.

For the small percentage of patients, 14% overall for all sizes, in whom the facial nerve has been taken, end-to-end intracranial anastomosis has been performed where the available facial nerve ends are long enough. A single sling suture is all that has been used, with no attempt at precise fascicular anastomosis. This procedure has been carried out in 26 patients, with good results in 23. There have been two failures, and one patient has not had sufficient time for regeneration.

Where facial nerve resection has not left an available area for anastomosis, I have preferred a hypoglossal–facial nerve anastomosis done prior to the patient's discharge, about 4 or 5 days postoperatively. It has provided a fairly satisfactory, retrainable level of facial function, though it scarcely approaches the normal face of the preserved facial nerve patient.

HEARING PRESERVATION

In the entire series of 504 operative patients, only 118 had reasonably good hearing preoperatively, and this was able to be preserved at a satisfactory level in 54. Satisfactory hearing can be defined in many different ways. For this purpose, I am restricting it to those patients who, with complete masking in the other ear, have no more than a 35 dB decrease in the midrange and have speech discrimination of at least 75%. As a group, these patients continue to use the telephone in the operated ear. Although lesser degrees of hearing may well be worth preserving since a hearing level that permits stereolocalization will be appreciated by the patient, it would not meet any ordinary classification of useful hearing. As with the facial nerve, hearing preservation has been best in those patients with the least preoperative deficit and the smallest tumors. Marked prolongation of the interval between peaks 1 and 3 in the brain stem auditory evoked response has been a predictor of poor prognosis for hearing preservation. Tumors that did not originate far laterally in the canal and did not erode the crista tended to have better hearing preservation.

All of my resections have been considered to be complete, and there has been 1 recurrence among the 504 operated patients. No other patient has demonstrated any evidence of recurrent or persistent tumor. In the one recurrent case operated on prior to CT scanning, the presence of invasion into the vestibule and cochlea in a 7 cm tumor was not recognized. The recurrence took place entirely within the petrous bone and was demonstrated by loss of facial nerve function several years after the initial removal. The secondary procedure revealed a totally intrapetrosal tumor replacing much of the middle and inner ear structures, with no new extension into the posterior fossa. In the CT and MRI era, such extension would have been recognized and recurrence prevented, since the apparently complete resection would have been carried into the vestibule and an actual complete resection achieved.

Secondary removals are significantly more difficult than primary because of scarring, adherence, violation of the capsule, and fungating tumor. In addition, damage from an inadequate removal may have already occurred and be unrepairable. Eight percent, 39 of my operative patients, have had a prior attempt at removal that was partial or unsuccessful. All of these were able to be completely removed at a secondary procedure, though with considerable more difficulty than would have occurred had they been primary, with poorer results regarding preservation of facial nerves or hearing compared with equivalent-sized primary tumors. Particularly distressing was the case of a patient who had been deaf since childhood in the opposite ear and who now developed a small acoustic neuroma in his only hearing ear. The decision had been made elsewhere to do a partial removal on the tumor to preserve hearing. Two years later, with hearing failing, I operated on the patient only to find a situation where I was virtually certain that I could have preserved the hearing except for the scarring of the prior partial removal.

A special problem exists in patients with central neurofibromatosis, now referred to by the National Institutes of Health consensus (for no apparent reason that I can accept) as *neurofibromatosis II*. These genetic, familial bilateral acoustic neuroma patients have, as a rule, multiple additional central nervous tumors with multiple neuromata of the ninth and tenth nerves and of the fifth nerve, as well as multiple tumors within the spinal canal including intramedullary tumors and extramedullary neuromas, neurofibromas, and meningiomas. They also have multiple intracranial meningiomas rather frequently. Their major presenting syndrome may be due to a supratentorial meningioma, or it may be the bilateral acoustic neuromas.

The preservation of hearing in these patients is exceedingly difficult because they may have multiple tumors within the auditory canal. I have seen tumors arising from all four nerves in the canal, that is, the superior vestibular, the inferior vestibular, the auditory, and the facial nerves. Growth rates in these tumors in this disease do not present any reasonable pattern. One tumor may grow rapidly, with the three adjacent tumors showing no change over many years, and the tumor on one side may grow quickly, whereas the tumor on the other side remains static for long periods.

In my hands the preservation of hearing in the bilateral acoustic neurofibromatosis patient has been significantly less than in the single acoustic neuroma patient. I believe this is the result of the multifascicular origin of the tumors and the multiplicity of tumors in the angle in each of these cases. It becomes the most difficult single decision for me in all of neurosurgery when a patient with bilateral acoustic neurofibromatosis already deaf in one ear presents with the problem of what to do about the tumor in the only hearing ear. Delay leads to further hearing loss in that ear and a poor chance of preserving the hearing. Aggressive intervention destroys the hearing earlier if it fails in the goal of preserving hearing. In this special group of patients

I have been able to preserve good hearing in only 10% of the operated ears. This may be due partially to greater delay in operating on a remaining hearing ear as well as to the anatomic problem of the multiple involvements. One of my patients whose hearing had been preserved after removal remained with good hearing for 12 years and then presented with failing hearing and, on reexploration, had a completely separate tumor of the auditory nerve.

This remarkable group of bilateral acoustic neuroma patients (of which I now care for 26 very special people) makes up a whole separate discussion. Their ability to continue to function with their multiple cranial and spinal tumors, operations, and disabilities is to me a most humbling yet inspiring lesson, and a most formidable challenge.

CHAPTER 7

Nondestructive Surgery for Vertigo

Approach of

I. Kaufman Arenberg, M.D.

and

W. P. R. Gibson, M.D.

Currently most of us have a first-option surgical bias for either nondestructive or destructive surgery in patients with refractory Meniere's disease. If we could significantly enhance the success rate of nondestructive inner ear surgery and actually alter in a positive direction the natural course of the disease over time, surely most of us would opt for a nondestructive procedure, as would have Sir Terrence Cawthorne. Cawthorne[1] gave support to this idea in 1965 by stating:

> Although I have played a small part in the development of destructive operations of the labyrinth in patients with intractable Meniere's disease, it is my hope that drainage of the endolymphatic sac [system] will eventually prove to be the operation of choice in Meniere's disease.

1. Does inner ear surgery performed at the endolymphatic sac (ELS) and duct (ELD) really work?

2. Does it work sometimes and not other times? If so, why?

3. Can the otologic surgeon really, anatomically and physiologically, decompress the hydropic labyrinth, analogous to the decompression of the glaucomatous eye by the ophthalmic surgeon?

4. Is it possible to determine if the ELS to mastoid shunt, with or without a valve, is correctly seated and hydrodynamically coupled?

5. Can any of these questions be answered? If so, can they be answered during surgery?

OVERVIEW

Meniere's disease, which includes endolymphatic hydrops (ELH), is a common disorder of the inner ear afflicting as many as an estimated 7 million Americans.[2] The disease is characterized by episodic vertigo, fluctuating hearing loss, tinnitus, and pressure or fullness of the ear. The most widely accepted definition of Meniere's disease was developed in 1972 by the American Academy of Otolaryngology: "a disorder of the membranous inner ear characterized by deafness, vertigo and usually tinnitus and has as its pathophysiologic correlate distention of the endolymphatic system."[3]

Classic Meniere's disease is a fluctuating or progressive but nonfluctuating, sensorineural hearing loss with episodic vertigo, tinnitus, and aural fullness or pressure. Other forms or variants of Meniere's disease include cochlear hydrops, in which there is no vertigo, and vestibular hydrops, in which patients do not exhibit sensorineural hearing loss (although cochlear duct changes, e.g., hydropic distortion can be objectively documented by electrocochleography [ECoG]).[4] It should be noted, however, that recent (1985) American Academy of Otolaryngology-Head and Neck Surgery criteria for reporting results do not accept these previously accepted variants because of lack of histopathologic confirmation of ELH.[5]

All types of Meniere's disease are thought to be caused by excess fluid volume in the inner ear under pressure (hydrops).[6] This increased pressure or rupture of the membranous endolymphatic fluid system can produce any or all of the associated symptoms: episodic vertigo, dysequilibrium, imbalance, hearing loss, tinnitus, pressure, and related disability.

The most common mechanism of ELH is thought to be a malfunction of the ELS (from a variety of factors and etiologies that are often idiopathic). When the ELS is functioning properly, it resorbs endolymph from within the inner ear. The ELS also acts as a pressure regulator of endolymph. Malfunctions can be caused by epithelial damage or subepithelial fibrosis and scarring or other factors that affect resorption and cause a backup of endolymph within the endolymphatic system.[7] Endolymphatic hypertension is analogous to glaucoma in the eye, a similar pathophysiologic process of excess of fluid under pressure causing sensory neural deficits in a closed fluid system. As in the early stages of glaucoma, ELH can cause a reversible sensory system deficit in both the vestibular and auditory systems.

HISTORICAL PERSPECTIVE

The first inner ear surgery was performed on the ELS in 1925 by Dr. Georges Portmann[8] using neither an operating microscope nor microsurgical instruments.* It is amazing that with these technical limitations he was able to find the ELS and decompress it. Yamakawa and Naito[9] and House[10] reintroduced and modified Portmann's ELS surgery using the operating microscope and microsurgical instruments. Once modern instrumentation became readily available, microsurgery on the ELS could be routinely performed.

In the early days of inner ear surgery, reports of inability to find the ELS at surgery varied from 5% to 30%.[11] Two anatomic studies by Arenberg, et al.[11] and Shea and Paparella[12] in the mid-1970s demonstrated that the ELS in Meniere's disease patients was far inferior to Donaldson's line and anterior to where it was most often found in patients without Meniere's disease.

These surgical and cadaver studies corroborated what was suggested by tomographic studies[13–15] of the vestibular aqueduct and its external aperture, namely, that the external aperture in 65% of patients with Meniere's disease is not in the "normal" anatomic position. In many Meniere's disease patients, the vestibular aqueduct cannot be visualized at all, an infrequent occurrence in "non-Meniere" or "normal" individuals.[15] Extensive studies of congenital and developmental anomalies and abnormalities of the ELS and vestibular aqueduct have also been done.[16–20]

By 1980, when these basic anatomic facts had been extensively assimilated, there were no further reports in the literature of inability to find the ELS. Unfortunately, the tendency to mistake a "false lumen" for the true lumen of the ELS was not really understood, discussed, or appreciated until 1986.[21]

TREATMENT GOALS

The primary goal of any long-term treatment of Meniere's disease is to attempt to positively alter the natural history of the

*The International Meniere's Disease Research Institute now has a videotape of Georges Portmann's first type of inner ear surgery with mallet and gouge, circa 1930.

disease, not just to suppress the most troublesome symptoms. The obvious goal is to control or completely eliminate vertigo as well as adjunctive spells of imbalance and positional dysequilibrium. In the long term, however, improvement or even real stabilization of the hearing can be more important in calculating the overall success and in assessing a real alteration in the natural history of Meniere's disease. It is virtually impossible to have recurrent vertigo in an operated ear that has resulted in a real improvement in hearing.

One way or another, the vertigo coming from only one ear can be eliminated or controlled, even if destructive surgery is required. However, once the hearing deficit loses its reversible component, chances for improved hearing and speech discrimination are, at best, marginal. The best treatment not only addresses the short-term, symptomatic relief of vertigo but also attempts to preserve or improve both auditory and vestibular system function for the long term. These long-term goals, when effected, actually can alter in a positive direction the natural history and course of Meniere's disease. Therefore, since bilateral disease is much more common than was previously thought,[22] the "good ear" should be checked periodically. Recurrent symptoms are routinely attributed to the bad ear until it becomes obvious that the good ear has also become affected.

TREATMENT CONCEPTS

1. Most patients with Meniere's disease get better without surgery. Sixty percent to 80% respond to conservative treatment by a variety of medical, dietary, and allergic regimens.[23] It is important to realize that many patients who seem to get better, may only, in fact, be experiencing fewer disabling attacks of vertigo. Although the vertigo is gone or significantly lessened, the acute attacks are exchanged for some form of chronic, often disabling, disequilibrium. Vestibular tests show that these patients continue to lose balance and auditory function even though vertigo is dissipiated. In fact, as vestibular function continues to deteriorate over time and there is burnout with the clinical absence of vertigo, loss of auditory function tends to decrease in a parallel manner. Therefore, these patients continue to lose balance function over time just as they continue to lose hearing.[24] If these patients are considered successes, they can distort the apparent success rate and undermine the concept of real changes in the natural history of Meniere's disease. The clinical absence of vertigo is not necessarily a good indicator of a successful treatment.

2. More than 50% of patients will develop measurable bilateral involvement; in other words, the disease will be present and measurable in the other ear in the next 5 to 15 years.[22] The bilateral involvement may or may not be clinically significant. The other 20% to 40% are patients who continue to experience acute attacks of vertigo and are considered medical treatment failures.

MEDICAL TREATMENT FAILURE

Medical treatment failure is defined as recurrence of symptoms despite adequate patient compliance with the various and preferred medical treatments. A 3- to 6-month trial is considered sufficient. If the patient has recurrent attacks of vertigo, fluctuating hearing loss, or both despite medical treatment compliance, the patient is deemed a medical treatment failure. If patient compliance is nil, medical treatment will not be helpful.

If medical failure is suspected and documented, one must determine whether vertigo or sensorineural hearing loss is the primary basis for surgical intervention, keeping in mind the importance of the functional and clinical status of the patient's other ear. The degree of work and social disability should also be critically assessed in evaluating medical treatment failure.[25]

Remember, it is important to be aware of those patients who appear clinically better, in whom attacks of vertigo are fewer and less severe but who still experience chronic imbalance, dysequilibrium, and possibly progressive sensorineural hearing loss with or without fluctuations. To reiterate, clinical absence of vertigo may often be mistaken for a medical treatment success when it is, in fact, the natural course of the disease.

STRATEGIES OF SURGERY ON THE ENDOLYMPHATIC SAC AND DUCT

In the following demonstration, drawings of intraoperative procedures (Appendix) are used to clarify the fine points of the microsurgical technique, including those pertinent to intraoperative ECoG monitoring. This description focuses on identifying the real ELS lumen and avoiding the false lumen of the ELS. Further, it emphasizes cannulating more proximally to or into the ELD at the external aperture of the vestibular aqueduct so that whatever implant is used can be seated correctly.

It is important to put nondestructive inner ear surgery for the treatment of vertigo and hearing loss in Meniere's disease and ELH into proper perspective. Surgery on the inner ear is done to treat the medically uncontrolled ELH causing the inner ear symptoms of Meniere's disease, most commonly the vertigo. Inner ear surgery treats only the hydrops from whatever etiology and does not correct or "cure" the underlying pathology or cause of the ELH itself. The goal of nondestructive inner ear surgery is only to shunt excess endolymph volume presumably under pressure from a neurosensory area where the hair cells are affected (damaged or partially destroyed) to an area where effects of the hydrops are minimized or eliminated (i.e., to the mastoid or subarachnoid space). With any nondestructive inner ear surgery, the ELS should be used as a safe, nonsensory anatomic point of entry into the distal endolymphatic system to tap into and decompress the more proximal excess endolymph under pressure in the proximal endolymphatic system. This same surgical technique should be used whether one wishes to implant a one-way escape valved shunt,[26] a nonvalved, capillary shunt with a fluid chamber,[27] or a simple capillary tube[28–30] or sac enhancement.[31] In our experience, neither Portmann's original procedure of opening and draining the ELS itself[8] (excluding the ELD), Shambaugh's simple uncovering of the ELS without opening it ("decompressing the sac"),[32] nor insertion of a plastic drain[32–35] is as likely to result in a real improvement in hearing, although it can happen. Intraoperative

ECoG is helpful in demonstrating these changes, especially if one is trying to achieve real hearing improvement not only for pure tones but, most important, in the patient's ability to understand speech (speech discrimination). The hearing result is the best way to assess real change, positive or negative, in the natural course of Meniere's disease. Merely draining the ELS is probably less likely to lead to improvement in hearing and vertigo, because the histopathologic changes in the ELS epithelium and perisaccular connective tissue are severe.[36] These changes can be best appreciated at the light and ultrastructural levels by the pathologist rather than intraoperatively by the surgeon (Table 7–1).[37]

The relatively low success rate for hearing improvement in all nondestructive inner ear surgeries (Table 7–2) is most likely the result of (1) misplacing the valved shunt into the false ELD lumen, (2) not placing the shunt far enough proximally into the ELS to decompress the hydropic labyrinth physiologically, or (3) not being able to cannulate the ELD sufficiently proximal to enter the hydropic endolymphatic system and attain a hydrodynamic coupling (Fig 7–1) of inner ear fluid with the

TABLE 7–1.
Nondestructive Surgical Treatments

I. Distal endolymphatic system surgery
  A. Endolymphatic system surgery without implant or shunt
    1. Endolymphatic sac decompression and drainage procedure into mastoid (G. Portmann–M. Portmann)
    2. Endolymphatic sac decompression and drainage procedure into subarachnoid space (Naito)
    3. Simple endolymphatic sac decompression only (Shambaugh)
  B. Endolymphatic system surgery with implant from endolymphatic sac; drainage into the mastoid cavity
    1. Silastic sheeting shunt and endolymphatic sac enhancement (Shea, Paparella, Arenberg-Spector, Arenberg-Stahle)
    2. Capillary tube shunt (Morrison, Austin)
    3. Capillary tube with fluid chamber (Gibson)
    4. Pressure-sensitive unidirectional inner ear valved shunt (Arenberg, Wright-Hicks, Huang)
  C. Endolymphatiac system surgery with implanted shunt from the endolymphatic sac; drainage to the subarachnoid space
    1. Subarachnoid shunt (House)
    2. Angled subarachnoid shunt (Brackmann-DeLaCruz, Gardner)
II. Proximal endolymphatic system surgery
  A. Endolymphatic system surgery involving stapes footplate
    1. Sacculotomy (Fick)
    2. Tack procedure (Cody)
    3. Sacculocentesis (Shea)
    4. Perilymph fistula repair/grafting (Stroud-Calcaterra, Tonkin-Fagan, Lesinski, Black)
  B. Endolymphatic system surgery involving the round window
    1. Sodium chloride osmotic diuresis (Arslan)
    2. Cochleostomy (Morrison)
    3. Cochleosacculotomy (Schuknecht)
    4. Otic-periotic shunt (House-Pulec)
    5. Intracochlear shunt (Shea)
    6. Cochlear dialysis (Morrison)
    7. Perilymph fistula repair and grafting (Arenberg-May-Stroud, Fagan, Tonkin, Black)

TABLE 7–2.
Classic Meniere's Disease: Results of Valved Shunts for Hydrops (Compared with worst preoperative baseline audiogram by ≥15 dB/16% SDS)

	A	B	C	D
(n = 214)	(83) 38.8% Hearing Improved	(46) 21.5% Hearing Stabilized	(29) 13.5% Hearing Worse	Recurrent Vertigo
Hearing	(129) 60.3% Hearing Improved or Stabilized			
Vertigo	(158) 73.8% Complete absence of vertigo and adjunctive spells		(56) 26.2%	

fluid in the valved shunt. There are, however, other reasons for failure of inner ear surgery[38, 39]

Identification of the Real Lumen of the Endolymphatic Sac

In any type of distal nondestructive inner ear surgery, it is important to identify and open the real lumen of the ELS. Failure to identify the real lumen may be one of the most common, technical causes of failure in nondestructive inner ear surgery. Unfortunately, the real lumen of the ELS can be very difficult to identify anatomically. This problem is exacerbated if there is significant fibrosis of the ELS or ELD, as is often seen with Meniere's disease. Furthermore, an anterior projecting sigmoid sinus sufficient to cause an exposure or access problem to the ELS and ELD occurs approximatley 50% of the time, but it is easily overcome, however, by decompressing the sigmoid sinus using Bill's island technique.[39]

The false lumen, however, is easy to identify and mistake for the "correct" anatomic structure.[40] If (1) the ELS is used as the anatomic point of entry into the endolymphatic system and

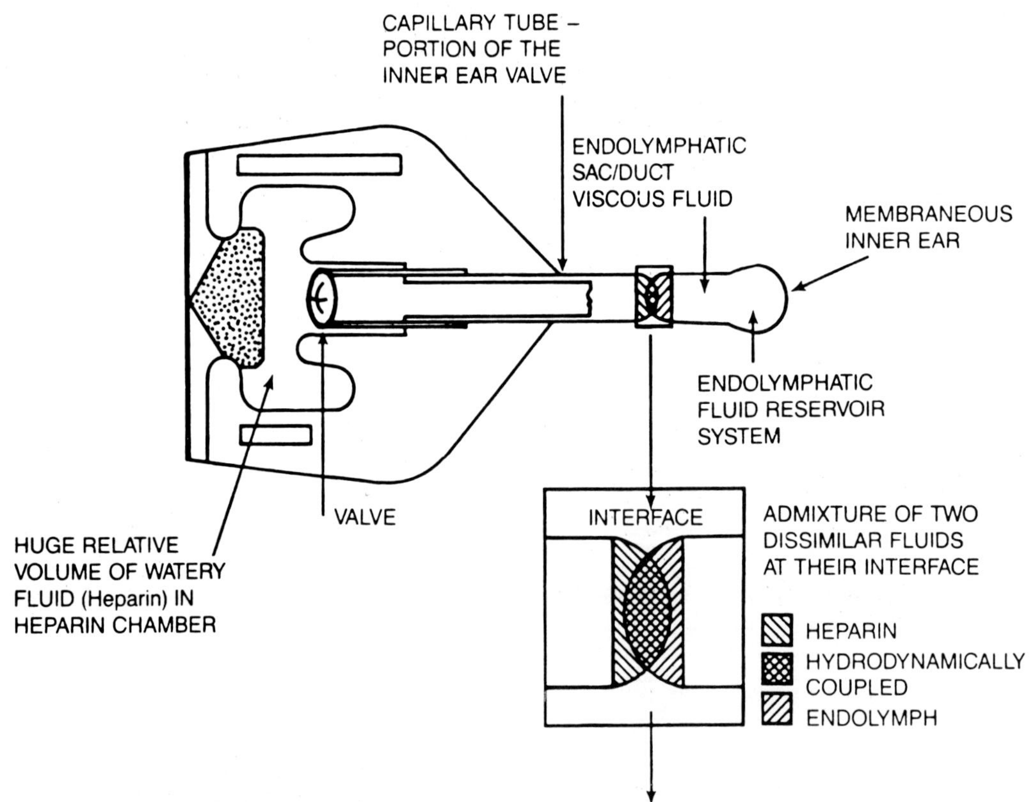

FIG 7–1.
Concept drawing of hydrodynamic coupling of inner ear fluid with fluid in the valve shunt.

(2) the inner ear implant is thought to be correctly placed or cannulated into or through the real lumen of the ELS into the ELS or the point of narrowing, (when, in fact, it is actually being placed into the false ELS lumen, which is outside the inner ear), the results that are theoretically and clinically possible obviously will not be achieved.[41–44]

What is the false ELS lumen, and why is it so easy to mistake this nonfunctional anatomic plane for the true ELS lumen, which is a true anatomic space? The false ELS lumen is the space between the lateral and medial wall of the ELS and either side of the posterior fossa dura. However, the true lumen of the ELS is the anatomic space between the lateral and medial walls of the ELS proper, or a functional lumen. It is easy to enter the anatomic space deep to the ELS and create a false lumen, which is, in fact, an anatomic plane, and thereby creating a false space that looks like the lumen of the ELS. The surgeon can, therefore, easily create a nonfunctional space leading nowhere without realizing the anatomic mistake. In the case of a double wall biopsy of the ELS for EM, developing this false lumen is done on purpose to obtain a specimen for pathologic study.[37] Color differences between the real lumen (pinkish gray) and false lumen (grayish blue) can be helpful. However, the posterior fossa dura, which is the medial wall of the false ELS lumen, can also look like a grayish "mucosa" through a small ELS incision. Another complicating factor is that the real ELS lumen, especially in cases of Meniere's disease, is often narrowed and scarred with avascular or atrophic walls.[7] Sometimes, the surgeon may inadvertently penetrate both the lateral and medial walls of the ELS because they may be atrophic. This can be better appreciated at the light microscopic level[7] and ultrastructural (electron microscopic) level[37] based on our understanding of normal human histology of ELS.[42] Therefore, even using the microsurgical approach, which is familiar, the surgeon must maintain a microanatomic, histopathologic concept of the anatomic facts.

The significance of surgically implanting any ELS device into the real lumen, as opposed to the false lumen, cannot be overemphasized in terms of achieving a positive clinical result.

A variety of congenital, developmental, or acquired anomalies and anatomic variants of the ELS or ELD and external aperture of the vestibular aqueduct are observed in about 10% of the cases[41] but are beyond the scope of this chapter. The reader is referred to references 16 through 19.

Importance of Hydrodynamic Coupling

When the ELS is used as the anatomic point of entry into the ELD, not identifying the true ELS lumen or correctly cannulating the ELD or hydrodynamically coupling (see Fig 7–1) the inner ear fluids within the implant are thought to be the major technical causes of failure in inner ear surgery.[40] It is imperative to realize that even if the real lumen of the ELS has been identified, the inserted device must break through to the excess endolymph for the proximal inner ear to be decompressed (if a valve is used, it can be hydrodynamically coupled with the excess endolymph more proximally). Hydrodynamic coupling is necessary to decompress the endolymphatic system and therefore maintain an effective decompression in the nor-

mal or physiologic range of volume or pressure dynamics in the inner ear.

Cannulation of the Real Lumen of the Endolymphatic Sac and Duct

It must be emphasized that the pressure-sensitive unidirectional inner ear valve represents a major conceptual and technical departure from other surgical procedures on the ELS. The primary technical goal of all other ELS surgeries from Portmann[8] on was to drain the ELS. Excess endolymph under presumed, increased pressure was drained into either the subarachnoid space or the mastoid cavity. In valve implant surgery, the ELD is cannulated, bypassing the entire diseased ELS. The valved shunt with its fluid reservoir hydrodynamically coupled to the proximal endolymphatic fluid reservoir acts by draining the excess endolymph through the pressure-sensitive and pressure-regulating valve and out into the mastoid cavity. In other words, with the valve implant, one is trying first to decrease or decompress the hydropic labyrinth and then to maintain decompression with normal endolymph volume and pressure. The valved shunt can effectively bypass the volume and pressure regulating functions of the (diseased) ELS. Therefore, the valve implant does not drain the ELS, rather, the ELS is only the anatomic point of safe entry into the endolymphatic fluid system reservoir.

These three major causes of inner ear surgery failure may account in part for the wide range in success rates reported for the various inner ear endolymphatic system operations. ELS surgeries have not been so successful either numerically or statistically as had been hoped, particularly for hearing, although elimination of vertigo has been achieved more consistently. Additional intraoperative time may be required to verify that the real lumen of the ELS has been located (see Appendix). Recent advances in intraoperative ECoG monitoring[45, 46] aid the surgeon, as electrophysiologic changes confirm when the real lumen is entered and the hydropic inner ear is effectively decompressed.

If these specific microsurgical techniques are followed, a reasonable level of success may be achieved with any implant or material the surgeon chooses. Dr. George E. Shambaugh, Jr. has always been a staunch advocate of adherence to the fine points of any microsurgical procedure. It is his firm conviction that if you do not faithfully reproduce the fine points and pay attention to the microsurgical details, you will be unable to reproduce the clinical results you seek. The advantages, techniques and examples of intraoperative electrophysiologic monitoring for nondestructive inner ear surgery are discussed in another section of this chapter.

Biopsy of the Endolymphatic Sac

We know from histopathologic[7, 42] and ultrastructural studies[36, 37] of the epithelium that lines the ELS that perisaccular fibrosis is often present in cases of Meniere's disease and that there is significant damage, whatever the etiology, to the resorptive capabilities and functional surface area of the ELS epithelia available for fluid transport. When the capillary tube portion of the valve implant is appropriately seated into the ELD, it effectively bypasses a nonfunctioning ELS. Therefore, a biopsy of the distal ELS[37, 47] can be taken because the pressure-regulating function[48] is now handled by the valve implant.

Complications

Long-term shunt extrusion, with or without infection, and traumatic fenestration of the posterior semicircular canal (PSSC) is known to have occurred in only 6 cases out of 900 and 4 cases out of 900, respectively, over 12 years. The complete loss of hearing can occasionally be avoided if it is immediately recognized and if only the perilymphatic space rather than the endolymphatic compartment of the PSSC is not violated. If this fenestra is immediately grafted and sealed, it is theoretically possible to save the inner ear. This is the only obvious way to fix this problem, other than alternatively going ahead with a complete labyrinthectomy. Intraoperative ECoG monitoring can be extremely helpful in this situation. A complete list of complications of inner ear surgeries that I have encountered is given in Table 7–3.

Destructive Procedures

Destructive procedures should be considered only if more conservative procedures have failed. Only in rare instances in Meniere's disease should it be the primary surgical intervention. The procedures available are vestibular nerve section (VNS), which can usually preserve existing hearing but rarely improves hearing over long-term follow-up,[49, 50] or labyrinthectomy, which will eliminate both auditory and vestibular function.

It is now possible to determine during surgery those patients who may really benefit from a primary destructive procedure. When the surgeon cannot document objectively that the hydropic labyrinth was effectively decompressed nondestructively by an appropriate change in ECoG intraoperatively, destructive surgery may be warranted. In other words, if the surgeon cannot decompress the labyrinth nondestructively, he or she can, at the same surgery, proceed to a destructive procedure depending on the residual hearing, either a labyrinthectomy or VNS. This approach should increase the success rate for nondestructive inner ear surgery at the endolymphatic ELS and ELD and also decrease the need for a labyrinthectomy or VNS as a primary surgery.

Value of Intraoperative Monitoring

Electrocochleography has proved to be a very powerful tool in assessing inner ear function, hydrops, or cochlear duct distortion.[4] Most researchers who study Meniere's disease agree that the parameters measured by ECoG, namely, the enhancement of the summating potential/action potential (SP/AP) ratio to clicks and tone burst SP recordings, indicate the presence (or absence) of ELH. Furthermore, EcoG may be beneficial in aiding surgeons estimate patient prognosis following inner ear surgery. The reversible component, or cochlear reserve, can often be better estimated with the use of transtympanic ECoG

TABLE 7–3.

Complications in the First 900 Valve Implant Operations

Complications	n	%
"Dead" ear		
Retrofacial air cell tract fenestration of the posterior semicircular canal	4	0.44
Endolymphatic duct probing too far into vestibule	1	0.11
	1	0.11
Technical problems suspected but unconfirmed;		
duct probing into vestibule		
Profound serous labyrinthitis	3	0.33
Postoperative inner ear infections (suppurative labyrinthitis)	3	0.33
Total	12	1.33
Facial nerve damage		
Complete and permanent facial paralysis	0	0
Transient facial paresis with essentially full recovery	6	0.67
Total	6	0.67
Cerebrospinal fluid (CSF) leaks		
Persistent leaks requiring surgical closure	3	0.33
Other instances of CSF leakage Minor leaks less than 0.5 mm	29	3.22
Total	32	3.55
Postoperative wound infection not involving the inner ear (three of these resulted in a dead ear and are not separate cases)	10	1.11
Valve implant extrusion*		
Infection	3	0.33
Noninfection	3	0.33
Total	6	0.6
Meningitis	0	0
Malignant hyperthermia (successfully treated with intravenously administered dantrolene)	1	0.11
Death	0	0

*Three of these were related to immediate or delayed postoperative wound infections and are not separate cases. In three other cases, spontaneous extrusion occurred postoperatively with no evidence of infection.

rather than audiometric preoperative urea or glycerol dehydration testing.[51] The ECoG abnormalities seen in baseline testing can be reversed acutely within 1 or 2 hours after urea or glycerol ingestion.[51] These observations suggested that surgical decompression of the hydropic labyrinth can be demonstrated intraoperatively. Surgeons then began to make comparisons between preoperative and postoperative ECoG tracings, and improvements were often seen. Figure 7–2 shows a markedly abnormal baseline ECoG in the preoperative workup, which became normal after inner ear valved shunt surgery; repeat ECoGs in this patient have remained normal. The patient has experienced excellent and sustained hearing improvement since nondestructive inner ear surgery and has been free of vertigo for 7 years. Critics contend, however, that such changes between preoperative and postoperative ECoG tests are unrelated to the surgery and reflect only the natural fluctuation of the disease.

The only way to prove or disprove the reality of these apparent changes was to bring ECoG into the operating room.

A

PT __PM__ AGE __27__ SEX __M__ DURATION OF SYMPTOMS __3 Yrs__
DIAGNOSIS __Classical Meniere's__ EAR __R__
PROCEDURE __ELS Valve__ DATE __10-29-80__

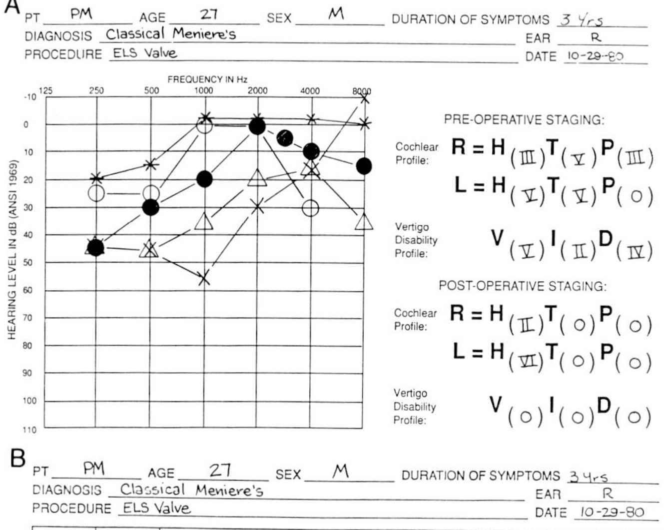

PRE-OPERATIVE STAGING:

Cochlear Profile:
$$R = H_{(III)} T_{(V)} P_{(III)}$$
$$L = H_{(V)} T_{(V)} P_{(o)}$$

Vertigo Disability Profile:
$$V_{(V)} I_{(II)} D_{(IV)}$$

POST-OPERATIVE STAGING:

Cochlear Profile:
$$R = H_{(II)} T_{(o)} P_{(o)}$$
$$L = H_{(VI)} T_{(o)} P_{(o)}$$

Vertigo Disability Profile:
$$V_{(o)} I_{(o)} D_{(o)}$$

B

PT __PM__ AGE __27__ SEX __M__ DURATION OF SYMPTOMS __3 Yrs__
DIAGNOSIS __Classical Meniere's__ EAR __R__
PROCEDURE __ELS Valve__ DATE __10-29-80__

KEY	DATE	CLINICAL STATUS	AC MPTA	SRT	RH	CID
○–○	10-27-80	Best Pre-Op	23	20	DNT	DNT
X–X	10-21-80	Worst Pre-Op	48	30	DNT	DNT
△–△	10-28-80	Pre-Glycerol	42	18	DNT	100%
□–□	10-28-80	Post-Glycerol	27	5	DNT	88%
◇–◇	10-29-81	1 yr. Post-Op	13	10	76%	100%
✳–✳	7-11-86	6 yr. Post-Op	17	10	60%	100%
●–●	5-9-88	8 yr. Post-Op	33	25	76%	100%

Intraoperative ECoG:

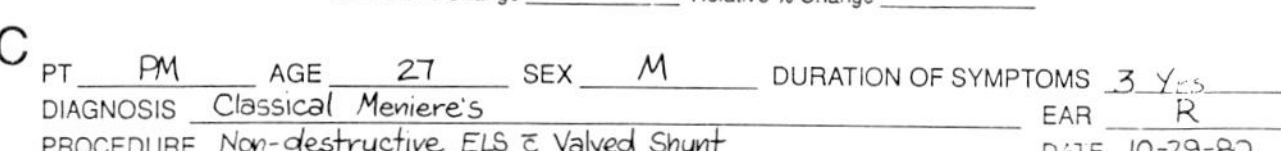

Baseline __________ Sac opened __________ Duct probed __________ Final Seating of Shunt __________
Absolute % Change __________ Relative % Change __________

FIG 7–2.
A 27-year-old man had intractable vertigo and Meniere's disease, with positive glycerol test results and significantly enhanced summating potential/action potential (SP/AP) ratio before surgery. Eight years after surgery the patient is free of vertigo and hearing is better than the worst preoperative rating. **A,** plotted serial audiometric curves. **B,** key to audiometric curves in **A. C,** preoperative and postoperative ECoG. Note that the SP/AP ratio and waveform morphology are normal 2 years after surgery.

C

PT __PM__ AGE __27__ SEX __M__ DURATION OF SYMPTOMS __3 Yrs__
DIAGNOSIS __Classical Meniere's__ EAR __R__
PROCEDURE __Non-destructive ELS c̄ Valved Shunt__ DATE __10-29-80__

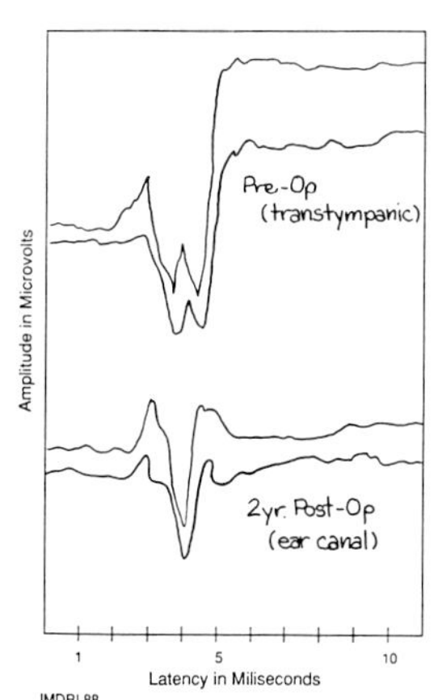

By using ECoG intraoperatively, the surgeon is able, for the first time, to successfully monitor electrophysiologic changes as they occur during nondestructive inner ear surgery with sac to mastoid shunts.

Electrocochleography was first brought into the operating room in 1961 when Ruben et al. attempted to study cochlear potentials and eighth nerve action potentials intraoperatively with otosclerotic patients.[52–55] These researchers used a ball-tipped Teflon-insulated, platinum wire electrode placed against the round window membrane. Utilizing click and pure tone sound stimulus via a loud speaker through a flexible tube situated at the external auditory orifice, they were able to elicit cochlear potentials (CPs) both before and after stapes mobilization. Due to the limitations of their recording equipment (oscilloscope to tape recorder), the patients' CPs were saved on tape for study at a later time. They found that following successful mobilization of the stapes, a significant increase in CP amplitude was observed, whereas the eighth nerve action potential failed to show the same increase in amplitude. This is consistent with a later finding by Dallos et al.[56] Their studies revealed that in guinea pigs the microphonic CP of the inner ear is represented, in part, by the displacement of the basilar portion of the basilar membrane, which is proportional to the velocity of stapes movement into the oval window. Although results were positive in demonstrating a change in CP amplitude that correlated with postoperative improvements in hearing, the surgeon was not able to assess the status of this electrophysiologic correlate during the surgical process.

Ruben et al. also cited other technical limitations to intraoperative recordings:[52–55] (1) stimulus intensities at the ear were limited to 80 dB; (2) electrical interference was often excessive while recording in a general operating room; and (3) the anatomy of the human middle ear often made it difficult to seat the round window electrode since it often lies deep within the round window niche.

It was not until the advent of the biomedical signal averager in the late 1960s that successful recordings of human CPs were made readily available. Several reports emerged simultaneously from various laboratories in 1967 reporting ECoG recordings obtained in humans with a minimum of surgical intervention.[57–60] Since this time, many authors have tried to understand CPs and their relation to inner ear function or dysfunction. From their studies, various techniques and electrode types have emerged in attempts to simplify the acquisition of these potentials.

It was not until 1987 that Gibson and Arenberg[45] improved and revised the basic intraoperative technique set down by Ruben et al. more than 20 years ago.[52–55] However, the major goal of this new technique was not to merely study the CP and eighth nerve action potentials but to continually monitor the electrophysiologic parameters of the SP/AP ratio and document the changes effected by any mechanical or neural manipulation of the auditory system during nondestructive inner ear surgery. Thus, providing almost "real time" feedback information to the surgeon concerning the effects of each surgical step or manipulation.

Decisions for the best surgical treatment for Meniere's disease patients refractory to medical therapy have rarely been based on objective data. Until recently, nondestructive inner ear surgeries performed proximally at the endolymphatic sac relied on anatomic, visual, and palpation techniques for assessing intraoperative success. There was no objective intraoperative feedback to confirm successful decompression of the hydropic labyrinth.

Currently it is possible to take ECoG into the operating room and effectively use it to monitor the presence of ELH through the use of silver, ball-tip, round window membrane electrode and a special sound delivery system. This sound delivery system includes the use of a Cadwell 8400 biomedical signal averager. (However, any advanced biomedical signal averager with low internal impedance may be adapted for use in the operating room.) This is coupled to a standardized length of suction tubing extending from a hearing aid button type of receiver to the ear canal. This setup allows the maintenance of a sterile surgical field while creating a sound delivery system for auditory evoked potentials. With this system we can directly measure, monitor, and continue to compare the baseline enhanced and abnormal SP/AP ratio of a click stimulus to any subsequent change. In addition, we can isolate the SP from the AP intraoperatively and subsequently measure this distortion potential using 20-ms fast-rate tone bursts.

A stable, enhanced ECoG ratio baseline can be established, and intraoperative electrophysiologic changes can be easily monitored. When the hydropic inner ear is decompressed, dramatic and rapid changes can occur in less than 30 seconds, from a stable abnormal baseline to normal, indicating that nondestructive inner ear surgery for hydrops can work. Therefore, the surgeon can readily monitor changes almost as soon as they occur. This provides the surgeon for the first time objective feedback that the hydropic labyrinth has been decompressed and during exactly which surgical maneuver.

Overall, when the SP/AP ratio at closing is compared to the surgical baseline data, a 10% absolute improvement is considered a significant intraoperative change in the presence of an abnormal surgical baseline ratio greater than or equal to an absolute measurement of 33%. It is believed that the relative percentage changes rather than the absolute percentage changes are probably more significant clinically.

It is now possible to determine during surgery those patients who may really need a primary destructive procedure. If one believes that the hydropic labyrinth is decompressed but there is no change from the abnormal but stable baseline ECoG, the inner ear can be reapproached to try to decompress the hydropic system from a different incision or to probe differently in the ELD. If after due diligence a nondestructive approach to the hydropic inner ear is not successful according to changes in ECoG parameters, the surgeon can proceed during the same surgery to a destructive procedure, either a labyrinthectomy or VNS, based on the residual hearing present in the contralateral ear.

The surgeon now no longer has to rely on only surgical anatomic observations for determining the end point of the surgery. If one uses this intraoperative algorithm, the success rate of nondestructive inner ear surgery should be improved and the need for (primary) destructive procedures minimized. This intraoperative use of ECoG should document (1) a successful endolymphatic system decompression of the hydrops, (2) that the ELS and ELD surgery can work, (3) how the surgery works, (4) when the surgery works, and (5) why the surgery works.

A prototype study was set up at the University of Sydney in March of 1987. A specially designed silver ball-tip round window electrode was used to monitor the inner ear to mastoid shunt surgeries with valve on six patients. Preliminary results from Australia are encouraging and support our hypothesis that the positive electrophysiologic changes seen in Meniere's disease patients could represent a decrease or improvement in the hydropic condition. This may result in actual hearing and vestibular improvements postoperatively. Intraoperative ECoG changes following very stable baselines were, in fact, demonstrated in the patients in this prototype study. One year postoperatively, all of the patients except one are free of vertigo and have demonstrated and maintained improved ECoG ratios in follow-up. These results, if continued long term, should contribute to the success rate of nondestructive inner ear surgery.

Since the prototype study in Australia, we have monitored 57 cases during surgery for Meniere's disease with ELH. Using a silver ball-tip electrode, described previously, against the round window membrane may yield excellent and stable evoked responses in the 50- to 80-μV range.

CONCLUSION

The ELD and ELS offer a safe but difficult point of entry to the inner ear. It has been known for many years that occasional dramatic improvements could follow nondestructive inner ear surgery at the ELS, but the efficacy of this approach was clouded by the uncertainty that the inner ear had truly been affected by the surgery and by the natural history of hydrops, which is so prone to fluctuations.

New developments previously detailed as to the understanding of the pathophysiology and the etiology coupled with electrophysiologic monitoring of the inner ear using intraoperative ECoG can at least indicate when the physical goal of decompression of the hydropic inner ear has been accomplished. Perhaps now the surgery of the ELS and, more important, of the ELD needs more careful evaluation.

ACKNOWLEDGMENT

We extend our sincere gratitude and appreciation to Holly K. H. Bohlen, M.A., CCC-A, and Stephanie Norman for their dedication to this project; without them this chapter would not have been completed.

Intraoperative ECoG and Surgery Technique

NOTE: All drawings are from the surgeon's viewpoint and for a right ear.

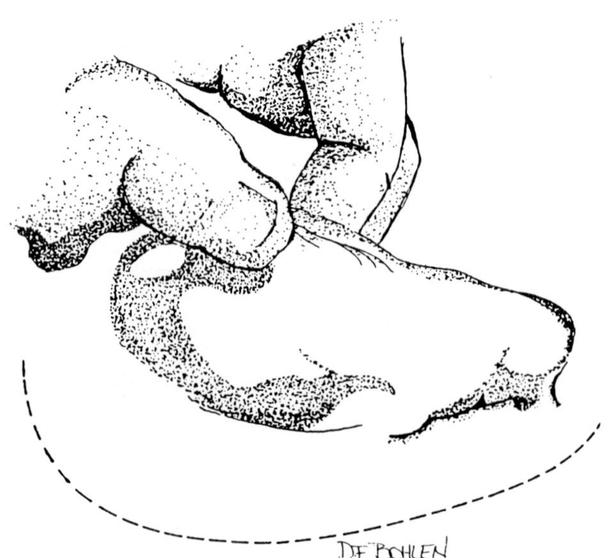

FIG 7A–1.
Postauricular incision.

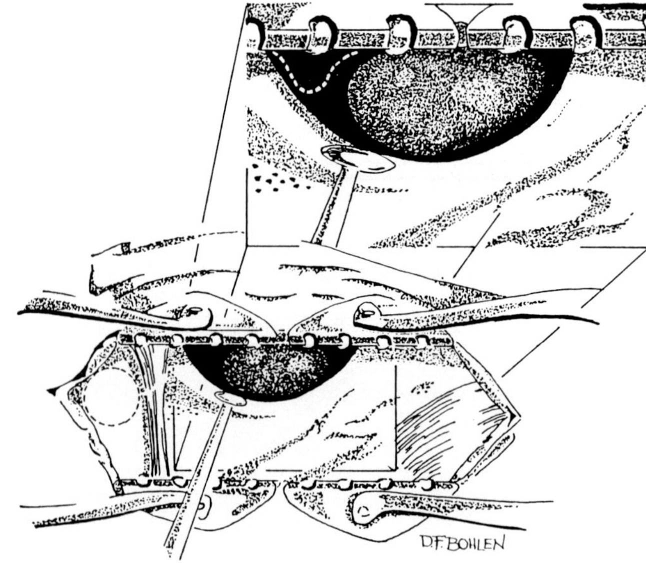

FIG 7A–2.
Elevation of posterior ear canal skin to tympanic sulcus from post-auricular incision.

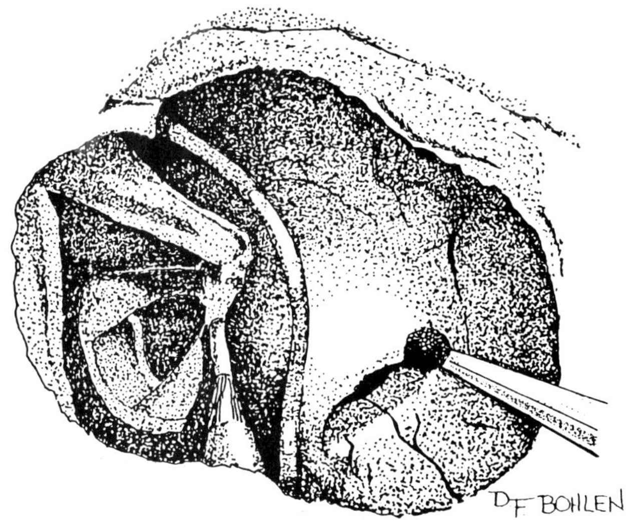

FIG 7A–3.
Microdrilling of lateral anterior bony ledge of round window membrane.

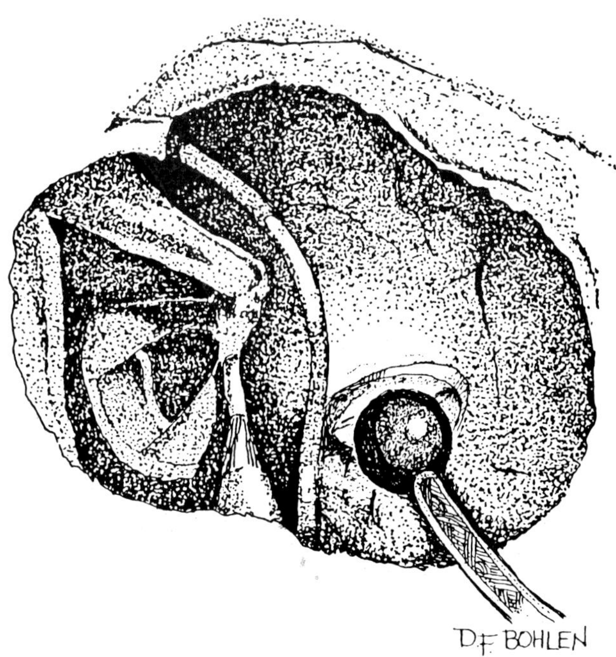

FIG 7A–5.
Silver ball-tip electrode in place.

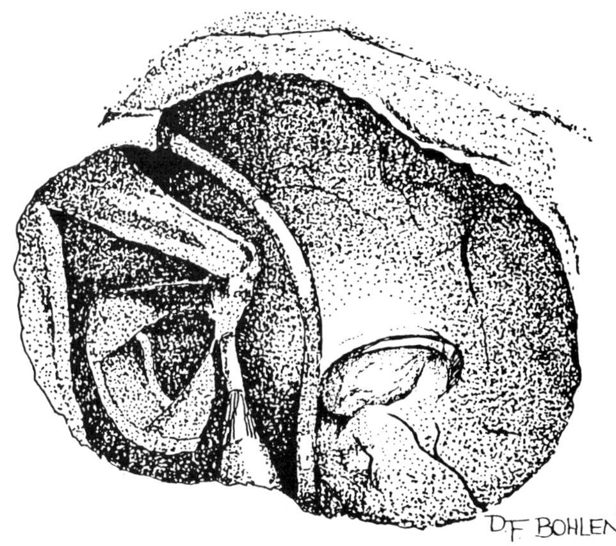

FIG 7A–4.
Drilled off lateral anterior bony ledge over round window niche.

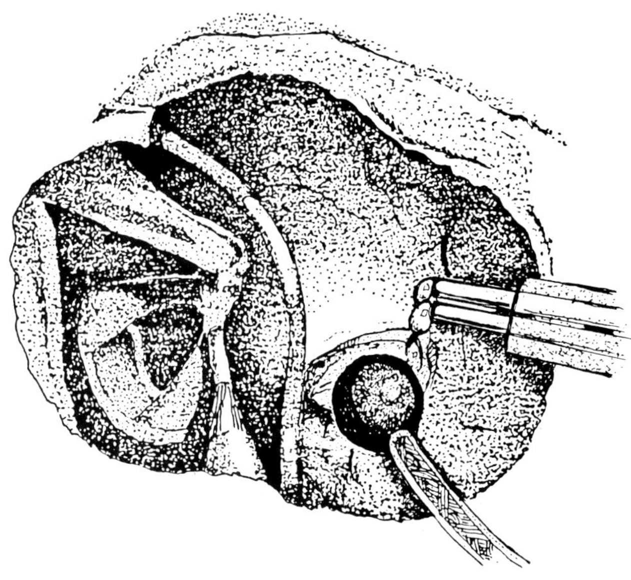

FIG 7A–6.
Autologous fibrin glue used as a sealant to anchor and isolate electrode from middle ear space.

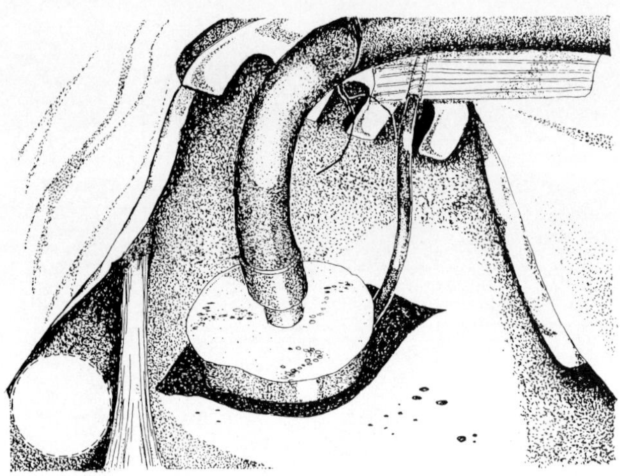

FIG 7A–7.
Sound delivery tube in place secured to retractor. Round window membrane electrode secured to retractor with Steri-Strip tape.

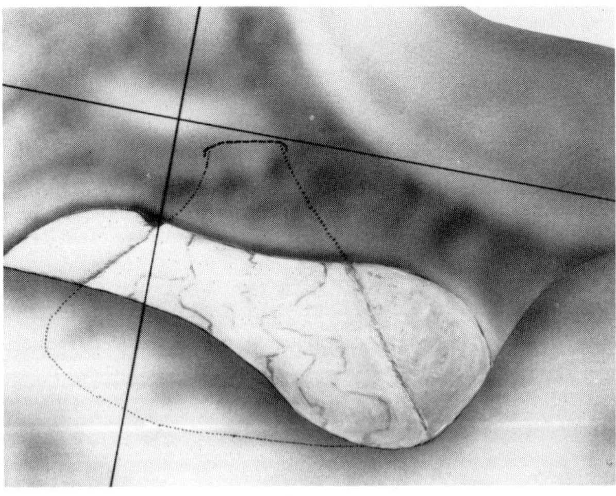

FIG 7A–8.
Surgical type I: Superior edge of the endolymphatic sac (ELS) is crossed by Donaldson's line. (Donaldson's line is the continuation in the mastoid of the horizontal semicircular canal as it bisects the posterior semicircular canal.

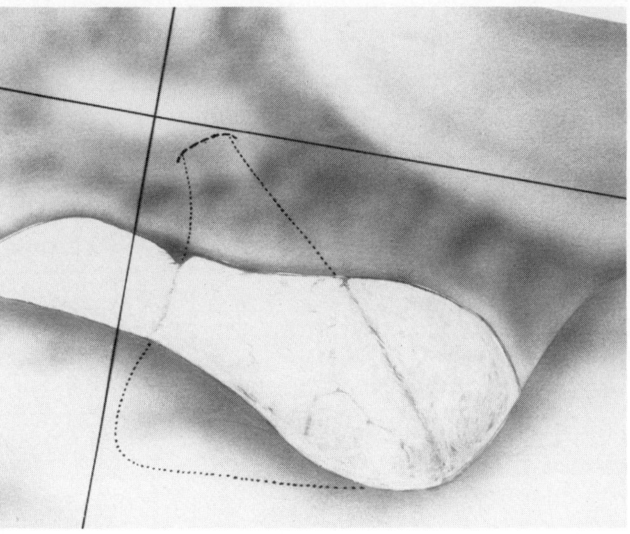

FIG 7A–9.
Surgical type II: Superior edge of the ELS is not crossed by Donaldson's line by at least 2 to 3 mm. Types I and II are most frequently seen in normal ears and infrequently in patients with Meniere's disease.

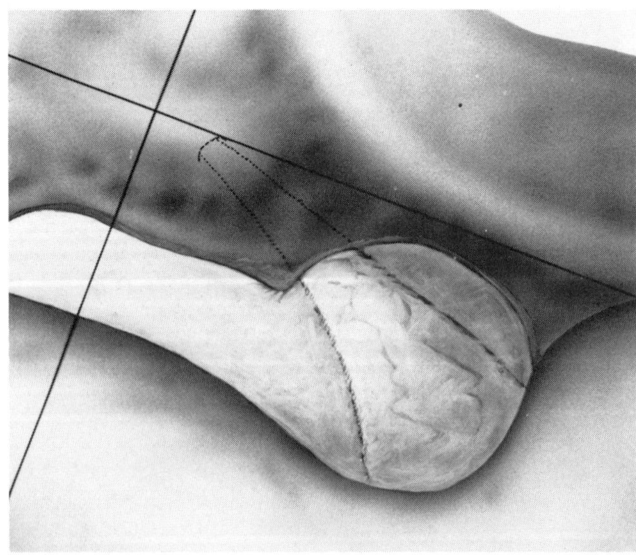

FIG 7A–10.
Surgical type III: The ELS is far inferior and anterior to Donaldson's line and often requires exenteration of the retrofacial air cell tract for surgical access.

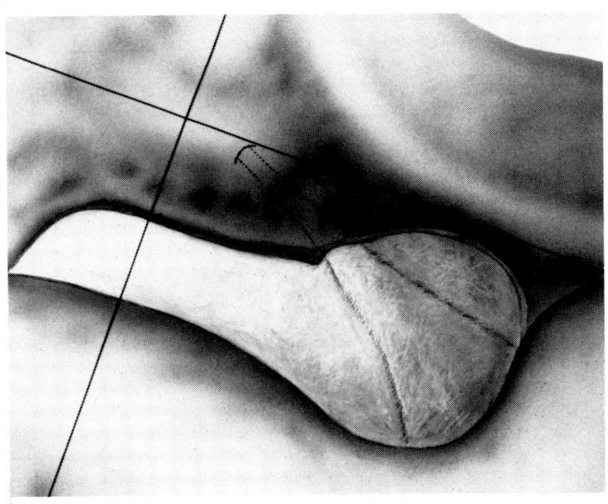

FIG 7A–11.
Surgical type IV (Shea): The ELS is so far anterior and inferior from the more normal type I or II positions that it is often on the jugular bulb rather than the sigmoid sinus. It is characteristically medial to the facial nerve.

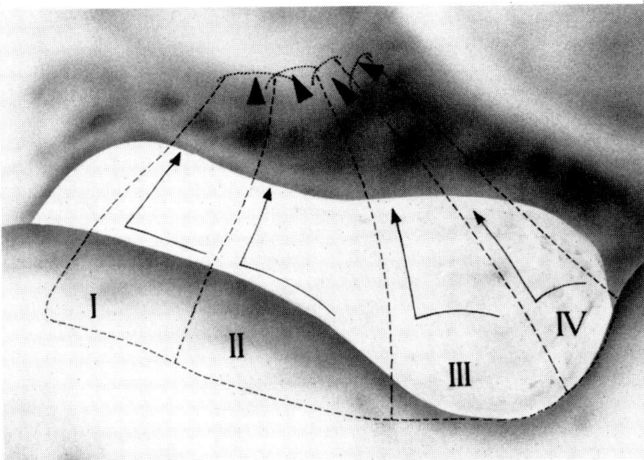

FIG 7A–12.
Composite drawing of surgical types I through IV shows their sizes and positions relative to each other, from a large ELS adjacent to Donaldson's line to smaller ELSs far from Donaldson's line. The external aperture of the vestibular aqueduct (EA/VA) is ghosted in, and it can be appreciated that this aperture also becomes smaller. Most important, the angulation of the EA/VA rotates away from the surgeon's direct access or cannulation. This is why it is advantageous to create an inferiorly based lateral ELS wall flap, which allows the surgeon to approach the EA/VA directly as it moves away into a technically more difficult position, for a direct shot at accurate cannulization.

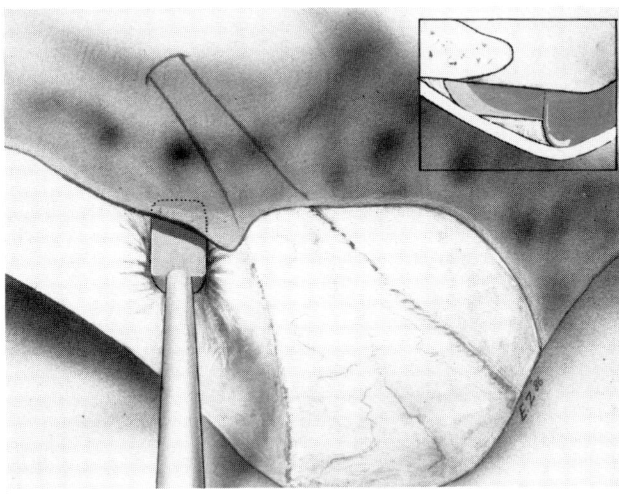

FIG 7A–13.
Endolymphatic sac is identified by color difference, thickness, and palpation for the point of attachment at the EA/VA. A superiorly based medial projection of the EA/VA, when identified accurately, defines the superior edge of the ELS. A special dural palpator elevator is designed to facilitate this demarcation by safely depressing the posterior fossa dura with the rounded head of the instrument while carefully separating the dura-ELS from its attachment to the otic capsule bone by the semisharp dissector edge (*inset*).

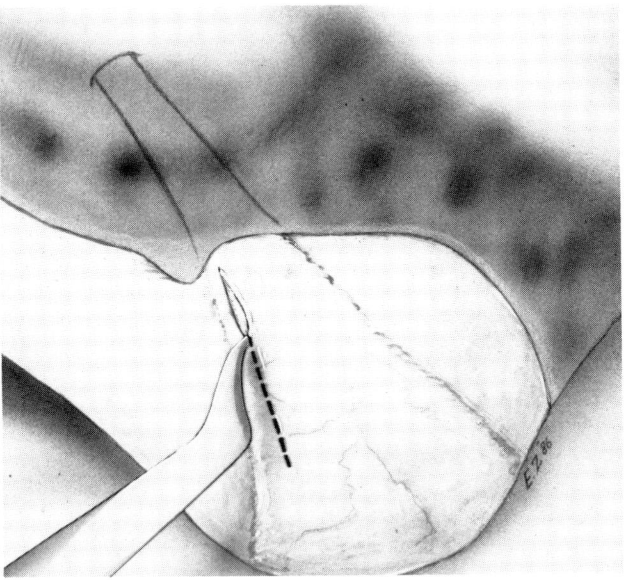

FIG 7A–14.
A specially designed ELS knife makes opening the ELS easier, particularly if it is thin and atrophic. Note that the first cut is made near the superior margin of the ELS, usually the thickest area of the ELS and hence the easiest in which to find the real lumen.

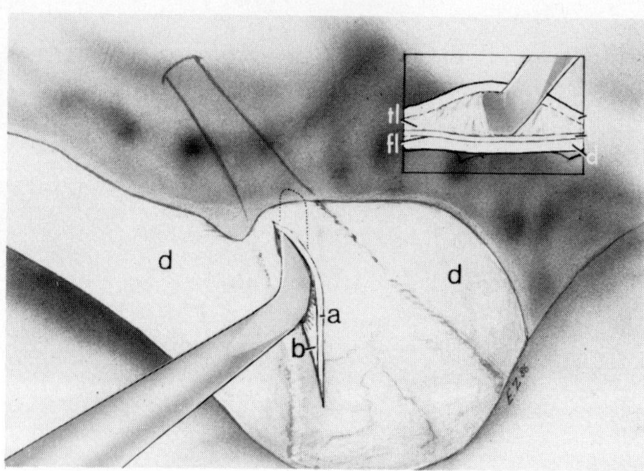

FIG 7A–15.
A 120- or 160-degree crabtree-type dissector is used to develop the opening into the ELS to determine if the opening is in the real lumen, the false lumen, or a created lumen. The real lumen is between the medial (*a*) and lateral (*b*) walls of the ELS. The 120-degree dissector will help break any adhesions in the real lumen (*inset*). *d* = posterior fossa dura.

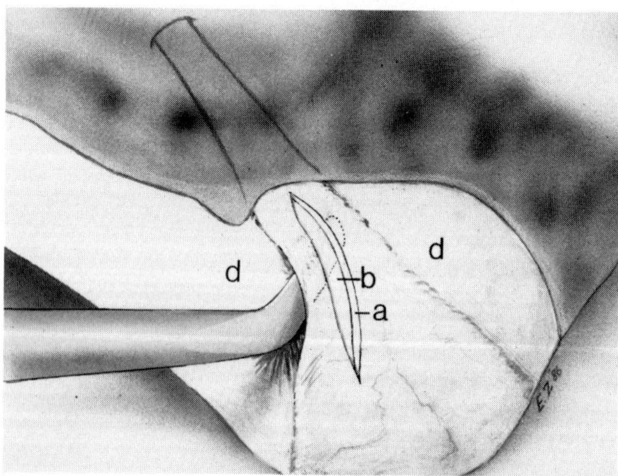

FIG 7A–16.
If the 120-degree dissector opens into a lumen more medial than both the lateral ELS wall (*a*) and the medial wall (*b*), it is in the false lumen. The false lumen is much easier to open and has fewer adhesions, because it is only an anatomic plane. Once entered, it is very easy to separate (*inset*).

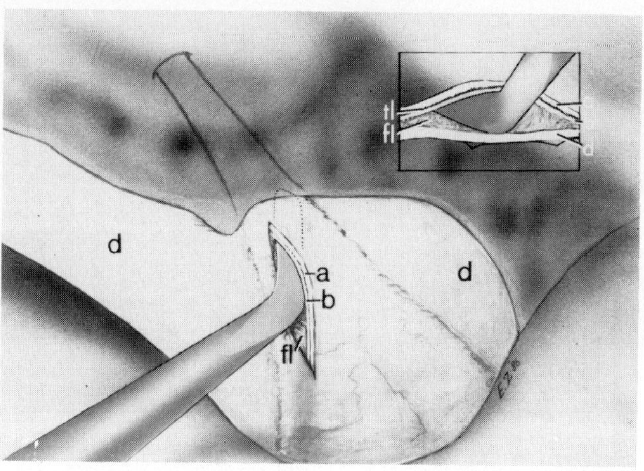

FIG 7A–17.
Entrance into the false lumen is anatomically resolved by making an additional ELS incision with the sac knife along the superior margin of the sac at its junction with the superior posterior fossa dura. The 120-degree dissector is used to elevate the entire ELS (both medial and lateral walls) off the posterior fossa dura. This is the basic technique for the double-wall ELS biopsy.[36] A special wedge dissector is most helpful for lifting the ELS off the dura once the true lumen is accurately entered. With the 120-degree dissector, if the false lumen has been entered and the medial wall of the ELS covers the dissector through the original incision (see Fig 7A–7) *then the original incision and dissection (see Fig 7A–8) has anatomically identified the real lumen of the ELS.)*

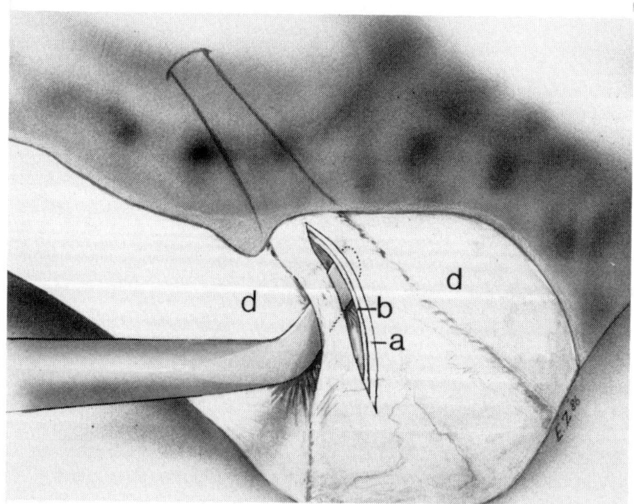

FIG 7A–18.
If the 120-degree dissector, passing along the posterior fossa dura under the entire ELS, and in the false lumen, is easily seen (no medial wall of the ELS covering the dissector) then the original incision (see Fig 7A–7) has cut through both lateral (*a*) and medial (*b*) walls of the ELS. When this occurs it is often better to make a new incision (see Fig 7A–7) in an area 1 mm from the original incision. It is also important in this situation to angle the sac knife on a greater bias so as to make an even thinner cut into the lateral wall of the ELS and enter the real lumen without cutting into or through the medial wall. The anatomic confirmation procedure (see Fig 7A–10) is repeated until the surgeon is satisfied that the real lumen has been found.

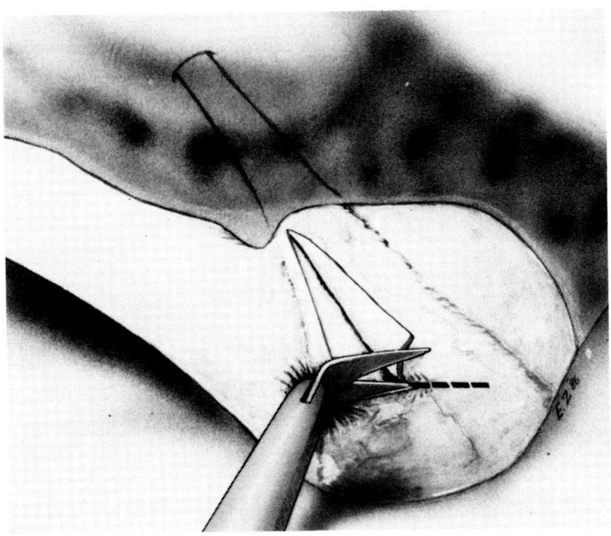

FIG 7A–19.
Once the real ELS lumen is anatomically identified, it can be most helpful, particularly in types III and IV ELS, to rotate an inferiorly based lateral ELS wall flap. This is accomplished with a special scissors, angled upward 30 degrees (and to the right for a right ear) so that the surgeon's hand is in a normal position and the cutting blades are parallel to the posterior fossa dura.

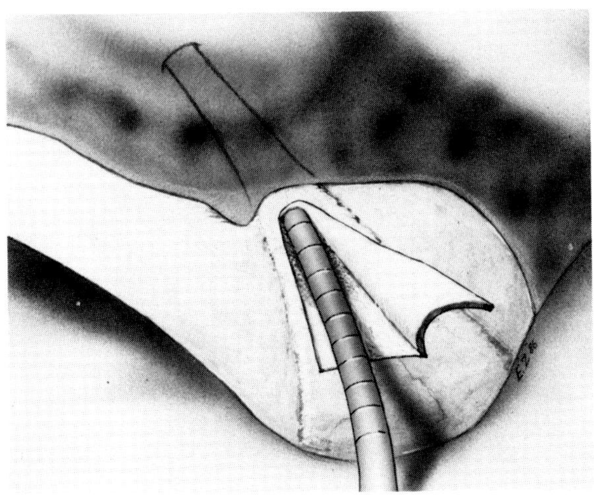

FIG 7A–20.
Once the inferiorly based lateral ELS wall flap is created, there is a much greater range of access to cannulate the endolymphatic duct (ELD) directly up to, and often through, the EA/VA (see Fig 7A–5). After the duct is palpated with the 120- or 160-degree dissector to try to feel for the bony EA/VA, a standard 6 or 10 mm duct probe is used to cannulate and measure the necessary length of the capillary tube portion of the valved shunt. Note that the outside diameters of the duct probe and of the capillary tube portion of the valved shunt are identical. Therefore, as far anteriorly as the ELD probe passes, so will the capillary portion of the implant.

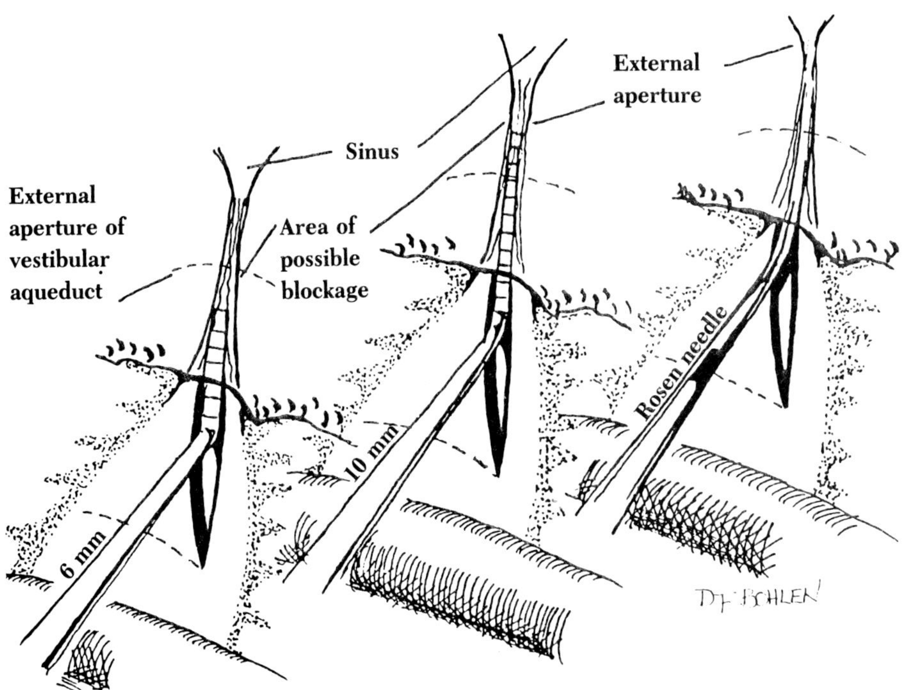

FIG 7A–21.
If the 6 mm probe is not sufficient, use the 10 mm duct probe and take the reading at the lateral bony surface, not at the opening of the ELS. Do not probe more anterior than 10 mm, particularly in a large VA, because the risk of intralabyrinthine damage increases dramatically past that point if you are entering just at the posterior surface of the posterior semicircular canal. With the inferiorly rotated flap, the surgeon can probe all along the EA/VA to find the largest, widest, highest opening into the proximal ELD.

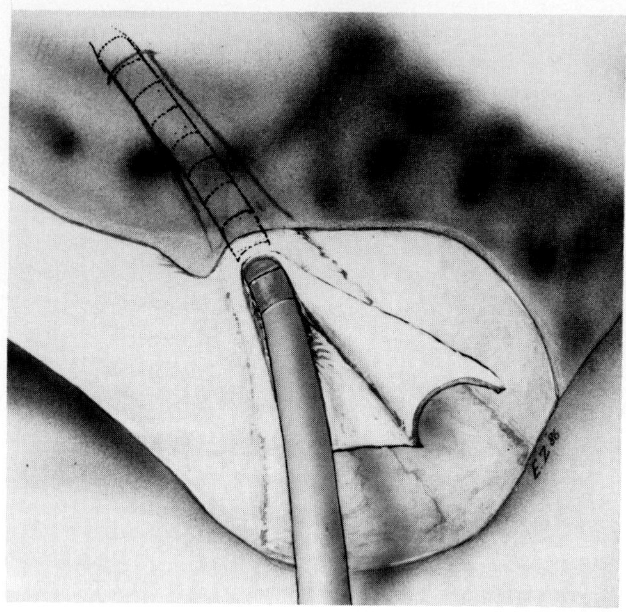

FIG 7A–22.
If there is a narrowed or "obstructed" area in the ELD and no ECoG confirmation of physiologic decompression of the labyringh (abnormal ECoG dramatically and quickly improves toward normal), very carefully try a sharp Rosen-type needle, carefully following the ELD up to the point of "blockage." It is essential to use intraoperative monitoring to safely and correctly do this. It is necessary to decompress the labyrinthine physiologically, with ECoG confirmation. The best anatomic dissection may be ineffective physiologically.

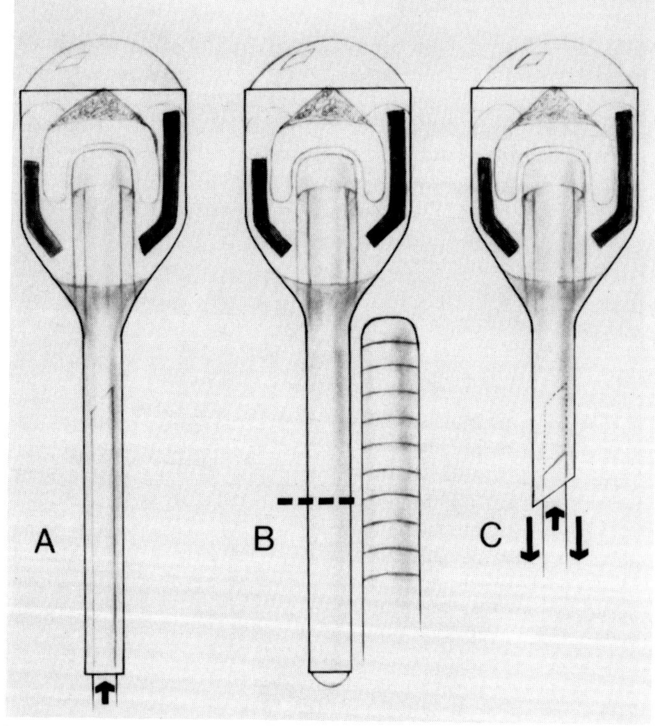

FIG 7A–23.
Once the ELD has been anatomically probed and decompression has been electrophysiologically confirmed by ECoG, the valved shunt is primed with heparin (or hyaluronidase; John Tonkin, personal communication, 1988) and the tail or wick is removed and used to facilitate mastoid aeration. The capillary tube portion is trimmed 1 to 2 mm *longer than measured (see Fig 7A–14), because its seating may be enhanced by the soft, tubular proximal end compared with the* solid duct probe. After trimming, it is essential to reprime the valve to make sure there are no air bubbles that could interfere with hydrodynamic coupling. Reprime the valve while simultaneously injecting the heparin as the priming needle is withdrawn.

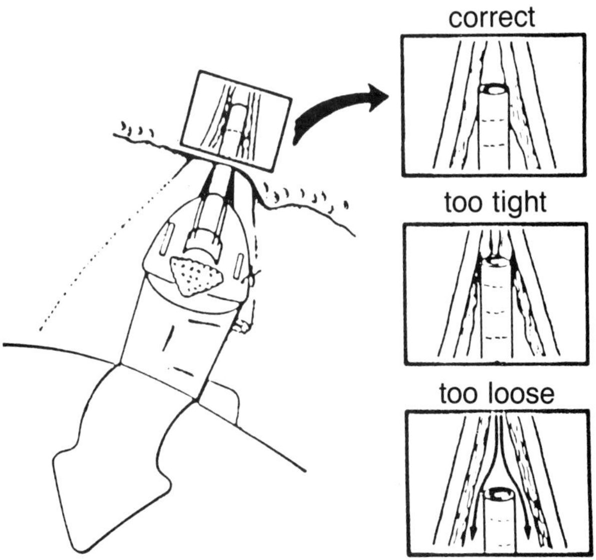

FIG 7A–25.
Anatomically and by palpation there is "correct seating." The surgeon must be careful to avoid a "too tight" seating so that ELD mucosa cannot block the inflow tract. On the other hand, a "too loose" valve seating will allow excess endolymph under pressure to escape around the capillary tube, undermining the effectiveness of the unidirectional valve implant. In some cases, there may be additional ECoG confirmation of correct valve seating and hydrodynamic coupling.

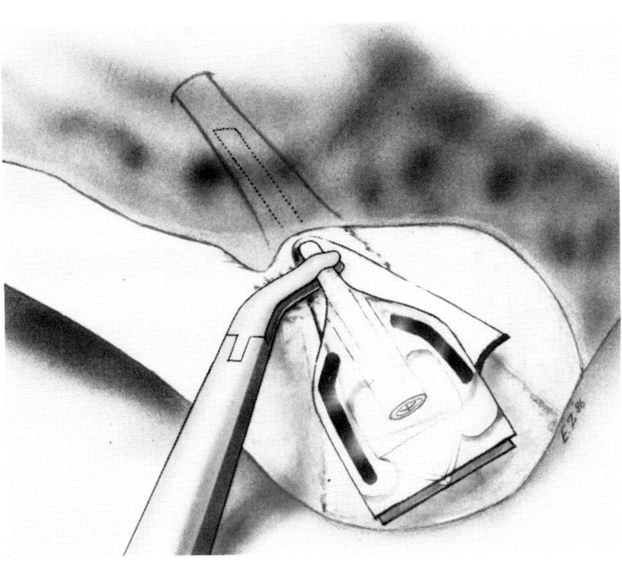

FIG 7A–24.
A special valve introducer (to the right for right ears) can be used to safely and securely grab the capillary tube portion of the valved implant *without* crimping, kinking, or pumping it, thus preventing any bubbles from getting into the system. If bubbles are visible, redo the above steps. It is helpful to fill the area around the ELS opening with heparin or dexamethasone so that the primed capillary tip of the valve with its meniscus is less likely to be dislodged once it is introduced into a fluid-fluid environment. Gently cannulate the capillary tube portion of the valve up the predetermined tract (as developed with the ELD probe) until it is accurately seated anatomically. There will routinely be almost no resistance if the same tract as the duct probe is followed (see Figs 7A–13 and 7A–14).

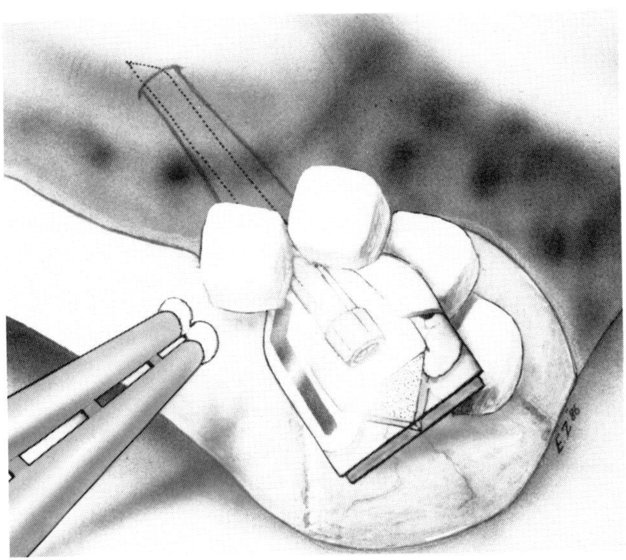

FIG 7A–26.
After the valve is anatomically and physiologically seated and hydrodynamically coupled, the ELS defect at the implant site is closed with anterior flap or fascia and autologous fibrin glue. A special bitubular delivery system is available. The glue is then used as a sealant over the open ELS. Small pledgets of absorbable sponge (Gelfoam) soaked in dexamethasone are placed around the implant to pump it up until the onflow tract is held up in the middle of the air-containing space of the mastoid cavity, as far from any surface as possible.

REFERENCES

1. Cawthorne T: Discussion. *Acta Otolaryngol (Stockh)* 1965; 59:152.
2. Stahle J, Stahle, C, Arenberg IK: Incidence of Meniere's disease. *Arch Otolaryngol* 1978; 104:99–102.
3. Alford BR: Report of Subcommittee on Equilibrium and Its Measurement. Meniere's disease: Criteria for diagnosis and evaluation of therapy for reporting. *Trans Am Acad Ophthalmol Otolaryngol* 1972; 76:1462–1464.
4. Gibson WPR, Moffat DA, Ramsden RT: Clinical ECoG in diagnosis and management of Meniere's disorder. *Audiology* 1977; 16:389–401.
5. Brackmann D, Jahrsdorfer R: Meniere's disease: Criteria for diagnosis and evaluation of therapy for reporting. *AAO-HNS Bull* July 1985, pp 6–7.
6. Shambaugh GE Jr, Glasscock ME: *Surgery of the Ear,* ed 3. Philadelphia, WB Saunders Co, 1980, pp 519–559.
7. Shambaugh GE Jr, Clemis JD, Arenberg IK: The endolymphatic duct and sac in Meniere's disease. I: Surgical and histopathologic observations. *Arch Otolaryngol* 1969; 89:816–825.
8. Portmann G: Vertigo: Surgical treatment by opening the saccus endolymphaticus. *Arch Otoloaryngol* 1927; 6:309–315.
9. Yamakawa K, Naito T: The modification of Portmann's operation for Meniere's disease (Yamakawa-Naito's operation) *Med J Osaka Univ* 1954; 5:167–175.
10. House WF: Subarachnoid shunt for drainage of hydrops: A report of 63 cases. *Arch Otolaryngol Head Neck Surg* 1964; 79:338–342.
11. Arenberg IK, Rask-Andersen H, Wilbrand H, et al: The surgical anatomy of the endolymphatic sac. *Arch Otolaryngol Head Neck Surg* 1977; 103:1–11.
12. Shea JS, Chole R, Paparella MM: The endolymphatic sac: Anatomical considerations. *Laryngoscope* 1979; 89:88–94.
13. Stahle J, Wilbrand H: The vestibular aqueduct in patients with Meniere's disease. *Acta Otolarynol (Stockh)* 1974; 78:36–48.
14. Sackett JF, Kozarek JA, Arenberg IK: The clinical significance of tomographic visualization or nonvisualization of the vestibular aqueduct. *Otolaryngol Clin North Am* 1980; 13:657–665.
15. Oigaard A, Thomsen J, Jensen J, et al: The narrow vestibular aqueduct: An unspecific radiologic sign? *Arch Otorhinolaryngol* 1975; 211:1–8.
16. Arenberg IK: Abnormalities, congenital anomalies, and unusual anatomic variations of the endolymphatic sac and vestibular aqueduct: Clinical, surgical, and radiographic correlations. *Am J Otol* 1980; 2:118–149.
17. Arenberg IK: Abnormalities, congenital anomalies, and unusual anatomic variations of the endolymphatic sac and vestibular aqueduct: Clinical, surgical, and radiographic correlations, Group I anomalies. *Am J Otol* 1981; 2:248–268.
18. Arenberg IK: Abnormalities, congenital anomalies, and unusual anatomic variations of the endolymphatic sac and vestibular aqueduct: Clinical, surgical, and radiographic correlations, Group II anomalies. *Am J Otol* 1981; 2:368–386.
19. Arenberg IK: Abnormalities, congenital anomalies, and unusual anatomic variations of the endolymphatic sac and vestibular aqueduct: Clinical, surgical, and radiographic correlations, Group III, IV, V anomalies. *Am J Otol* 1982; 3:221–240.
20. Jackler RK, Luxford WM, House WF: Congenital malformations of the inner ear: A classification based on embryogenesis. *Laryngoscope* 1987; 97(suppl 40):2–15.
21. Arenberg IK, Jackson CG, Gardner G, et al: The surgical anatomy and fine points of endolymphatic system surgery. A panel discussion at the 2nd International Symposium and Workshops on Surgery of the Inner Ear *Am J Otol* 1987; 8:345–354.
22. Balkany TJ, Sires B, Arenberg IK: Bilateral aspects of Meniere's disease: An underestimated clinical entity. *Otolaryngol Clin North Am* 1980; 13:603–611.
23. Torok N: Old and new in Meniere's disease. *Laryngoscope* 1977; 87:1870–1877.
24. Friberg U, Stahle J, Svedberg A: The natural course of Meniere's disease. *Acta Otolaryngol (Stockh)* 1984; 406:72–77.
25. Arenberg IK, Stahle J: Staging Meniere's disease (or any inner ear dysfunction) and the use of the vertigogram. *Otolaryngol Clin North AM* 1980; 12:643–657.
26. Arenberg IK, Stahle J, Newkirk JB: Unidirectional inner ear valve implant: Utilization in endolymphatic sac surgery for hydrops. Presented at the American Academy of Ophthalmology Otolaryngology Meeting, Section on New Instruments and Devices, Dallas, Oct 1977.
27. Gibson WPR: A study of endolymphatic sac surgery: The results after reconstructing the sac versus those in operations that fail to open the lumen and satisfactorily insert a Silastic implant. *Otolaryngol Clin North Am* 1983; 16:181–188.
28. Morrison AW: The surgery of vertigo: Saccus drainage for idopathic endolymphatic hydrops. *J Laryngol Otol* 1976; 90:87–93.
29. Austin DF: The endolymphatic shunt operation. *Otolaryngol Clin North Am* 1968; 1:589–606.
30. Paparella MM, Hanson DG: Endolymphatic sac drainage for intractable vertigo (method and experience) *Laryngoscope* 1976; 86:697–703.
31. Shambaugh GE Jr: Decompression of the endolymphatic sac for hydrops. *Otolaryngol Clin North Am* 1968; 1:607–611.
32. Shea JJ: Surgery of the endolymphatic sac. *Otolaryngol Clin North Am* 1968; 1:613–621.
33. Arenberg IK, Spector GJ: Endolymphatic sac surgery for conservation of hearing in Meniere's disease. *Arch Otolaryngol Head Neck Surg* 1977; 103:268–270.
34. Arenberg IK, Stahle J: Endolymphatic sac operations for Menieres disease: A comparison of the pressure-sensitive unidirectional inner ear valve and Silastic sheeting in patients with a minimum one-year follow-up. *Am J Otol* 1981; 2:329–334.
35. Arenberg IK, Wackym PA, Shambaugh GE Jr, et al: Comparative ultrastructure of the human endolymphatic sacs from normal and Meniere's disease patients: Spectrum of epithelial and subepithelial pathology. Presented at the 2nd International Symposium on Meniere's disease, Cambridge, Mass, June 20–23, 1988.
36. Arenberg IK, Norback DH, Shambaugh GE Jr: Ultrastructural analysis of endolymphatic sac biopsies: Biopsy technique and identification of endolympathic sac epithelium. *Arch Otolaryngol Head Neck Surg* 1982; 108:292–298.
37. Arenberg IK, Balkany TJ: Revision endolymphatic sac and

duct surgery for recurrent Meniere's disease. I: Failure analysis and technical aspects. *Laryngoscope* 1982; 92:1279–1284.

38. Arenberg IK: The fine points of valve implant surgery for hydrops: An update. *Am J Otol* 1982; 3:359–374.

39. Arenberg IK: Endolymphatic sac surgery (technique and long-term results). Presented at the 6th International Symposium on Neurological Surgery of the Ear and Skull Base, Zurich, Switzerland, May 29, 1988.

40. Arenberg IK: Results of endolymphatic sac to mastoid shunt surgery for Meniere's disease refractory to medical therapy. *Am J Otol* 1987; 8:335–344.

41. Huang T-S: Valve implants compared to other surgical methods. *Am J Otol* 1987; 8:301–306.

42. Wright WJ, Hicks GW: Valved implants in endolymphatic sac surgery. *Am J Otol* 1987; 8:307–312.

43. Stahle J, Arenberg IK: Ten year follow-up on the first five inner ear valve implants for intractable vertigo in Sweden. *Am J Otol* 1987; 8:287–293.

44. Arenberg IK, Gibson WPR: Non-destructive inner ear surgery for treatment of Meniere's disease and hydrops: The value of intraoperative electrocochleographic monitoring. Presented at the Sixth International Symposium on Neurological Surgery of the Ear and Skull Base, Zurich, Switzerland, May 28–June 2, 1988.

45. Arenberg IK, Gibson WPR: Improvements in audiometric and electrophysiologic parameters following non-destructive inner ear surgery utilizing a valved shunt for Meniere's disease. Presented at the 2nd International Symposium on Meniere's Disease, Cambridge, Mass, June 20–23, 1988.

46. Arenberg IK, Marovitz WF, Shambaugh GE Jr: The role of the endolymphatic sac in the pathogenesis of endolymphatic hydrops in man. *Acta Otolaryngol (Stockh) [Suppl]* 275:1–49.

47. Gibson WPR, Arenberg IK, Best L: Intraoperative electro-cochleographic monitoring of nondestructive inner ear surgery for hydrops: The intraoperative technique and preliminary clinical results. *Otolaryngol Head Neck Surg* 1988; 99:170–171.

48. Boyce SE, Mischke RE, Goin DW: Hearing results and control of vertigo following retrolabyrinthine vestibular nerve sections. *Laryngoscope* 1988; 98:251–261.

49. Glasscock ME III, Johnson GD, Poe DS: Long term hearing results following middle fossa vestibular nerve sections. Presented at the American Neurotology Society, Palm Beach, Fla, April 21–24, 1988.

50. Moffat DA, Gibson WRP, Ramsden TR, et al: Transtympanic electrocochleography during glycerol dehydration. *Acta Otolaryngol (Stockh)* 1978; 85:158–166.

51. Ruben RJ, Knickerbocker GG, Sekula J, et al: Cochlear microphonics in man. *Laryngoscope* 1959; 69:665.

52. Ruben RJ, Bordley JE, Lieberman AT: Cochlear potentials in man. *Laryngoscope* 1961; 71:1141–1163.

53. Ruben RJ, Lieberman AT, Bordley JE: Some observations on cochlear potentials and nerve action potentials in children. *Laryngoscope* 1962; 72:545–553.

54. Bordley JE, Ruben RJ, Lieberman AT: Human cochlear potentials. *Laryngoscope* 1964; 74:463–478.

55. Dallos P, Schoeny ZG, Cheatham MA: Cochlear summating potentials: Descriptive aspects. *Acta Otolaryngol (Stockh) [Suppl]* 1972; 302:1–45.

56. Portmann M, Aran J-M, LeBert G: Electro-cocleogramme humain endehors de toute intervention chirurgicale. *Acta Otolaryngol (Stockh)* 1967; 71:253–261.

57. Yoshie N, Ohashi T, Suzuki T: Non-surgical recordings of auditory nerve action potentials in man. *Laryngoscope* 1967; 77:76–85.

58. Sohmer H, Feinmesser M: Cochlear action potentials recorded from the external ear in man. *Ann Otol Rhinol Laryngol* 1967; 76:427–435.

59. Spreng M, Keidel WD: Separeirung von cerebroaudiogram (CAG), neuroaudiogramm (NAG) und otoaudiogramm (OAG) in der objecktiven audiometrie. *Arch Klin Exp Ohren-Nasen-Kehlkopfheik* 1967; 189:225–246.

Nondestructive Surgery for Vertigo

Approach of

Michael M. Paparella, M.D.

Michael S. Morris, M.D.
and
Sady S. daCosta, M.D.

ENDOLYMPHATIC SAC SURGERY

Paparella Technique

The Paparella procedure is begun with a curvilinear postauricular incision from the mastoid tip inferiorly toward the temporal line superiorly arcing 1.5 to 2.0 cm posterior to the postauricular crease. This incision is carried down to the level of the mastoid periosteum, and an anteriorly based flap is elevated in the subperiosteal plane. A complete mastoidectomy is carried out. The region of the aditus is widened, and the incus is exposed within the context of the fossa incudis.

The depth of drilling in the mastoid cavity is never taken below the level of the dome of the horizontal semicircular canal. The purpose for complete mastoidectomy is to gain good exposure that will facilitate steps taken later in the procedure. Exposure of the incus and horizontal semicircular canal is necessary for orientation and for taking measurements that will be described. Drilling below the dome of the horizontal semicircular canal endangers the posterior semicircular canal. Enlargement of the aditus facilitates transfer of air between middle ear and mastoid and prevention of a postoperative aditus block syndrome.[1]

The next step involves determination of the location of the posterior semicircular canal to avoid compromising this important structure. Using the fenestrometer, the surgeon takes the first measurement from the short process of the incus in the fossa incudis 10 mm inferiorly along the axis of the horizontal semicircular canal. The second measurement is started at the same point and taken in an inferoposterior direction at an angle of approximately 45 degrees to the linea temporalis. The zone of the solid angle is demarcated so that further surgery will not compromise the proposed location of the posterior semicircular canal. These measurements are based on anatomic studies and create a demarcated zone that will facilitate protection of the labyrinth.[2]

The lateral sinus is skeletonized and decompressed throughout its length in the mastoid, and bone overlying Trautmann's triangle is thinned and removed with mastoid curettes or a rongeur. Decompression of the lateral sinus enhances subsequent decompression of Trautmann's triangle and the contiguous dura below the solid angle. Immediately below the demarcated bony zone, an infralabyrinthine cell tract is searched for. Purposeful, exaggerated drilling of bone is done toward the jugular bulb to expose as much dura as safely as possible in this area. The anteriorly located facial nerve should be cautiously watched for and avoided.

Exposure of infralabyrinthine dura is important in that the sac and its lumen often lie within this area and not posterior to the posterior semicircular canal. The dura contiguous with the decompressed lateral sinus is firmly decompressed, especially below the solid angle. Care must be taken not to traumatize the dura above the sac, which is thin. This can lead to leakage of CSF.

The sac is entered beneath the solid angle. Epithelium of the sac is visualized, and a Whirlybird instrument is inserted to help to bluntly and safely identify the lumen. The entrance to the sac should not be opened to the mastoid cavity, so as to prevent fibrosis or granulation tissue from invading the sac. One or two silicone rubber (Silastic) T struts 0.005 in. thick are placed within the sac. Spacers or strips of a similar material are folded above and below the sac and between the dura and the overlying temporal bone to decompress the dura and contiguous lateral sinus more permanently. These strips serve as a soft, springlike mechanism for decompression of dura and sac. The T struts within the sac enlarge the lumen and help the passive transfer of nanoliters of endolymph.

A Silastic apron of the same thickness used previously in the procedure is placed over this region, followed by a sizable piece of absorbable gelatin sponge (Gelfoam) dipped in a steroid antibiotic solution. This holds the apron in place. The purpose of this apron is to help keep fibroblasts from invading the region of the endolymphatic sac.

The mastoid cavity and surrounding wound are meticulously cleaned of debris and bone dust. The wound is closed in a careful triple-layered fashion. A small Penrose drain is placed in the inferior aspect of the wound leading from the mastoid cavity outward. This drain is removed on the morning of the first postoperative day. A myringotomy is carried out in the tympanic membrane, and the middle ear is irrigated in such a way as to remove with care any bone dust that may have accumulated. A ventilation tube is placed. If, however, during the course of the procedure, leakage of CSF has developed, the ventilation tube is not placed. The tube helps to promote ventilation in the middle ear and mastoid, to ensure a more successful healing result, and to prevent otitis media postoperatively.[1]

Indications

Our philosophy and policy is that conservative treatment comes first. Medical treatment with psychologic support precedes any consideration of surgery. With medical therapy, we treat the symptoms, thus circumstantially improving conditions for the patient. Since most drugs act on an empirical basis, our policy is not to discourage the use of any of them if the treatment employed minimizes the symptoms and improves the quality of life for the patient.

In those cases in which the deafness or vertigo (or both) become intractable despite medical therapy or the symptoms progressively worsen, a conservative surgical procedure — ELS enhancement — is considered. We consider this surgical option for patients with intractable Meniere's disease, typical or atypical. The primary indications are vertigo and vestibular dysfunction; a secondary indication is deafness. The results are much better for vertigo than for improvement of hearing; however, there is evidence to suggest that approximately one patient of three does have improvement of hearing. The likelihood of improving vertigo or vestibular upset is 90%, of eliminating vertigo or vestibular upset is 70%, of retaining hearing 90%, and of improving hearing is 30% to 40%. The risk of deafness is 2%, and this is usually related to infection of the wound and aditus-block syndrome.[3] Other investigators have estimated that approximately one of four patients with Meniere's disease may eventually be a candidate for surgical therapy[4]; however, our ratio in a referral practice is closer to one in eight.

Another way of defining intractability is when nonprogressive Meniere's disease becomes progressive Meniere's disease, as determined by vertigo or deafness, in spite of prolonged medical therapy. The best and only way to determine progressive or intractable vertigo and vestibular dysfunction is via the history, which is capsulized in the record. The best way to document progressive or intractable hearing loss is with audiometry or preferably serial audiograms. In our previous studies, the average duration of disease before ELS enhancement was 6 years, with a minimum of 1 year.[1,3] Although uncommon, certain patients with Meniere's disease have a rapid downhill course. We have seen patients evolve into intractable, incapacitating vertigo and profound deafness within a 3-month period.

Endolymphatic sac enhancement as a conservative surgical treatment for Meniere's disease has stood the test of time for more than 60 years. It is conservative, since it is a temporal bone procedure, the purpose of which is to preserve and enhance labyrinthine function, as contrasted to destructive procedures, such as intracranial vestibular nerve section, which have greater morbidity and risk. Contraindications for ELS enhancement in patients with intractable Meniere's disease are few and in the main include systemic illnesses that contraindicate the use of general anesthesia. Endolymphatic sac enhancement has been successful in retaining or improving hearing of all degrees, including mild, moderate, or severe (profound) sensorineural hearing loss. Compared with intracranial vestibular nerve section, this conservative ear procedure requires only an overnight stay in the hospital and has been used successfully to treat incapacitating prolonged vertigo in patients of all ages, including children and elderly adults in their 80s and even 90s.

Problems in Achieving Exposure

Medial and Anterior Sigmoid Sinus

Previous clinical experience with nearly 900 cases of ELS enhancement has revealed that the sigmoid sinus is in an abnormal position in patients who have Meniere's disease. A prospective study of 23 consecutive surgeries on the ELS and 15 normal pneumatized temporal bones was undertaken, along with radiographic analysis of mastoid x-ray films from ten normal individuals, to analyze the position of the sigmoid sinus in patients with Meniere's disease. In most patients with Meniere's disease who underwent surgery on the ELS, the sigmoid sinus is located closer to the area of the ELS and closer to the semicircular canals, in a more anterior and medial location than in normal individuals.[5] Surgical management of an anteriorly or medially placed sigmoid sinus includes skeletonization and decompression of the sinus throughout its length in the mastoid. Bone over Trautmann's triangle is thinned and removed with mastoid curettes or a rongeur. Since the sigmoid sinus is often associated with hypopneumatization of air cells and a small or nonexistent Trautmann's triangle, decompression of the lateral sinus enhances subsequent decompression of Trautmann's triangle and the contiguous dura below the solid angle where the sac is entered.

Anomalies of the Endolymphatic Sac

In all conservative operations on the ELS, the sac must be safely identified without inadvertent injury to the structures of the inner ear or the mastoid segment of the facial nerve. It serves well to remember that the sac is not merely a dilation of the ELD but a distinct anatomic structure with average measurements of 8.9 by 9.0 mm. Following anatomic studies in human temporal bones, the ELS is consistently located below the bony capsule of the posterior semicircular canal, which appears not more than 11.5 mm inferior to the dome of the short process of the incus. The main body of the sac is found between 11.5 and 19.0 mm from the short process of the incus.[2] Measurements are made with the fenestrometer from the fossa incudis 10 mm along the axis of the horizontal semicircular canal and 12 mm (approximately 45 degrees) from the linea temporalis. The zone of the solid angle (containing the canals) is demarcated so that further surgery will not enter this zone.

This observation makes it unnecessary to risk exposure of the blue line of the posterior semicircular canal; using measurements taken following a complete mastoidectomy will avoid injury to this vulnerable structure. Purposeful exaggerated drilling of bone is done toward the jugular bulb to expose as much dura as safely as possible in this area. Often infralabyrinthine cells do not exist, and this exposure is done through solid bone. In restrictive mastoids (sclerotic or diploic), the anteriorly located facial nerve should be watched for and avoided. The purpose is to expose infralabyrinthine dura because the main body of the sac and its lumen often lie within this area and not posterior to the posteroinferior semicircular canal. The lumen of the sac is always entered and identified. In patients with Meniere's disease, the sac may be hypoplastic and may occupy a more inferior and anterior position than is customarily expected.

Endolymphatic Sac Enhancement

The method for ELS enhancement includes placement of Silastic T-struts (0.005 in. thick) within the lumen of the sac. Passive diffusion of endolymph is allowed to take place along inert alloplastic surfaces of Silastic placed in the expanded lumen of the sac. This procedure creates primarily decompression but also an extracellular electrolytic environment of sodium ions, which, in turn, creates an osmotic pull on endolymph from the opposite vestibular end of the ELD, which is high in potassium. Shunts or valves themselves are not used.[1,6]

In patients undergoing revisions of procedures on the ELS (approximately 5% of our ELS enhancement patients), extrusion of Silastic is not usually found. Instead, revisional procedures have revealed extrasaccular fibrosis or granulation tissue, osteoneogenesis, and aditus-block syndrome resulting in saccular obstruction and a tight contiguous dura. Meticulous removal of obstructive fibrosis and bony overgrowth in the region of the sac is undertaken, and the intraluminal Silastic T-strut is removed and replaced. After this obstruction is alleviated and the absorption of endolymph is once again enhanced, most patients return to a symptom-free state.[6] Exaggerated attempts are made to prevent further formation of bone and scar tissue.

Immediate Recurrent Vertigo

Wound Infection

At least 2 months of postoperative time is necessary to allow the ear to settle down after ELS enhancement. During this time, a small percentage of patients may have vertigo or hearing loss, only to develop a long-term good result. Indeed, we have seen many patients develop improved and sustained hearing years after ELS enhancement. A small subset of patients has been noted to develop vertigo or further sensorineural deafness following surgery on the ELS. Occasionally, these symptoms develop in the perioperative period, days to weeks following surgery.

In our experience, the main cause for immediate iatrogenic postoperative symptoms is infection of the wound, which occurs in less than 2% of patients. This wound infection is usually visible on the surface but may be invisible and subcutaneous. The danger is that inflammation of the postoperative mastoid can result in labyrinthitis and deafness. Other causes are once again looked for, including central disorders such as tumors of the cerebellopontine angle. If a pathologic condition is suspected to lie in the middle ear or mastoid, the operated ear is explored. On occasion, aditus block syndrome has been found with granulation tissue obliterating the mastoid cavity. In such a case, the aditus is widened, the mastoid cavity is cleared, and decompression of the sac is checked; if necessary, intraluminal Silastic is replaced in the sac.[6] Of course, the patient is treated with appropriate intravenous antibiotic therapy. We also routinely use a ventilation tube in these patients. The tube acts as a drain for the middle ear cleft, which assists the postoperative healing process and helps prevent otitis media in the immediate postoperative phase or, if the patient travels by air, for weeks subsequent to the procedure.

Delayed Recurrent Vertigo

Delayed onset of these symptoms is found in a group of patients with intractable Meniere's disease who have a good result for months or years following ELS enhancement, only to develop recurrent symptoms of Meniere's disease, including vertigo and deafness. In these cases, we consider ELS revision. The decision is made by the patient after careful discussion of the pros and cons of the procedure. To date, ELS revisions have been done for 5% of our patients who have had ELS enhancements.

The ear undergoing revisional surgery is found to have development of extrasaccular fibrous tissue, osteoneogenesis, and aditus block syndrome, all resulting in obstruction of the sac with an adjacent tightly compressed contiguous dura. This subset of patients provides a built-in control with which we can compare the "before" and "after" of a pathologic, iatrogenic lesion causing malabsorption of endolymph and symptoms of Meniere's disease. Then, on reversal of that lesion (enhancing absorption of endolymph), improvement of Meniere's disease and its symptoms often occurs. Results are better for vertigo and deafness from ELS revision than from initial ELS enhancement procedures. This is because the patient has had a good result from the primary procedure, and then iatrogenically induced bone and scar tissue have recreated the pathogenesis years later. Correction of these iatrogenic secondary lesions provides a better chance for a beneficial result than with the initial procedure.[6]

Traumatic Fenestration of the Semicircular Canal

The best possible management of traumatic injury involving the labyrinth is to avoid it by correctly knowing the normal anatomy and fully expecting and preparing for wide variations in anatomic relationships in the mastoid and labyrinth in patients with Meniere's disease. A key point in surgery on the ELS is to identify correctly the location of the sac. The close proximity of the posterior semicircular canal puts this extension of the labyrinth at risk for injury. Earlier in the chapter, we outlined a technique for reliable identification of the sac while safely locating and avoiding the posterior canal. Skeletonizing the periotic capsule and exposing the blue line of the posterior semicircular canal can result in unnecessary sensorineural hearing loss. The technique for taking anatomic measurements avoids this potential complication while reliably directing the surgeon away from injury to the canal. To date we are not aware of a single complication resulting from accidental fenestration.

With our method of demarcating the solid angle with the measurements described, entering the posteroinferior semicircular canal has not been a problem. Treatment of the sac takes place beneath the solid angle in the posteroinferior semicircular canal and not in the mastoid cavity. Spacers of silicone rubber are used to decompress permanently the dura from the bone. The posterior bony canal wall is carefully thinned for anterior exposure, and the dome of the horizontal semicircular canal, short process of the incus, and posterior incudal ligament in the fossa incudis are always identified. In rare cases where there is no mastoid and only a large sigmoid (lateral) sinus, this important landmark cannot be identified, and the sinus is decompressed, allowing for access to contiguous dura that contains the sac beneath the solid angle.

We have observed the aditus ad antrum in patients with Meniere's disease to be narrowed; exaggerated attempts are made to enlarge the aditus, and often a posterior atticotomy is done to permit and enhance aeration and healing of the mastoid cavity posteroperatively. The dome of the horizontal semicircular canal and the fossa incudis are important landmarks; while performing mastoidectomy and before demarcating the bone containing the posteroinferior semicircular canal, the surgeon never extends the depth of drilling below the dome of the horizontal semicircular canal. This is the best way we have found to avoid injury to the posteroinferior semicircular canal. If the posteroinferior semicircular canal is inadvertently entered or injured, the best policy is to identify it, protect it with a small fascial graft, and avoid further injury via irrigation, bone dust, and so forth, and then to quickly complete the procedure. Antibiotics are provided with the hope of preventing diffuse labyrinthitis. A drain may be helpful.

Bilaterality in Meniere's Disease

In a group of patients with clinical Meniere's disease, 32% were found to have evidence of bilateral disease based on a clinical picture that included several audiograms in conjunction with histories and vestibular tests. When studied further, 78% were found to have some abnormality in pure-tone audiograms for the ear contralateral to that initially diagnosed as having Meniere's disease. It is likely that the proportion of patients with bilateral disease would increase with continued follow-up. A conservative estimate would suggest that at least one half of all patients with Meniere's disease will develop bilateral disease during their lifetime. Kronenberg, in a long-term postoperative study of vestibular nerve section, found that 67% of patients with Meniere's disease developed bilateral involvement.[7] Several senior authorities have suggested that Meniere's disease is bilateral in "all patients," and this may be theoretically true if patients were to survive long enough to allow observation of this clinical manifestation.[8, 9]

The risk of involvement for the second ear is significant enough to influence the selection of a mode of therapeutic intervention, especially with regard to surgery and the choice of operation. A conservative procedure that would place cochlear function at little risk should be first considered. For this and other reasons, whenever medical treatment fails and the disease becomes intractable, we practice an extension of conservative therapy, the ELS enhancement. If the contralateral ear becomes involved subsequently, we are grateful for every attempt made to preserve and improve function in the first ear.

We have had occasion successfully to use ELS enhancement in patients with bilateral Meniere's disease, usually patients with classical or typical Meniere's disease but also occasionally in patients with vestibular Meniere's disease and prolonged incapacitating intractable vertigo. Vestibular Meniere's disease is characterized by episodic vertigo, aural pressure, tinnitus, intolerance for loudness, and diplacusis.[10] The primary indication is vertigo; the secondary indication is progressive and fluctuating deafness. The ear with the most involvement by history that accompanies attacks of vertigo, including hearing loss (documented by audiograms), aural (head and neck) pressure, headache, tinnitus, intolerance for loud sounds, and diplacusis, is the one for which ELS enhancement should be considered. In most patients, a procedure on the most symptomatic or involved ear suffices to eliminate or control vertigo, and hearing loss stabilizes or does not progress bilaterally, so that the other ear need not receive a procedure. In some patients, the opposite ear worsens, and months or years later ELS enhancement may need to be considered to stabilize or improve labyrinthine function on the opposite side.

Because of the high incidence of bilaterality, every attempt is made to avoid labyrinthectomy. We have treated a small subset of patients who received labyrinthectomy for Meniere's disease, only to develop progressive sensorineural deafness in the opposite, only hearing ear. Most patients with Meniere's disease will progress to a hearing level of 50 to 60 dB, with comparably reduced discrimination scores; however, we have observed some patients (20%) to progress to a severe or profound sensorineural hearing loss or even complete deafness from progressive Meniere's disease. A carefully described and performed ELS enhancement has been performed in the only hearing ear of such patients to stabilize and improve hearing. Although the major risk of 2% deafness for conservative ELS enhancement is lower than that for other procedures for treating Meniere's disease, we are pleased to report that this complication has not occurred in this difficult to treat subset of patients, and all patients to date have retained or improved hearing.[11]

REFERENCES

1. Paparella MM, Sajjadi H: Endolymphatic sac enhancement: Principles of diagnosis and treatment. *Am J Otol* 1987; 8:292–299.
2. Shea DA, Chole RA, Paparella MM: The endolymphatic

sac: Anatomical considerations. *Laryngoscope* 1979; 89:88–94.

3. Paparella MM, Goycoolea MV: Endolymphatic sac enhancement surgery for Meniere's disease: An extension of conservative therapy. *Ann Otol Rhinol Laryngol* 1981; 90:610–615.

4. Gacek RR: Surgery of the vestibular system, in Cummings CW, et al (eds): *Otolaryngology — Head and Neck Surgery.* St Louis, CV Mosby Co, 1987, pp 3333–3351.

5. Paparella MM, Sajjadi H, daCosta SS, et al: Significance of the lateral sinus and Trautmann's triangle in Meniere's disease. Paper presented at the 2nd International Symposium on Meniere's Disease. Cambridge, Mass, June 1988.

6. Paparella MM, Sajjadi H: Endolymphatic sac revision for recurrent Meniere's disease. *Am J Otol* (in press).

7. Kronenberg J: Long term hearing results after transtemporal supralabyrinthine vestibular neurectomy. Paper presented at the 2nd International *Symposium on Meniere's Disease,* Cambridge Mass, June 1988.

8. Paparella MM, Griebie MS: Bilaterality of Meniere's disease. *Acta Otolaryngol (Stockh)* 1983; 9:233–237.

9. Paparella MM, McDermott JC, deSousa LCA: Meniere's disease and the peak audiogram. *Arch Otolaryngol* 1982; 108:563–566.

10. Paparella MM, Mancini F: Vestibular Meniere's disease. *Otolaryngol Head Neck Surg* 1985; 93:148–151.

11. Paparella MM, Nissen RL: Primary surgery for Meniere's disease. Destructive surgery versus conservative surgery. *Am J Otol* 1987; 8:66–67.

CHAPTER 8

Destructive Procedures for Vertigo

Approach of

Harold F. Schuknecht, M.D.

Ablation or destruction of vestibular function is a rational therapy for some patients with intractable and disabling vertigo. Meniere's disease is the most common disorder for which vestibular ablation is used; however, the procedure may be indicated for other conditions, such as the episodic vertigo of delayed endolymphatic hydrops, intractable vertigo (and deafness) complicating stapes surgery, and unremitting vertigo complicating chronic otitis media.

Ablation surgery dates back to 1903 when Eugene Crockett at the Massachusetts Eye and Ear Infirmary reported curing two patients suffering with severe episodes of vertigo by simply removing the stapes.[1] In 1943, Cawthorne described a technique for destroying the labyrinth by an approach through the mastoid whereby the semicircular duct was avulsed.[2] Other methods of ablating the labyrinth via the semicircular canals consisted of electrocoagulation[3] and the use of barbed instruments.[4] In 1948, Lempert introduced an endaural approach with removal of the stapes and round window membrane.[5] In 1957, following the advent of stapes surgery for otosclerosis, Schuknecht described the transcanal approach to the oval window via a tympanomeatal flap and emphasized the importance of systematic ablation of the vestibular sense organs.[6]

It would be ideal if a simple, ablative procedure could be developed that would achieve consistent relief of vertigo while preserving hearing. This objective has been elusive. It is a well-established clinical observation that surgical attacks on the vestibular membranous labyrinth carry a high risk of injury to the auditory system.

Extra-labyrinthine procedures such as ultrasound or cryosurgery probably achieve some reduction in vestibular sensitivity, because reports show that relief of vertigo is achieved in many patients.[7–9] Although some success with these procedures cannot be denied, there are also many failures.[10] It seems doubtful that prolonged relief of vertigo can be expected without a more complete ablation of vestibular sense organs than is possible with these methods.

Labyrinthectomy is a highly successful procedure that is relatively free of complications. Success in relieving vertigo by labyrinthectomy depends on the total destruction of peripheral vestibular sensory function. The destruction of any remaining hearing is an unavoidable consequence of labyrinthectomy, and for this reason, it should not be done when hearing is serviceable or when there is evidence of disease in the opposite ear. The transcanal labyrinthectomy is the simplest and most direct approach to accomplish this objective.[11, 12]

CRITERIA FOR LABYRINTHECTOMY

Under what conditions would labyrinthectomy be a reasonable therapeutic option?

1. Hearing loss. Although no strict criterion can be set for levels of loss for pure-tone thresholds and word discrimination, the auditory function of the ear should be characterized as severely compromised. The opposite ear should have hearing that is normal or nearly normal with no evidence of disease.

2. Vertigo. The vertigo should be handicapping to occupational and social activities. It should be restrictive to life-style. When vertigo is accompanied by falling attacks, the need for definitive therapeutic action is strengthened.

3. Diagnosis. The history of episodic vertigo and fluctuat-

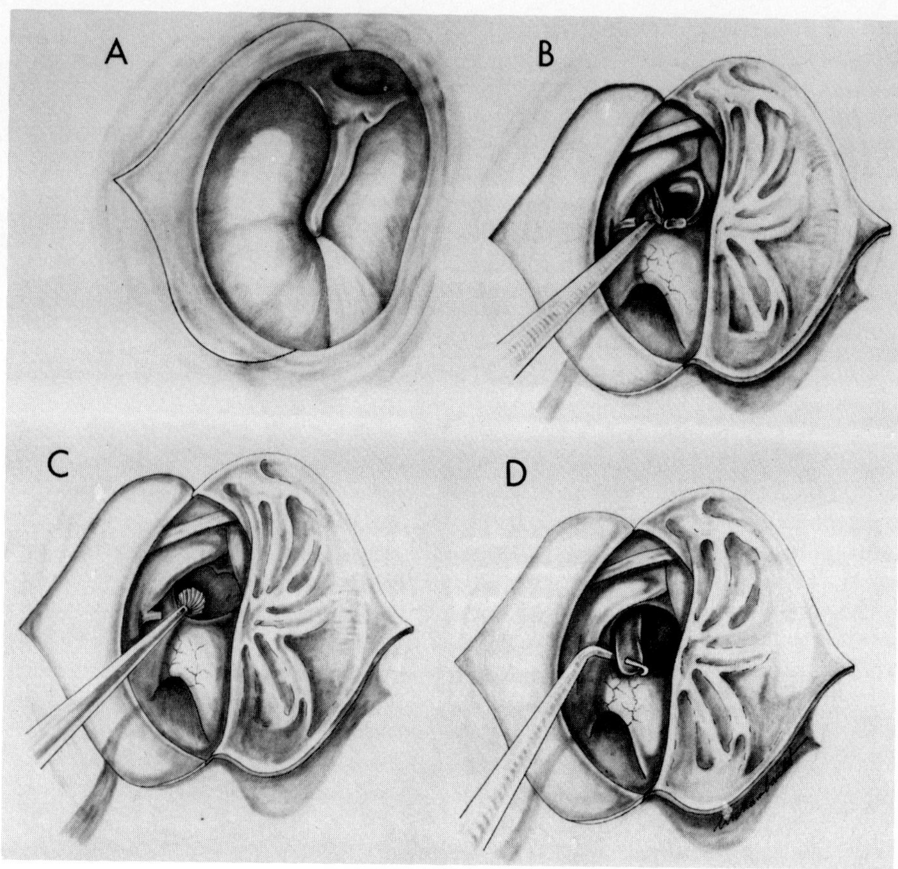

FIG 8–1.
Method of performing the transcanal labyrinthectomy. **A,** a tympanomeatal flap is elevated. **B,** the incus and stapes are removed. **C,** the oval window can be enlarged if so desired. **D,** the saccule is aspirated, and the utricular macula is engaged with a 3 mm hook and removed. The ampullae are macerated with a 3 mm hook.

ing hearing loss, often temporarily related sometime during the course of the disease, is diagnostic of idiopathic progressive endolymphatic hydrops (Meniere's disease). Diagnosis of other disabling vestibular disorders (e.g., surgical injury, delayed hydrops syndrome) also relies heavily on history. In addition, the etiology for the hearing loss and vertigo should be supported by reliable auditory and vestibular test data and computed tomography (CT) or magnetic resonance imaging (MRI), or both, of the temporal bone and cerebellopontine angle. Support of a second opinion may be advisable.

4. Age. The incidence of uncompensated dysequilibrium following labyrinthectomy (or any other ablative procedure) is directly related to the age of the patient. Patients in the older age group (>60 years) should be counseled regarding the possibility of permanent mild unsteadiness.

5. General health. Patients with low vision, neurologic disease, lower limb disorders, psychiatric disorders, or otherwise poor health are not candidates for ablation therapy. Patients should be psychologically motivated to get well.

6. Occupation. The patient's life-style, occupation, and avocations should be given careful study. A determination should be made as to what effect uncompensated postoperative dysequilibrium might have on these activities, should it occur.

METHOD OF TRANSCANAL LABYRINTHECTOMY

With the patient under general anesthesia, a tympanomeatal flap is elevated and reflected forward to expose the posterior mesotympanum (Fig 8–1). If necessary, bony annulus is removed to provide full visualization of the oval window region. The incus is disarticulated and removed. The stapedius tendon is sectioned, and the stapes is mobilized and removed. In cases of endolymphatic hydrops, a fibrous membrane is occasionally seen bridging the oval window. This condition is known as *vestibular fibrosis.*[13] The membrane, if present, is removed.

The otolithic membrane of the saccular macula should now be clearly in view. It appears as a white patch on the anterior part of the medial wall of the vestibule. The utricular macula is also sometimes visible at the superior margin of the oval window. The saccular macula has a bright white appearance because its otoconial surface is exposed to view, whereas the utricular macula has a whitish gray appearance because its neural surface is exposed to view (Fig 8–2). There is no objection to enlarging the oval window, although it is usually not required. If endolymphatic hydrops is present, the utricular macula is often displaced into the superior part of the vestibule by an enlarged saccule or cochlear duct.

The saccular macula is removed by aspiration. The utricular macula is engaged with an appropriate hook with the simultaneous assistance of an aspiration tube. A 3 mm right-angle hook is usually adequate for this purpose; however, I have fabricated a "utricular hook," which is a 3 mm right-angle hook with a second 0.6 mm hook at its end. Several passes with the hook along the medial and lateral walls as well as the anterior and posterior parts of the vestibule may be necessary to locate the utricular macula. Visual confirmation of removal of the utricular macula is an essential feature of vestibular ablation. Aspiration tubes larger than 24 gauge size are to be avoided, because the utricular macula may unknowingly disappear into the aspiration tube.

The hook is now used to probe the ampullae and thus blindly macerate the cristae. All manipulations in the vestibule must be gentle to avoid fracturing the cribrose areas, because to do so will result in a flow of cerebrospinal fluid (CSF).

There is nothing to be gained by removing the round window membrane or removing bone between the oval and round windows. The vestibule is now filled with pledgets of absorbable gelatin sponge (Gelfoam) that have been saturated in a solution of streptomycin sulfate (250 mg/mL).

The operation is completed by returning the tympanomeatal flap to its original position and packing it in place with silk strips and a piece of synthetic sponge.

RESULTS

Our results to date reflect the experiences reported in 1977.[11] From 1964 to 1975, transcanal labyrinthectomies were performed on 63 patients, of which 47 were for intractable vertigo of Meniere's disease, 7 for dysequilibrium following stapedectomy, 5 for the delayed hydrops syndrome, and 4 for dysequilibrium following healed chronic otitis media. In six patients the symptoms included falling attacks (Tumarkin's otolithic catastrophe[14]).

Of the 47 labyrinthectomies for Meniere's disease, 7 had previous labyrinthectomy failures done by others, of which 5 were transmastoid procedures and 2 were transcanal procedures. All but one of these patients retained caloric response in the operated ear. In each case the revision procedure was performed under local anesthesia to permit the monitoring of vertigo during surgery as an indicator of persisting vestibular sensory function. All but one experienced vertigo during and after revision surgery and were eventually relieved of disabling vertigo. The single patient who had no caloric response and no relief from a constant feeling of unsteadiness was found to have bone and fibrous tissue filling the vestibule.

The mean age of the patients was 53 years. The duration of hearing loss ranged from 7 months to 50 years. For the total material, the mean speech reception level was 78 dB, and the mean word discrimination score was 45%. Cold caloric responses, when compared with the opposite ear, were diminished 25% or more in duration in 48 (76%) and were totally absent in 7 (11%).

Three of the 63 patients complained of continuing dysequilibrium following surgery. Two of these had constant unsteadiness, one being the individual previously mentioned and

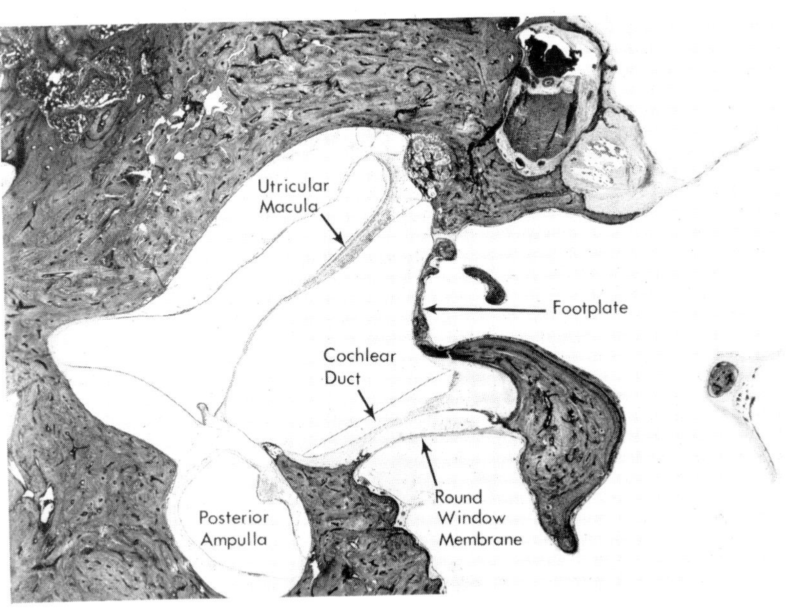

FIG 8–2.
Photomicrograph showing the normal relationship of the utricle to the oval window.

the other a person with considerable psychogenic overlay who eventually improved. It was determined that the third patient whose vertigo was episodic had developed Meniere's disease in the opposite ear.

The vertigo that follows labyrinthectomy subsides over a period of several weeks, although some unsteadiness, particularly on head movements, may persist for a few months. In older patients, a mild sense of dysequilibrium may persist indefinitely. Information on the time of return to full employment is known for 33 patients and ranged from 2 to 24 weeks (average 5 weeks).

Since 1975, I have performed an additional 47 transcanal labyrinthectomies, for a total of 110 cases. Several of the patients have developed Meniere's disease in the opposite ear, and a study is to be undertaken to determine what impact the prior labyrinthectomy may have had on the extent of their final disability.

OTHER METHODS OF ABLATION

Transmastoid Labyrinthectomy.—In this method the semicircular canals and vestibule are entered from posteriorly. The procedure is more time consuming than the transcanal method, but when properly performed, it is as successful as the transcanal procedure.[15, 16] The surgeon should be aware, however, that drilling away the semicircular canals in itself accomplishes little; it is the vestibular sense organs that must be targeted for destruction.

Vestibular Neurectomy.—Nerve section may be considered when intractable and disabling vertigo occurs in association with serviceable hearing.[17–22] The presumed advantage is that hearing can be preserved; however, this objective is not routinely achieved. The vestibular nerve can be reached via the posterior fossa by suboccipital or mastoid (retrolabyrinthine) approaches. It can also be exposed via the middle fossa. Each method has its advocates, but there are many otologists who prefer not to subject their patients to the risk of serious complications, however rare, that can occur with intracranial procedures.

Surgeons who advocate vestibular nerve section believe that persisting vestibular neurons can be responsible for dysequilibrium, even though the sense organs have been ablated. In addition, it has been proposed that amputation neuromas of the vestibular nerves can develop after labyrinthectomy and act as a nidus for continuing dysequilibrium. After labyrinthectomy in the cat, the vestibular nerves undergo slow atrophy with losses reaching only 53% after 3 years and no evidence of regeneration.[23] Yet temporal bone studies of postlabyrinthectomy ears of human patients show inner ear neuromas.[24] It is not known, however, whether these traumatic neuromas would be capable of producing vertigo.

The translabyrinthine vestibular neurectomy is, in essence, a combination of labyrinthectomy and nerve section.[17, 25] Although there is no clinical or experimental evidence that translabyrinthine vestibular nerve section has any therapeutic ad-

vantage over a well-performed labyrinthectomy, those surgeons who advocate the procedure believe that it provides a more certain total ablation of vestibular function. If we assume this is true, the translabyrinthine vestibular neurectomy might be a reasonable approach for failed labyrinthectomies when no caloric reaction is present. It has the same disadvantage of other nerve section procedures of opening into the subarachnoid space.

Chemical Ablation.—A discussion of ablation therapy for vertigo would not be complete without mentioning the methods of chemical ablation. Streptomycin sulfate can be given parenterally to ablate vestibular sensory function without a risk of hearing loss.[26] Because the effects are bilateral, there is severe posttreatment ataxia, sometimes with oscillopsia, that may require several weeks or months to subside and in some cases is permanent. For the reason that the treatment and recovery period are arduous for the patient, it should be reserved for those patients having bilateral disabling disease. Unilateral Meniere's disease is better treated by methods that limit their action to the diseased ear. Several authors have reported administering the drug for shorter periods of time to achieve partial ablation and claim good therapeutic results with less posttreatment ataxia.[27, 28]

Both streptomycin[29, 30] and gentamycin[30, 31] have been injected into the middle ear in attempts to accomplish unilateral vestibular ablation while preserving hearing. Chemical labyrinth ablation has also been done by placing salt crystals on the round window membrane[32] as well as into the inner ear.[33] Although some success has been reported, it has not been established that consistently good results can be achieved by these methods.

CONCLUSIONS

When the criteria for therapeutic labyrinthectomy have been met, the simplest, safest, and most predictable method is the transcanal procedure. Vestibular neurectomy may be indicated for patients with intractable vertigo when hearing is serviceable; however, some otologists, including myself, are reluctant to recommend an intracranial invasive procedure for a condition that in itself is not a risk for life expectancy.

REFERENCES

1. Crockett EA: The removal of the stapes for the relief of auditory vertigo. *Ann Otol Rhinol Laryngol* 1903; 12:67–72.
2. Cawthorne T: The treatment of Meniere's disease. *J Laryngol Otol* 1943; 58:563–571.
3. Day K: Surgical destruction of the labyrinth for Ménière's disease. *Laryngoscope* 1952; 62:547–555.
4. Lindsay JR, Siedentop K: Labyrinthine surgery in the treatment of Ménière's disease. *Ann Otol Rhinol Laryngol* 1955; 64:69–79.
5. Lempert J: Lempert decompression operation for hydrops of the endolymphatic labyrinth in Meniere's disease. *Arch Otolaryngol* 1948; 47:551–570.
6. Schuknecht HF: Ablation therapy in the management of Ménière's disease. *Acta Otolaryngol (Stockh)* 1957; 132(suppl):1–42.

7. Angell-James J: Erfahrungen bei der Behandlung der Menièreschen Krankheit mit Ultraschall. *HNO* 1970; 18:202–205.

8. Basek M: Ultrasound for Meniere's disease. Lateral canal vs round window approach. *Arch Otolaryngol* 1973; 97:133–134.

9. Stahle J: Ultrasound treatment of Meniere's disease. Long-term follow-up of 356 advanced cases. *Acta Otolaryngol (Stockh)* 1976; 81:120–126.

10. Peron DL, Kitamura K, Carniol PJ, et al: Clinical and experimental results with focused ultrasound. *Laryngoscope* 1983; 93:1217–1221.

11. Schuknecht HF, Hammerschlag PE: Transcanal labyrinthectomy, in Silverstein H, Norrell H (eds): *Neurological Surgery of the Ear*. Birmingham, Ala, Aesculapius Publishing Co, 1977, pp 172–175.

12. Glasscock ME III, Hughes GB, Davis WE, et al: Labyrinthectomy versus middle fossa vestibular nerve section in Menière's disease. A critical evaluation of relief of vertigo. *Trans Am Otol Soc* 1980; 68:42–48.

13. Schuknecht HF: *Pathology of the Ear*. Cambridge, Mass, Harvard University Press, 1974.

14. Tumarkin I: Otolithic catastrophe; a new syndrome. *Br Med J (Clin Res)* 1936; 2:175.

15. Graham MD, Colton JJ: Transmastoid labyrinthectomy indications. Technique and early postoperative results. *Laryngoscope* 1980; 90:1253–1262.

16. Graham MD: Transmastoid labyrinthectomy: Further experience with the indications, complications and early post-operative results. *J Laryngol Otol* 1981; 95:1205–1211.

17. Silverstein H, Silverstein D: Analysis of surgical procedures in patients with vertigo. *Otolaryngol Head Neck Surg* 1984; 92:225–228.

18. Glasscock ME III, Kveton JF, Christiansen SG: Middle fossa vestibular neurectomy: An update. *Otolaryngol Head Neck Surg* 1984; 92:216–220.

19. House JW, Hitselberger WE, McElveen J, et al: Retrolabyrinthine section of the vestibular nerve. *Otolaryngol Head Neck Surg* 1984; 92:212–215.

20. McElveen JT Jr, House JW, Hitselberger WE, et al: Retrolabyrinthine vestibular nerve section: A viable alternative to the middle fossa approach. *Otolaryngol Head Neck Surg* 1984; 92:136–140.

21. Kemink JL, Hoff JT: Retrolabyrinthine vestibular nerve section: Analysis of results. *Laryngoscope* 1986; 96:33–36.

22. Silverstein H, Norrell H, Smouha E, et al: Retrolabyrinthine or retrosigmoid vestibular neurectomy: Indications. *Am J Otol* 1987; 8:414–418.

23. Schuknecht HF: Behavior of the vestibular nerve following labyrinthectomy. *Ann Otol Rhinol Laryngol* 1982; 91:16–32.

24. Linthicum F Jr, Alonso A, Denia A: Traumatic neuroma. A complication of transcanal labyrinthectomy. *Arch Otolaryngol* 1979; 105:654–655.

25. Antoli-Candela F Jr, Alvarez de Cozar F, Antoli-Candela F: Transvestibular approach to the internal auditory canal. *Ann Otol Rhinol Laryngol* 1975; 84:145–151.

26. Wilson WR, Schuknecht HF: Update on the use of streptomycin therapy for Meniere's disease. *Am J Otol* 1980; 2:108–111.

27. Silverstein H, Hyman SM, Feldbaum J, et al: Use of streptomycin sulfate in the treatment of Meniere's disease. *Otolaryngol Head Neck Surg* 1984; 92:229–232.

28. Graham MD, Sataloff RT, Kemink JL: Titration streptomycin therapy for bilateral Meniere's disease: A preliminary report. *Otolaryngol Head Neck Surg* 1984; 92:440–447.

29. Stange G, Schmidt CL, Orthenberger H: Schadigung gleich- und gegenseitiger Hörpotentiale des Meerschweinchens nach intratympanaler Applikation von Streptomycinsulfat. *Arch Otorhinolaryngol* 1977; 217:361–368.

30. Beck C, Schmidt CL: 10 years of experience with intratympanally applied streptomycin (gentamycin) in the therapy of morbus Meniere. *Arch Otorhinolaryngol* 1978; 221:149–152.

31. Ödkvist LM, Bergholtz LM, Lundgren A: Topical gentamycin treatment for disabling Ménière's disease. *Acta Otolaryngol (Stockh)* 1984; 412(suppl):74–76.

32. Arslan M: Symposium on Meniere's disease. Treatment of Meniere's disease by apposition of sodium chloride crystals on the round window. *Laryngoscope* 1972; 82:1736–1750.

33. Colletti V, Fiorino FG, Sittoni V, et al: Chemical labyrinthectomy with NaCl. Meniere's disease treatment with deposition of NaCl in the vestibule. *Acta Otolaryngol (Stockh)* 1987; 104:7–12.

Destructive Procedures for Vertigo

Approach of

John T. McElveen, Jr., M.D.

and

Anthony E. Magit, M.D.

The term "labyrinthectomy" encompasses several procedures designed to ablate the vestibular receptors of the involved ear. Despite variations in technique, each of these procedures destroys residual hearing in the operated ear. This should be given serious consideration before recommending labyrinthectomy for any patient at risk for contralateral inner ear disturbances. However, if the patient is carefully selected and the procedure properly performed, labyrinthectomy can be a reliable means of eliminating incapacitating ear-related vertigo.

HISTORICAL PERSPECTIVE

Labyrinth surgery was first described by Jansen[1] (1895), who opened the lateral semicircular canal after performing a radical mastoidectomy because of a suppurative lesion. Lake[2] (1904), removed the lateral semicircular canal to treat unilateral vertigo, but he credited Milligan[3] (1904) for first using this operation in a nonsuppurative lesion. Neumann[4] (1905) used an intracranial approach to remove the semicircular canals, whereas Richards[5] (1907) used a transmeatal approach to open the three semicircular canals and the cochlea. A subtemporal approach was used by Putnam[6] (1938) to open the superior semicircular canal and introduce a coagulating current to destroy the labyrinth. Neville[7] (1935) and Mollison[8] (1939) injected alcohol into the lateral semicircular canal; Wright[9] (1935) and Peacock[10] (1938) injected alcohol through the oval window to perform chemical labyrinthectomies. Day[11] (1943), after completing a simple mastoidectomy, opened the lateral semicircular canal and introduced a coagulating current and sulfonamide crystals. thorne[12] (1943) created a lateral semicircular canal fistula with a transmeatal approach; whereas Lempert[13] (1948) used a transcanal approach to perform one of three procedures: fenestration of the lateral semicircular canal, opening of the round window or removal of the stapes, and aspiration of the vestibular contents.

Schuknecht[14] (1956) and Cawthorne[15] (1957) used a transcanal approach with a tympanomeatal flap to remove the stapes, extract the membranous labyrinth with a hook, and fill the bony labyrinth with Gelfoam. Armstrong[16] (1959) modified this technique by removing the promontory between the round and oval windows.

Pulec[17] (1969) combined transmastoid ablation of the intralabyrinthine space with translabyrinthine sectioning of the eighth cranial nerve. Antoli-Condela and House[18] (1969) performed separate series of total labyrinthectomy, including ablation of the utricle and saccule. Silverstein[19] (1976) detailed transmeatal labyrinthectomy with cochleovestibular neurectomy. Cole[20] (1982) described evacuation of the vestibular contents with introduction of streptomycin via the oval window.

INDICATIONS AND TECHNIQUE

The indications as well as the technique for labyrinthectomy have been modified since Jansen's[1] description. Whereas Jansen used labyrinthectomy to exteriorize and drain an infected labyrinth, currently the more common indication for this procedure is to relieve incapacitating ear-related vertigo by ablating the vestibular end organ. Consequently the technique has been changed in an attempt to more completely remove the vestibular receptors within the inner ear.

Despite some variations in technique, the labyrinthectomy procedures presently used can be divided into two major categories: transcanal procedures and transmastoid procedures.

Transcanal Technique

The transcanal technique, described independently by Schuknecht[14] in 1956 and Cawthorne[12] in 1957, gained widespread popularity because of its technical ease and limited morbidity. The operative procedure is usually performed after

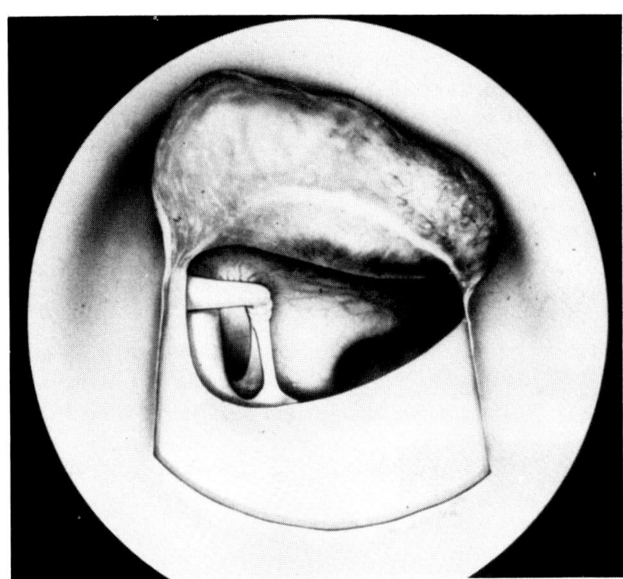

FIG 8–3.
Standard tympanomeatal flat in a right ear.

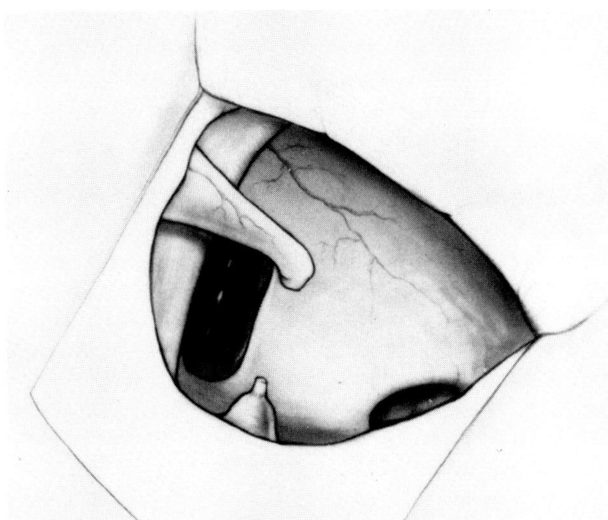

FIG 8–4.
Right middle ear with stapedius tendon sectioned and stapes re-moved.

administration of a local anesthetic. A standard tympanomeatal flap is elevated (Fig 8–3) and bone is curetted from the posterosuperior aspect of the bony external canal, facilitating the exposure of the stapes and oval window. The incudostapedial joint is separated and the stapedius tendon is sectioned. The stapes is completely mobilized and then removed from the oval window (Fig 8–4). At this point in the procedure a hook can be passed into the oval window and the membranous labyrinth extracted; however, complete removal may be difficult because of limited exposure. I prefer to use the Armstrong[16] modification

and drill off the bone between the oval window and the round window. Although Armstrong used a curette to remove this bone, the stapes drill with a diamond burr affords the surgeon greater control and precision (Fig 8–5). Once this bone has been removed, a 3 mm hook is introduced into the vestibule and the saccule, utricle, and receptors in the ampullated portion of the semicircular canals are removed (Fig 8–6). Gelfoam packing soaked in streptomycin sulfate is then placed in the vesti-

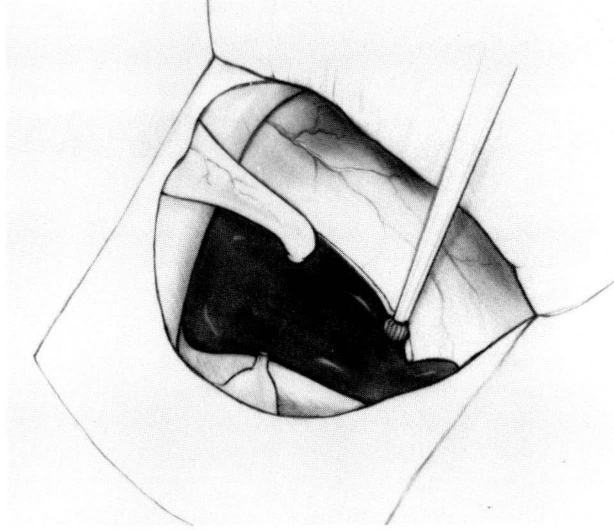

FIG 8–5.
Bone is removed between the oval window and round window regions in a right ear.

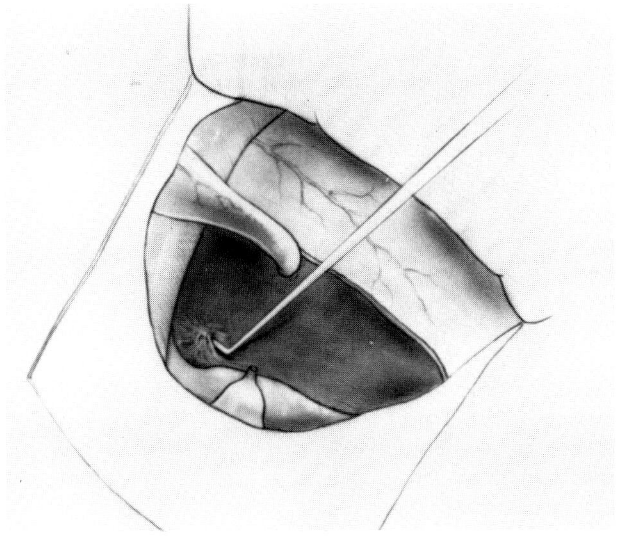

FIG 8–6.
Membranous labyrinth is removed from the vestibule.

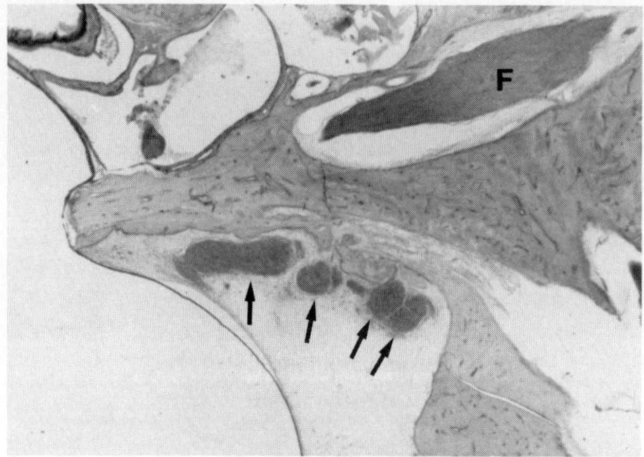

FIG 8–7.
Histologic section demonstrates traumatic neuroma (*arrows*) subsequent to labyrinthectomy. Facial nerve (*F*) is seen in this section.

bule. The tympanomeatal flap is returned to its normal position and the ear canal packed with Gelfoam.

The success rate of transcanal labyrinthectomy varies from 50% to 100%. The variability in results may be secondary to what I consider the pitfalls of this procedure: incomplete labyrinthectomy and traumatic neuroma formation. The risk of incomplete labyrinthectomy is inherent in the transcanal technique because the removal of the vestibular end organs is done blindly. In addition, excess scraping or drilling on the floor of the vestibule may traumatize the nerve endings, resulting in neuroma formation (Fig 8–7). Once these traumatic neuromas have formed, they are very difficult to eliminate, and result in persistent vertigo. In light of these pitfalls, what are the present indications for transcanal labyrinthectomy? I reserve this procedure for the elderly and for the patient who is a poor surgical risk. The hearing in the involved ear should have a pure tone average (PTA) worse than 80 dB with a speech discrimination score less than 20%. As with all labyrinthectomy procedures, any residual hearing is lost in the operated ear; consequently the patient must have adequate hearing and vestibular function in the contralateral ear.

Transmastoid Technique

Many of the pitfalls inherent in transcanal labyrinthectomy are circumvented with the transmastoid procedure. The operation is usually performed with the patient under general anesthesia. For hemostasis, the postauricular area is infiltrated with 1% lidocaine with 1:100,000 epinephrine. The incision is made approximately 2 cm behind the postauricular crease. A cortical mastoidectomy is performed and the lateral semicircular canal identified. The facial nerve is skeletonized in its mastoid segment (Fig 8–8). (Failure to identify the facial nerve in the mastoid risks injury to the nerve and an inadequate labyrinthectomy.) Although it is tempting to begin the labyrinthectomy on the upper surface of the lateral semicircular canal (Fig 8–9, A), it is more expedient to begin in the solid angle using the side of

the burr to open into the membranous portion of the lateral semicircular canal. The initial dissection proceeds inferiorly, following the course of the lateral semicircular canal toward the posterior semicircular canal (Fig 8–9, B). On opening the posterior semicircular canal, one follows it posteriorly and then superiorly to the common crus. From the common crus the superior canal is exteriorized from an inferior to superior direction. When performing a labyrinthectomy on a right ear, the drill should be reversed while drilling in the vicinity of the ampullated portion of the superior semicircular canal and the superior portion of the lateral semicircular canal. This minimizes the likelihood of the drill catching an edge of bone and flipping into the tympanic segment of the facial nerve. Once the ampullated ends of the superior and lateral semicircular canals are opened, one follows the crus of the posterior semicircular canal to its ampullated end. Great care is needed to ensure that the ampulla is adequately exposed without inadvertently undercutting the facial nerve with the upper surface of the burr. Once the ampullated ends of the semicircular canals are exteriorized, the vestibule is opened. It is important not to place the drill into the vestibule; this risks traumatic neuroma formation and inadvertent injury to the tympanic portion of the facial nerve. Once the vestibule is opened, under direct vision a small footplate hook is used to remove the neuroepithelium from the ampullated regions of the posterior, superior, and inferior semicircular canals. The utricle and saccule are then removed from the vestibule (Fig 8–10). Once this is completed, Gelfoam soaked in streptomycin sulfate is placed in the vestibule. The ear is returned to its normal position and the postauricular incision is closed in the standard fashion.

Some otologists supplement this procedure with a vestibular neurectomy, sectioning the superior and inferior vestibular nerves within the internal auditory canal. I reserve the transmastoid labyrinthectomy with vestibular neurectomy for those patients in whom previous transmastoid labyrinthectomy

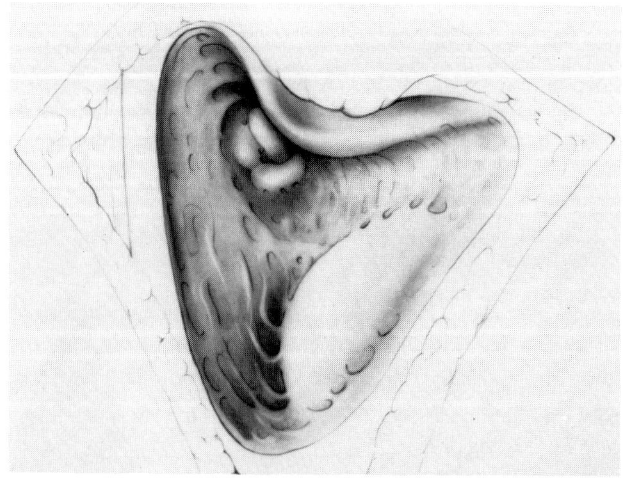

FIG 8–8.
Right mastoid cavity after cortical mastoidectomy. Facial nerves and semicircular canals are identified.

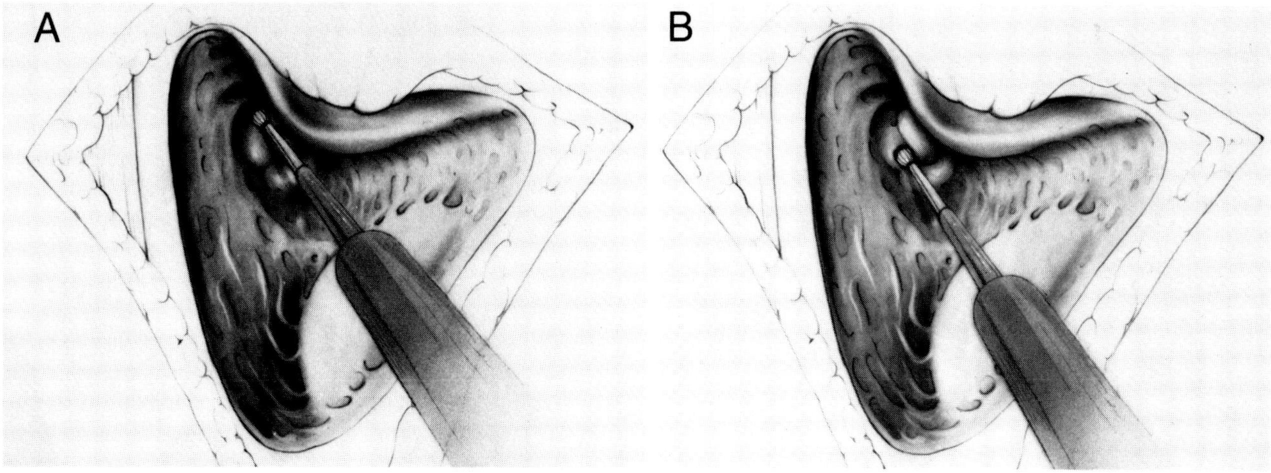

FIG 8–9.
Right mastoid cavity. **A,** incorrect drill position. **B,** correct drill position for initiating labyrinthectomy.

was not successful. With the success rate of transmastoid labyrinthectomy varying from 86% to 97%, supplementing this procedure with a vestibular neurectomy is seldom necessary.

The more consistent results with transmastoid labyrinthectomy underscores the advantage in removing the vestibular end organs under direct vision. Although this approach for labyrinthectomy is more dependable than the transcanal procedure, it is not without its problems. The transmastoid labyrinthectomy is usually done with the patient under general anesthesia and requires more time for dissection, making it unsuitable for the patient who is at poor surgical risk. The procedure requires greater dissection adjacent to the facial nerve, putting the nerve at increased risk. Such an injury was reported by Graham and Kemink.[21] The patient eventually had partial return of function. It is essential that the surgeon adequately identify the facial nerve, not only to lessen the likelihood of inadvertent injury but also to avoid the last pitfall of transmastoid labyrinthectomy, incomplete labyrinthectomy. In my experience it is often the neuroepithelium of the posterior canal ampulla that is inadequately removed. Usually in such cases the facial nerve has been inadequately skeletonized, making the surgeon hesitant to dissect further in the region of the posterior semicircular canal ampulla for fear of inadvertent facial nerve injury. As a consequence, neuroepithelium is left behind and the patient experiences eventual recrudescence of symptoms.

CONCLUSION

Labyrinthectomy remains a cornerstone in the treatment of incapacitating ear-related vertigo. However, increasing concern for hearing preservation and the advent of alternative treatment options have limited its use. Despite this, it is essential that the otologic surgeon be well versed in the current indications and techniques for labyrinthectomy.

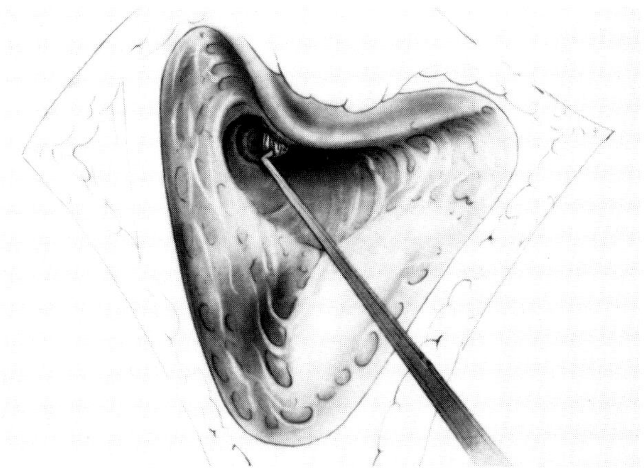

FIG 8–10.
Right mastoid cavity after transmastoid labyrinthectomy. Membranous labyrinth is removed under direct vision.

REFERENCES

1. Jansen A: Referat ueber die Operationsmethoden bei den verschiedenen otitischen Gehirnskomplicationen. Verhandl d deutsch otol Gesellsch. *Jena* 96, 1895, cited in Pulec J: Labyrinthectomy: Indications, techniques and results. *Laryngoscope* 1974; 84:1552–1573.
2. Lake R: Removal of the semicircular canals in a case of unilateral aural vertigo. *Lancet* 1904; 1:1567–1568.
3. Milligan W: Meniere's disease: A clinical and experimental inquiry. *J Laryngol Otol* 1904; 19:440.
4. Neumann H: Sitzungsb der oesterr otol Gesellsch, 1905. Monatsschr ohrenh (Berl Wein) 1905; 39:469, cited in Pulec J: Labyrinthectomy: Indications, technqiues and results. *Laryngoscope* 1974; 84:1552–1573.

5. Richards JD: Surgery of the labyrinth. *Trans Am Laryngol Rhinol Otol Soc* 1907; 161–188.

6. Putnam TJ: Treatment of recurrent vertigo by subtemporal destruction of the labyrinth. *Arch Otolaryngol* 1938; 27:161.

7. Neville WT: Four cases of vertigo treated by operation. *Proc R Soc Med* 1935; 28:1509–1600.

8. Mollison WW: Surgical treatment of vertigo by opening the external semicircular canal and injecting alcohol. *Acta Otolaryngol* 1939; 27:222–226.

9. Wright AJ: Aural vertigo: Alcohol injection through the oval window. *Proc R Soc Med* 1935; 28:1600–1601.

10. Peacock R: Alcoholic labyrinthine injection through the oval window in the treatment of aural vertigo. *Lancet* 1938; 1:421–423.

11. Day KM: Labyrinth surgery for Meniere's disease. *Laryngoscope* 1943; 53:617–630.

12. Cawthorne TE: The treatment of Meniere's disease. *J Laryngol Otol* 1943; 58:363–371.

13. Lempert J: Lempert decompression operation for hydrops of the endolymphatic labyrinth in Meniere's disease. *Arch Otolaryngol* 1948; 47:551–570.

14. Schuknecht HF: Ablation therapy for the relief of Meniere's disease. *Laryngoscope* 1956; 66:859–870.

15. Cawthorne TE: Meniere's disease. *Ann Otol Rhinol Laryngol* 1957; 56:18–38.

16. Armstrong BW: Transtympanic vestibulectomy for Meniere's disease. *Laryngoscope* 1959; 69:1071–1074.

17. Pulec JL: The surgical treatment of vertigo. *Laryngoscope* 1969; 79:1783–1822.

18. Antoli-Candela F, House W: Surgery for hydrops. *Arch Otolaryngol Head Neck Surg* 1969; 89:141–147.

19. Silverstein H: Transmeatal labyrinthectomy with and without cochleovestibular neurectomy. *Laryngoscope* 1976; 86:1777–1791.

20. Cole JM: Labyrinthectomy. *Laryngoscope* 1982; 92:1324–1325.

21. Graham MD, Kemink JL: Transmastoid labyrinthectomy: Surgical management of vertigo in the nonserviceable hearing ear. *Am J Otol* 1984; 5:295–299.

CHAPTER 9

Vestibular Nerve Section

Approach of

Herbert Silverstein, M.D.

and

Raleigh O. Jones, Jr., M.D.

Vestibular neurectomy (VNS) is being accepted as the procedure of choice to relieve intractable vertigo associated with unilateral vestibular disorders. The most common indication for this procedure is Meniere's disease. When the vertigo associated with Meniere's disease has been refractory to medical treatment (e.g., diuretics and antihistamines) and a sufficient time has elapsed to determine that vertigo attacks are a recurrent problem (minimum of 3 months), vestibular neurectomy is the procedure of choice to relieve vertigo and preserve hearing.

INDICATIONS

Although unilateral Meniere's disease is the most common indication, the procedure can be useful in selected cases of recurrent vestibular neuronitis, traumatic labyrinthitis, and vestibular Meniere's disease. Patient choice is a strong consideration in the decision of when to operate. Some patients may have one or two severe episodes each month and not have their life-style sufficiently affected to warrant a major surgical procedure to correct the problem. Other patients with only two or three attacks yearly can be so severely affected that they live in constant fear of the next recurrence. There should be objective evidence of unilateral inner ear disease. Unless the patient is experiencing an acute Meniere's attack, he or she should be able to perform a tandem gait test reasonably well.

Contraindication to VNS include bilateral vestibular disease, physiologic old age, poor medical condition, ataxia or other indications of possible significant central involvement, and vertigo from an only hearing ear. Vertigo from an ear with very poor hearing (80 dB speech perception threshold; <20% discrimination) is usually more appropriately treated with a destructive procedure such as labyrinthectomy and eighth nerve section. Our preferred approach is a transmeatal, transcochlear approach to the internal auditory canal with sectioning of the vestibular and cochlear nerves.

Previous mastoid or endolymphatic sac surgery is not a contraindication, nor is old age when the patient is healthy and has good balance function. Vestibular neurectomy has been done successfully in patients in their 70s, with excellent results and no additional morbidity. Elderly people usually take longer to regain good balance function than do younger individuals.

OPERATIVE APPROACHES

Middle Fossa Vestibular Nerve Section

From 1963 to 1978, the middle fossa approach was used to section the vestibular nerve. Results for vertigo control were good, but the procedure was formidable, anatomic landmarks were difficult, and complications such as facial nerve weakness or deafness did occur.[1] Patients more than 60 years of age were generally not candidates because it was difficult to elevate thin dura from the skull. Because the procedure was difficult and had a high risk of complications, many patients who had significant disability were not offered a middle fossa VNS with much enthusiasm.

Retrolabyrinthine Vestibular Nerve Section

In 1978, Silverstein and Norrell developed the retrolabyrinthine approach to the posterior cranial fossa for VNS (or

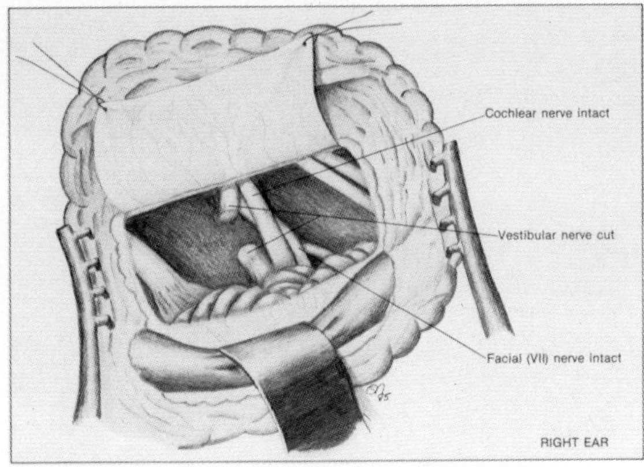

FIG 9–1.
Right RVNS. The vestibular fibers have been cut after the cochleo-vestibular cleavage plane was identified and separated.

RVN).[2,3] Although the approach had been previously described for use in trigeminal neuralgia procedures,[4] its application for selective VNS had not been described. Since the first report, we have performed this approach with good results in 78 patients; others have reported their series with similar good results.[5,6]

In this procedure, a simple mastoidectomy is performed, and the lateral sinus and posterior fossa dura just behind the sinus and in front of it are exposed. The endolymphatic sac is widely exposed and the posterior semicircular canal identified. The sigmoid sinus is collapsed with the lateral sinus retractor (Silverstein lateral sinus retractor, Storz Instruments, St. Louis), and the dura is incised in a C-shape fashion anterior to the sigmoid sinus based on the labyrinth. Intravenous mannitol is given when the drilling begins (1.5 gm/kg to a maximum of 1,000 gm), which causes contraction of the cerebellum and a wider exposure of the cerebellopontine (CP) angle. In 75% of cases, a good anteroposterior cleavage plane exists between the cochlear and vestibular fibers in the CP angle, with the cochlear fibers comprising the inferior portion of the eighth cranial nerve[7] and the vestibular fibers comprising the superior portion. This orientation is important; therefore, we routinely identify the fifth cranial nerve superiorly and the ninth, tenth, and eleventh nerve inferiorly. After the cleavage plane is visualized under high-power magnification, an incision is made in the cleavage plane, the cochlear and vestibular fibers are separated, and the vestibular nerve is transected (Fig 9–1). There are helpful landmarks in finding the cleavage plane. For instance, there is a slight color difference; the cochlear nerve appears whiter, and the vestibular fibers appear grayer. The cochlear fibers are more numerous (average 31,000) than the vestibular fibers (average 18,000). A fine blood vessel may be seen running on the surface between the cochlear and vestibular fibers. A mirror can be used to view the eighth nerve from the anterior surface, since the cleavage plane is sometimes more visible from this surface. The nervus intermedius, which usually lies in the cleavage plane, can also be seen anteriorly. The superior half of the eighth cranial nerve is transected when a cleavage plane cannot be readily identified. Most vestibular fibers will be cut and most cochlear fibers spared using this technique.

Results of this procedure have been good. In a review of our 78 patients, 83% were completely cured of their vertigo, and 9% were substantially improved; only 5% noted no change postoperatively. Overall patient satisfaction with the procedure has been 93%; sensorineural hearing has been maintained to within 20 dB, with 20% discrimination in 80%. Some patients experienced a conductive loss.

Retrosigmoid Internal Auditory Canal Vestibular Nerve Section

In 1985, in an attempt to improve these results, Silverstein et al. introduced the retrosigmoid internal auditory canal (IAC) approach to the IAC for VNS (Fig 9–2).[8] Because the cleavage plane between cochlear and vestibular fibers is more completely developed within the IAC, a more complete and selective vestibular neurectomy can be performed by cutting the nerves within the IAC. During this procedure, a posterior fossa craniotomy is made posterior to the lateral sinus, and the cerebellum is gently retracted to give exposure to the seventh and eighth cranial nerves and the IAC. The posterior wall of the IAC is removed to the singular canal, thereby exposing the branches of the eighth cranial nerve. The superior vestibular nerve is sectioned, and the singular nerve is divided. The inferior vestibular fibers that innervate the saccule are not divided because of their close association with cochlear fibers. The saccule has no known vestibular function in humans, so sparing these fibers will not result in vertigo attacks postoperatively.

This procedure has produced a 95% cure rate in our 14 patients, and hearing results are similar to those of the RVN. This procedure offers several advantages over the RVN. No abdominal fat is needed to fill the defect; thus, the procedure can be performed on thin patients. Since the exposure does not enter the mastoid, patients who have had chronic mastoiditis or a sclerotic mastoid or those with an anteriorly located sigmoid sinus can be candidates for the retrosigmoid IAC approach.[9,10] Complications have been infrequent; however, severe postoperative headache has been a problem for 75% of the patients. Fifty percent of the patients have had significant headaches, which are difficult to control with nonnarcotic analgesics and last many months. Four of the 14 patients (25%) still have severe headaches requiring continuous medication after 2 years. We have been unable to determine a cause for this problem, particularly since this approach has been used successfully for fifth nerve section and vascular decompression and is quite similar to the suboccipital approach often used for acoustic neuroma surgery. The postoperative headaches remain a major concern and have tempered our enthusiasm for the classic retrosigmoid IAC VNS.

Combined Retrosigmoid Retrolabyrinthine Vestibular Nerve Section

A further evolution of the VNS procedure was developed in 1987: the combined retrosigmoid and RVN.[11] This procedure incorporates the advantages of both the RVN and the retrosigmoid IAC approach. This approach allows the surgeon to assess the cochleovestibular cleavage plane in the posterior fossa and

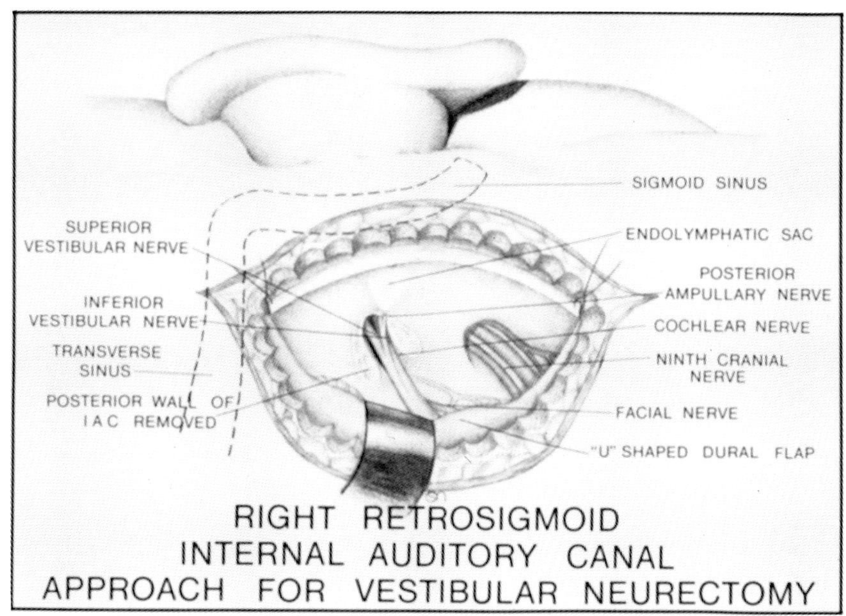

FIG 9–2.
Right retrosigmoid IAC VNS. The superior vestibular nerve is to be cut and the posterior ampullary nerve avulsed.

decide where the nerve section should be performed. If a good cochleovestibular cleavage plane exists, the VNS will be done in the CP angle. If not, the IAC can be opened and the superior vestibular and posterior ampullary nerves sectioned within the IAC.

In the combined retrosigmoid and RVN approach, a limited mastoidectomy is done. The lateral venous sinus is exposed from the transverse sinus to near the jugular bulb, and the posterior fossa dura is exposed for 1.5 cm posterior to the lateral venous sinus. The dural incision is made 3 mm behind the lateral venous sinus (Fig 9–3), and the lateral venous sinus is retracted anteriorly using stay sutures placed in the dural cuff. After the arachnoid is bluntly divided, the eighth nerve is examined and a cleavage plane sought between the cochlear and vestibular fibers. If the plane is present, the VNS is performed in the CP angle, as in the RVN. If no cleavage plane is identified, the dura is reflected off the temporal bone, the IAC is opened with a diamond burr, and the superior vestibular and posterior ampullary nerves are divided as in the retrosigmoid approach (Fig 9–4).

The development of the combined retrosigmoid and RVN represents a significant improvement over the two previous procedures. Much less bone removal is needed than in the RVN approach, which shortens surgical time. In addition, the surgeon has the option of opening the IAC and cutting the vestibular nerve more laterally where the cleavage plane is better defined. The advantage over the retrosigmoid approach is the cerebellar retraction is not necessary, and the moderate headache has occurred in only 2 of the 40 patients in whom this approach has been used with excellent results. Although follow-up is short (on average 12 months), no patient has had recurrent vertigo attacks postoperatively. Hearing has been preserved within 20

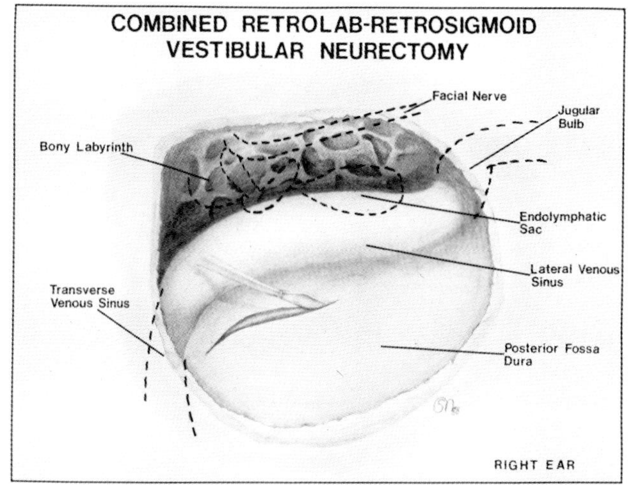

FIG 9–3.
Right retrosigmoid and RVNS. Dural incision is made 3 mm posterior to the lateral venous sinus.

dB of preoperative levels in 93%, and discrimination has been within 15% in 85% of patients.

COMPLICATIONS AND MANAGEMENT

Complications encountered in RVN are listed in Table 9–1. Cerebrospinal fluid (CSF) leaks occur in 10% because a tight closure of the posterior fossa dura is not possible. Cerebrospinal fluid leaks are easily managed with the placement of a contin-

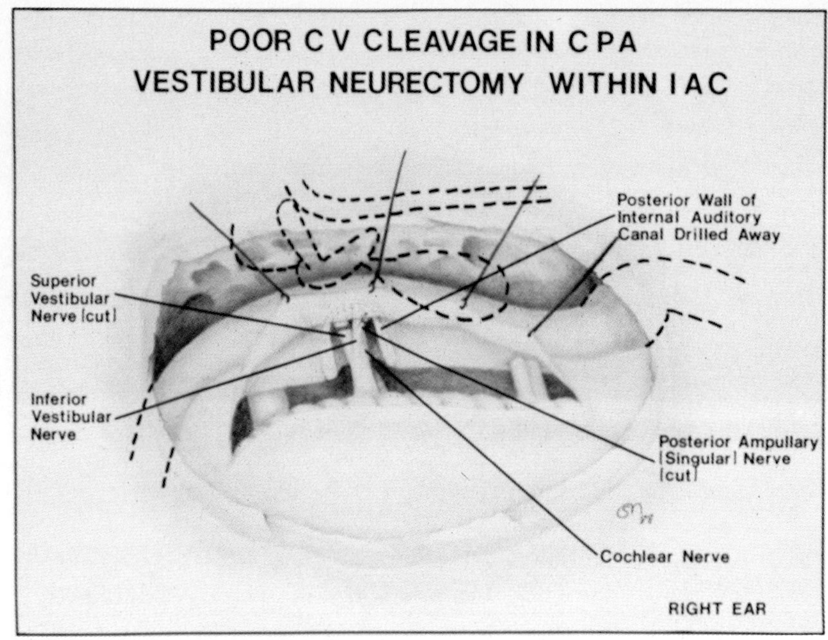

FIG 9–4.
Combined retrosigmoid and RVNS in cases when good cleavage plane between cochlear and vestibular *(CV)* fibers cannot be identified in the CP angle *(CPA)*. The IAC is opened and the nerve section done in a manner similar to the standard retrosigmoid approach.

TABLE 9–1.
Complications in Retrolabyrinthine
Vestibular Nerve Section

Complication	%
CSF leak	10
Superficial wound infections	3
Meningitis	0
Facial paralysis	0
Significant headaches	0

uous lumbar drain for 2 to 5 days to reduce CSF pressure. We have used this technique for the past 8 years, and no patient has required a second operation to close a postoperative CSF leak. Wound infection rate has been drastically reduced since we began using perioperative antibiotics. No antibiotics were used in the first 40 cases of RVN, and the infection rate was 20%. All infections were superficial and responded rapidly to local treatment and oral antibiotics, but this rate was regarded as unacceptably high. The use of nafcillin in a three-dose regimen (2 gm intravenously on call preoperatively, 2 gm intravenously in the operating room at the start of the procedure, and 2 gm intravenously 6 hours later) has reduced the infection rate to 3.3% in the last 28 cases. In cases of penicillin sensitivity, 600 mg of clindamycin is used in a similar dosage schedule. No cases of meningitis or infections caused by resistant microorganisms have been encountered.

No cases of facial paralysis or death have occurred. Postoperative unsteadiness is expected (as seen after labyrinthec-

tomy), but it improves with central compensation and is generally well tolerated and accepted.

Complications after retrosigmoid IAC VNS are listed in Table 9–2, and those of the combined retrosigmoid-RVNS approach are listed in Table 9–3.

TABLE 9–2.
Complications of Retrosigmoid–Internal
Auditory Canal Vestibular Nerve Section

Complication	%
Inadvertent opening labyrinth (1/14)	7
CSF leak	0
Postoperative infection	0
Facial paralysis	0
Meningitis	0
Headache (significant)	50

TABLE 9–3.
Complications of the Combined
Retrosigmoid and Retrolabyrinthine
Vestibular Nerve Sections

Complication	%
Postoperative headache	0.5 (2/40)
Facial paralysis	0
CSF leak	0
Meningitis	0
Wound infection, fat graft	0
Significant headache	10

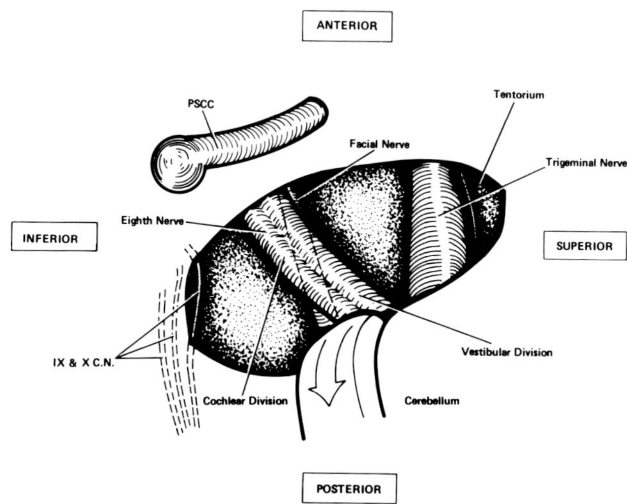

FIG 9–5.
View into the posterior fossa through the RVNS approach.

The cause of headaches after the retrosigmoid IAC VNS approach remains a mystery. Possibilities include cerebellar retraction, occipital neuralgia, drilling the IAC, and bone dust arachnoiditis.

The incidence of headache has been greatly reduced using the combined retrosigmoid and RVNS approach.

SUMMARY

Vestibular nerve section performed in the posterior fossa has gone through an evolution since we first described RVN in 1978. Ten years later we believe we have arrived at a procedure, the combined retrosigmoid and RVNS, that offers good results and the advantages of both the retrosigmoid and RVN approaches with minimal complications or morbidity.

REFERENCES

1. Silverstein H, Norell H, Haberkamp T: A comparison of retrosigmoid IAC, retrolabyrinthine and middle fossa vestibular neurectomy for treatment of vertigo. *Laryngoscope* 1987; 97:165–173.
2. Silverstein H, Norrell H: Retrolabyrinthine surgery: A direct approach to the cerebellopontine angle. *Otolaryngol Head Neck Surg* 1980; 88:462–469.
3. Silverstein H, Norrell H: Retrolabyrinthine vestibular neurectomy. *Otolaryngol Head Neck Surg* 1982; 90:778–782.
4. Hitselberger WE, Pulec JL: Trigeminal nerve (posterior root) retrolabyrinthine selective section. *Arch Otolaryngol* 1972; 96:412–415.
5. Kemink JL, Hoff JT: Retrolabyrinthine vestibular nerve section: Analysis of results. *Laryngoscope* 1986; 96:33–35.
6. House JW, Hitselberger WE, McElveen J, et al: Retrolabyrinthine section of the vestibular nerve. *Otolaryngol Head Neck Surg* 1984; 92:212.
7. Silverstein H: Cochlear and vestibular gross and histologic anatomy (as seen from the postauricular approach). *Otolaryngol Head Neck Surg* 1984; 92:207–211.
8. Silverstein H, Norrell H, Haberkamp T: A comparison of retrosigmoid-IAC, retrolabyrinthine, and middle fossa vestibular neurectomy for treatment of vertigo. *Laryngoscope* 1987; 97:165–173.
9. Silverstein H, Norrell H, Smouha E; Retrosigmoid-internal auditory canal approach vs. retrolabyrinthine approach for vestibular neurectomy. *Otolaryngol Head Neck Surg* 1987; 97:300–307.
10. Silverstein H, Norrell H, Smouha E, et al: Retrolabyrinthine or retrosigmoid vestibular neurectomy: Indications. *Am J Otol* 1987; 8:414–418.
11. Silverstein H, Norrell H, Jones R, et al: Combined retrolab-retrosigmoid vestibular neurectomy: An evolution in approach. *Am J Otol* 1989; 10:166–169.

Vestibular Nerve Section

Approach of

John L. Kemink, M.D.

Surgical management of patients with disabling vertigo and dysequilibrium is considered after patients fail to respond to appropriate expectant medical therapy. For vertigo of otologic origin, the offending peripheral vestibular system can generally be identified through the clinical history, physical examination, and appropriate audiologic, vestibular, and radiologic tests. The decision to proceed with surgery and the choice of the surgical procedure are based on a combination of factors. These factors include the etiology, bilateral hearing level and vestibular function, and the experience of the surgeon. There are numerous surgical procedures advocated to relieve vertigo of otologic origin, including endolymphatic sac surgery, repair of perilymphatic fistula, neurovascular decompression, and singular neurectomy, but transmastoid labyrinthectomy, and RVNS remain the mainstays of my surgical armamentarium for definitive management of vertigo.

An RVNS is an effective surgical approach to ablate vestibular function in the offending ear while preserving hearing. Experience with the RVNS procedure has proved it to be a reliable method of controlling episodic vertigo from peripheral vestibular dysfunction of many causes without undue morbidity.

INDICATIONS

In most series of RVNS, the most common indication has been intractable Meniere's disease. However, RVNS may also be performed for many other diagnoses, such as uncompensated vestibular neuritis, trauma (including neurosurgery or otologic surgery), vestibular hydrops, vertigo associated with suppurative otitis media, benign positional vertigo, and idiopathic progressive or sudden sensorineural hearing loss (SNHL) with persistent vertigo. In my experience, the presence of a unilateral SNHL correlates strongly with peripheral vestibular dysfunction. On many occasions, in cases with conflicting audiometric and vestibular findings, proceeding with an RVNS in the ear with poorer hearing has resulted in relief of vertigo. Therefore, the presence of an asymmetric SNHL preoperatively strongly suggests that symptoms are produced by the poorer hearing ear. One should remember that in occasional cases of

bilateral Meniere's disease or Meniere's disease in the only hearing ear, the better hearing ear may be the one responsible for the symptoms. Usually this will be easily confirmed by the typical history of active symptoms such as fluctuating hearing loss, tinnitus, and fullness predominating in that ear. With this unusual exception noted, in our experience, a unilateral SNHL is the most reliable indicator of the offending labyrinth.

In patients with symmetric cochlear function, the surgeon relies on subjective historical findings of fullness or tinnitus (or both) in the ear. On occasion, vestibular testing alone will clearly demonstrate the offending side. However, in this setting, localizing vestibular test results should be clearly reproducible before surgical intervention is considered. As a general rule, three or four bithermal caloric test results demonstrating a reduced vestibular response in the same ear are considered to be a reliable indicator of unilateral vestibular pathology. Other historical factors such as previous otologic surgery or a significant otologic trauma can be helpful in determining the offending side in some cases.

There continues to be a divergence of opinion as to when a hearing conservation procedure such as RVNS should be performed instead of labyrinthectomy. This decision should be individualized and based on a review of the diagnosis and residual hearing sensitivity. The final decision regarding the sacrifice of hearing must be guided by the desires of the patient. Nevertheless, certain guidelines and recommendations can be made. In general, the additional morbidity of an RVNS is indicated only in those patients who have useful hearing. Although 60-dB SRT and 50% discrimination have been used as a benchmark level, some patients find that this hearing level is not useful to them and would prefer labyrinthectomy to RVNS. Other patients surprisingly find much poorer levels of hearing useful, and I would, within reason, follow their wishes. In general, the older the patient, the more likely one would opt for the less extensive procedure, labyrinthectomy. I rarely perform RVNS in patients more than 65 years of age.

In the preoperative discussion with patients, all surgical options are presented. The advantages and disadvantages of each procedure are noted, and if, for instance, a patient has nearly normal hearing, a labyrinthectomy is excluded on that basis alone. Endolymphatic sac surgery is still performed in selected cases of Meniere's disease. My impression is that this procedure has a legitimate role in the management of vertigo, recognizing that there is approximately only a 50% long-term improvement rate. Furthermore, experience suggests that endolymphatic sac surgery is more effective for patients with an "active" ear (i.e., one that fluctuates substantially in SNHL, tinnitus intensity, and pressure sensation). In patients who have a long-standing, relatively fixed 50- to 70-dB SNHL with brief sudden onset attacks of vertigo, endolymphatic sac surgery appears to be unsatisfactory, and RVNS is preferred.

Retrolabyrinthine VNS is frequently offered as the primary surgical procedure for the control of intractable Meniere's disease. It is my experience that approximately 50% of patients will opt for this more definitive method of management. When hearing preservation is desired, RVNS is the procedure of choice for peripheral vestibular dysfunction of all diagnoses other than Meniere's disease.

SURGICAL CONSIDERATIONS

My surgical exposure of the vestibular nerve was originally through the middle cranial fossa. The retrolabyrinthine route was adopted because of increasing dissatisfaction with the small but troublesome incidence of sensorineural hearing loss (SNHL) and transient facial nerve paralysis. I also believed that the retrolabyrinthine approach would be technically less demanding. In all cases, surgical access was accomplished effectively without undue difficulty or excessive blood loss. In four cases, a large and anteriorly placed sigmoid sinus prompted a retrosigmoid approach, which was easily performed through the same scalp incision. Facial paralysis has not occurred, and the incidence of SNHL has been negligible (7%).

The retrolabyrinthine approach is potentially complicated by the difficulty of separating the cochlear and vestibular fibers. In all cases in this series, the eighth cranial nerve was a single nerve, although in 75% of patients I considered there to be a clear surgical septum between the cochlear and vestibular fibers. Previous histologic studies have shown that this septum may not precisely separate cochlear and vestibular fibers. In 25% of cases a clear surgical septum was not present, and in these cases the superior 50% of the nerve trunk was sectioned. The obvious undesirable consequence that may result from these anatomic variances is the sparing of vestibular fibers or sectioning cochlear fibers.

A potential solution might be sought by the retrosigmoid VNS advocated by Silverstein et al.[1] This procedure has the advantage of identifying vestibular fibers where they are more anatomically distinct from the cochlear fibers. Because of the limited number of patients who have undergone this procedure, it is unclear whether the morbidity associated with the additional cerebellar retraction required for this procedure will be acceptable. Certainly, it makes the procedure more technically demanding. An additional concern with the suboccipital approach has always been an increased incidence of troublesome postoperative headache, which I believe is unacceptable. Although the headaches usually resolve spontaneously, the symptoms may persist for 2 to 5 years and dominate the patient's life-style during this period.

SURGICAL APPROACH

My present method employs the RVNS approach. The patient is placed in a supine position, and electrodes for monitoring auditory brain stem response (ABR) are placed. A wide area of postauricular scalp is shaved, prepped, and draped. A curved incision begins above the temporal line anteriorly, proceeds posteriorly to the retrosigmoid region, then proceeds inferiorly toward the skull base posterior to the mastoid tip. An anteriorly based scalp flap is elevated, including the mastoid periosteum bone but lateral to the temporalis fascia superiorly. A wide area of temporalis fascia is harvested. A wide complete mastoidectomy is performed, with removal of the mastoid tip. The sigmoid sinus is decompressed, and approximately 1 to 2 cm of bone posterior to the sigmoid sinus is removed. The entire sinus can then be compressed posteriorly. The posterior fossa dura is exposed from the sinodural angle down into the retrofacial air cells inferiorly. Adequate exposure requires removal of retrofacial air cells well medial to the facial nerve to the level of the jugular bulb. In addition, the posterior half of the tegmen mastoideum is removed. A dural incision is performed parallel and approximately 0.5 to 1 cm medial to the sigmoid sinus. In 4 of 100 patients a retrosigmoid dural incision was performed because of an anteriorly placed sigmoid sinus. The anteromedial dural flap is held anteriorly with a silk suture, and the incision is continued parallel to the superior petrosal sinus if additional relaxation is needed for adequate exposure. An Apfelbaum retractor is then inserted to retract the cerebellum. After the position of the tentorium is noted, the neurovascular bundle exiting the porus acousticus of the IAC is identified. Frequently the cisterna magna needs to be opened and a portion of the cerebellar flocculus retracted posteriorly for better exposure of the nerve bundle. The eighth cranial nerve is then identified. The facial nerve is positively identified by gentle inferior retraction of the eighth nerve. The eighth nerve is viewed carefully for any differences in color and for the septum that may divide the cochlear and vestibular portions of the nerve. A Rosen needle is frequently used to establish this plane, and the nerve is sectioned with fine neurosurgical scissors. The retractor is removed, and the dural incision is closed with 4-0 interrupted silk sutures. This closure is usually not watertight and is covered with a piece of temporalis fascia. A previously harvested bone chip is used to block the aditus ad antrum. Care is taken not to allow it to rest against the ossicular chain. A second piece of temporalis fascia is placed superficial to the bone chip to seal the aditus ad antrum from the mastoid cavity, which is then obliterated with abdominal fat. The incision is closed with interrupted 2-0 chromic suture in the periosteum and subcutaneous tissue and a running locked 2-0 Prolene suture in the skin. A snug mastoid dressing remains in place for 5 days postoperatively, at which time it is removed and the wound inspected. An additional dressing is left on for another 3 to 5 days.

A number of additional techniques and medications that

facilitate successful neurotologic surgery are used routinely. Prophylactic antibiotics are given on call to the operating room and for 24 hours afterward. When the drilling begins on the mastoid, the anesthesiologist is instructed to hyperventilate the patient to P_{CO_2} of 25 to 30. Mannitol (25 to 50 gm) is also given at this time to accomplish a brisk diuresis.

ELECTROPHYSIOLOGIC MONITORING

The RVNS approach entails the risk of injury to the cochlear nerve. The RVNS procedure requires cerebellar retraction, blunt separation of the vestibular and cochlear branches of the eighth nerve, and the section of the vestibular fibers. All of these manipulations place the cochlear division of the eighth nerve at risk. Monitoring options include the ABR, round window electrocochleography, direct eighth nerve recording, or a combination of all of these modalities. Although, in general, hearing preservation rates without monitoring during this procedure were excellent, intraoperative monitoring is now performed to optimize the hearing results.

In our practice, a combination of ABR and direct eighth nerve recording are used to monitor RVNS procedures. The ABR monitoring is carried out using subdermal needle electrodes, with the reference electrode introduced anterior to the tragus, parallel to the external auditory meatus. After exposure of the neural bundle, a hand-held bipolar electrode is introduced to confirm the identity of the cochlear and vestibular divisions.

The great majority of patients undergoing VNS demonstrate normal hearing to moderate sensorineural hearing impairment and have normal ABRs preoperatively. Most of the ABR or eighth nerve response changes seen during this procedure are related to traction of the eighth cranial nerve medially from the acoustic meatus. This may be induced by cerebellar retraction or direct surgical manipulation of the nerve. The separation of vestibular and cochlear divisions may bring about further changes, especially an increase in wave V latency and a reduction of its amplitude. Usually, there is a partial or complete restoration of the ABR configuration following completion of the VNS and after the removal of the cerebellar retractor. In our experience, if wave V is preserved and the transient intraoperative latency shift does not exceed the preoperative baseline by 1.0 ms, hearing is preserved to within 5 to 10 dB of the preoperative level.

Eighth cranial nerve action potentials can be directly recorded by means of a hand-held bipolar recording electrode on the intracranial portion of the nerve. This technique assists in the identification of the cochlear and vestibular branches whenever the septum separating the two branches is absent or attenuated or when there are other deviations from normal anatomy. In my experience, the amplitude of this action potential (which is equivalent to the far field scalp-recorded ABR wave II) exhibits a 3:1 ratio between the cochlear and the vestibular branches, respectively. It is important to note that due to volume conduction facilitated by the ever-present thin film of CSF coating the neural bundle, the response will always be present even when recording from the vestibular branch. Therefore, this procedure is of limited value and should be used only as an adjunct to other means of identification.

CLINICAL EXPERIENCE

From 1983 through 1985, 60 patients underwent RVNS for treatment of disabling labyrinthine dysfunction. They have been followed up for a minimum of 3 years. In this series, 29 patients (48%) had a diagnosis of Meniere's disease with the complete syndrome of fluctuating SNHL, episodic vertigo, aural fullness, and tinnitus. In 31 patients (52%), labyrinthine dysfunction was attributed to other causes. Fifteen patients had a diagnosis of uncompensated vestibular neuritis as determined by a compatible history and a reproducible and significantly reduced vestibular response (RVR) on repeated electronystagmography (ENG) evaluations. Six patients had labyrinthine dysfunction due to temporal bone trauma or previous neurologic or neurootologic surgery, including anterior craniotomy, stapedectomy, tympanoplasty, singular nerve section, and temporal bone fracture (two patients). Five patients had vestibular hydrops with vertigo associated with aural fullness and pressure. Three of these patients also demonstrated a reproducible RVR by ENG. Other diagnoses included an Arnold-Chiari malformation with progressive SNHL (one) benign positional vertigo (one), sudden hearing loss while under general anesthesia for parotid surgery (one), and vertigo after acute suppurative otitis media (two).

All patients underwent full neuro-otologic and metabolic evaluations and a radiologic examination.

Audiologic assessment was performed for both pure-tone and speech discrimination ability. Hearing was normal preoperatively in 29 patients. In 18 patients the hearing acuity was between 20 and 40 dB SRT, and in 13 patients it was between 40 and 60 dB SRT in the involved ear. Twenty-five patients with Meniere's disease had SRTs greater than 20 dB, and four had SRTs between 0 and 20 dB. Four patients with a diagnosis other than Meniere's disease had SNHLs less than 20 dB SRT. These patients' diagnoses were suppurative otitis media associated with transient facial paralysis and mild SNHL, progressive SNHL, sudden hearing loss under general anesthesia, and temporal bone fracture with moderate SNHL. Two patients had a preoperative conductive hearing loss, one after a previous tympanoplasty and one after stapedectomy.

Electronystagmography was employed and showed a reproducible RVR in all but 13 patients. Of these patients, 10 had unilateral Meniere's disease, 2 had vestibular hydrops, and 1 had benign positional vertigo. One patient with Meniere's disease had a significant RVR in the opposite ear.

RESULTS

Vertigo.—Overall, 52 of 60 patients (87%) noted significant or complete control of their vestibular symptoms after RVNS. Seven of 60 (11%) noted improvement but had continuing complaints of dysequilibrium, and 1 patient was unchanged.

In the 29 patients with Meniere's disease, 24 patients (83%) considered themselves cured, and 5 (17%) considered themselves improved (Table 9–4).

Four of the patients with a diagnosis other than Meniere's disease had an SNHL in the involved ear, and all noted complete relief of vertigo postoperatively.

TABLE 9–4.
Results of Patients With Vertigo or Meniere's Disease

	No.	%
Vertigo (*N* = 60)		
Control of symptoms	52	60
Improved	7	11
Unchanged	1	2
Meniere's disease (*N* = 29)		
Complete control	24	83
Improved	5	17

The 27 remaining patients had normal preoperative bone conduction levels with clinical or ENG evidence suggesting a peripheral vestibular disorder. Twenty of these 27 patients (74%) noted relief of their vertigo postoperatively. Six patients (22%) noted no change in their symptoms postoperatively, and one patient believed that he was worse.

In this series, it appears that the presence of a unilateral SNHL is an important predictive correlate of peripheral labyrinthine dysfunction, since in every case, VNS benefited such individuals. Of the group that failed to improve, all had normal preoperative SNHL levels, and four of these patients had uncompensated vestibular neuritis. Overall, patients with uncompensated vestibular neuritis have done poorly after surgery, and vestibular rehabilitation therapy is recommended.

Hearing.—In this series of 60 patients, 3 (5%) demonstrated improvement in their hearing. All of these had Meniere's disease. One of these three demonstrated a substantial improvement of hearing to levels that had not been present during the past 2 years. Four (7%) patients noted an SNHL postoperatively, three of whom had Meniere's disease (Table 9–5). In the patients with Meniere's disease, the most significant hearing loss was a 40 dB SNHL across all frequencies. One patient demonstrated a 40 dB low-tone incremental SNHL, which subsequently improved by 20 dB. One patient in whom the nerve was generously sectioned to assure that all vestibular fibers were divided noted a marked decrease in discrimination. The only hearing loss in a patient with a diagnosis other than Meniere's disease was a moderate high-frequency SNHL. The remaining 53 (88%) patients had unchanged SNHLs, although 4 patients noted 5 to 10 dB conductive hearing losses, and 1 patient noted a 25 dB conductive hearing loss postoperatively. Blocking the attic during surgery preventing the accumulation of bone dust in the middle ear space has diminished this problem recently.

Complications.—Death, stroke, facial nerve paralysis, and meningitis did not occur. One patient had a transient sixth cranial nerve palsy from presumed increased intracranial pressure. Three patients required a second operation for closure of a CSF leak despite routine use of both temporalis fascia to reinforce the posterior fossa dural closure and abdominal fat to obliterate the mastoid cavity. One leak was associated with a wound infection and required subsequent drainage. Four other superficial wound infections occurred, only one of which required drainage. One wound infection occurred in the abdominal wound where fat was harvested. Postoperatively, the patient with an Arnold-Chiari malformation developed hydrocephalus, and one patient coincidentally developed the onset of myasthenia gravis.

CONCLUSION

I continue to recommend RVNS to my patients as an effective surgical approach to ablate vestibular function in a symptomatic ear while preserving hearing. It is a reliable method of controlling episodic vertigo from peripheral vestibular dysfunction of many causes without undue morbidity. It is a particularly effective procedure for patients with Meniere's disease or with an asymmetrical SNHL loss that indicates the involved peripheral labyrinth. Although I frequently offer RVNS as a primary surgical procedure for the control of vertigo in Meniere's disease, I continue to perform endolymphatic sac surgery and transmastoid labyrinthectomy in appropriate cases. In general, the surgical approach is uncomplicated and is enhanced by the addition of intraoperative electrophysiologic monitoring of auditory function.

REFERENCE

1. Silverstein H, Norrell H, Smouha EE: Retrosigmoid–internal auditory canal approach vs. retrolabyrinthine approach for vestibular neurectomy. *Otolaryngol Head Neck Surg* 1987; 97:300–307.

CHAPTER 10

Cochlear Implants

Approach of

Thomas Balkany, M.D.

INDICATIONS AND IMPLANT TYPE IN ADULTS

Indications

The clinical use of implantable electronic devices to stimulate the auditory systems of profoundly deaf individuals has been a relatively recent advance. This development is a result of both medical and technologic advances within the past 20 years.

Only 10 years ago, a predominant opinion among otolaryngologists was that long-term electrical stimulation of the auditory system was impossible or unworkable. Few, if any, at that time speculated that open-set speech discrimination would ever be possible with such a device. Yet today, open-set speech discrimination can be expected in a majority of selected postlinguistically deafened adults, and clinical trials are rapidly proceeding in prelinguistically deafened adults. A large body of experience has been developed and continues to develop for the use of cochlear implants in children as well.

In general terms, candidates for cochlear implantation without restriction by the Food and Drug Administration (FDA) include those who (1) are healthy, postlinguistically deafened adults (18 years of age or older); (2) are profoundly or totally bilaterally deaf; (3) do not benefit from high-power hearing aids; (4) have been deaf for a minimum of 12 months to allow time for spontaneous recovery of hearing; and (5) are medically, psychologically, and emotionally stable. Previous restrictions, absence of middle ear pathology, and total patency of the cochlea are no longer considered absolute contraindications.

Under specific FDA protocols, both prelinguistically deafened adults and prelinguistically or postlinguistically deafened children may be considered candidates (investigational device exemption stage). At least 30 centers around the country are performing clinical trials in these groups.

Prelinguistically deafened adults should use an auditory-verbal or auditory-oral approach to communication and show little or no benefit on closed-set segmental subtests of the MAC (minimal auditory capabilities) and THRIFT (three interval forced choice test of speech pattern contrast perception) batteries with hearing aids. The MAC and THRIFT were developed for evaluating cochlear implant candidates and others with profound hearing loss.

After an initial screening, which may be conducted in person or through correspondence (e.g., review of medical and audiologic records, completion of questionnaires), suitable candidates are generally evaluated through a multispecialty team approach. Evaluation includes otologic, audiologic, psychologic, speech and language, and radiologic evaluation.

The medical evaluation is essential to rule out ongoing or acute processes, as well as the suitability of the temporal bone for electrode implantation.

The audiologic evaluation establishes baseline data and, in a surprisingly large percentage of cases, has indicated that patients are not candidates and may be significantly helped with conventional amplification. (In these cases a trial of hearing aids is mandatory.)

Type

At the present time, our preferred cochlear implant is the Nucleus Mini-22 device. In our experience with 56 cases, this device has proved to be generally reliable and effective.

We have also used the University of California at San Francisco cochlear implant with good results in the past and look forward to its clinical availability in the future for controlled testing. The House/3M implant currently is not available.

The development of cochlear implant devices is an ongoing process. Great credit must be given to William House and other pioneers who proceeded in the face of widespread resistance to establish the safety and efficacy of the single-channel devices.

Based on their success, multichannel devices were developed later and, we believe, are proving to be more effective as a general rule. Early multichannel work by Robin Michaelson has also overcome obstacles, leading to the current success of the devices.

Certainly manufacturers of all devices, both single channel and multichannel, can point to "star patients" within their groups. However, as an overall experience, we believe the multichannel device will prove to be superior for most postlinguistically deafened patients.

At this time, single-channel cochlear implants are available in Europe for intracochlear and extracochlear insertion and use a variety of processing strategies. Some European colleagues have stressed development of low-cost devices that could be made available in spite of the restrictions of their socialized systems of medical care.

Multichannel devices are also available for intracochlear as well as extracochlear use, though the majority of multichannel devices are intracochlear.

A variety of processing and transmission strategies are available with cochlear implants as well. The Symbion cochlear implant is a percutaneous device in which a biocompatible pedestal is anchored to the skull and extends through the postauricular skin for a hard wire connection. The other internal devices are powered and provided with information through transcutaneous radio frequency stimulation or magnetic induction.

INDICATIONS AND IMPLANT TYPE IN CHILDREN

As mentioned earlier, the indications for cochlear implants in children are similar to those of other deaf patients. Limitations on very early insertion of cochlear implants are primarily the ability of audiologists to confirm profound or total deafness in infants. Thus, at the present time, in spite of early identification of presumed deafness, a long-term trial of a hearing aid remains necessary to determine whether speech and language and auditory development will proceed.

Children who are candidates for cochlear implantation should demonstrate profound to total, bilateral sensorineural hearing loss. Radiologic contraindications to placement of the receiver-stimulator or the electrode array should not be present. Medical contraindications to implant surgery and rehabilitation should not be present. Families and (if possible) candidates should be well motivated and possess appropriate expectations. Candidates, families, and education facilities should be prepared and willing to participate in and cooperate with preoperative and postoperative training and assessment programs. Children in fully manual programs are not candidates at this time and should be placed on a waiting list. Children should demonstrate little or no benefit from a hearing aid for the implanted ear.

Less of a consideration is the size of the middle ear and mastoid. The cochlea is not a consideration due to its development in utero. It is widely agreed that by 2 years of age, the mastoid, including the facial recess, is well developed enough to permit straight forward implantation. By age 2 years, only 2 cm of further growth will occur in the mastoid bone, and the head is 50% adult size.

We use the Nucleus Mini-22 device for children as well as adults. This device is significantly larger, both in thickness and surface area, than the 3M/House device currently undergoing clinical trials in children. It requires a larger scalp flap to be elevated. Nonetheless, in our experience with 13 children (2 were 3 years of age), we have not encountered surgical difficulties. In fact, as in certain other otologic circumstances, the surgery appears to be somewhat easier in children than in adults.

Children being implanted with the Nucleus Mini-22 device are controlled under an FDA protocol that requires a 6-month trial of habilitation (or rehabilitation) therapy using a method designed by Ling along with powerful hearing aids.

If the patient makes uninterrupted progress with this method, it is continued indefinitely, and the patient may not be a candidate. If the patient plateaus with this method, he or she is then considered to be a candidate if all other criteria are met.

ROUND WINDOW OBLITERATION

Obliteration of the round window by bone or fibrous tissue is not uncommonly experienced during cochlear implant surgery. Preparation by the surgeon, however, renders this an annoyance rather than a surgical contraindication in most cases.

If obliteration is to occur, it most commonly occurs in the area of the hook portion of the cochlea and round window niche. This is thought to occur due to the proximity of the distal end of the cochlear aqueduct. Inflammatory meningitic changes are thought to proceed through the cochlear aqueduct to this area of cochlea. Thus, the surgeon must be prepared to remove this obstruction to enter the patent portion of the basal turn of the cochlea.

Balkany et al.[2] have described the techniques and results of radiologic imaging of the cochlea. In most cases it is possible to predict narrowing, fibrous, or bony obstruction to the basal turn. In some cases, however, the surgeon may encounter fibrous obstruction of the basal turn that is not radiographically evident.

Insertion of long cochlear electrodes has been accomplished in spite of "total" obliteration of the cochlea by bone. Good results have occurred in one of two cases in which this has been attempted and reported. However, in less than total obliteration of the inferior segment of the basal turn of the cochlea, excellent results can be expected when insertion is performed by experienced operators.[3] In short, obliteration of the round window or inferior segment of the basal turn is not a contraindication for insertion of long intracochlear electrodes.

MONDINI DEFORMITY

Congenital anomalies are most frequently encountered in deaf children and prelinguistically deaf adults. The Mondini deformity may be recognized by imaging and currently is a term used to describe a wide variety of labyrinthine dysplasias.

We (and other centers as well) have inserted electrodes into cochleas that had radiographic evidence of absent bony partitioning. This has been done with both single-channel and multichannel devices, and results are consistent with those obtained by implantation of deaf patients who have radiographically normal cochleas. Nonetheless, it is important to inform the family of the added risk to the facial nerve and the failure to stimulate when congenital anomalies are identified.

Radiographic absence or diminutive size of the internal auditory canal has been associated with failure of the auditory system to stimulate in the past. This deformity probably has greater significance than the Mondini deformity.

ELECTRODE FAILURE

All forms of cochlear implants have undergone mechanical failure. A widespread recall of the 3M/House device occurred when cable breakage was noted in a number of patients. The cable was then "stress relieved" as it left the titanium case, and the device is apparently quite reliable at this time.

A number of multichannel devices have also failed, although most mechanical failures appeared to occur within the electronics package of the Nucleus device rather than in the cable. It would be expected, however, that over the years mechanical failures of many types will be encountered.

Both single-channel and multichannel intracochlear and extracochlear devices have been removed and new devices inserted. Our experience with two patients, one with a single-channel device and one with a multichannel device, as well as several cases reported by others, indicates that removal and reinsertion can be performed with relative simplicity.

It should be remembered that the bone of the facial recess overlying the facial nerve is usually very thin after surgery, and if a soft tissue graft has been placed into the facial recess, removal may put the facial nerve at additional risk.

CEREBROSPINAL FLUID LEAKS AT THE INNERCOIL SITE

Our clinical experience and that of others has indicated that leakage of perilymph or cerebrospinal fluid (CSF) from the round window area where the electrode was inserted is rare.

Research with cats indicates that a soft tissue seal in this area forms rapidly and becomes water tight as well as highly resistant to penetration by experimental otitis media.[4]

A seat in the mastoid or parietal bone is routinely drilled for the implantable package of the device. It is frequently sutured in place through drill holes placed in the skull. Cerebrospinal fluid leaks may occur in this area; however, we have not encountered any. Great care should be taken when one is drilling the seat and the tie down holes. The thickest bone in the area is located at the sinodural angle, and as the drilling proceeds superior and posterior, the bone may become thin, especially in young children. Nonetheless, surgical diligence and painstaking technique have avoided problems in this area.

INFECTION

Infection has not been a reported complication of cochlear implants except in difficulties that occur with the design or surgical creation of the scalp flap. The incision should be 1 to 2 cm peripheral to the outer circumference of the cochlear implant.

This incision is planned so that it has a very wide base superiorly for the temporal vessels and inferiorly for the occipital vessels. Unfortunately, adults may have skin thick enough to cause difficulty with magnetic attraction and radio frequency transmission. Thus, thinning of these flaps is necessary and may result in reducing the vascular supply to the flap as well as creating a potential breakthrough over the device itself.

Intraoperatively we administer intravenous cephalosporin. We use a closed (Jackson-Pratt) drainage system for approximately the first 24 hours and continue antibiotic coverage while the drain is in place.

Copious irrigation with normal saline is used throughout the procedure, and gentle retraction of the flap with sutures rather than relying solely on self-retaining retractors may also be helpful.

We have implanted multichannel devices in two patients with chronic inflammatory disease of the middle ear.

In these patients, a radical mastoidectomy was performed, the eustachian tube, mastoid cavity, and external auditory canal were obliterated with muscle and fascia, and the external auditory canal skin was everted, closed with a pursestring suture, and returned to position. This has been done as a one-stage procedure during implantation without complication.

OTHER CONSIDERATIONS

The hypotympanic air cell tract may easily be confused with the round window niche by the inexperienced surgeon. The round window membrane rarely lies more than 2 mm inferior to the pyramidal process. This distance should be verified whenever doubt exists.

In cases in which electrode placement is uncertain, a simple anteroposterior transorbital film can be taken while the patient is on the operating table to confirm position. Poor placement may then be corrected prior to awakening the patient.

Most profoundly deaf implant recipients have little vestibular function preoperatively. However, in those with combined responses to warm and cool caloric stimulation of more than 20 degrees of second slow-phase velocity, postoperative vertigo is often experienced.

REFERENCES

1. Ling D: *Speech and the Hearing Impaired Child: Theory and Practice.* Washington, DC, AG Bell Assoc, 1976.
2. Balkany TJ, Dreisbach JD, Cohen NL, et al: Surgical anatomy and radiographic imaging of cochlear implant surgery. *Am J Otol* 1987; 8:195–200.
3. Balkany TJ, Gantz BJ, Nadol JB: Multichannel cochlear implants and partially ossified cochleus. *Ann Otol Rhinol Laryngol* 1988; 97(suppl 135):3–8.
4. Brennan WJ, Clark GM: An animal model of acute otitis media and the histological assessment of a cochlear implant in the cat. *J Laryngol Otol* 1985; 99:851–856.

Cochlear Implants

Approach of

William M. Luxford, M.D.

and

William F. House, M.D.

Many centers throughout the world have investigated the cochlear implant. In the United States, the FDA has monitored these investigations. The FDA has approved the 3M/House and the Nucleus 22-channel devices for general use in adults. Other devices, including the San Francisco, Symbion, and the 3/M Vienna are undergoing investigational clinical trials in adults controlled by the FDA. The FDA is also monitoring clinical studies of the 3M/House and the Nucleus 22-channel devices in children. The FDA criteria for these groups include adults 18 years of age or older and children 2 to 17 years old. In general, patients have a bilateral profound-total sensorineural hearing loss, are unable to benefit from conventional hearing aids, are in good physical and mental health, and have the motivation and patience to complete a rehabilitation program.

PATIENT SELECTION

Selection criteria of an appropriate implant candidate vary from group to group. As each implant center gains more experience, they may modify the audiologic and medical criteria.

Audiologic Criteria

An audiologic assessment is the primary means of determining implant suitability, and audiologic results are the most common reason for rejection of a candidate, that is, the patient would perform better with an appropriate hearing aid than he or she would with a cochlear implant. A potential implant candidate has bilateral, profound to total sensorineural hearing loss, usually with a three-frequency average (500, 1,000, and 2,000 Hz) pure-tone unaided threshold in the better ear equal to or greater than 95 dB. Audiologic testing procedures differ between adults and children.

Adults

A prospective candidate is evaluated with appropriate powerful hearing aids. Factors regarding function with a hearing aid, such as recruitment and discomfort, are considered when one evaluates the likelihood of the patient performing better with an implant than with a hearing aid.

If the patient cannot obtain an aided speech detection threshold of 70 dB sound pressure level (SPL), approximately a 53 dB hearing level or better, or performs very poorly on the discrimination test with conventional amplification, a cochlear implant is likely to provide greater benefit.

In the past, most investigators believed that prospective patients should have zero open-set word scores. As more knowledge is gained about the effectiveness of the different cochlear implants and their ability to provide awareness of speech, perhaps particular patients with scores as high as 10% on the W-22 word list may be candidates for a cochlear implant.[1]

A full list of test procedures and criteria for patient selection recommended by the device manufacturers and principal investigators are typically specified in the product labeling or in the training manuals.

In an attempt to standardize the reporting of cochlear implant results across the different investigators, the American Academy of Otolaryngology-Head and Neck Surgery formed an ad hoc subcommittee of cochlear implants. A minimum protocol developed by the subcommittee for cochlear implant research in adults containing descriptions of unaided and aided preimplant tests has been published.[2]

Children

Children evaluated for the cochlear implant undergo an extensive audiologic assessment.[3] Tympanometry and otoscopy are performed to rule out middle ear pathology at the time of testing. Acoustic reflexes are measured. In children less than 6 years of age, auditory brain stem response testing is required to confirm a profound hearing loss. Traditional behavioral audiometry or play audiometry with visual, social, or tangible reinforcers are used as needed. If there is no response to sound at maximal levels through the head phones, the child is conditioned to respond to a hand-held bone oscillator to ensure that he or she understands the task.

Discrimination tests are performed with the aid that provides the best warble-tone threshold. With an appropriate hearing aid, the child's performance on the discrimination tests in the ear selected for implantation must be poorer than or equal to the average test results obtained from children using a cochlear implant. The audiologically poorer ear is usually chosen for implantation.

Parent and teacher reports of the child's auditory ability must be consistent with the measured severity of the hearing loss. The child must also have a history of an appropriate hearing aid trial. If recent hearing aids or ear molds have not been optimal, and if testing reveals that usable hearing may remain, a 3- to 6-month trial with appropriate aids and molds is required before a decision on the implant is made. In these cases, the parents and school are encouraged to provide intense auditory training during the trial period.

Medical Evaluation

The medical evaluation includes a complete history and physical examination to detect problems that might interfere with the patient's ability to complete either the surgical or rehabilitative measures of implantation. Appropriate laboratory studies should be ordered to eliminate any suspected medical disorder.

In adults and children receiving the cochlear implant, the etiology of deafness has varied. From the variety of responses to cochlear implantation of patients with the same etiology, the etiology of hearing loss would not seem as important as the onset of loss.

For cochlear implant candidates, the onset of profound hearing loss is best described as congenital (hearing loss present at birth) or acquired (hearing loss occurring after birth).

Adults deafened prior to acquisition of verbal language skills (congenital and early acquired) are considered prelingually deaf. Those adults deafened after the acquisition of verbal language skills (late acquired) are considered postlingually deaf.

Acquired deafness in children can be further defined by age of onset as prelingual (≤ 1 year), perilingual (1 to 5 years), and postlingual (≥ 5 years).[4] Naturally, the later the onset of profound hearing loss the greater the chance that the child will develop an auditory memory and realize the benefit of sound.

The majority of implant groups have limited their patients to adults. Many programs select only postlingual deaf adults, whereas others include prelingual deaf adults. Experience indicates that prelingual and postlingual deaf adults gain similar auditory information through the cochlear implant, but the prelingual deaf adults cannot use the information as effectively. Probably because of the lesser benefits derived, prelingual deaf adults have a higher nonuser rate.[5]

Physical Examination

It is important to identify preoperatively any external or middle ear disease, including perforations of the tympanic membrane, that must be treated prior to cochlear implantation.

For young children it is important to evaluate the size of the implant in relation to the size of the child's skull and to consider the issues involved with skull maturation.[6] The distance between the cochlear promontory and the mastoid cortex, the approximate sites of the electrode array, and the receiver-stimulator increases about 1.7 cm from birth to adulthood, with one half of the increase occurring during the first 2 years of life.[7] The electrodes must be long enough to tolerate the increase in height and width of the skull that will occur with the child's growth. The accommodation occurs through the gradual straightening of the excess electrode length within the air-containing mastoid cavity.

Radiologic Evaluation

High-resolution computed tomography of the temporal bone is performed in all cases to identify partial or complete ossification of the scala tympani, soft tissue obliteration of the scala, congenital malformation of the inner ear, and surgical landmarks.[8] Complete agenesis of the cochlea and an abnormal acoustic nerve, the result of either congenital malformation, trauma, or surgery, are contraindications for cochlear implant placement.[9]

Cochlear hypoplasia (Mondini deformity) is not a contraindication for cochlear implantation. Children with incomplete congenital cochlear malformations implanted with the 3M/House single-channel device are successful users, and one adult Mondini patient implanted with the Nucleus 22 channel is a successful user.[10–12]

Ossification of fibrous occlusion of the cochlea or the round window does not exclude a patient from implantation, but it may influence which implant system is used. Patients with occlusion of the cochlea are at a higher risk of not responding to electrical stimulation and may require substantially higher power output from the signal processor than patients with little or no bone growth.[13]

Magnetic resonance imaging (MRI) is not practical for evaluating implant candidates. It shows little bony detail and, as yet, not enough of the membranous inner ear. With improvements in the use of surface coils, MRI may become more useful in evaluation of the membranous inner ear in detecting cochlear fibrosis.

Promontory Evaluation

Nearly all implant teams perform an electrical stimulation test. A positive response is a perception of sound when either the round window membrane or the promontory is stimulated. Some investigators no longer feel promontory stimulation is critical in the selection of candidates because patients with a negative response, as well as a positive promontory test, respond to intracochlear stimulation.

Psychologic Criteria

Children who are potential candidates for a cochlear implant undergo a detailed psychologic assessment.[14]

In the past, adult cochlear implant candidates also underwent a detailed psychologic assessment.[15] However, very few of the deaf patients evaluated failed to meet the criteria. Those with severe psychopathology were nearly always detected before the psychologic assessment; therefore, only those adult patients who cause concern are psychologically assessed. Counseling is provided to families who have misconceptions or unrealistic expectations regarding the benefits and limitations of the cochlear implant.

DEVICE CHARACTERISTICS

Extracochlear Versus Intracochlear Device

The extracochlear device has the theoretical advantage of safe placement of the electrode; however, there are potential disadvantages for efficacy. In some cases of calcification of the basal turn of the cochlea, the voltage requirement for the extracochlear device may exceed the ability of the device to provide the necessary current. Another disadvantage is that anchoring the electrode is more difficult in most extracochlear designs, a critical problem in children because a young child will experience an increase in the distance between the electrode tip and the receiver-stimulator package with age. If the extracochlear device is not well anchored at the round window, there will be movement of the electrode from its original site that will affect performance.

Single-Channel Versus Multichannel Device

Though the cochlear implant systems present a wide range of processor or electrode alternatives, they all work by electrically stimulating viable neural elements of the inner ear. From examination of temporal bones from nine patients with cochlear implants, Linthicum believes that ganglion cells are the structures of the inner ear that are being stimulated and that response to stimulation may occur with as few as 5% of the normal population of ganglion cells.[16] At present, there is no preoperative test to predict the number or place of viable neural elements within the cochlea. In patients with few surviving ganglion cells, there may be no difference in efficacy between single-channel and multichannel devices. If there is no difference in efficacy, since single-channel systems can be simpler and less expensive than multichannel systems, a single-channel system could provide the same benefit at the lower cost.

Factors other than surviving neural elements may play a part in determining efficacy between single-channel and multichannel devices, namely, onset of hearing loss, ossification of cochlea, congenital malformations of the ear, and size of the internal receiver package. Studies suggest that a postlingually deafened adult and possible a prelingually deafened adult would do better with a multichannel device.[17–19] Information on the use of single-channel and multichannel devices in children is being gathered. Multichannel devices with long intracochlear electrodes are usually contraindicated in patients with total ossification of the cochlea. Patients with congenital malformations of the cochlea have received effective stimulation from either a single-channel or multichannel device. Redesigning of the internal receiver package used in adults may be required for use in young children.

Induction Coil Versus Percutaneous Plug

In some stimulation strategies, such as those with simultaneous stimulation of more than one electrode pair, there is an advantage to the percutaneous plug. However, because of safety considerations of infection of tissue around the plug, percutaneous plugs in children are relatively contraindicated in favor of a totally implanted induction coil.

SURGICAL TECHNIQUE

Techniques of implantation differ in detail from prosthesis to prosthesis. The cochlear implant should be implanted only by qualified surgeons specifically trained to perform the procedure. Surgeons should avoid having any prosthetic material in contact with the skin of the external ear canal. Therefore, the preferred procedure for placement of an implant in a patient with a normal external ear canal is via the transmastoid facial recess approach to the round window–scala tympani. In patients with mastoid cavities where the posterior external ear canal is absent, the preferred procedure is total obliteration of the mastoid with closure of the external ear meatus.

The external ear canal approach to the round window is acceptable in adults. The initial problems of electrode extrusion have been overcome by formation of a deep groove in the external canal and encasing the electrode in bone. This procedure, however, is not acceptable in children. With the electrode encased in the external ear canal, no accommodation for skull growth would occur. Therefore, the electrode would be displaced from its original intracochlear position over time.

The placement of a cochlear prosthesis in the child is essentially the same as in the adult, because the key anatomic structures, including the cochlea, middle ear, ossicles, and tympanic membrane, are in place and in their adult configurations at birth. By age 2 years, the mastoid antrum and facial recess, which provide access to the middle ear for active electrode placement, are adequately developed. A few modifications are required to accommodate these smaller dimensions of the mastoid process and the thinness of the scalp and temporal squama. The induction coil is firmly anchored to the squamous portion of the temporal bone, and the active electrode is sealed at the round window with connective tissue. Because the same electrode is used in children as in adults, the accommodation for skull growth occurs through gradual straightening of the excess electrode length left within the air-containing mastoid cavity. Fortunately, growth-related problems have not been identified in children with implants.[20]

Operative Procedure

The position of the receiver-stimulator varies among devices. To prevent receiver-stimulator extrusion through the incision, one must make the incision at least 1 to 2 cm wider than

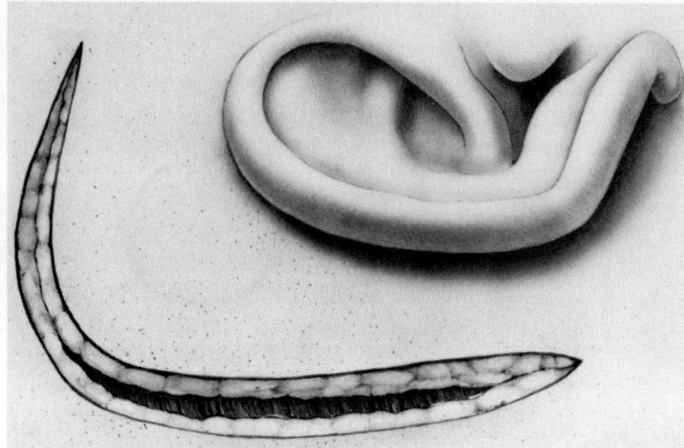

FIG 10–1.
The postauricular incision is made at least 1 to 2 cm beyond the edge of the internal receiver.

the expected receiver-stimulator (Fig 10–1). It is important also to maintain good vascular supply to the flap to decrease the chance of the wound not healing.

In adults and older children, the anterior postauricular flap is then elevated in the avascular plane between the scalp and temporalis muscle. Pieces of temporalis muscle are removed at and around the site of the receiver-stimulator. Postoperatively, the scalp heals down against the bone around the receiver-stimulator, minimizing the thickness of the scalp over the internal device. As a result, the power required to transfer the stimulus from the external transmitter transcutaneously to the internal receiver is decreased. The decreased distance between the external transmitter and the internal receiver also improves the magnetic attraction between the two devices for those systems using magnets. In young children with thin scalps, the postauricular incision is carried down to bone. The temporalis muscle is elevated off the parietal portion of the skull with the skin as a single-layer flap forward to the spine of Henle.

The site for the internal receiver in the skull is created at the position previously determined so that there is a separation of at least 1 cm between the incision and the edge of the receiver-stimulator. Suture tunnel holes created on either side of the seat with a guarded burr will be used to help hold the receiver-stimulator in place. The Symbion implant is the only hard-wired device (i.e., there is a direct connection between the external transmitter and the internal receiver). The percutaneous plug is held in place with bone screws.

The mastoidectomy is done using conventional burrs and suction irrigation techniques (Fig 10–2). Different from chronic ear surgery, the superior and posterior mastoid cortical margins should not be saucerized. The margins can be undercut to create a bony overhang that will stabilize the coiled electrode within the mastoid cavity. The bone removal extends back to the sigmoid, but retraction of the sigmoid is not required unless it is far forward. Enough of the bone in the attic is removed so that the top of the incus can be clearly seen. The incus should not be dislocated or removed because this does not increase surgical exposure. The short process of the incus and its buttress are important landmarks in development of the facial recess.

Posterior bony ear canal wall is thinned without exposing the overlying vascular strip tissue. Thinning of the bony ear canal is necessary, because in viewing the round window area, one will find that the direction of vision is parallel to the external auditory canal.

The facial recess is then opened. The facial nerve is carefully skeletonized at the mastoid genu to avoid exposure of the nerve sheath. Once the facial recess is opened, the lip of the round window niche is usually visible just inferior to the stapedius tendon and oval window. To get a good look at the round window, one must open the facial recess more inferiorly and posteriorly. Usually it is not necessary to remove the chorda tympani to adequately visualize the round window niche area. If the facial recess is very restricted, the chorda can be removed, but since the chorda enters the middle ear at the level of the annulus, one must be careful not to damage the tympanic membrane.

With a small diamond stone and intermittent suction-irrigation, the lip of the niche is removed, and the round window membrane comes into clear view. To avoid possible damage to the facial nerve, one must not rotate the diamond stone when passing it through the facial recess to the round window area. In cases where the round window niche is almost hidden under the pyramidal process, one must drill forward and thin the promontory until the scala tympani is entered.

In approximately 50% of the cases, the round window niche and membrane are replaced with new bone growth. This condition is more frequent in patients whose deafness is attributable to meningitis rather than to other diseases. In these cases, a surgeon must drill forward along the basal coil for as much as

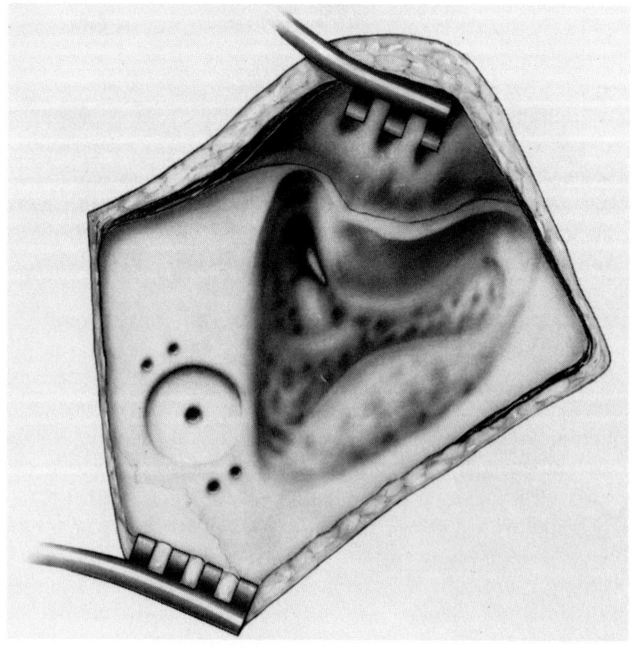

FIG 10–2.
Internal receiver seat superoposterior to the simple mastoidectomy.

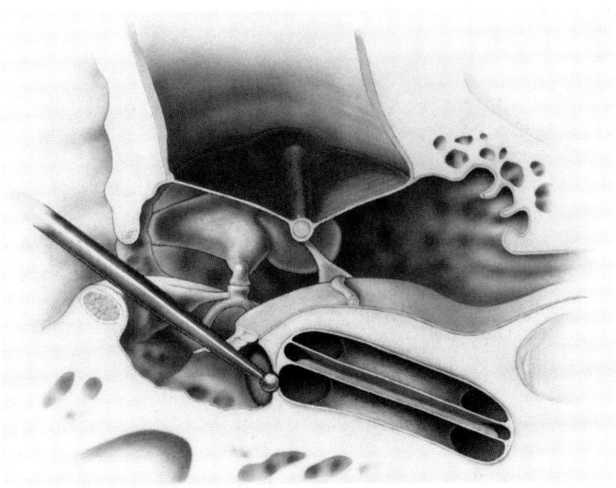

FIG 10–3.
Creating the opening into the scala tympani.

4 to 5 mm. Usually the new bone is white and can be demarcated from the surrounding otic capsule. Following this white plug of bone with the drill will usually lead to the patent scala, allowing placement of the electrode array. If new bone growth completely obliterates the scala, the surgeon drills forward 6 or 7 mm into the white new bone for replacement of the electrode. Complete ossification of the cochlea may alter the effectiveness of multichannel systems, whose electrodes are usually inserted 15 to 25 mm from the round window. In cases of complete ossification, an alternative short electrode device may be more beneficial.

When drilling the round window niche or attempting to create an opening into the scala tympani through new bone growth, one must direct the burr anteriorly toward the nose (Fig 10–3). Drilling superiorly may lead to damage to the basilar membrane and osseous spiral lamina, which may result in the loss of ganglion cells. If the surgeon directs the burr inferiorly, a hypotympanic air cell may accidentally be entered, and the active electrode will be placed improperly into this area. Postoperatively, these cases may fail to stimulate. Temporal bone imaging will show that the active electrode is extracochlear. Revision surgery with placement of the electrode array into the scala tympani will remedy this situation. If the surgeon is uncertain of the placement of the electrode, an intraoperative anteroposterior transorbital plane film can be taken to check the electrode position.

Extracochlear electrodes are usually stabilized at the round window. Intracochlear electrodes, both short and long, are advanced carefully into the scala tympani (Fig 10–4). Either smooth thumb forceps or small two-prong guides are used to direct the electrode tip into the scala tympani. Most important, force must not be used when the electrode is advanced. Force not only may lead to insertion trauma to the inner ear structures but also may distort the shape of the electrode. Both of the problems will affect adversely the outcome.

If electrocautery is used after placement of the internal receiver, bipolar electrocautery is recommended because it minimizes the possibility of passing current through the receiver. Postauricular flap is closed in layers occasionally over a drain.

Surgery routinely takes $1\frac{1}{2}$ to $2\frac{1}{2}$ hours. Patients are usually discharged home the day following surgery, returning for their first postoperative visit in about 1 week. Approximately 4 to 6 weeks pass, allowing for resolution of the edema in the postauricular flap, before one begins fitting the patient with the signal processor.

COMPLICATIONS

The risks of the implant procedure are the same as those for chronic ear surgery: infection, facial paralysis, CSF drainage, meningitis, and the usual risks of anesthesia. All of these risks are remote in chronic ear surgery and have proved to be so in implant surgery as well.

Failure of healing of the incision and associated minor infections would seem to be the most common problem associated with implant surgery. In a few patients where the internal receiver has been placed too close to the wound's edge or in patients where the flap over the internal receiver is too thin, the internal receiver extruded. As mentioned, it is important to maintain at least 1 to 2 cm between the incision and the edge of the internal receiver. The ideal thickness for the flap is 6 to 7 mm. Although too thin a flap may necrose, too thick a flap may diminish device performance by decreasing the transcutaneous transmission of information.

Problems with the facial nerve can occur as the result of both surgery and stimulation. It is important to maintain good surgical landmarks when the facial recess is created. Though the facial nerve is identified, it usually does not have to be uncovered with the facial recess approach. It is important to maintain adequate irrigation at the facial recess to help dissipate the heat generated by the turning shaft of the diamond burr that is being used to create the exposure of the round window

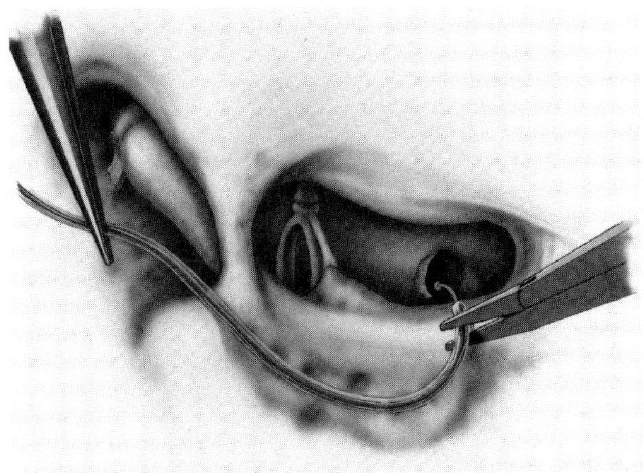

FIG 10–4.
Placing an intracochlear device.

and entrance into the scala tympani, especially in drill out cases. To help alleviate the problem of the drill shaft turning against the facial nerve, one could use a drill like the Treace Skeeter. The width of the drill bit shaft is smaller, and a sleeve around most of the length of the shaft protects the surrounding tissues as well.

Cerebral spinal fluid drainage has occurred at both the internal receiver site and the cochlea. In some patients, especially postmenopausal women and young children, the temporal squama can be quite thin. In these cases, to create an adequate seat for the internal receiver package, one must carry the bony dissection down to the dura. If small dural tears do occur, they should be covered with temporalis fascia, and the fascia should be supported with the internal receiver. After insertion of the intracochlear electrode to prevent perilymphatic fistulae, close the cochleastomy with strips of temporalis fascia. A gusher of CSF is more likely in patients with congenitally malformed inner ears. After insertion of the intracochlear electrode, carefully plug the cochleastomy with fascia.

In adults, the possible effects of the implant on the vestibular system and on tinnitus have been evaluated by clinical monitoring, patient questionnaires, and objective study.[21] There is no evidence that the implant has any significant negative impact in these areas.

One concern in extending the cochlear implant program to children was the risk of increased incidence or severity of otitis media, to which children are more prone than adults. It was conceivable that otitis media could cause the implanted internal coil and the electrode in the mastoid and middle ear to become an infected foreign body. Further, the infection might extend along the electrode into the inner ear, possibly resulting in meningitis and further degeneration of the auditory system. A recent study found that the short 6 mm intracochlear electrode of the 3M/House cochlear implant did not increase the incidence or severity of otitis media in children of otitis media-prone age. Children with implants who subsequently had a middle ear infection did not develop meningitis or any other evidence of inner ear infection.[22] Studies are under way to determine if longer intracochlear electrodes of the multichannel devices will increase the incidence of inner ear infections. At this time most of the otitis-prone children implanted with the Nucleus 22 channel electrode, inserted 15 to 25 mm, have had their implant for only about one year. Fortunately, there has been no reported cases of postoperative meningitis.

REVISION SURGERY

There are two primary reasons for revision surgery: (1) to replace a failed device and (2) to upgrade a system. Revision is possible because human and animal temporal bone studies have shown the following problems either do not occur or are not significant when the correct surgical technique for implanting electrodes of the different devices is used: degeneration of the remaining viable neural elements due to mechanical trauma to the organ of Corti during insertion or removal of the electrodes, osteogenesis, degeneration of the neural tissue by electrical

stimulation, and spread of infection from the middle ear into the inner ear.

For those patients undergoing revision surgery of a failed device, either a similar device or an upgrade can be reimplanted in the same ear. But which ear should be implanted in those patients with a functioning device? The rationale for revising the already implanted ear is that the contralateral ear would be saved for the so-called ideal implant. However, in other otologic elective surgery, the better hearing ear and certainly the only hearing ear is not operated. We do not, as yet, have a test that allows us to determine preoperatively that a new device, an upgrade, will actually provide more benefit for the patient than the older functioning implant. Since the animal and human studies have suggested that correctly placed implants do not have significant adverse effect on viable neural elements within the cochlea, I believe the possible risks to the contralateral ear are outweighed by the benefits of maintaining the patient's only source of hearing. My preference, in most cases with functioning devices, is to place the upgrade in the unimplanted contralateral ear. Several years later, if the patient was again interested in an upgrade, I would reimplant the worst hearing ear, using the side that provided the least benefit (presumably the side with the oldest implant). I would reimplant the ear with the functioning device if the contralateral unimplanted ear had changes on radiographic studies that would hinder the placement of the electrode.

Most patients who have undergone revision implant surgery have had a failed device. A few patients have had a functioning single-channel intracochlear system removed and replaced with a multiple-electrode intracochlear device. Most patients are using their new devices. One or two patients who were nonusers of the single-channel system are also nonusers of the multichannel implant. Two patients who underwent revision of failed devices with another implant system (failed 3M/House revised to a Nucleus 22 channel), both early in their rehabilitation period, believe they received more benefit from the original system. Hopefully, as they become accustomed to the output of the new device, they will both determine that they receive as much benefit, if not more, from it.

Not all upgrades will require surgery. Upgrades have and will be made in the external portion of the system (microphone, external transmitter, and signal processor).

COMMENT

Two studies have looked at what factors might provide prognostic indicators for identifying patients most likely to benefit from a cochlear implant. One study reviewed children using the 3M/House device,[23] and the other study examined adults using the Nucleus 22 channel.[24]

Eisenberg et al., in their review of children, believed that a later age at onset of deafness, a shorter duration of auditory deprivation, and an educational program with special emphasis of auditory-only training were important prognostic indicators.[23]

Dowell et al., in their review of adult patients, found no correlation between age and performance but a highly significant negative correlation between the length of profound deafness and performance.[24] For their patients the performance was worse if the hearing was lost more than 13 years before implantation. A review of three patients who each had profound hearing loss of more than 30 years noted that although the patients received similar information as others, they were not able to use it as effectively in the recognition of running speech. Dowell et al. believed that this was possibly due to loss of central auditory processing resulting from the long period of sound deprivation.[24]

Even though a shorter duration between onset of hearing loss and implantation is beneficial, it is very important that the interval be long enough to be certain of the degree of hearing loss, to determine the full benefits of hearing aids of tactile devices, and to be sure that the profound loss has been accepted by both the patients and family. The interval is at least 6 months for most adults and often as long as 1 year for children.

In adult patients, I occasionally use the 3M/House single-channel implant, but I prefer to use a multichannel transcutaneous device. The Nucleus 22 channel device is the only device presently available. I have not used a multichannel percutaneous device (Symbion implant). In children, only two devices, the 3M/House and the Nucleus, are approved presently for investigation by the FDA. Since the approval of the Nucleus investigation, I have used the Nucleus device more often in an attempt to learn if it will provide more benefit for the child than the 3M/House device. When other devices, such as the multichannel transcutaneous San Francisco implant, are approved for investigation in adults and children, I plan to use them more frequently.

Results of cochlear implant stimulation have been documented. Although an implant does not as yet restore normal hearing, it provides in adults an awareness of environmental sounds, improves speech reading, and, in many patients, allows them to partially understand speech without the aid of visual cues. Children also experience an improvement in auditory skills, and because of the improvement, many of them increase their speech and language skills, especially those who are in an educational program with special emphasis on auditory-only training.

The patient, adult or child, likely to receive the most benefit from a cochlear implant is one who acquires deafness after developing verbal language skills and is implanted within a few years of the onset of deafness.

REFERENCES

1. Gantz BJ: Cochlear implants: An overview, in Myers EN (ed): *Advances in Otoloryngology — Head and Neck Surgery*. Chicago, Year Book Medical Publishers, 1987, vol 1, pp 171–200.
2. Brackmann DE: Recommendations for the reporting of preoperative testing and postoperative results in cochlear implantation. *Otolaryngol Head Neck Surg* 1987; 97:519–521.
3. Thielemeir MA, Tonokawa LL, Petersen B, et al: Audiological results in children with a cochlear implant. *Ear Hear* 1985; 6(suppl 3):27S–35S.
4. Boothroyd A: Issues of pre- and postimplant evaluation regarding cochlear implants in children, in Mecklenburg D (ed): *Seminars in Hearing*. New York, Thieme Medical, 1986, vol 7, pp 349–359.
5. Eisenberg LS: Use of the cochlear implant by the prelingually deaf. *Ann Otol Rhinol Laryngol* 1982; 91(suppl 91):62–66.
6. Mangham CA, Luxford WM: Cochlear prosthesis surgery in children, in Mecklenburg D (ed): *Seminars in Hearing* New York, Thieme Medical, 1986, vol 7, pp 361–369.
7. O'Donoghue GM, Jackler RK, Jenkins WM, et al: Cochlear implantation in children: The problem of head growth. *Otolaryngol Head Neck Surg* 1986; 94:78–81.
8. Jackler RJ, Luxford WM, Schindler RA, et al: Cochlear patency problems in cochlear implantation. *Laryngoscope* 1987; 97:801–805.
9. Shelton C, Luxford WM, Tonokawa LL, et al: The narrow internal auditory canal in children: A contradiction to cochlear implants. *Otolaryngol Head Neck Surg* 1989; 100:227–231.
10. Miyamoto RT, McConkey AJ, Myres WA, et al: Cochlear implantation in the Mondini inner ear malformation. *Am J Otol* 1986; 7:258–261.
11. Jackler RJ, Luxford WM, House WF: Sound detection with the cochlear implant in five ears of four children with congenital malformations of the cochlea. *Laryngoscope* 1987; 97(suppl 40):15–17.
12. Mischke RE: Personal communcation, 1988.
13. Eisenberg LS, Luxford WM, House WF, et al: Electrical stimulation of the auditory system in children deafened by meningitis. *Otolaryngol Head Neck Surg* 1984; 92:700–705.
14. Tiber N: A psychological evaluation of cochlear implants in children. *Ear Hear* 1985; 6(suppl 3):485–515.
15. Crary WG, Wexler M, Berliner KI, et al: Psychometric studies and clinical interviews with cochlear implant patients. *Ann Otol Rhinol Laryngol* 1982:91 (Suppl 91):55–58.
16. Linthicum FH: Personal communication, 1988.
17. Schindler RA, Kessler DK: The UCSF/Storz cochlear implant: Patient performance. *Am J Otol* 1987; 8:247–255.
18. Franz BK, Dowell RC, Clark GM, et al: Recent developments with the Nucleus 22-electrode cochlear implant: A new two format speech coding strategy and its performance in background noise. *Am J Otol* 1987; 8:516–518.
19. Gantz BJ, McCabe BF, Tyler RS, et al: Evaluation of four cochlear implant designs. *Ann Otol Rhinol Laryngol* 1987; 96(suppl 128):145–147.
20. Luxford WM, House WF: Cochlear implants in children: Medical and surgical consideration. *Ear Hear* 1985; 6(suppl):20S–23S.
21. Eisenberg LS, Nelson JR, House WF: Effects of the single electrode cochlear implant on the vestibular system on the profoundly deaf adult. *Ann Otol Rhinol Laryngol* 1982; 91(suppl 91):47–54.
22. House WF, Luxford WM, Courtney B: Otitis media in children following the cochlear implant. *Ear Hear* 1985; 6:24S–26S.
23. Eisenberg LS, Kirk KI, Thielemeir MA, et al: Cochlear implants in children: Speech production and auditory discrimination. *Otolaryngol Clin North AM* 1986; 19:409–421.
24. Dowell RC, Mecklenburg DC, Clark GM: Speech recognition for 40 patients receiving multi-channel cochlear implants. *Arch Otolaryngol* 1986; 112:1054–1059.

CHAPTER 11

Glomus Tumors

Approach of

Derald E. Brackmann, M.D.

Since first described in 1945 by Rosenwasser,[1] therapy of glomus tumors of the temporal bone has been controversial. Some have advocated no treatment in that these tumors may be very slow growing and produce minimal symptoms, others have advocated surgical removal, and still others have recommended x-ray therapy as the primary treatment modality. It is difficult to evaluate the efficacy of the various forms of therapy since the clinical course and growth rate of these tumors are quite variable. Patients who have survived more than 40 years with these tumors without treatment have been reported.[1a, 2] That all such tumors are not clinically benign is shown by the studies of Brown,[3] Spector et al.,[4] and Rosenwasser,[5] who found mortality rates ranging from 5% to 13% with glomus jugulare tumors.

In general, I favor surgical treatment of glomus tumors of the temporal bone. In this chapter, I will outline the surgical therapy that I employ and then discuss this treatment compared with radiotherapy.

EVALUATION OF GLOMUS TUMOR

Great strides in the evaluation of patients with glomus tumors have been made in recent years. New techniques have allowed accurate assessment of the size and involvement of the temporal bone and skull base with glomus tumors. These new techniques allow preoperative planning and assessment of the risk of surgery. Following are the tests routinely used in the evaluation of patients with glomus tumors of the temporal bone:

1. Routine hearing tests. Routine air, bone, and speech hearing tests are performed to assess the degree of both conductive and sensorineural hearing impairments.

2. Polytomography. This technique was once our mainstay for the assessment of the degree of involvement of the temporal bone by glomus tumors. It has now been replaced by cranial computed tomography (CT) and is no longer used routinely in the assessment of glomus tumors.

3. Cranial computed tomography. Thin-section (1.5-mm thick) cranial CT using the bone algorithm has become the standard method of assessment of glomus tumors of the temporal bone. Tumors confined to the middle ear and mastoid are delineated from those tumors that involve the jugular bulb. Extensive lesions that extend onto or medial to the internal carotid artery (ICA) and those that extend transdurally are also defined by this technique. In many cases cranial CT is the only examination that is necessary for planning of treatment. As will be described shortly, involvement of the jugular bulb is the major consideration in preoperative planning. Rarely is it necessary to perform retrograde jugular venography since the advent of cranial CT.

4. Magnetic resonance imaging (MRI). I do not find MRI as useful as cranial CT in the assessment of glomus tumors. Because bone is not demonstrated on MRI, it is difficult to assess the involvement of the temporal bone by the tumor. Demonstration of the jugular bulb and vein on MRI indicates occlusion of these structures since they do not produce signals if there is normal blood flow. Thus, MRI may provide additional information, but I prefer CT for the routine evaluation of glomus tumors.

5. Arteriography. Four-vessel angiography is used when cranial CT has demonstrated a large glomus tumor. There are several justifications for this examination. The first is to assess the involvement of the ICA by tumor, which is necessary to assess the advisability of surgery. If surgery is undertaken, planning for management of involvement of the carotid artery must be made.

Cross compression studies are performed. The carotid artery on the involved side is occluded during injection of the contralateral ICA. Perfusion of the ipsilateral cerebral cortex is studied to assess cross blood flow. Good contralateral perfusion is an indication that ligation of the involved carotid artery may be well tolerated.

In some cases where tumor completely surrounds the ICA, planning for sacrifice of the artery must be made. We perform balloon occlusion of the ICA just below the origin of the ophthalmic artery. Electroencephalographic (EEG) monitoring is performed. The patient's neurologic status is carefully and frequently monitored. Xenon perfusion studies of the brain may be used when this technique is available. If the patient tolerates the balloon occlusion well, the balloon is detached and left in place in the ICA, which then allows sacrifice of the carotid artery at surgery. If the patient does not tolerate balloon occlusion of the artery, plans must be made for saphenous vein graft replacement of the ICA at the time of its resection.

With four-vessel angiography, one can also assess the blood supply to the tumor, particularly studying the vessels arising from the ICA or from the vertebral artery in tumors that extend intracranially. Finally, at the time of angiography, embolization is routinely employed. Embolization may be used as preoperative adjunctive therapy, as the primary treatment modality, or as a combination and will be discussed further later.

Based on the findings of these studies, accurate classification of the extent of the glomus tumor of the temporal bone is made.

CLASSIFICATION

Several schemes for classification of glomus tumors of the temporal bone have been proposed. At the Otologic Medical Group, we use a classification developed by my associate Antonio De la Cruz. It is a clinical surgical classification. The extent of the tumor is described by the involvement of structures of the temporal bone and skull base. A series of operations that correspond with the extent of the tumor is used.

Tympanic Tumor

The tympanic tumor is a tumor that has arisen from the glomus tympanicum body of the promontory along Jacobson's nerve. This tumor is confined entirely to the mesotympanum. All of its borders can be seen with routine otoscopy. In tumors of this type, no other studies are necessary. One knows that this small tumor could not arise from the jugular bulb, or it would extend beyond the inferior margins of the tympanic annulus. One consideration in this tumor or any other vascular tumor of the middle ear is to rule out an aberrant carotid artery or a dehiscent jugular bulb. The aberrant carotid artery lies more anteriorly and is paler than the glomus tumor. The jugular bulb lies more posteriorly and is darker blue. If there is any question about the existence of either of these lesions, cranial CT must be done to exclude them.

Tympanomastoid Tumor

The tympanomastoid tumor arises from the glomus body on the promontory but has enlarged so that it extends beyond the tympanic annulus either inferiorly or posteriorly. Once a tumor has reached this size, there is no way clinically to delineate its true extent. Any patient with a tumor that extends beyond the tympanic annulus must have thorough radiographic evaluation. Studies will show this tumor to not involve the jugular bulb. It may extend into the mastoid and into the retrofacial air cells, but the jugular bulb itself is not involved.

Jugular Bulb Tumor

The jugular bulb tumor arises from the glomus body on the dome of the jugular bulb. It then extends into the middle ear to a variable degree and also into the jugular bulb. By definition, this tumor is limited to involvement of the middle ear, mastoid, and the jugular bulb. It does not extend onto the carotid artery or medially into the skull base or intracranially.

Carotid Artery Involvement Tumor

The carotid artery involvement tumor has arisen from the jugular bulb but has extended beyond the confines of the jugular bulb and vein and is contacting the carotid artery. Smaller tumors of this type may contact the ICA only at the skull base. Larger tumors may extend far medially and involve not only the ascending but also the horizontal portion of the ICA and the petrous apex.

Transdural Tumors

Transdural tumors arise from the jugular bulb and extend not only onto the ICA as just described but also extend through the jugular foramen intracranially to a variable degree.

Glomus Vagale Tumors

Glomus vagale tumors are not actually tumors of the temporal bone but are tumors of the skull base. They arise from the glomus body along the vagus nerve at the base of the skull. When first detected, glomus vagale tumors are often larger than glomus tumors of the temporal bone because they produce symptoms of pulsatile tinnitus and hearing loss later. One may often distinguish a glomus vagale tumor by the production of a vocal cord paralysis prior to the onset of hearing loss or tinnitus or the appearance of a vascular mass in the ear. Almost always, glomus tumors of the temporal bone will produce otologic symptoms prior to the onset of vocal cord paralysis.[6]

The treatment of glomus vagale tumors is usually the same as for a large glomus jugulare tumor since they involve the temporal bone and the ICA in the same way. Occasionally, a glomus vagale tumor will arise lower in the neck, in which case an approach from below may be used rather than the lateral infratemporal fossa approach. These tumors are unusual in my experience.

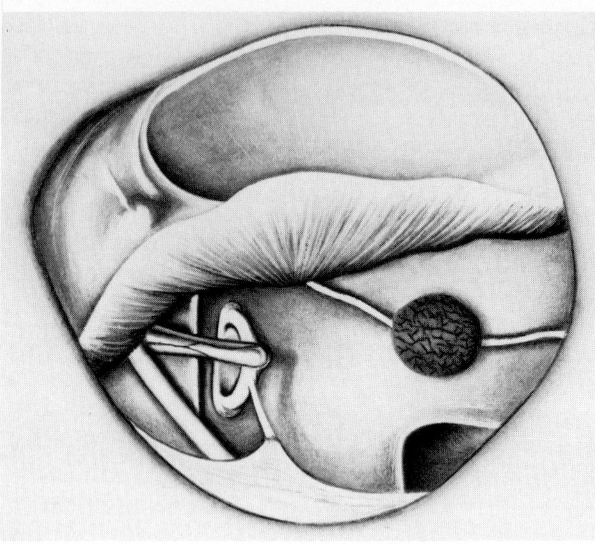

FIG 11–1.
Transcanal exposure of glomus tympanicum tumor.

SURGICAL APPROACHES

A series of operations are used at the Otologic Medical Group for removal of glomus tumors of the temporal bone.[7] The extent of the surgery is determined by the preoperative evaluation and classification of the tumor as described earlier.

Transcanal Approach

The transcanal approach is used for small glomus tympanicum tumors that are limited to the mesotympanum. The surgery is performed under local anesthesia with preparation as for a stapes operation. The tympanomeatal flap is elevated. The inferior incision should extend more anteriorly so that the inferior aspect of the tympanic membrane can be elevated. The tumor is identified on the promontory (Fig 11–1). As previously noted, one must always consider the possibility of an aberrant ICA in these cases. That possibility should have been excluded by preoperative evaluation if there is any doubt.

The blood supply to the glomus tympanicum tumor is the inferior tympanic branch of the ascending pharyngeal artery. This vessel may be bipolarly coagulated, or a small piece of oxidized cellulose (Surgicel) may be used to occlude the bony canaliculus from which it arises. The tumor is then removed with a cup forceps. There is often brisk bleeding from the distal end of the artery anterior to the stapes near the cochleariform process. It is difficult to control this artery directly, but if left alone, it will usually clot readily. It is important not to use monopolar cautery on the promontory because it may produce damage to the inner ear. Additional small pledgets of Surgicel may be placed over the promontory. When hemostasis is secure, the tempanomeatal flap is replaced and the ear canal packed. The patient is discharged from the hospital the following day. This operation should produce no morbidity.

Mastoid Approach

The mastoid approach is used for glomus tumors of the tympanomastoid variety. The tumor may extensively involve the middle ear and mastoid, but it has arisen from the glomus tympanicum body and does not involve the jugular bulb.

Hair is removed from approximately 6 cm about the ear, and the incision is made 1.5 cm posterior to the postauricular sulcus. A simple mastoidectomy is completed, and the facial recess is opened. The surgeon then extends the facial recess opening inferiorly by severing the chorda tympani nerve and following the fibrous annulus of the tympanic membrane as a landmark. This is referred to as the extended facial recess approach and allows complete exposure of the middle ear and the hypotympanum.

After the tumor is exposed, Surgicel packs are used to tamponade the main arterial supply in the hypotympanum, and the tumor is removed with cup forceps. The tumor can be stripped from the ossicles if necessary.

Glomus tympanicum tumors often spread into the retrofacial air cells. A cutting burr is used to remove the air cells inferior to the labyrinth beneath the facial nerve, thereby leaving the facial nerve suspended within a thin layer of bone to allow the surgeon access to the entire hypotympanum (Fig 11–2). A small curette is used to remove bits of tumor from crevices in the hypotympanum. The dome of the jugular bulb can be inspected to be certain that it is free of tumor.

If the ossicles are involved by the tumor, they may be removed and ossicular reconstruction accomplished from the posterior tympanotomy. Some tumors extend through the tympanic membrane. In that case, a tympanoplasty and ossicular reconstruction may be accomplished in the routine manner.

In some cases there is extensive destruction of the canal wall by large glomus tympanicum tumors. In these cases it may

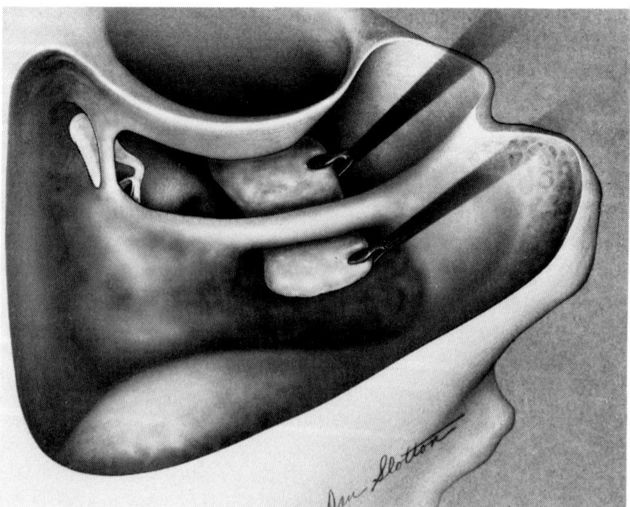

FIG 11–2.
Transmastoid exposure of large glomus tympanicum tumor.

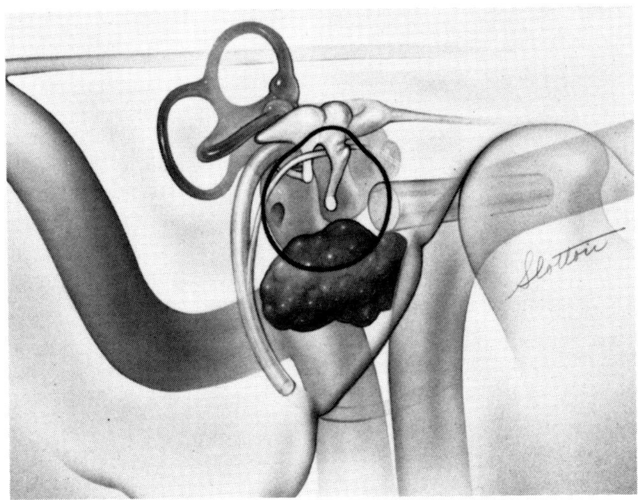

FIG 11–3.
Diagram of glomus jugular tumor contacting ICA. The overlying tympanic ring and facial nerve prevent adequate exposure of the tumor and carotid artery.

be better to use a canal wall down technique combined with tympanoplasty and mastoid obliteration following complete tumor removal.

Mastoid and Neck Approach

The mastoid and neck approach is used for small glomus jugulare tumors. By definition these tumors involve the jugular bulb but do not extent onto or medial to the ICA or into the neck or posterior fossa. The approach for removal of these tumors is to first complete the dissection described earlier. The next step is to amputate the mastoid tip, which is most easily done by identifying the periosteum of the digastric groove and following this forward until it turns abruptly superiorly at the stylomastoid foramen. Drilling laterally, both anteriorly and posteriorly, frees the entire mastoid tip.

The incision is then carried into the neck along the anterior border of the sternocleidomastoid muscle. The sternocleidomastoid muscle is freed from the mastoid tip and retracted posteriorly. The mastoid tip is then removed. The posterior belly of the digastric muscle is identified and freed from the digastric groove and retracted anteriorly to allow exposure of the neurovascular bundle in the neck. The internal jugular vein is identified and freed from surrounding tissues, and 2-0 silk sutures are placed around it. The jugular vein is followed over the transverse process of the first cervical vertebra into the base of the skull. The eleventh cranial nerve is identified (usually lying on top of the vein) and preserved.

This approach is used for limited tumors that do not extend into the neck or skull base and it is usually possible to preserve the ninth, tenth, and eleventh cranial nerves. The main reason for the neck exposure is to ligate the jugular vein.

Exposure of the sigmoid sinus and jugular bulb is then completed with diamond burrs. The limited tumors do not involve the medial wall of the jugular foramen. The proximal sigmoid sinus is controlled with extra luminal packing of Surgicel. The jugular vein is tied in the neck. The sigmoid sinus is

opened just distal to the proximal packing, and Surgicel is advanced into the jugular bulb to control bleeding from the inferior petrosal sinus. Care is taken not to pack this area too firmly, or a weakness of the ninth, tenth, and eleventh cranial nerves might result. Electromyographic (EMG) monitoring of activity in the sternocleido mastoid muscle is useful for detecting irritation of the eleventh cranial nerve during the dissection. A needle electrode is placed into the muscle preoperatively, and stimulation of the nerve will result in contractions. This monitoring is useful in identifying and preserving the function of the ninth, tenth, and eleventh cranial nerves. A similar electrode may be placed in the tongue to monitor the twelfth cranial nerve in larger tumors.

The dome of the jugular bulb is then excised along with the tumor. If the tympanic membrane or ossicles are involved, they may be reconstructed as described earlier. Closure is with subcuticular Dexon suture in layers. Usually there is no morbidity associated with this approach. If intact, the tympanic membrane and ossicular chain are preserved, as is the posterior canal wall. Unless there is preoperative involvement of the ninth, tenth, and eleventh cranial nerves, it is not necessary to sacrifice them in removal of this limited tumor.

Infratemporal Fossa Approach

The development of the infratemporal fossa approach by Fisch has been a significant advance in our ability to totally remove large tumors.[8] Previously used approaches that do not remove the external auditory canal (EAC) or reroute the facial nerve did not allow adequate exposure of the tumor or ICA (Fig 11–3). The infratemporal fossa approach is used for large glomus tumors that extend to the carotid artery, into the neck and skull base, or intracranially. This approach has allowed adequate exposure and control of vital structures so that tumors that previously were considered nonresectable can now be totally removed with safety and limited morbidity (Fig 11–4).

The dissection used in the mastoid and neck approach described earlier is first accomplished. After the facial recess is

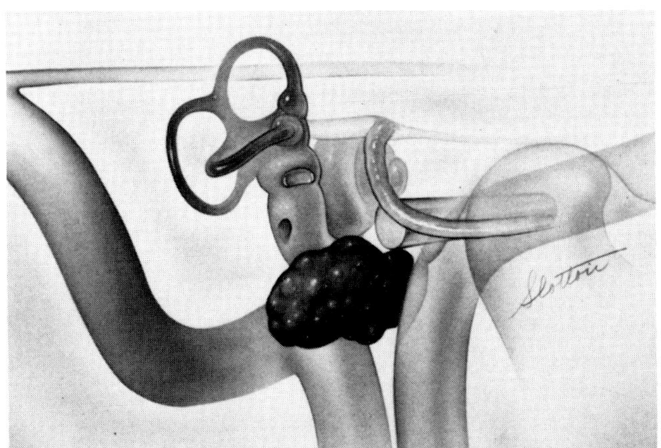

FIG 11–4.
Diagram of infratemporal fossa exposure. The tumor and carotid artery are exposed by removal of the tympanic ring and anterior rerouting of the facial nerve.

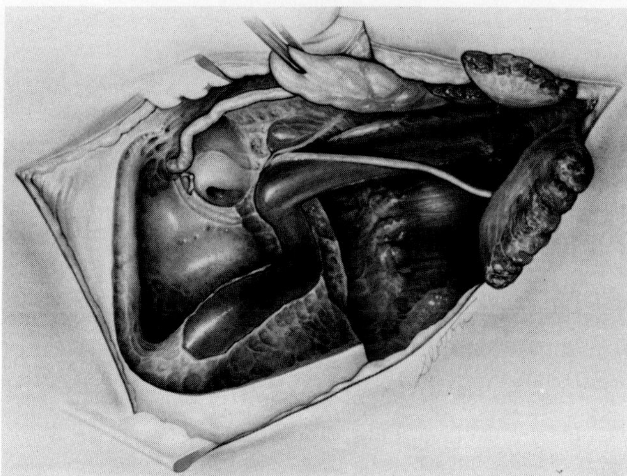

FIG 11–5.
Infratemporal fossa exposure. (See text for details.)

open, the incudostapedial joint is disarticulated. The EAC is then transected at the level of the bony cartilaginous junction. The skin of the meatus is everted and closed with 5-0 nylon sutures. The periosteum of the postauricular area is sutured behind the opening in the meatus to further reinforce the closure. The skin of the EAC is removed along with the tympanic membrane, malleus, and incus. The bony EAC is then removed. Following this, the facial nerve is freed of bone from the geniculate ganglion through the stylomastoid foramen. Fisch originally described exposure of the facial nerve through the stylomastoid foramen into the parotid with permanent anterior transposition of the facial nerve. In my experience, this always produced a temporary facial paresis and sometimes a minor permanent residual facial weakness. I have modified this approach as follows.

Rather than exposing the facial nerve into the parotid, I elevate the entire tail of the parotid along with the periosteum of the stylomastoid foramen along with the nerve.[9] I carefully free the facial nerve from the fallopian canal with sharp dissection. There are multiple fibrous connections, which I sharply incise in the descending portion of the nerve. In the tympanic portion of the nerve there are no adhesions, and this section elevates readily. I then elevate the entire tail of the parotid with the contained facial nerve lateral to the mandibular ramus (Fig 11–5). I place a large silk suture through the periosteum of the stylomastoid foramen and attach it to the soft tissue in the area of the root of the zygoma. This elevates the facial nerve and prevents its being stretched when retractors are placed.

For the past 18 months, I have been using continuous monitoring of facial nerve activity during this dissection. The EMG electrodes are placed into the facial musculature, and the activity of the muscle is continuously monitored. Even minor manipulation of the facial nerve produces activity in the facial muscles. This technique has significantly improved postoperative facial nerve function.[10]

After the facial nerve and parotid are elevated, I place a large Perkins retractor beneath the angle of the mandible and retract the entire mandible forward. I have not had to resect the mandibular condyle even in large tumors that extend into the infratemporal fossa extensively.

Transposition of the facial nerve allows exposure of the skull base in the area of the jugular foramen and carotid artery. The common carotid artery is identified, and the ECA ligated. The ICA is then followed through the skull base into its intratemporal course. The ninth, tenth, and eleventh cranial nerves are identified in the neck and followed into the jugular foramen. The twelfth cranial nerve is also identified and followed to its foramen.

The sigmoid sinus is doubly ligated with silk sutures. The jugular vein is elevated and the tumor freed inferiorly. The tumor is then freed from the carotid artery anteriorly. Bleeding caroticotympanic vessels are controlled with bipolar cautery. If the tumor is adherent to the ICA, it is best to leave a portion of it on the artery at this point and remove the bulk of the tumor. The removal of the last bit of the tumor from the artery is then saved for the conclusion of the procedure. The tumor is freed superiorly and posteriorly and then medially, and a total removal of the tumor is thus accomplished.

If there is intracranial extension of the tumor, a decision must be made at this point whether to attempt a total removal of the tumor. I base this decision on the amount of blood loss to this point. If blood loss has been limited to less than 3,000 mL, as is almost always the case, we proceed with removal of the intracranial extension of the tumor. If there has been greater than this amount of blood loss, one may encounter problems with bleeding despite the replenishment of the known clotting factors with fresh frozen plasma and platelet packs. In such a case, I prefer a two-stage procedure with removal of the intracranial portion of the tumor approximately 6 months after the primary surgery.

The removal of the intracranial portion of the tumor is often easier than the removal of that within the temporal bone. By the time one is ready for removal of the intracranial extension, the blood supply has often been controlled. The blood supply to the intracranial portion of the tumor is often discrete and can be controlled with bipolar cautery as with other cerebellopontine angle tumors.

If tumor has been left along the ICA, it is now removed. Closure is accomplished by obliterating the mastoid defect with strips of abdominal fat. If the cerebrospinal fluid (CSF) space has been entered, continuous lumbar drainage is used for approximately 5 days until the wound is sealed.

RISKS AND COMPLICATIONS OF SURGERY

There are considerable risks and complications to this extensive surgery. Large tumors, particularly those that extend transdurally, often intimately involve the ninth, tenth, eleventh, and twelfth cranial nerves. Total removal of the tumor requires sacrifice of these nerves. The approach itself produces a permanent conductive hearing impairment because of removal of the tympanic membrane and ossicles and blind sac closure of the EAC. With management of the facial nerve with the method described, without continuous EMG monitoring, approximately

50% of patients had no facial weakness at any time during their course. In the other half, a paresis resulted. I have had only 2 patients out of 50 who had an infratemporal fossa approach that have had a significant permanent facial weakness. Both of these patients had preoperative x-ray therapy as a curative measure but then had recurrence of tumor. This problem will be discussed further. The other patients have had excellent recovery of facial function or no weakness at all.[9]

Since continuous EMG monitoring has been used over the past 18 months on 20 patients undergoing an infratemporal fossa approach, none has developed a total paresis, and all have had perfect recovery of facial nerve function. The usefulness of this technique is obvious.[10]

The ICA is at risk in extensive tumor that involves its wall. Nearly always it is possible to remove the tumor from the artery and preserve it. The problem that I most commonly encounter is producing a defect in the ICA at the origin of the carotico-tympanic branch that is often very hypertrophied. I have been able to repair these small defects in the ICA, and none of the patients has had a stroke.

When extensive involvement of the carotid artery is demonstrated on preoperative studies, balloon occlusion tests as described are performed preoperatively. If balloon occlusion is not tolerated, a saphenous vein graft is inserted at the time of tumor resection if removal of the carotid artery is necessary for complete tumor removal.

Cerebrospinal fluid leak and infection are occasional problems. Continuous lumbar drainage has avoided the problem of persistent CSF leak, and appropriate antibiotics have quickly cleared the few cases of infection that have occurred.

I do not routinely perform a tracheotomy or gastrostomy on patients in whom we have had to sacrifice the ninth, tenth, or eleventh cranial nerves. Most patients can manage their secretions adequately. Teflon injection of the vocal cord is done in patients with permanent loss of vagus nerve function. Nasogastric feeding tubes are used early in the postoperative course. If patients are not able to maintain adequate nutrition by mouth, a percutaneous gastrostomy is performed as a temporary measure. Cricopharyngeal myotomy is a useful technique for patients who have persistent swallowing difficulty. All patients have eventually been able to maintain adequate nutrition by the oral route, and none has had a problem with persistent aspiration. There have been no deaths in my series.

MANAGEMENT OF SECRETING TUMORS

Patients with either sustained or intermittent hypertension or those with signs of a hypermetabolic state should raise suspicion of a secreting tumor. I do not evaluate all patients for a secreting tumor since it is uncommon in my experience. If a patient has hypertension, heat intolerance, palpitations, or a history of diaphoresis, I then order appropriate studies.

Twenty-four-hour urine specimens are collected for examination for vanillylmandelic acid (VMA) and metanephrines. Some drugs may cause false positives, and one should check with the laboratory to investigate that possibility. If results are abnormal, they should be repeated and the history reviewed for factors that may cause false positive reactions. If results again are abnormal, CT scan of the abdomen should be performed, as well as four-vessel angiography searching for multiple tumors.

A new sensitive and specific study for identification of secreting tumors will soon be available. This test involves the intravenous injection of meta-iodobenzylguanidine labeled with iodine 131. This substance tags adrenergic vesicles and allows identification on scintigraphic imaging.

When a secreting tumor is identified, treatment is begun 3 days preoperatively using 250 mg of α-methyl-*p*-tyrosine four times daily. This drug inhibits the hydroxylation of tyrosine to dopa, which is the initial and rate-limiting step in catecholamine synthesis. When it is used for sufficient duration preoperatively, catecholamine stores are depleted, making anesthetic management safer. Intraoperatively, adrenergic blockers such as phentolamine and dibenzyline are used to stabilize blood pressure. If adequate preoperative blocking has not been accomplished, enlargement of the vascular bed may occur when the tumor is removed, with resultant hypotension. In this case, administration of colloid might be necessary to maintain blood pressure.

Urinary catecholamines should be checked postoperatively to ensure that all secreting tumor tissue has been removed. If urinary levels of catecholamines do not fall to normal, further investigation should be carried out to identify other secreting tumors.[11]

EMBOLIZATION

Embolization is a relatively new modality for treatment of glomus tumors. Large glomus tumors are routinely embolized with polyvinyl alcohol sponge 24 hours preoperatively. We have found this to reduce blood loss and greatly facilitate total tumor removal.

In very large tumors where total removal cannot be accomplished, embolization provides palliation by reducing tumor blood flow.

X-RAY THERAPY

Besides surgery, the most commonly used modality for therapy of glomus tumors is irradiation. Fifteen years ago we performed a study of the effect of x-ray therapy on glomus tumors.[12] Seven patients who had received irradiation for glomus jugulare tumors subsequently were operated on by members of the Otologic Medical Group. We compared the preirradiation biopsy specimen with the biopsy taken following various doses of x-ray therapy. The effect of irradiation that was apparent in these cases was on the blood vessels and fibrous elements of the tumor rather than on the tumor cells themselves. We found that the effect of 2,000 to 3,000 rad was very similar to the effect of 4,000 to 6,000 rad in these cases. Following this study, we developed a protocol that uses relatively small doses of external irradiation in the 2,000 to 3,000 rad range for patients who have nonresectable tumors or for the elderly or those in poor health. The palliation afforded by this small dose of irradiation appears to be equal to that obtained with the larger dose with much less morbidity. With this smaller dose of irradiation, it is possible to administer a second course if the tumor revascularizes and shows renewed growth.

DISCUSSION

From the previous description of techniques available for treatment of glomus tumors, one can see that smaller tumors can be removed with a minimum of morbidity, and there is little argument that that is the preferred method of management of glomus tympanicum tumors and smaller jugulare tumors. Where the debate arises is in the treatment of larger tumors where surgery may produce morbidity in regard to hearing, facial nerve function, function of the ninth, tenth, eleventh, and twelfth cranial nerves, and risks to the carotid artery. It is interesting to review the radiotherapy literature that discusses the radiosensitivity of glomus jugulare tumors and at the same time describes radioresistance of the histologically identical carotid body tumor.[12] This misconception arose years ago when the surgical techniques in the temporal bone were not well developed, and attempts at removal of glomus tumors of the temporal bone were often disastrous. From our study of the effect of x-ray therapy on glomus tumors as well as those of others, it is apparent that the glomus tumor cell itself is not radiosensitive. What responds to external x-ray treatment is the blood supply to the tumor. A radiation vasculitis is produced, and it does result in shrinkage of the tumor and slowed growth. It does not, however, cure a glomus tumor.

I agree that in elderly patients or in those in poor health, x-ray therapy is a reasonable method of controlling a tumor. On the other hand, I believe that total excision is the preferred treatment in younger patients. Newer microsurgical techniques, particularly the infratemporal fossa approach, have now allowed total exposure of even large tumors and total removal with safety. Rehabilitative measures that provide good quality of life can be instituted when total tumor removal requires sacrifice of the involved cranial nerves.

One might argue that x-ray therapy might first be used to ascertain the biologic behavior of the tumor and its response to x-ray with reservation of surgery for those cases that do not respond well or exhibit aggressive growth. I have considered that argument and believe it reasonable in some cases, as in older patients where the expected 8 to 10 years of palliation corresponds with their normal life expectancy. On the other hand, in younger patients I do not think it is best, because if surgery is later necessary, it does increase the morbidity of the extensive surgical procedure. The only patients in whom I have encountered problems with wound healing or persistent facial paresis have been in patients who have received preoperative x-ray therapy. I thus agree with Brown[3] and Spector et al.,[4] who prefer surgery as the primary modality for glomus tumor treatment. X-ray therapy is reserved for those patients who have incomplete removal and show signs of recurrent tumor growth or for the elderly or those in poor health.

CONCLUSION

After a review of the literature as well as my personal experience in the management of glomus tumors, I agree with Rosenwasser, who stated, "Long-term follow-up of my cases of glomus jugulare tumors [30 years] and wide experience with cases referred to me have convinced me that surgery, when feasible, is the method of choice in treatment of this lesion."[5]

REFERENCES

1. Rosenwasser H: Carotid body–like tumor of the middle ear and mastoid bone. *Arch Otolaryngol* 1945; 41:64–67.
1a. Bickerstaff ER, Howell JS: The neurological importance of tumors of the glomus jugulare. *Brain* 1953; 76:576–593.
2. Steinberg, N, Holz WG: Glomus jugularis tumors. *Arch Otolaryngol* 1965; 82:387–394.
3. Brown JS: Glomus jugulare tumors revisited: A ten-year statistical follow-up of 231 cases. *Laryngoscope* 1985; 95:284–288.
4. Spector GJ, Fierstein J, Ogura JH: A comparison of therapeutic modalities of glomus tumors in the temporal bone. *Laryngoscope* 1976; 86:690–696.
5. Rosenwasser H: Long-term results of therapy of glomus jugulare tumors. *Arch Otolaryngol* 1973; 97:49–54.
6. Leonetti JP, Brackmann DE: Glomus vagale tumors: The significance of early vocal cord paralysis. *Otolaryngol Head Neck Surg* 1989; 100:533–537.
7. Sheehy JL, Brackmann DE: Technique of mastoidectomy, in English GM (ed): *Otolaryngology.* Philadelphia, Harper & Row, Publishers, 1984, Chapter 21.
8. Fisch U: Infratemporal fossa approach for glomus tumors of the temporal bone. *Ann Otol Rhinol Laryngol* 1982; 91:474–479.
9. Brackmann DE: The facial nerve in the infratemporal approach. *Otolaryngol Head Neck Surg* 1987; 97:15–17.
10. Leonetti JP, Brackmann DE, Prass RC: Improved preservation of facial nerve function in the infratemporal approach to the skull base. *Otolaryngol Head Neck Surg* 1989; 101:74–78.
11. Cantrell RW, Kaplan MJ, Winn HR, et al: Catecholamine-secreting infratemporal fossa paraganglioma. *Ann Otol Rhinol Laryngol* 1984; 93:583–588.
12. Brackmann DE, House WF, Terry R, et al: Glomus jugulare tumors: Effect of irradiation. *Trans Am Acad Ophthalmol Otolaryngol* 1972; 76:1423–1431.

Glomus Tumors

Approach of

C. Gary Jackson, M.D.

Glenn D. Johnson, M.D.
and
Dennis S. Poe, M.D.

Glomus tumors, or paragangliomas, are benign, well-vascularized tumors of the extra-adrenal paraganglia. Paraganglia resemble carotid bodies and are composed of two cell types: a granule-storing chief cell and a Schwannlike satellite cell.[1] The jugulotympanic and intravagal paraganglia give rise to the three types of glomus tumors that involve the skull base: the glomus jugulare, glomus tympanicum, and glomus vagale tumors. Although they are relatively rare tumors, the glomus tumor is the most common neoplasm of the middle ear and is the second most common after the neurilemmoma in the temporal bone.[2]

Although benign, these lesions may cause significant morbidity due to cranial nerve involvement and intracranial extension. Definitive treatment is by surgical resection. The development of modern techniques of infratemporal surgery had allowed definitive resection of these skull base tumors with control of the carotid artery and jugular system under direct visualization. Palliative treatment with radiation therapy is reserved for those patients for whom the risk of surgery exceeds the expected morbidity of the unresected tumor.

ASSOCIATED LESIONS

Lesions occurring in association with craniocervical paragangliomas have been estimated to occur with an incidence of 5% to 25%. Paragangliomas of the head and neck have a proclivity toward multicentricity. Synchronous tumors have been reported to occur approximately 10% of the time.[3,4] Bilaterality of glomus jugulare tumors have been reported in 1% to 2% of cases.[5] Glomus jugulare tumors are more likely to have associated lesions than tympanicum or vagale tumors.[2] Glomus tumors have also been found to be associated with other neoplasms such as thyroid carcinoma, pheochromocytoma, other neurogenic disorders, and the multiple endocrine neoplasia.[3]

If an ipsilateral carotid body tumor or glomus vagale tumor is detected in a patient with a glomus jugulare tumor, we usually excise the neck lesion first, followed by the skull base procedure for the jugulare tumor approximately 7 to 10 days later. If a contralateral glomus-vagale tumor is present, the most clinically dangerous lesion is resected first. The other lesion is removed later, with special care taken to preserve function of the vagus. A tracheotomy is essential when the possibility of a bilateral vagus nerve palsy exists.

Early methods to detect catecholamines, such as chromaffin staining, suggested that glomus tumors were nonhormonally active.[1] Newer methods, such as formaldehyde-induced fluorescent microscopy, have shown that all glomus tumors contain catecholamines. All reported glomus tumors have secreted norepinephrine except one, which secreted dopamine.[6]

Although only 1% to 3% of glomus tumors secrete catecholamines in large enough quantity to cause clinical symptoms, an unrecognized secreting tumor could cause disastrous intraoperative or anesthetic complications.

Preoperative assessment for the presence of a hormonally active tumor, either the primary glomus tumor or an associated pheochromocytoma, is therefore essential to avoid intraoperative complications related to excessive catecholamine secretion. An obvious pheochromocytoma syndrome may be caused by an independently secreting glomus tumor with peripheral catecholamine levels elevated as high as a thousand-fold.[4] If the patient is found to have an independently secreting glomus tumor, our protocol has been to use preoperative pharmacologic alpha and beta blockade. We have used propranolol and phenoxybenzamine for approximately 1 week, followed by closely monitored surgery. Another option is the use of hypotensive anesthesia.

In this sense, independent secretion of vasoactive substances by glomus tumors has been widely recognized. We have

TABLE 11–1.
Glasscock-Jackson Classification of Glomus Tumors

Type	Physical Findings
Glomus tympanicum	
Type I	Small mass limited to the promontory
Type II	Tumor completely filling middle ear space
Type III	Tumor filling middle ear and extending into mastoid
Type IV	Tumor filling middle ear, extending into mastoid or through tympanic membrane to fill external auditory canal (EAC); may also extend anterior to ICA
Glomus jugulare	
Type I	Small tumor involving jugulare bulb, middle ear, and mastoid
Type II	Tumor extending under IAC; may have intracranial extension
Type III	Tumor extending into petrous apex, may have intracranial extension
Type IV	Tumor extending beyond petrous apex into clivus or infratemporal fossa; may have intracranial extension

recently generated the hypothesis that these tumors are capable of secreting neuropeptides such as cholecystokinin (CCK) in addition to catecholamines. The identification of gastrointestinal complications, notably postoperative ileus, far in excess of what is usually expected for this type of skull base surgery prompted study of these patients for such secretion. The chief cell, as a member of the DNES, is certainly capable. We found that glomus tumor surgery was associated with prolonged postoperative ileus, regardless of status of the vagus nerve. Hypothetically, data were generated to implicate the secretion of CCK by the tumor and subsequent depletion with resection as etiologic. This role of CCK in the production or prevention of ileus is uncertain at this time. Clearly, the histochemistry of glomus tumors appears complex.

The presence of associated lesions is more than just of academic interest. An ipsilateral carotid body tumor may complicate the skull base resection of a glomus jugulare tumor by interfering with identification of cranial nerves IX and X in the neck as well as compromising control of the carotid artery and jugular vein. A contralateral glomus jugulare or vagale tumor could increase the patient's chances for developing bilateral 10th nerve palsies.[7] Traditionally, bilateral carotid arteriography is the most accurate approach for the diagnostic search for these associated lesions in the neck. Modern imaging techniques are supplanting angiography for this purpose.

CLASSIFICATION

Tumor classifications have been developed to assist in surgical planning and to provide standards for reporting. Olding and Fisch proposed a system in 1979 dividing glomus tumors into four categories: A, B, C, and D.[8] A tumors were limited to the middle ear cleft. B tumors extended to the tympanomastoid

area without destruction of bone in the infralabyrinthine compartment of the temporal bone. C tumors extended into and destroyed bone of the infralabyrinthine and apical compartment of the temporal bone. D tumors had intracranial extension. In 1982, subdivisions were proposed, adding three subclassifications to categories C and D.[9] The Glasscock-Jackson classification, described in 1982, maintains the tympanicum-jugulare differentiation (Table 11–1).[10] This system was developed to be directly applicable to surgical planning (Table 11–2) as well as to provide a standard form for analysis and reporting of treatment results. To date, no uniform nomenclature exists for this purpose.

DIAGNOSIS

The extent of the glomus tumor, both in the temporal bone and extratemporally, is usually not evident by clinical examination alone. The surgical approach used is vastly different for a glomus tympanicum tumor than for a glomus jugulare tumor, even if the jugulare tumor is fairly small. Patients who present with otoscopic findings suggestive of a glomus tumor require thorough evaluation for extent of the lesion prior to surgical resection.

We cannot overemphasize the need for a thorough, systematic evaluation of every suspected glomus tumor. Conceptually, there are several purposes to this evaluation. A vascular appearing mass in the middle ear must first be differentiated from a vascular anomaly such as an abberant carotid artery of high, dehiscent jugular bulb. If the mass is radiologically consistent with a glomus tumor, it should be classified as to type (tympanicum, jugulare, or vagale) and extent (see Table 11–1) for purposes of therapeutic planning. If the tumor extends into the jugular bulb, it is considered a glomus jugulare tumor. If a clear bony separation can be demonstrated between the tumor and the jugular bulb, the tumor is considered a glomus tympanicum. As discussed previously, associated lesions may affect surgical planning and so should be thoroughly evaluated prior to any definitive surgical procedures.

Whenever one is contemplating resection of a glomus jugulare or vagale tumor, the relationship of the tumor to the ICA and jugular vein must be determined. Adequacy of the collateral arterial system should be investigated if any chance for ligation of the ipsilateral ICA exists.

Once these steps have been taken, the appropriate approach for surgical resection can be planned. The patient's med-

TABLE 11–2.
Glomus Tumors: System of Surgical Procedures*

Glomus tympanicum
    Transcanal (type I)
    Extended facial recess (types II, III, and IV)
Glomus jugulare
    Traditional skull base dissection (types I and II)
    Modified infratemporal fossa approach (types III and IV)

*Modified from Jackson CG, Glasscock ME, Harris PF: Glomus tumors: Diagnosis, classification, and management of large lesions. *Arch Otolaryngol* 1982; 108:401–406.

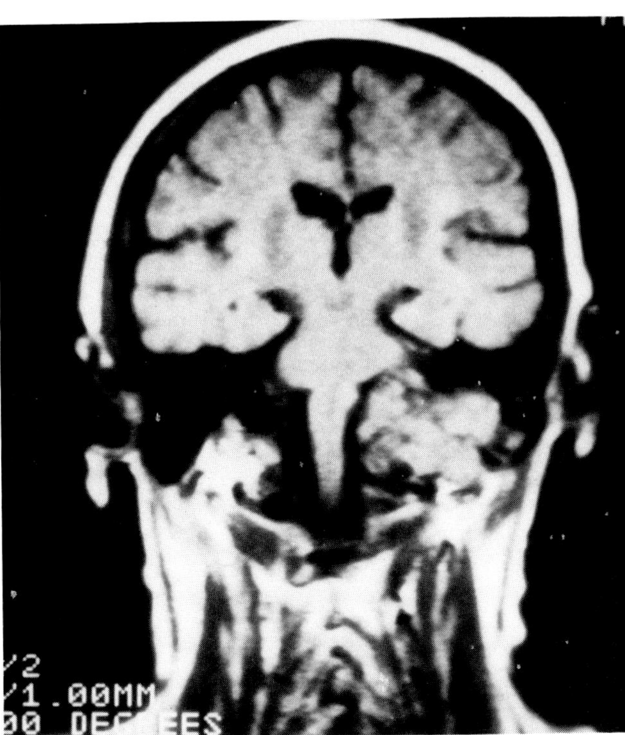

FIG 11–6.
MRI demonstrates a large skull base glomus tumor with intracranial extension.

ical condition must be thoroughly evaluated if a skull base procedure is planned to determine if the patient can reasonably be expected to tolerate the procedure and adequately compensate from expected cranial nerve deficits. In general, patients older than age 60 to 65 years tolerate this surgery and its attendant problems poorly. Unless circumstances demand it, tumors in this group are better palliated. Because of slow growth rates, it is unlikely that the patient will suffer from this tumor in the natural course of his or her remaining life. This slow grow rate argument is not applicable to younger patients with similar lesions.

We mention the use of a myringotomy or tympanotomy for biopsy only to condemn it. The diagnosis of glomus tumors is made by the presence of characteristic findings on imaging studies. A biopsy is almost always unnecessary, subjects the patient to the risk of potentially massive bleeding, and unnecessarily extends the limits of definitive resection. When tissue is essential, a formal postauricular, wide-field approach exposing all anatomy is recommended.

Our diagnostic evaluation consists of a combination of high-resolution, thin-section, CT of the temporal bone, skull base, and intracranial cavity; MRI of the head; and carotid arteriography with cross-compression studies. These three studies are complimentary to each other and demonstrate different aspects of the glomus tumor. Computed tomography scanning is best for showing bony erosion of the skull base and temporal bone as well as defining soft tissue within the temporal bone in relationship to the temporal bone anatomy. Magnetic resonance imaging shows the intracranial and infratemporal fossa exten-

sion with better definition than CT imaging (Fig 11–6). It also can define whether the jugular vein is patent or occluded. Soft tissue detail is also superior. This is particularly useful for judging tumor involvement of the ICA. Carotid arteriography is necessary to define the status of the intracranial circulation. It is important for preoperative planning to know if the tumor is fed entirely by the external carotid system or if it receives some feeding branches from the ICA. This is especially important in recurrent tumors. One should also look at the adequacy of the contralateral lateral sinus and jugular vein, especially if the ipsilateral jugular vein is not completely occluded by the tumor. Surgical resection of a glomus tumor will leave the contralateral jugular system as the dominant venous drainage of the intracranial cavity, and if it is very small or absent, significant brain edema could result postoperatively.

Arteriography, although not 100% accurate, is helpful in evaluating tumor involvement of the intratemporal or extratemporal carotid artery. If ICA involvement is suspected, resection of the ICA with possible grafting must be considered. The complications that must be considered when this is performed are major neurologic deficits resulting from insufficient perfusion of the ipsilateral hemisphere. We are presently routinely using cross-compression studies as a screening evaluation of the contralateral circulation but with the realization that adequacy of circulation so demonstrated does not guarantee that the patient will not develop retrograde thrombosis and significant neurologic sequella from interruption of the ICA. Other methods available for evaluation of the adequacy of contralateral circulation include balloon occlusion with EEG monitoring and xenon perfusion studies. The soft tissue detail affordable by MRI is also useful to assess tumor extent relative to ICA but is of no use in predicting an uncomplicated interruption of flow (Fig 11–7).

Preoperative screening for a secreting tumor or an associated pheochromocytoma should consist of serum epinephrine and norepinephrine levels and a urinary catecholamine screen. A 24-hour urine collection is analyzed for epinephrine, norepinephrine, metanephrine, normetanephrine, and vanillylmandelic acid (VMA). If any of these levels are elevated, a thorough search for a pheochromocytoma is indicated. Selective venous samples are taken from the venous drainage of the tumor as well as the adrenal area and analyzed for catecholamines. Thyroid screening is done only when clinical circumstances warrant it. Search for other neuropeptides at this time is "experimental" or "investigational."

OPERATIVE APPROACHES

The surgical approach used to resect a glomus tumor is determined by several factors: the type of tumor (tympanicum, jugulare, vagale), extent of disease, the need for identification of cranial nerves IX through XII, and the necessity for proximal and distal control of the carotid artery. The following series of surgical approaches are designed to match the type and extent of disease as determined by diagnostic investigation (see Table 11–2).

Glomus Tympanicum

A small glomus tympanicum tumor confined to the promontory with margins completely visualized through the tympanic membrane (type I) can be surgically removed through a tympanotomy approach. Once the tumor extends beyond view, past the annulus of the tympanic membrane, it becomes a type II lesion and requires a posterior approach using a mastoidectomy with extended facial recess for resection.

Tympanotomy Approach (Type I)

A tympanomeatal flap is elevated as in stapes surgery. The superior limb of the tympanomeatal incision is then extended anteriorly and the tympanic membrane dissected off the malleus to give exposure of the anterior mesotympanum. The facial nerve and ossicular chain are examined, and if involved by tumor, they are freed from the tumor mass. Once the entire margins of the tumor are visualized, the tumor is grasped by a cup forceps and removed. Bleeding is usually controlled by packing the middle ear with an absorbable gelatin sponge (Gelfoam) soaked with epinephrine 1:1,000 or with bone wax. When bleeding is controlled, the tympanomeatal flap is returned and the external canal filled with ointment (Fig 11–8).

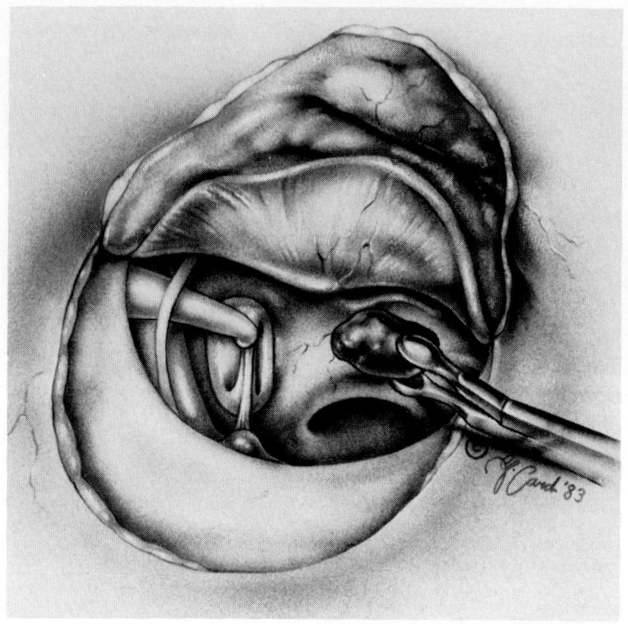

FIG 11–8.
Tympanotomy exposure is adequate for the removal of tympanicum tumors whose margins are visible 360 degrees.

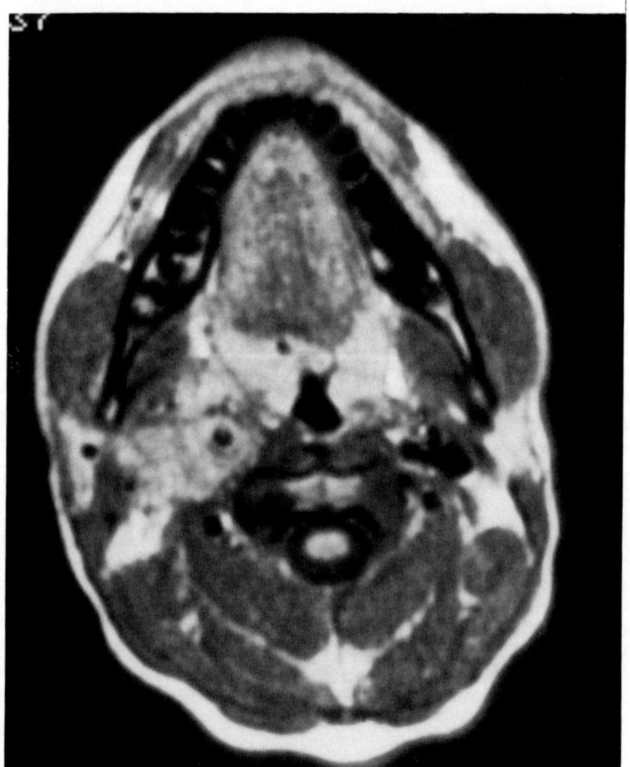

FIG 11–7.
MRI illustrates aggressive involvement of ICA circumferentially by a right-sided glomus tumor.

Extended Facial Recess Approach (Types II Through IV)

This approach, used for types II through IV tympanicum lesions, gives good visualization of the middle ear, facial nerve, ossicular chain, hypotympanum, and eustachian tube. A standard postauricular incision is made, followed by a complete mastoidectomy using a microsurgical drill and continuous suction-irrigation. The facial nerve is identified from the fossa incudus to the stylomastoid foramen. With a small diamond burr, the chorda tympani is identified and the facial recess opened. The chorda tympani is sharply transected close to the facial nerve. The facial recess is then extended by removing bone between the facial nerve posterior medially, the stylomastoid foramen inferiorly, the middle ear anteriorly, and the tympanic annulus laterally. Bleeding is controlled with Gelfoam soaked in epinephrine 1:1,000 and bipolar cautery. The tumor, as well as all vital anatomy, needs to be completely exposed before removal is attempted (Fig 11–9). Even though one has radiologic evidence of a bony partition between the glomus tympanicum tumor and the jugular bulb, one should identify the bony floor of the hypotympanicum when the tumor is removed to confirm the absence of extension into the bulb. The carotid artery may be dehiscent into the middle ear, so the anterior aspect of the medial wall of the middle ear should be carefully inspected to determine the presence or absence of a bony covering to the carotid artery before tumor is removed in this area. The tumor is then removed with cup forceps (Fig 11–10). The hypotympanic air cells should be curetted or drilled out to remove all tumor extension into this area. Bleeding can usually be controlled by packing the middle ear with Gelfoam soaked with epinephrine 1:1,000 or using bone wax packed into the inferior tympanic canaliculus where the inferior tympanic artery enters the middle ear cavity. The postauricular wound is closed routinely and a mastoid compression dressing applied.

Glomus Jugulare and Skull Base Vagale Tumors

A glomus jugulare tumor involves the jugular bulb and as such cannot be completely excised without removing the bulb or the position of the jugular bulb involved by tumor. The presence of cranial nerves IX, X, and XI in the pars nervosa of the jugular bulb makes identification of these nerves essential to their preservation. The proximity of the jugular bulb to the carotid artery dictates an approach that allows dissection of tumor off the carotid under good visualization with proximal and distal access to the carotid should cross clamping be required. The importance of this step cannot be overemphasized and can be considered the rate-limiting step of skull base surgery for glomus tumors. Glomus tumors can usually be sharply dissected off the ICA. The first step is to definitively identify the carotid by separating the artery in its adventitial plane from the surrounding fibromuscular tissue in the neck and at the skull base. Sharp scissor dissection is used to peel the tumor off the carotid. Bleeding is often encountered as the caroticotympanic artery is separated from the ICA. If a stub of the caroticotympanic artery is left, it can be bipolared, otherwise the opening in the ICA needs to be oversewn.

If the media of the carotid appears involved by tumor, a small layer of tumor is left on the carotid and the remaining tumor resected. The involved portion of carotid is then resected and vein grafted over an internal shunt. Although there is no fool proof method of preoperatively evaluating the adequacy of collateral circulation, this should be evaluated if there is evidence on arteriography that the carotid is involved by tumor. We routinely employ a cross-compression study regardless of

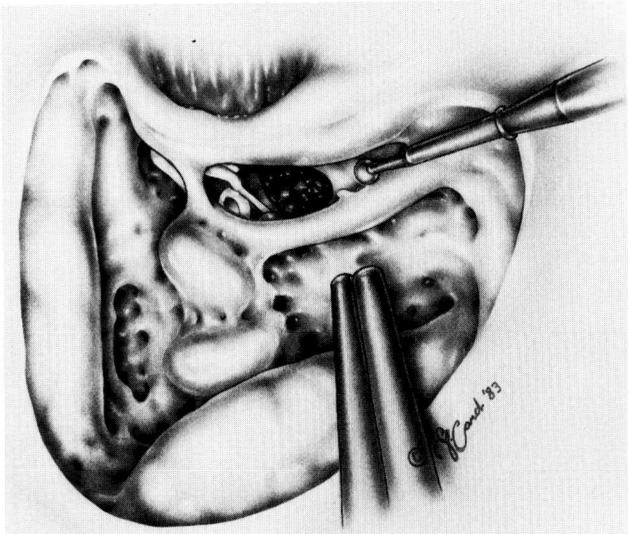

FIG 11–9.
All vital anatomy is identified and the facial recess extended prior to tumor removal.

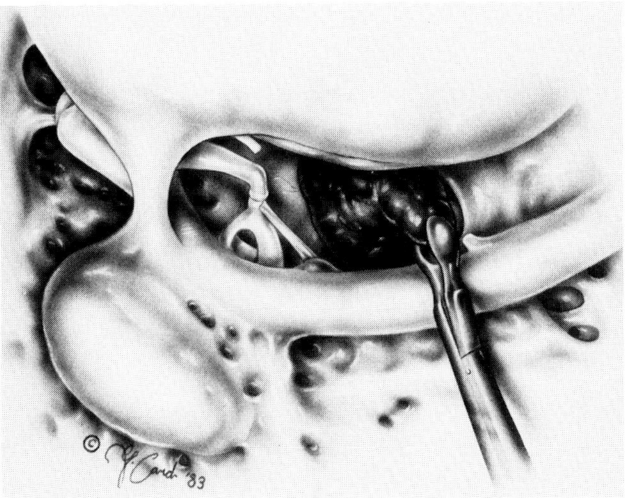

FIG 11–10.
Once the jugular bulb and ICA are free of tumor, removal can begin. Additional exposure can be obtained transcanal.

angiographic evidence of carotid involvement. This study will at least demonstrate whether there is adequate flow through the circle of Willis to feed the ipsilateral cerebral arteries from the contralateral carotid. It does not, however, guarantee adequacy of perfusion to the ipsilateral hemisphere. If there is angiographic evidence of carotid involvement by the tumor, further investigation for adequacy of contralateral flow is advisable. Balloon occlusion with EEG monitoring in an awake patient[11] and xenon perfusion studies give additional information regarding the chances for major neurologic sequellae should the involved carotid be temporarily or permanently occluded.

The technique used for management of the facial nerve will depend on the size and location of the glomus tumor. The facial nerve can be left in its fallopian canal when small tumors are removed; however, larger glomus tumors will require either mobilization or transection of the facial nerve to achieve adequate exposure of the jugular bulb area and anterior intratympanic carotid artery. Preoperative facial palsy is an extremely poor prognostic sign. All 18 of our patients with this finding required facial nerve resection as a result of nerve involvement. The jugular vein is controlled distally by ligation in the neck. Proximal control is achieved by intraluminal packing of the lateral sinus with Surgicel. Bleeding that occurs from the multiple lumens of the inferior petrosal sinus is managed by packing the lumen with Surgicel once the tumor is removed.

When one is working around the many neurovascular structures at the skull base, control of bleeding is essential for visualization. Hemostasis is achieved throughout the skull base procedure by the use of constant irrigation, bipolar coagulation, and periodic use of epinephrine-soaked Gelfoam packing. Embolization is not recommended purely on risk benefit assessment.

Glomus vagale tumors often extend superiorly to involve the skull base. Their resection follows the same principles as jugulare tumors. The following lateral skull base approaches differ primarily in the degree of anterior exposure that is afforded (see Table 11–2).

Extended Facial Recess–Skull Base Approach (Types I Through II)

Lesions confined to the jugular bulb, middle ear, and mastoid (types I and II) can often be resected by an approach that preserves the EAC. This has the obvious advantage of leaving hearing acuity intact. A Y-shaped incision is used (Fig 11–11). It starts with a postauricular incision that is extended inferiorly in the neck along the anterior border of the sternocleidomastoid muscle to the greater horn of the hyoid. A preauricular limb is then incised; it starts at the inferior margin of the tragus and extends inferiorly to join the postauricular incision just below the lobule. An anterior flap is developed just superior to the parotid fascia. The posterior flap is developed superficial to the fascia overlying the sternocleidomastoid muscle and mastoid pericranium. The anterior aspect of the auricle is retracted superiorly to expose the inferior and anterior aspect of the tympanic bone. The developed flaps are retracted with dura hooks.

The fascia overlying the sternocleidomastoid muscle is grasped with clamps and elevated anteriorly and superiorly. The posterior belly of the digastric muscle is identified. The facial nerve is then identified as it exits from the stylomastoid foramen just superior to the insertion of the posterior belly of the digastric muscle into the mastoid tip. The facial nerve is followed into the parotid until it branches at the pes anserinus.

The internal jugular vein is then identified in the upper neck. Cranial nerve XI is identified as it courses just anterior to the lateral process of the second cervical vertebra. The carotid sheath is opened, and the common carotid artery, ICA, ECA, and 10th cranial nerve are dissected from the area of the carotid bifurcation to the region under the posterior belly of the digastric. The 9th cranial nerve is usually too high to identify at this point. All of these structures are isolated, marked with vessel loops, and represent "distal control" for nerves and vascular "proximal" control.

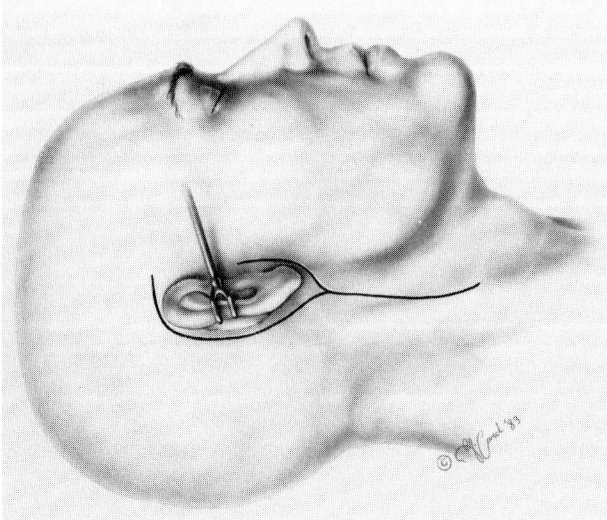

FIG 11–11.
An adapted parotidectomy incision is used to gain access to the temporal bone and neck.

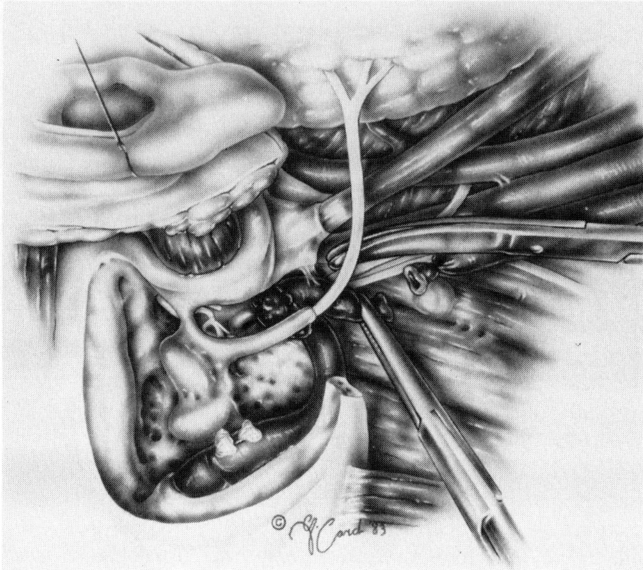

FIG 11–12.
Contents of the skull base lateral to the jugular bulb are removed for exposure. Here cranial nerve VII is left in its fallopian canal for small tumor removal.

A T-shaped incision is made over the mastoid. With the facial nerve in view, the sternocleidomastoid muscle and posterior belly of the digastric are dissected off the mastoid tip. A complete mastoidectomy is then performed using a microsurgical drill and continuous suction-irrigation. The middle fossa and sigmoid sinus are skeletonized. Care is taken to preserve a thin layer of bone over the sigmoid. The digastric ridge is identified. The facial nerve is exposed from the fossa incudis to the stylomastoid foramen. The chorda tympani is identified and the facial recess opened. An extended facial recess approach is then performed as previously described. The mastoid tip is amputated. Bone is drilled away inferior and anteroinferior to the EAC. The tympanic membrane annulus, which was exposed in the extended facial recess exposure, is followed all the way to the area of the eustachian tube. The styloid process is amputated. Bone lateral to the anterior aspect of the jugular bulb is removed (Fig 11–12). The carotid artery from the skull base to the area of the eustachian tube is exposed. Enough bone is removed from around the carotid artery so that a bulldog clamp can be placed around the artery should distal control of a ruptured carotid be needed. At this point, the amount of anterior exposure is assessed. If the carotid artery that is exposed in the anterior mesotympanum is free of tumor and the anterior margin of tumor is clearly visible, no further anterior exposure is necessary. If more anterior exposure is necessary, the EAC must be taken down, the external meatus closed over, and a maximal conductive hearing loss accepted.

If anterior exposure is deemed adequate, the facial nerve is mobilized at this point. It is left in its bony canal until now to minimize chances for catching it in the drill burr during the anteroinferior bone removal. First the bone covering the facial nerve from the second genu to the stylomastoid foramen is "egg shelled." The thin bone is then removed with a no. 1 knife. The

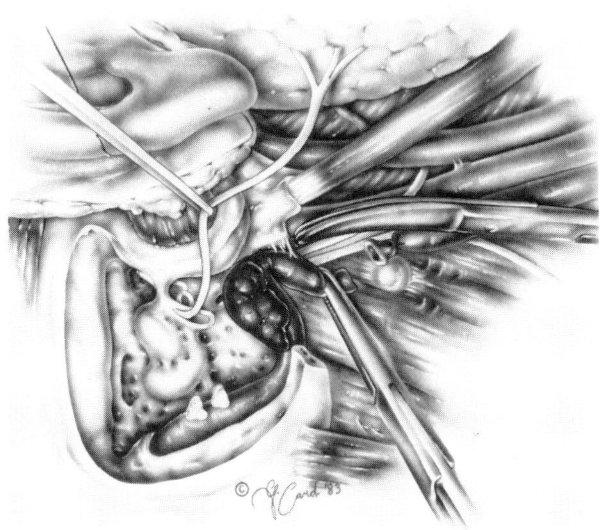

FIG 11–13.
With cranial nerve VII mobilized and EAC maintained, tumor dissection off ICA is begun.

nerve is lifted out of the fallopian canal as atraumatically as possible. The fibromuscular tissue at the stylomastoid foramen is sharply dissected off the area of the facial nerve without trying to get too close to the nerve. This decreases chances for injuring the nerve and also leaves a clump of fibromuscular tissue attached to the nerve that can be used as a handle when the nerve is transposed. The facial nerve is then rotated anteriorly and draped over the lip of the EAC. The bone that was inferior to the facial nerve can now be removed and the jugular bulb completely exposed. Brackmann has presented an important new technique in which nerve VII can be mobilized yet remain functionally intact. We have found the technique useful but inadequate when upper exposure limits are required for larger tumors. The jugular vein is ligated below the level of the second cervical vertebra. A 2-cm area of bone overlying the sigmoid sinus is removed. Surgicel is packed extraluminally superiorly and inferiorly through the bony opening. The lumen of the sigmoid is then opened with a no. 11 blade and the sigmoid packed intraluminally with large pieces of Surgicel. The extraluminal Surgicel is eased out as more intraluminal packing is placed. Any remaining bone around the jugular bulb is then removed.

The cut end of the jugular vein is grasped with a clamp and retracted superiorly. Using sharp dissection, the surgeon separates the jugular vein from the ICA and cranial nerves IX, X, and XI. Dissection is carried superiorly until tumor is encountered (Fig 11–13).

Working in the adventitial plane of the carotid artery, the surgeon separates the fibromuscular tissue at the skull base from the carotid so that the artery's anatomy is clearly defined from the bifurcation to its anterior extent of exposure at the region of the eustachian tube. Cranial nerve IX is by necessity transected as it crosses the ICA at the level of the stylopharyngeus. Scissor dissection is then used to strip the tumor off the carotid.

Once the tumor is clearly freed from the carotid, the resection can proceed. The jugular vein and bulb with the contained tumor are sharply dissected out of the skull base. The pars nervosa is kept in view during the resection to avoid unnecessary injury to cranial nerves IX, X, and XI. If the tumor involves the pars nervosa of the jugular bulb, the cranial nerves must be resected with the tumor. Brisk bleeding from the inferior petrosal sinus is controlled by packing the sinus lumen with Surgicel. Once bleeding is controlled, the defect is thoroughly examined, and any residual tumor is removed (Fig 11–14). Drains are placed, and the wound is closed in two layers. If cranial nerve X had to be resected in a patient with normal vocal cord mobility preoperatively, a tracheotomy is performed. A bulky compression dressing is applied.

Infratemporal fossa approach (Types III and IV)

Larger glomus jugulare tumors that fall into the Glasscock-Jackson type III and IV categories require more anterior exposure than that afforded by the previously described procedure. To adequately visualize the entire intratemporal portion of the carotid artery, one must remove the tympanic bone and bone of the glenoid fossa and infratemporal fossa.

A large C-shaped incision is used, starting from the temporoparietal region about 3 cm anterior to the helical root, progressing 5 cm posterior to the postauricular crease, and ending in the neck 2 cm below the angle of the mandible (Fig 11–15). The incision is carried down to the temporalis fascia and mastoid periosteum and through the platysma. An anterior flap is developed superficial to the temporalis fascia and periosteum and deep to the platysma. The EAC is transected at the bony-cartilagenous junction and the dissection carried anteriorly superficial to the periparotid fascia. The external meatus is oversewn with everting absorbable sutures. The facial nerve

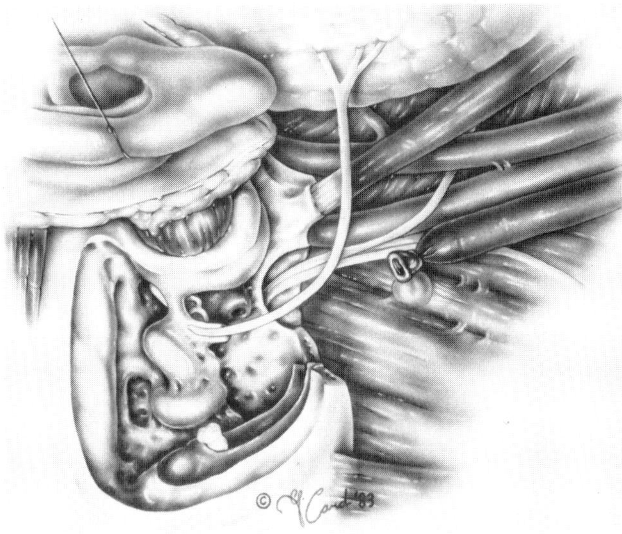

FIG 11–14.
Total tumor removal. Note the intraluminal packing of the lateral sinus and EAC preservation.

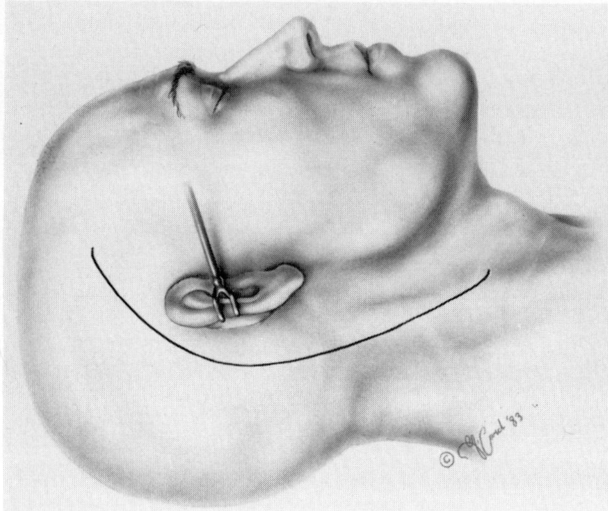

FIG 11–15.
An anteriorly based flap allows access to the neck, temporal bone, and infratemporal regions.

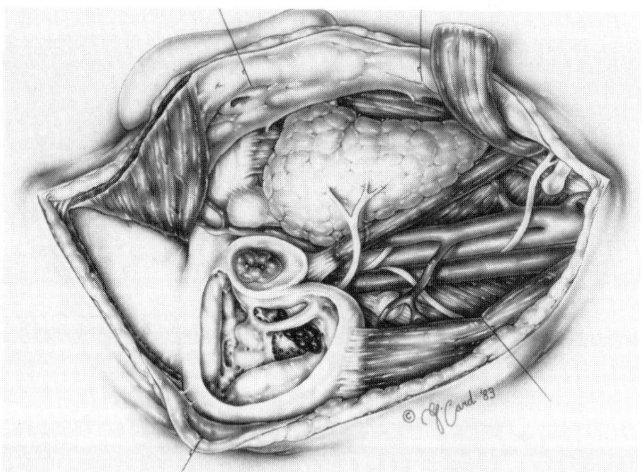

FIG 11–16.
The EAC is transected and neck with mastoid exposure done.

is identified and followed into the parotid to the pes, and the neurovascular structures in the neck are identified as previously described.

A T-shaped incision is made over the mastoid, and the sternocleidomastoid and posterior belly of the digastric are dissected off the mastoid tip. A complete mastoidectomy with extended facial recess approach is performed (Fig 11–16). The incudostapedial joint is disarticulated. The external canal skin and tympanic membrane are sharply dissected out of the canal, and the posterior bony canal wall is removed with a mastoid rongeur. The incus and malleus are removed. The mastoid tip is amputated. The bone of the anterior external canal wall and glenoid fossa is drilled away, exposing the capsule of the temporomandibular joint. The bone lateral to the jugular bulb is removed to expose tumor.

The facial nerve is mobilized and transposed anteriorly at

this point. The nerve is mobilized up to the geniculate ganglion as previously described. The petrosal nerves are sectioned for enhanced mobility. The nerve is then transposed anteriorly and held along the posterosuperior surface of the parotid gland. The remaining bone lateral to the jugular bulb and sigmoid sinus is removed.

Transposition of the facial nerve now allows downward and anterior dislocation of the mandible, which gives adequate exposure for further anterior removal of bone along the horizontal course of the intratemporal carotid artery. The limit of anterior bone removal is reached when there is adequate exposure to allow placement of a bulldog clamp around the carotid anterior to the anterior margin of tumor. When extreme anterior exposure is required, the mandibular condyle can rarely be resected to give unrestricted anterior dislocation of the mandible. Transection of the facial nerve after its branching at the pes is preferable to excessive stretching of the nerve. The nerve endings are tagged and reanastomosed at the completion of the procedure. This is rarely necessary (Fig 11–17).

The jugular vein is ligated in the neck. The sigmoid is first extraluminally, then intraluminally, packed with Surgicel. The jugular vein is retracted superiorly and separated from the carotid and cranial nerves X, XI, and XII to the level of the tumor. The ICA is separated from the fibromuscular tissue at the skull base. The tumor is then sharply separated from the carotid. The lateral jugular bulb is excised and the tumor removed from the skull base. Cranial nerves X, XI, and XII are kept in view during the dissection and spared unless involved by tumor. Cranial nerve XII can usually be spared if there is no preoperative evidence of dysfunction. A large suction allows identification of the multiple openings of the inferior petrosal sinus, which are packed with Surgicel (Fig 11–18). The wound is closed in multiple layers, and a bulky compression dressing is applied.

Vagale

The surgical approach to glomus vagale tumors uses the same principles described for glomus jugulare lesions. The exposure used is dictated by the tumor extension superiorly. Prox-

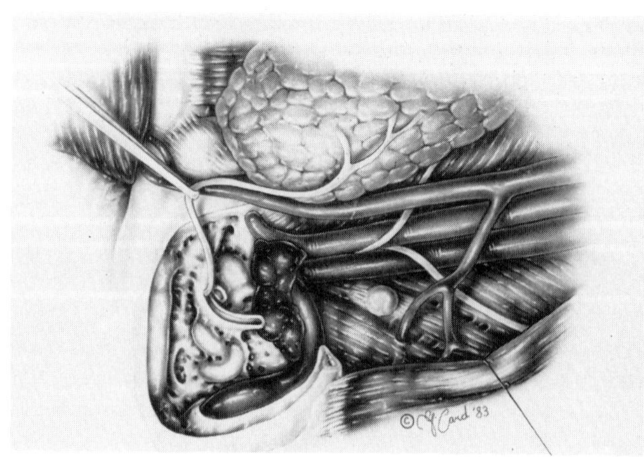

FIG 11–17.
The facial nerve is mobilized from the internal genu to allow mandibular anterior dislocation. Note proximal and distal ICA control.

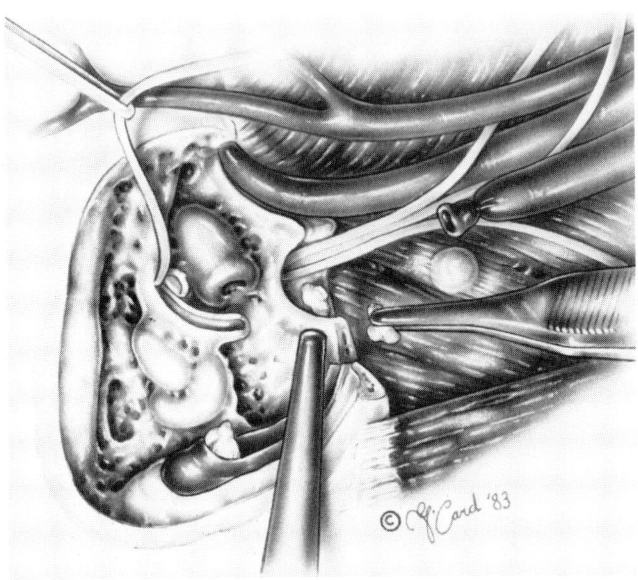

FIG 11–18.
Tumor removal is complete. Packing occludes the inferior petrosal sinus.

imal and distal control of both the jugular vein and ICA are mandatory. These tumors in general have a more tenacious attachment to the carotid than jugulare lesions and are more difficult to separate from cranial nerves X, XI, and XII.

Intracranial Extension

Intradural extension of glomus tumors usually occurs into the posterior fossa by tumor growth at the jugular fossa and hypoglossal foramina. Direct intracranial intradural posterior fossa extension is preceded by extradural erosion of the temporal bone by tumor with the dura pushed ahead of it into the intracranial space. Imaging studies cannot be uniformly relied on to differentiate between these two entities preoperatively. Traditionally, the tumor with its intracranial extension has been regarded as two separate lesions. In point of fact, they are single. Intracranial extension is best managed by a one-stage removal. Success of this single-stage protocol is dependent on successful closing of the defect to prevent CSF leakage. A two-stage approach, advocated to reduce the occurrence of postoperative CSF leak,[12] makes total tumor removal more difficult. The well-defined dissection planes that are present during the first stage are partially obscured by the inevitable fibrosis that occurs between the two stages.

The operative exposure afforded by the skull base approach is optimal for removal of intracranial extension with only minor additional bone removal. Identification of the cranial nerves in the neck and skull base affords the best opportunity for preservation of these nerves when the intracranial extension is excised.

Under certain circumstances, a two-stage procedure may offer certain advantages. When there is overt EAC involvement by the tumor with probable bacterial contamination, a two-stage approach may be elected to reduce the risk of intracranial in-

fection. When a procedure has lasted an extraordinary amount of time, a second stage may be preferable to the compromise of the skull base team's efficiency. Other factors, such as a critical change in the patient's vital signs, may force a two-stage approach.

After the appropriate skull base approach, the tumor is separated from the ICA and removed from the temporal bone to the level of the intradural extension. Bleeding is controlled by packing the multiple openings of the inferior petrosal sinus with Surgicel and judiciously using bipolar cautery. Additional bone removal is then done depending on the location of the intracranial extension.

If intracranial extension is small, a retrolabyrinthine approach to the posterior fossa may be adequate. Posterior fossa involvement up to and including the IAC may be approached by a classical translabyrinthine approach when hearing is not a concern. For involvement of the cochlea and clivus, a translabyrinthine approach is followed by mobilization of the labyrinthine portion of the facial nerve and ICA. Transcochlear removal of bone will usually afford adequate exposure into the anteromedial petrous apex and clivus. For more posteriorly extensive intracranial extension, a suboccipital approach may be required. Bone is removed from the retrosigmoid area and the dura anterior and posterior to the occluded sigmoid is opened. The intracranial extent of the tumor can then be removed. This approach gives good exposure for visualization of the roots of nerves IX, X, XI, and XII (Fig 11–19). However, it is unlikely that tumor sufficiently large to extend intracranially will spare these nerves.

The most difficult aspect of surgery for intracranial extension of skull base tumors is the management of the dural defect. Avoidance of a major CSF leak is critical to the success of this procedure. Our present technique uses autogenous fascia (temporalis or fascia lata) placed over the defect and secured to the dural or bony margins. For small defects, a local flap such as a rotated temporalis muscle flap is used to fill the operative defect (Figs 11–20 and 11–21). For larger defects, a free microvascular

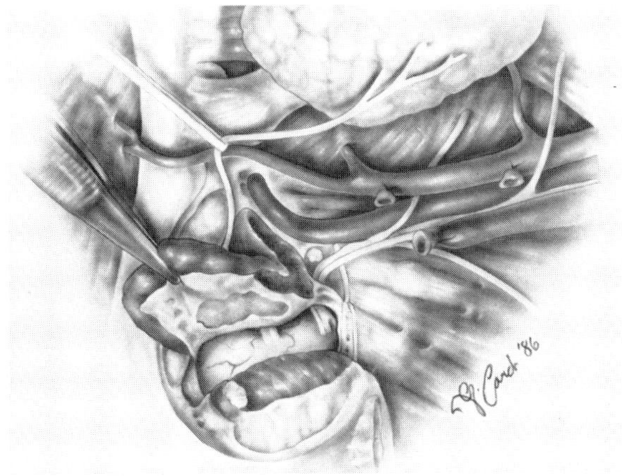

FIG 11–19.
The combined approach to the ICE of a glomus tumor is exhibited. Tumor is off the ICA and debulked from the temporal bone to afford mobility.

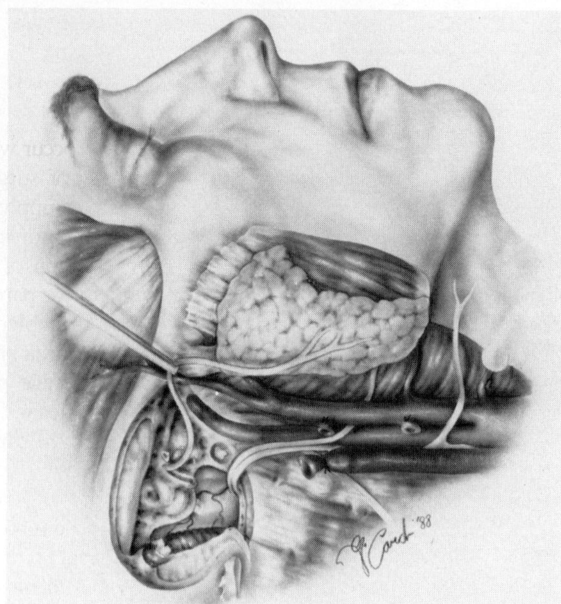

FIG 11–20.
A small to medium dural defect is shown.

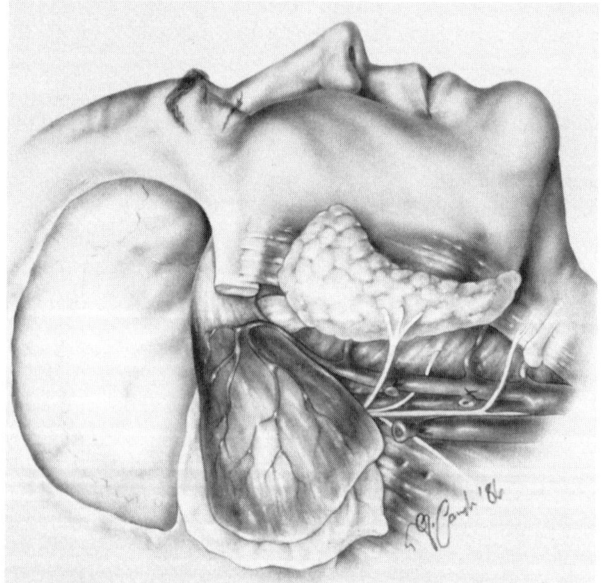

FIG 11–21.
Temporalis fascia and a muscle flap rotated on its axis reconstruct the defect. A lumbar drain augments this reconstruction.

rectus abdominus free lap is used to cover the fascia graft and fill the defect (Figs 11–22 to 11–24). The flap is trimmed to slightly overfill the defect because the muscle mass will lose about 50% of its bulk over 3 to 4 months. The wound is closed in two layers over closed suction drains. A lumbar drain is then placed and kept in for 1 week as long as it continues to drain and there is no sign of infection. The patient who has a recurrent tumor after full-course radiation therapy will have diminished wound healing in the radiated field, making successful repair

of the dural defect more difficult. In all such cases, free flap reconstruction is preferred.

Extended Infratemporal Fossa Exposure

On occasion, large glomus tumors extend beyond the limits of the temporal bone anteriorly into the deep confines of the infratemporal fossa. The anterior limits of ICA to the cavernous sinus must be accessed. Maximum facial nerve mobilization and anteroinferior mandibular displacement is required for access. The zygoma must be detached and reflected with the temporal

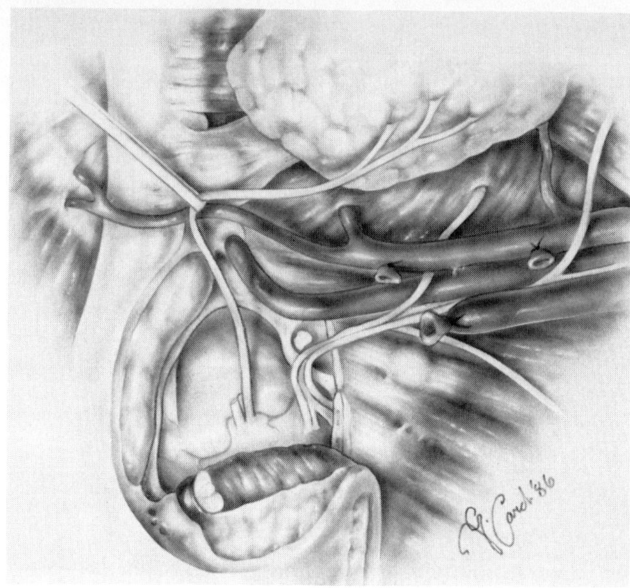

FIG 11–22.
A larger dural defect is shown.

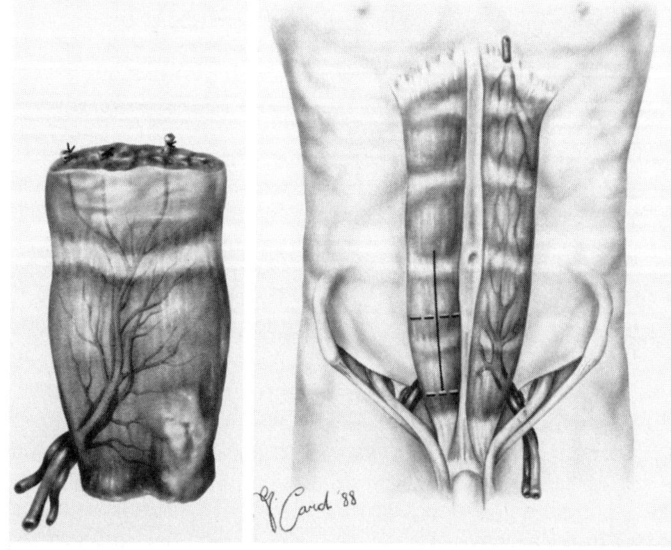

FIG 11–23.
The rectus abdominus is a utilitarian donor site for the free flap.

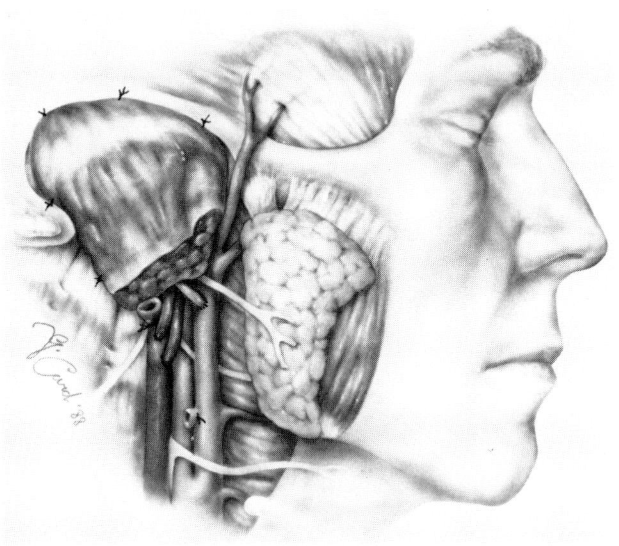

FIG 11–24.
The free flap is shown positioned. It should be bulky, because shrinkage up to 50% of its original volume can be anticipated.

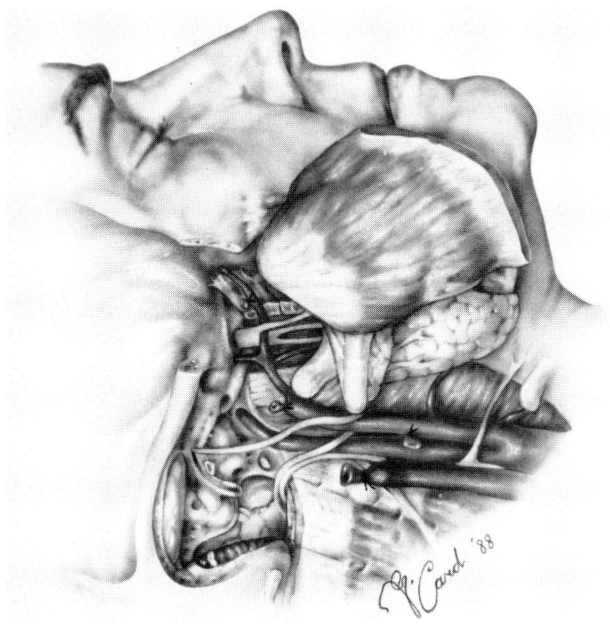

FIG 11–25.
Note the anatomy of the infratemporal fossa, which must be managed to access this area.

musculature inferiorly. To achieve this exposure, the surgeon must sacrifice the eustachian tube, contents of the foramen spinosum, the mandibular division of cranial nerve V, the pterygoid plates, and occasionally V_2 (Figs 11–25 and 11–26). Access to the floor of the middle cranial fossa is likewise available by removal of the tegmen. The nasopharynx is readily exposed.

More utilitary for diverse cranial base problems, this exposure is not often required for glomus tumors except the most extensive of the largest.

CRANIAL NERVE INJURY AND POSTOPERATIVE MANAGEMENT PROTOCOLS

Cranial Nerve VII

Optimal postoperative facial nerve function will occur when the facial nerve is treated with the least amount of surgical trauma and when minimal interruption of its blood supply occurs during mobilization. There is probably some individual variation in the arterial supply to the vertical portion of the fallopian canal that affects the degree of postoperative paresis. We have noted that when there has not been an arterial bleeder at the posterior surface of the fallopian canal in the area of the stapedius muscle, the patient has a better than average postoperative facial nerve function. The surgical techniques we employ to minimize surgical trauma to the facial nerve during removal of skull base tumors include the following:

1. If the glomus jugulare lesion is small, it may be removed without transposing the facial nerve out of the canal.
2. The facial nerve is left in its bony canal until most of the bone is removed at the skull base to minimize chances for the nerve to get caught in the burr.
3. It is better to transect the nerve after it branches at the pes if extreme anterior exposure is needed rather than to excessively stretch the nerve.
4. When the nerve is mobilized at the stylomastoid foramen, a small amount of fibromuscular tissue is left attached to the nerve. The nerve is very adherent to the soft tissue at the area of the foramen, and excessive nerve trauma is more likely to occur if an attempt is made to strip the nerve clean. This fibromuscular tissue also serves as a handle to use when the nerve is mobilized, avoiding the need to handle the nerve itself. Preoperative facial palsy in glomus tumors in 100% of our cases has meant nerve involvement and consequent facial nerve resection. Facial nerve monitoring is not regarded as essential.

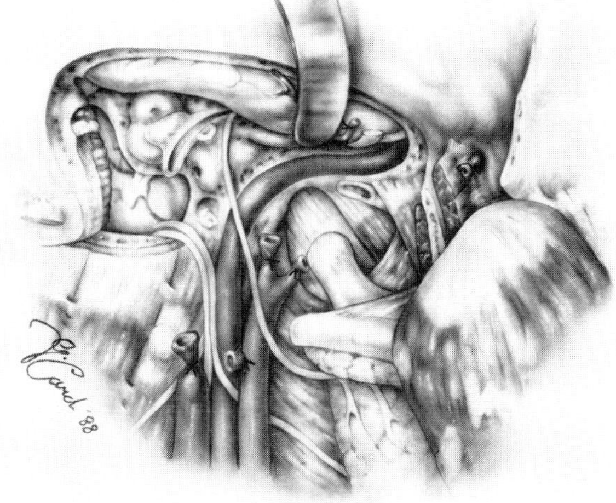

FIG 11–26.
The extended infratemporal fossa exposure affords access to IAC, all divisions of cranial nerve V, the middle fossa, and deep regions of the infratemporal fossa.

Postoperative care of the patient with facial paresis or paralysis involves primarily care of the eye. The patient wears a moisture chamber over the eye at night and uses artificial tears and lubricating ointment frequently enough to keep the eye moist. The ophthalmologist sees all patients with facial paresis and evaluates their need for an upper lid gold weight insertion or lateral canthoplasty.

Cranial Nerves IX, X, XI, and XII

Identification of the cranial nerves in the neck and following them superiorly to the inferior extent of the tumor is the first step in preserving the integrity of these nerves. Cranial nerve IX is often transected during development of the advential plane of the carotid at the skull base. The nerve is encountered as it crosses laterally over the carotid at the level of the stylopharyngeus muscle. When the lateral jugular bulb is opened to remove the tumor, profuse bleeding occurs. A large-bore suction is used to clear the blood sufficiently to visualize the pars nervosa and avoid transecting the nerves as the tumor is excised. If the tumor involves the nerves in the area of the bulb, the nerves have to be sacrificed to completely resect the tumor. Overpacking the lumens of the inferior petrosal sinus or sinuses in the bulb should be avoided, because this can put excessive pressure on cranial nerves X and XI and cause postoperative weakness or paralysis. As the hypoglossal nerve exits the skull base from a separate foramen, it is usually possible to preserve its function as long as there is no preoperative evidence of hypoglossal dysfunction to indicate tumor involvement.

Transection of cranial nerve IX without transection of X does not cause any adverse effects. If cranial nerve X is unexpectedly transected in a patient who had normal function preoperatively, a tracheotomy is performed at the conclusion of the procedure. If the tumor is large and one believes that there is very little chance of saving the vagus nerve, a tracheotomy is performed at the beginning of the procedure. The tracheotomy helps prevent the pulmonary complications of an incompetent larynx in a patient who has just undergone a prolonged surgical procedure and anesthetic. A Teflon cord is injected or phonosurgery is performed by 1 week postoperatively. When the patients are able to handle their secretions adequately, they are progressively decannulated over the next few days.

Parenteral nutrition is employed until the patient can support his or her own caloric intake. Gastrointestinal decompression is necessary until the ileus abates. Once the patient is decannulated, the occupational or speech therapist uses a video barium swallow to evaluate the patient's ability to handle various food consistencies. The effect of head positioning maneuvers to close off the denervated pyriform sinus can be evaluated directly by this study. The occupational therapist then coaches the patient through the first few meals and advances the diet as the patient's progress dictates. Close supervision of the patient during the early phase of swallowing rehabilitation is critical to prevent the patient from aspirating and help the patient avoid the frustration that often accompanies slow progress. This attention to detail has eliminated the problem of aspiration.

INTRAOPERATIVE HYPOTENSION (CATECHOLAMINE WITHDRAWAL)

Intraoperative catecholamine withdrawal is best prevented by diagnosing the presence of a secreting glomus tumor preoperatively and administering a pharmacologic blockade prior to performing surgical excision. This is more thoroughly discussed in the section on diagnosis.

Massive Hemorrhage

Glomus vagale and all but the smallest glomus jugulare tumors are adjacent or adherent to the adventitia of the carotid artery at the skull base. Avoidance of catastrophic blood loss is dependent on several operative principles. A vessel loop is placed around the ICA in the neck, and the carotid proximal to the tumor is exposed sufficiently to allow a bulldog clamp to be placed around the artery prior to any attempt to remove the tumor. The carotid is clearly defined at the skull base by separating it from the fibromuscular tissue at the skull base in the artery's adventitial plane. Tumor removal is begun by separating the tumor from the carotid while working in a relatively bloodless field.

Opening the jugular bulb for final tumor removal always results in brisk bleeding. The jugular vein is ligated in the neck, and the sigmoid sinus intraluminally packed with Surgicel prior to this step. As much bone lateral to the sigmoid and jugular bulb should be removed prior to tumor removal to give unobstructed visualization of the bulb anatomy during tumor removal. We do not employ preoperative embolization of glomus tumors. We believe that any decrease in intraoperative blood loss is offset by the potential risks of the embolization procedure.

INDICATIONS FOR NONOPERATIVE MANAGEMENT

The preferred treatment of a glomus tumor is surgical excision. In those cases where the tumor occurs in an elderly patient or a patient with a serious medical illness, the difficulty of the patient's accommodating to the postoperative cranial nerve deficits, and the risks of a skull base procedure must be weighed against the potential risk to the patient of the untreated tumor. Radiation therapy is recommended as palliative treatment in those patients who are considered nonsurgical candidates.

TEAM APPROACH

Surgery of this magnitude cannot be performed without the interdisciplinary support of several specialists who constitute the team. Neurotology heads the team and collaborates closely with head and neck surgery, neurosurgery, plastic surgery, general surgery, and anesthesiology. Critical care nurse specialists, physical therapists, dieticians, psychiatrists, radiology, and the patient's family are integral. Without such a team approach, this surgery should not be attempted.

REFERENCES

1. Batsakis JG: Paragangliomas of the head and neck, in *Tumors of the Head and Neck: Clinical and Pathologic Consideration,* ed 2. Baltimore, Williams & Wilkins Co, 1979, pp 289–380.
2. Spector GJ, Ciralsky RH, Ogura JH: Glomus tumors in the head and neck: III. Analysis of clinical manifestations. *Ann Otol* 1975; 84:73–80.
3. Smith PG, Schwaber MK, Goebel JA: Clinical evaluation of glomus tumors of the ear and the base of skull, in Thawley SE, et al (ed): *Comprehensive Management of Head and Neck Tumors.* Philadelphia, WB Saunders Co, 1987, pp 207–218.
4. Spector GS, Giralsky R, Maisel RH, et al: Multiple glomus tumors in the head and neck. *Laryngoscope* 1975; 85:1006–1075.
5. Zak FG, Lawson W: *The Paraganglionic Chemoreceptor System, Physiology, Pathology and Clinical Medicine.* New York, Springer-Verlag New York, 1982.
6. Schwaber MK, Glasscock ME, Jackson CG, et al: Diagnosis and management of catecholamine secreting glomus tumors. *Laryngoscope* 1984; 94:1008–1015.
7. Jackson CJ, Glasscock ME, Nissen AJ, et al: Glomus tumor surgery: The approach, results, and problems. *Otolaryngol Clin North Am* 1982; 15:897–916.
8. Oldring D, Fisch U: Glomus tumors of the temporal region. *Arch Otolaryngol* 1981; 107:209–213.
9. Fisch U: Infratemporal fossa approach for glomus tumors of the temporal bone. *Ann Otol Rhinol Laryngol* 1982; 91:474–479.
10. Jackson CG, Glasscock ME, Harris PF: Glomus tumors: Diagnosis, classification, and management of large lesions. *Arch Otolaryngol* 1982; 108:401–406.
11. Fisch U, Fagan P, Valavanis A: The infratemporal fossa approach for the lateral skull base. Symposium on skull base surgery. *Otolaryngol Clin North Am* 1984; 17:513–549.
12. Fisch U: Infratemporal fossa approach for extensive tumors of the temporal bone and base of the skull. *J Laryngol Otol* 1978; 92:949–967.

CHAPTER 12

Pituitary Tumors

Approach of

Louis G. Petcu, M.S., M.D.

and

Clarence T. Sasaki, M.D.

Disorders of the pituitary gland have been amenable to surgical treatment for nearly 100 years. Although other transcranial approaches have enjoyed popularity in the past and are occasionally indicated today, it is the consensus among otolaryngologists and neurosurgeons that the transseptal transsphenoidal procedure is the preferred surgical approach to the management of pituitary lesions. This procedure involves close cooperation between otolaryngologists and neurosurgeons and in most institutions can be performed with an operative mortality of less than 1% to 2%.

An aggressive approach to the treatment of pituitary lesions has been warranted by both advances in surgical technique and understanding of pituitary pathology. Advances in neuroradiology and neuroendocrinology have allowed more complete understanding of the role of the pituitary in various endocrine syndromes and have permitted earlier diagnosis. Combined with the low morbidity and mortality of the transseptal transsphenoidal technique, this has increased the number of lesions that can be surgically managed.

HISTORICAL NOTE

The first surgical approaches to the pituitary gland predated the complete understanding of the endocrine nature of this organ and were attempts to address the problem of an expanding intracranial mass. As a result, they were intracranial approaches. The earliest (1893) reported attempt, by Caton and Paul,[1] was a middle cranial fossa approach, first suggested by Sir Victor Horsely,[2] who later utilized this approach on a series of 10 patients. Giordano[3] is credited with the first extracranial approach to the pituitary, which was the transseptal transsphenoidal approach. It was successfully modified by Schloffer[4] in 1907 by using a dorsal nasal split with wide resection of the septum and medial orbital walls, resulting in markedly altered nasal physiology. At the same time, Moszkowicz[5] devised a technique that utilized a forehead flap transposed into the sphenoid sinus to prevent cerebrospinal fluid (CSF) rhinorrhea.

In 1905, Krause[6] used the transfrontal approach, and Kanavel[7] described an intranasal approach utilizing a U-shaped subnasal incision allowing upward rotation of the nose and improved exposure. Halstead,[8] in 1910, proposed the sublabial incision, and it was adopted by Cushing[9] in 1912. This approach allowed good exposure while permitting conservation of nasal function and avoiding a facial scar, and it was used by Cushing in 231 pituitary procedures, despite inadequate magnification or illumination.[10] It was later abandoned, however, as experience with transcranial approaches grew and as a result of Henderson's[11] analysis of Cushing's series of patients, which seemed to indicate that the transcranial approaches had a lower incidence of recurrence.

In the period following World War II, the transseptal transsphenoidal approach was revived because of several factors. Perioperative antibiotics, intraoperative fluoroscopy, and the operating microscope made this approach relatively safer than the transcranial approach. Variations of this technique exist, including the transethmoidal transsphenoidal approach,[12] and the triangulation method of Angell-James,[13] which utilizes a transethmoidal approach for exposure and a transnasal approach for instrumentation.

INDICATIONS

There are many indications for the transseptal approach to the skull base, but resection of pituitary adenomas is the most common, representing 66% to 83% of all hypophyseal procedures.[14, 15] Of these, greater than one half of the tumors are endocrinologically active. A prolactin-secreting adenoma, producing the amenorrhea-galactorrhea syndrome, is the most common type of functioning adenoma.[16] An adrenocorticotropic hormone-secreting adenoma tends to assume smaller size and can be enucleated with preservation of pituitary function, although the Cushing's syndrome that marks this tumor may result in wound-healing complications. Growth hormone-secreting adenomas prove to be uniquely challenging since they produce acromegalic changes in the operative field, such as septal irregularities and a thickened calvarium. Hyperostotic changes in the frontal sinus make anterior transcranial approaches to the sella less desirable than the transsphenoid approach. Tumors that secrete luteinizing hormone and follicle-stimulating hormone, though described, are relatively rare.

A second major group of patients require total hypophysectomy for control or palliation of endocrine-responsive tumors.[17] Selection of patients is usually based on demonstration of previous response to endocrine manipulation (hormonal therapy or castration) or those who have failed to achieve effective tumor palliation by other means. Endocrinologically significant hypophysectomy requires resection of at least 90% of functioning pituitary tissue.

Total hypophysectomy is effective in palliation of advanced breast carcinoma,[18] particularly if the tumor is estrogen receptor positive. Often, oophorectomy is the initial endocrine manipulation, with hypophysectomy reserved for patients who fail to respond to this measure or to administration of androgens or estrogens. There is additional evidence that a decrease in growth hormone levels is associated with a decrease in skeletal pain due to metastases.[19]

Likewise, total hypophysectomy has been shown to be efficacious palliation in selected cases of prostatic carcinoma.[20] Patients most likely to benefit in this group are those with painful skeletal metastases and obstructing pelvic or urinary masses after failure of initial measures, such as estrogen therapy, castration, or radiation. Of note, hypophysectomy has reduced skeletal pain from endocrine-insensitive tumors in some patients. The mechanism of this effect is not understood.

Another indication for hypophysectomy is the control of diabetic retinopathy. Although laser photocoagulation is currently the mainstay of therapy, hypophysectomy is the treatment of choice for rapidly progressive multifocal retinopathy. Comparative studies indicate that hypophysectomy is more effective in preventing blindness than photocoagulation.[21, 22]

The transseptal transsphenoidal approach to the pituitary is additionally indicated for nonpituitary parasellar tumors (meningiomas, craniopharyngiomas, chordomas) empty sella syndrome, CSF rhinorrhea, and sphenoid sinus lesions (mucocoeles, sphenoid sinusitis, and sphenoid sinus carcinomas).

OPERATIVE TECHNIQUE

The patient is anesthetized through an orotracheal tube and moved to a semi-Fowler position. The vibrissae are trimmed. The sublabial mucosa, anterior nasal spine, and membranous septum, including the floor of the nose, are injected with 10 mL of 0.5% lidocaine (Xylocaine) hydrochloride with epinephrine 1:200,000. The surgeon begins the scrub and prepares the operative area with povidone-iodine (Betadine) soap and solution, including the area of the face and right thigh. A fat and fascia graft is taken from the right thigh and preserved in saline for later use. The operative field is triangulated with towels, which are sutured to the skin. Draping is completed with an abdominal drape. Cocaine flakes (approximately 80 mg) are applied with four wire applicators to the sphenopalatine ganglia bilaterally and the anterior ethmoid nerves for mucosal decongestion. The surgeon and assistant drape the microscope, ensuring that it is equipped with a 300 mm objective lens and straight eye pieces. Local anesthesia for hemostasis is reinforced with a subsequent 10 mL of 0.5% lidocaine with epinephrine 1:200,000 delivered to the sublabial tissues and anterior nasal spine. The cocaine applicators are removed at this time. A horizontal, sublabial incision from canine ridge to canine ridge is made, angling superiorly toward the pyriform crests. Richardson retractors are used for exposure by the assistant who stands at the patient's head. Elevation of the periosteum is facilitated by using a Mackenty elevator to expose the anterior nasal spine and pyriform crests. Attachment of the anterior spine to the caudal edge of the septal cartilage is temporarily preserved. This maintains a certain degree of septal stability, which facilitates elevation of the mucoperichondrial septal mucosa. The caudal edge of the nasal septum is exposed with a double hook by the assistant, and a longitudinal incision is made along its free edge with a no. 15 blade. The subperichondrial space is identified using a Cottle knife, and anterior tunnels are performed sublabially with a Cottle elevator. To avoid perforating the septal flaps, we recommend visualization through the nose using a Cottle speculum for exposure (Fig 12–1). The pyriform crests are conservatively removed with a Kerrison rongeur. All bleeders are electrocoagulated at this time. Complete hemostasis is essential to the ease of further dissection. The surgeon performs inferior tunnels with a Mackenty elevator from vomeral ridge to lateral nasal wall. The superior and inferior tunnels are connected by sharp dissection using the spaded end of the Cottle elevator. The quadrangular septal cartilage is disarticulated from its attachment to the vomer inferiorly and the ethmoid plate posteriorly, leaving the septal cartilage hinged superiorly.

The surgeon inserts a Hubbard hypophysectomy speculum, displacing the septal cartilage to the left (Fig 12–2) and exposing the perpendicular ethmoid plate and vomer between its blades (Fig 12–3). The sphenoid rostrum will now be revealed (Fig 12–4). The surgeon follows the vomer to the sphenoid rostrum,

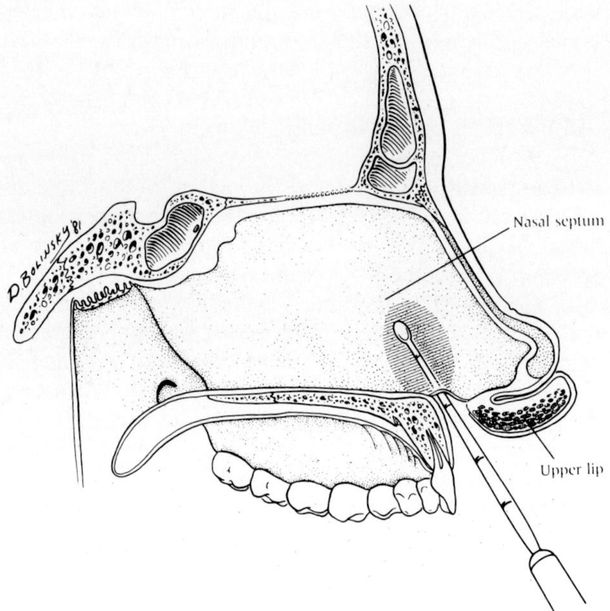

FIG 12–1.
Visualization through the nose using a Cottle speculum for exposure.

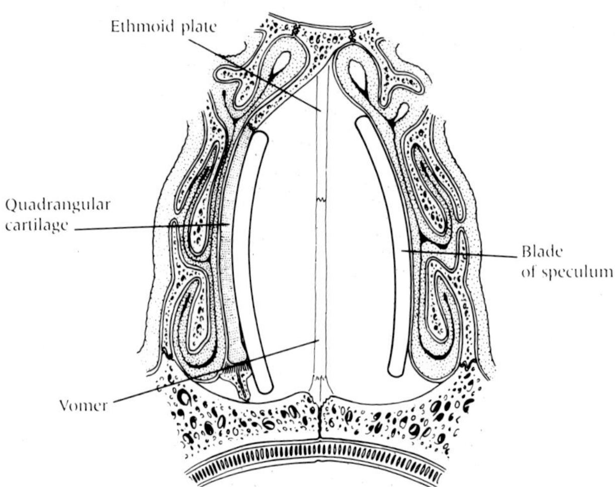

FIG 12–2.
Insertion of Hubbard hypophysectomy speculum, displacing the septal cartilage to the left.

gentle bulge of the sella turcica may be identified with use of the operating microscope. Bone overlying the sella is characteristically thin and may be removed with a stapes curette. With the Angell-James dissectors, the dura may be dissected from this thin plate of bone to be removed with Kerrison rongeurs. Should the bone at this point appear thickened, the surgeon should suspect that he or she may, in fact, be opening into the anterior cranial fossa and should prepare to obtain intraoperative lateral roentgenograms for purposes of reorientation (Fig 12–6). On the other hand, when the anterior sella wall is thick, an air drill is of distinct advantage in obtaining a safe exposure.

After the sphenoidotomy has been enlarged, the disposition of the sella within the sphenoid sinus can be assessed. Three major variants determine the ease with which the anterior and inferior walls of the sella can be identified.[23, 24] The most common (85%) and most favorable configuration is the sellar

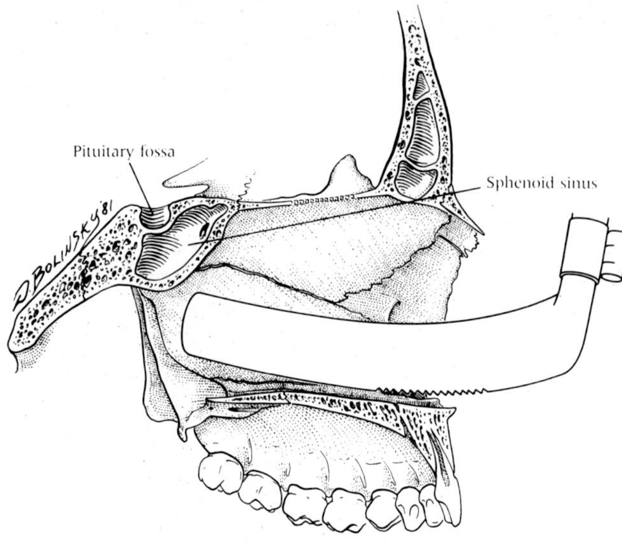

FIG 12–3.
Exposure of the perpendicular ethmoid plate and vomer between blades of Hubbard hypophysectomy speculum.

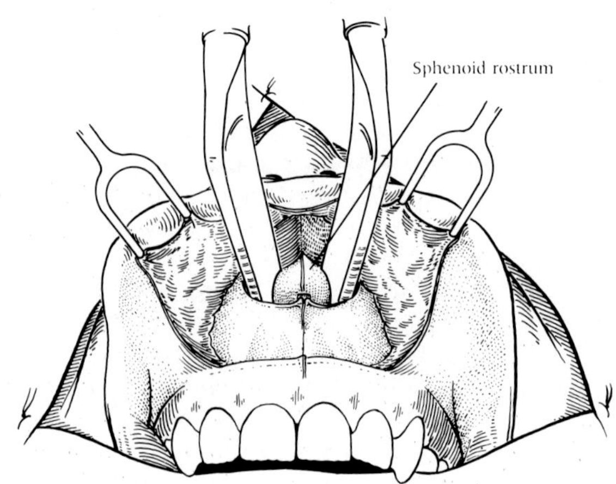

FIG 12–4.
The sphenoid rostrum is revealed.

removing perpendicular ethmoid with heavy pituitary forceps. Remnants of the perpendicular ethmoid superiorly and vomer inferiorly are intentionally left for purposes of midline orientation. The sphenoid sinus is entered by grasping the remnant of bony septum on the rostrum of the sphenoid with a heavy pituitary forceps, applying a circular twisting motion. When an opening has been effectively created in the rostrum of the sphenoid, it may be enlarged using Kerrison rongeurs (Fig 12–5). The mucosa is carefully removed from the sphenoid sinus by traction using Angell-James dissectors and pituitary forceps. Curettage is avoided to spare injuring dehiscent carotid arteries or optic nerves. After the sphenoid septum is removed, the

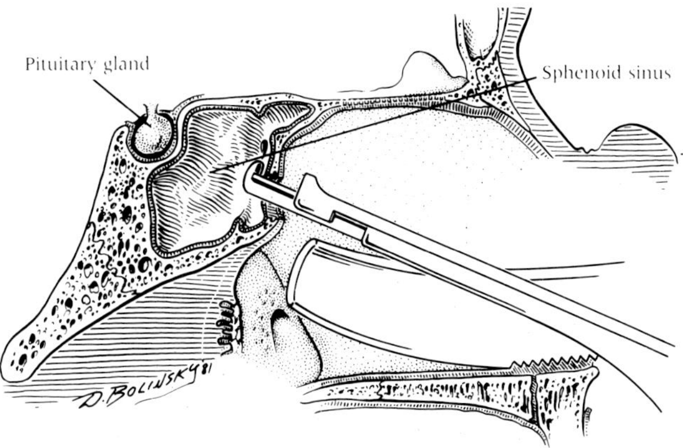

FIG 12–5.
Enlargement of sphenoid using Kerrison rongeurs.

type, in which the sphenoid sinus envelops the anterior and inferior portions of the sella, which can be clearly identified bulging downward from the superior and posterior portion of the sinus. The second most common and less favorable configuration is the presellar (12%). This type consists of a sphenoid that is only partially pneumatized, with cancellous bone obscuring surgical landmarks at the basisphenoid. The least common configuration is the chonchal configuration (3%), where the sphenoid sinus is only rudimentary or is completely absent, with the sella covered with cancellous bone. This type is often encountered in children. These sellar variations underscore the importance of preoperative computed tomography (CT) and on-table videofluoroscopy. The presellar and conchal variants can be safely approached in the sagittal plane by a diamond-tipped air-driven drill under fluoroscopic control.

Common pitfalls in entering the sella are (1) the failure to recognize the midline after sphenoidotomy has been made and (2) variation in the shape of the sellar floor that may direct the surgeon into the anterior cranial fossa superiorly or into the clivus inferiorly. This occurs with a shallow, flat sellar floor that creates an obtuse angle with the posterior wall of the sphenoid sinus. The midline problem can be averted if midline surgical landmarks are carefully identified.[11] In this regard, it is important to note that the intersphenoid septum is on the midline only 53% of the time and is absent in 28% of cases. The sphenoid rostrum and the vomer provide the most reliable midline surgical indicators. The problem of superior or inferior penetration can be ameliorated, again, by the use of sagittal videofluoroscopic views. Often, however, the floor of the sella (normally about 1 mm thick) is obvious. A thick sella floor is present in 18% of cases.[25]

Entry into the sella is achieved by thinning the anterior wall with the air-driven drill in the midline. The opening may be enlarged to 1 to 1.5 cm square dimensions with the 2 mm Kerrison rongeurs. A small-gauge needle is first introduced into the gland to preclude the possibility of a cavernous carotid aneurysm or a tortuous carotid artery. The dura enveloping the hypophysis may then be entered by making a cruciate incision through the anterior dura. Occasionally at this point profuse hemorrhage occurs. This is due to the existence of a venous

plexus called the intercavernous, or circular, sinus, which provides a communication between the cavernous sinuses laterally in 76% of the cases studied. This plexus is embedded in the leaves of the dura and is subject to considerable anatomic variation. It is located anterior to the hypophysis in 9% of the patients who underwent hypophysectomy, existing superior or inferior to the plane of dissection or completely enveloping the gland. Bipolar cautery is often sufficient to seal the leaves of the dura. In a reported series of 38 patients, hemorrhage from the anterior intercavernous sinuses was profuse enough in two patients to abort the hypophysectomy.[26] Also of note with regard to the dural structure of the pituitary is that the pia and arachnoid mater are usually confined to the area of the infundibulum above the diaphragma sellae. Hence, the CSF space is theoretically never penetrated if dissection is limited to the sella, and CSF leakage should not occur. In practice, however, 20% of autopsy specimens had prolapse of arachnoid into the sella,[27] thus providing potential for CSF leakage.

Excision of the adenoma or total hypophysectomy can then proceed according to plan. The most common location for a pituitary microadenoma is superficial, anterior, and inferior. Careful dissection with Angell-James dissectors will free the gland from the anterior and lateral dural sheaths. Suction is set

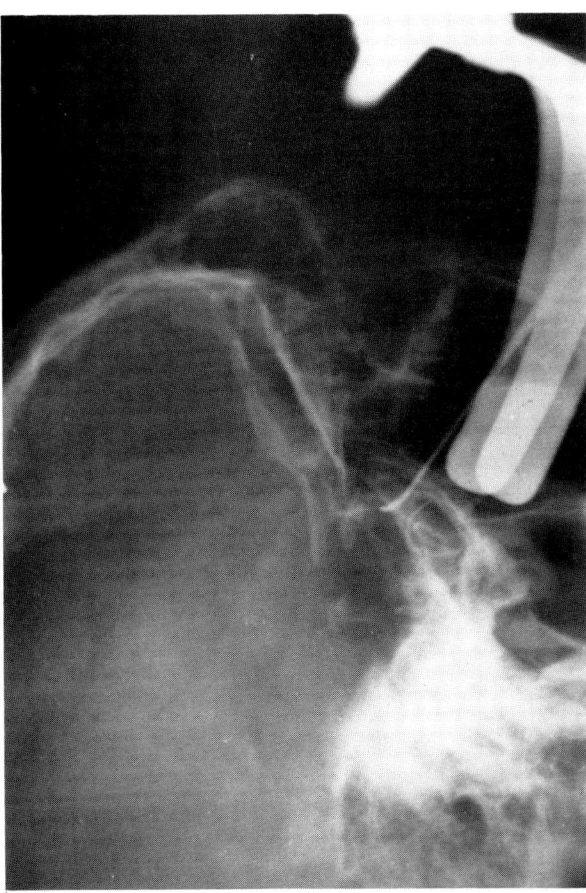

FIG 12–6.
Intraoperative lateral roentgenogram for purposes of reorientation.

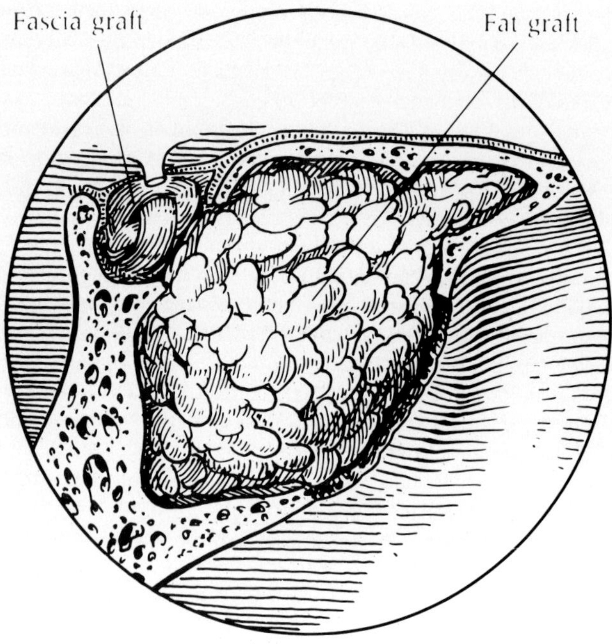

FIG 12–7.
Following removal of tumor, closure is done using fascia lata and fat to fill the empty sella turcica.

at 100 to 120 mm Hg to prevent damage to the normal gland and suprasellar structures.[28] An attempt to elaborate a plane between the gland and the normal tissues is made, unless the tumor is adherent to vascular or suprasellar structures. The anesthesiologist may perform a Valsalva maneuver, or air may be injected via an intrathecal catheter to prolapse the gland into the sella. No traction must be applied to the gland, since damage to the neurons of the neurohypophysis may lead to permanent diabetes insipidus. Similarly, traction may tear suprasellar arterial structures or lead to damage of the optic nerve. In a series of 30 patients, two deaths were attributed to subarachnoid hemorrhage and hemorrhage from the anterior cerebral artery, respectively.[29] The extent of the resection can total 60% to 70% of the adenohypophysis with preservation of normal pituitary function.[28]

Following tumor removal, closure consists of fascia lata and fat to fill the empty sella turcica (Fig 12–7). The sphenoid is also filled with fat and absorbable cellulose sponge. The surgeon removes the Hubbard speculum, and bacitracin-impregnated gauze is packed bilaterally to prevent septal hematoma formation. In general, one length of nasal petrolatum gauze will be necessary for each nasal chamber. The sublabial incision is closed with interrupted 3-0 chromic catgut sutures (Fig 12–8). A standard submucosal resection dressing is then applied. The packing may be removed on the fifth postoperative day.

Carotid Artery

Caution must be exercised along the lateral walls of the sella to avoid encroachment on the cavernous sinus, which contains cranial nerve VI, the cavernous venous plexus, and the internal carotid artery. Imbedded in the lateral wall of the cavernous sinus are cranial nerves III, IV, and VI. The carotid artery follows a very tortuous course through this area, forming an S-shaped curve in both coronal and sagittal planes. At both the entry point to the sinus (foramen lacerum) and the exit point (dural reflection off the anterior clinoid process), the artery is firmly tethered, but in the intervening course, it is unsupported within the sinus.[30, 31] Traction on the cavernous portion of the carotid can therefore cause lacerations in these two areas.

Anatomic studies have described variations in the course of the cavernous carotid artery. The artery may approach as close as 4 mm to the midline in 10% of cases.[27] The average intercarotid distance is 14 mm; however, a wide range of 4 to 23 mm exists. The carotid artery is dehiscent into the sphenoid sinus without bony protection in approximately 4% of cases[23] and in the sella in 6% of cases.[24]

The cavernous carotid artery is therefore at risk in dissections of the sella, particularly in the case of a large adenoma where erosion of the bony landmarks has taken place. A cavernous or paraclinoid carotid artery aneurysm may present as a lesion requiring preoperative bilateral carotid angiography or intraoperative needle aspiration, as discussed earlier, for diagnosis. Pia described no intracavernous aneurysms and only four paraclinoid aneurysms in his series of 450 aneurysms.[32] Nutik[33] described successful clipping of 15 paraclinoid aneurysms in 13 patients utilizing a transcranial approach, with 1 patient sustaining a cerebrovascular accident. Damage to the carotid artery can be circumvented by enucleation of the tumor mass. Baker and Bridges[34] reported an incidence of two cavernous carotid hemorrhages in a series of 18 patients, and Macbeth and Hall[35] reported 1 in a series of 36 patients. Significant mortality and morbidity may be expected as a result of carotid ligation in this area.[36–38]

Only anecdotal reports of intraoperative laceration of the cavernous carotid artery exist. Parkinson and West[39] have described three patients in whom intracavernous carotid artery aneurysms were cross-clamped and the carotid lumens reconstructed. They used a transcranial approach and profound hy-

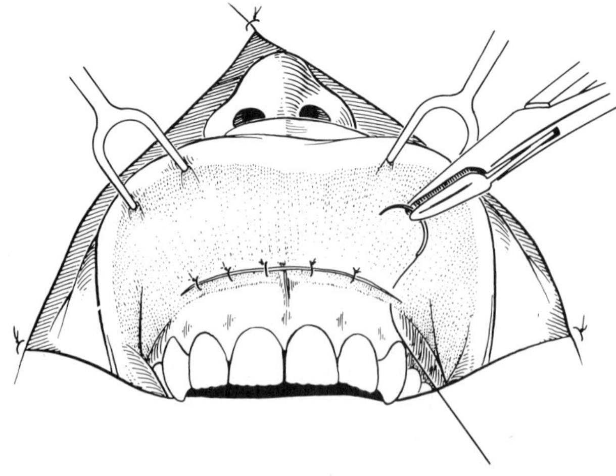

FIG 12–8.
Sublabial incision closed with interrupted 3-0 chromic catgut sutures.

pothermia with temporary circulatory arrest. Even under these ideal circumstances, one of the patients died. From our personal experience, intraoperative carotid laceration can be controlled by pressure, offering the possibility of permanent balloon occlusion for control of hemorrhage. In our institutional experience of more than 500 cases, this complication occurred only once. The patient survived with no neurologic sequelae.

Optic Nerve

The position of the optic nerve and chiasm is relevant in large tumors that extend above the diaphragma sellae. The optic nerves lie encased in the sphenoid bone in canals that diverge posteromedially to anterolaterally and can usually be identified as bulges in the lateral portion of the anterior sellar floor. In 80% of autopsy specimens, the chiasm lies directly superior to the diaphragma sellae.[27] The remainder of specimens are equally divided into chiasms displaced anteriorly over the tuberculum sellae or displaced posteriorly over the dorsum sellae. The dimensions of the diaphragma sellae average 8 mm in length and 11 mm in width.[23] Posteriorly along the diaphragm there is a hiatus for the pituitary stalk that creates an opening greater than 5 mm in approximately 50% of patients. It creates an opening large enough to permit herniation of arachnoid into the sella after removal of the adenoma or after total hypophysectomy. The incidence of ophthalmic complications has been reported as 2 of 345 patients[13] and 2 of 67 patients[12] in transethmoidal-transsphenoidal procedures, compared with 1 in 38 patients[26] in transseptal-transsphenoidal procedures. This rate compares with a 6% to 7% visual loss encountered in the transcranial approach.[40] This, in turn, compares with improvement in visual symptoms (typically bilateral temporal hemianopsia) in 42% to 83% of patients undergoing transcranial resection and 71.7% to 81% of patients undergoing transsphenoidal resection.[41] In our institutional experience of more than 500 cases, no visual complications occurred using the transseptal transsphenoidal approach.

COMPLICATIONS

Empty Sella Syndrome

Empty sella syndrome refers to prolapse or extension of subarachnoid space into the sella. Often this extension causes a flattening of the pituitary gland against the walls of the sella and sometimes expanding the bony confines of the sella itself. It is generally classified into two groups, primary and secondary, according to etiology. The former is used to denote those empty sellae due to defects in the diaphragma sellae, whereas the latter denotes a prolapse of the subarachnoid space into a sella that has been evacuated by surgery, infection and necrosis, or irradiation. Empty sella syndrome is part of the differential diagnosis of enlarged sella turcica that includes neoplasm, aneurysm, arachnoid cyst, granuloma, or chronically increased intracranial pressure.

Primary empty sella syndrome may occur as a result of increased CSF pressure, as encountered in hypertension, congestive heart failure, pseudotumor cerebri, or the pickwickian syndrome. Of interest is the fact that anatomic defects in the diaphragma sellae occur six times more frequently in females than in males.[42-44] Erosion of the sellar floor may establish a communicating sinus between the subarachnoid space and the sphenoid sinus, resulting in CSF rhinorrhea and potential for meningitis.[45] Of note, remodeling of the pituitary gland does not generally result in clinical endocrinopathies.

Secondary empty sella syndrome occurs infrequently as a complication of hypophysectomy, whether surgical, cryologic, or radiologic, and frequently presents with visual field changes due to downward tenting of the chiasm.[46] This is sometimes interpreted as evidence of tumor recurrence because this phenomenon occurs several months to years after treatment. Small, peripheral, and stable visual field defects may be followed conservatively; however, progressive lesions should be aggressively managed. Indications for surgical repair of the empty sella syndrome are basically CSF rhinorrhea with or without attendant meningitis or progressive visual field changes.

The surgical treatment of secondary empty sella syndrome may be similar to the original procedure.[47, 48] In one published series of patients who underwent revision transsphenoidal surgery after prior treatment, 3% had empty sella syndrome. One of these patients presented with visual field changes, and three presented with CSF rhinorrhea. Although these authors found that two thirds of their operative deaths occurred in transsphenoidal surgery following prior therapy (surgery, radiation, or combination) and complications such as visual field changes, cranial nerve damage, and arterial injuries were more frequent, they noted a 60% improvement in visual loss and 70% success in repair of CSF rhinorrhea. In all cases, complications and mortality were higher when the initial procedure was transcranial compared with transsphenoidal.

Cerebrospinal Leak

Cerebrospinal fluid rhinorrhea is a complication of both surgical and radiotherapeutic treatment of pituitary lesions. In a review of 11 series of transsphenoidal hypophysectomies involving 783 patients, the incidence of CSF rhinorrhea was 10.3%, and the incidence of secondary meningitis was 5.4%.[49] Anatomic factors involving the diaphragma sellae, already discussed, may play a role in etiology. The postsurgical knowledge of the patient's anatomy and probable source of CSF leak may simplify subsequent surgical repair. Depending on the clinical situation, a short period of medical therapy may be warranted, but surgical treatment for persistent leak should take place before fibrosis between tissue planes has occurred. If medical management is elected, the patient must remain at bed rest with the head elevated to 20 to 30 degrees. Repair of the fistula may be best accomplished by fascia packing of the sella and fat or muscle packing of the sphenoid sinus. It can be augmented in the case of large CSF leaks by duraplasty with lyophilized cadaveric dura and tissue adhesive. Overpacking of the sella must be avoided because of possible compression of the carotid artery and cranial nerve VI in the cavernous sinus.

Other Complications

Other complications encountered are meningitis, hemorrhage, septal perforation, numbness of the upper incisors, and permanent diabetes insipidus. Although the incidence of meningitis in the pre-1978 series reported by Lee[39] was 5.4%, later series have reduced rates to less than 1%. Probably this reduction is multifactorial, depending on more powerful antibiotics and earlier diagnosis (smaller tumor size at surgery resulting in less frequent penetration of the subarachnoid space) and other factors. Hemorrhage may occur as a result of manipulations of the lateral walls of the cavernous sinus (discussed earlier) or traction or blind manipulation of the suprasellar structures. Strict intraoperative hemostasis is important in prevention of the postoperative complication of subarachnoid hemorrhage and hematoma formation. Septal perforations occur in 1% to 3% of patients and are avoided by conservative septal dissection along recognized anatomic planes. The complication of upper incisor numbness can be reduced by limiting dissection of the pyriform crest bone and thus avoiding the anterosuperior alveolar nerve.[50] Finally, permanent diabetes insipidus may develop in 1% to 2% of cases and can be managed with the use of vasopressin analogues.

CONCLUSION

Much progress has been made in the reduction of the operative mortality of 5.6% in Cushing's early series. This progress has been achieved by the use of antibiotics, the operating microscope, preoperative neuroradiologic evaluation, operative videofluoroscopy, and a more complete knowledge of parasellar anatomy. Similar reductions in the complication rates have been realized. More complete understanding of the physiology of the hypophysis in normal and disease states has expanded the indications for hypophyseal surgery. Mortality rates have now been reduced to less than 2% in several series.[50, 51] These factors in combination have made transseptal transsphenoidal surgery an important component in managing pituitary disease.

REFERENCES

1. Caton R, Paul FT: Notes of a case of acromegaly treated by operation. *Br Med J* 1893; 2:1421–1423.
2. Horsley V: Address in surgery: On the technic of operations on the central nervous system. *Br Med J* 1906; 2:411–423.
3. Giordano: *Comendio Chir Operat Ital* 1897; 2:100.
4. Schloffer H: Erfolgreiche Operation eines Hypophysentumors auf rasadern Wege. *Wien Klin Wochenschr* 1907; 20:621–624.
5. Moszkowicz L: Zur Technik der Operationen an der Hypophyse. *Wien Klin Wochenschr* 1907; 20:792–795.
6. Krause F: Hirnchirurgie (Freilegung der Hypophyse). *Deutsche Klin* 1905; 8:1004.
7. Kanavel AB: Removal of tumors of the pituitary body by an infranasal route. *JAMA* 1909; 53:1704–1707.
8. Halstead AE: Remarks on the operative treatment of tumors of the hypophysis: With a report of two cases operated on by an oronasal method. *Surg Gynecol Obstet* 1910; 10:494–502.
9. Cushing H: *The Pituitary and Its Disorders.* Philadelphia, JB Lippincott Co, 1912, p 300.
10. German WJ, Flanigan S: Pituitary adenomas: A follow-up study of the Cushing series. *Clin Neurosurg* 1962; 10:72–81.
11. Henderson WR: The pituitary adenomata: A follow-up study of the surgical results in 338 cases. *Br J Surg* 1939; 26:811.
12. Kirchner JA, Van Gilder JC: Transethmoidal hypophysectomy. *Trans Am Acad Ophthalmol Otolaryngol* 1975; 80:391–396.
13. James JA: Transethmoidsphenoidal hypophysectomy. *Arch Otolaryngol* 1967; 86:256–264.
14. Kenan PD: The rhinologist and the management of pituitary disease. *Laryngoscope* 1979; 89(suppl 4):1–26.
15. Kern EB, Pearson BW, McDonald TJ, et al: The transeptal approach to lesions of the pituitary and parasellar regions. *Laryngoscope* 1979;89(suppl 15):1–34.
16. Pearson OH, Brodkey JS, Kaufman B: Endocrine evaluation and indication for surgery of functional pituitary adenomas. *Clin Neurosurg* 1974; 21:26–38.
17. Collins WF, Sasaki CT: Transsphenoidal surgery for endocrine-inactive tumors of the pituitary, in Ronsokoff J (ed): *Encyclopedia of Modern Techniques in Surgery.* Mt Kisco, NY, Futura Publishing Co, 1981.
18. Pearson OH: Endocrine treatment of breast cancer. *CA* 1976; 26:165.
19. Chan L, O'Malley BW: Mechanism of action of sex steroid hormones. *N Engl J Med* 1976; 294:1322–1328, 1372–1381, 1430–1437.
20. Schoomes R, Bourke RS, Reynoso G, et al: Hypophysectomy for reactivated disseminated prostatic carcinoma. *S Afr Med J* 1972; 46:1278–1285.
21. Kohner EM, Hamilton AM, Joplin GF, et al: Florid diabetic retinopathy and its response to treatment by photocoagulation or pituitary ablation. *Diabetes* 1976; 25:104–110.
22. Balodimos MC: Treatment of diabetic retinopathy. Pituitary ablation and retinal photocoagulation. *Med Clin North Am* 1971; 55:989–999.
23. Renn WH, Rhoton AL Jr: Microsurgical anatomy of the sellar region. *J. Neurosurg* 1975; 43:288–298.
24. Hardy J, Maira G: Microsurgical anatomy in transsphenoidal hypophysectomy. *J Neurol Sci* 1977; 21:151–157.
25. Rhoton AL Jr, Harris FS, Renn WH: Microsurgical anatomy of the sella region and the cavernous sinus. *Clin Neurosurg* 1977; 24:54–85.
26. Hudson WR, Kenan PD: Transsphenoidal management of pituitary adenomas and other selected lesions of the sella turcica. *Laryngoscope* 1974; 84:1159–1169.
27. Bergland RM, Ray BS, Torack RM: Anatomic variations in the pituitary gland and adjacent structures in 225 human autopsy cases. *J Neurosurg* 1968; 28:93–99.
28. Spencer DD: Resection of pituitary tumors, in Sasaki CT, McCabe B, Kirchner JA (eds): *Surgery of the Skull Base.* Philadelphia, JB Lippincott Co, 1984.
29. Bateman GH: Transsphenoidal hypophysectomy, a review of 70 cases treated in the past two years. *Trans Am Acad Ophthalmol Otolaryngol* 1962; 63:103–110.
30. Parkinson D: Collateral circulation of the cavernous carotid artery: Anatomy. *Am J Surg* 1964; 7:251–268.
31. Parkinson D: A surgical approach to the cavernous por-

tion of the carotid artery. Anatomical studies and case report. *J Neurosurg* 1965; 23:474–493.

32. Pia HW: Classification of aneurysms of the internal carotid system. *Acta Neurochir* (Wien) 1978; 40:5–31.

33. Nutik SL: Ventral paraclinoid carotid aneurysms. *J Neurosurg* 1988; 69:340–344.

34. Baker DC, Bridges TJ: Transantrotrosphenoidal hypophysectomy. *Trans Am Acad Ophthalmol Otolaryngol* 1964; 68:60–64.

35. MacBeth R, Hall M: Hypophysectomy as a rhinological procedure. *Arch Otolaryngol* 1962; 75:440–450.

36. Lombardi G, Passerini A, Migliavacca F: Intracavernous lesions of the internal carotid artery. *AJR* 1963; 89:361–371.

37. McKinney J, Acree T, Soltz SE: Syndrome of unruptured aneurysm of the intracranial portion of the internal carotid artery. *Bull Neurol Inst NY* 1936; 5:247–277.

38. Wilson CB, Myers FK: Bilateral saccular aneurysms of the internal carotid artery in the cavernous sinus. *J Neurol Neurosurg Psychiatry* 1963; 26:174–177.

39. Parkinson D, West M: Lesions of the cavernous plexus region, in Youmans JR (ed): *Neurological Surgery*. Philadelphia, WB Saunders Co, 1982, pp 3004–3023.

40. Landolt AM, Wilson CB: Tumors of the sella and parasellar areas in adults, in Youmans JR (ed): *Neurological Surgery*. Philadelphia, WB Saunders Co, 1982, pp 3107–3162.

41. Laws ER, Trautman JC, Hollenhorst RW: Transsphenoidal decompression of the optic nerve and chiasm. *J Neurosurg* 1977; 46:717–722.

42. Kaufman B, Chamberlain WB Jr: The ubiquitous "empty" sella turcica. *Acta Radiol (Diagn) (Stockh)* 1972; 13:413–425.

43. Neelon FA, Goree JA, Lebovitz HE: The primary empty sella, clinical and radiographic characteristics and endocrine function, *Medicine (Baltimore)* 1973; 52:73–92.

44. Jordan RM, Kendall JW, Kerber CW: The primary empty sella syndrome: Analysis of the clinical characteristics, radiographic features, pituitary function, and cerebrospinal fluid adenohypophyseal hormone concentrations, *Am J Med* 1977; 62:569–580.

45. Weiss MH, Kaufman B, Richards DE: Cerebrospinal fluid rhinorrhea from an empty sella. Transsphenoidal obliteration of the fistula: Technical note. *J Neurosurg* 1973; 39:674–676.

46. Lee WM, Adams JE: The empty sella syndrome. *J Neurosurg* 1968; 28:351–356.

47. Laws ER Jr, Keen EB: Complications of transsphenoidal surgery. *Clin Neurosurg* 1976; 23:401–416.

48. Laws ER Jr, Fode NC, Richmond MJ: Transsphenoidal surgery following unsuccessful prior therapy. *J Neurosurg* 1985; 63:823–829.

49. Lee KJ: The sublabial transseptal transsphenoidal approach to the hypophysis. *Laryngoscope* 1978; 88(suppl 7):1–65.

50. Sasaki CT: Transseptal transsphenoidal approach to the sella, in Sasaki CT, McCabe B, Kirchner JA (eds): *Surgery of the Skull Base*. Philadelphia, JB Lippincott Co, 1984, pp 79–93.

51. Kern EB: Transnasal pituitary surgery. *Arch Otolaryngol* 1981; 107:183.

Pituitary Tumors

Approach of

Jonas T. Johnson, M.D.

and

Ellen Tabor, M.D.

The otolaryngologist is ideally suited to perform transnasal surgery on the sphenoid sinus. The indication most commonly encountered is a request by a neurosurgical colleague to assist in the transnasal exposure of the sella turcica. This approach has been demonstrated to be a direct, safe, and rapid approach to the pituitary gland. Less commonly, acute and chronic inflammatory lesions or neoplastic changes may require access to the sphenoid to afford specimens for both bacteriologic and histologic evaluation as well as to effect drainage.

TABLE 12–1.
Differential Diagnoses of Sellar and Parasellar Lesions*

Chromophobe adenoma (80% of pituitary adenomas)
Eosinophilic adenoma (15% of pituitary adenomas)
Basophilic adenoma (5% of pituitary adenomas)
Craniopharyngioma
Aneurysm of the internal carotid artery
Empty sella syndrome
Metastatic tumors
Optic and/or hypothalamus glioma
Hamartoma of the hypothalamus
Ectopic pinealoma, teratoma, dermoid, epidermoid
Meningioma
Prepontine lesions (chordoma)
Mucocele of the sphenoid sinus
Sellar abscess secondary to sphenoiditis
Fibrous dysplasia
Granulomatous disease
Bony tumors of the sphenoid
Rathke's cleft cyst
Arachnoid cyst
Schwannoma associated with cranial nerves II–VI

*From Lee KJ: The sublabial transseptal transsphenoidal approach to the hypopharynx. *Laryngoscope* 1978; 88 (suppl 10): 1–65. Used by permission.

INDICATIONS

Pituitary surgery may be performed for removal of pituitary tumors or to palliate patients with metastatic breast or prostate carcinoma, and it has been recommended for the control of diabetic retinopathy. In addition, transsphenoid pituitary surgery may be indicated for patients with symptomatic empty sella syndrome.

Chromophobe adenoma is the most common type of pituitary tumor, constituting 10% of all intracranial tumors.[1] The chromophobe adenoma is not hormonally active; however, tumor expansion may compromise other pituitary functions with resultant endocrine dysfunction. Encroachment by tumor on the optic chiasm causes bitemporal hemianopsia. A multitude of other conditions may affect the sellar region (Table 12–1). The details of the diagnostic evaluation of patients with these various endocrinologic tumors is beyond the scope of this chapter.

The most common nontumorous cause of sellar enlargement is the empty sella syndrome.[2] Normally, the sella turcica is completely filled by the pituitary gland. The sellar diaphragm attaches to the tuberculum sellae anteriorly and to the clinoid processes posteriorly. It is intact with the exception of a midline opening through which the pituitary stalk passes. The diaphragm prevents CSF from entering the sella.

A defect in the diaphragm may result in prolapse of the subarachnoid space through the diaphragm into the sella (Figs 12–9 and 12–10). Alternatively, this condition may develop subsequent to pituitary surgery or irradiation therapy of a pituitary tumor. A defect in the diaphragm may then allow the subarachnoid space to herniate into the sella. In either case, gradual expansion of the sella occurs as the CSF-filled pulsatile mass compresses residual pituitary gland.

In rare instances, erosion of the floor of the sphenoid sinus may occur, which may result in CSF rhinorrhea. Visual defects may be an indication that the optic chiasm has prolapsed into

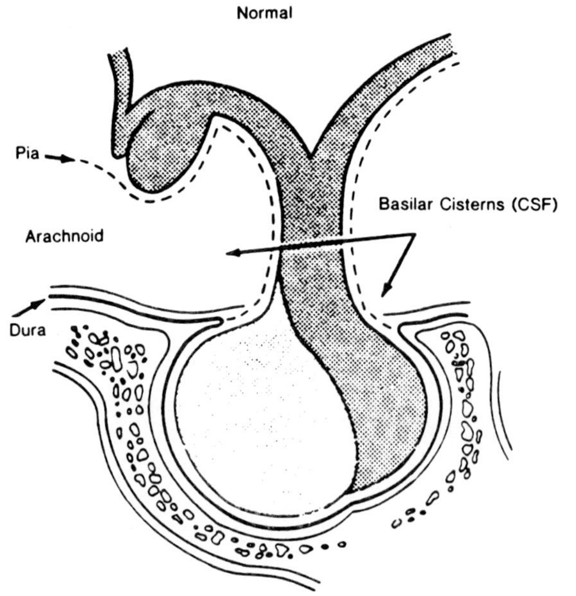

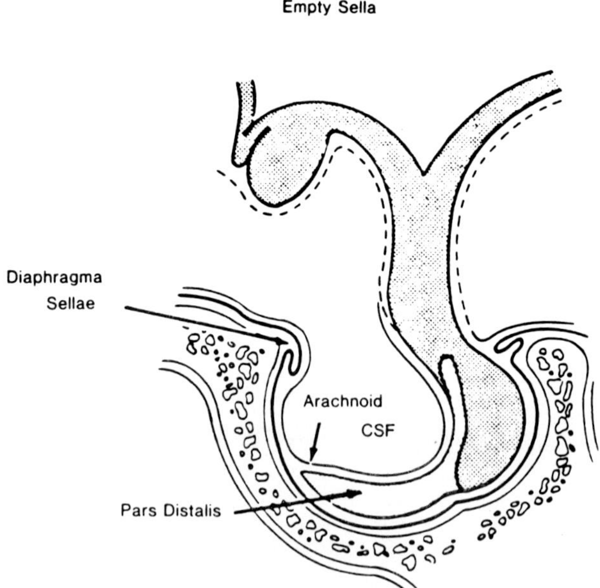

FIG 12–9.
The normal relationship of the meninges to the pituitary gland *(left)* in empty sella syndrome *(right)*. Herniation of the arachnoid membrane through the diaphragma sellae allows CSF to compress the pituitary. (From Browne JD, Kohut RI: Headache and the primary empty sella syndrome. *Arch Otolaryngol Head Neck Surg* 1986; 112:883–885. Used by permission.)

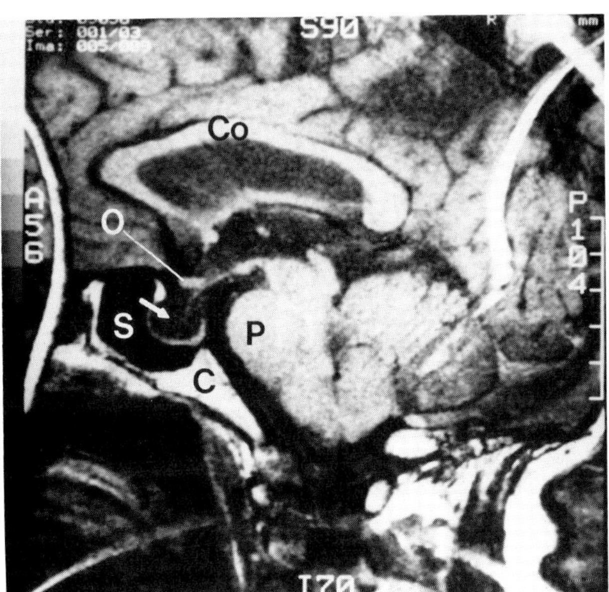

FIG 12–10.
Empty sella. Sagittal T_1-weighted magnetic resonance image (MRI) shows CSF herniating into the sella turcica *(arrow)*. The CSF gives intermediate signal intensity. The air in the sphenoid sinus *(S)* is black (no signal). Fat within the marrow space of the clivus *(C)* is white. *O* = optic chiasm; *P* = pons; *Co* = corpus callosum.

the empty sella, with resultant visual field defects. It, however, rarely occurs. Headache has been reportedly associated with empty sella syndrome, but many patients with this condition do not have headache.[2] In general, patients with idiopathic empty sella syndrome do not have endocrine abnormalities. Uncomplicated, the empty sella syndrome requires no treatment. However, CSF rhinorrhea and disturbance of vision are indications for surgery.

Choice of Technique

Transnasal exposure of the sphenoid sinus may be accomplished along the midline transseptal route, laterally via the transethmoid route, or obliquely via the transantral route. In our experience, the latter transantral route is seldom indicated.

The procedure most commonly employed today is the midline transnasal approach to the sphenoid sinus. When sphenoid sinus surgery is undertaken for removal of pituitary tumors, the procedure is most often performed in corroboration with a neurosurgeon.

The transseptal-transsphenoid approach to the pituitary gland offers a safe, rapid midline access to the sellar region. This operation is an extension of the maxilla-premaxilla-septal procedure commonly undertaken by rhinologists today. Avoidance of a facial incision with preservation of the nasal spine, septal cartilage, and mucosa results in maintenance of both cosmesis and function. The risk of injury to the brain, optic nerve, or major vascular structures is low, and craniotomy can be avoided. Transseptal sphenoidotomy is limited due to the deep and narrow operating field and the possibility of postoperative CSF rhinorrhea.

Transethmoid sphenoidotomy has been espoused by some as a technique of choice for pituitary surgery because it affords a shorter route to the sella, allowing the operator to place the instruments transnasally while observing them through the transethmoid exposure.[3] This approach has the advantage of avoiding the risk of nasal or septal perforation, especially in patients who have had prior transseptal procedures. Contamination from the oral cavity is avoided, and devitalization of the teeth is not a factor.

The disadvantage of the transethmoid procedure is clearly related to the oblique approach, which increases the opportunity for the operator to become disoriented. Access to pituitary tumors with suprasellar extension is also compromised by this oblique approach. The transethmoid procedure requires an external scar. The procedure should not be used in cases in which there is underpneumatization of the sphenoid sinus.

When chronic polypoid degeneration of the paranasal sinus mucosa requires surgical therapy, transethmoid sphenoidotomy is a safe and effective means to improve the nasal airway, irradicate diseased mucosa, and afford satisfactory drainage. The transethmoid approach offers the advantage of exenteration of the ethmoid sinuses in conjunction with sphenoidotomy. This, however, is a relative contraindication for the transethmoid approach when pituitary surgery is contemplated. As in other forms of transnasal sphenoidotomy, every attempt should be made to clear up the sinus infection prior to the intracranial procedure.

Preoperative Assessment

Preoperative evaluation includes careful nasal and sinus history and physical examination. Active infection in the sinonasal tract is a relative contraindication to transnasal pituitary surgery. Infection should be treated and resolved prior to sphenoidotomy. Prior transseptal sphenoidotomy makes a secondary procedure more difficult inasmuch as elevation of mucoperichondrial flaps is frequently complicated by adhesions, and septal perforation may occur. Under these circumstances, some consideration should be given to transethmoid sphenoidotomy, which affords an alternative direct route.

Preoperative evaluation should include CT or magnetic resonance imaging (MRI) to afford the operator a clear understanding of the patient's intranasal, sphenoid, and sellar anatomy. Preoperative radiographic evaluation greatly enhances our understanding of individual anatomic variability and can improve our ability to undertake sphenoid surgery without undue risk. The intrasinus septum is off the midline in nearly 50% of patients.[4] Therefore, correlation with imaging techniques is a must prior to sphenoid surgery (Fig 12–11). The cavernous sinuses are lateral to the sella and sphenoid sinus and contain cranial nerves III, IV, V, and VI and the internal carotid artery (Figs 12–12 and 12–13). The optic nerves, carotid arteries, and the maxillary branches of the trigeminal nerve produce bulges on the lateral wall of the sphenoid sinus.

In a study of cadaveric specimens, Fujii et al. noted that the optic canals protrude into the superolateral part of the sphenoid sinus in greater than 90% of cases (Fig 12–14).[5] Complete bony dehiscence was noted in 4% of optic nerves that

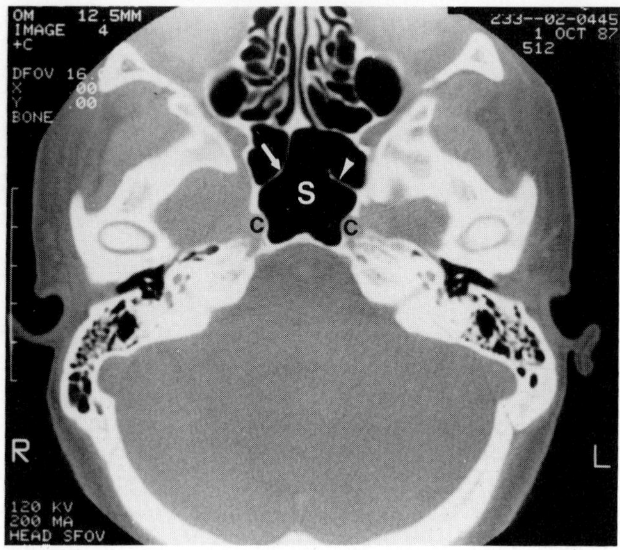

FIG 12–11.
Bony algorithm on an axial CT slice shows the intrasinus septum *(arrow)* on the right dividing the sphenoid *(S)* asymmetrically. There is a partial septation on the left (arrowhead). *C* = internal carotid artery.

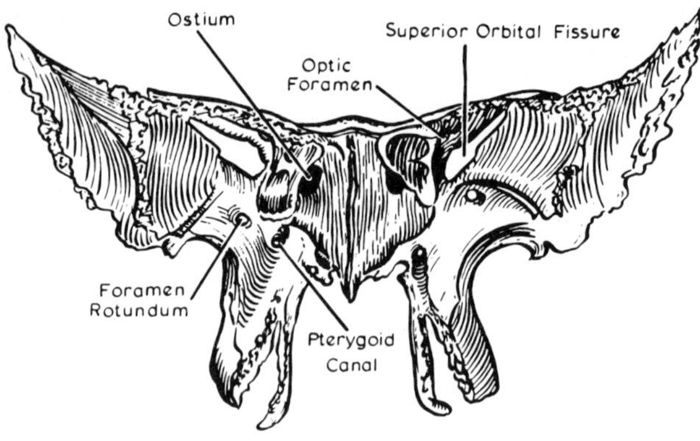

FIG 12–12.
Anterior of sphenoid bone demonstrating relationship of sphenoid ostium to major skull base foramen. (From Lee KJ: The sublabial transseptal transsphenoidal approach to the hypophysis. *Laryngoscope* 1978; 88(suppl 10):1–65. Used by permission.)

were covered by only the optic sheath and sinus mucosa. In 78% of cases, less than 0.5 mm thickness of bone separated the nerve from the sinus. Similarly, the carotid artery produces a prominent bulge in the lateral wall of the sphenoid sinus in greater than 90% of cases. Once again, Fujii et al. note that 8% of cases demonstrated no bone overlying the carotid artery.[5] The carotid artery passes within 4 mm of the midline in approximately 10% of cases (Fig 12–15). The maxillary branch of the trigeminal nerve bulges into the inferolateral part of the sphenoid sinus commonly. This nerve may be covered with an extremely thin portion of sphenoid bone or may be completely dehiscent as well.

Hamberger et al. report that in 11% of cases, only the presellar sphenoid is pneumatized and no pituitary bulge can be noted within the sphenoid sinus (Fig 12–16).[6] Another 3% of patients have only conchal pneumatization in which there is a thick bone between the sinus and sella (Fig 12–17). This situation is a relative contraindication to the transsphenoid procedure; however, some authors describe sellar drill out using video fluoroscopic control.[7]

OPERATIVE TECHNIQUE

Transseptal Sphenoidotomy

The patient is positioned in the supine position on the

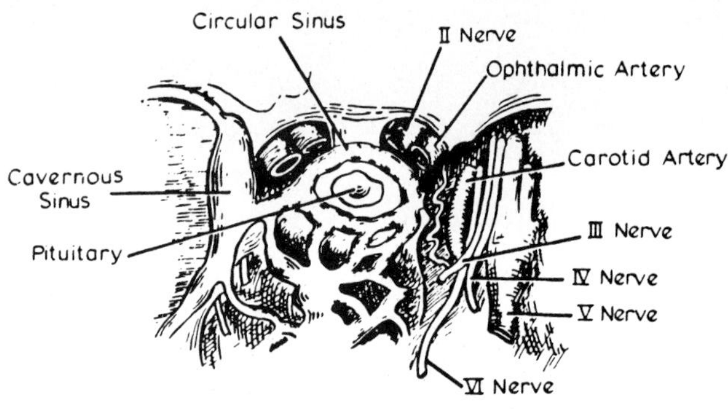

FIG 12–13.
Schematic of the sellar area demonstrating important anatomic relationships. (From Lee KJ: The sublabial transseptal transsphenoidal approach to the hypophysis. *Laryngoscope* 1978; 88(suppl 10):1–65. Used by permission.)

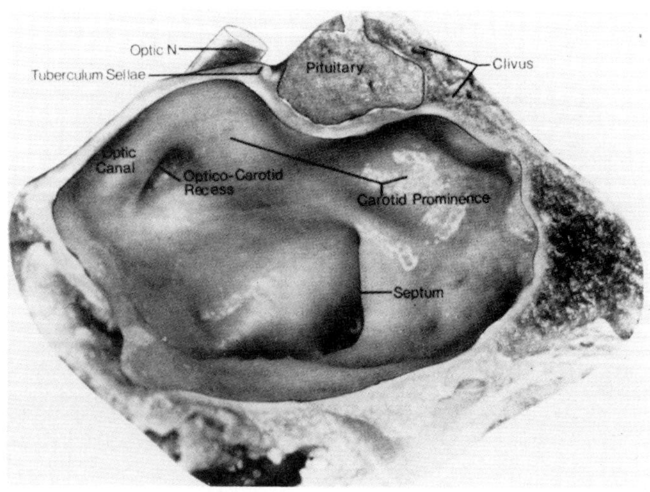

FIG 12–14.
Dissection of the lateral wall of the right side of the sphenoid sinus and sella in a midsagittal plane. Note the bulging of the optic canal and carotid artery in the cavernous sinus. (From Fujii K, Chambers SM, Rhoton AL Jr: Neurovascular relationships of the sphenoid sinus: A microsurgical study. *J Neurosurg* 1979; 50:31–39. Used by permission.)

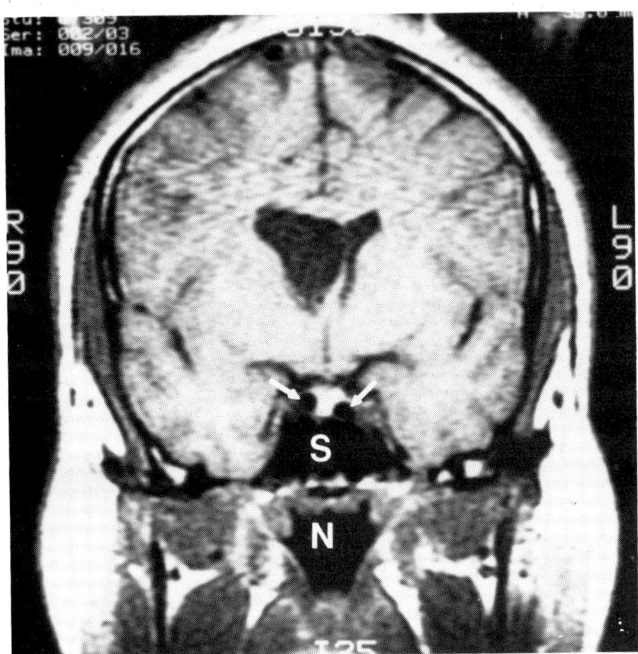

FIG 12–15.
Coronal T₁-weighted MRI demonstrates the intercarotid artery distance is approximately 4 mm. The centimeter scale is on the right side of the scan slice. The carotid arteries *(arrows)* are black (no signal). *S* = sphenoid sinus; *N* = nasopharynx.

operating table, following which general endotracheal anesthesia is undertaken. The patient is subsequently placed in a Mayfield skull clamp, and the head is turned approximately 30 degrees toward the surgeon situated on the right side. The field is then prepped and draped. When a pituitary procedure is anticipated, a separate abdominal or thigh area should be prepped and draped for harvesting of fat and fascia to be used for sinus obliteration at the completion of the case. Some authors have indicated that adipose may be safely harvested from abdominal procedures being undertaken in adjacent operating rooms from other patients; however, the advisability of this practice must be questioned in view of current guidelines for prevention of transmittable disease.

The nose is subsequently topically cocainized employing 200 mg of cocaine solubilized in 8 to 10 mL of normal saline solution. Cotton pledgets are soaked and subsequently wrung out, following which they are carefully placed in the nose to afford complete nasal vasoconstriction. When septal deviation limits access to the nasal cavity, the anterior nose may be vasoconstricted preliminarily, following which a pledget can be introduced into the sphenoethmoid recess. The mucoperiosteum of the nasal septum is then infiltrated with 1% lidocaine with epinephrine 1:100,000 to facilitate subperichondrial dissection. Effective vasoconstriction requires 5 to 10 minutes.

A hemitransfixion incision is developed on the left side. Submucoperichondrial, submucoperiosteal dissection is then carried back along the nasal septum, emphasizing the technique

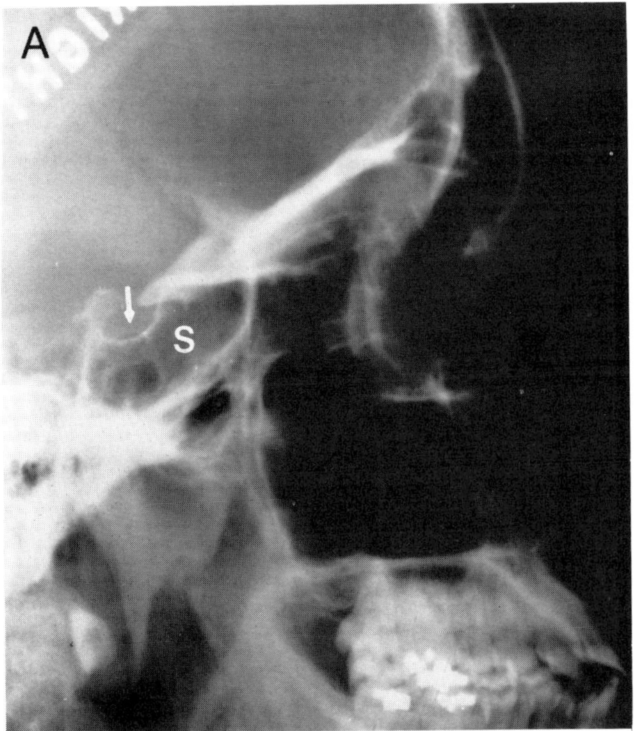
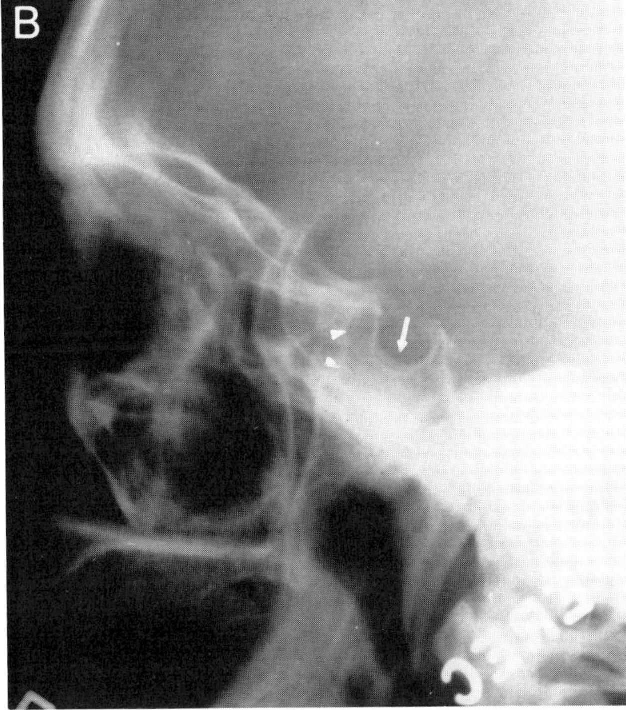

FIG 12–16.
Sphenoid sinus pneumatization. **A,** lateral plain film of the sinuses demonstrates a well-pneumatized sphenoid *(S).* **B,** conchal pneumatization results in bone separating the pneumatized sinus anteriorly from the sella *(arrow).* Arrowheads demonstrate the posterior margin of the sphenoid.

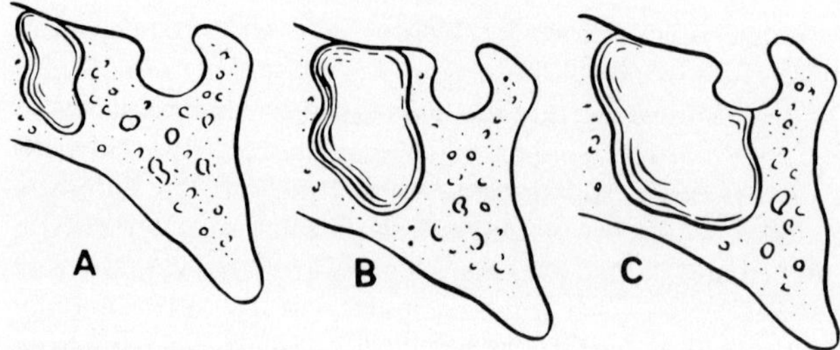

FIG 12–17.
Schematic representation of variable sphenoid aeration. *A*, conchal; *B*, presellar; *C*, sellar. (From Lee KJ: The sublabial transseptal trans-sphenoidal approach to the hypophysis. *Laryngoscope* 1978; 88(suppl 10):1–65. Used by permission.)

familiar to rhinologists known as the maxilla-premaxilla approach. Dissection is carried from the nasal dorsum to the maxillary crest. Inferior tunnels are elevated bilaterally. This requires that the mucoperiosteum of the floor of the nose be gently elevated posteriorly. Desiccating fibers of the nasal septum are carefully separated from the maxillary crest employing sharp and blunt dissection, with care taken to avoid septal perforation. The quadrangular cartilage is then separated from the maxillary crest by carefully scoring the cartilage as it attaches to the maxillary crest. A narrow (1 to 2 mm) strip of quadrangular cartilage left attached to the maxillary crest is dissected free and removed. The quadrangular cartilage is separated from the ethmoid bone posteriorly, and the composite quadrangular cartilage-mucosal septal flap is reflected to the right to afford more complete exposure of the midline perpendicular plate of the ethmoid and vomer, which are dissected out as the mucoperiosteum is elevated bilaterally.

Ethmoid and vomer are removed posteriorly to the face of the sphenoid. The superiormost ethmoid bone should be cut sharply with rongeurs to avoid unnecessary torque on the cribriform plate. Subsequently, the ethmoid plate should be removed in as large a piece as possible so it can be used for reconstruction of the sphenoid or replaced in the perichondrial pocket at the completion of the procedure. When the face of the sphenoid is encountered, mucoperiosteum is reflected laterally on either side, affording visualization of the sinus ostium. The middle turbinates may be out-fractured to facilitate exposure.

At this point, the lip is retracted superiorly, and a sublabial incision is made from canine to canine and connected to the intraseptal envelope with elevation of the mucoperiosteum. The piriform aperture is widened with rongeurs to afford improved exposure. If a prominent nasal spine compromises visibility, it may be narrowed without creating postoperative deformity; however, its removal is unnecessary and should be avoided. Following removal of the perpendicular plate of the ethmoid and vomer back to the face of the sphenoid, a self-retaining retractor is inserted and opened (Figs 12–18 and 12–19). The position of the retractor is confirmed under fluoroscopic control.

Under most circumstances, the sphenoid can be entered directly with gentle palpation of the sphenoid ostium employing a blunt elevator. The opening is then enlarged with pituitary forceps or Kerrison punch rongeurs. The sphenoid septum is identified and removed, as is the sphenoid sinus mucosa.

When one is operating for pituitary tumors, the sella turcica is opened using a sella punch. Dura is coagulated with electrocautery and then incised. This maneuver and the subsequent hypophysectomy are undertaken by the neurosurgeon.

At the completion of pituitary tumor removal, the sella is

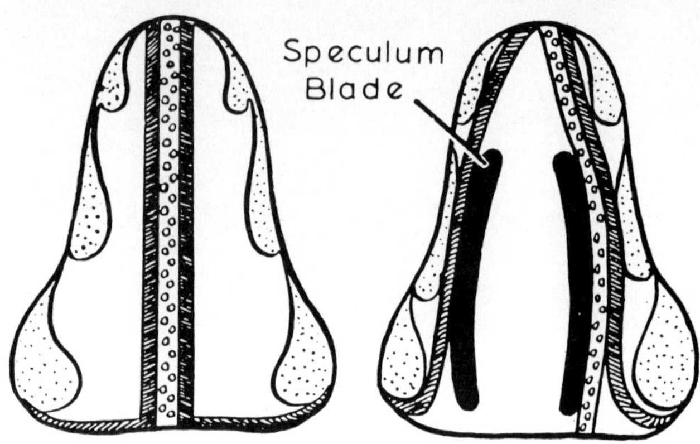

FIG 12–18.
The mucoperichondrial flap is elevated unilaterally, allowing displacement of the quadrangular cartilage with the self-retaining retractor. (From Lee KJ: The sublabial transseptal transsphenoidal approach to the hypophysis. *Laryngoscope* 1978; 88(suppl 10):1–65. Used by permission.)

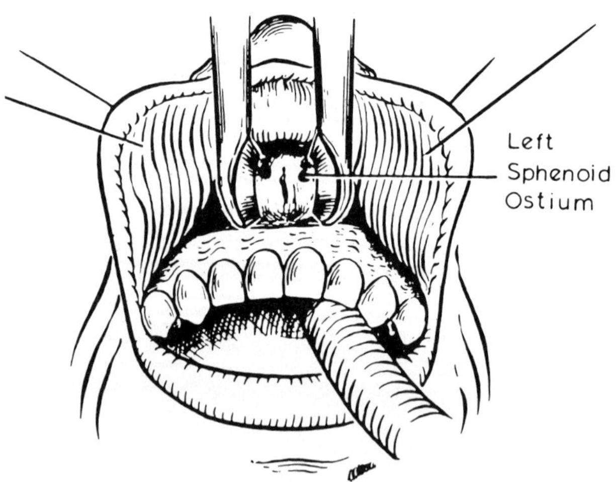

FIG 12–19.
Surgical exposure with self-retaining retractor is demonstrated here. (From Lee KJ: The sublabial transseptal transsphenoidal approach to the hypophysis. *Laryngoscope* 1978; 88(Suppl 10):1–65. Used by permission.)

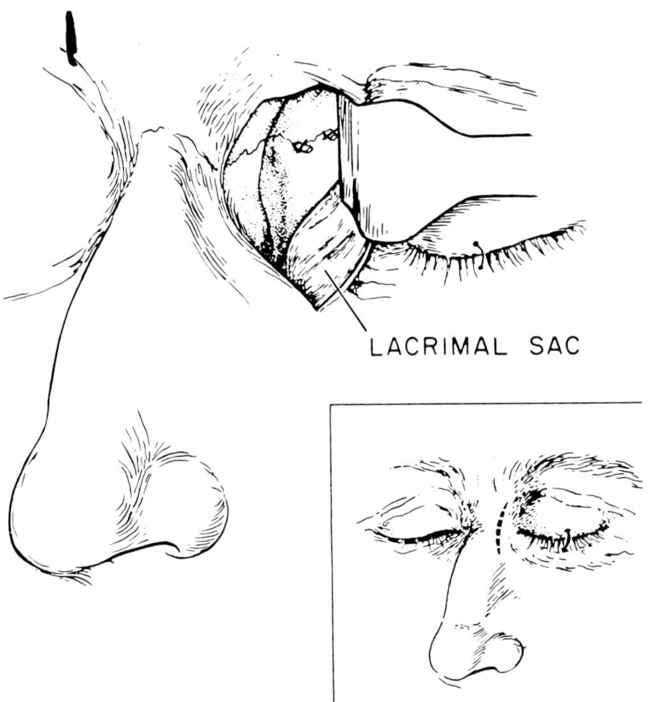

FIG 12–20.
A curvilinear incision is employed to allow elevation of the medial periorbitum with subsequent ligation of the anterior and posterior ethmoid arteries. (From Schmidek HH, Sweet WH (eds): *Operative Neurosurgical Techniques.* New York, Grune & Stratton, 1982. Used by permission.)

packed with adipose tissue. It frequently is possible to employ a strut of septal cartilage to wedge into the residual sella, forming a firm floor for the adipose pack. The sphenoid sinus is then packed with a second piece of adipose tissue, once again held in place with a cartilaginous strut. Some divergence of opinion exists concerning obliteration of the sella and sphenoid. Many authors recommend muscle,[7–9] whereas others achieve similar results with adipose tissue.[3, 4, 10, 11]

The nasal septal mucoperiosteal flaps are then returned to their anatomic position. Replacement of the residual perpendicular plate of the ethmoid may facilitate reoperation should it be necessary. If septal perforation has occurred, the laceration should be repaired with chromic sutures on mini-Keith needles. The caudal nasal septum is fixed to the anterior nasal spine with absorbable suture. The sublabial incision is loosely closed with interrupted chromic suture. The hemitransfixion incision is then closed with interrupted 4-0 chromic suture.

Silicone rubber (Silastic) or plastic sheets are employed to fashion nasal septal splints held in place with a single 2-0 silk suture passed through and through. These septal splints tend to compress and coapt the mucoperichondrial flaps, reducing the risk for postoperative hematoma and decreasing postoperative edema. The nasal cavities are then packed bilaterally with gauze impregnated with antibacterial ointment. The

packing is left in place for 5 days; the nasal splints are routinely maintained 10 to 14 days.

In 1979, Kern et al. reviewed their experience with more than 500 transseptal transsphenoidal hypophysectomies.[8] Intraoperative mortality of 1.39% was encountered. Deaths were associated with meningitis, carotid vascular occlusion, intracranial hemorrhage, and injury to the hypothalamus.

Kern et al. stress that CSF leakage in the postoperative period is best treated by early reexploration.[8] This allows repacking of the sella and sphenoid with allograph tissue. Operative complications included postoperative visual decrease, subarachnoid hemorrhage, transient oculomotor injury, meningitis, nasal-septal perforation, CSF rhinorrhea, and permanent diabetes insipidus. Each of these complications occurred in less than 2% of cases.

Romanowski et al. reviewed 98 patients undergoing transsphenoidal hypophysectomy.[12] Meningitis developed in 6%. Sixty four of these patients had received prophylactic antibiotics, in whom 5 (7.8%) developed meningitis. In contrast, meningitis developed in only 1 of 34 patients (2.9%) who did not receive perioperative antibiotics. The risk of postoperative meningitis is increased with CSF leakage.

Transethmoid Sphenoidotomy

Following induction of general endotracheal anesthesia, the patient is prepped and draped to expose the upper two thirds of the face. The head is placed in a Mayfield headholder and elevated approximately 20 degrees. The eyes are protected with either a tarsorrhaphy suture or plastic eye shields. The area of incision, approximately midway between the dorsum of the nose and the medial canthus, is infiltrated with 1% lidocaine with epinephrine 1:100,000. The incision is then begun approximately 1 cm superior to the medial canthus and carried inferiorly to a total length of 3 cm (Fig 12–20). The medial palpebral ligament is elevated with the periosteum over the anterior lacrimal crest. The lacrimal sac is retracted laterally, and the periosteum of the lamina papyracea is elevated gently and retracted laterally. The anterior and posterior ethmoid arteries are then subsequently identified, clipped, and ligated as they are identified in the frontoethmoid suture line. Care is taken to mark this area such that no bony resection is carried superior to the frontoethmoidal suture line inasmuch as this may result in inadvertent entry into the anterior cranial fossa.

The posterior ethmoid artery is the posterior limit of dissection of the ethmoid. The optic foramen is 4 to 7 mm posterior to the posterior ethmoid artery. This artery also traverses the roof of the posterior ethmoid cell, thereby allowing the operator to identify the posterior ethmoid cell. The posterior wall of the ethmoid cell is, in fact, the anterior wall of the sphenoid sinus.

The lamina papyracea is taken down beginning first in the lacrimal fossa (Fig 12–21). The dissection is then extended to the posterior ethmoid cell. An incision is made through the lateral nasal mucosa, and the middle turbinate is identified. The middle turbinate is removed, as is the entire ethmoid mucosa to the posterior ethmoid cell. The sphenoid ostium is then

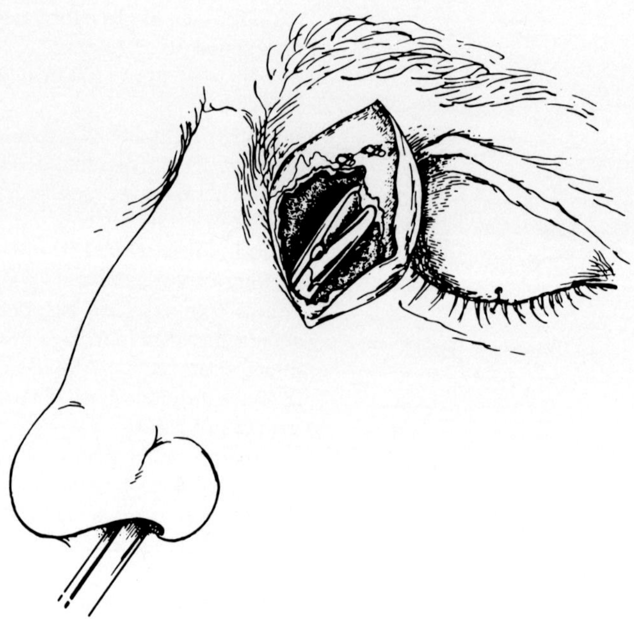

FIG 12–21.
The ethmoid air cells are removed transnasally under direct visualization from the external ethmoidectomy exposure. (From Schmidek HH, Sweet WH (eds): *Operative Neurosurgical Techniques.* New York, Grune & Stratton, 1982. Used by permission.)

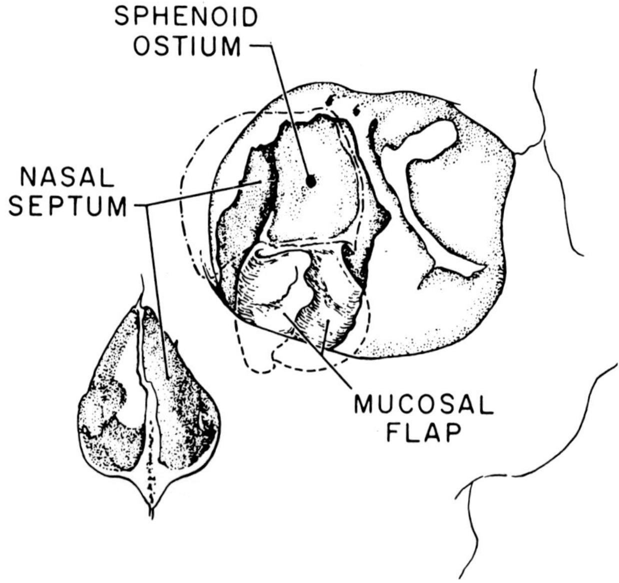

FIG 12–22.
The nasal-septal mucosal flap, based inferiorly, is reflected down allowing exposure of the sphenoid ostium. (From Schmidek HH, Sweet WH (eds): *Operative Neurosurgical Techniques.* New York, Grune & Stratton, 1982. Used by permission.)

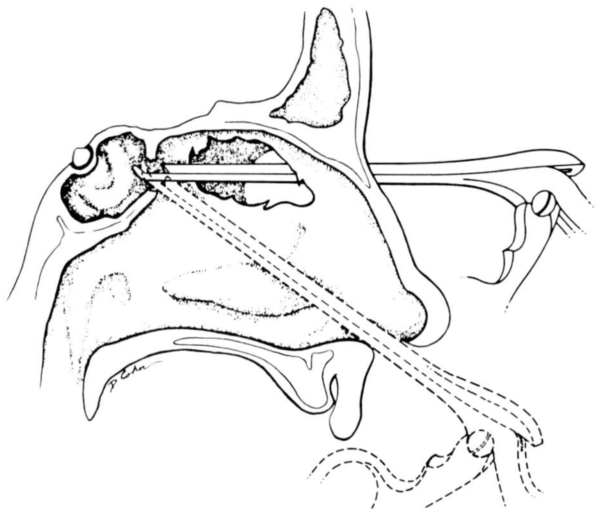

FIG 12–23.
Surgical instruments can be passed either through the ethmoidectomy defect or transnasally, thereby allowing the surgeon a better view of the work area. (From Schmidek HH, Sweet WH (eds): *Operative Neurosurgical Techniques.* New York, Grune & Stratton, 1982. Used by permission.)

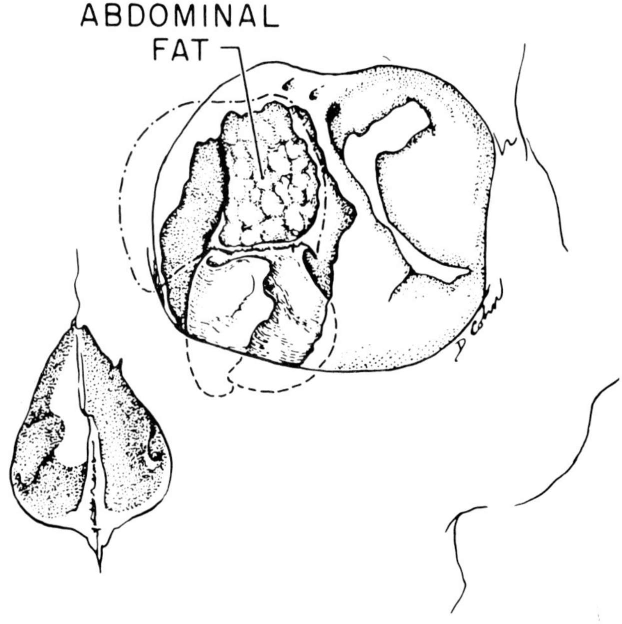

FIG 12–24.
Abdominal fat is used to obliterate the sphenoid sinus, following which the mucosal flap is repositioned and the nasal cavity packed. (From Schmidek HH, Sweet WH (eds): *Operative Neurosurgical Techniques.* New York, Grune & Stratton, 1982. Used by permission.)

identified on the anterior wall of the sphenoid sinus and its position corroborated by fluoroscopy (Fig 12–22). From this point on, instruments are passed through the nares as the surgeon observes through the ethmoidectomy defect (Fig 12–23). The anterior wall of the sphenoid is taken down, and the internal anatomy of the sphenoid sinus identified much as one identifies this anatomy following a transseptal sphenoidotomy. Medial projection of the carotid canals may be visualized and should not be confused with the sella. Aspiration with a thin needle has been advocated when doubt arises.

During transethmoidal sphenoidotomy, the midline can be localized by passing an instrument through the nose along the nasal septum into the sphenoid. One must remember that the sphenoid septum does not necessarily represent the midline and is of no value in identifying the midline without prior radiographic confirmation.

Following completion of the pituitary surgery, the sella is obliterated with abdominal fat, the sphenoid is obliterated with fat, and nasal packing is employed similar to that following transseptal surgery (Fig 12–24). The intercanthal incision is closed in two layers, care being taken to approximate the medial palpebral ligament to the periosteum of the nasal bone.

COMPLICATIONS

Transnasal sphenoidotomy carries with it certain risks. By virtue of the nature of the procedure undertaken in a deeply seated sinus, anatomic disorientation carries with it the risk of injury to numerous vital structures in the immediate area. The most important includes injury to the optic nerve by inappropriate dissection of the superolateral aspect of the posterior ethmoid cell or sphenoid sinus. Injury to the optic chiasm can occur by carrying dissection too far superiorly through the roof of the sphenoid or if the chiasm has prolapsed into the sella, as in the empty sella syndrome. Injury to the carotid artery may occur as it traverses the lateral wall of the sphenoid sinus. Recall that in some cases, the intercarotid distance may be 4 mm. Careful preoperative evaluation of the radiographic studies will help the operator to recognize anatomic variants and prepare accordingly.[13]

Intranasal complications may occur as a result of the surgical approach chosen for access to the sphenoid sinus. The transseptal sphenoidotomy is most commonly associated with nasal septal perforation. When the sublabial approach is employed, devitalization of the teeth commonly occurs. Overzealous resection of quadrangular cartilage may be associated with saddle deformity of the nose. However, preservation of the quadrangular cartilage as previously described will avoid this complication.

Transethmoid sphenoidotomy may result in inadvertent injury to the lacrimal system or perforation of the periorbital tissues. This, in turn, may result in retrobulbar hematoma and, potentially, blindness. Gentle handling of tissues and careful attention to the anatomic landmarks will result in avoidance of

undue risks to the optic nerve or inadvertent violation of the fovea ethmoidalis. With either technique, nasal synechiae may develop between septum and turbinates. The use of postoperative splints effectively prevents this problem.

When sphenoidotomy is employed for hypophysectomy, the potential for additional complications ensues. The most common of these is transient diabetes insipidus, which may occur in 15% of cases. Cerebrospinal fluid leakage and meningitis occur less commonly.

CONCLUSION

Many institutions favor a team approach to transnasal pituitary surgery. The otolaryngologist is ideally suited, by virtue of his or her expertise in rhinology and familiarity with microsurgery, to play a prominent role in the management of lesions of the sphenoid and sella turcica. The importance of a comprehensive knowledge of sphenoid anatomy and careful preoperative evaluation with modern imaging techniques cannot be overestimated.

REFERENCES

1. Hayes TP, Davis RA, Raventos A: The treatment of pituitary chromophobe adenomas. *Radiology* 1971; 98:149–153.
2. Randall RV: Empty sella syndrome. *Compr Ther* 1984; 10:57–65.
3. Cummings CW, Johnson JT: Transethmoidal approach to the pituitary, in Schmidek HH, Sweet WH (eds): *Current Techniques of Operative Neurosurgery.* New York, Grune & Stratton, 1977, pp 173–180.
4. Lee KJ: The sublabial transseptal transsphenoidal approach to the hypophysis. *Laryngoscope* 1978; 88 (suppl 10):1–65.
5. Fujii K, Chambers SM, Rhoton AL Jr: Neurovascular relationships of the sphenoid sinus. *J Neurosurg* 1979; 50:31–39.
6. Hamberger CA, Hammer G, Norlen G, et al: Transsphenoidal hypophysectomy. *Arch Otolaryngol* 1961; 74:2–8.
7. Papel ID, Kennedy DW, Cohn E: Sublabial transseptal transsphenoidal approach to the skull base. *Ear Nose Throat J* 1986; 65:20–31.
8. Kern EB, Pearson BW, McDonald TJ, et al: The transseptal approach to lesions of the pituitary and parasellar regions. *Laryngoscope* 1979; 69 (suppl 15):1–34.
9. Sherwen PJ, Patterson WJ, Griesdale DE: Transseptal, transsphenoidal surgery: A subjective and objective analysis of results. *J Otolaryngology* 1986; 15:155–160.
10. Moskowitz D, Sasaki CT: Transseptal approach to the skull base, in Cummings CW, Fredrickson JM, Harker LA, et al. (eds): *Otolaryngology — Head and Neck Surgery.* CV Mosby Co, 1986, pp 945–958.
11. Hashimoto N, Handa H, Yamagami T: Transsphenoidal extracapsular approach to pituitary tumors. *J Neurosurg* 1986; 64:16–20.

12. Romanowski B, Tyrell DL, Wein BK, et al: Meningitis complicating transsphenoidal hypophysectomy. *Can Med Assoc J* 1981; 124:1172–1175.
13. Roppolo HMN: Intrasellar and parasellar abnormalities, in Latchaw RE (ed): *Computed Tomography of the Head, Neck and Spine.* Chicago, Year Book Medical Publishers, 1985, pp 329–355.

CHAPTER 13

Skull Base Tumors

Approach of

Harold C. Pillsbury III, M.D.

There is perhaps no area of greater controversy than the management of a malignant neoplasm at the skull base. The surgeon confronting malignancies in this area has to deal with two issues. The first involves whether a large resection encompassing reasonable margins is acceptable for a patient with poor prognosis given that these procedures are often deforming. The second issue is whether, after radiation therapy, a smaller procedure that is not deforming but that will, in most instances, lead to a less than satisfactory local cure rate can be done. Treatment planning often involves the series of compromises between these two alternatives. Some nonmalignant neoplasia in this area will also be considered since management options are often similar.

TRANSSEPTAL APPROACH TO THE SPHENOID SINUS

Several points in the transseptal approach to the sphenoid sinus are important for the surgeon. The least important of these is the open rhinoplasty vs. sublabial approach. Which approach is appropriate depends on the preference of the surgeon. I prefer to use the sublabial approach because of the problem of the columellar scar. Those who advocate the open rhinoplasty approach prefer it because they can maintain the integrity of the nasal spine. Theoretically it prevents drooping of the nasal tip. In my experience, this has not been a problem, with up to a 5-year follow-up on individual cases. More important, wide exposure of the rostrum of the sphenoid is needed so that the approach to the sella will be adequate.

The importance of the intrasphenoid sinus septum cannot be overstressed. The posterior terminal end of the midline intrasphenoid sinus septum can be the carotid canal. If the sphenoid sinus is not well pneumatized, there is a considerable block of bone between the septum and the carotid canal. In a well-pneumatized or hyperpneumatized sphenoid where the clivus is very thin, the terminal end of the intrasphenoid sinus septum can be adherent to a thin bony wall of the carotid canal (Fig 13–1). In this situation, torsion on the intrasphenoid sinus septum can result in a tear in the carotid wall. This is a very dangerous situation that can be best managed by packing the sinus and floating an occluding balloon into the carotid artery angiographically.

Knowledge of the anatomy of the cavernous sinus is critical when one is operating in the sphenoid sinus. The bulge of the carotid artery in the lateral wall of the sinus is well known. Superior to this can be found the optic nerve as it progresses anterior from the chiasm. The relationship between cranial nerves III and IV, and the second division of V and VI, also is important in the cavernous sinus (Fig 13–2). The transseptal, transsphenoid approach to the pituitary can be used for tumors of the clivus, including chordomas. It also is useful for exploration for cerebrospinal fluid (CSF) leaks in this area.

APPROACH TO THE MIDSKULL BASE AND CLIVUS

Transpalatal Approach

Indications for the transpalatal approach are tumors of the nasopharynx, including chordomas, and angiofibromas. The approach often is part of a more major exposure of the skull base in this area. It also is used for repair of choanal stenosis, as either a primary or secondary procedure, and in cases of cervical spine decompression.

Two basic types of palatal incisions are in common use. One is a U-shaped incision slightly anterior to the junction of the soft and hard palates. The soft palate is separated from the

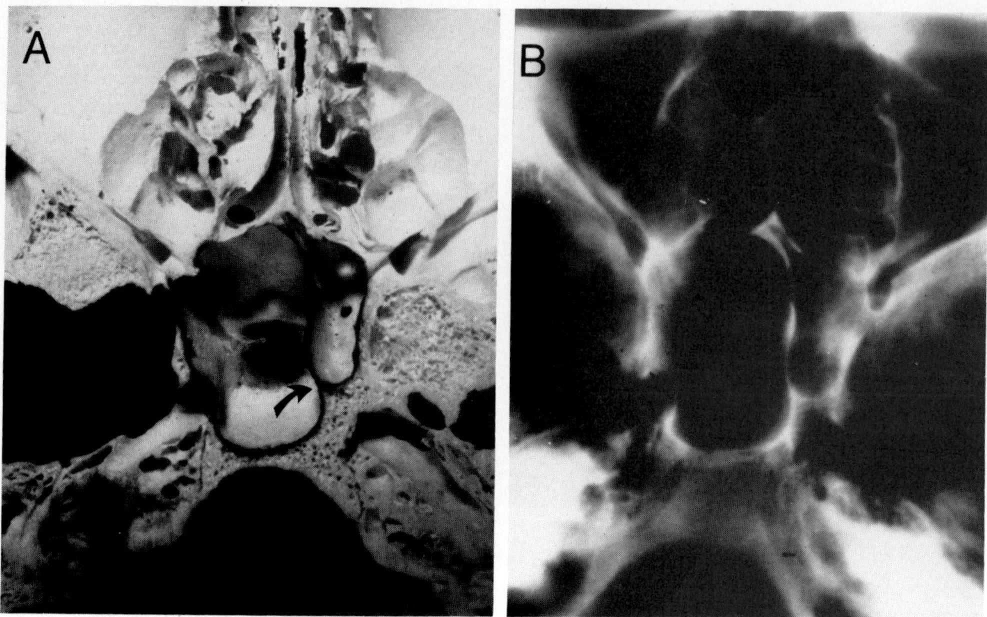

FIG 13–1.
A, intrasphenoid sinus septum terminating at the carotid canal *(black arrow)*. **B**, radiograph from the specimen in **A** showing the termination of the intrasphenoid sinus septum at the carotid canal.

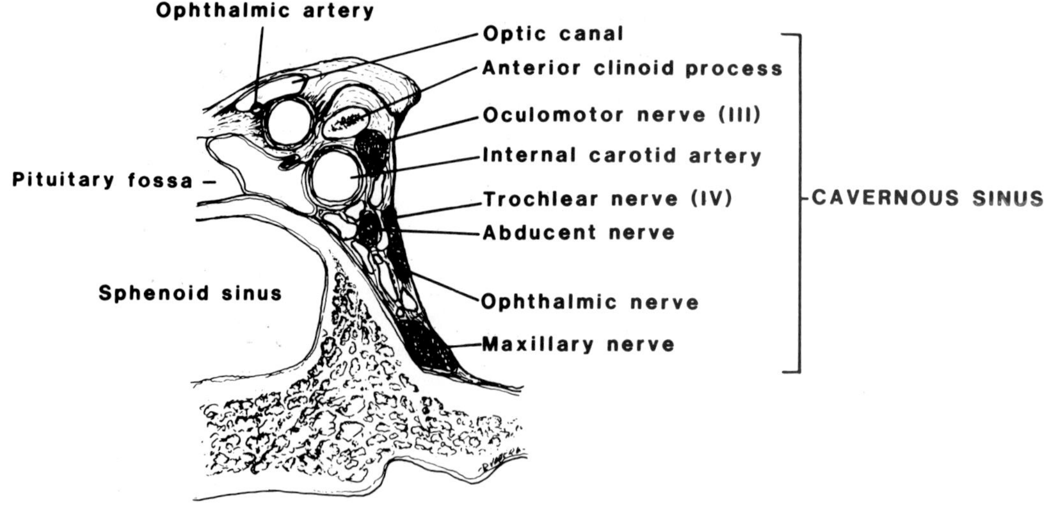

FIG 13–2.
Schematic of the cavernous sinus showing the relationships of neurovascular structures to the sphenoid sinus.

hard palate at its attachment with the palatal aponeurosis. The soft palate is then retracted inferiorly, and portions of the hard palate are resected as needed for exposure.

A slightly more versatile approach is the midline incision that extends just lateral to the uvula. This incision can be carried on midline anteriorly just posteriorly to the incisive canal. Kennedy et al.[1] and Kennedy[2] have recently described a variation of this incision. The soft palate incision is the same as just described, but as the incision reaches the junction of the posterior one third and the anterior two thirds of the hard palate, it is carried over in a gentle curve to one side, approximately at the level of the second premolar. It then courses anteriorly for another centimeter, curves around to the contralateral side posterior to the incisive canals, and then turns posterior, lateral, and anterior to the palatine artery. The authors believe that this prevents problems with the tendency toward shortening of the palate.[1,2] Once the mucoperiosteum of the hard palate is retracted laterally, exposure is easily developed by resection of necessary portions of the hard palate.

Cervical Approach to the Midskull Base

The midskull base area also can be reached through the neck, as has been well described by Stevenson et al.[3] and Cloward and Passarelli.[4] Advantages of the cervical approach include better exposure inferiorly and laterally and the fact that it is an extraoral procedure. The exposure of the midskull base is not as good as the midline approaches. After intubation and endotracheal anesthesia, I perform a tracheotomy; I believe this allows better retraction of the larynx and pharynx and a more controlled postoperative airway. The head is turned to the opposite side.

The initial incision begins at the mastoid tip and then follows a standard submandibular gland incision to the midline. Superior and inferior subplatysmal skin flaps are elevated. Sharp and blunt dissection expose the internal and external carotid arteries, superior thyroid and arteries, the hypoglossal nerve, and the digastric muscle. The hypoglossal nerve is mobilized from the styloid to the mylohyoid groove. I have elected to remove the submandibular gland, separate the lateral hyoid muscular attachments, resect the lateral hyoid, and retract the hypoglossal nerve, digastric, and suprahyoid soft tissues superiorly. However, Cloward and Passarelli retract these tissues inferiorly,[4] thus preserving even the superior thyroid and lingual arteries, which I divide. At this point the lateral vertebral body can be palpated and easily exposed. A plane is then created between the prevertebral and buccopharyngeal fascia as far superiorly as the attachment of the pharyngeal constrictor muscle on the pharyngeal tubercle. If necessary, an elongated styloid process is resected because further lateral exposure encroaches on the parapharyngeal space. This exposure is facilitated by incising the fascial band from the styloid to the posterior pharyngeal wall. A subperiostial dissection of the pharyngeal mucosa superior to the pharyngeal tubercle as far as the vomer exposes the ventral clivus. Deep retractors are necessary for the remainder of the procedure. Inferiorly the prevertebral fascia and midline cervical musculature is split in the midline. An operating microscope is then brought into the field. Vertebral bodies can be removed with a drill as needed. Lateral dissection is limited inferiorly by the internal carotid artery and more superiorly by the inferior petrosal sinuses, which are on level with the jugular tubercle.

If the pharynx and dura have not been inadvertently opened, closed suction drains can be placed, which help to approximate the pharynx in its anatomic position. Otherwise, deep sutures are placed from the buccopharyngeal to the prevertebral fascia. A nasopharyngeal pack also is placed, along with a Penrose drain in the neck. Cervical stabilization may be required.

Ancillary Procedures for Inferior or Lateral Exposure in Association With Other Approaches to the Midskull Base and Clivus

The most versatile of the ancillary procedures is the median labiomandibulotomy with perilingual dissection (mandibular swing). It is easily combined with a radical neck dissection (RND) with good lateral exposure and with control of the extracranial carotid system. By following the lingual nerve, the surgeon approaches the infratemporal fossa inferiorly. Exposure inferiorly of the posterior wall of the pharynx requires division of the lingual nerve. This procedure will be discussed in more detail in the section of anterolateral approaches to the infratemporal and pterygomaxillary fossae.

The midline labiomandibulotomy with midline glossotomy is another procedure allowing quick access to the posterior pharyngeal wall without neural injury. In combination with the transpalatal approach, it gives excellent exposure from the sphenoid to about the fourth cervical vertebral body. However, lateral exposure is limited, and control of the intracranial portion of the carotid is not possible. I have performed tracheotomies on patients with this approach and with the mandibular swing.

The degloving midfacial approach (sublabial Denker-type Caldwell-Luc procedure) easily can be combined with transpalatal approaches for lateral exposure.

ANTERIOR AND ANTEROLATERAL APPROACHES TO THE INFRATEMPORAL AND PTERYGOMAXILLARY FOSSAE

In a manner similar to that for craniofacial resection, head and neck surgeons have approached malignancies extending into the infratemporal and pterygomaxillary fossae with the concept of en bloc resection. In 1969, Terz and co-workers espoused the need for en bloc resections for tumors invading the pterygoid fossa.[5] They even advocated initial exposure of the middle cranial fossa to facilitate the excision. Biller and associates[6] and Krespi and Sisson[7] have described techniques using wide-field exposure for composite resection of tumors invading the infratemporal fossa, the pterygoid, or the nasopharynx. Spiro et al. combined the idea of the median labiomandibulotomy and paralingual dissection in continuity with control of the great vessels in the upper neck.[8] In addition, the standard maxillectomy approach has been added to these procedures to achieve the desired en bloc resection. The key is complete exposure of the carotid from the lower portion of the neck to the temporal bone. Undoubtedly, current enthusiasm about such aggressive approaches has been bolstered by the development of myocutaneous flaps[9,10] and microvascular techniques. These powerful reconstructive tools allow one-stage repair of extensive head and neck defects. Although no large series with long-term follow-up have been reported, Krespi and Sisson's initial report with short-term follow-up is impressive and encouraging, with 11 of 14 patients free of disease.[7]

Preoperative Considerations

Evaluation of the extent of a malignancy of the upper aerodigestive tract has been facilitated by the use of flexible and rigid nasopharyngoscopes. Computed tomography (CT scanning) has greatly improved our ability to further assess tumor extent. Magnetic resonance imaging (MRI) may offer advantages for soft tissue delineation. I often use both. Angiographic procedures may occasionally be useful in lesions of the anterior skull base but, in general, are less necessary than for those of the middle and posterior fossae.

After a careful head and neck examination, CT or MRI (or both) and routine laboratory studies, including a chest radiograph, liver function tests, and alkaline phosphatase enzyme determinations, should be used to evaluate potential metastatic lesions. Because of the propensity for multiple carcinomas in patients with head and neck malignancies, esophagoscopy, laryngoscopy, and bronchoscopy are indicated for most patients.[11] Heavy smokers should have pulmonary function tests. Careful assessment of the nutritional status of debilitated patients is essential. If preoperative or postoperative radiation therapy is considered, a dental consultation is required. A Panorex view is indicated even in edentulous patients, since retained tooth roots may be present. If maxillectomy is considered, dental impressions should be made and a palatal prosthesis fabricated.

I generally recommend surgical excision combined with postoperative irradiation for T3 and T4 carcinomas of the upper aerodigestive tract. I believe that combined therapy is indicated for these extensive lesions and that its use postoperatively as opposed to preoperatively avoids potential problems with healing and infection that are often associated with preoperative irradiation.[12] A more conservative approach of using radiation therapy only in the presence of positive margins[13] may be as effective.

In general, if one has a question about the need for a larger rather than smaller resection, one should err on the side of the larger resection.

Most surgeons would consider unresectable those tumors that have invaded the clivus or the vertebral bodies or those with more than superficial involvement of the sphenoidal sinus.[7, 14] Although tumor extension into the floor of the middle cranial fossa may be excised en bloc through an initial craniotomy, results have been disappointing and morbidity unacceptably high.[15] Thus, such extension should be considered a relative contraindication to excision until more experience is gained. A portion of the eustachian tube and much of the nasopharynx can be excised en bloc with the infratemporal fossa, pterygoid and pterygopalatine fossae, and portions of the maxilla. An aminoglycoside and clindamycin or cefazolin are given just prior to the procedure and are generally continued until 24 hours after the last drain is removed. Tracheotomy is mandatory.

I generally use postoperative radiation therapy. Krespi and Sisson combined preoperative chemotherapy with their surgical procedure.[7] Again, one cannot make definitive statements about the best combination of therapies, since to date there are no series large enough, nor is there adequate long-term experience to substantiate such statements.

Procedure

My procedure is essentially that described by Biller and co-workers[6] and Krespi and Sisson.[7] The patient's face, neck, and portion of the chest or back as needed for possible my-

ocutaneous flap reconstruction are prepared in the usual manner. After draping, I generally use the Conley modification of the Schobinger incision for neck exposure. The horizontal limb begins at the mastoid tip and extends two finger breadths below the angle of the mandible, gently curving upward and around the chin to split the lip in the midline. The vertical limb is placed so that it begins behind the carotid and gently curves inferiorly to the midportion of the clavicle.

A radical neck dissection is then performed. The accessory nerve may be spared if there is no significant jugulodigastric adenopathy. Complete exposure is facilitated by removal of the sternocleidomastoid and internal jugular vein and the posterior belly of the digastric muscle. The external carotid is followed superiorly and ligated just distal to its lingual branch. In general, it may be best to remove the neck contents en bloc with the local excision, but the neck contents can be removed separately. Injections of local anesthetic with epinephrine are carried out along the lines of the intraoral incision. After the lip is divided with a V-shaped incision, the next decision is where to divide the mandible. If there is a question of mandibular involvement, the osteotomy is performed just anterior to the mental foramen. The posterior mandible may thus be removed as indicated by tumor involvement. For larger tumors, it is best excised to allow for better exposure and en bloc resection. In smaller tumors when the mandible may be preserved, I prefer a midline or parasymphyseal osteotomy to a lateral osteotomy, since the exposure is as good or better, and the osteotomy will be out of the field of radiation. The advantage of the parasymphyseal osteotomy as opposed to the midline one is that the mylohyoid muscle does not need to be incised, thus preserving the integrity of the anterior floor of the mouth.[16] Although beveled and stepped osteotomies have been successfully used with wiring of the segments, I prefer using a compression plate system. I position and apply the plate, drilling and tapping screw holes prior to a straight osteotomy. This reliably preserves the preoperative occlusion, shortens closure time, and probably hastens and improves healing of the bone. Whether midline, parasymphyseal, or lateral osteotomy is used, the mucosal incision will continue along the floor of the mouth until the margin of resection is encountered. If the patient has had recent dental extraction, the incision is best carried along the alveolar ridge through the same incision through which the teeth were extracted. Otherwise the floor of the mouth incision would cut off most of the blood supply to the lingual gingiva on this side. With splitting of the mandible and incision along the floor of the mouth, the parapharyngeal space is opened like a book, thus exposing the anterolateral aspect of the infratemporal fossa as well as the posterior oral cavity and area of resection.

For en bloc excision of large tumors, the mandible will be excised, and thus a large cervicofacial flap is elevated with stripping of the masseter muscle, incising the temporalis attachments to the coronoid, and cutting across the neck of the mandible or disarticulating the condyle. In addition to excision of the mandible, the posterior belly of the digastric muscle, the stylohyoid ligament, and the styloglossus and stylopharyngeus muscles are removed, and, if necessary, an elongated styloid process is shortened. This maneuver facilitates exposure of the internal carotid artery to the skull base.

For large squamous cell carcinomas of the tonsillar fossa with soft palate or lateral pharyngeal wall involvement, Krespi and Sisson believe that one should extend the dissection superiorly to remove the retropharyngeal nodes.[7] The aim is to excise all structures medial to the internal carotid artery at the skull base, including the infratemporal fossa. Necessary portions of the soft and hard palate follow, thus variably excising the pterygoid and pterygopalatine fossae. Blunt finger dissection is easily carried out in the retropharyngeal space to the cartilaginous eustachian tube, which is divided medial to the internal carotid artery.

Reconstruction is usually performed with a pectoralis major myocutaneous flap, but smaller resections may be handled with posteriorly based tongue flaps. Ventilation tubes in the eardrum and prefabricated palatal prostheses complete early rehabilitation. To facilitate swallowing, a cricopharyngeal myotomy is generally recommended in the larger excisions or when a large portion of the soft palate is excised.[7]

Although the emphasis here has been on larger excisions, the median labiomandibulotomy and mandibular swing approaches are also extremely useful in exposure of portions of the skull base for benign tumors of the parapharyngeal space, infratemporal fossa, and area of the clivus. These will often include such tumors as schwannomas, glomus tumors, and midline chordomas. In the case of a chordoma without significant lateral extension, the simplest procedure is the median labiomandibular glossotomy. With soft palate splitting and removal of the posterior hard palate, exposure can be obtained from the sphenoid to the fourth cervical vertebrae, thus allowing tumor excision or cervicomedullary decompression.[17] Although Stevenson and colleagues have described a transclival approach to the ventral surface of the brain stem without entering into the oral cavity,[3] I would agree with Biller and co-workers that oral contamination has not been a problem since the use of prophylactic antibiotics.[6] Of note is the fact that with the paralingual dissection, if the excision is to be carried below the level of the tongue base, the lingual nerve will need to be divided. For benign tumors, I reanastomose the lingual nerve, and I have seen some apparent return of sensory function.

Complications

To date, complications have been few and not different from those accompanying other large series of such procedures that have yet to be published. Discovery of residual disease at the bony skull base and abnormal nodes of Ranvier are to be considered complications unless these events are anticipated preoperatively. I have also had the experience of tumor ascending the trigeminal nerve up the foramen ovale. Injury to the carotid artery and CSF leaks are also possible, although I have not encountered these complications in our series.

Comments regarding nutritional status, need for triple endoscopy, and routine blood tests already have been alluded to in the section on anterolateral approaches to the infratemporal and pterygomaxillary fossae.

ANTERIOR SKULL BASE

Historical Perspectives

The resection of anterior skull base neoplasia involves primarily an extension of the maxillectomy first performed by Lizars in 1826. The next significant contribution to this field was by Ohngren, who in 1933 described an oblique line extending from the medial canthus to the pterygoid plates. The prognosis for sinus malignancy behind this line was dim.[18] Ohngren advocated partial resection of these lesions, followed by radiotherapy for the unresected posterior superior extent of tumor.[18] This resulted in such poor survival that radiotherapy as a primary modality was increasingly advocated. Not until 1963, when Ketcham et al.[19] reported craniofacial resection, was survival for patients with sinus malignancy improved from 20% to between 50% and 70%. Recent enthusiasm for more aggressive resection of intracranial tumor, including vital structures in the cavernous sinus, has not appreciably increased the long-term survival of patients with significant intracranial extension. The unfortunate association of sinus malignancy with chronic sinusitis has led to a delay in diagnosis until secondary symptoms such as orbital or intraoral invasion become manifest. Perhaps the advent of endoscopic sinus surgery, including maxillary sinoscopy, will have an impact on the earlier diagnosis of malignant neoplasia in this area.

Physical Examination

The tragedy of sinus neoplasia is the delay from the onset of symptoms to diagnosis, which averages 6 months. Common presenting symptoms include nasal obstruction, epistaxis, and anesthesia of the second to third division of the fifth cranial nerve. More advanced malignancies involving the cavernous sinus will result in ophthalmoplegia, followed by proptosis and chemosis. Posterior involvement beyond the maxillary sinus involving the pterygoids results in trismus. Frank involvement of the anterior cranial fossa results in headaches and occasionally meningitis.

Pathologic Considerations

Squamous cell carcinoma accounts for an overwhelming percentage of sinus neoplasia. Other less common tumors include esthesioneuroblastoma, adenocarcinoma, adenocystic carcinoma, lymphoma, sarcoma, melanoma, and juvenile angiofibroma. To some extent, treatment planning is dependent on histology. In patients with squamous cell carcinoma, whenever the ethmoid is extensively involved, the craniofacial resection is generally employed. The concept of achieving an adequate margin around squamous cell carcinoma is difficult to imagine without an en bloc resection of the ethmoid including the superior margins. A craniofacial resection is always performed for esthesioneuroblastoma where the site of origin is the cribriform plate. The same approach can be used for the sinonasal undifferentiated carcinoma, another variety of small

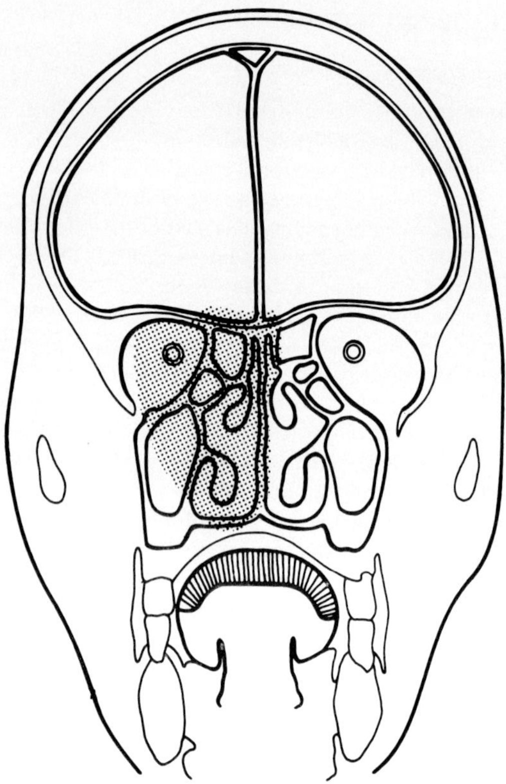

FIG 13–3.
Right ethmoid-orbital tumor and the area comprised in the resection.

cell cancer commonly found in the cribriform ethmoid area. This lesion is highly malignant and also requires a craniofacial resection for adequate surgical margins. Although the lesion is radiosensitive, the prognosis seems to be sufficiently dim that there is some question as to whether surgery at all will be an option for this lesion in the future. Adenocarcinoma often arises in the ethmoid and is commonly seen among woodworkers.[20] This lesion is aggressive, and since radiotherapy offers little in the way of additional therapy, the craniofacial resection with a wide margin is recommended. Those who have sarcomas and melanomas also are poor candidates for radiation and chemotherapy. Thus, when these lesions abut the anterior cranial fossa, a craniofacial resection for an adequate surgical margin is recommended. Adenocystic carcinoma presents a unique challenge. When there is no known intracerebral invasion, a craniofacial resection is a viable approach for management of this lesion. Unfortunately many adenocystic tumors do involve intracranial structures, and when this is the case, the prognosis is sufficiently dim for the craniofacial option to be abandoned. A more limited resection, followed by radiotherapy, is considered acceptable. Lymphomas are seldom, if ever, considered surgical candidates. The diagnosis of a lymphoma in this area is sufficiently uncommon that the surgeon must consider the possibility of sinonasal undifferentiated carcinoma or esthesioneuroblastoma whenever a small cellular tumor is diagnosed. Juvenile angiofibroma, though not a malignant neoplasm, is a benign disease that may require a malignant operation for extirpation of the tumor. My experience with this lesion is that a craniofacial resection is seldom, if ever, indicated. I resect lesions that do not show intracranial invasion and irradiate those that do. My results from this form of therapy have been gratifying.

Radiographic Considerations

At this time, high-resolution CT with contrast taken in the axial and coronal planes is the method of choice for assessing tumor extent. Bone and soft tissue algorithms are used to ascertain both the tumor mass and sites of bony erosion. Three-dimensional CT enhancement of the two-dimensional data may provide help in determining the sites and extent of skull base involvement. Magnetic resonance imaging is not as helpful in sinus malignancy due to the inadequacy of fine bony detail presently available in magnetic resonance images. The only area where MRI may be valuable is in the differentiation between tumor and soft tissue inflammation seen in conjunction with sinus malignancies. This, however, is a relatively small point since bony destruction is the hallmark of lesions in this area. One of the areas where CT has been helpful is in the determination of involvement of the sphenoid sinus and nasopharynx. These two areas are particularly noteworthy, because when tumor invades them, the prognosis is universally dismal. Most important, we have a significant tendency to underestimate tumor involvement in this area. Robins et al. recently reported a 30% incidence of underestimation of tumor extent in sinus malignancies.[21] When operative intervention of this magnitude is considered, it is prudent to assume that any questionable areas are malignant and should be dealt with accordingly.

Adjunctive Radiotherapy

In lesions where radiotherapy is deemed to be helpful, I employ it preoperatively. Since, for the most part, craniofacial resections incorporate an anatomic resection, the opportunity to improve the control of microscopic disease is better in my opinion when radiotherapy is given preoperatively than when it is given postoperatively. This is not a unique view and is employed by many others.[22–24]

Surgery

Tumors are believed to be inoperable when there is involvement of the greater wing of the sphenoid, optic chiasm, sphenoidal sinus or nasopharynx, frontal lobes, or sphenopalatine fossa, as indicated by extensive erosion of the pterygoid plates.[10, 13, 19, 25–27] The presence of neck metastases is also a relative contraindication, although in selected cases resection is indicated for palliation or as the only chance for cure.[15] Patient philosophies influence individualized approaches. The limits of anterocranial floor excision are the entire ipsilateral cranial floor with orbitomaxillectomy, the opposite ethmoidal sinuses, the planum sphenoidale posteriorly, and as much of the anterior cranial vault as indicated (Fig 13–3). Orbital exenteration is usually indicated and should be performed when there is anterior ethmoidal involvement. This is underscored by the high

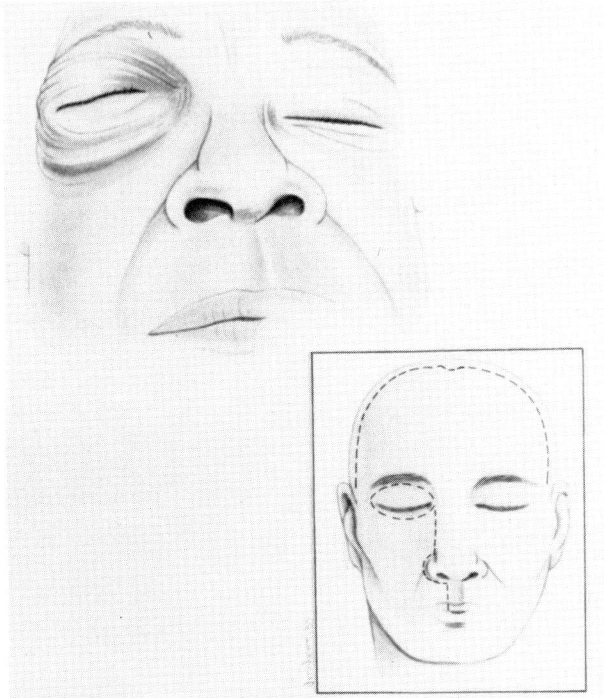

FIG 13–4.
Skin incisions for extirpation of a right ethmoid-orbital tumor.

recurrence rate when the orbit was preserved in Ketcham's large series.[13]

A tracheotomy should be considered in patients requiring maxillectomy as part of the craniofacial resection. This should be an individualized decision based on the patient's age, general medical condition, and the extent of the resection. If its use is questionable, I believe it is most conservative to perform the tracheotomy at the time of the craniofacial resection.

Perioperative antibiotics are chosen in conjunction with the neurosurgical team. I generally use a third-generation cephalosporin.

Procedure

A lumbar CSF drain is placed. The patient's head is shaved, followed by preparation of the head, face, and neck as indicated. The entire face and anterior cranium are draped, and the drapes are sutured into place. A second towel is then draped over the face, with its superior extent just below the area for the placement of the most inferior burr hole. This towel helps isolate the cranial and facial fields as much as possible. The neurosurgeon begins with a bifrontal craniotomy. After the coronal incision (Fig 13–4), the anterior skin flap is developed by dissection just deep to the galea aponeurotica, as far as the supraorbital ridge, with care taken to preserve the supraorbital vessels. By initial dissection close to the galea, the underlying pericranial flap will have some extra soft tissue superficially. The pericranium is incised 1 to 2 cm more posterior to the skin incision to provide additional length (Fig 13–5). The pericranial flap is then elevated to the supraorbital rim and held anteriorly with towel clips and rubber bands. Burr holes are then per-

formed, and a bone flap is incised, with care being taken to preserve its attachment laterally to the temporalis muscle (Fig 13–6). Anteriorly, the dura is often tightly adherent to the cranial vault and is carefully elevated away from it. The lumbar drain is opened, allowing enough CSF drainage to give good exposure of the floor of the anterior cranial fossa without undue pressure on the frontal lobes (Fig 13–7). At this point, resectability can be determined, as previously discussed. Extension through the cribriform area necessitates dural excision to maintain the specimen en bloc. The dural defect can be closed with temporalis fascia, fascia lata, or lyophilized dura. This graft is reinforced by the pericranial flap.[28, 29] If there has not been cribriform breakthrough, inferior dissection is continued posteriorly past the cresta galli. Dural sleeves with olfactory nerves are transected. Sometimes, it is possible to clip the sleeves before the transection, but at other times the sleeves first must be cut and repaired later in the procedure.

The posterior bony cut should be just anterior to the sphenoidal sinus area, which can be seen as a gentle upsloping posterior to the cribriform plate. I like to perform the initial bone cuts with a hand-held drill and complete them with osteotomes. The lateral extent is determined by the tumor size, which often extends into the ipsilateral orbit, and at minimum should include the medial aspect of the contralateral ethmoidal system. The anterior cut should be made so as to remove the posterior wall and floor of the frontal sinus, allowing subsequent "craniotomy" of the frontal sinus area.[30] The posterior cut ideally would enter just anterior to or into the sphenoidal sinus. When these cuts are completed, the neurosurgeon takes a break. A large cottonoid is placed between the specimen and the remaining dura to protect it from facial resection. The flaps are temporarily replaced and the facial towel flipped back over the craniotomy site to further protect it. During either the cranial or facial portion of the procedure, frozen sections should be liberally taken to ensure normal margins.[31]

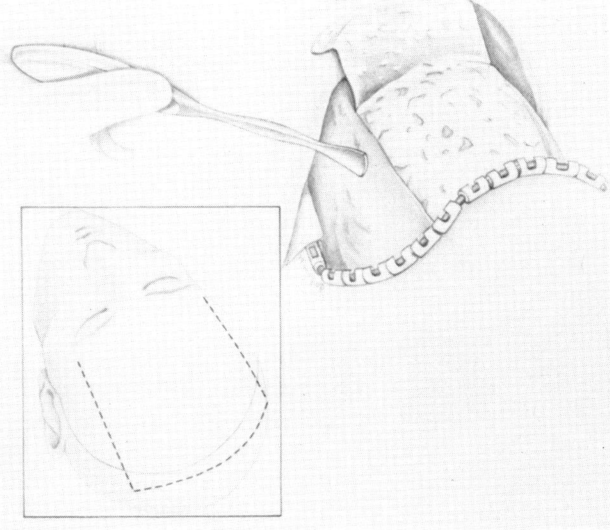

FIG 13–5.
Elevation of the coronal incision with a pericranial flap extending above the level of the coronal incision.

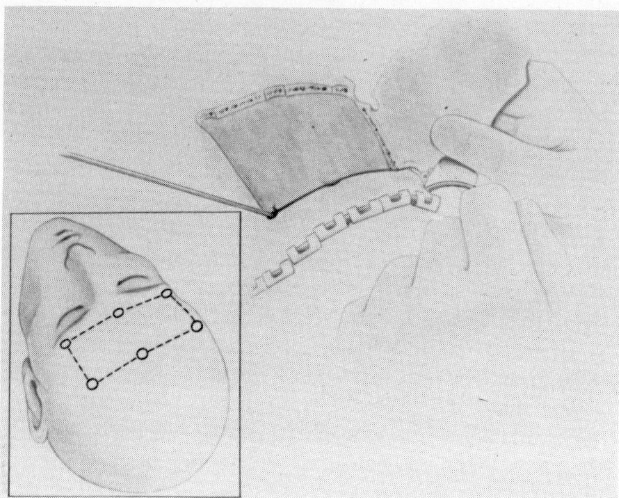

FIG 13–6.
Elevation of the craniotomy flap attached to the right temporalis muscle.

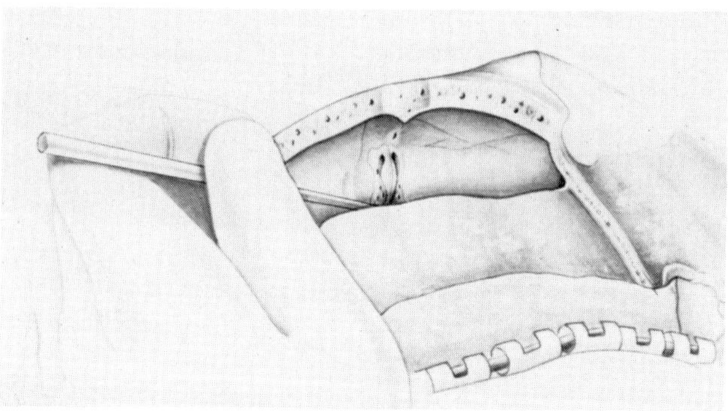

FIG 13–7.
Elevation of the dura from the cribriform plate and cresti galli.

The extent of the facial resection will depend on the extent of the lesion. Unfortunately, in most cases, it necessitates a Weber-Ferguson type of incision, with combined orbitomaxillectomy. Occasionally, however, one may need to perform only a lateral rhinotomy with medial maxillectomy.[32] The maxillectomy procedure is routine. The septum is removed if there is any involvement of this mucosa. If there is no septal involvement, removal of the septal bone and cartilage and ipsilateral mucoperiosteum and mucoperichondrium then can be cut at the level of the maxillary spine from anteriorly to posteriorly and rotated superiorly to further reinforce the cribriform defect.

At the completion of the facial portion of the procedure, attention is turned toward reconstruction. Although fascia lata galea, iliac bone crest, or septal bone grafts have been used to fill the cribriform defect,[12,32] I believe that the pericranial flap best achieves this goal.[27,29] It is placed through the lower portion of the bone flap. Wires placed inferiorly in the bone flap must thus be placed through this flap. The pericranial flap is sutured as far posteriorly as possible, with several tacking sutures between the pericranial flap and dura to obliterate any dead space and reinforce any dural grafts or previously sutured defects (Fig

13–8). The cranial incision is closed and drained. Attention is then turned to the facial defect. As noted previously, a septal flap may be used to reinforce the cribriform defect. I routinely use split-thickness skin grafts to line the cavities and to resurface the orbital floor if the orbit has not been exenterated. I generally do not use flaps for reconstruction of the defect. If the patient desires, I would recommend waiting 1 to 2 years prior to doing so. The latissimus dorsi[10] and pectoralis major flaps appear to have the most versatility.[9,10] However, temporalis, forehead, and cheek flaps are good local alternatives in specific situations. The palatal prosthesis is inserted, followed by packing, which is left in place for 7 days.

Although the craniofacial resection is usually performed at a single sitting, there may be a reason in some cases to delay the extracranial portion. This may apply especially in benign tumors when, in addition to excising the cranial portion of the tumor, tying off the intracranial blood supply to the extracranial portion of the tumor may allow ischemia, infarction, and tumor shrinkage. Most surgeons, however, would rather use preoperative embolization techniques, especially in vascular tumors such as nasopharyngeal angiofibromas, to achieve a one-stage resection.[33]

Complications

The most common complication of craniofacial resection has been CSF leakage.[12,27,32] The routine use of the pericranial flap may decrease the occurrence of this problem and thus concomitantly reduce the incidence of meningitis.[28,29] Osteoradionecrosis, oteomyelitis, loss of the dural graft, contusion of the frontal lobes from retraction, delayed bleeding, local abscesses, and the syndrome of inappropriate antidiuretic hormone secretion have all been reported.[5,12,27,32] However, these problems appear to be unusual in current reports, since experience has accumulated, and the technique has been refined.

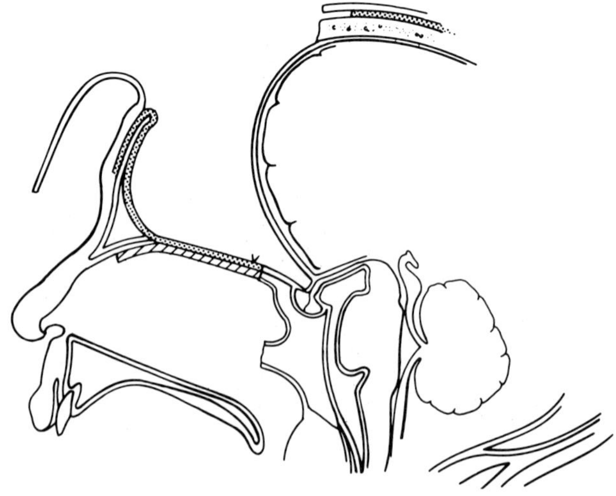

FIG 13–8.
Placement of the pericranial flap attaching it to the dura at the planum sphenoidale. The pericranial flap is spiculed, with the skin graft on the nasal surface being demonstrated using interrupted lines.

Mortality in current large series has ranged from 4% (2 of 54)[15] to 11% (3 of 22).[27]

SUPERIOR LATERAL APPROACH TO THE INFRATEMPORAL FOSSA

Preoperative Considerations

Obwegeser has described a superior approach to the infratemporal fossa area.[34] This procedure can be used for exposure of the lateral orbital wall and orbital cone area, the temporomandibular joint, the infratemporal fossa, pterygomaxillary space, nasopharynx, and the upper parapharyngeal space for benign or malignant lesions. The limitations of his procedures include difficulty with exposure past the midline, and it is my belief that exposure of the carotid is not as good as through the anterolateral approach when the carotid artery is kept in view during the whole procedure.

The major advantages of the procedure include the fact that there are no facial incisions and the facial nerve is protected without being rerouted.

Procedure

The procedure begins with a coronal type of incision in the hairline. The incision is carried all the way across to the contralateral side if more inferior exposure is needed. On the ipsilateral side, the incision inferiorly is carried to just posterior to the pinna and then anteriorly over the superior aspect of the pinna and in the preauricular crease inferiorly just below the level of the ear canal. In the midline, the dissection is carried out deep to the pericranium and more laterally is carried out just superficial to the temporalis fascia until the zygomatic arch is reached. Here the dissection is continued deep to the periosteum onto the masseter muscle. The next steps depend on what kind of exposure is needed. The zygomatic arch can be reflected inferiorly pedicled onto the masseter muscle. Either the coronoid process alone or the coronoid and condyle can be pedicled on a temporalis muscle and reflected superiorly. In this manner, exposure is easily attained through the infratemporal fossa more medially into the pterygomaxillary fossa.

It is important during the dissection to avoid the temporal branch of the facial nerve because it crosses the zygoma. The facial nerve must also be protected during the inferior retraction necessary to expose the infratemporal fossa area. The procedure may very easily be combined with a lateral rhinotomy or a wide Caldwell-Luc procedure with removal of the posterior maxillary sinus and pterygoid plates for complete exposure in this area. Obviously, combined with use of a midfacial degloving procedure, large tumors can be removed from the pterygomaxillary space without any facial incisions at all.

If there is any question of extension into the middle cranial fossa, one should be prepared to perform a temporal craniotomy to achieve an en bloc resection.

Complications

The most common complication is pain involving the temporomandibular joint. Obwegeser describes maneuvers to combat this problem.[34] There are many situations here where an oral surgeon or a dental colleague could be of assistance. Injury to the facial nerve can occur unless careful attention is taken to avoid stretching the nerve during the inferior exposure. If stretching cannot be avoided, the nerve should be cut distal to its branching point and reanastomosed at the end of the case to minimize synkinesis.

LATERAL APPROACH TO THE INFRATEMPORAL FOSSA

Preoperative Considerations

This lateral approach to the infratemporal fossa was popularized by Fisch and Pillsbury[14] and incorporates three contiguous areas. The first of these is the jugular bulb and is most commonly used for approaching glomus jugulare tumors. The second wider approach encompasses the sphenoid sinus and can be used for approaching chordomas in the region of the clivus. The third region incorporates the nasopharynx and can be used for the occasional incidence of carcinoma of the nasopharynx where a lateral surgical approach is indicated.[35] I would be more likely to approach the nasopharynx through a midline labiomandibulotomy, as popularized by Krespi and Sisson.[36]

Procedure

All approaches to the lateral skull base incorporate mastoidectomy with anterior transposition of the facial nerve. This allows exposure to the jugular bulb and facilitates exposure of the carotid in the temporal bone. In this dissection, the carotid artery becomes the landmark for approaching the cavernous sinus. For tumors in the infratemporal fossa, including sarcomatous lesions and lesions of the fifth nerve, a resection of the mandibular condyle is necessary, and this can be accomplished after anterior transposition of the facial nerve. When anterior transposition does not afford adequate exposure, the facial nerve should be cut after the division into several of its branches. If the nerve is incised after the division into various branches, there is less synkinesis once nerve reanastomosis and regeneration occur. The internal maxillary artery is followed, and the takeoff of the middle meningeal is noted, following this to the foramen spinosum. The leaves of the lateral pterygoid are dissected free from the mandible and the muscle itself sacrificed in the approach. The medial pterygoid is likewise sacrificed so that surgical exposure is facilitated. The pterygoid plexus of veins are encountered in this exposure, and the control of this area is sometimes difficult. I routinely use the Malis bipolar coagulator in this part of the dissection. In approaching the foramen ovale, I identify the lingual and inferior alveolar nerves as well as the buccal branch at nerve V. Frequently, tumors in this area originate from the fifth cranial nerve. Should there be an indication for a combined approach, a transtemporal craniotomy is performed so that the lesion can be exposed above and below the foramen ovale. Commonly, errors in judgment are made when tumors are encountered in the infratemporal

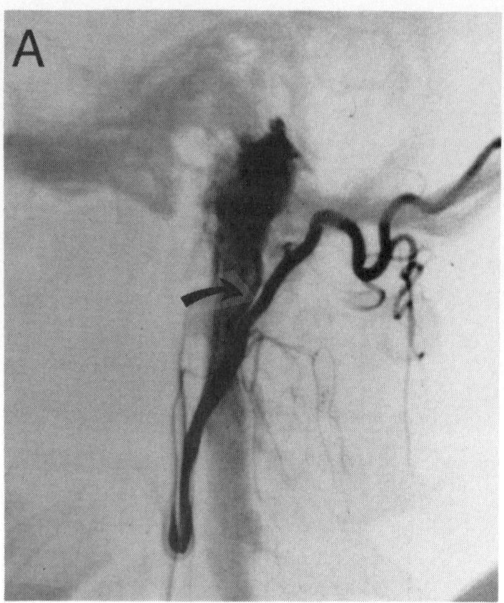

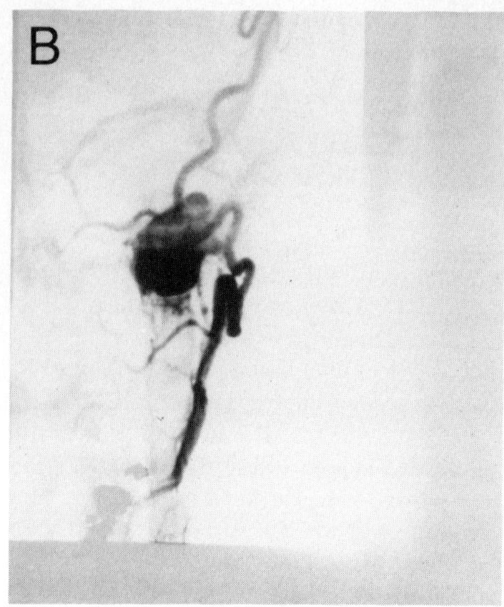

FIG 13–9.
A, glomus jugulare tumor with a feeder from the occipital artery *(black arrow).* **B,** another view of the tumor in **A** showing complete filling of the jugular foramen with neoplasm.

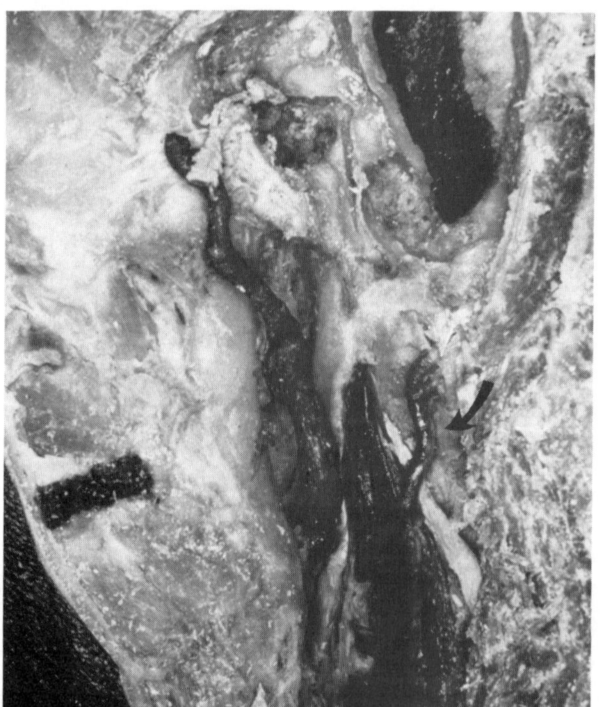

FIG 13–10.
Cadaveric dissection of the left skull base. Note the occipital artery going toward the region of the jugular bulb *(black arrow),* which is the point of the dissection where the sigmoid sinus has been uncovered and the styloid process is still in place.

fossa and the surgeon is unprepared to follow them intracranially. This should obviously be well planned in advance of any surgical undertaking.

The classic glomus jugulare tumor is seen in Figure 13–9. The tumor is fed by the occipital branch of the external carotid artery as shown by the arrow on Figure 13–9 and the cadaveric dissection in Figure 13–10. The incision I prefer is seen in Figure 13–11 and is rather an unusual approach, allowing for good cosmesis and exposure. The external auditory canal is closed as a blind sack (Fig 13–12), with the remaining external canal wall skin and tympanic membrane removed to prevent subsequent cyst formation. The facial nerve is then identified in the parotid (Fig 13–13).

The jugular vein and carotid artery are identified, and umbilical tape keepers are placed around each vessel (Fig 13–14). A radical mastoidectomy is performed (Fig 13–15), and the sigmoid sinus is tied off using temporalis fascia to patch the resulting dural defect (Fig 13–16). The facial nerve is anteriorly transposed from the fallopian canal over the root of the zygoma as shown on the cadaveric dissection (Fig 13–17). The jugular vein is then tied off and the jugular bulb opened. The tumor is resected, and the inferior petrosal sinus is packed with oxidized cellulose (Surgicel). The facial nerve is then returned to its anatomic position (Fig 13–18), and the wound is closed. A closed suction catheter drainage system is always employed (Fig 13–19). The patient always experiences a temporary facial palsy (Fig 13–20), which recovers nicely if the facial nerve has not been interrupted (Fig 13–21).

An important point in resecting tumors of the jugular bulb is the ligation of the sigmoid sinus. I generally perform this by exposing the dura in front and behind the sinus. An incision is then made posterior to the sinus and the brain pushed out of the way, following which a double ligature is placed around the sinus. Once the sinus is ligated, the defect in the posterior dura is patched with temporalis fascia. A muscle plug is used to reinforce the closure of the sigmoid sinus, always allowing for flow through the superior petrosal sinus. This lessens the

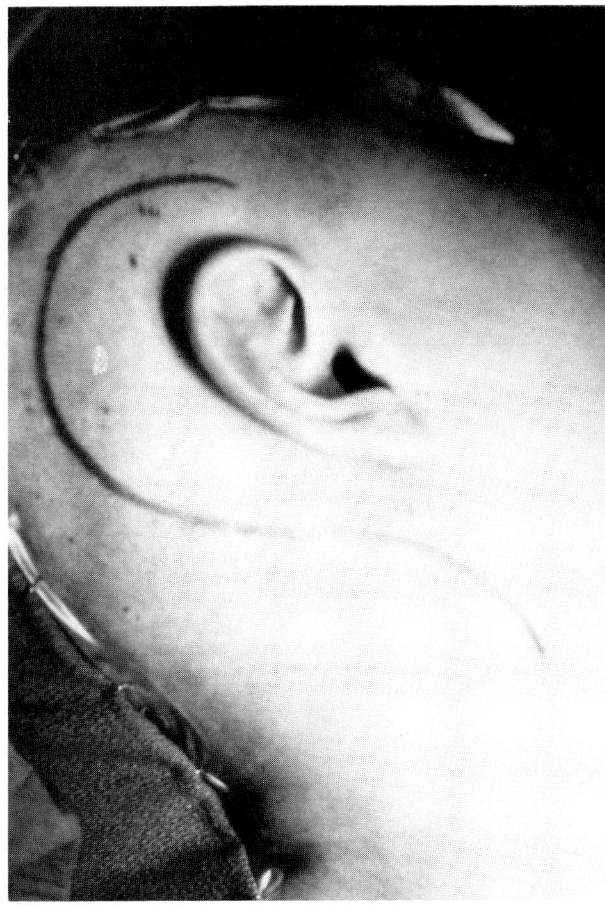

FIG 13–11.
Proposed incision for a left glomus jugulare tumor as shown in Figures 13–9 and 13–10.

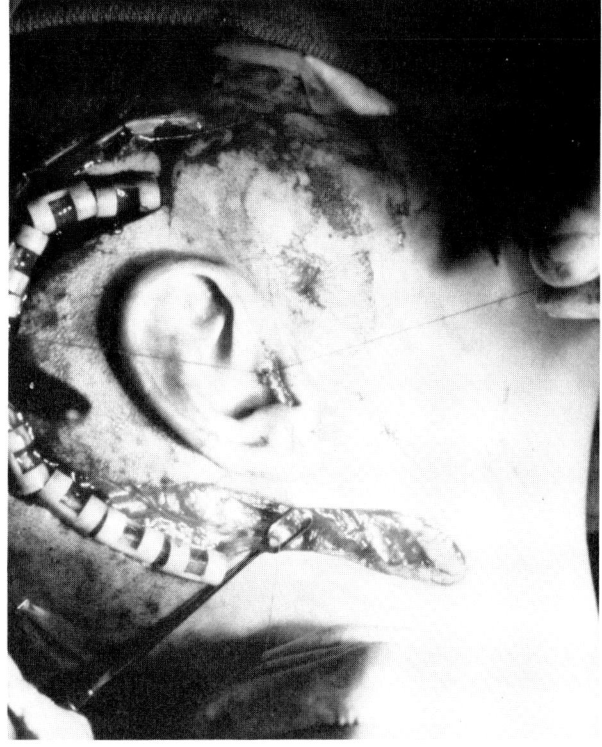

FIG 13–12.
Blind sack closure of the external auditory canal, following which the entire external auditory canal and tympanic membrane were excised.

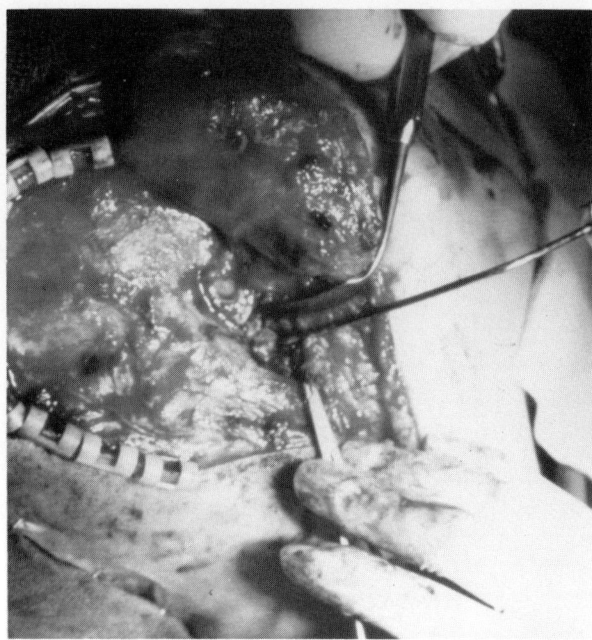

FIG 13–13.
Isolation of the facial nerve and the parotid prior to the mastoidectomy portion of the procedure.

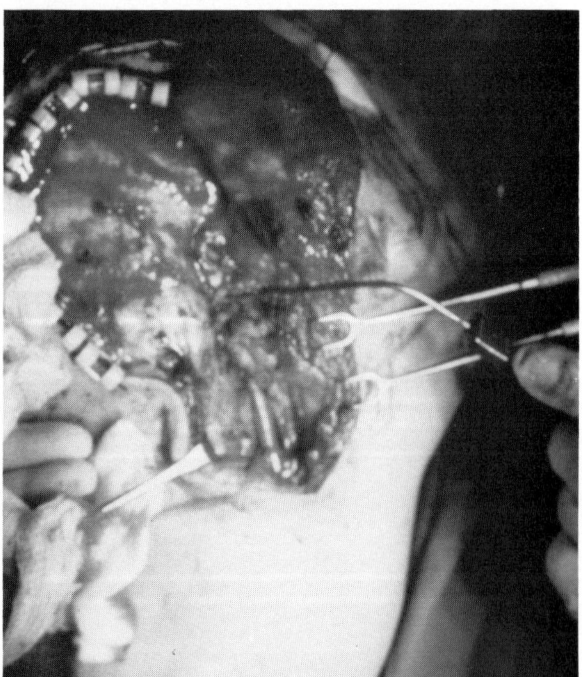

FIG 13–14.
Isolation of the jugular vein, carotid artery, and cranial nerves XI and XII in the neck.

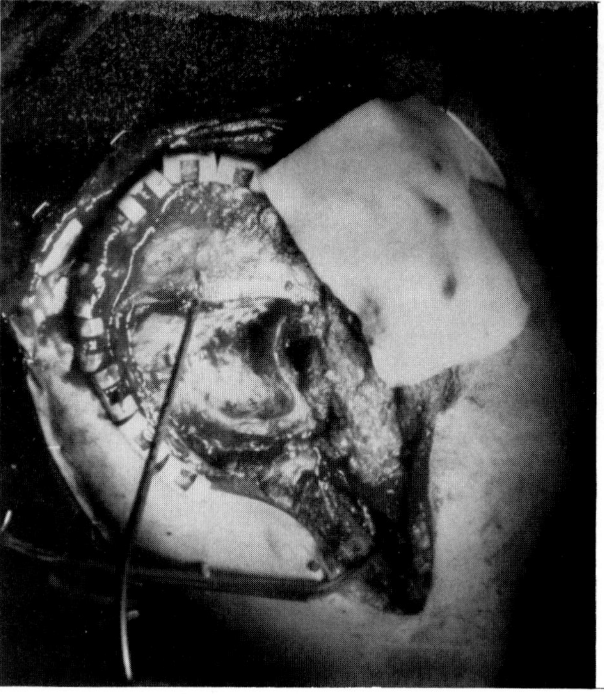

FIG 13–15.
Mastoidectomy completed with saucerization of the mastoid cavity allowing for elimination of the defect in the postoperative period.

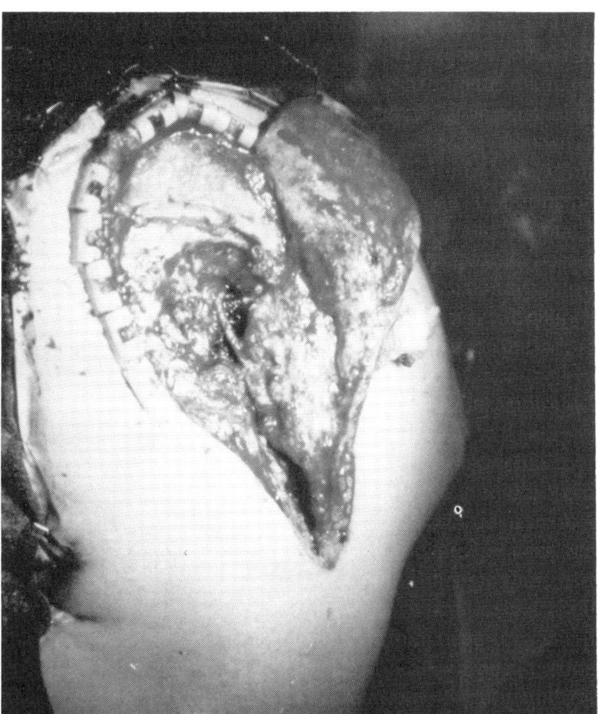

FIG 13–17.
Operative site after removal of the tumor, with Surgicel placed in the petrosal sinus and the facial nerve returned to its normal anatomic position.

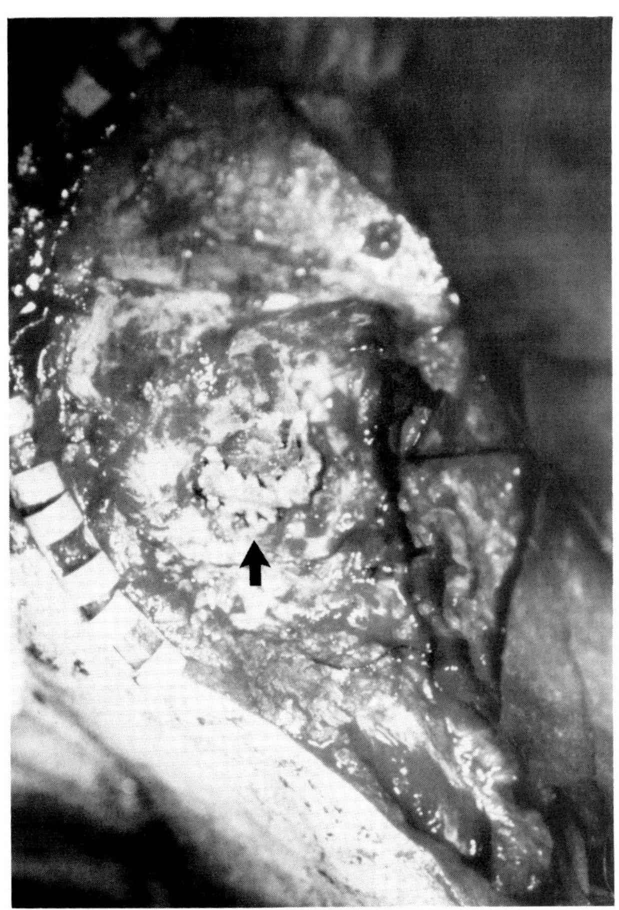

FIG 13–16.
Temporalis fascia graft over the dural defect created by ligation of the sigmoid sinus high in the mastoid.

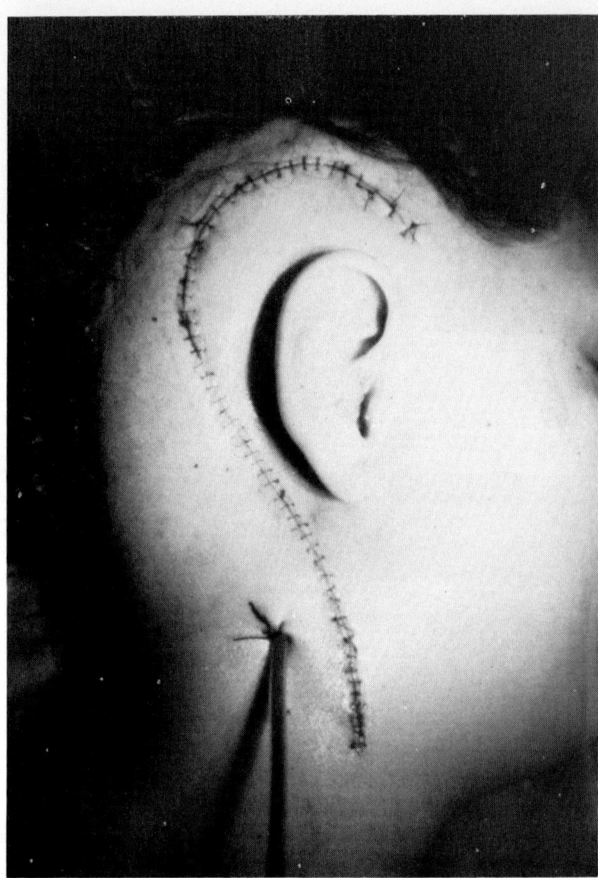

FIG 13–18.
The skin incision is closed with drain, and a suction catheter is in place.

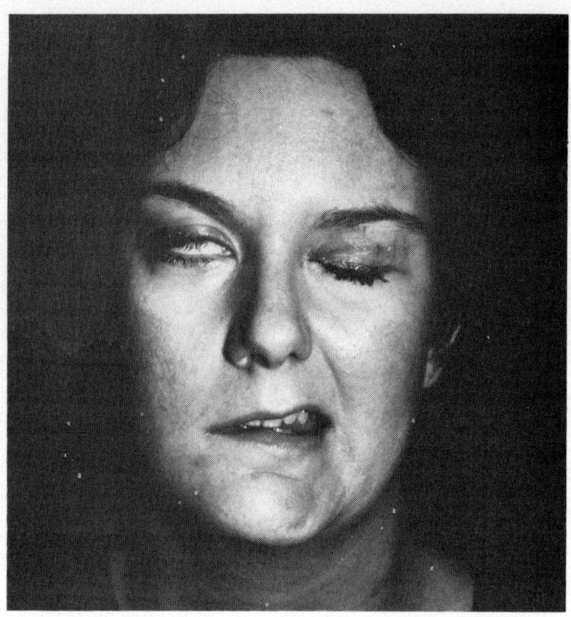

FIG 13–19.
Patient's appearance 1 week postoperatively with paralysis of the right facial nerve.

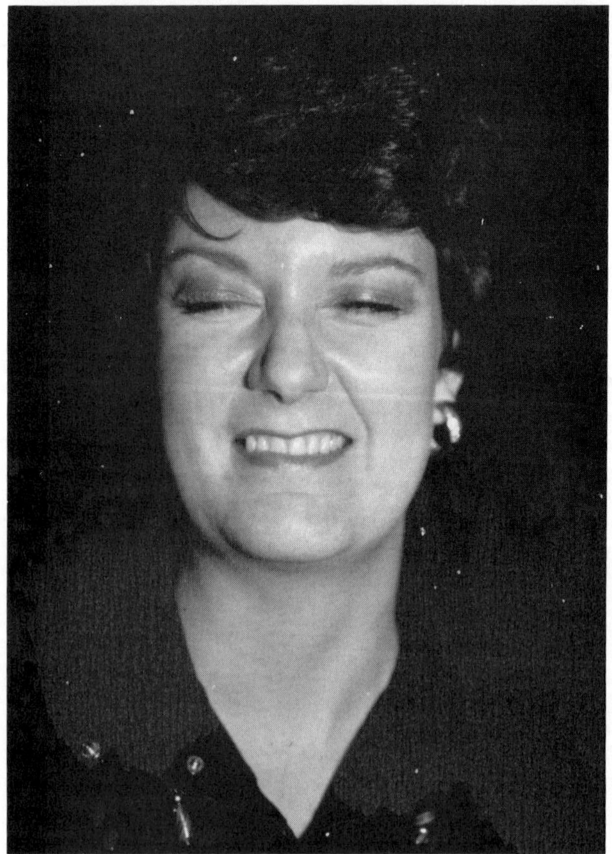

FIG 13–20.
Patient's appearance 3 months postoperatively with return of facial nerve function.

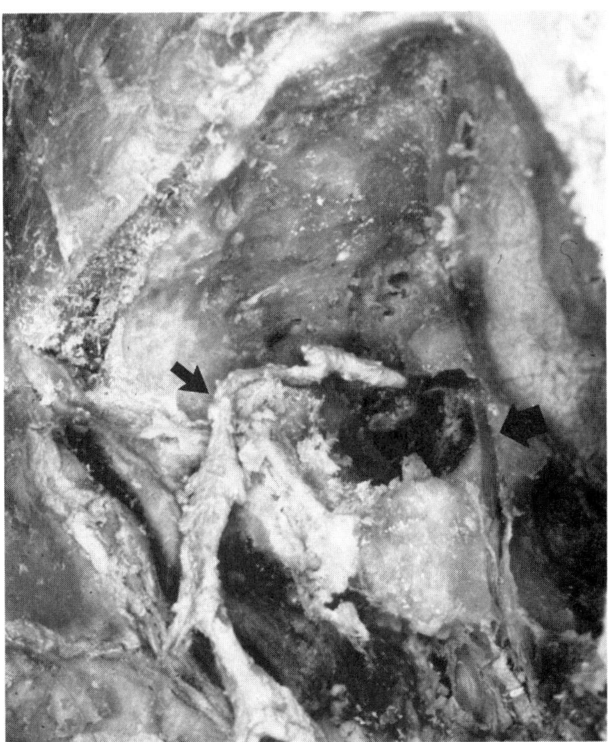

FIG 13–21.
Anterior transposition of the facial nerve over the root of the zygoma *(narrow black arrow)* and the fallopian canal from which the nerve was taken *(wide black arrow)*.

incidence of cerebral venous hypertension by allowing for drainage of the blood via the superior petrosal sinus to the cavernous sinus and then down to the opposite jugular vein. Once a tumor is removed, I generally use Surgicel to pack the inferior petrosal sinus, which may have multiple ostea. Dissection of cranial nerves IX, X, XI, and XII is imperative if one is to preserve these, and dissection should be one of the surgical goals in removing early glomus jugulare tumors. Clearly it is more difficult after radical radiotherapy and is a case for direct surgical extirpation of these tumors. In approaching large glomus jugulare tumors, I have, in the past, believed that a one-stage approach was preferable. Having encountered several large CSF leaks and two episodes of significant meningitis, I have begun using a two-stage approach, with the intracranial approach being done first, after which a fascia lata dural patch is placed. The inferior approach is then done using a lateral skull base dissection. This latter technique has been employed by Fisch and Pillsbury[14] for years and is, in our opinion, the preferred technique to lessen the morbidity of this surgical undertaking.

Complications

The most frequent complication of these procedures is CSF fistulae. They can be prevented by providing a meticulous dural closure and doing the large resections using a two-stage procedure.

The second most frequent complication for the lateral approach is inadequate tumor resection. This technique is not suitable for malignancies and should be used with caution when one approaches lesions in the clivus and nasopharynx.

CONCLUSION

The choice of an approach for resection of a skull base lesion rests on the surgeon's experience and the location of the lesion. Many approaches with their particular advantages and disadvantages have been discussed. A familiarity with all of these gives the surgeon the flexibility to adjust his or her approach to the lesion rather than struggling with the risks and heartaches of inadequate exposures and suboptimal control of vital structures.

REFERENCES

 1. Kennedy DW, Papel ID, Holliday M: Transpalatal approach to skull base. *Ear Nose Throat J* 1986; 65:48–60.
 2. Kennedy DW: Skull base surgery: 1–3. *Ear Nose Throat J* 1986; 65:2–4.
 3. Stevenson AC, Sidney RJ, Perkins RK, et al: A transclival approach to the ventral surface of the brainstem for removal of a clivus chordoma. *J Neurosurg* 1966; 24:544–551.
 4. Cloward RB, Passarelli P: Removal of giant clival chordoma by an anterior cervical approach. *Surg Neurol* 1979; 11:129–134.
 5. Terz JJ, Alksne JF, Lawrence W Jr: Craniofacial resection for tumors invading the pterygoid fossa. *Am J Surg* 1969; 118:732–740.
 6. Biller HF, Shugar JM, Krespi YP: A new technique for wide-field exposure of the base of the skull. *Arch Otolaryngol* 1981; 107:698–702.
 7. Krespi YP, Sisson GA: Skull base surgery in composite resection. *Arch Otolaryngol* 1982; 108:681–684.
 8. Spiro RH, Gerald FB, Strong EW: Mandibular "swing" approach for oral and oropharyngeal tumors. *Head Neck Surg* 1981; 3:371–378.
 9. Ariyan S, Cuono CB: Myocutaneous flaps for head and neck reconstruction. *Head Neck Surg* 1980; 2:321–345.
10. Savage RC: Orbital exenteration and reconstruction for massive basal cell and squamous cell carcinoma of cutaneous origin. *Ann Plast Surg* 1983; 10:458–466.
11. Gluckman JL, Crissman JD, Donnegan JO: Multicentric squamous cell carcinoma of the upper respiratory tract. *Head Neck Surg* 1980; 3:90–96.
12. Sisson GA, Bytell DE, Becker SP, et al: Carcinoma of the paranasal sinuses and craniofacial resection. *J Laryngol Otol* 1976; 90:59–68.
13. Ketcham AS, Chretien PB, Van Buren JM, et al: The ethmoid sinuses: A re-evaluation of surgical resection. *Am J Surg* 1973; 126:469–476.
14. Fisch U, Pillsbury HC: Infratemporal fossa approach to lesions in the temporal bone and base of skull. *Arch Otolaryngol* 1979; 105:99–107.
15. Terz JJ, Young HF, Lawrence W: Combined craniofacial resection for locally advanced carcinoma of the head and neck: I. Tumors of skin and soft tissue. *Am J Surg* 1980; 140:163.

16. McGregor IA, MacDonald DG: Mandibular osteotomy in the surgical approach to the oral cavity. *Head Neck Surg* 1983; 5:457–462.
17. Wood BG, Sadar ES, Levine HL: Surgical problems of the base of the skull: Interdisciplinary approach. *Arch Otolaryngol* 1980; 106:1–5.
18. Ohngren LG: Malignant tumors of the maxillo-ethmoidal region: A clinical study with special reference to the treatment with electrocautery and irradiation. *Acta Otolaryngol* 1933; 19(suppl):1–476.
19. Ketcham AS, Wilkins RH, Van Buren JM, et al: A combined intracranial facial approach to the paranasal sinuses. *Am J Surg* 1963; 106:698–703.
20. Acheson ED: Nasal cancer in the furniture and boot and shoe manufacturing industries. *Prev Med* 1976; 5:295–315.
21. Robins PE, Powell DJ, Stansbie JM: Carcinoma of the nasal cavity and paranasal sinuses: Incidence and presentation of different histological types. *Clin Otolaryngol* 1979; 4:431–456.
22. Jackson RT, Fitz-Hugh GS, Constable WC: Malignant neoplasms of the nasal cavities and paranasal sinuses (a retrospective study). *Laryngoscope* 1977; 87:726–736.
23. Sisson GA, Becker SP: Cancer of the nasal cavity and paranasal sinuses, in Suen JY, Myers EN (eds): *Cancer of the Head and Neck*. New York, Churchill Livingstone, 1981, pp 242–279.
24. Cheng VST, Wang CC: Carcinoma of the paranasal sinuses. A study of sixty-six cases. *Cancer* 1977; 40:3038–3041.
25. Eilber F, Zanem HA: Pterygoid dissection for extensive cancer. *Plast Reconstr Surg* 1977; 9:545–550.
26. Supance JS, Seid AB: Craniofacial resection for ethmoid carcinoma in children. *Int J Pediatr Otorhinolaryngol* 1981; 3:185–194.
27. Terz JJ, Young HF, Lawrence W: Combined craniofacial resection for locally advanced carcinoma of the head and neck: II. Carcinoma of the paranasal sinuses. *Am J Surg* 1980; 140:618.
28. Johns ME, Winn HR, McLean WC, et al: Pericranial flap for the closure of defects of craniofacial resection. *Laryngoscope* 1981; 91:952–959.
29. Shah JP, Galicich JH: Craniofacial resection for malignant tumors of ethmoid and anterior skull base. *Arch Otolaryngol* 1977; 103:514–517.
30. Malecki J: New trends in frontal sinus surgery. *Acta Otolaryngol* 1959; 50:137–140.
31. Wilson JS, Westbury G: Combined craniofacial resection for tumor involving the orbital walls. *Br J Plast Surg* 1973; 26:44–56.
32. Schramm VC, Myers EN, Maroon JC: Anterior skull base surgery for benign and malignant disease. *Laryngoscope* 1979; 89:1077–1091.
33. Waldman SR, Levine HL, Astor F, et al: Surgical experience with nasopharyngeal angiofibroma. *Arch Otolaryngol* 1981; 107:677–682.
34. Obwegeser HL: Temporal approach to the TMJ, the orbit, and the retromaxillary-infracranial region. *Head Neck Surg* 1985; 7:185–199.
35. Wiet RJ, Pillsbury HC, Postma DS, et al: Anterior and lateral approaches for tumors of the skull base, in English GM (ed): *Textbook of Otolaryngology*. Philadelphia, Harper & Row, Publishers, 1987, pp 1–27.
36. Krespi YP, Sisson GA: Transmandibular exposure of the skull base. *Am J Surg* 1984; 148:534–538.

Skull Base Tumors

Approach of

Yosef P. Krespi, M.D.

The overall medical management of skull base cancer can be one of the most frustrating conditions faced by the modern otolaryngologist. Improvements and modifications of treatment modalities and advances in extirpative and reconstructive surgery have markedly altered the natural history of advanced head and neck cancer.[1–6] Vikram reported that about twice the number of patients die from distant metastasis from primary tumors in the head and neck region than from uncontrolled disease.[7] These findings were not present 15 to 20 years ago.[8] The percentage of deaths from uncontrolled local disease and distant metastasis has reversed largely because of the common use of multimodality agents in the treatment of head and neck cancer. The ability of head and neck surgeons to successfully palliate the individual patient with disease beyond the possibility of cure has improved. Modern anesthesia and surgical resection with primary (immediate) or secondary (delayed) reconstructive techniques give the patient immediate relief of pain caused by the cancer with acceptable appearance.[1,9–12] Surgeons specializing in the same region of the body may disagree philosophically as to the extent that one should palliate advanced tumors. Specialists should be aware of the modern technical methods that have been developed to remove these deadly tumors from complex locations such as the lateral skull base.[13–17]

Since the majority of patients with persistent or recurrent skull base tumors have usually reached the tolerable limits of other treatment options, one is faced with a choice between no intervention and aggressive surgery. The patient with recurrent disease has already failed one or two different treatment modalities, usually surgery or irradiation or both. Future treatment with radical surgery should be undertaken only after considerable attention is given to the patient's medical and social history. There is ample evidence that one can provide satisfactory palliation to these patients through the proper use of additional surgery.[16,18–20] Since the possibility of cure is less than 20%, if one cannot offer significant palliation, radical surgery should not be performed. It is far better to let such high-risk patients live out their remaining months in relative comfort. Medical support using tranquilizers and narcotics will keep the terminal patients comfortable. In hopeless cases it is far more important that the time and energy of the surgical team be spent directing attention to relieving the stress and emotional tension of the patient and his or her family than attempting unwarranted surgical heroics. On the other hand, the patient with unresectable cancer who is receiving heavy narcotics may be removed from any social contact with friends, relatives, and hospital personnel. A carefully planned surgical procedure on persistent or recurrent skull base cancer can successfully palliate most of the patients and cure a small number of them. The tremendous pain secondary to cancer is usually reduced or eliminated. With modern reconstructive and rehabilitation techniques, the surgical site can be improved to such a degree that very little nursing care is required.[21,22] The advantages of surgery for malignant lesions extending and involving the lateral skull base are clearly prolonged survival, decrease or elimination of facial and cranial pain, and tremendous ease in nursing care requiring relatively short-term hospitalization in the majority of cases.[23] Death in these patients usually occurs from recurrent aspiration, pneumonia, distant metastasis, local or intracranial tumor recurrence, and, rarely, major vessel blowout.

Malignancies involving the lateral skull base, including the infratemporal fossa, pterygomaxillary fossa, and parapharyngeal space, are commonly associated with trismus and severe pain. Seven patients with malignant tumors of the infratemporal fossa were presented by Shapshay et al.[24] All of the patients in this series had persistent, incapacitating facial pain. Trismus, sensory loss along the trigeminal nerve, and middle ear effusion were also present in about one half of the patients. Other pathologic conditions may present in similar fashion and are usually included in the differential diagnosis. These are (1) trigeminal neuralgia, (2) glossopharyngeal neuralgia, (3) neuritis secondary to herpes zoster and sarcoidosis of other inflammatory conditions, (4) sinusitis, (5) temporomandibular joint syndrome, (6) elongated styloid (Eagle's syndrome), and (7) intracranial tumors of vascular lesions.

Patients with primary or secondary malignant tumors of the lateral skull base can remain undiagnosed for extended periods. The most important factor in making the proper diagnosis is a high index of suspicion.[25,26] Malignant tumors of the lateral skull base often are declared inoperable or noncurable. Difficulties in the past were related to (1) the fact that one could not obtain adequate surgical margins, (2) excessive blood loss due to difficulty in exposure of great vessels, (3) surgical resection resulting in considerable cosmetic and functional deformity, and (4) unsatisfactory palliation. Lateral skull base resection will be described in detail. This procedure provides an en bloc resection of tumor with relatively low morbidity and appears to accomplish excellent palliation and, in some instances, cure. The majority of the patients operated had persistent or recurrent malignancies following failure of an earlier surgical resection or radiation therapy. Squamous cell carcinoma has a known propensity to spread along the lymphatics, fascial planes, and nerve sheaths. It is evident that unless complete en bloc lateral skull base resection is performed, adequate surgical margins cannot be obtained. Several reports confirm this concept in which attempt of an incomplete surgical resection without removal of lateral skull base structures may result in local recurrence in more than 80% of the cases.[27–30] The survival rate for patients with tumors in this area is dismal when standard limited operative approaches or primary radiation therapy are used.

EMBRYOLOGY OF THE SKULL BASE

The skull begins to appear at the end of the first month as mesenchymal condensations surround the developing brain. The first part that is evident is the occipital region, forming the occipital plate from which two extensions on each side grow laterally to complete the foramina around the hypoglossal nerve. At the same time, the mesenchymal condensations extend forward, dorsal to the pharynx, to reach the primordium of the hypophysis. These will then establish the clivus of the cranial base and the dorsum sella of the future sphenoid bone.

Early in the second month, the hypophysis is surrounded by mesenchymal condensation, which extends ventrally to form the anlage of the ethmoid bone and the nasal septum.

During the fifth week, the two otocysts become enclosed in their mesenchymal otic capsules, which soon differentiate into dorsolateral (vestibular) and ventromedial (cochlear) parts enveloping the primordia of semicircular canals and cochlea. Between these two regions, the facial nerve lies in a deep grove. The otocyst fuses with the lateral process of the occipital plate, leaving a wide hiatus through which the internal jugular vein and cranial nerves IX, X, and XI will exit the skull. At this stage, the mesenchyme around the hypophysial stalk spreads out laterally to form the greater sphenoid wings. The smaller processes located ventrally indicate the lesser sphenoid wings.

The first signs of the vault, or neurocranial part of the skull, appear about the 30th day. They consist of curved plates of mesenchyme at the sides of the skull, gradually extending cranially to blend with each other; they also extend downward to reach the base of the skull.

The chondrification of the skull base begins in the second month. The chondrification centers at the mesenchymal condensations are named mainly in relation to the notochord: parachordal or prechordal.

The first cartilaginous foci appear in the occipital plate, one on each side of the notochord, and they fuse at the end of the seventh week. At the same time, the cartilaginous basal plate is formed, through which the notochord, hypoglossal nerve, and the hypophysis will pass. The otic capsules become cartilaginous and begin to fuse with the lateral aspect of the basal plate.

The cartilage of the posterior part of the sphenoid is formed from two hypophyseal centers. At first they unite behind and later in front, finally enclosing the craniopharyngeal canal containing the hypophyseal diverticle. The canal is usually obliterated by the third month.

Around the eighth week, the basioccipital cartilage (plate) joins with the basisphenoid cartilage, which develops from the hypophyseal cartilage. More anteriorly, the trabecular cartilage becomes a vertical cartilagenous plate within the nasal septum called mesethmoid. This cartilage separates the epithelium of each side of the nasal cavity and connects the nasal capsule cartilage with the basisphenoid.

Ossification commences before the chondrocranium has fully developed, and on completion, bone overtakes cartilage until only small sections of the chondrocranium remain.[31, 32]

General Characteristics In Development of the Skull Base

1. The base of the skull develops from mesenchymal cells located between the cranial part of the neural tube and the foregut during the fourth week.

2. Mesenchymal cells originate from both primitive streak and cranial neural crest.

3. During the fifth to sixth week, mesenchymal cells collect in certain areas to form condensations, collectively referred to as the desmocranium or the blastemal stage of skull development. Some of the condensations will differentiate directly into membranous bone, whereas others will develop into cartilage, most of which subsequently ossifies.

4. Cartilage formation is evident by the seventh week, and the chondrocranium reaches its height of development during the third month.

5. Ossification begins during the latter part of the second month.

6. Many bones are partly membranous and partly cartilaginous, especially in the base of skull.

7. Most individual bones of the skull arise from two or more centers of ossification.

SURGICAL ANATOMY OF THE SKULL BASE

Surgical exposure of the extracranial surface of the middle cranial fossa presents a difficult problem to the otolaryngologist-head and neck surgeon. Guidelines or mapping of the structures are not readily available to assist the surgeon during lateral skull base resection. Knowledge of the surgical anatomy of the middle fossa skull base is very important. The various surgical techniques leading to lateral skull base resection were developed following extensive cadaver dissections. Anatomically, this portion of the skull base can be divided into two lateral and one midline compartment. The imaginary borders between the compartments are made by the petrous portion of the internal carotid arteries traversing the temporal bone and the pterygoid plates. This represents a convenient surgical and anatomic separation. Each compartment presents its own problems of surgical exposure for tumor resection (Figs 13–22 and 13–23).

The lateral compartment is composed of a portion of the greater wing of the sphenoid bone and the under surface of the petrous portion of the temporal bone. Together they form the roof of the infratemporal fossa. Limited or wide surgical access to the lateral compartment can be obtained with a variety of surgical techniques designed particularly for the temporal bone. The transcervical transmastoid, translabyrinthine, transcochlear, and infratemporal fossa approaches all have been described.[18, 33, 34] Each of these techniques expose the skull base from the lateral direction via the temporal bone. The medial extent of the dissection does not allow safe and ready access to the midline compartment. The structures that limit exposure are the facial nerve, the mandibular ramus, the temporomandibular joint, and the internal carotid artery. Critical anatomic structures such as the foramen lacerum and pterygomaxillary space fall into the line separating the midline and lateral compartments. Separation of the middle fossa skull base into three compartments provides an anatomic and radiologic convenience; however, surgeons must be prepared to cross these imaginary lines as indicated by the pathologic condition.

FORAMINA AND CANALS

Anterior to the Petrous Bone

Here the foramina can be roughly joined by an imaginary crescentic line. The foramen lacrimale is in the anterolateral corner of the middle cranial compartment. Anastomotic vessels between the lacrimal and middle meningeal arteries traverse through this small foramen. Medial to the foramen lacrimale, and occupying most of the anterior border of the middle cranial compartment, is the superior orbital fissure. Through this fissure will pass the ophthalmic vein, branches of the middle meningeal (orbital branch), the lacrimal arteries, the ophthalmic division of the fifth cranial nerve, and cranial nerves III, IV, and VI. When viewed directly from above, both the foramen lacrimale and the superior orbital fissure are hidden by the lesser sphenoid wing. Therefore, the first foramen to be seen from above is the foramen rotundum. The foramen rotundum is in a general anteroposterior direction and opens into the upper-

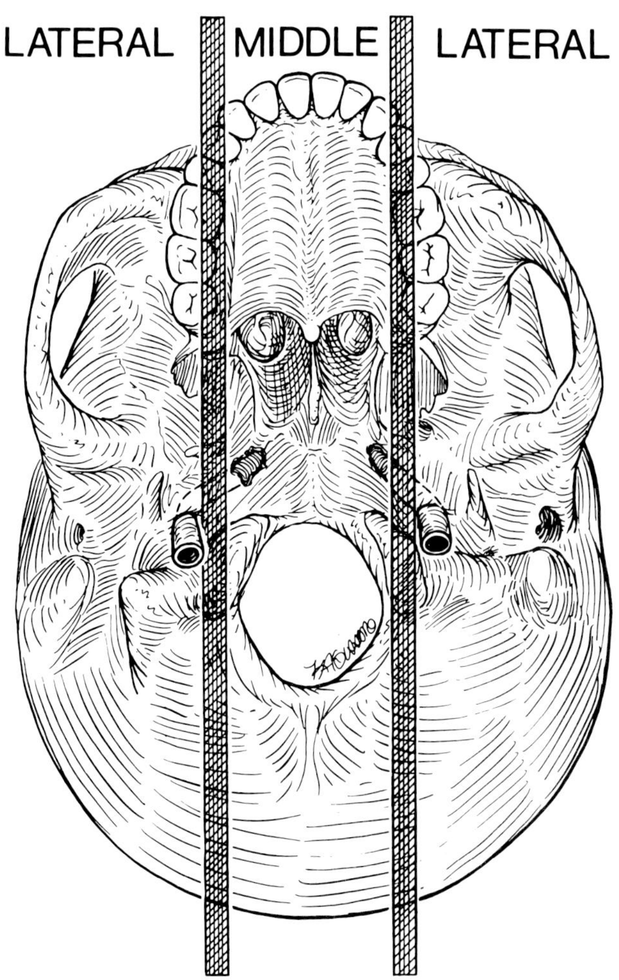

FIG 13–22.
Two ventrical lines divide the middle fossa skull base into three compartments. These imaginary lines traverse through the petrous carotid artery and pterygoid plates.

most region of the pterygopalatine fossa. It contains the maxillary division of the fifth cranial nerve. The foramen rotundum is surrounded posteriorly by two large foramina, medially by the foramen lacerum and the carotid canal, and laterally by the foramen ovale. Foramen lacerum is a gap between the petrous apex and the body of the sphenoid bone. The foramen itself is the anterosuperior opening of the distal end of the carotid canal that passes through the petrous bone. The foramen lacerum also contains the greater superficial petrosal nerve, which joins here with the deep petrosal nerve arising from the carotid's sympathetic plexus. The meningeal branch of the ascending pharyngeal artery also enters the skull through foramen lacerum. Small lymph nodes in this region provide a channel for tumor spread from the nasopharynx and pharyngeal walls into the skull. Lateral to the foramen lacerum and the carotid canal is the foramen ovale, through which pass the mandibular division of the fifth cranial nerve and an accessory meningeal artery. Next to the foramen ovale is the foramen spinosum, which the middle meningeal artery and the recurrent branch

of the mandibular nerve pass. Two tiny holes on the anterior surface of the petrous bone contain the greater and the lesser superficial petrosal nerves. The first nerve originates in the geniculate ganglion within the temporal bone. After it emerges through the "facial hiatus," it lies in a small groove that ends in the foramen lacerum. The lesser superficial petrosal nerve enters into the temporal bone through the tympanic canaliculus, which is infralateral to the first foramen.

Posterior to the Petrous Bone

The main foramen in this region is the jugular foramen. It is bounded by the temporal bone laterally and the occipital bone medially. The foramen is divided into a medial compartment that contains cranial nerves IX, X, and XI as well as the inferior petrosal sinus. The lateral compartment contains the internal jugular vein and the meningeal branches of the occipital and ascending pharyngeal arteries. The internal jugular vein is formed by the transverse and inferior petrosal sinuses. The hypoglossal canal is posteromedial to the jugular foramen. It contains a small meningeal artery, an emissary vein, and cranial nerve XII, which leaves the skull above the occipital condyle to join the neurovascular complex of the jugular foramen. The internal acoustic meatus is in the posteromedial surface of the petrous bone. It transmits the seventh and eighth cranial nerves as well as the internal auditory blood vessels.[35, 36]

All of the foramina discussed so far were described according to their position in the intracranial surface of the skull base. They all have corresponding openings on the external surface of the skull base. Their exact relation to other extracranial structures such as muscles or blood vessels will be described in three separate sections: (1) the infratemporal fossa, (2) the parapharyngeal space, and (3) the pterygopalatine fossa.[37]

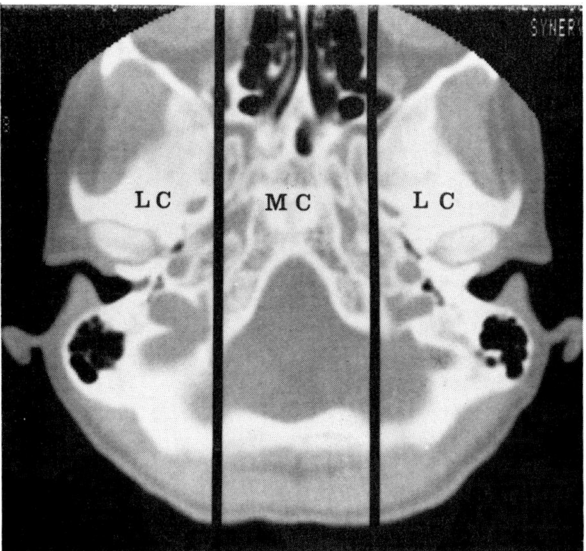

FIG 13–23.
Axial CT scan with bone windows demonstrating the lines dividing the middle fossa skull base into lateral *(LC)* and midline *(MC)* compartments.

Infratemporal Fossa

The roof of the infratemporal fossa consists of the skull base area, the sphenoid bony crest laterally, the inferior orbital fissure anteriorly, a line joining the foramen spinosum, the foramen ovale and the origin of the lateral pterygoid plate medially, and a line joining the foramen spinosum and the articular tubercle posteriorly. The anterior wall is formed by the posterior wall of the maxillary sinus and the pterygoid plates.

The infratemporal fossa contains three muscles of mastication: the medial and lateral pterygoid muscles and the lower part of the temporalis muscle inserting onto the coronoid process of the mandible. The main artery in the infratemporal fossa is the maxillary artery with its branches. This artery courses through the infratemporal fossa to reach the pterygopalatine fissure. It enters the pterygopalatine fossa and gives off its terminal branches. In the infratemporal fossa, the artery gives off a number of branches to the masticatory muscles. In addition, its deep auricular branches and the anterior tympanic branches supply the external and middle ear. The middle meningeal and accessory meningeal arteries ascend vertically to enter the skull through the foramen spinosum and the foramen ovale, respectively. These arteries are accompanied by nerves throughout their course in the infratemporal fossa.

The chorda tympani leaves the skull through the petrotympanic fissure (with the anterior tympanic artery), courses through the infratemporal fossa, and joins the lingual nerve. The auriculotemporal nerve arises by two sensory roots from the mandibular nerve. Each root receives parasympathetic secretomotor fibers from the otic ganglion. After surrounding the middle meningeal artery, the two roots unite around the posterior surface of the mandibular neck to supply the parotid gland. Superiorly, the auriculotemporal nerve gives its general sensory branches to the temporal region of the scalp. The otic ganglion lies in close contact with the mandibular nerve, immediately below the foramen ovale.

Preganglionic parasympathetic fibers of the lesser petrosal nerve synapse in the otic ganglion to give the postganglionic secretomotor fibers to the parotid gland. The nerve fibers traversing the otic ganglion are the sympathetic fibers from the plexus on the middle meningeal artery, the motor fibers to the medial pterygoid, tensor palatini and tensor tympani muscles, and some sensory fibers from the fifth and ninth cranial nerves.

The pterygoid plexus is the main venous structure in the infratemporal fossa. This plexus is formed by veins around the lateral pterygoid muscle adjacent to the maxillary artery. The plexus drains into the maxillary vein. It is anatomically and clinically significant that the pterygoid plexus has widespread communications with many surrounding veins that pass through the foramina and the sphenoidal emissary foramen to reach the cavernous sinus intracranially.

The tensor palatini muscle arises between the eustachian tube medially and the foramen ovale and foramen spinosum laterally. The muscle hooks around the pterygoid hamulus and then spreads medially into the soft palate. Parotid tissue that lies medial to the ascending mandibular ramus (deep lobe) is also in the infratemporal fossa.[38]

Parapharyngeal Space

The parapharyngeal space has a shape of an inverted pyramid. The base is the external surface of the skull base and the apex of the pyramid in the hyoid bone. Anteriorly, the upper portion of the parapharyngeal space is limited by the pterygoid plates. The spine of the sphenoid and the posteromedial aspect of the mandibular condyle lie laterally. The vertebral column and the prevertebral muscles are located posteriorly. The medial wall of the parapharyngeal space is the superior pharyngeal constrictor muscle and the tonsillar fossa.

The parapharyngeal space is usually divided into two main compartments by its fascial planes: the anterior (prestyloid) and the posterior compartments. The prestyloid compartment is in direct continuity with the infratemporal fossa, and it contains mainly the styloid muscles and the tensor and levator palatini muscles.

Three muscles and two ligaments have their origin in the styloid process. The stylopharyngeus muscle, the longest of the three muscles, runs between the internal and external carotid arteries into the pharyngeal wall between the superior and middle pharyngeal constrictors. This muscle is innervated by the ninth cranial nerve, and it acts to elevate and dilate the pharynx as well as move the epiglottis during swallowing and speaking. The styloglossus is one of the four extrinsic muscles of the tongue. It is innervated by the twelfth cranial nerve, and it retracts and elevates the tongue. The stylohyoid muscle runs to the greater cornu of the hyoid bone, where it divides to surround the central tendon of the digastric muscle. This muscle is innervated by the seventh cranial nerve and elevates and pulls the hyoid bone backward during swallowing. The ligaments attached to the styloid process are the stylomandibular and the stylohyoid. The first is formed by the thickening of the investing fascia of the neck, and it separates the parotid from the submandibular gland. The second runs into the lesser cornu of the hyoid bone and may be partly ossified.

In the prestyloid compartment of the parapharyngeal space, two arteries ascend toward the base of the skull accompanied by their veins. These are the ascending palatine artery (from the facial artery) and the ascending pharyngeal artery (from the external carotid artery), both of which eventually penetrate the skull base supplying the meninges. All of the structures in the prestyloid compartment are embedded in connective fatty tissue and a few lymph nodes.

The close relationship between the prestyloid compartment with the infratemporal fossa explains the fact that disease in this region may present with trismus, bulging of the lateral pharyngeal wall, and neurologic symptoms caused by mandibular nerve involvement.

The posterior compartment of the parapharyngeal space is divided further into the retropharyngeal (medial) and the retrostyloid (lateral) spaces. The retropharyngeal space is important in various disease processes, where it provides a route for the inflammatory process to extend both upward and downward. The retropharyngeal space contains very important lymph nodes that receive drainage from the nasopharynx, nose, paranasal sinuses, and oropharynx. The retrostyloid compartment contains mainly the carotid sheath. The carotid sheath is formed under the petrous bone by condensation of the different cervical fasciae. They are joined immediately by the twelfth cranial nerve, which exits the skull through the hypoglossal canal. Thus, four cranial nerves are found within the carotid sheath at its uppermost part. Three of these nerves leave the sheath on its way through the neck.

The eleventh cranial nerve (spinal part) runs with the internal jugular vein in a general posteroinferior direction to enter the sternocleidomastoid muscle.

The glossopharyngeal nerve accompanies the stylopharyngeus muscle in an anteroinferior direction. It passes between the internal and external carotid arteries and into the pharyngeal wall between the superior and middle constrictor muscles, where it lies closely lateral to the tonsillar fossa. The twelfth cranial nerve joins the vagus and adheres to its lateral surface immediately below the skull base, exiting at the level of the posterior belly of the digastric muscle. It curves anteriorly, superficial to both internal and external carotid arteries but deep to the occipital artery. At this level the hypoglossal nerve splits to the motor branch of the tongue muscles and to the superior root of the ansa cervicalis.

The vagus nerve leaves the skull with the accessory nerve through the jugular foramen. It gives two small branches: the meningeal branch, which passes back into the skull, and the auricular branch (Arnold's nerve), which passes through the tympanomastoid fissure into the external ear canal. Immediately below the skull base arises the pharyngeal branch, which runs between the carotid arteries to form the pharyngeal plexus over the middle constrictor muscle. The superior laryngeal branch arises inferior to the pharyngeal branch and runs toward the larynx deep to both carotid arteries. The main trunk of the vagus continues in the carotid sheath throughout the neck.

The sympathetic chain, which is formed by the ascending upper thoracic preganglionic fibers as well as the cervical sympathetic ganglia, is located immediately posterior to the carotid artery. The chain itself ends at the base of the skull, but its fibers on the internal carotid artery enter the skull. The three sympathetic ganglia lie on the prevertebral muscles. The superior ganglion lies between the internal carotid artery and the longus capitis muscle at the level of C2-3. The middle cervical ganglion lies at the level of C6. The inferior ganglion is at the root of the neck.

The retrostyloid compartment also contains lymph nodes. These are found in the upper most part of the retrostyloid compartment (node of Krause) in the skull base. The node of Rouvier is more medial in the skull base, relating closely to the superolateral corner of the nasopharynx and the fossa of Rosenmuller.

Pterygopalatine Fossa

The pterygopalatine fossa (sphenopalatine fossa) is the main neurovascular "relay box" of the midface. The bony walls and structure of the pterygopalatine fossa are the posterior wall of the maxillary sinus anteriorly; the perpendicular plate of the palatine bone and its orbital and sphenoidal processes medi-

ally*; the pterygoid process and the greater wing of the sphenoid bone posteriorly; and the body of the sphenoid bone and inferior orbital fissure, which forms a communication between the pterygopalatine fossa and the infratemporal fossa, superiorly. Inferiorly, the pterygopalatine fossa has no floor; it has the shape of an inverted irregular pyramid. The apex of this pyramid is formed by the posterior wall of the antrum and the pterygoid process of the sphenoid.

Foramina and Canals

In the posterior wall, the foramen rotundum connects with the middle cranial fossa. Through it pass the second division of the trigeminal nerve and a small artery. The pterygoid canal (vidian canal), through which pass the vidian nerve and the vidian artery, is also located posteriorly. The bony ridge between these two openings has a great surgical importance. In the anterosuperior wall, the inferior orbital fissure contains the terminal portion of the maxillary nerve with its branches, the zygomatic and infraorbital nerves, the infraorbital blood vessels, and the inferior ophthalmic veins. In the medial wall, the sphenopalatine foramen brings the sphenopalatine artery and nerve into the nasal cavity. The foramen of Juvara is below the sphenopalatine foramen, about halfway to the apex of the pterygopalatine fossa. It contains the neurovascular supply to the nasal cavity. In the lateral wall, the pterygomaxillary fissure contains the superior posterior alveolar artery, nerves to the posterior upper jaw and teeth, and the sphenopalatine vein. The third part of the maxillary artery also enters the pterygopalatine fossa through this fissure. Inferiorly (apex), the greater and lesser palatine foramina bring the corresponding arteries and nerves to the hard and soft palate, respectively.

The venous drainage is mainly into the pterygoid venous plexus in the neighboring infratemporal fossa. The sphenopalatine vein is situated on the posterior surface of the posterior maxillary sinus wall, the greater palatine vein, and the inferior ophthalmic vein from the orbital floor drain into the pterygoid plexus.

The neural structures are located posteriorly in the pterygopalatine fossa. The pterygopalatine ganglion is situated in the superior part of the pterygopalatine fossa near the sphenopalatine foramen. It receives general sensory fibers from the maxillary nerve, sympathetic fibers from the vidian nerve, and parasympathetic fibers also from the vidian nerve. Only the preganglionic parasympathetic fibers traverse the ganglion. The sympathetic fibers originate in the internal carotid plexus, where they form the deep petrosal nerve to join the parasympathetic fibers of the greater superficial petrosal nerve. These sympathetic and parasympathetic fibers accompany the general sensory fibers of the different branches of the maxillary nerve to reach and supply the lacrimal gland as well as the minor salivary glands of the nose, palate, and pharynx, which gives the auto-

---

*These processes articulate with the body of the sphenoid bone, which forms the roof of the pterygopalatine fossa. This articulation leaves a foramen, the sphenopalatine foramen, situated in the posterosuperomedial corner of pterygopalatine fossa.

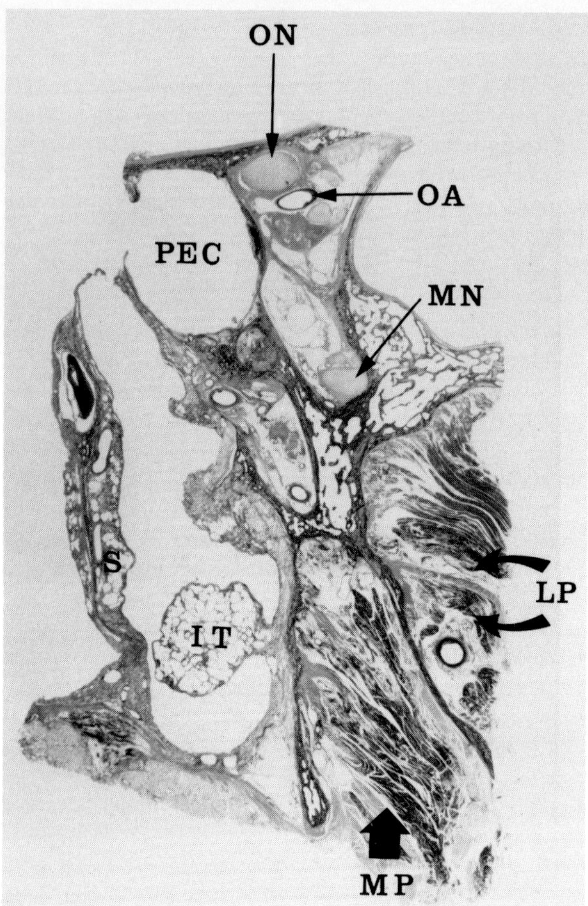

FIG 13–24.
Coronal section of the middle cranial fossa skull base at the level of posterior nasal cavity (posterior to the maxillary sinus). *PEC* = posterior ethmoid cells; *S* = septum; *ON* = optic nerve; *OA* = ophthalmic artery; *MP* = medial pterygoid muscle, *LP* = lateral pterygoid muscle; *IT* = inferior turbinate; *MN* = maxillary nerve.

nomic vascular control in these regions. These branches are the sphenopalatine, greater and lesser palatine, lateral and posterior nasal, nasopalatine, pharyngeal, infraorbital, zygomatic, and superoposterior aveolar.

The sphenoid sinus and the nasopharynx, which is located at the midline compartment of the middle fossa skull base, will be discussed shortly.[39]

The sphenoid sinus is a midline structure divided into two unequal cavities by a septum. Its anatomic relationships make the sphenoid sinus a critical structure when one attempts to assess the resectability of a skull base tumor. Superiorly, the sinus borders the pituitary gland, frontal lobes, and the cavernous sinus. The pons and the basilar artery are located behind the posterior wall; the nasopharynx is inferior. The carotid arteries lie lateral to the sphenoid sinus and may be dehiscent within the sinus, protected only by dura and sinus mucoperiostium. Superomedial to the carotid arteries and anterior to the pituitary gland is the optic chiasm. Drainage into the nasal cavity is through the sphenoid ostium at the anterior wall.

The nasopharynx is a complex structure with important

anatomic relationships. The anterior wall of the nasopharynx contains the two openings for the posterior choanae. The inferior wall is comprised of the soft palate and communicates with the oropharynx through the pharyngeal isthmus. The two lateral walls are penetrated by the eustachian tube orifices. Only the superior and posterior walls contain no ostia (Figs 13–24 to 13–28).

Superiorly, the nasopharynx is lined with pseudostratified ciliated columnar epithelium. However, this changes to stratified squamous epithelium inferiorly as the oropharynx is approached. The mucosa of the nasopharynx contains goblet cells, minor salivary glands, and lymphoid tissue. The adenoids are located on the upper posterior wall of the nasopharynx and usually involute before adolescence. The nasopharynx has abundant bilateral lymphatic drainage. The primary drainage site is the nodes of Rouviere, located in the lateral pharyngeal space at the skull base. Secondary drainage is to the jugulodiagastric nodal group.

The nasopharynx is suspended from the skull base by the pharyngeal aponeurosis. Because of its location, there is early involvement of adjacent structures by tumors of the nasopharynx. The carotid artery, cavernous sinus, and cranial nerves III, IV, V_1, V_2, and VI are frequently involved. The abducens nerve

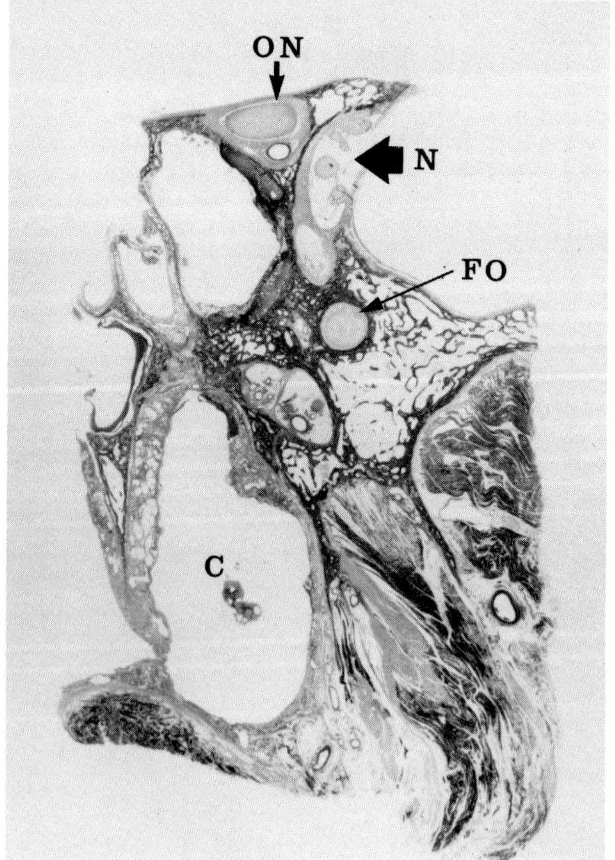

FIG 13–25.
C = choana; *FO* = foramen rotundum; *ON* = optic nerve; *N* = cranial nerves III, IV, and VI.

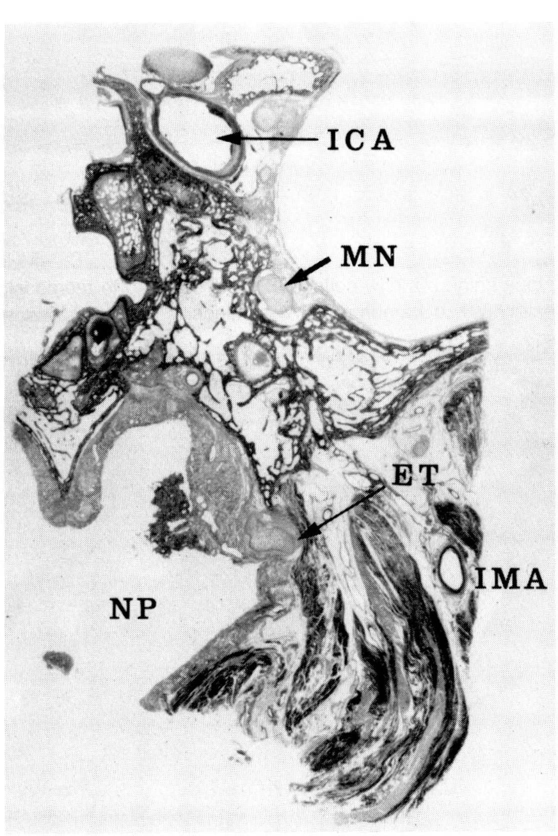

FIG 13–26.
NP = nasopharynx; *MN* = maxillary nerve; *ICA* = internal carotid artery; *IMA* = internal maxillary artery; *ET* = eustachian tube.

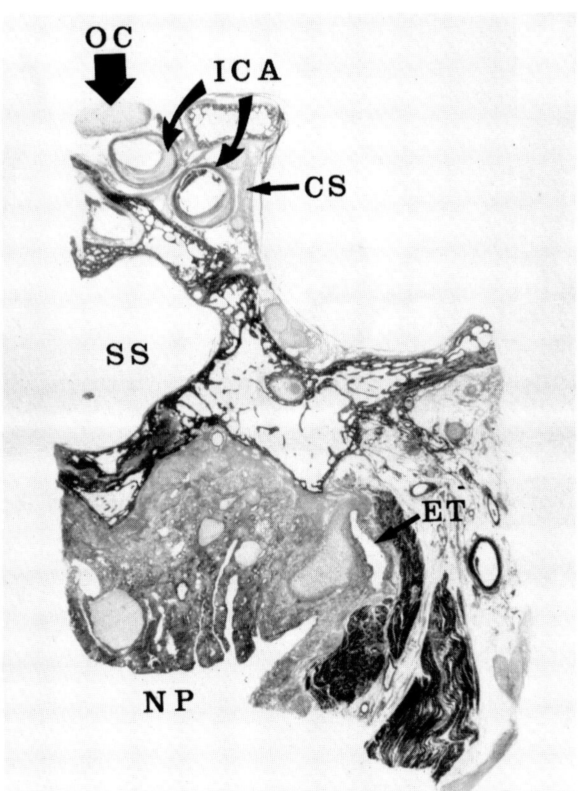

FIG 13–27.
ICA = internal carotid artery; *OC* = optic chiasm; *ET* = eustachian tube; *SS* = sphenoid sinus; *NP* = nasopharynx; *CS* = cavernous sinus.

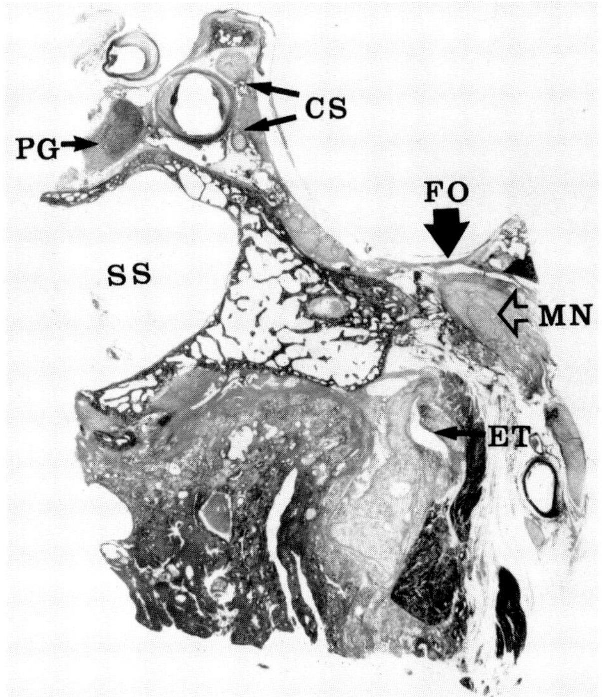

FIG 13–28.
PG = pituitary gland; *CS* = cavernous sinus; *FO* = foramen ovale; *MN* = mandibular nerve; *ET* = eustachian tube; *SS* = sphenoid sinus.

is involved earliest. Extension of tumor into the middle fossa can occur through the foramen lacerum located on the nasopharyngeal side of the pharyngeal aponeurosis. Although cervical metastasis is uncommon in sinonasal malignancy, it is often the presenting symptom in nasopharyngeal carcinoma. Therefore, the neck should be carefully examined, including the posterior triangles.

PREOPERATIVE EVALUATION

Complete neurotologic and head and neck examination is performed on each patient prior to surgery. Computed tomography of the involved region to determine the resectability of the tumor is very important. It allows a three-dimensional mapping of the tumor.[40, 41] Coronal and axial sections produced by high-resolution CT make it possible to assess the tumor size, location, and involvement of vital structures with great accuracy. The results of the CT scan also assist the surgeon in tayloring the operative approach to a given lesion. Magnetic resonance imaging was not routinely available in our institution during the period of this study. However, its ability to contrast different soft tissue may make it an attractive contribution in the preoperative evaluation of these lesions.[42, 43]

Computed tomography has been used extensively in the diagnostic evaluation of lesions of the skull base and has become the standard radiologic examination in this region. As knowledge of radiologic anatomy and resolution of CT have improved, so have surgical techniques advanced. We are performing extensive procedures today on patients who would have been deemed inoperable only a few years ago. Computed tomography enables the physician to accurately stage disease prior to treatment and to follow patients who have undergone treatment to determine the response to therapy or to discover recurrence at the earliest possible time, in some cases before the presence of clinical signs.[25, 44–46]

In the middle fossa skull base, just as in the anterior fossa, soft tissue reconstruction and postoperative radiation therapy may make interpretation of CT scans difficult postoperatively. It is important to obtain early postoperative images to have a baseline for later comparison. Serial changes such as thickening or nodularity of soft tissue, displacement of the pharynx or major blood vessels, development of fluid collections, or bone changes each may signify recurrent disease.

Computed tomography scanning has proved to be extremely helpful in the preoperative assessment and postoperative follow-up of patients with skull base lesions.[46] Postoperative CT enables the physician to obtain a baseline study and then to serially follow the patient's anatomy in regions that may be clinically silent. It is recommended that all such patients undergo CT scanning twice yearly for at least the first 3 years postoperatively.

Each patient with extensive lateral skull base malignancy must have bilateral carotid angiography with cross-compression testing to predict the patient's tolerance to temporary or permanent carotid artery ligation. The internal carotid artery is located at the center of the surgical dissection and is at risk of direct or indirect injury, which may result in debilitating or fatal stroke. To obtain oncologic margins in some patients, one may resect the carotid artery to be included in the surgical specimen. Therefore, preoperative assessment of both carotid systems is of fundamental importance. Intracranial crossflow from one hemisphere to the other with demonstration of patent anterior and posterior communicating vessels in the circle of Willis is a favorable sign. The patient may also be studied with oculoplethysmography to determine back pressure from the contralateral carotid system. The external and internal carotid systems and the vertebral system are individually studied bilaterally. In some cases, a temporary balloon catheter is introduced via the transfemoral approach and is positioned in the internal carotid artery distal to the bifurcation and inflated under electroencephalographic (EEG) control.[13] The balloon is filled with 2 mL of contrast material and left in position for approximately 1 minute. During this time, contrast injections of the contralateral carotid artery and vertebral artery are performed to determine the extent of collateral circulation to the occluded sides. Fisch[13, 14] reported that 16 out of 17 patients tested tolerated the occlusion without any clinical signs or symptoms and without EEG changes. In one patient, a hemiparesis began to develop immediately after balloon inflation. The balloon was immediately deflated, and all neurologic signs returned to normal within 1 or 2 hours. The potential complications with this procedure may include balloon rupture, distal migration of the balloon, intimal damage due to balloon, overdistention, and thrombosis below the balloon with subsequent embolism following deflation. Therefore, the procedure must be carried out under temporary heparinization. A Silverstone clamp (Codman and Shurtleff, Inc.) for gradual occlusion over 3 to 5 days prior to the definitive procedure is advised by others.[47] The clamp is gradually occluded while the patient is awake and alert. This is recommended when the carotid artery is intimately involved with the tumor and must be resected en bloc with the lateral skull base dissection.[19, 48, 49]

Intractable pain, trismus, serous otitis media, and multiple cranial nerve paralysis are not considered contraindications to surgery. However, the presence of intracranial tumor and extensive erosion of bony structures of the skull base, especially the posterior and lateral walls of the sphenoid sinus, cavernous sinus, foramen lacerum, and vertebral bodies, are considered contraindications to tumor resectability.

Following completion of the evaluation, patients and their families must be informed of the extent of the cancer and the unpredictable, low cure rate that is associated with this type of extensive surgery. A thorough informed consent must be obtained in each case.

SURGERY

There are several important factors to consider and steps to take in the preoperative preparation of the patient in any skull base procedure. Preoperative preparation of the patient is vital in any skull base procedure. If brain or dura exposure is anticipated, a lumbar subarachnoid drain is placed preop-

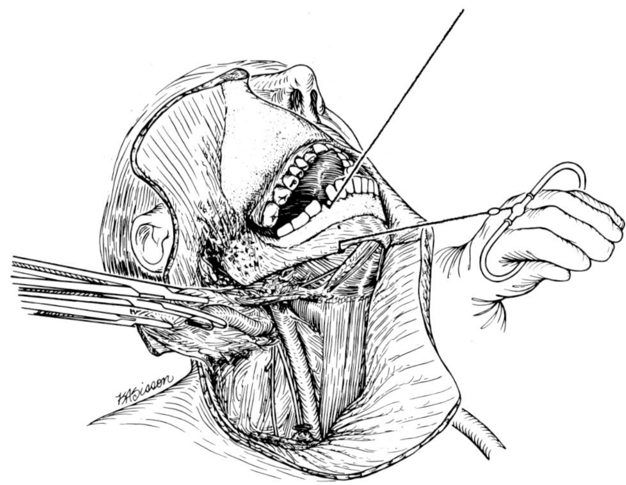

FIG 13–29.
Division of the mandible at the level of the mental foramen with a Gigli saw.

eratively, and approximately 50 to 60 mL of CSF is withdrawn during the operation. It is not necessary to reinfuse the CSF after the procedure is terminated as was once thought. If further exposure and frontotemporal lobe retraction is required, mannitol may be infused in a dosage of 1 to 1.5 mg/kg of body weight. This dosage will reduce the brain water content and provide greater exposure. An excellent neuroanesthetic technique is hyperventilation. It produces a respiratory alkalosis that results in cerebral vasoconstriction and ultimate decrease in intracranial pressure. Because surgery is lengthy and because of the length of time that variable blood loss occurs, placement of urethral catheter, central venous pressure catheter, and arterial line is recommended preoperatively. Temporary tarsorrhaphy is placed to prevent inadvertent damage of orbital contents. The thigh is always shaved and prepared for fascia lata, dermis, or skin graft to be used during the reconstruction.[10, 47]

Lateral skull base surgery provides wide exposure to both midline and lateral compartments of the middle cranial fossa skull base with maximum vascular control and exposure of most cranial nerves. A midline lip-splitting incision exposes the mandible. Lateral mandibulotomy at the angle of the jaw is performed when the ascending ramus is removed with the specimen. (Fig 13–29). If the mandible is to be saved, midline mandibulotomy is preferred.

The dissection is along the lateral floor of the mouth, which enables the surgeon to swing the mandibular ramus laterally, thus exposing the midline and lateral compartments of the extracranial skull base. Division of the styloglossus, stylopharyngeus, stylohyoid, and pterygoid muscles exposes the parapharyngeal space and infratemporal fossa (lateral compartment). By mobilization of the palate and the oropharynx medially and detaching the nasopharynx and pharyngeal walls from the skull base with division of the veli palatini muscles and the cartilaginous eustachian tube, the clivus and the cervical spine (midline compartment) can be exposed. Both compartments may be joined by removing the pterygoid plates and the

posterior walls of the maxillary sinus, thus gaining wide exposure of two thirds of the extracranial surface of the middle cranial fossa. In the past, a major criticism of this technique was the potential for meningitis resulting from oral flora contamination.[50, 51] Today this is no longer a concern because prophylactic antibiotic coverage begun preoperatively and continued for 72 hours postoperatively prevents oral flora contamination. If a portion of the nasopharynx or pharyngeal walls is resected, the possibility of a pharyngeal fistula may exist (Fig 13–30). Resurfacing the pharynx with a myocutaneous flap may be necessary in the event of a large pharyngeal defect. For smaller defects, a tongue flap may be used, and dermal graft is recommended to protect the carotid artery, especially in an irradiated patient.

Tumors involving the infratemporal fossa and the pharyngeal space can be removed via lateral skull base resection. Lesions in these areas can be metastatic from or a direct extension of primary tumors of the nasopharynx, tonsil, palate, sinuses, temporal bone, and parotid gland. The lateral skull base approach provides wide exposure for tumors located at the lateral and midline compartment of the middle cranial fossa skull base. The concept is en bloc removal of the lateral skull base.[52–57]

The facial skin can be removed if it is directly involved. The facial nerve is usually sacrificed if the tumor extends lateral to the mandible to involve the parotid gland. The zygomatic arch and the zygomatic buttress are removed with the temporalis muscle, which provides an adequate superior tumor margin. Posterior extension of the tumor requires partial or total removal of the temporal bone. From bifurcation to the carotid canal, the internal carotid artery is identified and preserved. The tumor usually can be safely separated from the internal carotid artery. In cases when it is not possible to separate the tumor from the internal carotid (e.g., due to direct extension or dense adhesions), one can attempt to sacrifice the internal carotid. Safely removing the internal carotid relies on adequate

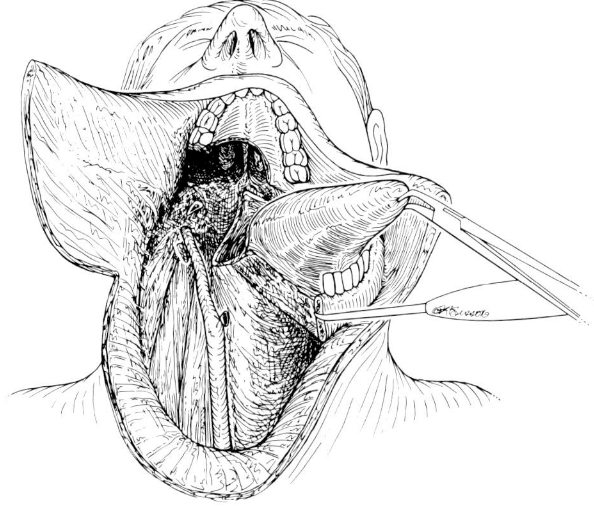

FIG 13–30.
Surgical defect following removal of larger oropharyngeal tumor extending superiorly to the nasopharynx.

preoperative bilateral evaluation of the carotid and vertebral systems.

The decision whether or not to sacrifice the internal carotid artery is best made during surgery. Following proximal occlusion of the vessel, a needle is placed into the internal carotid artery to measure back pressure. If the back pressure is more than 40 mm Hg, the internal carotid artery may be safely ligated and excised with the tumor. I have done this in four cases without any morbidity. In rare cases where the internal carotid artery involvement is very close to the bony skull base, the carotid canal may be drilled out.[14, 58, 59] After the carotid foramen is identified by drilling medially and anteriorly along the under surface of the petrous bone, the petrous portion of the internal carotid is identified and mobilized from its canal. This will allow a sufficient distal stump of the internal carotid for ligation or maybe even bypass.[49] In some cases, even without carotid involvement, the drill out and mobilization of the internal carotid can be performed to gain access superiorly and medially to the carotid artery.

In the absence of pharyngeal wall involvement, the oral cavity is entered at the retromolar area adjacent to the mandibular ramus. The resulting mucosal defect is small and may be closed primarily. Extensive pharyngeal wall involvement may require resection of the tonsilar fossa, nasopharynx, and the large areas of posterior or lateral pharyngeal walls. The reconstruction of such pharyngeal defects is performed primarily with a myocutaneous flap. Tumors involving the pharynx and the skin through and through may require two flaps for reconstruction. The deltopectoral flap is used for replacing the cutaneous defect, and the pectoralis myocutaneous flap is used for reconstructing the pharyngeal defect.[60]

Consideration for total laryngectomy is given if the patient loses a significant portion of pharyngeal or tongue musculature. Laryngectomy will prevent debilitating and dangerous complications such as persistent aspirations and pneumonia.

Complications

Complications that may occur from transmandibular transcervical lateral skull base resection for middle fossa malignancies are as follows: unilateral or bilateral serous otitis media, orocutaneous fistula, cervical skin flap necrosis, malunion of mandibulotomy, chronic aspiration or dysphagia, and facial nerve paralysis (permanent). In my experience, the pharyngocutaneous or orocutaneous fistulization have not been common. Even if there is communication between the lateral wall of the nasopharynx and the neck, high output salivary fistulae do not occur.

NASOPHARYNGEAL CARCINOMA

There is considerable disagreement in the world literature as to the proper classification of nasopharyngeal carcinomas, which makes analysis of survival statistics difficult. Carcinomas comprise 98% of all malignant neoplasms of the nasopharynx. Eighty percent of these tumors are either keratinizing or, more frequently, nonkeratinizing squamous cell carcinoma and are undifferentiated with an accompanying lymphocytic component.[61] This tumor deserves special classification because of its high radiosensitivity.[47, 62–64]

There appears to be a racial susceptibility to nasopharyngeal carcinoma. In Hong Kong, nasopharyngeal carcinoma represents 18% of all malignancies compared with 2% in New York City.[65] This susceptibility is probably due to both environmental and genetic factors.[66] It has been demonstrated that Chinese born in the United States have a 20 times greater chance of dying from cancer of the nasopharynx than whites. Chinese immigrants have a 30 to 40 times greater chance.[67–69]

Epstein-Barr virus (EBV) has been implicated as a causative factor in acquiring nasopharyngeal carcinoma. High titers of EBV antigens are found in nasopharyngeal carcinomas but are not found in other squamous cell tumors of the head and neck. Antibodies against EBV early antigen and viral capsid antigen are found in poorly differentiated and lymphoepithelial nasopharyngeal carcinomas. Their titers are roughly proportional to the tumor burden. In patients with consistently low anti-EBV antibody levels, a sudden increase in these levels is presumptive evidence of recurrent or metastatic disease.[70]

The presenting symptom of nasopharyngeal carcinoma in 50% of all cases is a cervical node metastasis. The extent of nodal metastasis gives no indication of the size of the primary tumor. The most commonly involved nodes are the jugulodigastric (70%), upper deep cervical (66%), omohyoid (34%), spinal accessory (28%), and inferior cervical (20%). In patients with an isolated posterior triangle nodal metastasis, the most common primary site is the nasopharynx. Patients with cervical nodal metastasis with an unknown primary site demand blind biopsies of the nasopharynx to rule out an occult primary.

Serous otitis media in the ear ipsilateral to the tumor is almost as common a presenting symptom as cervical node metastasis; unfortunately, its significance is often overlooked. Other symptoms are halitosis secondary to interference of the mucosal ciliary function by tumor and epistaxis and nasal obstruction. The primary lymphatic drainage of the nasopharynx is through the retropharyngeal system. Nodal metastasis in this area can cause compression near the jugular foramen and result in a jugular foramen syndrome (paralysis of cranial nerves IX to XII and the carotid sympathetics).

Until recently, treatment of nasopharyngeal carcinoma consisted of surgical biopsy and radiation therapy. For lymphoepitheliomas, radiation therapy is beneficial, with 5-year survival rates of greater than 30%.[71] The presence of nodal metastases decreases the survival rate for all types of nasopharyngeal carcinomas. Distant metastases occur in 20% of patients. Of these, 50% have bony involvement, and in 30%, the lungs and liver are involved.[72] The presence of distant metastases is not related to control of the local disease and has a 91% 1-year mortality rate.

For small tumors, surgical excision may be attempted. When CT and MRI scanning are used, the tumor can be mapped out, and resectability can be assessed more accurately. The approach to most of these tumors without infratemporal fossa involvement would be through a transmandibular exposure. Lesions extending to the infratemporal fossa require lateral skull base resection with or without mandibulectomy. Whether surgical

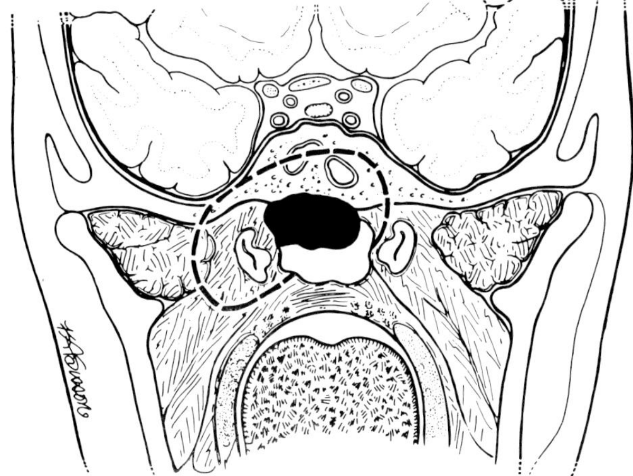

FIG 13–31.
Nasopharyngeal tumor involving the roof and one lateral wall.

excision improves survival or not is so far not determined, since radiation therapy is always used with surgery.[17, 58, 73–75]

Surgical Technique

The transcervical-transmandibular approach to the skull base, as described by Biller and Krespi,[17, 33] offers wide exposure of the middle cranial fossa skull base with the advantage of proximal vascular control. It is useful for approaching tumors of the clivus and nasopharynx. The transmandibular transcervical approach via a midline mandibulotomy provides wide exposure to the midline compartment of the skull base, nasopharynx, clivus, anterior foramen magnum, and the upper cervical spine (see Fig 13–29).

With the patient under general anesthesia, in a supine position and the neck slightly extended, a tracheotomy is performed. After the tracheotomy, a curvilinear incision is made extending from the mastoid tip and passing 4 to 5 cm below the mandible to the submental region. The inferior border of the submandibular gland is identified. The digastric tendon and stylohyoid muscle are released from their hyoid attachment and reflected superiorly with the submandibular gland. The major neurovascular structures are identified and followed toward the skull base as they pass deep to the posterior belly of the digastric muscle.

The common and internal carotid arteries, the internal jugular vein, and the cranial nerves X, XI, and XII are preserved. The external carotid artery is ligated and divided distal to the superior thyroid artery. The skin incision is then extended toward the lower lip. A midline lip-splitting incision is made, and the anterior mandibular periosteum is elevated. An oscillating power saw is used to mark a stair-step anterior mandibulotomy. Four drill holes for wire closure are made before the mandibulotomy. The mandible can be divided with the oscillating saw or a Gigli wire saw. Care should be taken not to damage the apices of the anterior central incisors (see Fig 13–30).

The tongue is retracted contralaterally, and an incision is made in the floor of the mouth extending toward the anterior tonsillar pillar. The lingual nerve is identified and preserved,

except for its postganglionic fibers to the submandibular and sublingual glands, which are divided. Further retraction of the hemimandible together with the submandibular triangle contents is achieved by dividing the external carotid artery distal to the lingual artery. This allows the hemimandible to swing further laterally and distal to the lingual artery. The styloid musculoligamentous complex is also divided (Fig 13–31).

The oral and neck incisions are connected, thus creating one surgical space. Depending on the exact location of the lesion and the procedure to be performed, the surgeon may elect to extend the oral incision onto the soft and hard palates, follow the medial border of the maxillary teeth, and raise a hemipalatal mucoperiosteal flap. An osteotome or a rongeur is used to remove portions of the hard palate and posterior maxilla if additional exposure to the clivus or nasopharynx is needed (Fig 13–32). Blunt dissection is used to separate the pharyngeal constrictors from the prevertebral fascia. The entire oropharynx and nasopharynx are retracted contralaterally, maintaining their circumferential integrity. The contralateral retraction of the nasopharynx is limited superolaterally by the cartilaginous eustachian tube and the tensor and levator palatini muscles. Division of these structures provides detachment of the nasopharynx from the skull base. Following this, the pharynx is pushed to the contralateral side, and the anterior surface of the clivus and C1 is exposed. To reach the vertebrae themselves, the prevertebral fascia, longus colli muscles, and anterior periosteum have to be incised.

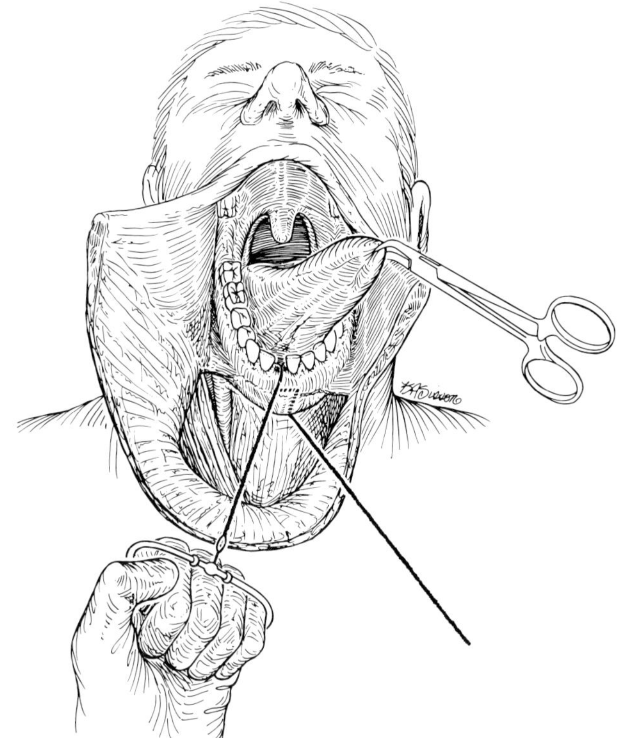

FIG 13–32.
Midline mandibulotomy in stair-step fashion. Note that one medial incisor is removed, and the mandibulotomy cut is performed through the tooth socket.

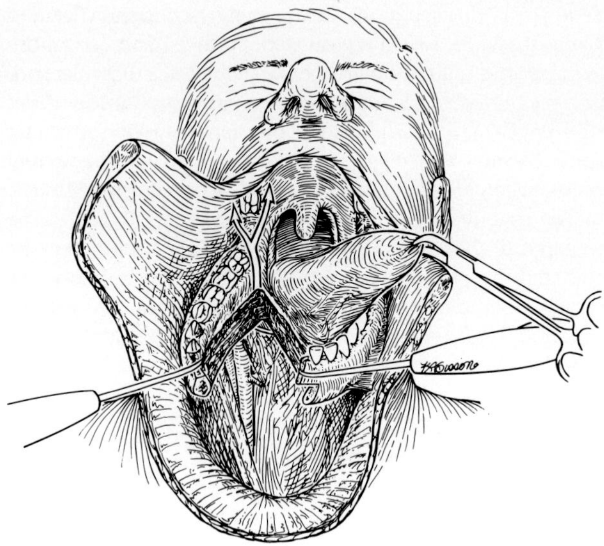

FIG 13–33.
Midline mandibulotomy and lateral floor of mouth incision. The dissection can be extended medially to the midline compartment or laterally toward the lateral compartment of the skull base.

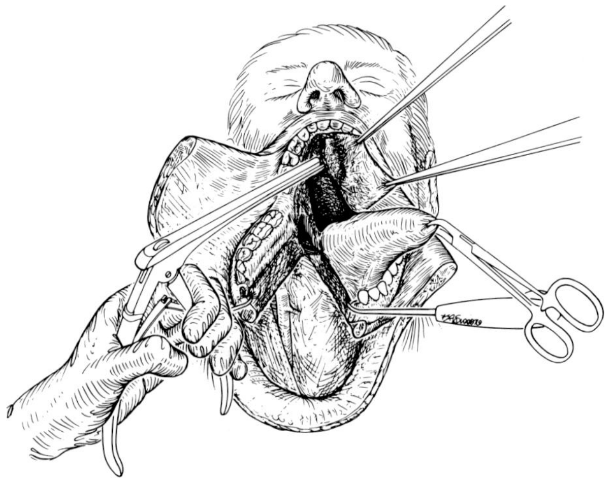

FIG 13–34.
Removal of hard palate after the hemipalate mucosal flap is elevated.

To excise a malignant nasopharyngeal tumor, the surgeon must extend the incision onto the soft palate, following the medial border of the maxillary dentition. The soft tissues of the palate are elevated to expose the nasopharynx and the bony palate. Exposure can be improved by removing the hard palate with Kerrison rongeurs. At this point the entire nasopharynx is exposed, and resection of nasopharyngeal tumors can be accomplished (Figs 13–33 and 13–34).

Further dissection is required to remove tumors arising from the clivus, such as chordomas. With blunt dissection, a space is created between the superior constrictor muscles and the prevertebral fascia superior to the hypoglossal nerve. The styloglossus, stylopharyngeus muscles, and glossopharyngeal nerve are divided. The oropharynx can now be retracted to the contralateral side. The eustachian tube is transected under direct vision by placing scissors medial to the internal carotid artery. This detaches the mucosa of the nasopharynx from the skull base. Once the nasopharynx has been retracted to the contralateral side, the prevertebral fascia is incised. Retraction of the prevertebral musculature exposes the clivus and upper cervical spine. Removal of chordomas can be accomplished under direct visualization with conventional instruments or laser.

This approach is also used for removal of nasopharyngeal carcinomas. A minimum of 1 to 1.5 cm of mucosal margin is obtained. Bony skull base is removed together with the tumor to obtain deep margins (Fig 13–35). The posterior pharyngeal and lateral nasopharyngeal walls and the ipsilateral eustachian tube are included in the specimen (Fig 13–36). Tumor involvement of both lateral nasopharyngeal walls with extension into the infratemporal fossa bilaterally limits resectability of this lesion. Extensive involvement of the infratemporal fossa to one

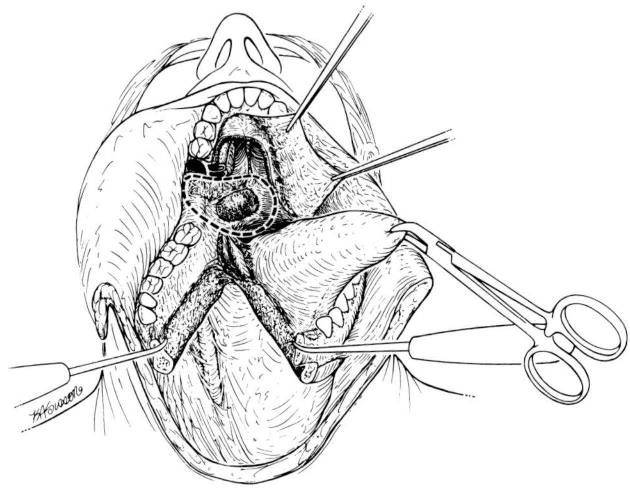

FIG 13–35.
Surgical margins are outlined around the nasopharyngeal lesion.

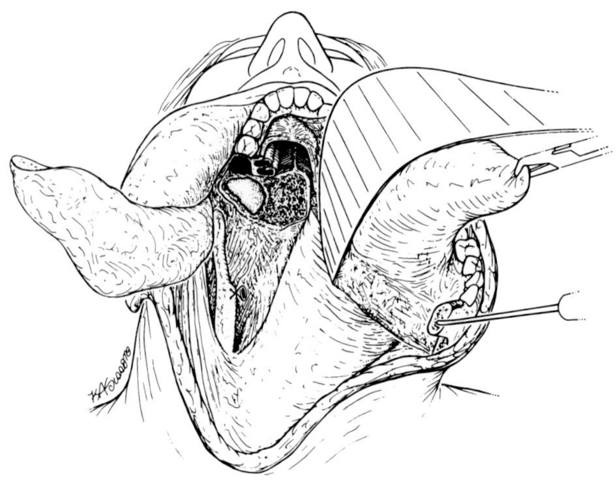

FIG 13–36.
Surgical defect at the nasopharynx following transmandibular resection of a nasopharyngeal tumor.

side requires lateral skull base resection. The ramus of the mandible may or may not be included in the resection. However, mandibulotomy with a lateral swing will provide wide access to the infratemporal fossa.

The closure begins by resuspending the remaining nasopharynx and replacing the hemipalate flap. A cricopharyngeal myotomy is performed, and the soft tissue closure is performed routinely. In dentulous patients, lingual splints may be required to prevent nonunion of the mandibulotomy. Although the approach itself does not involve the sacrifice of any cranial nerves, removal of the tumor is often associated with the sacrifice of one or more of these nerves. As a result, these patients may have swallowing difficulties and aspiration postoperatively.[76–80]

FUNCTIONAL PROSTHETIC REHABILITATION OF ORAL CAVITY FOLLOWING SKULL BASE SURGERY

Frequently, patients undergoing major resections for malignancies of the infratemporal fossa, nasopharynx, and related structures, face the unfortunate prospect of prolonged multiple reconstructive procedures to establish oral function and acceptable cosmesis.

The development of prosthetic materials and their use together with the widespread adoption of the myocutaneous flap enable the surgeon to perform single-stage reconstruction of skull base defects with rapid return of oral cavity and oropharyngeal function. Postoperative problems are resolved by a multidisciplinary team consisting of the head and neck surgeon, the prosthodontist, and the speech therapist. Lateral skull base resection for cancer may affect the neurologic function of the oral cavity, pharynx, and larynx. The neurologic deficit coupled with anatomic defects enhance the oral, pharyngeal, and laryngeal disability. The planned reconstruction of the oral cavity and vocal tract may be divided into five functional valves: (1) the lips, (2) the tongue, (3) the hard and soft palates, (4) the velopharyngeal port, and (5) the larynx.

Lateral skull base resection may affect the function of all five of these valves. The velopharyngeal port and the hard and soft palates play a larger role in speech production. Defects of these areas are more readily rehabilitated prosthetically than defects of the mobile tongue or tongue base. Classification of the maxillary obturators also aids in selection of the appropriate reconstructive methods. The available choices of obturators consist of the palatal obturator, the palatal lift prosthesis, and the palatal reshaping prosthesis. Modification of these basic types are made to suit the individual defect. Some general factors that affect the functional return of the oral cavity and oropharynx postoperatively are (1) patient and family motivation, (2) acceptance of prosthesis, (3) previous experience with dentures, (4) manual dexterity, (5) absence of tremors, and (6) articulation abilities.

The prosthodontist will make preoperative impressions of the patient's oral cavity, and, if necessary, moulage of the facial structures is obtained. The head and neck surgeon may desire a surgical obturator for immediate placement at the time of closure, particularly if portions of the hard and soft palates are included in the resection. This enables the patient to gain oral competence quickly and may delay scarring and retraction of the defect. A definitive obturator may be placed at a later date following maturing of the maxillary cavity.

Hemimandibulectomy patients may benefit from attachment of a guidebar prosthesis to correct resultant muscle imbalance and malocclusion. With the aid of this guidebar, the patient may chew relatively tough foods.

Finally, it remains essential that a cooperative multidisciplinary effort by the head and neck surgeon, the prosthodontist, and the speech therapist be expended. Each specialty lends expertise that ultimately ensures a better result for the patient.[81, 82]

DISCUSSION AND REVIEW OF THE LITERATURE

Tumors of the paranasal sinuses were described by Hippocrates and Galen, who believed that treatment only spread the tumor and shortened the patient's life. Rogers, in 1824, was the first American to partially remove the upper jaw maxilla. In 1827, the French surgeon Gensoul performed the first maxillectomy in a patient with osteogenic sarcoma. At the turn of the century, the use of cautery to destroy tumors in the paranasal sinuses was described. Radiation therapy was introduced after 1910 and was used in combination with electrocautery.[83]

The management of tumors of the sinonasal tract has undergone significant evolution since 1955. During the first half of this century, antrostomy with curettage and cauterization or radiation was the treatment of choice. Martin remarked on the poor salvage rate for carcinoma of the paranasal sinuses treated with curettage and recommended initial radical surgical removal of the tumor.[84]

In 1954, Smith et al. reported the first series of cases involving craniofacial resection for carcinoma of the paranasal sinuses.[85] Of their three patients, one was unresectable at the time of operation, one was considered palliated, and the other was disease free at follow-up 1 year later. Since that time, radical surgical excision has become the preferred treatment modality.

Only recently, lesions of the lateral skull base have been accessible to the head and neck surgeon. The difficulty associated with this type of surgery was the complex anatomy of this region, which includes the internal carotid artery, the great venous sinuses, and cranial nerves VII, IX, X, and XII. The infratemporal fossa approach described by Fisch et al.[13, 14] provided surgical access to the infratemporal fossa with exposure of major blood vessels and cranial nerves. Usually the facial nerve was dissected and mobilized; also the intrapetrous portion of the internal carotid artery is drilled out and exposed. By Fisch's classification, the type A infratemporal fossa approach provides access to the temporal bone and its infralabyrinthine and apical compartments. The type B infratemporal fossa approach provides access to the clivus, and the type C infratemporal fossa approach provides access to the parasellar-parasphenoid region and the nasopharynx. It should be noted that the access in type C infratemporal fossa approach, allowing exposure of the nasopharynx, is quite lengthy and has certain limitations as far as resecting large malignant tumors, usually malignant ones. The type C infratemporal fossa approach permits access to lesions of the nasopharynx, pterygomaxillary fossa, eustachian tube, parasellar region, sphenoid sinus, and maxillary sinus. This approach was used most frequently for squamous cell carcinoma that failed radiation therapy, adenoid cystic carcinoma around the eustachian tube orifice, and advanced juvenile nasopharyngeal angiofibromas. According to Fisch,[13] nasopharyngeal carcinoma can be removed en bloc along with the eustachian tube, levator and tensor palatine muscles, pharyngobasilar fascia, and pterygoid muscles. A plane of cleavage is developed along the clivus as far as the vomer anteriorly and as far as the atlas posteriorly.

In general, it was thought that there were no surgical options to treat recurrent carcinoma of the nasopharynx, which was reinforced because of the proximity of the carotid arteries and brain stem. Most surgeons debated the issue that the nasopharynx does not lend itself to en bloc surgical resection.[30, 64, 86] In this region, a deep invasion of the skull base is common, with early multiple cranial nerve involvement early in the process. Repeated radiation therapy as described by McNeese and Fletcher in 1981 can result in extended palliation, but the tremendous risks of radionecrosis of the skull base and mandible exist. Palliative chemotherapy may provide another option, but to date, no large series have been reported.

Fisch reported effective palliative removal of T4 nasopharyngeal lesions and radical removal of T1 and T2 nasopharyngeal carcinomas.[58] He utilized the type C infratemporal fossa approach for excisions of these lesions. All of the T4 patients died within 2 to 3 years because of tumor persistence. These patients presented preoperatively with extensive neurologic defects involving cranial nerves IV, V, VI, X, and XII. Radical removal of these lesions obviously is impossible due to infiltration of dura and multiple cranial nerves; therefore, they must be considered unresectable. However, he reported six patients with persistent T1 and T2 tumors who underwent radical surgical resection and were alive without evidence of disease 2 to 5 years following surgery. He concluded that radical removal of recurrent T4 nasopharyngeal carcinoma through the infratemporal fossa approach is impossible. However, palliation in these patients was excellent, specifically, relief from trigeminal pain. The results following removal of T1 and T2 nasopharyngeal tumors were gratifying according to Fisch.[58]

Terz et al. recommended a combined intracranial-extracranial approach to such cases.[87, 88] Goepfert et al. recommended postoperative radiation as an alternative to combined intracranial-extracranial approach in patients with abnormal margins or in patients with perineural involvement around the foramina at the skull base.[19] Fairbanks-Barbosa described an operative technique for the section of the pterygoid musculature in patients with advanced cancer of the paranasal sinuses.[89] Because of frequent metastasis to retropharyngeal lymph nodes and the fact that squamous cell carcinoma spreads along the fascial planes, Fairbanks-Barbosa thought it was necessary to remove pterygoid musculature with the entire contents of the infratemporal fossa to obtain adequate surgical margins. Eilber and Zarem reported a series of 14 patients who underwent resection of malignancies of the infratemporal fossa.[90] This was the first systematic approach to the en bloc resection of the malignancies of this region. In a median follow-up of 20 months, local control was

achieved in 10 out of 14 patients. Friedman[60] et al. reported a procedure designed for en bloc resection of infratemporal fossa structures and named it "stylo hamular dissection."[60] They utilized this procedure in eight patients with advanced malignancies of the infratemporal fossa with encouraging results and excellent palliation. In this series, two of the patients sustained immediate postoperative strokes, and five out of seven surviving patients were disease free between 5 and 42 months postoperatively.[60] Close et al.[91] reported two patients who underwent resection of posterior nasal and nasopharyngeal carcinomas with a modified infratemporal fossa approach.[13, 58] One patient died of meningitis 7 months after incomplete resection, and the other patient was without evidence of disease 6 months following surgery and radiation therapy.[91]

Squamous cell carcinoma of the tonsillar fossa and pharyngeal pillars, with extension superiorly to the posterior and lateral pharyngeal wall and soft palate, requires special attention at the skull base.[6, 20, 28] The limits of standard composite resection for such lesions must be extended to include the lateral skull base structures. Following the internal carotid artery to the skull base, exposure and protection of this vessel during resection are the keys to this operation. The distal external carotid is routinely ligated and included in the surgical specimen. Structures medial to the mandible, including the pterygoid muscles, levator and tensor veli palatine muscles, styloid complex muscles, cartilaginous portion of the eustachian tube, and pterygoid plates all are resected. As described by Biller et al. previously,[33] the cartilaginous eustachian tube and levator veli palatine muscles must be divided to detach the superior constrictor muscle and the nasopharynx from the skull base. This facilitates en bloc and safe resection of malignant tumors that have originated or extended to this area.

Retropharyngeal nodes are usually present in tonsillar lesions with extension toward the soft palate and posterolateral pharyngeal wall. As noted by Ballantyne,[20] metastatic retropharyngeal lymph nodes were found in 44% of the patients with cancer of the pharyngeal walls. These nodes are located between the superior constrictor and the prevertebral muscles. They consist of two main groups. The superolateral nodal group (Rouviere) is present at the skull base, close to the internal carotid foramen and jugular foramen. The inferomedial group is located at the level of the oropharynx, deep to the superior constrictor muscle. Dissection of the retropharyngeal lymph nodes at the skull base should be carried out in tumors of the tonsillar fossa with superior extension with lateral and posterior pharyngeal wall involvement and in nasopharyngeal tumors. This dissection is done safely by following the internal carotid artery to the skull base and resecting the structures medial to this vessel, including the prevertebral fascia and pharyngeal wall.

Lateral skull base resection provides access to surgical clearance of lymphatics and fascial planes. Also, this kind of en bloc resection, including muscles and cranial nerves, may eliminate perineural tumor spread. Since this is the feature of cancer spread within the infratemporal fossa, pterygomaxillary fossa, and the parapharyngeal space, lateral skull base resection with reliable reconstructive methods can achieve a higher survival rate and improve the quality of life in patients affected with these aggressive lesions.

REFERENCES

1. Conley JJ, Schuller DE: Reconstruction following temporal bone resection. *Arch Otolaryngol* 1977; 103:34–37.
2. Jesse RH, Shugarbaker EV: Squamous cell carcinoma of the oropharynx: Why we fail. *Am J Surg* 1976; 132:435–438.
3. Johns ME, Winn HR, McLean WC, et al: Pericranial flap for the closure of defects of craniofacial resection. *Laryngoscope* 1981; 91:952–959.
4. Ketcham AS, Chretien PB, Van Buren JM, et al: The ethmoid sinuses: A re-evaluation of surgical resection. *Am J Surg* 1973; 126:469–476.
5. Schramm VL, Myers DN, Moroon JC: Anteior skull base surgery for benign and malignant disease. *Laryngoscope* 1979; 89:1077–1084.
6. Wilson JS, Westbury G, Richardson AE: Craniofacial resection of the anterior and middle cranial fossae en bloc with the hemi face and repair by multiple flaps, in Chambers RG (ed): *Cancer of the Head and Neck.* Amsterdam, Excerpta Medica, 1975.
7. Vikram B: Changing patterns of failure in advanced head and neck cancer. *Arch Otolaryngol* 1984; 110:564–575.
8. Goepfert H: Are we making any progress? *Arch Otolaryngol* 1984; 110:562–563.
9. Baker SR: Surgical reconstruction after extensive skull base surgery. *Otolaryngol Clin North Am* 1984; 17:591–599.
10. Myers DL, Sataloff RT: Spinal fluid leakage after skull base surgical procedures. *Otolaryngol Clin North Am* 1984; 17:601–612.
11. Sataloff RT, Myers DL, Roberts BR: Pain following surgery of the skull base. *Otolaryngol Clin North Am* 1984; 17:613–625.
12. Tenta LR, Caldarelli DD, Keys GR: Surgical palatomaxilloschisis: An avenue to the pterygomaxillary space. *Otolaryngol Head Neck Surg* 1981; 89:59–61.
13. Fisch U, Fagan P, Valavanis A: The infratemporal fossa approach for the lateral skull base. *Otolaryngol Clin North Am* 1984; 17:513–552.
14. Fisch U, Oldring DJ, Senning A: Surgical therapy of internal carotid artery lesions of the skull base and temporal bone. *Otolaryngol Head Neck Surg* 1980; 88:548–554.
15. Glasscock ME, Miller GW, Drake FD, et al: Surgery of the skull base. *Laryngoscope* 1978; 88:905–923.
16. Kinney SE, Wood BG: Surgical treatment of skull-base malignancy. *Otolaryngol Head Neck Surg* 1984; 92:94–99.
17. Krespi YP, Sisson GA: Transmandibular exposure of the skull base. *Am J Surg* 1984; 148:534–538.
18. Fisch U, Pillsbury HC: Infratemporal fossa approach to lesions in the temporal bone and base of skull. *Arch Otolaryngol* 1981; 107:698–702.
19. Goepfert H, Jesse RH, Lindberg RD: Arterial infusion and radiation therapy in the treatment of advanced cancer of the nasal cavity and paranasal sinuses. *Am J Surg* 1973; 126:464–468.
20. Krespi YP, Sisson GA: Skull base surgery in composite resection. *Arch Otolaryngol* 1982; 108:681–684.
21. Baker DC, Conley J: Surgical approach to retromandibular parotid tumors. *Ann Plast Surg* 1979; 3:304–314.
22. Caldarelli DD, Rejowski JE: Surgical management of recurrent or advanced squamous cell cancer of the head and neck. *Clin Plast Surg* 1985; 12:505–514.
23. Chandler R: Cryosurgery for recurrent cancer of the head and neck. *Otolaryngol Head Neck Surg* 1974; 7(suppl):193–204.
24. Shapshay SM, Elber E, Strong MS: Occult tumors of the infratemporal fossa: Report of seven cases appearing as preauricular facial pain. *Arch Otolaryngol* 1976; 102:535–538.
25. Noyek AM, Kassel EE, Wortzman G, et al: CT in occult disease of the skull base and basilar foramina. *J Otolaryngol* 1982; 11:419–427.
26. Shapshay SM, McCann CF, Ucmakli A, et al: Diagnosis of infratemporal fossa tumors using percutaneous core needle biopsy. *Head Neck Surg* 1979; 2:168–171.
27. Longacre JJ, Mayfield FH, Lotspeich ES, et al: Combined transoral, transcervical, and transosseous team approach to tumors of the nasopharynx and pharyngeal region. *Am J Surg* 1965; 110:644–648.
28. Palmer JA, Snell GE: Surgical treatment of extensive tumors of the lateral face and auricular area by radical soft tissue and subtotal temporal bone excision with deltopectoral flap coverage. *J Otolaryngol* 1979; 8:531–536.
29. Perez CA, Ackerman LV, Mill WB, et al: Malignant tumors of the tonsil. Analysis of failures and factors affecting prognosis. *AJR* 1972; 114:43–58.
30. Ross DE, Sukis AE: Nasopharyngeal tumors. A new surgical approach. *Am J Surg* 1966; 11:524–530.
31. Diewart VM: A morphometric analysis of craniofacial growth and changes in spatial relations during secondary palatal development in human embryos and fetuses. *Am J Anat* 1983; 167:495–522.
32. Roberts GJ, Blackwood HJ: Growth of the cartilages of the mid-line cranial base: A radiographic and histological study. *J Anat* 1983; 136:307–320.
33. Biller HF, Shugar JM, Krespi YP: A new technique for widefield exposure of the base of the skull. *Arch Otolaryngol* 1981; 107:698–702.
34. House WF, Hitselberger WE: The transcochlear approach to the skull base. *Arch Otolaryngol* 1977; 102:334–342.
35. Hitselberger WE, House WF: A system of operations for skull base tumors. *Adv Neurol* 1976; 15:275–280.
36. House WF: Transcochlear approach to the petrous apex and clivus. *Trans Am Acad Ophthalmol Otolaryngol* 1977; 84:927–931.
37. Goldenberg RA: Surgeon's view of the skull base from the lateral approach. *Laryngoscope* 1984; 94:1–21.
38. Van-Huijzen C: Anatomy of the skull base and the infratemporal fossa. *Adv Otorhinolaryngol* 1984; 34:242–253.
39. Takahashi R: The formation of the human paranasal sinuses. *Acta Otolaryngol* 1984; 408:1–28.
40. Som PM, Shugar JM, Parisier SC: A clinical-radiographic classification of skull base lesions. *Laryngoscope* 1979; 89:1066–1076.
41. Wiet RJ, Kazan R, Sacy G: Skull base mapping. *Laryngoscope* 1982; 92:515–523.
42. Doubleday LC, Jing BS, Wallace S: Computed tomography of the infratemporal fossa. *Radiology* 1981; 138:619–624.
43. Whelan MA, Reede DL, Meisler W, et al: CT of the base of the skull. *Radiol Clin North Am* 1984; 22:177–217.
44. Han JS, Huss RG, Benson JE, et al: MR imaging of the skull base. *J Comput Assist Tomogr* 1984; 8:944–952.
45. Mafee MF, Valvassor GE, Dobben GD: The role of radiology in surgery of the ear and skull base. *Otolaryngol Clin North Am* 1982; 15:723–753.
46. Som PM, Biller HF, Lawson W, et al: Parapharyngeal space masses: An updated protocol based upon 104 cases. *Radiology* 1984; 153:149–156.
47. Sataloff RT, Myers DL, Lowry LD, et al: Total temporal

bone resection for squamous cell carcinoma. *Otolaryngol Head Neck Surg* 1987; 96:4–14.

48. Glasscock ME, Smith PG, Bond AG, et al: Management of aneurysms of the petrous portion of the internal carotid artery by resection and primary anastomosis. *Laryngoscope* 1983; 93:1445–1453.

49. Urken ML, Biller HF, Haimov M: Infratemporal carotid artery bypass in resection of a base of skull tumor. *Laryngoscope* 1985; 95:1472–1477.

50. Ketcham AS: A combined intracranial facial approach to the paranasal sinuses. *Am J Surg* 1963; 106:698–703.

51. Sisson GA, Bytell DE, Becker SP, et al: Carcinoma of the paranasal sinuses and craniofacial resection. *J Laryngol Otol* 1976; 90:59–68.

52. Arena S, Hilal EY: Neurilemomas of the infratemporal space: A report of a case and review of the literature. *Arch Otolaryngol* 1976; 102:180–184.

53. Buchanan G: Two rare tumors involving the infratemporal fossa: Alveolar soft part sarcoma and hemangiopericytoma. *J Laryngol Otol* 1975; 89:375–389.

54. Clairmont AA, Conley JJ: Malignant fibrous histiocytoma of the parapharyngeal space. Case report. *Plast Reconstr Surg* 1977; 59:747–749.

55. Gay I, Elidan J, Kopolovic J: Chondrosarcoma at the skull base. *Ann Otol Rhinol Laryngol* 1981; 90:53–55.

56. Stell PM, Mansfield AO, Stoney PJ: Surgical approaches to tumors of the parapharyngeal space. *Am J Otolaryngol* 1985; 6:92–97.

57. Wetmore SJ, Suen JY, Snyderman NL: Preauricular approach to infratemporal fossa. *Head Neck Surg* 1986; 9:93–103.

58. Fisch U: The infratemporal fossa approach for nasopharyngeal tumors. *Laryngoscope* 1983; 93:36–44.

59. Lambert PR, Johns ME, Winn RH: Infralabyrinthine approach to skull base lesions. *Otolaryngol Head Neck Surg* 1985; 93:250–258.

60. Friedman WH, Katsantonis GP, Cooper MH, et al: Stylohamular dissection: A new method for en bloc resection of malignancies of the infratemporal fossa. *Laryngoscope* 1981; 91:1869–1879.

61. Batsakis JG: The pathology of head and neck tumors: Nasal cavity and paranasal sinuses, part 5. *Head Neck Surg* 1980; 2:410–419.

62. Einhorn J: Treatment of malignant nasopharyngeal tumours. *East Afr Med J* 1970; 47:403–409.

63. McNeese MD, Fletcher GH: Retreatment of recurrent nasopharyngeal carcinoma. *Radiology* 1981; 138:191–193.

64. Million RR: Cancer of the head and neck. Nasopharyngeal cancer. Management of neck node metastases. *JAMA* 1972; 220:402–405.

65. Digby KH, Fook WL, Che YT: Nasopharyngeal malignancy. *Br J Surg* 1941; 28:517.

66. Buell P: Nasopharyngeal cancer in Chinese in California. *Br J Cancer* 1965; 19:459.

67. Creely JJ Jr, Lyons GD Jr, Trial ML: Cancer of the nasopharynx: A review of 114 cases. *South Med J* 1973; 66:405–409.

68. Miller D: The etiology of nasopharyngeal cancer and its management. *Otolaryngol Clin North Am* 1980; 13:467–475.

69. Sofferman RA, Heisse JW Jr: Adenoid cystic carcinoma of the nasopharynx after previous adenoid irradiation. *Laryngoscope* 1985; 95:458–461.

70. Lynn TC, Hsieh RP, Chuang CY, et al: Epstein-Barr virus associated antibodies and serum biochemistry in nasopharyngeal carcinoma. *Laryngoscope* 1984; 94:1485–1488.

71. Bloom SM: Cancer of the nasopharynx: A study of ninety cases. *J Mt Sinai Hosp* 1969; 36:277.

72. Batsakis JG: *Tumors of the Head and Neck.* Baltimore, Williams & Wilkins Co, 1979, pp 264–268.

73. Kraus CJ, Baker SR: Extended transantral approach to pterygomaxillary tumors. *Ann Otol Rhinol Laryngol* 1982; 91:395–398.

74. Mesic JB, Fletcher GH, Goepfert H: Megavoltage irradiation of epithelial tumors of the nasopharynx. *Int J Radiat Oncol Biol Phys* 1981; 7:447–453.

75. Wood GD, Stoll PM: The LeForte I osteotomy as an approach to the nasopharynx. *Otolaryngol Clin North Am* 1984; 9:59–61.

76. Arbit E, Patterson RH Jr: Combined transoral and median labiomandibular glossotomy approach to the upper cervical spine. *Neurosurgery* 1981; 8:672–674.

77. De-Campora E, Camaioni A, Calabrese V, et al: Conservative trans-mandibular approach in the surgical treatment of tumors of the parapharyngeal space. *J Laryngol Otolaryngol* 1984; 98:1225–1229.

78. Delgado TE, Garrido E, Harwick RD: Labiomandibular, transoral approach to chordomas in the clivus and upper cervical spine. *Neurosurgery* 1981; 8:675–679.

79. Miller J, Parent AD: Microscopic decompression of the anterior upper cervical spine: A case of odontoid malunion to the atlas. *Neurosurgery* 1984; 14:583–587.

80. Sherk HH, Pratt L: Anterior approaches to the cervical spine. *Laryngoscope* 1983; 93:168–171.

81. Chalian VA, Drane JB, Standish SM: *Maxillofacial Prosthetics: Multidisciplinary Approach.* Baltimore, Williams & Wilkins Co, 1971.

82. Wurster CF, Krespi YP, Davis JW, et al: Combined functional oral rehabilitation after radical cancer surgery. *Arch Otolaryngol* 1985; 111:530–533.

83. Watson WL: Cancer of paranasal sinuses. *Laryngoscope* 1942; 52:22–42.

84. Martin H: Cancer of the head and neck. *JAMA* 1948; 137:1306–1376.

85. Smith RR, Klopp CT, Williams JM: Surgical treatment of cancer of the frontal sinus and adjacent areas. *Cancer* 1954; 7:991–994.

86. Goepfert H: The infratemporal fossa approach for nasopharyngeal tumors [letter]. *Laryngoscope* 1983; 93:1231.

87. Terz JJ, Alksne JF, Lawrence W Jr: En bloc resection of the pterygoid region in the management of advanced or pharyngeal carcinoma. *Surg Gynecol Obstet* 1970; 130:349–352.

88. Terz JJ, Alksne JF, Lawrence W Jr: Craniofacial resection for tumors invading the pterygoid fossa. *Am J Surg* 1969; 118:732–740.

89. Fairbanks-Barbosa J: Surgery of extensive cancer of the paranasal sinuses. Presentation of a new technique. *Arch Otolaryngol* 1961; 73:129.

90. Eilber FR, Zarem HA: Pterygoid dissection for extensive cancer. *Plast Reconstr Surg* 1977; 59:545–550.

91. Close LG, Mickey BE, Samson DS, et al: Resection of upper aerodigestive tract tumors involving the middle cranial fossa. *Laryngoscope* 1985; 95:908–914.

PART TWO

Nasal and Sinus Surgery

CHAPTER 14

Nasal Septal Reconstruction

Approach of

Richard J. Lipton, M.D.

and

Eugene B. Kern, M.D.

Septal surgery can be exceedingly challenging. The nasal septum is a complex structure, and the surgeon can be faced with a wide range of pathologic possibilities. Although patients may have a variety of septal deformities, the most prominent symptom is nasal airway obstruction. Nasal septal reconstruction (NSR) can produce a happy functional person, or it can result in chronic misery and even death. An operation on the nasal septum must never be taken with a cavalier attitude. The purpose of this chapter is to thoroughly yet succinctly discuss the evolution of modern physiologic nasal septal surgery.

In essence, septal deformities occur when there is too much skeletal structure for the overlying perichondrial or periosteal space. As far as the cartilage is concerned, resulting growth forces cause irregularities and bowing.[1] The situation can be considered as analogous to an overstuffed envelope (Fig 14–1). Trauma further complicates the situation by producing growth of the cartilage and bone in abnormal directions. Growth of the mucoperichondrium across a fracture site with adherence to the opposite side can make surgical dissection difficult. Carefully planned surgical access with excision of excess cartilage and bone will allow the septum to assume a more normal position, which usually improves nasal breathing.

The repair of nasal septal deformities has evolved over the past century as knowledge of nasal airway physiology has emerged. The first attempts at surgical correction involved the application of force to the deflected septum with a blunt instrument. Earliest surgical excision of a septal deformity was performed without regard for surrounding mucosal or skeletal structures. The concept was simply to relieve "rhinostenosis." Freer[2] and Killian[3] were among the first to recognize that repair

of the obstructing septum may be accomplished without sacrifice of mucosa. The introduction of a submucous resection (SMR) was both a monumental and positive step in the history of nasal septal surgery. Although the SMR operation remained the gold standard for many years, it became obvious to many rhinologists that there were still shortcomings:

1. Caudal end deformities are not corrected.
2. Access to the premaxilla and anterior nasal spine is limited.
3. Convexities of the nasal valve area are not addressed.
4. Submucous resection is not applicable to children.
5. Reoperation is difficult when no skeleton is replaced.

The inability to manage pathology at the caudal end (Fig 14–2) was a serious limitation of the SMR. This was addressed by Metzenbaum,[4] among others,[5–9] who proposed alternative methods for the management of these caudal end deformities.

A basic approach to nasal airway obstruction requires something more than the SMR. It requires the surgical ability to expose and completely uncover and reconstruct deformities of the nasal septum that are capable of producing nasal airway obstruction. This includes deficiencies at the caudal end and the dorsal portion of the quadrangular cartilage, the upper lateral cartilage, the anterior nasal spine, the maxillary crest, and the premaxilla, all of which are unapproachable and consequently untreatable by the approach advocated by the proponents of the SMR operation.

Cottle and Loring,[10] in 1948, introduced an integrated and comprehensive surgical approach to the entire nasal septum,

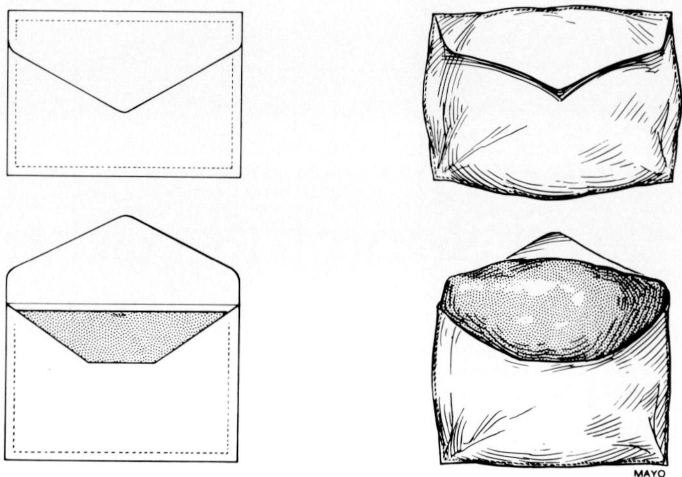

FIG 14–1.
The overstuffed envelope illustrates the irregularities that occur when there is too much cartilage for the perichondrial space.

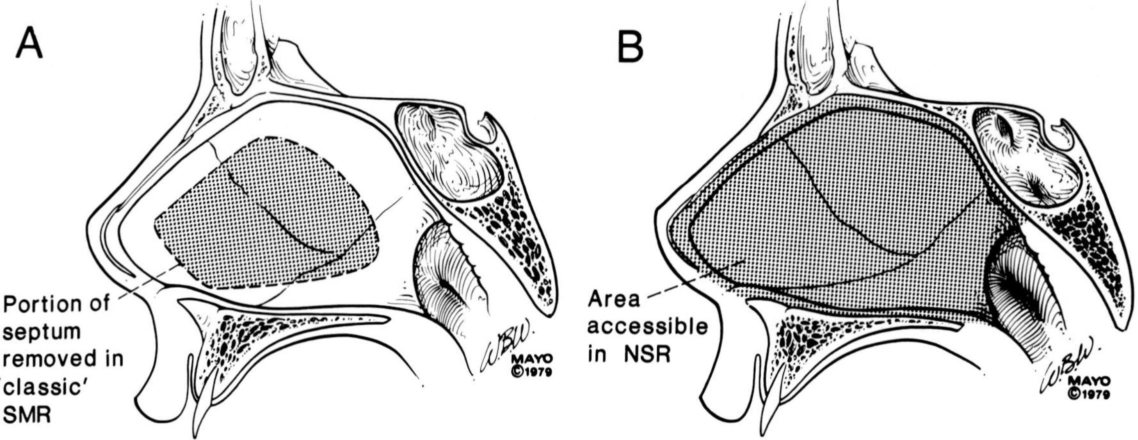

FIG 14–2.
A, shaded area represents the portions of the nasal septum that can be approached by SMR. **B,** structures of the nasal septum and upper lateral cartilage (ULC) that can be approached by the NSR concept using the maxilla-premaxilla, or M-P, approach. The shaded area represents the portions of the entire septum that can be exposed by this method. (From Kern EB: Nasal septal reconstruction vs. submucous resection, in Snow JB (ed): *Controversy in Otolaryngology.* Philadelphia, WB Saunders Co, 1980, p 336. Used by permission.)

which was subsequently referred to as the "maxilla-premaxilla," or M-P, approach to extensive nasal septal surgery.[11] The purpose and direction of NSR has been distilled by Cottle and summarized as the seven sine qua nones of septal surgery:

1. Continuing diagnosis
2. Maxilla-premaxilla approach
3. The reality of scar in that we operate through scar, because of scar, and despite scar
4. Mobilization of the entire septum when necessary
5. Preservation or replacement of the caudal end of the septum
6. Immediate repair of mucosal tears
7. The ability to perform a total septal reconstruction with or without pyramid surgery

Nasal septal reconstruction using the M-P approach has since replaced the classical SMR as the complete surgical technique for the repair of the nasal septum and its adnexae. Central to the new philosophy are the concepts of wide exposure, conservation of tissues, limited resection, and reconstruction by repositioning and replacing skeletal structure to reconstitute normality without sacrifice of mucosa. Additional important advantages of the M-P approach are sparing of mucosal incisions, elevation of mucosa from the floor of the nose, mobilization of the joint fascia at the anterior nasal spine, access to the posterior nose, and preservation of neurovascular bundles.

Since the restoration of normal nasal breathing is the primary goal of nasal septal surgery, a thorough understanding of nasal physiology is integral to the surgeon's practice. For a full discussion of nasal physiology, several excellent reviews are available.[12–15]

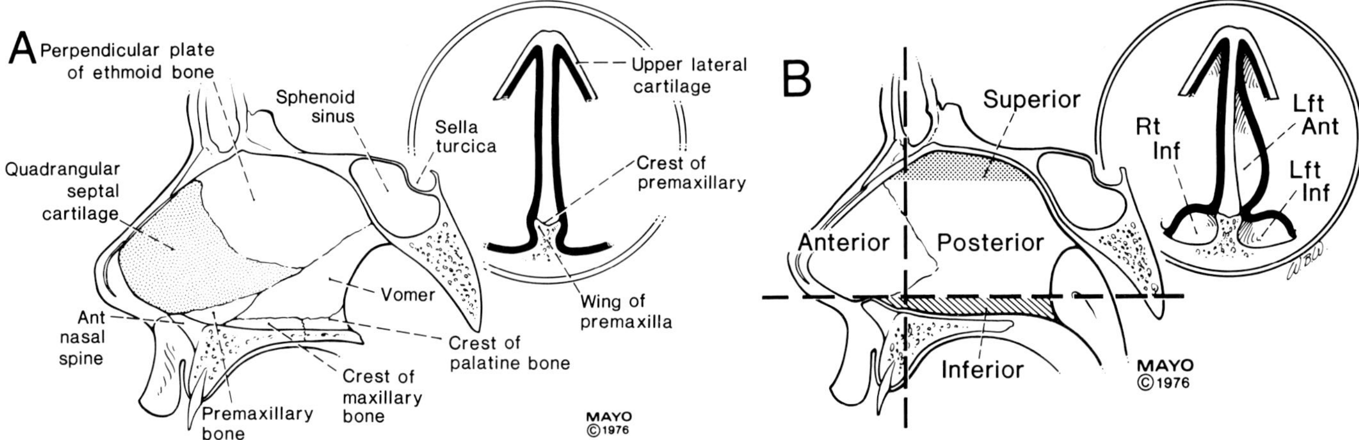

FIG 14–3.
A, pertinent anatomic terms and structures. **B**, the division of the nose and nasal septum into anterior, posterior, superior, and inferior portions. The anterior portion of the septum is that part of the nose anterior to an imaginary vertical line drawn from the proximal end of the nasal bones to the hard palate. The inferior portion is that area of the septum and the floor of the nose that lies below the articulation of the quadrangular septal cartilage with the anterior nasal (maxillary) spine and crest and wings of premaxilla. Superior refers to the portion of the septum in the region of the cribriform area. The left anterior tunnel wound be a mucosal flap elevated from the left side of the septum back to the imaginary line dividing the anterior portion from the posterior portion. Beyond that imaginary line, mucosal elevation on the same side would be the left posterior tunnel. Mucosal elevation from the floor of the nose up to the region of articulation of the quadrangular septal cartilage with the anterior nasal spine and premaxillary wings would be the inferior tunnel. (From Kern EB: Nasal septal reconstruction vs. submucous resection, in Snow JB (ed): *Controversy in Otolaryngology.* Philadelphia, WB Saunders Co, 1980, p 344. Used by permission.)

Conceptually, NSR using the M-P approach allows complete exposure of any surface of any structure that may require modification. Accordingly, functional surgery to improve nasal breathing can be performed on the septum, pyramid, and lobule all at the same operation. Although the technique must be tailored to each individual pathologic variation, the general principles and the sequence most frequently employed are described.

TECHNIQUE

Attention to patient comfort prior to, during, and following surgery is essential. Surgery truly begins with the preoperative examination and discussion. At that time, the details of the procedure and the expectations of the patient are thoroughly addressed. Most adults can be operated on with local anesthesia, though some prefer a general anesthetic. Premedication with a short-acting anxiolytic serves to reduce apprehension. Narcotics and additional benzodiazepines are administered and titrated intravenously during the procedure as needed for patient comfort.

ANESTHESIA

A most important step in the successful performance of NSR is vasoconstriction of the mucosa. Vasoconstriction minimizes bleeding, which, in turn, facilitates visualization of the pathology permitting precise surgical correction. The medications that will be described are used during both general and local anesthesia. Bleeding is the nemesis of exposure; therefore, optimum vasoconstriction is required. The nose is first sprayed with 0.5% phenylephrine hydrochloride solution, two puffs in each nostril. This is followed by the topical application of 4% lidocaine (Xylocaine) spray, which serves to minimize the discomfort experienced when the cocaine flakes are applied. Approximately 100 mg of cocaine flakes are delivered on moistened cotton tips directly to the regions of the sphenopalatine ganglion and the anterior ethmoid vessels. Cetacaine is then applied to the upper buccogingival fold. About 1 mL of 0.5% bupivacaine (Marcaine) with epinephrine 1:100,000 and 1% hyaluronidase (Wydase) is injected as a test dose through the upper buccogingival fold into the region of the floor of the nose, the premaxilla, and the anterior nasal spine. If there are no untoward reactions, an additional 4 mL of the anesthetic solution is injected into the regions of the sites of the hemitransfixion and intercartilaginous incisions, along both nasofacial grooves (below the infraorbital margin), at the nasofrontal angle, head of the inferior and middle turbinate, and finally, into the region of the incisive foramina bilaterally. The local anesthetic is given 10 minutes to attain a maximal vasoconstrictive effect. This combination will give the surgeon approximately 1.5 to 2 hours of vasoconstriction and anesthesia. Supplemental vasoconstriction can be obtained with temporary packs soaked in epinephrine 1:100,000 when necessary. Magnification of the surgical field is enhanced by the use of two-power optical loops and is strongly recommended to optimize atraumatic surgical technique.

MAXILLA-PREMAXILLA APPROACH

Pertinent anatomic terms and structures are illustrated for review in Figure 14–3.

A right hemitransfixion incision is made with a no. 15 blade

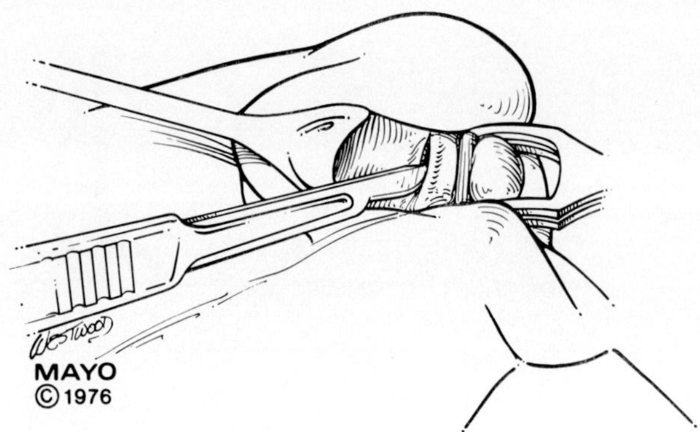

FIG 14–4.
A right-handed surgeon holds a Cottle columella clamp in the left hand, and the assistant holds an alar protector. After a columellar clamp has been applied to identify the caudal end of the septum, a right hemitransfixion incision is made about 1 to 2 mm behind the caudal end of the nasal septum with a no. 15 blade. (From Kern EB: Nasal septal reconstruction vs. submucous resection, in Snow JB (ed): *Controversy in Otolaryngology.* Philadelphia, WB Saunders Co, 1980, p 345. Used by permission.)

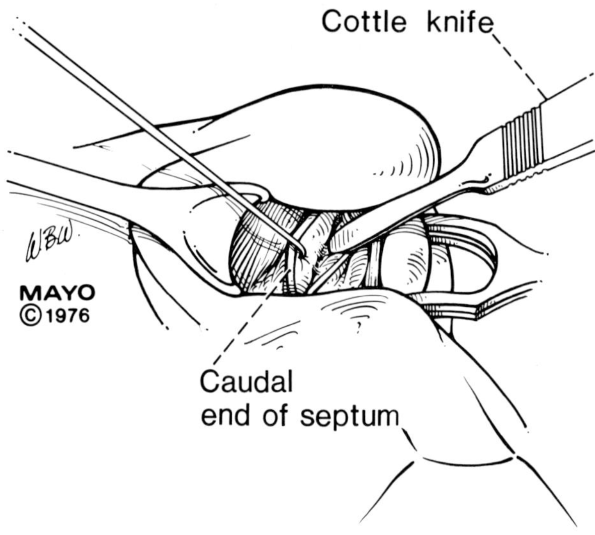

FIG 14–5.
Through the right hemitransfixion incision, the quadrangular septal cartilage is retracted to the right with a hook, and the Cottle knife is used to begin the left anterior tunnel by sharp dissection beneath the mucoperichondrium of the septal cartilage. (From Kern EB: Nasal septal reconstruction vs. submucous resection, in Snow JB (ed): *Controversy in Otolaryngology.* Philadelphia, WB Saunders Co, 1980, p 345. Used by permission.)

paralleling the caudal end of the septum (Fig 14–4). The incision is carried down to cartilage, and the Cottle knife is used to start the left anterior tunnel (Fig 14–5). The perichondrium is very tightly adherent to the cartilage anteriorly, and it is at this point that the surgeon scratches the cartilage to ensure a plane beneath the perichondrium. Bleeding is minimal, and dissection proceeds with alacrity when the submucoperichondrial plane is maintained (Fig 14–6). The left anterior tunnel is extended

beneath the periosteum of the bony septum to form a left posterior tunnel (Fig 14–7). The posterior dissection is carefully directed to avoid drifting superiorly toward the roof of the nose and the cribriform region. Elevation of the mucoperiosteum in this area may cause disturbances in olfaction and can produce a cerebrospinal fluid (CSF) leak, if the cribriform region is injured.

When the structure causing the nasal airway obstruction is located on the left side and it has been clearly exposed by this approach, it may be simply excised. Care should be taken not to injure the mucosa on the opposite side. Forces on the nasal

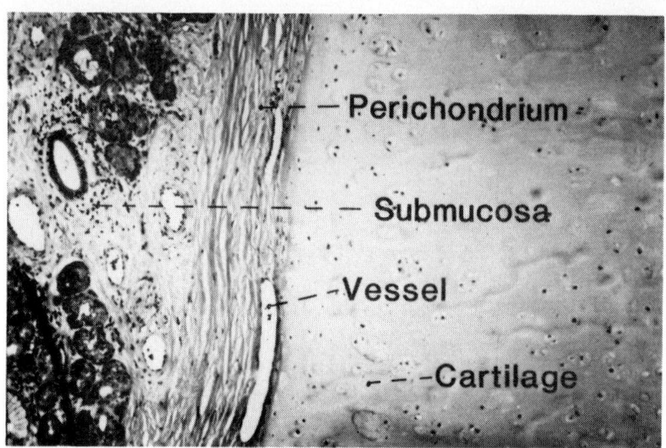

FIG 14–6.
Histologic section of human nasal septal cartilage and overlying perichondrium and submucosa. Note the presence of vessels in the perichondrium and their relationship to the septal cartilage (magnification × 100). (From Kern EB: Nasal septal reconstruction vs. submucous resection, in Snow JB (ed): *Controversy in Otolaryngology.* Philadelphia, WB Saunders Co, 1980, p 345. Used by permission.)

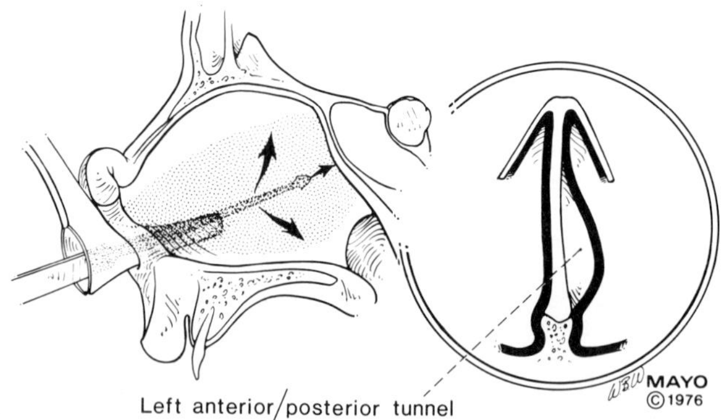

FIG 14–7.
As the dissection continues, the left anterior tunnel becomes a left anteroposterior tunnel, with elevation of the mucoperiosteum of the perpendicular plate of the ethmoid bone and the vomer in the posterior portion of the nose. With a nasal speculum placed through the hemitransfixion incision into the left anterior tunnel, a Cottle elevator is used to continue mucoperichondrial and mucoperiosteal elevation back to the face of the sphenoid. (From Kern EB: Nasal septal reconstruction vs. submucous resection, in Snow JB (ed): *Controversy in Otolaryngology.* Philadelphia, WB Saunders Co, 1980, p 346. Used by permission.)

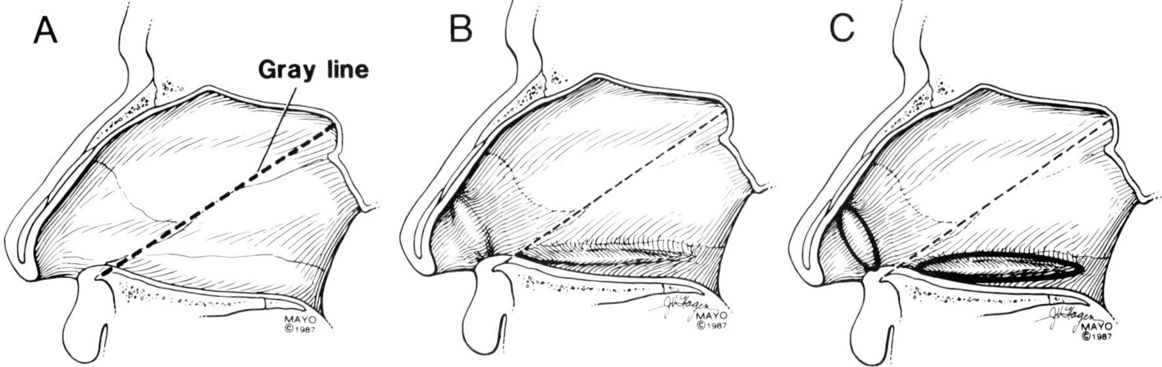

FIG 14–8.
A, the Gray line is an imaginary line drawn from the anterior nasal spine to the sphenoid rostrum. **B,** septal deformities that occur anterosuperior to this line are vertically oriented, whereas posterosuperior deformities are horizontally oriented. **C,** excision of septal deformities is outlined.

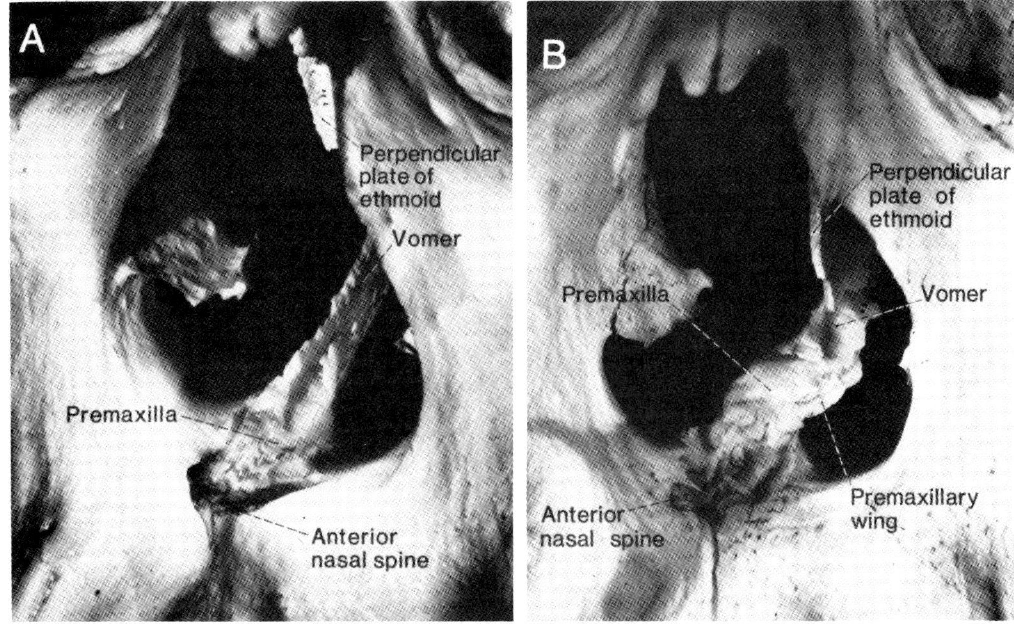

FIG 14–9.
A, normal bony anatomy in the region of the anterior nasal spine, premaxilla, and vomer. **B,** example of abnormal bony anatomy in the region of the anterior nasal spine, premaxilla, and vomer, which is approachable by the method with development of inferior tunnels. (From Kern EB: Nasal septal reconstruction vs. submucous resection, in Snow JB (ed): *Controversy in Otolaryngology.* Philadelphia, WB Saunders Co, 1980, pp 341–342. Used by permission.)

septum are such that when the deflection is located anterosuperior to a line drawn from the nasal spine to the sphenoid rostrum, the elliptical excision should be oriented vertically. When the deformity is posteroinferior to this line, the excision should be oriented horizontally (Fig 14–8). This line is named the Gray line after Vernon D. Gray, M.D., of Los Angeles, who first introduced this concept.

Premaxillary wing deformities and posterior septal spurs are both frequently encountered by the rhinologic surgeon. They tend to occur at the osseocartilagenous junction of the quadrangular cartilage and the vomerian crest (Fig 14–9). The mucosa overlying them has usually been thinned by the tur-

bulent air flow that they cause. These hot spots can be easily torn during surgical dissection. Inferior tunnels allow development of mucosal flaps beneath low septal spurs and premaxillary wing deformities, thereby minimizing tearing of nasal mucosa and the possible development of a septal perforation.

A left submucosal tunnel is created along the floor of the nose (left inferior tunnel) by undermining the upper lip through the right hemitransfixion incision (Fig 14–10). The anterior nasal spine and then the left piriform aperture are exposed through this incision. Full curve and half curve dissectors are used to elevate the mucoperiosteum off the floor of the nose posteriorly to the soft palate (Fig 14–11). This subperiosteal

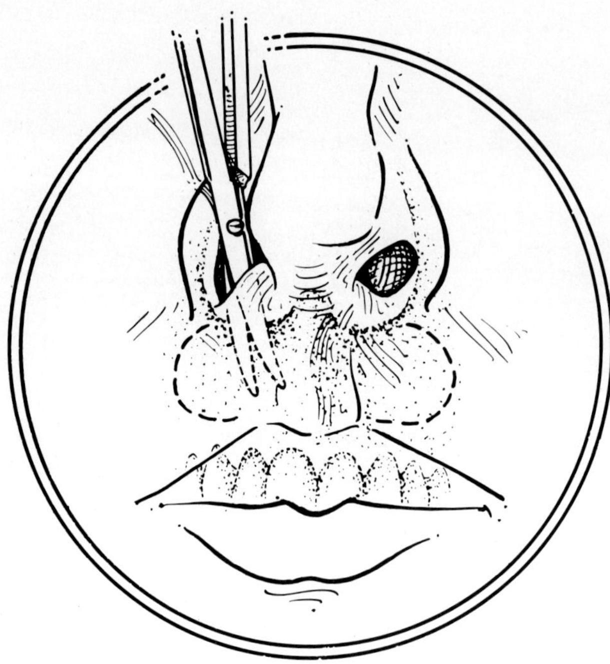

FIG 14–10.
The lip is undermined by elevating the tip of the nose with the left hand and placing a Knapp scissors into the hemitransfixion incision between the oral mucosa and the orbicular muscle anterior to the nasal spine. The nasal spine and the floor of the nose are exposed (within the limits of the dotted lines) so that a right inferior tunnel can be created. (From Kern EB: Nasal septal reconstruction vs. submucous resection, in Snow JB (ed): *Controversy in Otolaryngology.* Philadelphia, WB Saunders Co, 1980, p 346. Used by permission.)

tunnel is extended medially until resistance is met in the region of the maxillary crest. Posteriorly the periosteal fibers are less adherent to the bone, and the inferior tunnel is readily connected to the posterior tunnel. Anteriorly the perichondrial and periosteal fibers decussate at the osseocartilaginous junction to form the firm joint capsule of the septum. The surgeon must use sharp dissection to connect the inferior and anterior tunnels in the region of the anterior nasal spine to avoid a dehiscence in the mucosa (Fig 14–12). At this point, the entire left side of the septum is exposed from within the septal space (intraseptal).

If a posterior bony deformity needs removal, the cartilagenous septum is incised vertically at least 2 cm posterior to the caudal end without disrupting the right mucoperichondrium (Fig 14–13). A right posterior tunnel is created isolating the deformity (Fig 14–14). Angled scissors or rongeurs are used to safely separate the deformed bony septum, and it is removed with alligator (delicate otologic) forceps. Avulsion of the posterior septum can be dangerous, because while it is in direct continuity with the perpendicular plate of the ethmoid, manipulation may fracture the ethmoid complex and cribriform plate, producing a CSF leak.

Extensions of the maxilla-premaxilla approach are employed for caudal end and right anterior deformities. Following exposure of the left side of the septum, right anterior and posterior tunnels can be created in a similar fashion as the left side.

The entire septum can be skeletonized and widely uncovered for surgical correction. If the caudal end has been displaced from the anterior nasal spine, it is mobilized and trimmed as necessary to fit into the normal perichondrial space. A right inferior tunnel is employed for right anterior and posterior deformities primarily to elevate mucosa beneath the deformity and prevent dehiscence of the mucoperichondrium.

Early rhinologic surgeons did not believe that the septum contributed to the external nasal contour. Experience has taught that saddle nose deformities may ensue when the support of the caudal end of the septum is not adequately maintained.[16] Saddle nose deformities may even occur decades following SMR. Modification of the caudal end of the septum should not weaken its structure or disturb its relationship with the premaxilla and anterior nasal spine.

Tears in the mucosa will occur during dissection even in the most experienced hands. If unrecognized, these small mucosal tears can quickly become very large (>2 cm) and, if left unrepaired, may lead to a septal perforation. Prevention is the key to the avoidance of complications. Therefore, when NSR is performed, most mucosal tears should be repaired with absorbable suture. If tears occur on both sides of the septum, skeletal structure (bone or cartilage) is carefully placed intraseptally between the mucosal flaps, and the torn mucosa is sutured. Occasionally, absorbable gelatin film (Gelfilm) may be placed in the septal space to serve as a scaffold for the torn everted mucosal edges to heal and to help prevent septal perforation.

The cartilaginous septum derives its blood supply from the overlying perichondrium (see Fig 14–6). If the perichondrium remains elevated off the cartilage postoperatively, as when a septal hematoma is present, the cartilage can become infected and necrose, resulting in a septal perforation. Examination of the septal space and removal of blood plus the use of light pressure nasal packing most often prevent this complication. If

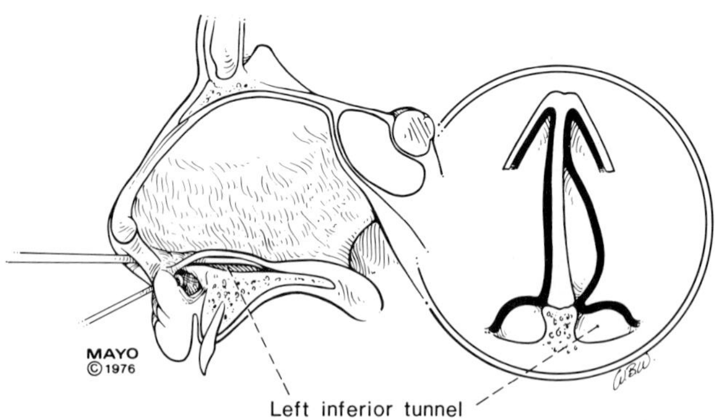

FIG 14–11.
Development of a left inferior tunnel. The crest of the piriform aperture is identified, and a curved Cottle elevator is used to elevate mucosa along the floor of the nose on the left. Three tunnels have now been developed; a left anteroposterior, a right inferior, and a left inferior. (From Kern EB: Nasal septal reconstruction vs. submucous resection, in Snow JB (ed): *Controversy in Otolaryngology.* Philadelphia, WB Saunders Co, 1980, p 347. Used by permission.)

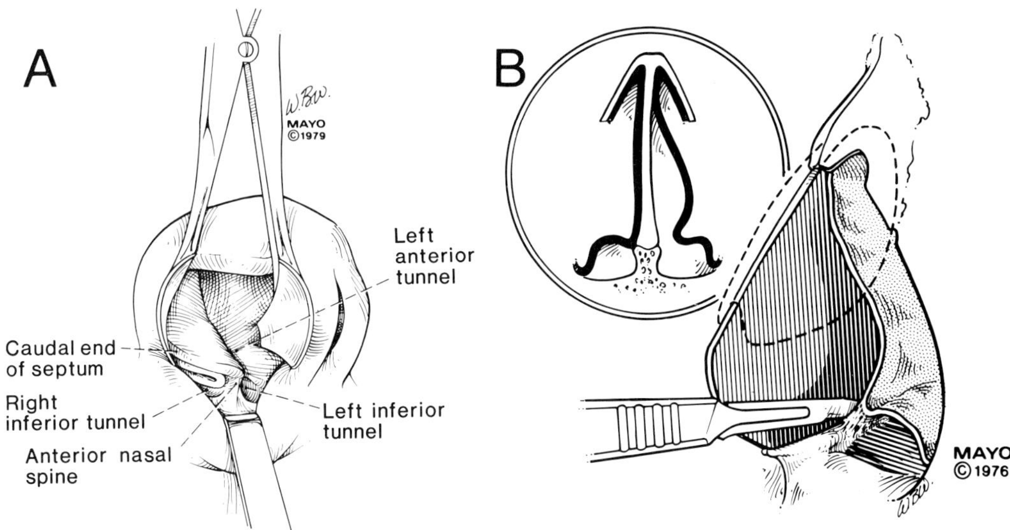

FIG 14–12.
A, left-sided tunnels are not connected; tissue is firmly adherent to the region of the osseous and cartilaginous joint between the quadrangular septal cartilage and the crest of the premaxilla. **B,** joining of the left anterior and left inferior tunnels by sharp dissection of the fibrous tissue that binds the mucosa in this area to the crest of the premaxilla. Care is taken not to perforate the mucosa. (From Kern EB, Pearson BW, McDonald TJ, et al: *Laryngoscope* 1979; 89(Suppl 15):1–34. Used by permission.)

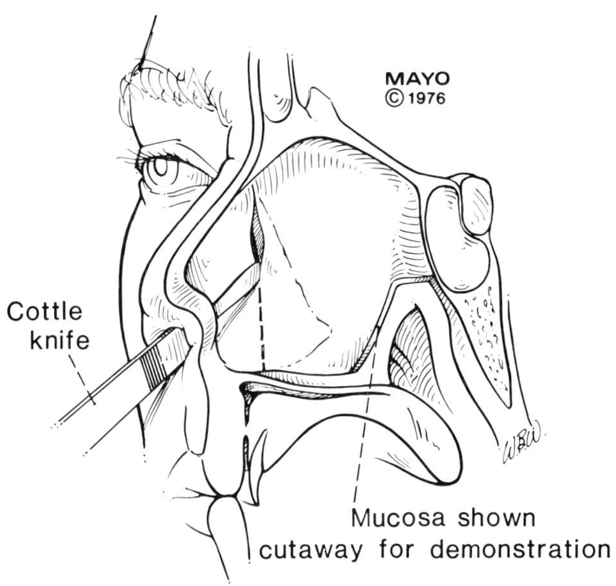

FIG 14–13.
With a Cottle knife in the left anterior tunnel, a vertical incision is made in the quadrangular septal cartilage caudal to the perpendicular plate of the ethmoid bone at a point about 2 to 3 cm behind the caudal end of the septum. Care is taken not to perforate the mucosa. This incision allows access to the right side of the septum so that the right posterior tunnel can be elevated before the posterior portion of the septum is removed, when desired. (From Kern EB: Nasal septal reconstruction vs. submucous resection, in Snow JB (ed): *Controversy in Otolaryngology.* Philadelphia, WB Saunders Co, 1980, p 348. Used by permission.)

bleeding in the intraseptal space is excessive, a drain (small rubber band) can be employed to prevent a hematoma.

Thin bone and lightly crushed cartilage are routinely replaced between the septal flaps (Fig 14–15, A) to help prevent a postoperative septal perforation and to facilitate surgical dissection if a second septal exploration is required. The replaced bone and cartilage also reduce the pulling force secondary to intraseptal cicatrization, which may later produce a saddle of the nasal dorsum. Maintaining a semirigid medial wall by replacing septal skeleton may offer a physiologic advantage over creating a flaccid septal membrane, as in the classic Killian operation. During inspiration, even slight differences in pressure between the nostrils may amount to a critical transseptal pressure difference sufficient to produce collapse of the septum into one nostril. This can impede nasal breathing.

Plastic nasal stents are cut and placed on either side of the septum. These stents help maintain the position of the healing septum and can prevent synechiae formation between the septum and the lateral nasal wall.[17] Antibiotic-impregnated petrolatum (Vaseline) gauze packs are first placed posteriorly on the pathologic side and then on the opposite side. The stents are secured anteriorly with a single silk suture after the hemitransfixion incision has been closed with one or two interrupted chromic sutures (Fig 14–15,B). The remaining internal nasal dressing (packing) is introduced, and then the external dressings and nasal cast are applied.

Prevention of complications begins with adherence to certain surgical tenets. The nasal mucosa is the organ of the nose. It must be handled carefully with a minimum of trauma. Where torn or incised, it should be repaired to heal by primary intention. Secondary intention healing should be avoided. If the submucosa is hypertrophied by chronic inflammation, it may need to be thinned. Raw surfaces should not be allowed to contact each other so as to prevent synechiae or a septal perforation.

The postoperative nose needs to heal, and it should be put at rest for this purpose. Occlusion of the nasal airway induces an outpouring of nasal secretions that serve to bathe the healing mucosa in physiologic solution. Internal nasal dressings (or packing) serve this purpose. They also keep the repaired septum properly aligned. These dressings are left in place for 6 days, and the nose is allowed to reject these dressings. The lubricated gauze packing is removed atraumatically (sometimes advanced over several days).

Postoperative hemorrhage is extremely rare when the integrity of the mucosa is maintained and nasal packing is removed gently. Early or aggressive removal of the packs before the nose is ready can cause shearing of crusts and epistaxis. Bleeding may also occur if the nose is injured by cleaning with suction. When hemorrhage does occur, the nose is simply vasoconstricted and examined for the bleeding site. Vasoconstriction will usually stop minor bleeding. If a specific site is identified, it is cauterized (carefully avoiding cauterization on both sides of the septum). Rarely is it necessary to repack the nose. If there is frank mucosal injury or loss, the nose is put to rest with small cotton balls placed in the nasal vestibule until healing occurs.

INFECTION

Infection following NSR is uncommon. Postoperative septal abscess can be avoided by making sure that blood does not accumulate within the septal space. If a dehiscence in the mu-

coperichondium does not occur during dissection, a low posterior drainage site may be indicated. The use of nasal stents and packing also helps to avoid this complication. Fever and increase in pain anytime from 3 to 10 days postoperatively

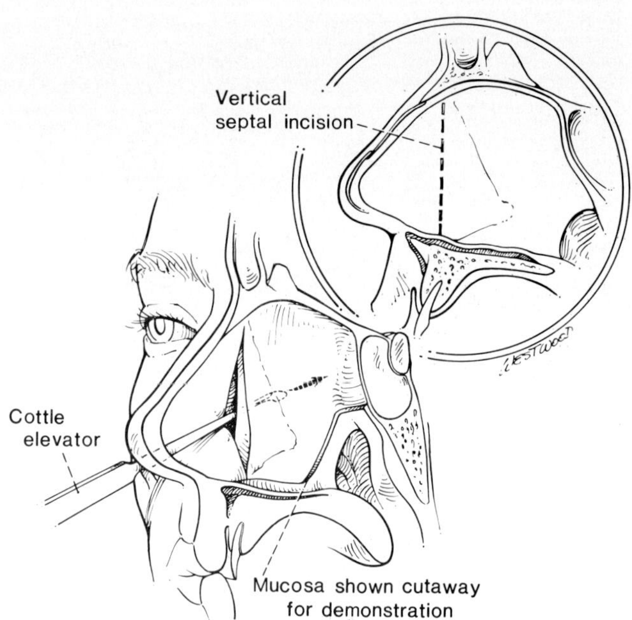

FIG 14–14.
Development of a right posterior tunnel. With a Cottle elevator placed through the vertical incision in the cartilage, elevation begins on the right side to create a tunnel beneath the mucoperichondrium and mucoperiosteum. (From Kern EB, Pearson BW, McDonald TJ, et al: *Laryngoscope* 1979; 89(Suppl 15):1–34. Used by permission.)

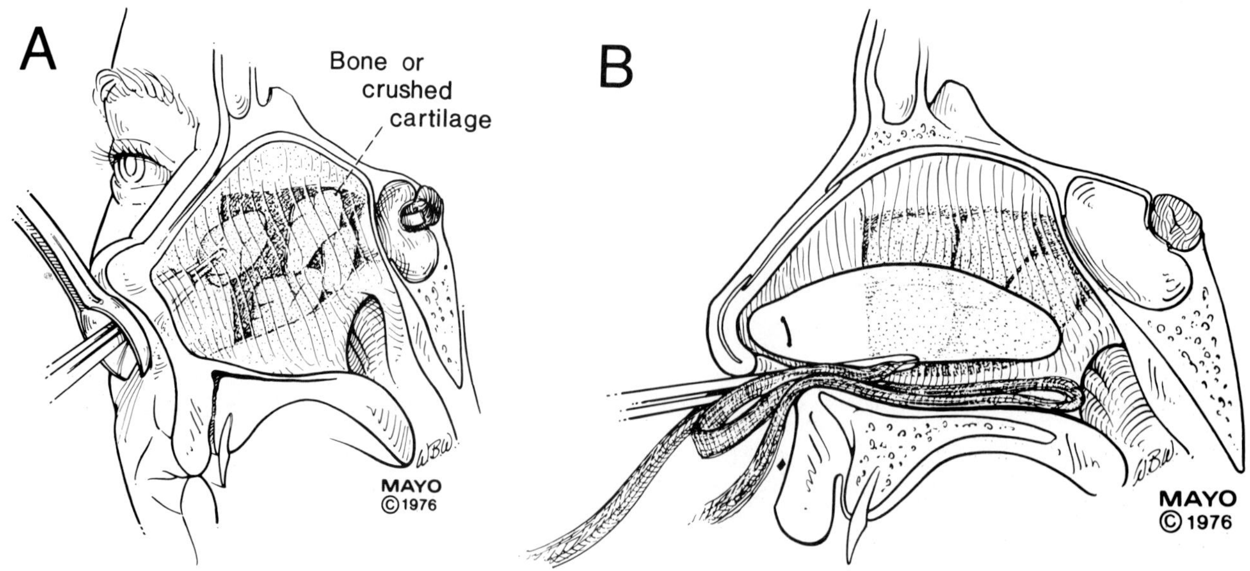

FIG 14–15.
A, crushed cartilage and bone are replaced within the septal space. **B,** nasal stents are secured on either side of the septum, and nasal packing is introduced to complete the closure of the procedure. (From Kern EB, Pearson BW, McDonald TJ, et al: *Laryngoscope* 1979; 89(Suppl 15):1–34. Used by permission.)

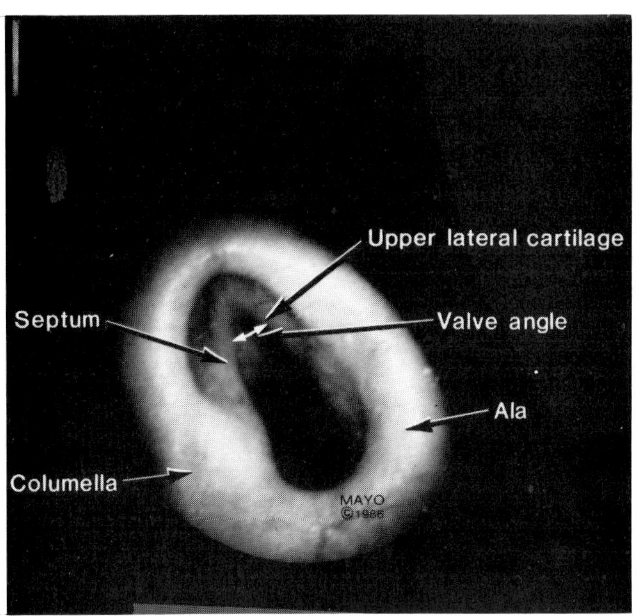

FIG 14–16.
Clinical view of nasal valve. When a nasal speculum is used, care must be taken not to obscure the nasal valve. Sometimes vibrissae may need to be trimmed to visualize the nasal valve. The nasal valve is perhaps best examined without any instrument in the nose. (From Kasperbauer JL, Kern EB: *Otolaryngol Clin North Am* 1987; 20:699–719. Used by permission.)

SURGERY OF THE NASAL VALVE AND VESTIBULE

Surgeons who operate on patients with nasal airway obstruction often confront those whose functional limitation is located in the nasal vestibule or the nasal valve (Fig 14–16). Nasal septal reconstruction must encompass repair of these structures as well.[22]

In the normal individual, the nasal valve is a dynamic flow-limiting portion of the nasal airway. It is an inverted cone-shaped region bounded by the caudal septum medially, the upper lateral cartilage (ULC) superiorly and laterally, the piriform margin inferiorly, and the head of the inferior turbinate posteroinferiorly (Fig 14–17). Abnormalities of any of these structures or the mucocutaneous lining of the valve may contribute to airway obstruction.

Aside from nonsurgical trauma, a common cause of nasal valve obstruction is nasal surgery, especially rhinoplasty. Therefore, a key to the management of nasal valve dysfunction is prevention. Numerous rhinoplastic techniques risk sacrifice of the functional integrity of the valve to achieve a particular cosmetic goal. When the nasal tip is modified, mucosa and skin of the nasal valve and vestibule must be preserved and adequate structural support maintained. A small amount of scar tissue contracture in this region can produce significant airway dysfunction. It is not the purpose of this discussion to promulgate rhinoplastic techniques; however, the rhinologist recognizes that almost all desired tip modifications may be accomplished

warrants a thorough examination. If an abscess is suspected, it may be necessary to return the patient to surgery for adequate examination and reexploration of the septal space, which will both confirm the diagnosis and serve as the first step in treatment. Purulent material is sent for culture and sensitivities. The septal space is thoroughly irrigated, and adequate skeleton is replaced to maintain the integrity of the septum.[18] Appropriate antibiotic treatment is instituted.

Blood-contaminated intranasal dressings are a perfect culture medium for bacteria. Impregnation of nasal packing with antibiotic ointment helps impede bacterial growth. Although no prospective clinical studies have proved the efficacy of perioperative oral antibiotics in nasal surgery, we routinely administer an antistaphylococcal cephalosporin while the nasal packing is in place.

Toxic shock syndrome is a toxin-mediated illness that has been reported in patients following nasal surgery.[19–21] Clinically it is characterized by fever, rash, hypotension, vomiting, and diarrhea in the absence of positive blood cultures. The toxin is produced by bacteria (most commonly *Staphylococcus aureus*) that grow in the nasal packing. Treatment involves supportive measures accompanied by removal and culturing of the nasal packing. Antibiotics, in general, do not play a large role in the management of these patients; however, an antistaphylococcal agent is usually administered.

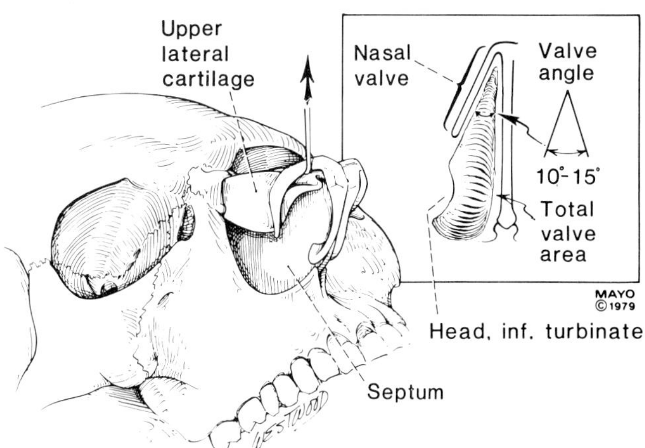

FIG 14–17.
The nasal valve area is bounded by the nasal septum, caudal end of the ULC, and soft fibrofatty tissue overlying the pyriform aperture and floor of the nose and posteriorly by the head of the inferior turbinate. This area is shaped like an inverted cone or teardrop, the slitlike apex of which is the nasal valve angle and normally subtends an angle of 10 to 15 degrees. (From Kern EB: Nasal septal reconstruction vs. submucous resection, in Snow JB (ed): *Controversy in Otolaryngology*. Philadelphia, WB Saunders Co, 1980, p 339. Used by permission.)

TABLE 14–1.
Nasal Valve Obstruction Pathologic Classification

I. Intramural
  A. Anatomic
    1. Mucosal
       a. Inflammatory
       b. Hypertrophy
    2. Submucosal
       a. Scar
       b. Hematoma
       c. Abscess
    3. Cutaneous
       a. Synechia (adhesions)
       b. Stricture
    4. Cartilage
       a. Septal
          (1) Absent
          (2) Thickened
          (3) Deflected
          (4) Twisted
       b. Upper Lateral
          (1) Absent
             (a) Complete
             (b) Incomplete
          (2) Thickened
          (3) Deflected
          (4) Twisted
          (5) Fixed collapse (secondary to nasal pyramid trauma)
          (6) Physiologic collapse
    5. Turbinate
       a. Bone (concha)
       b. Mucosal
          (1) Physiologic nasal cycle
          (2) Dependent (sleep position)
          (3) Vasomotor rhinitis
          (4) Allergic
          (5) Hyperplastic
  B. Pathophysiologic
    1. Turbulence
II. Extramural
  A. External pressure
  B. Intranasal space-occupying lesions
    1. Foreign body
    2. Growths

without unnecessary sacrifice of vestibular cutaneous lining. Furthermore, carefully planned intranasal incisions may prevent scar contracture in the region of the nasal valve and the resultant nasal airflow disturbances.

Causes of valvular obstruction include scarring of the mucocutaneous lining, caudal septal deformities, excess or returning ULC, inadequate cartilaginous support of the ala, narrowed piriform aperture, and turbinate hypertrophy. A classification of valve pathology has been reported[15] and is presented in Table 14–1.

Synechia in the nasal valve area is one of the most difficult surgical problems faced by the rhinologist (Fig 14–18). If the scar is thin, it can be divided and the valve stented with Silastic for several weeks until the raw surfaces reepithelializes. When the scar is thick, it can be excised and the defect grafted with

split-thickness skin or buccal mucosa (Fig 14–19). Long-term results with each of these techniques have been disappointing. Local skin flap repairs (Fig 14–20) and z-plasty techniques as

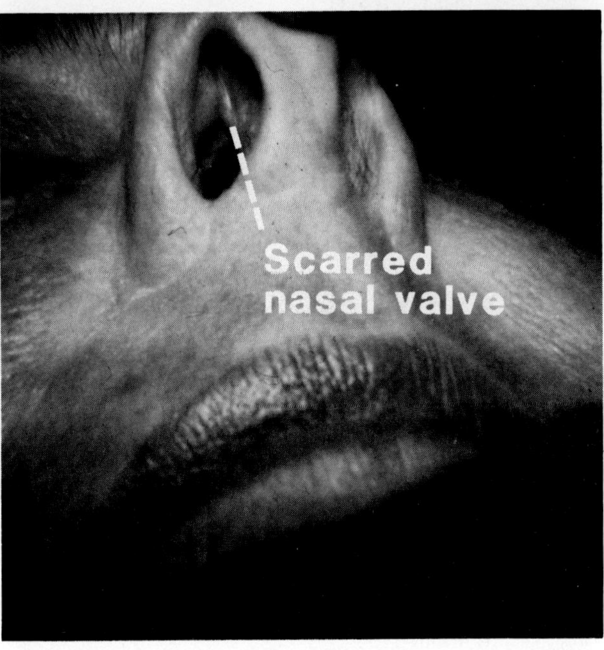

FIG 14–18.
Photograph of a postoperative mucocutaneous synechia of right nasal valve. (From Kern EB: Nasal septal reconstruction vs. submucous resection, in Snow JB (ed): *Controversy in Otolaryngology.* Philadelphia, WB Saunders Co, 1980, p 364. Used by permission.)

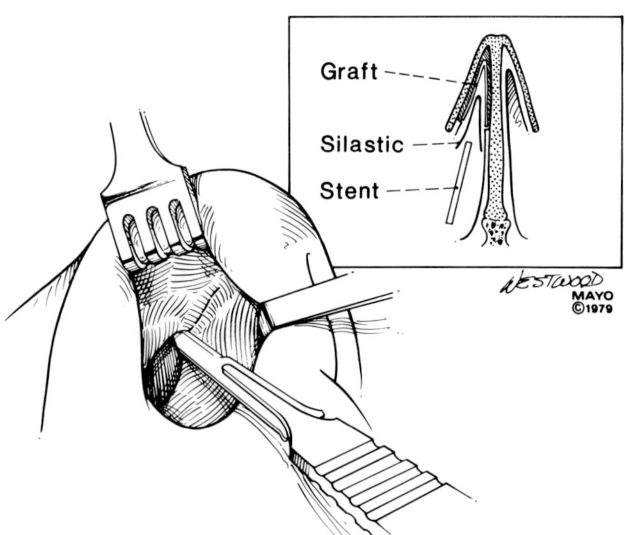

FIG 14–19.
Scar tissue can be removed, and Silastic sheeting can be folded and sewn, along with placement of plastic stent, to hold the graft in position to reconstruct a new nasal valve and prevent further scarring. (From Kern EB: Nasal septal reconstruction vs. submucous resection, in Snow JB (ed): *Controversy in Otolaryngology.* Philadelphia, WB Saunders Co, 1980, p 364. Used by permission.)

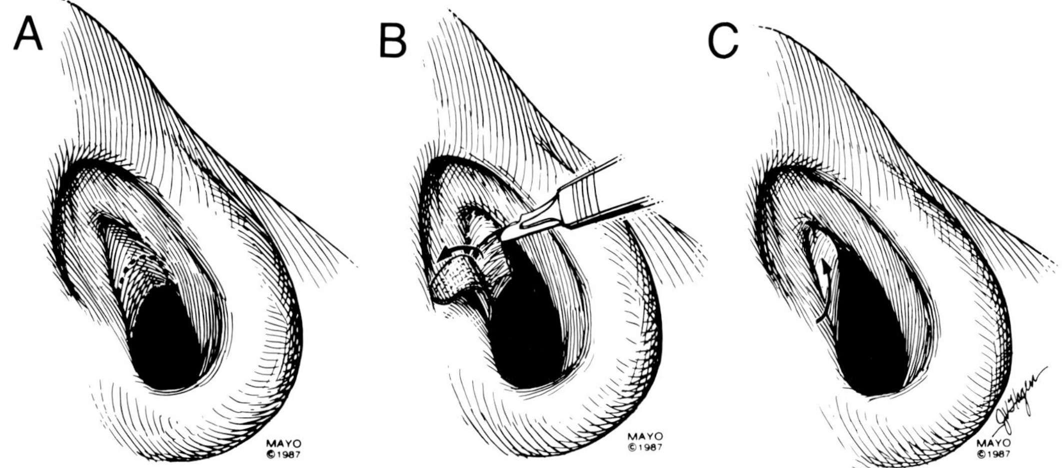

FIG 14–20.
Local flap repair of nasal valve synechia. **A**, incision is outlined on caudal side of synechia. **B**, flap is elevated, and subcutaneous scar tissue is excised. **C**, flap is shown sewn into place.

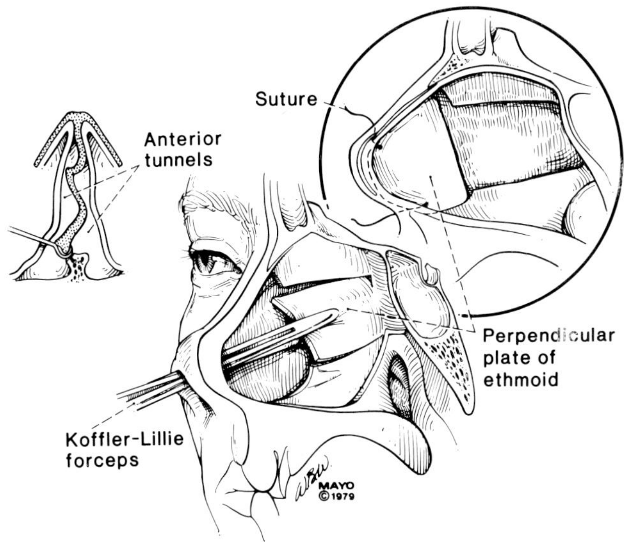

FIG 14–21.
Bilateral anterior tunnels have been created to allow removal and replacement of deformed caudal end of septum with autogenous bone graft from perpendicular plate of ethmoid. (From Kern EB: Nasal septal reconstruction vs. submucous resection, in Snow JB (ed): *Controversy in Otolaryngology.* Philadelphia, WB Saunders Co, 1980, p 359. Used by permission.)

well as composite alar swing flaps have also been used with variable success.

Occasionally the caudal septum may be so severely damaged that simple modification will be inadequate to solve the problem. This is sometimes the case with saddle nose deformities. The surgeon must be prepared to completely excise and replace the entire caudal end of the septum, if necessary, to reconstitute normality. The perpendicular plate of the ethmoid bone can be trimmed and used to reconstruct caudal septal defects (Fig 14–21).

The ULC is frequently the cause of valvular obstruction. Excess ULC returning may need to be excised to open the valve angle (Fig 14–22).[23] When the nose is cosmetically narrowed by aggressive removal of ULC and vestibular skin, the lateral wall of the nasal valve can scar toward the septum and narrow or close the liminal angle. Infracture of the frontal process of the maxilla (lateral osteotomies) can also cause a narrowing of the nasal valve area. When this results in nasal airway obstruction, the nasal valve needs to be reconstructed, which often means the resculpturing of the ULC to restore the normal re-

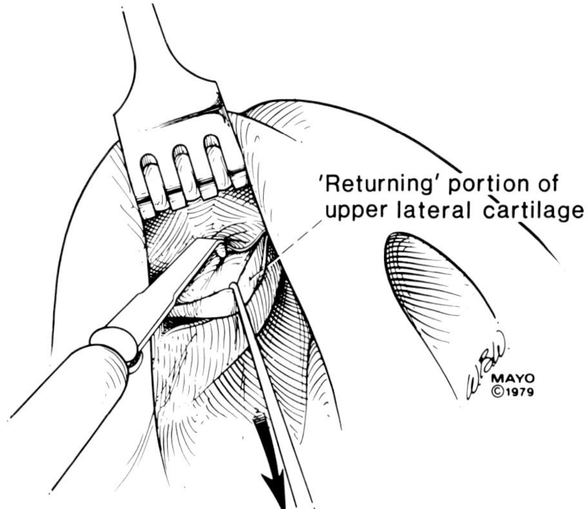

FIG 14–22.
Weighted hook is applied to cartilage for countertraction, with dissection with no. 66 Beaver knife blade down to perichondrium. Curling, or returning, of distal portion of upper lateral cartilage may be observed. (From Kern EB: Nasal septal reconstruction vs. submucous resection, in Snow JB (ed): *Controversy in Otolaryngology.* Philadelphia, WB Saunders Co, 1980, p 360. Used by permission.)

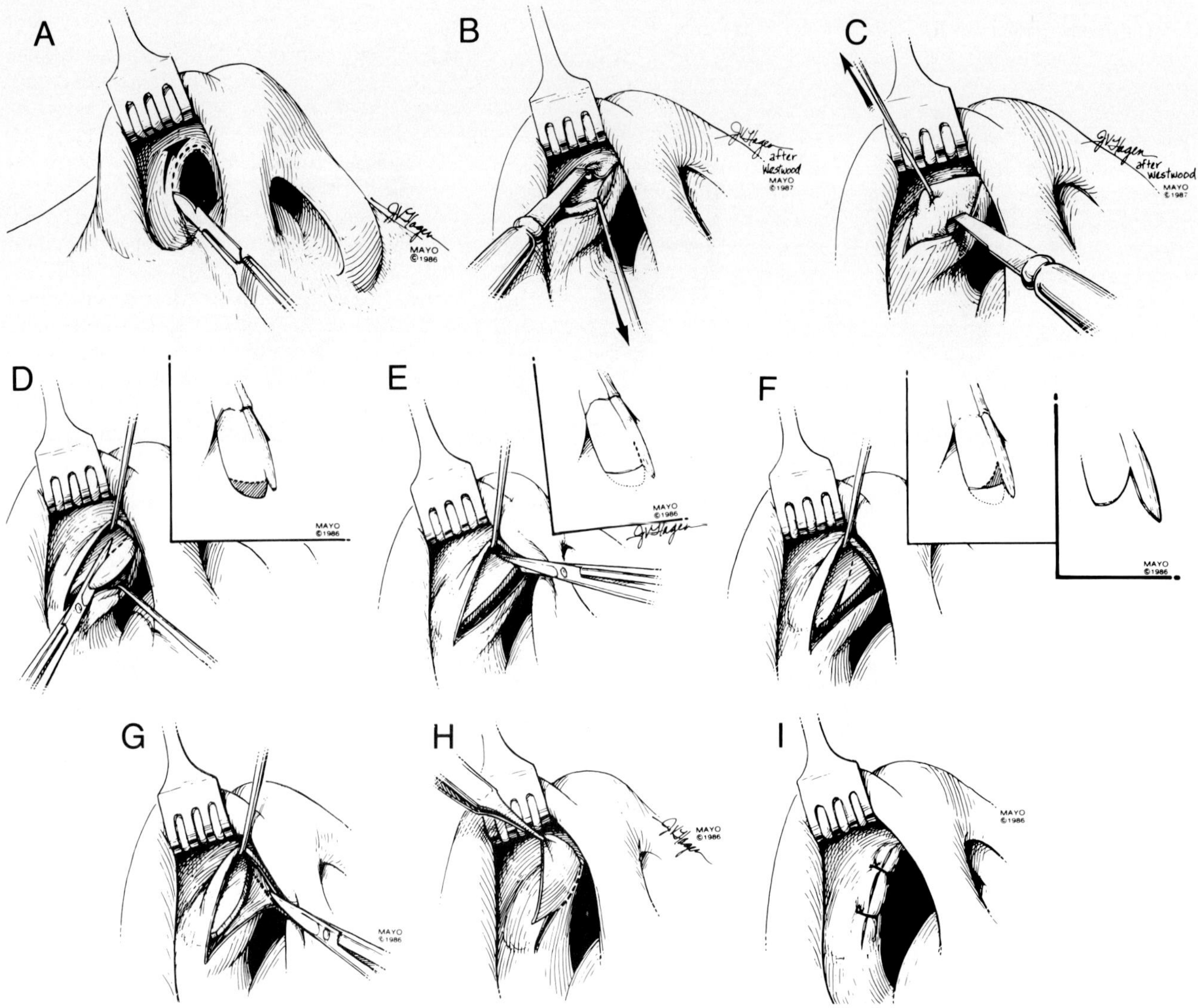

FIG 14–23.
A, intercartilaginous incision with no. 15 blade carried down just beneath the skin. **B,** weighted hook is applied to the ULC for countertraction, and dissection with a no. 66 Beaver knife blade is down to the perichondrium. **C,** the undersurface of the ULC may be exposed, preserving the skin. **D,** resection of the caudal end of the ULC may be carried out directly, and mucocutaneous tissue can be preserved. **E,** the ULC can be completely separated from nasal septum medially, and the submucosa can be preserved if desired. **F,** medial triangle of the ULC can be removed submucosally from its attachment to the septum. **G,** after the caudal end and medial triangle of the ULC have been removed, the mucocutaneous tissue is separated from the septum. **H,** the excess tissue is trimmed, and, **I,** the intercartilaginous incision is closed, thereby opening and widening the apex of the valve angle. (From Kasperbauer JL, Kern EB: *Otolaryngol Clin North Am* 1987; 20:699–719. Used by permission.)

lationship between this structure and the caudal septum. We use a flap technique described by Dr. Fausto Lopez-Infante of Mexico City (Fig 14–23).[24] The caudal edge of the ULC is trimmed through an intercartilaginous incision, and a triangle of cartilage is removed at its attachment to the septal cartilage. The excess vestibular skin is minimally trimmed, and the incision is closed. This maneuver takes advantage of the greater angle cephalad between the ULC and the septum and local skin flap rotation. Outfracture of the frontal process of the maxilla may also be needed to reopen the liminal angle.

Alar collapse occurs when the normal anatomic relation-ships that serve to support the nasal alae are disturbed.[25] The anterolateral vestibular wall is supported by the lateral crus of the lower lateral cartilage (LLC), which, in turn, derives its support from its relationship to the mesial crus of the LLC, the ULC, and the fibroareolar tissues of the ala nasal base, anterior nasal spine, and caudal septum. Simultaneous disruption of more than one of these relationships may lead to alar collapse. Conservative trimming of the nasal cartilages may help to prevent this complication. Vertical transection of the LLC along with vestibular skin coupled with aggressive shortening of both the LLC and the ULC can lead to alar collapse.

Management of alar collapse involves the restoration of the structural support of the anterolateral vestibular wall. Conchal cartilage grafts positioned cephalad to the LLC can provide some support. Repositioning of the LLC in relationship to the ULC may help to stent open the narrowed vestibule. The rhinolift is a procedure where the entire nasal dorsum is exposed through intercartilaginous incisions, and an ellipse of skin is removed transversely from the nasal dorsum. This rotates the tip and may restore a more normal relationship between the ULC and LLC. Composite alar swing flaps have also been used to correct this deformity.

SEPTAL PERFORATION

Perforation of the nasal septum may result from trauma (surgical or nonsurgical), infection, inflammatory diseases, or neoplasm. The most common cause, however, is surgical trauma.[26] Patients with septal perforation may experience dryness, crusting, epistaxis, whistling (particularly when small), or disturbed nasal breathing, or as is frequently the case, may be totally asymptomatic.

Prevention of septal perforation as a complication of nasal septal surgery begins with meticulous attention to details of surgical technique, including careful patient preparation, adequate anesthesia, vasoconstriction, atraumatic dissection, fixation of tissues, and appropriate closure. Repair of mucosal tears and replacement of intervening tissues will reduce the risk of perforation.

If a septal perforation is asymptomatic, no treatment is needed. If symptoms occur, saline irrigations and locally applied petrolatum may help decrease the crusting and superficial bleeding. Small perforations may be closed surgically through the use of local tissue advancement techniques.[27] More recently, use of a prosthetic Silastic septal button to close a perforation has obviated the need for surgery in many cases (Fig 14–24). Custom-made buttons may be created for even the largest perforation.

Septal perforations present particular problems in the correction of nasal septal deformities as well as other procedures that transverse the septal space (i.e., transseptal sphenoidotomy and transseptal hypophysectomy). Lack of a firm septal skeleton makes dissection hazardous, and preexisting septal perforations are more likely to enlarge. The use of inferior tunnels until more normal planes of dissection are reached has simplified revision surgery following extensive removal of septal skeletal structures by allowing access and mobilization of mucosal flaps with minimal tearing of the mucosa.

ATROPHIC RHINITIS

Atrophic rhinitis is a chronic degenerative disease of the nose characterized by chronic inflammation with atrophy of glandular elements and submucosal fibrosis. There is patchy squamous metaplasia with a reduction in the number and function of the nasal cilia.[28, 29] This impairs the nose's mucociliary clearance mechanisms. With impairment of the natural defenses, there is an overgrowth of bacteria and the production of a fetid odor.

Patients with atrophic rhinitis may be severely debilitated and socially withdrawn. They may have pain, crusting, epistaxis,

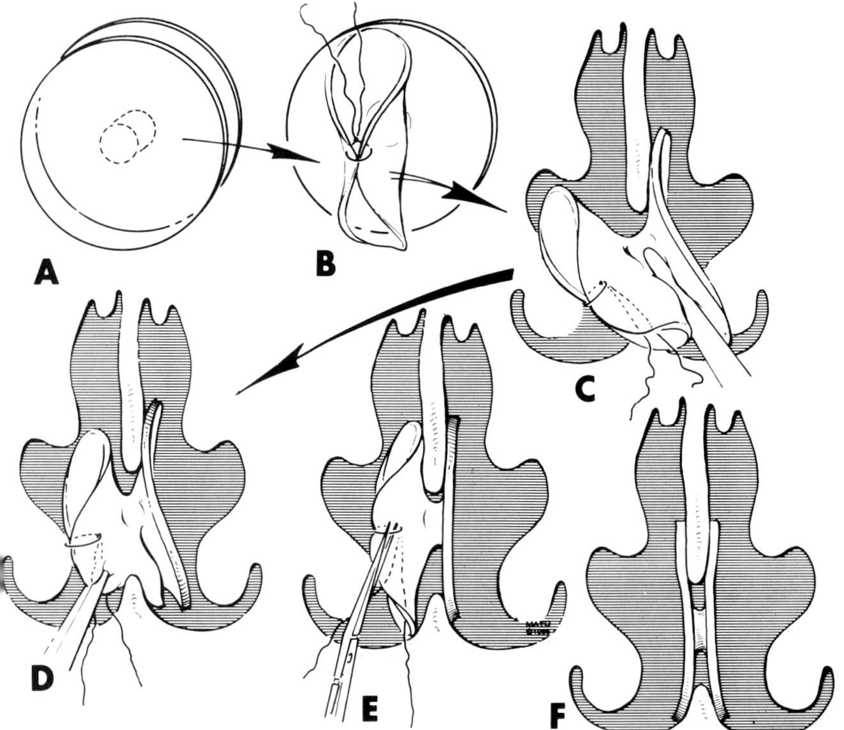

FIG 14–24.
A, insertion of the Silastic prosthesis. **B,** one flange is sutured together to aid placement. **C,** the central axle is grasped, and the prosthesis is advanced into the defect. **D,** the button is advanced into position, and **E,** the suture is snipped. **F,** the button is adjusted for maximal comfort and rests in position, occluding and covering the septal perforation. (From Hanson RD, Facer GW, Kern EB: *OTO '87* 1986; 1:2–5. Used by permission.)

and visual disturbance in addition to generalized malaise.

Surgical destruction of nasal mucosa can lead to atrophic rhinitis. It is not clear how much tissue must be preserved to prevent this complication, but it appears that a critical level is reached beyond which atrophy ensues. In the context of surgery for correction of nasal airway obstruction, turbinectomy can be considered an important cause of atrophic rhinitis.[30,31] Conservation turbinate surgery may be considered for irreversible mucosal disease, but complete turbinectomy should be avoided for nonmalignant disease. Electrocautery or cryodessication is not recommended for treatment of mucosal disorders. Medical diagnosis to determine the nature of mucosal pathology (vasomotor rhinitis or allergic rhinitis), followed by specific treatment (avoidance, antihistamines, or steroids) and limited focal turbinate surgery, is advised.

Numerous strategies have been proposed for the treatment of atrophic rhinitis. Patients who experience minor crusting and odor may benefit from the local application of streptomycin or Dabs* solution in the form of nasal douches to reduce bacterial overgrowth. Sesame oil with rose geranium is applied daily to loosen crusts, coat the injured mucosa, and reduce the fetid odor. Topical estrogen cream also helps the mucosa develop increased vascularity. Nasal occlusion helps to conserve nasal secretions that bathe the injured mucosa in physiologic fluids. We recommend the use of petrolatum-impregnated cotton balls in the nasal vestibule for temporary occlusion of the nasal airway. Patients customize this to their personal needs.

Surgery for atrophic rhinitis (endonasal microplasty) is directed at reducing the caliber of the nasal airway as well as increasing the vascularity and thickness of the submucosa.[32–34] Implantation of cartilage or bone beneath the mucosa on the lateral nasal wall, along the floor of the nose, and in the septal space has been advocated. Results with this procedure have been encouraging. Endonasal microplasty, however, is by no means a total solution of the problem of atrophic rhinitis, but it is a good beginning.

Another important aspect of the care rendered to the patient with atrophic rhinitis is continued psychologic support. The degree of debilitation this chronic condition can cause is very surprising. Frequent visits with adjustment of the medical regiment and counseling give the patients hope and encouragement.

SUMMARY

Nasal septal reconstruction is the complete surgical approach to the treatment of nasal airway obstruction resulting from deformities of the nasal septum and its adnexae. Adherence to principles of wide exposure, conservation resection, and restoration of normality without sacrifice of structure permit correction of the abnormality while minimizing complications.

*Dabs solution is composed of 1 L of saline solution, 80 mg of gentamicin, 100 mg of polymyxin B sulfate, and 500 mg of neomycin sulfate. The patient is instructed to irrigate each nostril with 20 mL of the solution as directed.

The maxilla-premaxilla approach is a technique that allows the surgeon access to all parts of the septum and pyramid. The surgeon may use the entire maxilla-premaxilla approach or modify it as needed. Today, the best functional results are achieved when the entire deformity is corrected without sacrificing the resilience and stability of the septum. This may require the reintroduction or reconstruction of the cartilaginous and bony structures that have been removed during the procedure. A thorough understanding of nasal physiology is crucial to the nasal surgeon and is the basis of modern septal surgery. Prevention is the key to the management of complications, whereas both anatomy and physiology are the keys to the success of NSR.

REFERENCES

1. Pirsig W, Lehmann I: The influence of trauma on the growing septal cartilage. *Rhinology* 1975; 12:39–46.
2. Freer OT: The correction of deflections of the nasal septum with a minimum of traumatism. *JAMA* 1902; 38:636–642.
3. Killian G: The submucous window resection of the nasal septum. *Ann Otol Rhinol Laryngol* 1905; 14:363–393.
4. Metzenbaum M: Replacement of the lower end of the dislocated septal cartilage versus submucous resection of the dislocated end of the septal cartilage. *Arch Otolaryngol* 1929; 9:282–296.
5. Peer LA: An operation to repair lateral displacement of the lower border of the septal cartilage. *Arch Otolaryngol* 1937; 25:475–477.
6. Salinger S: Deviation of the septum in relation to the twisted nose. *Arch Otolaryngol* 1939; 29:520–532.
7. Seltzer AP: The nasal septum: Plastic repair of the deviated septum associated with a deflected tip. *Arch Otolaryngol* 1944; 40:433–444.
8. Fomon S, Gilbert JG, Silver AG, et al: Plastic repair of the obstructing nasal septum. *Arch Otolaryngol* 1948; 47:7–20.
9. Fomon S, Bell JW, Berger EL, et al: New approach to ventral deflections of the nasal septum. *Arch Otolaryngol* 1951; 54:356–366.
10. Cottle MH, Loring RM: Surgery of the nasal septum: New operative procedures and indications. *Ann Otol Rhinol Laryngol* 1948; 57:705–713.
11. Cottle MH, Loring RM, Fischer GG, et al: The "maxilla-premaxilla" approach to extensive septum surgery. *Arch Otolaryngol* 1958; 68:301–313.
12. Cottle MH: The structure and function of the nasal vestibule. *Arch Otolaryngol* 1955; 62:173–181.
13. Ersner MS: Rhinoplastic procedures to establish normal physiologic nasal function. *Pa Med* 1948; 51:749–754.
14. Bridger GP: Physiology of the nasal valve. *Arch Otolaryngol* 1970; 92:543–553.
15. Kasperbauer JL, Kern EB: Nasal valve physiology. *Otol Clin North Am* 1987; 20:699–719.
16. Cohen S: Role of the septum in surgery of the nasal contour. *Arch Otolaryngol* 1939; 30:12–20.
17. Campbell JB, Watson, MG, Shenoi PM: The role of intranasal splints in the prevention of post-operative nasal adhesions. *J Laryngol Otol* 1987; 101:1140–1143.
18. Olsen KD, Carpenter RJ, Kern EB: Nasal septal trauma in children. *Pediatrics* 1979; 64:32–35.

19. Hull HF, Mann JM, Sands CJ, et al: Toxic shock syndrome related to nasal packing. *Arch Otolaryngol* 1983; 109:624–626.
20. Barbour SD, Shlaes DM, Guertin SR: Toxic-shock syndrome associated with nasal packing: Analogy to tampon-associated illness. *Pediatrics* 1984; 73:163–165.
21. Jacobson JA, Kasworm EM, Crass BA, et al: Nasal carriage of toxigenic *Staphylococcus aureus* and prevalence of serum antibody to toxic-shock-syndrome toxin 1 in Utah. *J Infect Dis* 1986; 153:356–359.
22. Kern EB: Surgical approaches to abnormalities of the nasal valve. *Rhinology* 1978; 16:165–190.
23. Gray VD: Physiologic returning of the upper lateral cartilage. *Int Rhinol* 1970; 8:56–59.
24. Lopez-Infante F: Personal communication, 1984.
25. Fomon S, Gilbert JG, Caron AL, et al: Collapsed ala. *Arch Otolaryngol* 1950; 51:465–484.
26. Fairbanks DNF, Fairbanks GR: Nasal septal perforation: Prevention and management. *Ann Plast Surg* 1980; 5:452–459.
27. Tipton JB: Closure of large septal perforations with a labial-buccal flap. *Plast Reconstr Surg* 1970; 46:514–515.
28. Cottle MH: Nasal atrophy, atrophic rhinitis, ozena: Medical and surgical treatment. *J Int Coll Surg* 1958; 29:472–484.
29. Sinha SN, Sardana DS, Rajvanshi VS: A nine years' review of 273 cases of atrophic rhinitis and its management. *J Laryngol Otol* 1977; 91:591–600.
30. Dawes PJD: The early complications of inferior turbinectomy. *J Laryngol Otol* 1987; 101:1136–1139.
31. Moore GF, Freeman TJ, Ogren FP, et al: Extended follow-up of total inferior turbinate resection for relief of chronic nasal obstruction. *Layngoscope* 1985; 95:1095–1099.
32. Young A: Closure of the nostrils in atrophic rhinitis. *J Laryngol Otol* 1971; 85:715–718.
33. Huizing EH: Surgery of the lateral nasal wall in atrophin rhinitis and ozena. *Rhinology* 1976; 14:79–81.
34. Gupta SC: Septoplasty in the unilateral atrophic rhinitis with deviated nasal septum. *J Laryngol Otol* 1985; 99:163–165.

Nasal Septal Reconstruction

Approach of

Fred J. Stucker, Jr., M.D.

Prior to addressing specific problems and suggested techniques, I will describe a routine, if such exists, septoplasty. This step-by-step detailing of the surgical maneuvers will serve as a reference point to alleviate the need to repeat specific techniques that we routinely use for specific problems or management of a complication.

SUGGESTED STEPS IN ROUTINE SEPTOPLASTY

Anesthesia

Five neurosurgical cottonoids saturated with a 5% cocaine solution, with the excess solution squeezed out, are placed for topical anesthesia and vasoconstriction. The total dose of cocaine is kept under 200 mg in adults. Two packs are placed intranasally on both sides. Cottonoids are positioned superiorly along the apex of the nose where the septum is joined by the lateral nasal wall, and a second pack is placed on each side along the floor, across and touching the septum and middle turbinate and in contact with the posterior wall in the region of the sphenopalatine ganglion. The fifth cottonoid is placed in the upper lip sulcus between the lip and the premaxilla. The cocaine packs are left in place for 10 minutes to allow adequate topical anesthesia and vasoconstriction. The majority of nasal procedures are carried out under local anesthesia using 1% lidocaine with epinephrine 1:100,000. Anesthesia personnel monitor the patient's vital signs and provide an appropriate level of intravenous sedation (although this is kept to a minimum). It is unusual to require more than 8 to 10 mL of local anesthesia for a nasal and septal reconstructive procedure.

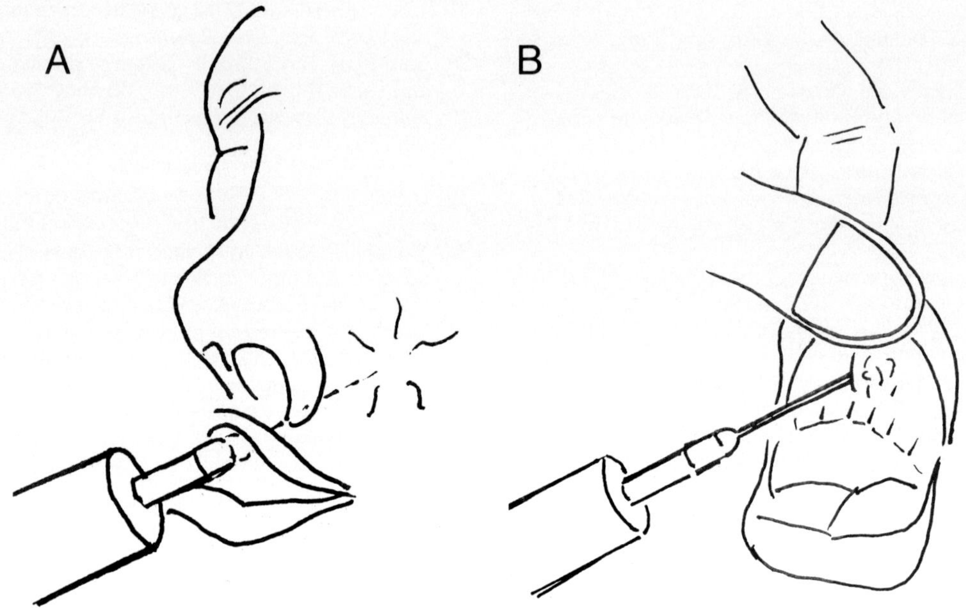

FIG 14–25.
A, sublabial injection site following 4% topical cocaine. **B,** infraorbital block via sublabial injection route.

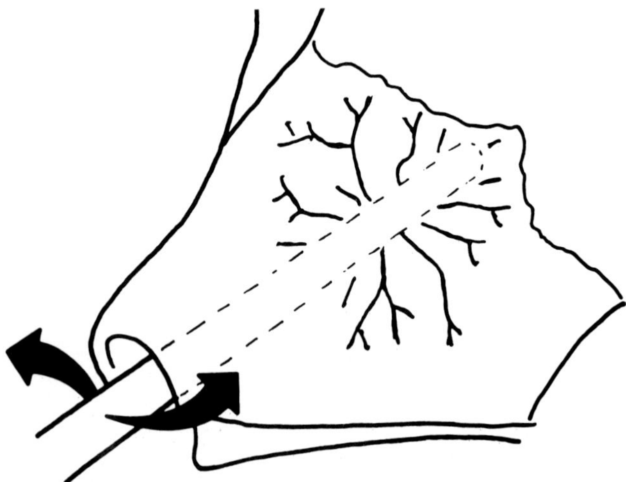

FIG 14–26.
Mobilization of bony septum with Sayer elevator. (From Stucker FJ Jr: *Laryngoscope* 1982; 92:129. Used by permission.)

The infiltration is commenced by removing the cottonoid beneath the upper lip and injecting approximately 0.5 mL through the mucosa at the base of the nose. The mucosa provides a relatively painless entry site, and the loose tissue in this region allows infiltration with less discomfort than the more commonly employed percutaneous or intranasal injection routes. From the same sublabial site, bilateral infraorbital and alar base blocks are carried out (Fig 14–25). The entire columella up to the tip is infiltrated via the sublabial route, as are the bony nasomaxillary grooves on both sides. These injections usually require approximately 5 mL of local anesthetic solution. The needle is withdrawn, and the septum and dorsum of the nose are injected intranasally. A most important injection site is the mucosal apex of the septum and lateral nasal wall. Here the infiltration commences where the nasal bones converge on the septum and advances posteriorly. This injection blocks the critical anterior and posterior ethmoidal nerves. This regional block precedes the draping and prepping, which ensures adequate time to elapse for the optimum anesthetic and vasoconstrictive effects.

Mobilization of Bony Septum

Fracturing and mobilization of the bony septum constitute the initial maneuver in all septoplasty procedures. A Sayer elevator is placed in the nose between the bony septum and nasal bones, and by employment of a rocking horizontal motion medial to lateral, the perpendicular plate and vomer are mobilized (Fig 14–26). This is carried out on both sides. It often greatly improves visualization and enhances the technical aspects of the cartilage work. Approximately 10% of septoplasty work is adequately completed with just this simple maneuver, primarily when the obstruction results from the bony septum being impacted against the lateral bony wall. If there is inadequate anesthesia, it will become apparent with the bony mobilization, and further local infiltrations or greater palatine foramen blocks are indicated. The fear of precipitating a CSF rhinorrhea has not materialized. This maneuver has been done as described in more than 3,000 cases with no known instances of CSF rhinorrhea or other complications.

Incisional Approach

There are three basic surgical approaches to septal work.

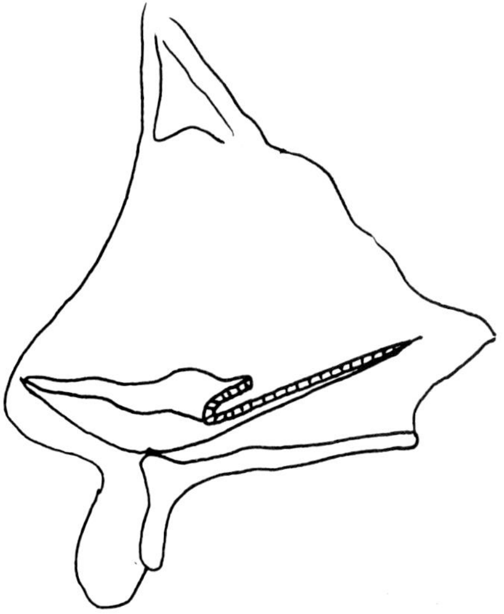

FIG 14–27.
Unilateral elevation of mucoperiochondrial and mucoperiosteal flap. Note inferior incision enhances access and prevents soft tissue avulsion with skeletal resection.

A hemitransfixion incision, a complete transfixion incision, and the external or open rhinoplasty approach. The specific case will dictate which of these is to be employed.

Unilateral Flap

In the majority of cases, regardless of which incisional approach is used, a unilateral mucoperichondrial or mucoperiosteal flap is developed with the thought of maintaining the integrity of the opposite side to enhance stability and minimize the chance of perforation. In patients such as those with a thickened quadrangular cartilage or trauma-induced reduplications of the septum, bilateral flaps may be required. A rather routine finding in septal flap elevation is the presence of a spur or inferior dislocation, which, combined with the tissue decussation along the maxillary crest, handicaps the smooth elevation of the mucosal flap. The hemi or complete transfixion incision on the side of the flap elevation is carried into the nose in this inferior location as far posteriorly as needed to completely expose the cartilage and bone to be surgically modified (Fig 14–27). This large superiorly and posteriorly based mucosal flap is reflected laterally, exposing the entire surgical field and avoiding the often damaging event of tearing or avulsing mucosa when one is working on the skeletal structures. At the completion of the bone and cartilage work, this mucosal flap drapes over the septum while providing a generous inferior drainage site. The caudal incision is always closed and sutured.

Spurs

The spurs determined to be obstructive are resected with a sharp chisel by removing bone, cartilage, and mucosa as a single entity. Since the opposite side is intact, this management of spurs has not resulted in a perforation or compromised healing in several hundreds of cases, and rapid epithelialization

has been routinely noted. Postoperative oozing may be slightly increased, but to date no patient has required postoperative packing. The mucosal flap, because it has been "stretched" to cover the hypertrophic lateralized spur or dislocated septum, most often adequately drapes over the denuded area where the spur has been resected.

Skeletal Management

Modifications of the cartilaginous septum can be accomplished by *resections of strips* in whatever area is required to allow reasonable straightening and provide a bilateral nasal airway (Fig 14–28). *Carving cartilage* is also a frequently employed technique to achieve straightening. The thickened anterior nasal spine region is frequently narrowed using a combination of knife, chisel, or rongeur to achieve thinning in this region. The junction of the quadrangular cartilage with the ULC and the perpendicular plate of the ethmoid bone is the thickest part of the normal septum. Resection with a Takahashi forceps or shave excision can be employed to open up the airway in the apex of the nasal valve. The bony septum can be fractured and will remain in the midline if forces of traction, such as the crooked cartilage or the tethering effect of soft tissues holding it in an abnormal position, are attended to. It is prudent to remember that resection of portions of the bony septum is not associated with the potential problems of injudicious resection of the cartilaginous septum.

Closure

The mucosal flaps are sutured once the septum is reasonably straight and in the midline and a bilateral airway assured. This is done with a running coaptation stitch of 4-0 chromic suture (Fig 14–29). This suture assures obliteration of the dead space, aids in strengthening the septum, and circumvents the

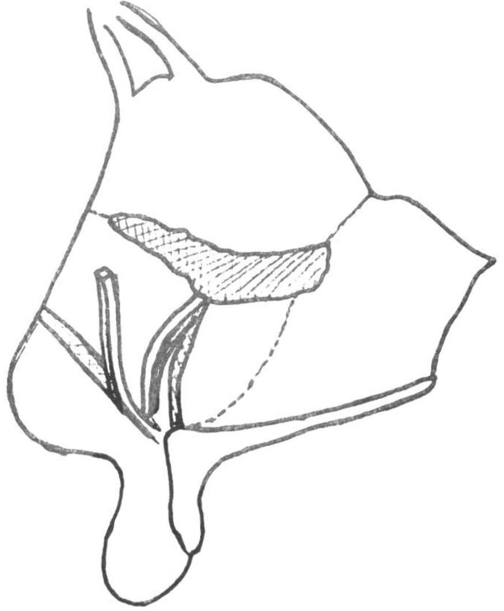

FIG 14–28.
Strategic resection of cartilage strips to allow straightening while maintaining support.

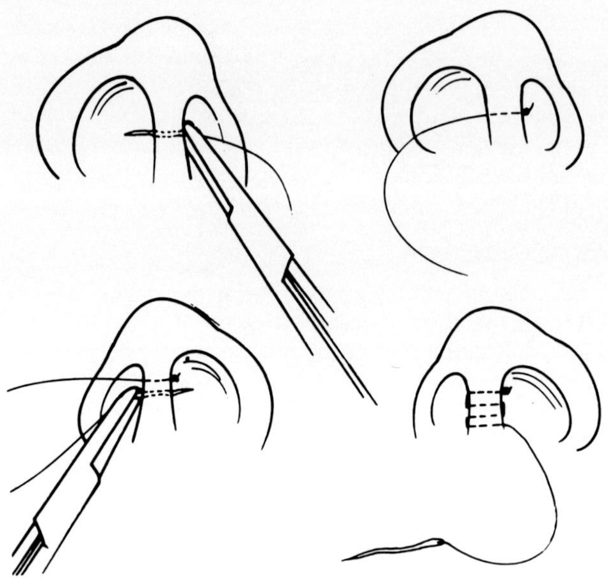

FIG 14–29.
Placement of running septal suture. (From Stucker FJ Jr: *Laryngoscope* 1982; 92:131. Used by permission.)

need for intranasal packs with their attendant morbidity and problems. The running whipstitch is a 4-0 chromic suture double knotted on its free end with a swedged on straight needle. The suture is passed back and forth from one side to the other of the septum, coaptating the mucosal flap. The final pass is cut and need not be tied. Since it is not tied, there are no strangled areas of tissue to necrose and lead possibly to a perforation. Ten to 15 passes are usually sufficient, and as stated, the need for packs is avoided. The caudal incision, whatever the approach, is sutured at this time or at the completion of the rhinoplasty portion if there is external nasal reconstruction done.

TECHNIQUES FOR SPECIFIC PROBLEMS

Caudal septal deformities can result from any number of anatomic malformations of the structures contributing to the position of the caudal end of the septum. Abnormalities in this region may contribute to a functional as well as a cosmetic deformity. Etiologies may be traumatic, congenital, or iatrogenic. Structures involved most commonly are the quadrangular cartilage and the nasal spine. Less often involved as contributing structures are the LLCs (primarily the medial crura), soft tissues of the columella, and lateral crura of the LLCs and the ULCs. Any structure attached to the caudal end of the septum and able to fix it in place by scarring or normal attachments in an abnormal position can contribute to a caudal septal deformity.

Fractures and dislocations of the anterior nasal spine, spurs, and scar tissue all may be repositioned, carved, fashioned, or excised to recreate a normal anatomic condition. Instruments most commonly used include knife, scissor, chisel, bone-biting forcep, and rongeur. It is not essential to provide epithelial coverage over bony areas, but healing occurs more quickly and predictably with less morbidity when mucosa and skin are pre-

served to cover denuded areas. It is my routine to surgically bare the bone and cartilage structures with sharp dissection before I embark on the carpentry shaping with chisels and rongeurs. This decreases the potential of avulsing important soft tissue coverage, and if significant bony bleeding occurs, it can be controlled with a bovie or bone wax. Commonly soft tissue at the base of the columella between the flaring feet of the medial crura can be removed to achieve adequate narrowing. A dislocated caudal septum often requires realignment and management of medial crura to achieve a symmetric columellar base (Fig 14–30). Plication with one or more Vicryl or Dexon mattress sutures is necessary to ensure permanent narrowing and symmetry in this region. The transfixion incision is always closed with a running absorbable suture. It is prudent to excise redundant mucosa but to err always on the side of conservatism. The elevated mucoperichondrial flaps are always coapted with a running septal whipstitch.

Deformities and dislocations of the caudal septum are fundamentally septal cartilage pathology with varying contributions from contiguous structures. The various combinations of specific corrections allow only generalized comments. Inspite of the myriad of conditions, in most cases a unilateral mucoperichondrial flap need only be elevated, and cartilage shaping, excising, and repositioning are carried out with a scalpel. The cartilage carpentry consists of judicious and strategic shave or strip excisions, thinning or carving with a knife blade to allow reasonable straightening. The peripendicular plate and vomer

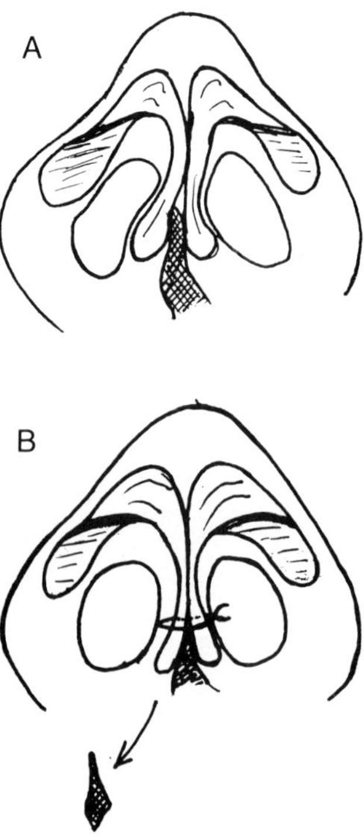

FIG 14–30.
A, dislocated caudal septum with columellar base asymmetry. **B,** symmetry created with septoplasty, partial resection of nasal spine, and plication with mattress suture.

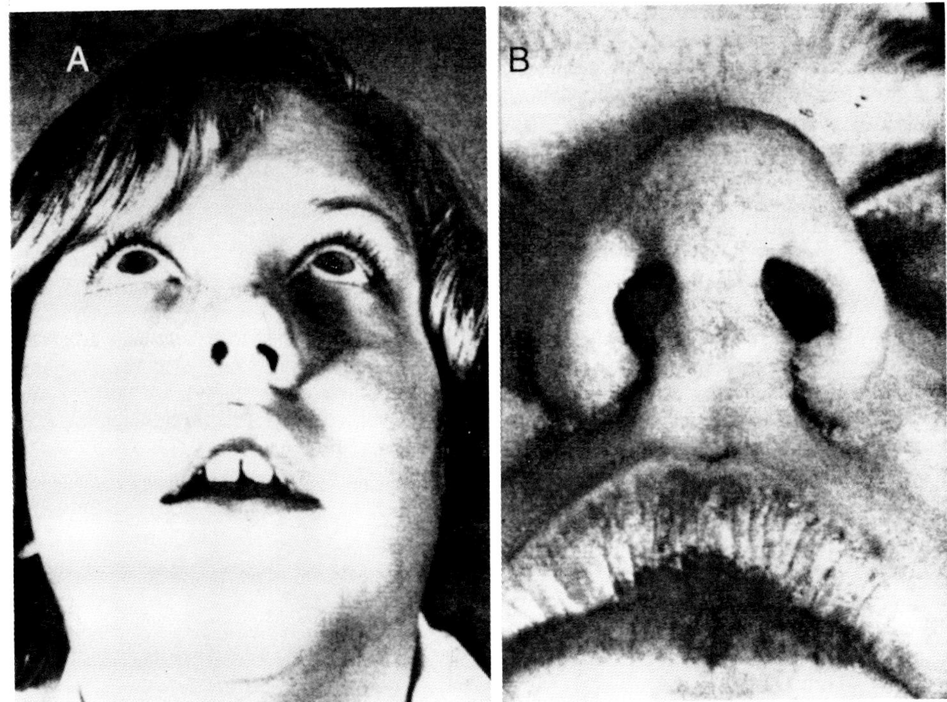

FIG 14–31.
A, 12-year-old girl with resulting alar asymmetry from a right lateral rhinotomy for teratoma resection at age 6 months. **B,** 4 months following left alar adjustment to achieve symmetry. (From Stucker F, Bryarly R Jr, Shockley W: Nasal surgery in the pediatric patient, in Ward P, Berman W (eds): *Plastic and Reconstructive Surgery in the Head and Neck: Proceedings of the Fourth International Symposium, American Academy of the Facial Plastic and Reconstructive Surgery.* St Louis, CV Mosby Co, 1984, vol 1, p 786. Used by permission.)

can be fractured, reserving removal for those sections not consistent with straightening.

Malpositioned medial crura secondary to previous surgery or trauma may contribute to a malaligned caudal septum. Direct visualization and exposure through an external rhinoplasty approach most effectively demonstrates the contribution of each component to the deformity and thus its correction.

Caudal spurs not only can contribute to caudal septal deformities but often are intimately associated with their etiology and thus also its correction. Those spurs not contiguous with the anterior nasal spine are expeditiously managed as suggested in the initial section of this chapter, that is, by en bloc resection following flap development. More anterior spurs require epithelial coverage following removal to prevent an unacceptable scar contraction and asymmetry of the columella or ala.

Soft tissue stenosis or scarring along the floor of the nose, alar base, or columella, as mentioned previously, is most commonly the result of injudicious resections or incisions in this region. Other causes are resection of a lesion without tension-free epithelial coverage, complication of a nasogastric tube, and catheters employed for epistaxis. Regardless of the etiology, a stenosis must be corrected by use of local flaps or grafts. Asymmetries require release of scar contractures and suture replacement to obtain improvement. It is often wise to imagine corrective steps on both sides since symmetry is always superior to a more normal but asymmetric appearance. This may result in surgical reconstruction on a normal side to match its opposite member

(Fig 14–31). Whenever operating in the floor of the nose, alar base, or columella, one must always be alert to the consequences of the resulting cicatrix. Avoid injudicious placement of incisions and excessive resection of tissues without the benefit of prudent preoperative planning.

Reduplication and Telescoping Injuries

Reduplications and telescoping injuries of the septum were as difficult a surgical problem as existed in nasal surgery prior to the popularization of the external rhinoplasty approach. The inordinately thickened septum has little potential for adequate thinning through conventional septal approaches. This relates to inability to diagnose as well as technical difficulties in thinning. Because bilateral flap elevation and midline perception are essential to thin the septum to normal proportions precisely in the midline, the external rhinoplasty approach is ideal (Fig 14–32). Often the cartilaginous septum can be thinned with a knife, but the mastoid drill provides propitious management of calcified cartilage, bone, and spurs. I sever the ULC from the septum to provide the necessary space for using the drill. The horizontally opened nasal speculum protects the mucosa from damage from the rotatory drill. The newly thinned midline septum is then sandwiched between bilateral mucosal flaps coapted with a running septal whipstitch, maintaining essential vertical and horizontal support.

Retraction

Retraction of the columella produces airway obstruction by circumventing the normal nasal air currents. The condition is commonly associated with an acute nasolabial angle and a ptotic tip. The nasal flow is not driven superiorly as is normal, and the usual complaint, the cosmetic deformity aside, is nasal obstruction. Superior traction on the soft tissue of the nose elevating the tip significantly improves nasal breathing in the absence of other obstructive problems. The cause is usually radical septal or spine resection and is aggravated by the aging process. There are instances where the problem is congenital. This anatomic configuration is commonly seen in the black nose but does not produce symptoms of nasal airway difficulties because of the more horizontal flow of the nasal air currents in people of color.

Correction is most expeditiously carried out via an external rhinoplasty approach using autogenous cartilage grafts to replace the spine and quadrangular cartilage deficiency (Fig 14–33). Correction of the ptotic tip and placement of a columellar strut are often indicated.

Alar Collapse

Alar collapse has many etiologic causes, essentially all of them surgical. The most common surgical misadventure is excessive resection of alar cartilage support. This is most apt to result from closed or blind resection techniques, as through transcartilage or retrograde resection of LLC techniques. Another cause includes resecting both perichondrial layers and attachments between the LLC and ULC. Other causes include incisions through or resection of the lateral nasalis and dilator nasi muscles. Disruption or resection of the lateral aponeurotic connection from the nasal process of the maxilla to the ULC can cause alar collapse. Endonasal scarring and contraction from excessive or inappropriate mucosal resection may also lead to this problem.

Treatment

Treatment is focused on correcting or replacing resected tissues aimed toward recreating the normal anatomy. Repositioning the lateral ala and soft tissue fixation with mattress sutures will suffice when the problem is not severe. These mattress sutures may be left in 5 days with no difficulty, provided they are oriented along relaxed skin tissue lines. More severe collapse will require autogenous cartilage battens from the septum or concha with mattress suture fixation for 3 to 5 days (Fig 14–34).

The acute superior mucosal angle between the septum and the lateral nasal wall is reconstructed by using through-and-through mattress sutures, once again being careful to orient them parallel to the relaxed skin tension lines. An alternative is the fixation of bilateral battens of cartilage with matress sutures through the mucosal apices tied over the septum, thus avoiding the external skin sutures.

Prevention

Prevention lies with a conservative resection of the cephalic margins of the LLC and especially to exercise caution in blind techniques. Although the dictum of never resecting mucosa is

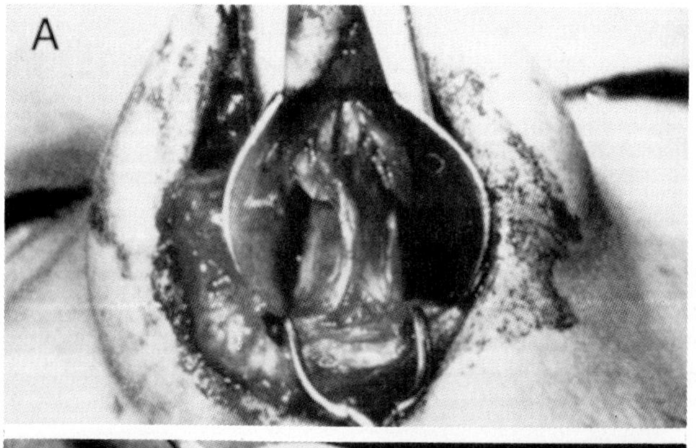

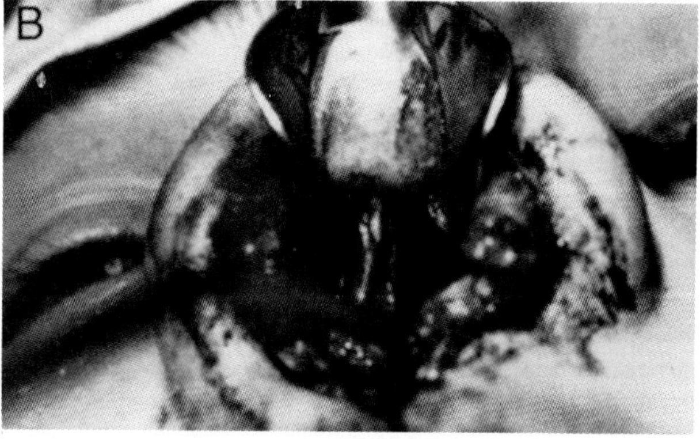

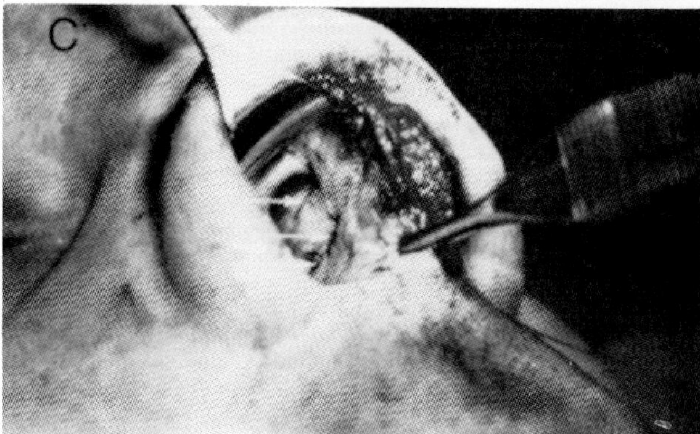

FIG 14–32.
A, thickened septal cartilage (10-mm ball retractor in photograph). **B,** septum thinned with carving, placing it precisely in midline. **C,** mucoperichondrial flaps coapted with continuous septal suture. (From *Laryngoscope* 1982; 92:131. Used by permission.)

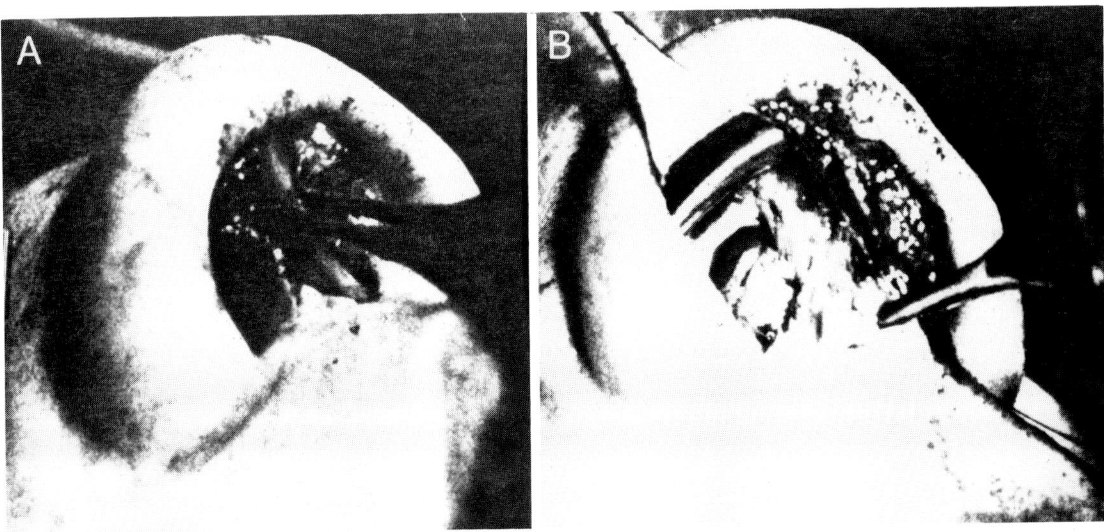

FIG 14–33.
A, placement of cartilage graft. **B,** fixation with a running septal whipstitch. (From Blitzer A, Lawson W, Friedman WH (eds): *Surgery of the Paranasal Sinuses.* Philadelphia, WB Saunders Co, 1985. Used by permission.)

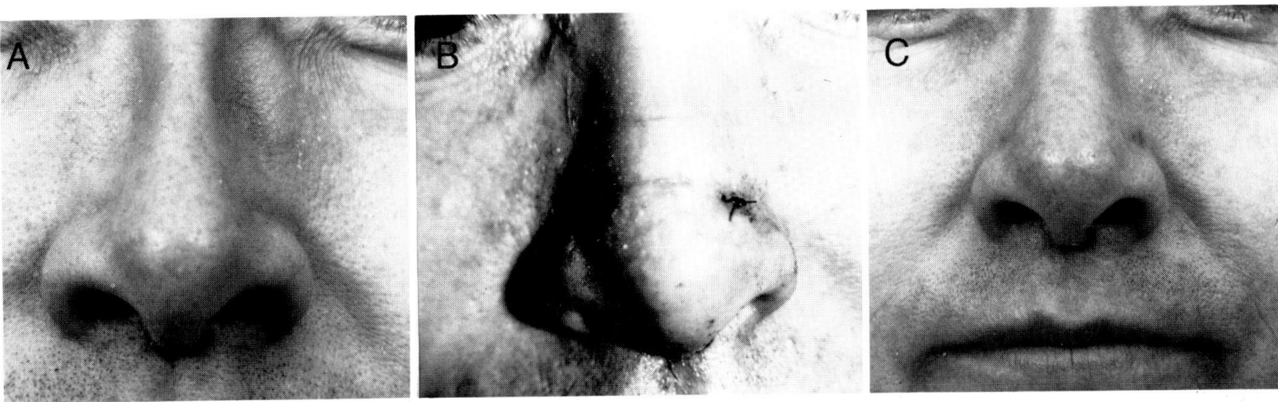

FIG 14–34.
A, preoperative bilateral total nasal obstruction from valve collapse. **B,** 6 days postoperatively with mattress suture fixation. **C,** 8 months postoperatively.

not true, the consequences of excessive removal indicates its probable origin. Preservation of all but redundant or excessive mucosa is a very wise maxim.

Careful layered reattachment of tissues in alotomy and rhinotomy incisions is necessary. Judicious conservative alar adjustment repair after incision and resections can eliminate an adynamic and flaccid alae.

VALVULAR PROBLEMS

For an adequate nasal airway, there must be approximately 2 to 4 mm of space from superior to inferior in the valve area. It is critical that the superor angle or apex be sharp. The potential areas contributing to valve obstruction include the septum, the mucosa, the ULC and its aponeurotic connections to the maxilla, the lateral nasal wall and the inferior turbinate. The most critical area and most frequently compromised is the apex superiorly.

Treatment

A septum that impinges on or into the valve region requires movement to the midline, shave excision, or resection. Mucosa can become thickened related to previous surgical procedures and may blunt the apex of the valve area. This is a common sequelae when scar contracture occurs along the transfixion incision as it connects with an intercartilaginous incision. This shortening of the scar blunts the sharp superior angle of the valve. A method of avoiding this common complication is to extend the transfixion incision 3 to 5 mm more superiorly and carry the intercartilaginous incision medially so as to meet the transfixion incision at a sharp angle (Fig 14–35). The commonly seen postoperative web of mucosa at the superior aspect of the valve area is avoided.

Prevention

The lateral nasal wall can impinge on the airway in the valve area by a careless surgical maneuver, especially if the lateral osteotomy produces collapse of the lateral nasal wall. This is one of the few indications for the use of packing: to support a collapsed nasal bone. Judicious management of the ULC and the incision placement must be such as to avoid compromise in this central region. I also recommend routine preservation of the mucosal integrity bridging beneath the septum and ULC. Most hump resections are easily carried out extramucosally when viewed from above with the aid of an Aufricht elevator.

I suggest leaving a bony strut when carrying out the lateral osteotomy with soft tissue attachments, including preserving the lateral nasalis muscle and aponeurotic attachments to the ULC (Fig 14–36).

Synechia

Synechiae are not always the result of a surgical misadventure. Carefully executed septal and turbinate surgery can, on occasion, result in the formation of mucosal bridges during the healing process. The floor of the nose may fill with clotted blood and other debris, affording the span for mucosal epithelialization. The unfortunate ramification of this complication is that the usual preventive measures are often morbid and can yield far more severe complications. These steps include nasal packs and various nasal splints. In my experience, the routine use of splints is not only uncomfortable and morbid but also associated with an unacceptable high incidence of septal perforation, a far more difficult and serious complications than synechiae. The septal whipstitch affords more support when associated with a judicious septoplasty while literally precluding the complications of septal hematomas, necrosis, perforations and all but eliminating the incidence of synechiae.

The most efficacious manner of avoiding synechiae is to stage septal and lateral (turbinate) nasal wall mucosal surgery. This, however, is expensive, often not possible, and in general not necessary. Over the past 4 or 5 years, I have employed carbon dioxide laser turbinectomy surgery, which when combined with routine septal and nasal reconstructive techniques,

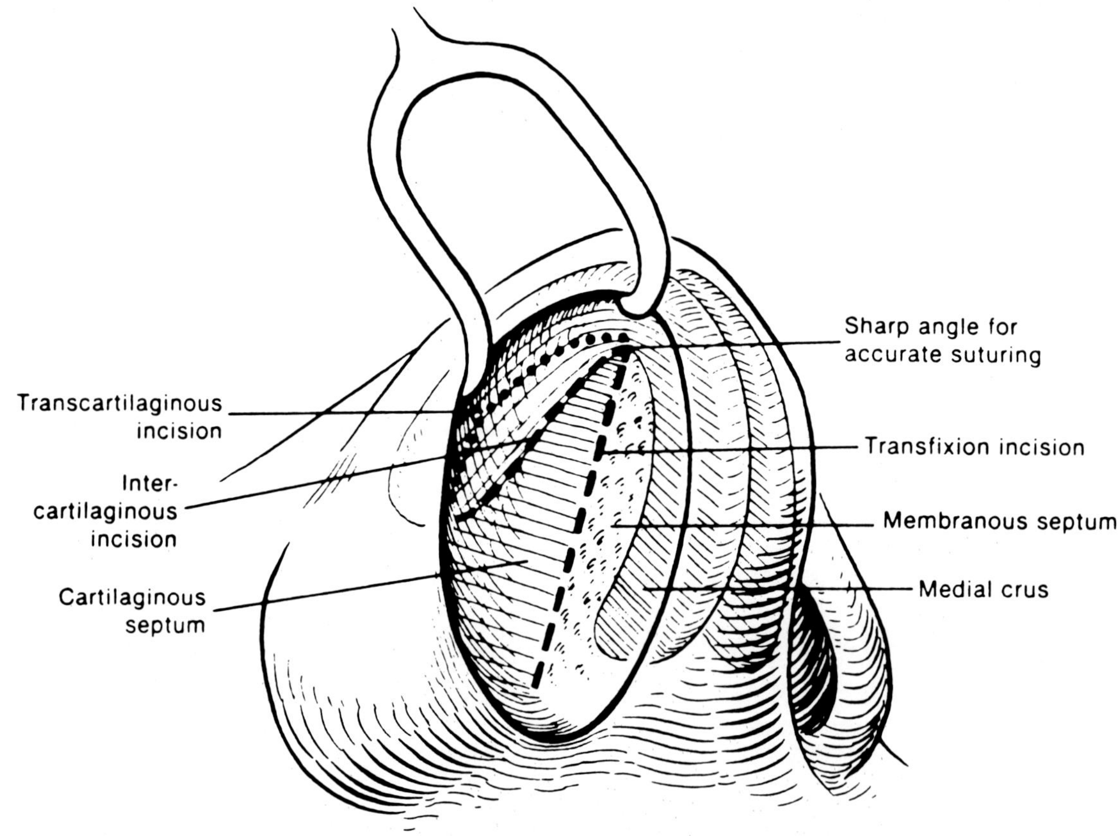

FIG 14–35.
Transfixion incision or intercartilaginous incision meet at an acute angle, ensuring proper reposition of mucosa and decreasing likelihood of scar contracture and blunting the apical valve angle. (From Cummings CW (ed): *Otolaryngology—Head and Neck Surgery.* St Louis, CV Mosby Co, 1986, vol I (Krause CJ, ed), p 786. Used by permission.)

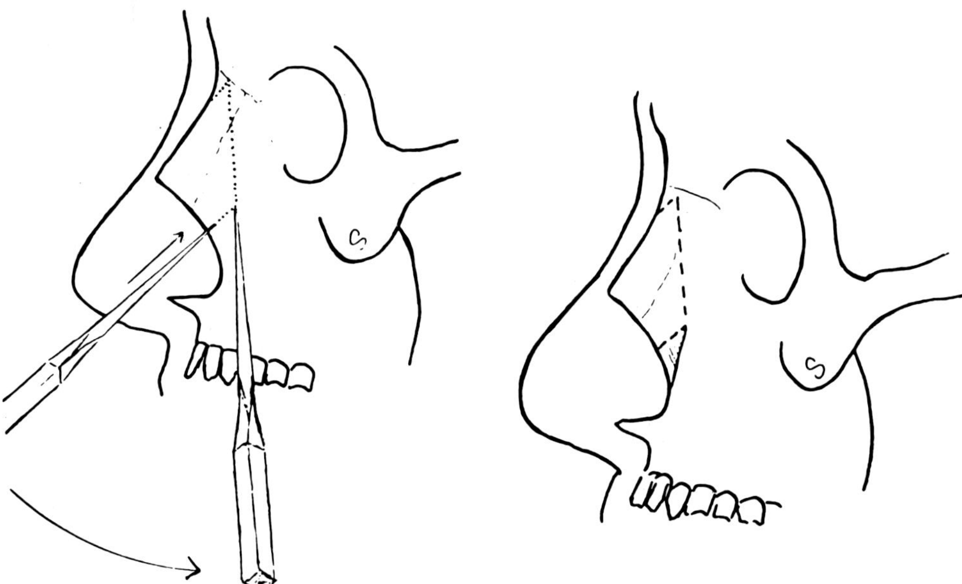

FIG 14–36.
Intact bony strut. (From Stucker FJ, Smith TE Jr: *Arch Otolaryngol* 1976; 102:695–698. Used by permission.)

has essentially eliminated the potential for synechiae. Because bone is not easily vaporized, it is often necessary to resect small segments of anteroinferior turbinate bone with a forcep. The septal whipstitch allows avoidance of intranasal packing and splints and their attendant morbidity. The CO_2 laser turbinectomy produces a dry wound with a physiologic dressing, which allows the operator to visualize with anterior rhinoscopy the surgically patent nasal valve area. The need to vaporize more than the caudal 25% of the inferior turbinate is very unlikely, thus avoiding the posterior region where troublesome bleeding is much more common.

In the event synechiae do occur, the management is often a relatively simple outpatient procedure. In the absence of the requirement for more extensive surgery, the CO_2 laser is employed after topical and local infiltration of anesthesia. These synechiae are readily vaporized, clearing the airway with little adjacent tissue reactions. Naturally the usual laser precautions must be observed, and there should be a moist pack placed in the posterior nose. The physiologic dressing following the CO_2 lasered tissue requires no postoperative use of packs or splints. Since there is most often no attendent bleeding, this airway is easily evaluated with anterior rhinoscopy in the postoperative period. Complete healing and mucosalizations occur within 10 days. The patient is usually asymptomatic and able to carry out most routine activities immediately following surgery.

Fenestra

The occurrence of a through-and-through hiatus in the septum during the operative procedure probably results more commonly from mucosal avulsion when cartilage or bone is resected. If a complete flap elevation and an inferior incision are used, this mishap can be avoided. Should one be faced with a perforation intraoperatively, the ideal situation is to have bi-

lateral flaps mobilized and covering an autogenous graft, preferably cartilage. The three-tissue sandwich is then coapted with 10 to 11 passes of the running septal whipstitch as described.

Septal Perforation

Substance abuse is rapidly replacing iatrogenic causes of septal perforation. Successful repair with the former category of patients is futile in the absence of drug rehabilitation. It is strongly recommended that one refrain from a mere surgical exercise in this type of patient. Repair of a septal perforation in a compliant patient is a much more rewarding surgical exercise since the popularity of the external rhinoplasty approach. Successful closure, often futile with closed techniques, is in excess of 90% of my cases since I have incorporated the open rhinoplasty techniques. In my experience, the use of splints over the past 20 years replaced radical cartilage resection as the most common iatrogenic cause of perforations.

Prevention of a septal perforation is almost assured in nasal surgery etiologies by using conservative techniques in septoplasty, along or associated with rhinoplasty surgery. These precautions include conservative flap elevation, and in most instances, this includes only a unilateral mucoperichondrial or mucoperiosteal flap with an inferior incision along the entire extent of intended septal surgery. This maneuver greatly increases visualization and surgical access and also affords drainage of any accumulated blood. Conservative resections of strips or portions of bone and cartilage to allow straightening without removal of the intrinsic structural support of the septum are advocated. This approach to septal surgery, when combined with the continuous septal whipstitch that coapts the mucosal flap while maintaining the structural integrity of the septum, affords maximal safety.

The repair of a septal perforation essentially attempts to

recreate the septoplasty situation by elevating the mucosal flaps and positioning autogenous graft material in the region of the septal cartilage dehiscence. The graft material may be septal cartilage or bone if this material is not lacking. Smaller perforations without saddling or dorsal collapses may be closed by using fascia or periosteum sandwiched between mobilized mucosal flaps. The most common tissue used for septal perforation repair is conchal cartilage shaved quite thin, morselized where necessary, and placed between the mucosal flaps. Usually adequate amounts of musoca can be mobilized from the floor of the nose and advanced superiorly on one side. The mucosa from its opposite side can be elevated from beneath the ULC and advanced inferiorly. All types or combinations of cephalic-caudal and inferior-superior advancements are possible. Complete mucosal coverage on one side is mandatory, but successful closure is more assured if mucosal closure exists bilaterally. Careful coaptations of flaps with a running septal whipstitch completes the surgical closure. Neurosurgical pads are placed along the septum, which are kept moist with saline solution and antibiotic drops for 48 to 72 hours. These wicks are completely saturated with saline solution prior to careful removal. This prevents avulsion of small mucosal flaps on removal of the pads if these wicks become dried out. This compromises the edges of the flaps, which already have a tenuous blood supply, and may ultimately doom the septal perforation closure. Desiccation and dehydration of the mucosal flaps compromise the healing process and likely contribute to surgical failure.

My success rate using the previously described techniques has risen to more than 90%. Failures were commonplace when I employed closed techniques. The external rhinoplasty allows access to the entire peripheral edges of even extremely large perforations.

Atrophic Rhinitis

Fortunately, this much described complication receives much less management energy than journal space. It is, in reality, a rare entity today and reflects the much more conservative approach to nasal surgery than in the past. Twenty percent to 30% of the caudal end of the inferior turbinate can in my experience be resected with impunity without fear of creating an atrophic mucosal (rhinitis). Judicious resection of middle turbinates can also be done by leaving the medial bony plates and mucosa. In the absence of radical and usually inappropriate endonasal surgery, the condition of atrophic rhinitis will likely remain uncommon.

Surgery for this condition except in marginal situations in my experience will remain unrewarding. Recreation of the mucosal mass and the proper valve resistance is likely not possible and thus likely to fail. Medical treatment by the topical toileting in the absence of a surgical breakthrough will probably remain the most successful form of treatment.

COMPLICATIONS OF SEPTAL SURGERY

Septal Hematoma

Septal hematoma, whether unilateral or bilateral, is a po-

tentially devastating postsurgical or traumatic event. The hematoma elevates the perichondrium from the cartilage, thus depriving it of its source of nourishment and removal of toxic catabolic products. The low metabolic rate of cartilage allows a period of time before the process is irreversible, usually 3 to 5 days. Bilateral hematomas are more dangerous than unilateral ones for obvious reasons, but both deserve emergent attention. In the event that an infection and abscess occur, the necrosis and dissolution of the cartilage are extremely rapid. There no longer is a 3- to 5-day period of reversible change.

The treatment of a hematoma is immediate drainage by an inferior incision and coaptation of the mucosal flaps with the running septal whipstitch. All patients are maintained on antibiotic therapy until the condition is resolved.

My recommended technique of septoplasty consisting of unilateral flap elevation, inferior incision, and coaptations of mucosal flaps with the running septal whipstitch fundamentally precludes a hematoma. The potential space is closed by sutures, and the inferior intranasal extension of the transfixion incision provides drainage for any bleeding.

Saddle Deformity

The type and degree of saddling dictate the techniques possible for its correction. Those secondary to the circumferential cicatrix of a septal perforation are best corrected by addressing the fundamental problem, the perforation. This has previously been discussed. Those saddle deformities resulting from or having contributions from excessive dorsal resection are best managed by dorsal augmentation. It is my recommendation that minor augmentation or effacement of 1 to 4 mm is best corrected with onlays of autogenous cartilage. This most often is harvested from the ear. Augmentations of 4 mm or more are routinely augmented with rolled polyamide mesh. Over the past 15 years in more than 300 cases, nasal dorsi have been augmented with this material, with removal of only 4 implants, all for infections. An interesting turn of events in correction of saddle deformities by augmentation is that it is more difficult to obtain a satisfactory cosmetic result for minor corrections than for more major deformities.

Cerebrospinal Fluid Leak

I routinely fracture the bony septum with a Sayer elevator (as the first maneuver) at the onset of all septoplasty and septorhinoplasty procedures. This medial to lateral rocking action is carried out on both sides of the septum, and I have done this in more than 3,000 cases without evidence of a single case of CSF rhinorrhea. The only exception to the routine use of this maneuver are those few patients with a previous history of CSF rhinorrhea secondary to trauma. My experience with more than 6,500 nasal procedures has likewise not yielded a single instance of CSF rhinorrhea. (CSF rhinorrhea resulting from trauma is outside the scope of this chapter.)

Epistaxis

Bleeding serious enough intraoperatively to compromise

the procedure is very unlikely, especially if certain routine precautions are followed. Bleeding and clotting abnormalities must be tested for and eliminated as potential problems in suspect patients. Using local anesthesia with vasoconstrictive drugs and waiting an appropriate period are routine, as is elevation of the head of the operating table to decrease venous bleeding. Certain other conditions such as hemangiomas and Osler-Weber-Rendu disease are hopefully detected preoperatively, and appropriate management decisions avoid a disastrous intraoperative accident. Turbinectomies in association with septal surgery can be a cause of troublesome bleeding. The use of the CO_2 laser has essentially eliminated intraoperative bleeding and the necessity of postoperative packing. Troublesome turbinate bleeding is uncommon when the posterior portion of the turbinate is avoided. In more than 6,500 nasal procedures, no patient has required intraoperative transfusions.

Serious bleeding following nasal surgery is extremely rare but always remains a possibility. I have seen two instances of severe postoperative bleeding requiring transfusions. Both were probably secondary to arterial bleeding, one at 3 days and the other at 5 days. Trauma precipitated one, and the other occurred without an obvious cause. Cautery and packing were required in both patients.

Minor mucosal bleeding has been recorded in a number of patients, but very few required packing for control. The majority stop spontaneously or respond to suctioning the clots from the nose. Bleeding and oozing are noticeably less common phenomena since the elimination of employing intranasal packs as a routine over the past 11 years. The trauma of removing packs and meticulous suturing both probably play a roll.

Postoperative Infection

Antibiotics are not routinely used but are reserved for cases where infection is more likely or the occurrence of an infection would have severe consequences. Reconstructive surgery using autografts or alloplasts and patients with rheumatic heart disease serve as indications for intraoperative and postoperative antibiotics. It appears to be a good policy in preventing infection to use sound surgical principles with alacrity and inflicting a minimum of surgical trauma on the tissues.

Postoperative infections are more common in augmentation procedures, those cases employing external incisions, and the use of endonasal to external nasal mattress sutures, such as those used in correcting valvular problems or alar abnormalities in the unilateral cleft lip nose. The need to address both septal and valvular abnormalities cannot be overemphasized.

The treatment of infection requires draining of the abscess collection, removal of any foreign body, and antibiotic coverage. A broad-spectrum antibiotic is instituted and changed only after cultures provide more information as to the proper drug.

Septal abscess is a particularly critical situation, often unrecognized in a timely manner, and if untreated, it can yield potentially severe consequences. An abscess collection is rapidly destructive to cartilage, with dissolution and collapse a likely scenario if untreated or belatedly treated. It is incumbent on anyone doing septal surgery to examine all patients postoperatively for this uncommon, but devastating complication. The routine use of a unilateral mucoperichondrial flap, incised inferiorly, and coapted to the septum with a running whipstitch, essentially eliminates the occurrence of septal hematomas or abscesses postoperatively.

Toxic Shock Syndrome

Toxic shock syndrome is estimated to occur in 1 of every 10,000 nasal operations. It is certainly a rare complication but is totally avoidable by the simple elimination of any intranasal tamponading device. The septal whipstitch and CO_2 laser turbinectomy avoid the necessity of packs and thus any concern for toxic shock syndrome. Those rejecting this advice might be wise to use Merocel intranasally in place of the usual packing.

CHAPTER 15

Intranasal Sinus Surgery

Approach of

Terry L. Fry, M.D.

and

Newton D. Fischer, M.D.

INDICATIONS

The most important key to successful sinus surgery is accurate preoperative assessment. This assessment is facilitated if the patient can be examined during both a quiescent period and an acute phase of the disease, and preferably prior to use of decongestants. Systematic decongestion of the mucous membranes often aids in localization of the pathologic etiology. Vasoconstrictive shrinkage of the middle turbinate away from the septum is occasionally effective in relieving a patient's periorbital headache. This complaint may be corrected by septoplasty in some cases or may require aggressive allergy management in another. More often, the headache persists until the area of the middle meatus is maximally vasoconstricted, indicating the need to address treatment to the osteomeatal complex. Endoscopic evaluation of the nasal cavity, area of the middle meatus, and sphenoethmoidal recess cannot be overemphasized.

Localized osteomeatal or early sinus disease can be handled in the outpatient clinic. This may be done directly, in the absence of septal deformity, or endoscopically if the surgeon has this expertise.[1]

The most important factor in safe sinus surgery is a thorough knowledge of the nasosinal anatomy. This is well described in texts and should be explored in a cadaver to reinforce the three-dimensional relationships (Fig 15–1).[2,3]

Radiologic examination or coronal computed tomography (CT) scan evaluation of the sinuses is helpful, but it should not supplant a thorough physical examination. These radiologic evaluations are crucial for appropriate preoperative planning for mucoceles or other complications of sinus disease (Fig 15–2).

The approach to sinal disease, whether via external, standard intranasal, or endoscopic techniques, should be determined by the extent of disease and by the expertise of the surgeon. The external approach is usually indicated for orbital abscess, chronic frontal sinusitis or mucocele, or in the patient lacking the crucial landmark, the middle turbinate. An external approach is indicated, if needed, for examination or exenteration of the entire maxillary or frontal sinus cavity. The intranasal approach, whether via standard or endoscopic method, is often dictated by the extent of disease. One of the more perplexing problems encountered is chronic nasal polyposis with secondary infection. Polypectomy, though a safe procedure, only briefly improves nasal obstruction; and it does very little to correct chronic ethmoid sinusitis. The surgical goal in the treatment of chronic nasal polyposis and sinusitis should be transformation of the diseased multi-air-celled ethmoid labyrinth into a clean single compartment through which any recurrent disease process is easily treated.

Endoscopic attack on pansinusitis secondary to generalized nasal polyposis is possible, but use of suction forceps and a laser is advocated.[1]

TECHNIQUE

We find the standard intranasal approach, with the prerequisite of an intact middle turbinate, very effective for simultaneous approach to extensive bilateral anterior and posterior ethmoids as well as sphenoid disease. A simultaneous septoplasty not only vastly improves visibility of these sinuses but

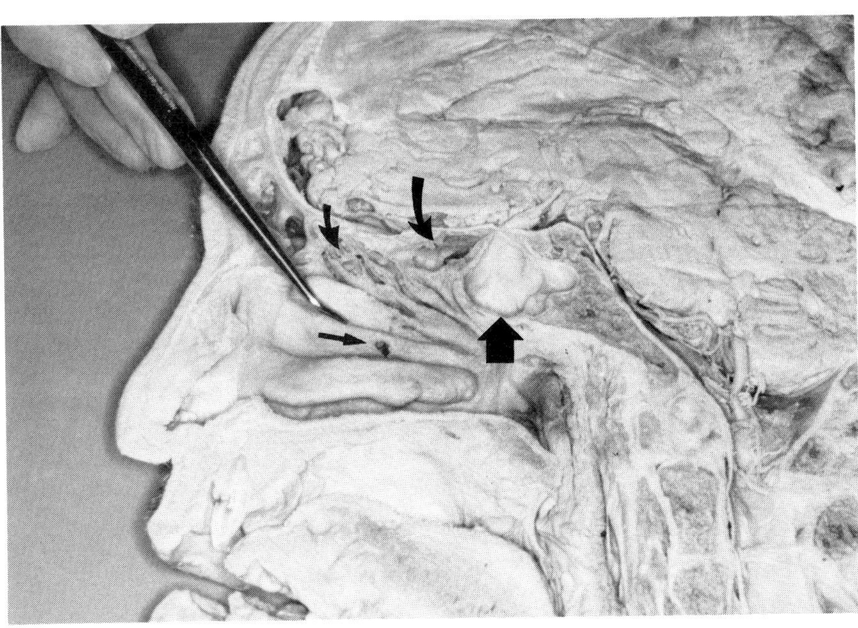

FIG 15–1.
Lateral nasal wall of cadaver. Note natural ostium *(small straight arrow)*, anterior ethmoid sinuses *(small curved arrow)*, posterior ethmoid sinuses *(large curved arrow)*, and sphenoid sinus *(large straight arrow)*.

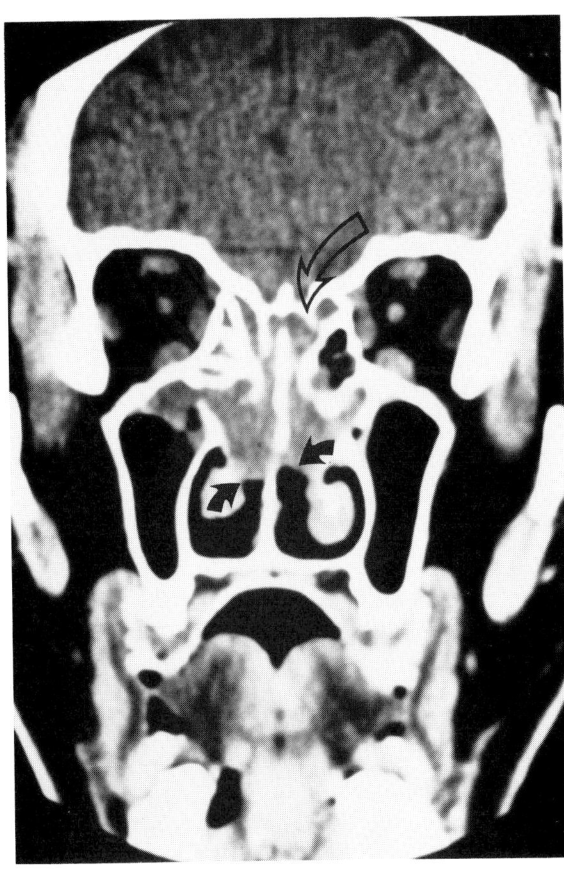

FIG 15–2.
Coronal CT of 63-year-old patient with chronic sinus disease 10 years after polypectomy. Note the absence of the left middle turbinate *(large arrow)* and synechia between septum and inferior turbinates *(small arrows)*.

also typically improves function and access to these areas for later care.

A second prerequisite for good visibility is adequate hemostasis. After topical application of no more than 100 mg of cocaine flakes, the middle turbinates and lateral nasal walls, as well as the pterygopalatine space, are injected with an anesthetic containing epinephrine 1:200,000. This is usually done during the nasal prep to ensure at least a 10-minute delay before the initial surgical incision. Should bleeding obscure the operative field at any point during the surgery, a 20 cm strip of nasal packing soaked in the same epinephrine-containing anesthetic is packed into the area while the surgeon turns his or her attention to the opposite side. In this way, one can alternate from side to side as needed throughout the case. A special point should be made concerning patient comfort throughout the procedure, either via intravenous medication or general anesthesia, because increases in blood pressure secondary to discomfort or anxiety will increase bleeding.

A last but equally important requirement for good visualization is adequate illumination of the surgical field. Today's standard bright fiberoptic headlights are ideal for tonsillectomy and so forth but actually produce a distracting field of reflected light when one is working through a nostril. We much prefer a headlight with a small, concentrated, and most important, paraxial beam, such that the light is directed into the field visualized by the surgeon's dominant eye. These advantages are available in the Goode headlight (Fig 15–3) and the fiberoptic Storz no. 085001 headlight. The latter also produces a larger than ideal pool of light that may be somewhat bothersome. It is, however, paraxial and brighter illumination than the former.

Following septoplasty-mobilization of the quadrilateral cartilage, one can easily see the entire middle turbinate. A scalpel (no. 15) is used to bisect the anterior two thirds of the turbinate vertically and with gentle rocking will easily fracture through

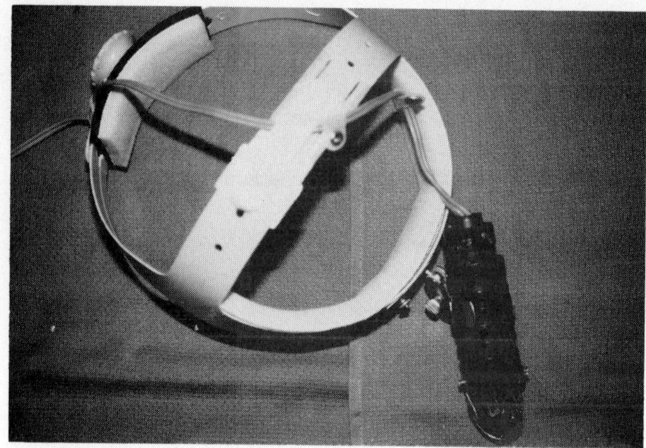

FIG 15–3.
The Goode headlight provides a small bright area of illumination directed paraxially.

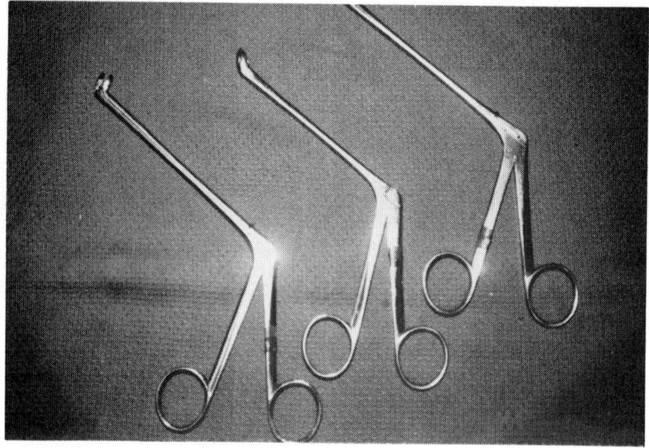

FIG 15–4.
Blakesly forceps: straight, oblique, and right-angled.

the bony air cells or bullae that are often contained within it. The lateral half of the middle turbinate is then grasped and removed with straight-ethmoid forceps, with care taken at all times to preserve, undisturbed, its medial half (Fig 15–4). The obliquely angulated forceps now facilitate gentle extraction of the anterior ethmoid air cells, which during exenteration give much the same sensation as collapsing tender popcorn. There should be no resistance encountered during gentle grasping and extraction of these air cells. Should bleeding impair visibility, the ethmoid cavity is packed with anesthetic-epinephrine strips of packing, which are left undisturbed while the same surgical maneuvers are undertaken in the contralateral nostril.

The anterior ethmoids and nasofrontal extension of the ethmoid air cells are safely removed if the surgeon will alternately visualize the intranasal area about to be grasped by the forceps and then using the eye unaided by the headlight to check the direction and angle of the forceps with reference to the orbit and the medial canthus. The nasofrontal pathway is anterior to the medial canthus and lateral to the middle turbinate, whose medial half and superior attachment is still completely intact. The remaining ethmoids are lateral to the middle turbinate and yet medial to the medial wall of the orbit. As a further measure of safety, we discard the extracted ethmoid contents into a small glass filled with saline solution, noting that ethmoid and polyp fragments sink, whereas any small fragments of periorbital fat will float. We continue these maneuvers posteriorly, remembering that if the more proximal extent of the forceps arm is resting on the pyriform aperture of the nasal floor, the face of the sphenoid is approximately 7 cm back, at a 30-degree angle. Of special note, it is also inferior to the posterior ethmoids (Fig 15–5).

Use of the same unaided eye to determine the area of the maxillary sinus allows placement of the 90-degree forceps, jaws open, into this sinus, thus creating a large opening in the area of the middle meatus or osteomeatal complex. Access through the markedly enlarged meatus (preferably 1 by 1 cm) allows

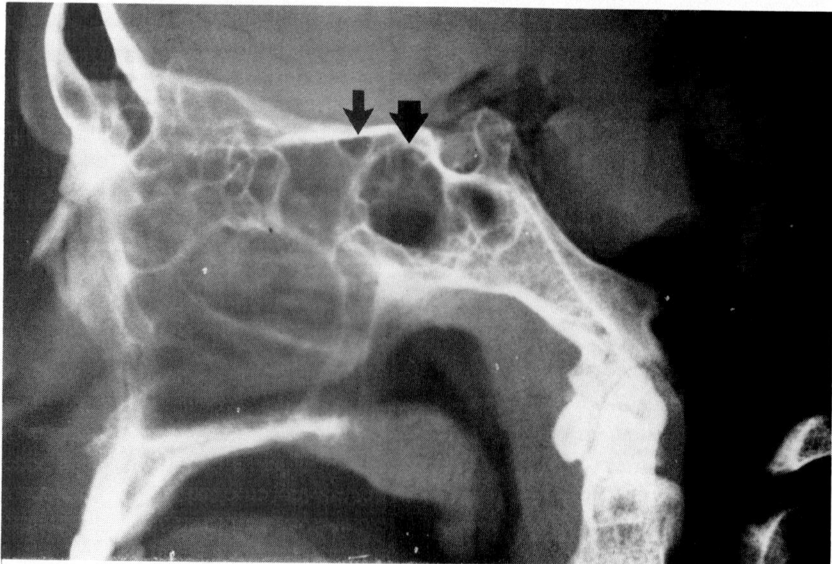

FIG 15–5.
Sagittal radiograph. Note that the roof of the sphenoid *(large arrow)* is lower than the roof of the posterior ethmoids *(smaller arrow)*.

removal of the uncinate process, extraction of polypoid mucosa, and drainage of contents, and yet this approach avoids the postoperative complaints inherent with a Caldwell-Luc procedure. This new middle meatal antrostomy accommodates endoscopic examination of the maxillary sinus both intraoperatively and in future follow-up visits.

It should again be stressed that the surgeon remove only those air cells superiorly, which are seen to extend from the intact bony roof and offer no resistance to gentle extraction. At the completion of the sphenoethmoid exenteration, any polypoid changes along the inferior margin of the remaining middle turbinate can be sharply trimmed. We have continually stressed the preservation of the medial half of the middle turbinate, which is a prerequisite for the safety of this approach and for future safe transnasal removal of any recurrent polyps, which can often be easily performed in the outpatient clinic. We also stress the importance of maintaining enough middle and inferior turbinal tissue to ensure proper humidification of the nasal cavity.

At the completion of the procedure, the septal pocket is aspirated free of blood, the septum is positioned midline, the incision is closed, and the septum is splinted. Strips of absorbable gelatin sponge (Gelfoam) covered with antibiotic ointment are placed lateral and medial to the middle turbinate. In patients with a greater tendency for bleeding, each nasal cavity is also packed with antibiotic-coated strips of $^1/_2$-inch gauze. Packing is removed at 48 hours, and splints and remaining Gelfoam are removed after 7 days.

The patient is advised against strenuous activity and is maintained on appropriate antibiotic therapy to cover *Staphylococcus,* anaerobes, and other organisms (dictated by culture) for the first postoperative week or longer, if indicated.

COMPLICATIONS

Epistaxis

Epistaxis, intraoperatively, is avoided by appropriate patient sedation and comfort as well as by careful injections of a vasoconstrictor (as described in the section on technique), with an adequate period of time prior to surgical manipulation. Injury to the ethmoidal arteries is avoided through good visibility and knowledge of the anatomic boundaries. In the event that ethmoidal bleeding is problematic, an injection of 1 mL of the same anesthetic-epinephrine solution (used preoperatively) beneath the medial orbital periosteum with a $1^1/_2$-inch 25-gauge needle produces sufficient vasoconstriction to allow completion of the surgery. Gelfoam packing should certainly be reinforced by antibiotic-saturated gauze packing for the first few days postoperatively if bleeding has been a problem intraoperatively. Appropriate antibiotics should be given to any patient requiring nasal packing postoperatively.

Injury to the internal maxillary artery is avoided by conservative surgical manipulation of the posterior one third of the middle turbinate. Injury to this vessel often requires transantral or transoral placement of vascular clips on the internal maxillary artery. Premature termination of extensive sphenoethmoid surgery because of bleeding is a rare event but a necessity if good

visibility is compromised. Occasionally, one has difficulty visualizing the sphenoid due to excessive bleeding. Again, the septoplasty, performed initially, gives an alternate approach to this area. Removal of the perpendicular plate of the posterior nasal septum reveals the bony rostrum of the sphenoid. This can be removed with heavy rongeurs, allowing inspection and drainage of the sphenoid. Should this approach be necessary, the posterior edge of the septal mucoperiosteal flaps should be divided to facilitate direct drainage of the sinus into the nasopharynx.

All patients should be screened preoperatively for coagulopathies or use of anticoagulants. They are additionally cautioned against the use of aspirin and nonsteroidal anti-inflammatory analgesics, which decrease platelet aggregation, in the week prior to and that following their surgery. Patients are also asked to avoid strenuous exercise, which may elevate blood pressure excessively in the initial postoperative week.

Cerebrospinal Fluid Leak

A dreaded complication of sphenoethmoidectomy performed through any approach is CSF leak. We again stress preservation of the undisturbed medial half of the middle turbinate as a crucial landmark with its superior attachment bordering the cribriform plate laterally. Therefore, with hemostasis and good illumination, gentle grasping of any nonresisting ethmoid contents lateral to this turbinate will render no such leak. However, should a CSF leak occur due to an overly aggressive, less cautious, or impatient attack on this area, the previously elevated mucoperiosteum from the superior aspect of the septum is readily transformed into a superiorly based flap and rotated to cover the area of dural interruption. This flap should be carefully positioned and held in place with Gelfoam, followed by antibiotic ointment–saturated gauze packing, which is left undisturbed with the patient resting, head elevated, for 1 week. If gentle removal of the gauze packing results in renewal of the CSF rhinorrhea, a coronal CT scan may indicate the need for craniofacial approach with a direct dural repair in conjunction with a neurosurgical colleague.

Orbital Complications

Surgical violation of the lamina papyracea is recognized when the extracted fatty debris is seen to float atop the saline in the small glass of ethmoid debris. Immediate recognition leads to no significant sequelae, because one prewarns the patient that periorbital ecchymosis is a possibility. Continued removal of lamina papyracea and periorbital fat, however, can lead to enophthalmos, diplopia, possible blindness, and certainly inability to visualize the more posterior sphenoethmoid areas due to prolapse of fatty tissue. Therefore, early recognition is paramount. As mentioned earlier, sighting the angle and length of the forceps relative to the orbit using the eye unaided by the headlight lessens this risk. Any resisting tissue such as orbital periosteum must be released and not removed. However, instruction of one's assistant to immediately inform the surgeon of fat floating in the glass of saline solution will avoid any further insult to this area. As has been continually stressed, good visibility will allow removal of ethmoid disease while preserving the smooth bony roof and walls of the labyrinth. Ethmoid disease does not resist gentle extraction. Any area of resistance should be released and reexamined. Injury to the medial canthus, optic nerve, or any significant insult to the orbit is avoided in this manner. Intraorbital hematoma resulting in blindness has been described with endoscopic ethmoidectomy.[4–6] This result can hopefully be minimized by avoidance of orbital patching and tight nasal packing if one has inadvertently violated the lamina papyracea.

ADVANTAGES

The intranasal approach to ethmoidectomy allows a simultaneous approach to both sides, exenteration of even the most anterior ethmoid air cells, and facilitation of later care of this area through the improved visibility offered by septoplasty.

The external scars, inherent postoperative periorbital ecchymosis, and swelling of an external approach are avoided. Correction of the area of the osteomeatal complex is also difficult through an external approach.

The facial swelling and dental hypesthesia of the transantral approach are avoided. This access may be necessary, however, for extensive chronic maxillary sinusitis such as that resulting from dental pathology.

The junior author (T.L.F.) believes that avoidance of an inferiorly placed nasal antral window is a significant benefit. Despite placing nasal antral windows posteriorly enough to avoid the cold air–induced toothache described by some patients, the majority of patients still have a chronic complaint. They are bothered by the frequent presence of an inspissated mucous plug either in the nasopharynx or, if dislodged, in the hypopharynx, where it often interferes with clear speech. Perhaps the natural (more superior) and the surgically created (inferior) openings that on the one hand improve sinus drainage, on the other hand provide a constant pathway for ventilation through this sinus. The result is a drying and therefore pooling of sinus secretions until this small mucous plug is dislodged to produce symptoms elsewhere. This transsinal route of airflow is avoided with enlargement of the sinal meatus lateral to the middle turbinate. Fry has also found the latter procedure the most beneficial in patients with frequent barotrauma and "sinus headaches" secondary to mild changes in pressure. This meatal enlargement is readily accomplished endoscopically. As

mentioned previously, however, this technique often is inadequate for complete mucosal exenteration of a severely diseased maxillary sinus. However, the new middle meatal window facilitates fiberoptic and rigid telescopic examination.

The most recent trend, endoscopic sinal surgery, certainly carries with it the same risks for complications inherent in any technique of intranasal sinal surgery. These risks are likewise minimized with the endoscopic technique by good visibility and hemostasis. We certainly practice the same careful endoscopic evaluation for diagnostic and any indicated intraoperative and postoperative follow-up. However, when extensive ethmoid exenteration is indicated, even a small amount of bleeding impairs visibility through this small endoscope, leading to premature termination of the procedure or excessive risks if it is continued. Extensive rhinolith disease can also be frustrating to the endoscopic surgeon. Less extensive or less inflamed pathologic conditions are readily treated with the endoscopic technique.

We do not wish to minimize the risks of a thorough sphenoethmoidectomy performed through any approach. However, one cannot overlook the risks of inadequately treated ethmoid, frontal, or sphenoid sinusitis. The safety of the approach is determined by the surgeon's familiarity with the technique and the patience and ever-present caution with which it is performed.

REFERENCES

1. Kennedy DW, Zinreich SJ: The functional endoscopic approach to inflammatory sinus disease: Current perspectives and technique modifications. *Am J Rhinol* 1988; 2:89.
2. Moss-Salentijn L: Anatomy and embryology, in *Surgery of the Paranasal Sinuses*. Philadelphia, WB Saunders Co, 1985, pp 1–22.
3. Montgomery WW: The management of the orbit in surgery of the paranasal sinuses. *Otolaryngol Clin North Am* 1983; 16:423–439.
4. Stankiewicz JA: Complications of endoscopic intranasal ethmoidectomy. *Laryngoscope* 1987; 97:1270–1273.
5. Kennedy DW: Endoscopic middle meatal antrostomy theory, technique and patency. *Laryngoscope* 1987; 97(suppl 43).
6. Stammberger H: Endoscopic sinus surgery: Complications and results. Paper presented at the American Rhinologic Society, Sept 18, 1987.
7. Stankiewicz JA: Complications of endoscopic nasal surgery: Occurrence and treatment. *Am J Rhinol* 1987; 1:45.

Intranasal Sinus Surgery

Approach of

David W. Kennedy, M.D.

INDICATIONS

If one accepts the premise that obstruction is the crucial event in the pathogenesis of sinusitis and that persistent obstruction is the usual cause of chronic disease, the indications for therapy aimed at the ostiomeatal complex are greater than was previously thought. Study of the pathogenesis of sinus disease, endoscopic evaluation, and CT evaluation all tend to support the hypothesis that most inflammatory sinus disease begins within the area of the anterior ethmoid. These studies also support the concept that persistent disease may remain in the ostiomeatal complex in patients with recurrent frontal and maxillary sinusitis (Fig 15–6).

Except in a case of a threatened complication, initial therapy in sinus disease is essentially always medical, using antibiotics, topical steroids, allergy hyposensitization, and oral steroids as appropriate. Patients who do not respond well to adequate medical therapy or who persist with recurrent bouts of acute sinusitis undergo diagnostic nasal endoscopy. A careful comprehensive examination is performed using deflected view telescopes. The entire nasal airway with its recesses is examined, but particular attention is paid to the middle meatus. The aim is to identify an underlying cause for the inflammation within the ostiomeatal complex, either anatomic or from persistent inflammation.

Patients are selected for CT evaluation if they have abnormal endoscopic findings or a well-documented past history. All patients undergo CT evaluation prior to surgical intervention, even if the underlying cause can be easily diagnosed by endoscopy alone. In these cases, CT provides information about the extent of disease and anatomic details that cannot be obtained from endoscopy alone.

Whenever possible, the CT evaluation is performed in the coronal plane. This plane provides the greatest degree of anatomic information, particularly with regard to variations within the ethmoidal roof. The presence of metallic dental artifacts is not a contraindication to coronal scanning because the scatter typically does not interfere with visualization within the ostiomeatal complex. However, some patients may not be able to assume the required prone, neck extended position. In this situation, an axial scan is performed and coronal reconstructions are performed. It is also important that sinus CT scans are photographed with appropriate magnification and soft tissue windowing if significant disease is not to be missed.

Patients selected for surgery are those who have symptomatic sinus disease with or without nasal polyposis and who have not responded well to medical therapy. In nasal polyposis, surgical intervention is not usually performed when the patient's symptoms are well controlled on medical therapy. These patients are typically followed, even if there is some persistence of the polyps. Similarly, the mere presence of sinus opacification on CT is not an indication for surgical therapy unless the disease correlates with history and endoscopic findings.

The ideal patient for functional endoscopic sinus surgery is one in whom a limited underlying cause can be identified for widespread disease. One such example is a patient with a frontal sinus mucocele in whom a limited underlying cause can be identified in the anterior ethmoid. In these situations, the problem may be resolved with a relatively minor outpatient operation under local anesthesia, greatly reducing the morbidity associated with traditional techniques. In diffuse nasal polyposis, the advantages of using endoscopes are less marked. However, they enable more complete removal of disease than is possible with other intranasal techniques. Deflective view telescopes create the ability to visualize into the recesses.

The maxillary sinus may be examined endoscopically by introducing a trocar and cannula sublabially (Fig 15–7). Although not used for routine diagnostic examination, this approach does allow for the direct visualization and biopsy of unusual radiographic lesions and for the removal of occasional symptomatic retention cysts. The cystic (intrasinus) portions of antral choanal polyps also can be removed through this approach. More diffuse chronic maxillary sinus disease or sinus polyposis may be treated by endoscopic removal of the associated ostiomeatal disease. After the natural ostium of the sinus is widened, obstructive polyps adjacent to the ostium can be removed with right-angle forceps, frequently avoiding the necessity for a Caldwell-Luc procedure.

In frontal sinusitis, the functional endoscopic approach provides an alternative to trephination or an external approach.

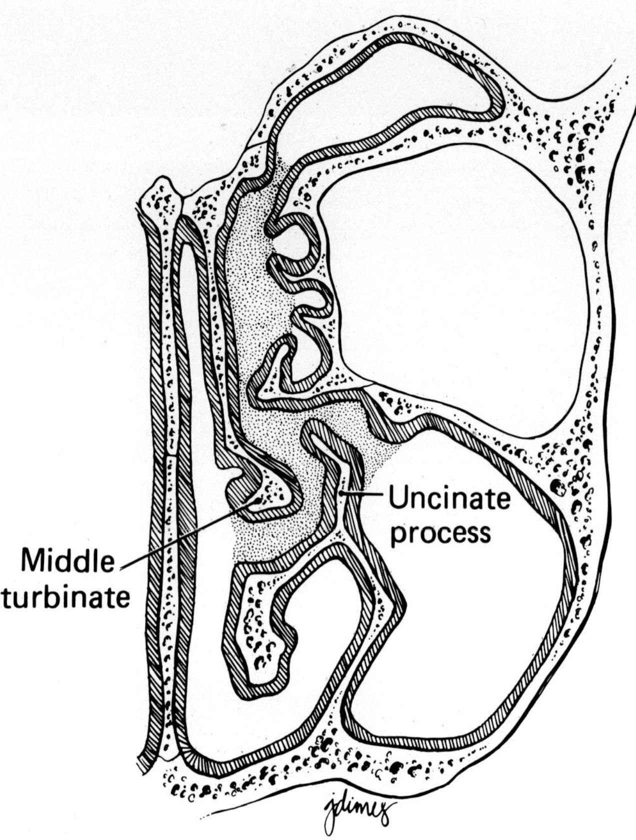

FIG 15–6.
Diagrammatic respresentation of the ostiomeatal complex *(shaded area)*. The maxillary and frontal sinuses are functionally dependent on this area for ventilation and drainage. Relatively minor swelling in the narrow ostiomeatal channels may cause obstruction and secondary sinus disease. Low-grade infection may persist in this area, causing recurrent infection. (From Kennedy DW, Zinreich SJ, Rosenbaum AE, et al: *Arch Otolaryngol* 1985; 111:576–582. Used by permission.)

Although these approaches may not offer the same success rate as a frontal sinus exenterative procedure, they can be performed with minimal morbidity in well-trained hands. In addition, the endoscopic approach, unlike obliteration, preserves the ability to image the sinus subsequently for residual disease. Contraindications to the technique include patients with intracranial complications or osteomyelitis and possibly patients with frontal sinus disease in whom marked bony narrowing of the internal os has occurred.

TECHNIQUE

The surgery is typically performed under local anesthesia and frequently as an outpatient. The patient usually does not receive preoperative sedation, but IV sedation and monitoring are performed in the operating room. Relaxing music is provided by headphones. The patient is positioned supine in a slightly head-elevated position with the head turned toward the

surgeon. The surgeon sits comfortably alongside the patient. Topical cocaine on nasal applicators is applied to nasal mucosa and middle meatal areas. After 5 minutes, the medial infundibular wall and the inferior aspect of the middle turbinate are injected with 1% lidocaine (Xylocaine) with adrenaline 1:100,000 under endoscopic visualization (Fig 15–8). Repeat nasal endoscopy is performed. If necessary, the middle turbinate is slightly subluxed medially to allow adequate visualization of the middle meatus. The patient is instructed to breathe through the mouth to avoid blowing blood droplets onto the lens during the surgery.

The operation is performed using rod optic telescopes with differing angles of deflection. Throughout the surgery, the 0-degree telescope is used whenever possible to increase the safety of the operation and simplify instrument manipulation. Deflected view telescopes are used only for access to the recesses of the operative field.

There is no standard operation with this approach, the aim of the surgery being to remove areas of obstruction, severely diseased mucosa, and underlying bony osteitis. The surgery is therefore tailored to each individual patient, based on accurate preoperative assessment and the operative findings. Thus, patients with maxillary sinus disease might require only infundibulotomy, or infundibulotomy and middle meatal antrostomy, and patients with frontal recess disease might require anterior ethmoidectomy and frontal recess exenteration. For the purposes of this description, a complete sphenoethmoidectomy

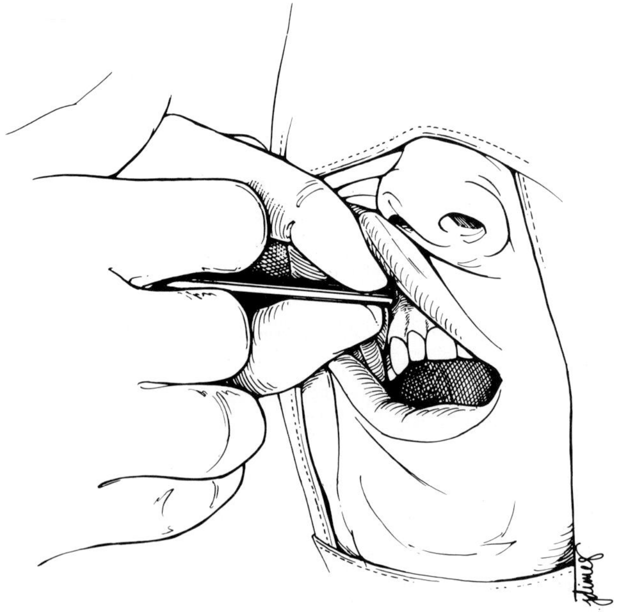

FIG 15–7.
Introduction of the trocar and cannula for maxillary sinuscopy. After the sublabial area is infiltrated with local anesthetic, the trocar is introduced into the upper lateral aspect of the canine fossa. The maxillary sinus is then examined with a 30-degree telescope. (From Kennedy DW, Zinreich SJ, Rosenbaum AE, et al: *Arch Otolaryngol* 1985; 111:576–582. Used by permission.)

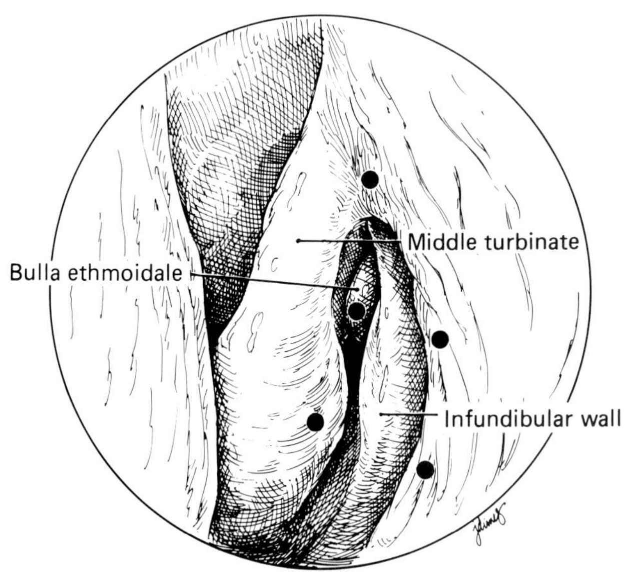

FIG 15–8.
The lateral nasal wall and inferior part of the middle turbinate are injected at various sites under endoscopic visualization *(black dots)*. Care is taken not to inject the head of the middle turbinate or other areas that will be in close proximity with the telescope lens, so as to avoid blood from the injection site obscuring visualization. (From Kennedy DW: *Arch Otolaryngol* 1985; 111:643–649. Used by permission.)

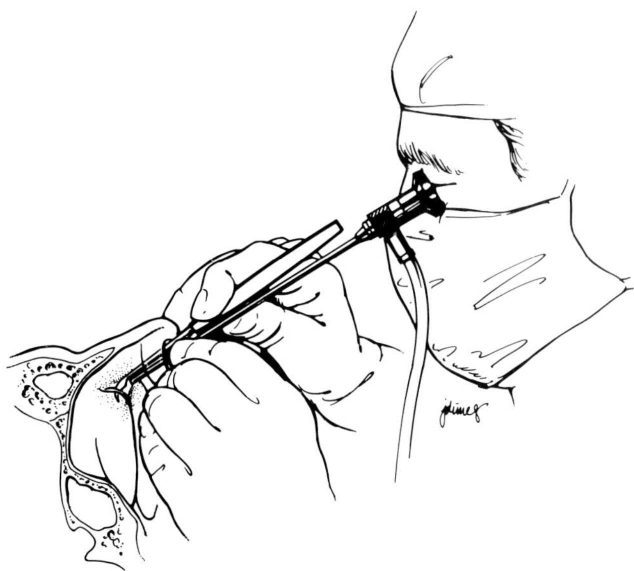

FIG 15–9.
A sickle knife is used to incise the uncinate process just posterior to its attachment to the lateral nasal wall. The attachment approximately parallels the free border of the middle turbinate. Throughout the dissection, the telescope is held rigidly by resting the hand holding it against the patient's face. The telescope lens is kept well back from the operative site. (From Kennedy D: Functional endoscopic sinus surgery: Technique. *Arch Otolaryngol* 1985; 111:643–649. Used by permission.)

will be described. However, it should be borne in mind that this is performed only in cases of diffuse pansinus disease.

An infundibulotomy is first performed by incising the mucosa of the lateral nasal wall around the attachment of the uncinate process. A sickle or Rosen knife may be used (Fig 15–9). The uncinate process is then subluxed medially and removed with forceps, allowing access to the infundibulum and ethmoidal bulla. The anterior ethmoid cells and bulla ethmoidale are removed with forceps (Fig 15–10). The bone of the medial orbital wall is identified and skeletonized. As the more superior cells are removed, the area of the roof of the ethmoid and the area of the anterior ethmoidal artery are identified. Once identified, the ethmoidal roof is used as the most important landmark during the dissection and is further skeletonized (Fig 15–11). If either the anatomy or the extent of the disease creates a situation where the roof of the ethmoid is not easily identified in this area, superior dissection is limited until the roof has been identified more posteriorly within the posterior ethmoid or sphenoid sinus.

The anterior ethmoidal artery passes across the ethmoid immediately inferior to the fovea ethmoidale. The vessel lies in a partial or complete bony conduit and is frequently attached to the ethmoidal roof by a bony septum. Dissection near the area typically results in some bleeding from adjacent increased vascularity. If visualized, the anterior ethmoid artery warns of the immediate vicinity of the ethmoidal roof. The bone of the roof of the ethmoid also has a slightly different color from and appears to be more sensitive to pain than the ethmoidal cell partitions. However, the surgeon must be aware that the roof may be thin or dehiscent in the area of the vessel. If bleeding is encountered from the artery, temporary local packing or microfibrillar collagen is applied. After the anterior ethmoid

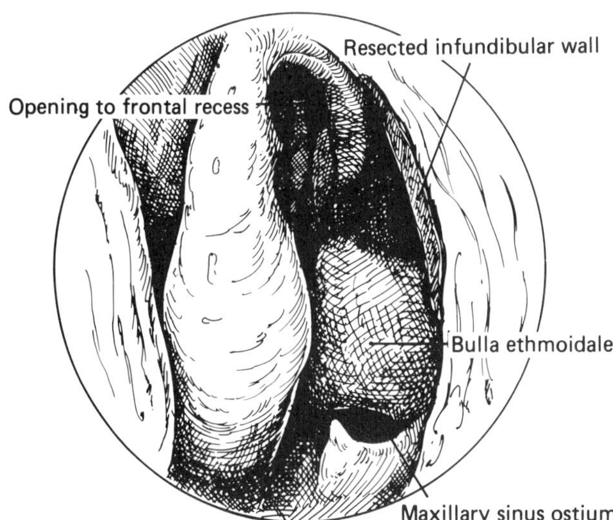

FIG 15–10.
View of the anterior ethmoid and bulla after removal of the uncinate process. When necessary, the next step would be infracture of the medial part of the bulla and its removal with forceps. (From Kennedy DW: *Arch Otolaryngol* 1985; 111:643–649. Used by permission.)

cells and bulla are removed and the ethmoidal roof is identified, the frontal recess may be explored if the skull base has been identified. In this area, the 30-degree or occasionally the 70-degree telescope is required for visualization. At the end of the dissection, it is usually possible to identify the internal os of the frontal sinus, and frequently an excellent view of the sinus mucosa is obtained (Fig 15–12).

The posterior ethmoid is entered by infracturing and removing the basal or ground lamella of the middle turbinate. This can be performed with safety inferiorly even if the ethmoidal roof has not yet been identified (Fig 15–13). Posterior ethmoid disease is then removed. If extensive ethmoid pneumatization is present, the optic nerve may occasionally be seen passing posteromedially as a convexity in the lateral wall of the posterior ethmoid sinus.

The sphenoid sinus may be entered either through the posterior ethmoid or by identifying the natural ostium medial to the middle turbinate. Since the most posterior ethmoid cell frequently pneumatizes toward the anterior clinoid, the sphenoid sinus bulge is identified in the inferomedial aspect of that cell. If clearly apparent, it is infractured and entered (Fig 15–14). If the anterior wall of the sinus is not easily identified, the telescope is reintroduced medial to the middle turbinate. The sphenoid sinus ostium is then identified and opened.

Finally, the maxillary sinus ostium is located either visually with the 30-degree telescope or by palpation. If the ostium is not easily seen, pressure on the medial wall of the maxillary sinus in the area of the fontanelle frequently reveals the site of the opening by causing a bubble of blood. If the opening is stenotic, it is widened posteriorly, anteriorly, and inferiorly (Fig 15–15). A good view of the maxillary sinus can then be obtained with the 70-degree telescope. If necessary, severe irreversible

mucosal disease can be removed from the sinus using angled forceps under direct vision.

Since the telescope is advanced during the dissection, the surgeon must keep in mind that it is easy to penetrate more deeply than is apparent by the endoscopic view. As the dissection is performed from anterior to posterior, it is helpful to identify the bony laminae that are entered (Fig 15–16). However, the medial orbital wall and the ethmoidal roof provide the most important landmarks when extensive surgery is required. Once these two landmarks have been identified, the remainder of the surgery becomes significantly easier.

The key to the surgery is meticulous atraumatic technique. Bleeding is minimized by avoiding trauma to the turbinates and more vascular mucosa of the lateral nasal wall. Nasal packing is usually not required. If persistent bleeding is present at the end of surgery, a small hemostatic sponge may be placed in the operative cavity lateral to the middle turbinate and secured in place by a suture taped to the cheek.

When massive nasal polyposis is present, sufficient nasal polyps are removed at the beginning of the surgery to allow visualization of the uncinate process. However, as soon as the uncinate process can be seen, infundibulotomy is performed. Early removal of the uncinate process aids in removing polyps attached to it with minimal bleeding. All polyp removal is performed under endoscopic visualization with meticulous atraumatic technique using Blakesly forceps or Kennedy-Blakesly suction forceps. In patients with severe or recurrent nasal polyposis, the KTP-532 laser has proved beneficial in allowing polyp removal with minimal bleeding. The laser fiber is attached to the outside of the telescope, and the laser is aimed by directing the telescope. The polyps may be grasped with suction forceps and cut at the base by bringing the laser fiber into contact with the tissue.

External or transantral ethmoidectomy are not chosen as a procedure of first choice in uncomplicated patients with inflammatory sinus disease. It is important, however, that the surgeon recognizes both the limits of the technique and his or her own limitations when performing intranasal ethmoidectomy. If the surgeon becomes unsure of the landmarks, or bleeding precludes visualization and cannot be controlled with temporary packing, the procedure should be discontinued. If required, the sinus can be exenterated later by a repeat endoscopic operation or via an alternative approach. Ethmoidectomy through an external incision remains the safest approach for difficult disease and should be the procedure of choice for surgeons who are not experienced in intranasal techniques.

POSTOPERATIVE CARE

Meticulous cleaning of blood and fibrin clots from the operative cavity is essential during the postoperative period so as to the avoid development of adhesions and renewed ostiomeatal obstruction. The patient is seen in the outpatient clinic 1 to 2 and 4 to 5 days following surgery and with decreasing frequency until the cavity is healed. At each visit the cavity is carefully cleaned under topical anesthesia and endoscopic control. Blood and mucus are suctioned from the ethmoid cavity

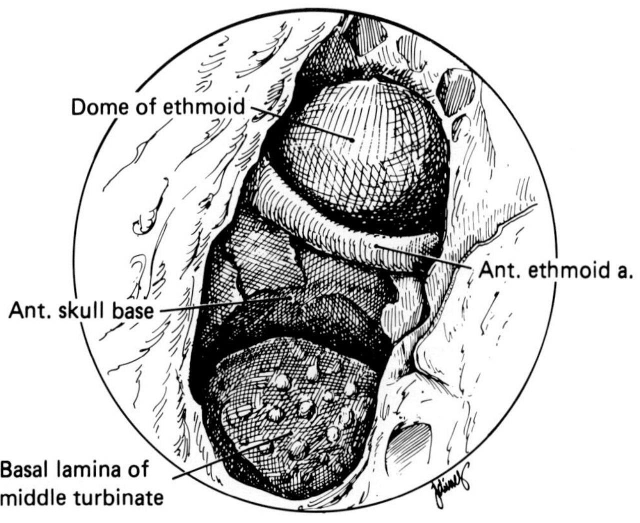

FIG 15–11.
View of the skull base and basal or ground lamella of the middle turbinate after removal of the anterior ethmoid cells. The anterior ethmoid artery is seen passing across the ethmoid in a bony canal immediately below the roof. (From Kennedy DW: *Arch Otolaryngol* 1985; 111:643–649. Used by permission.)

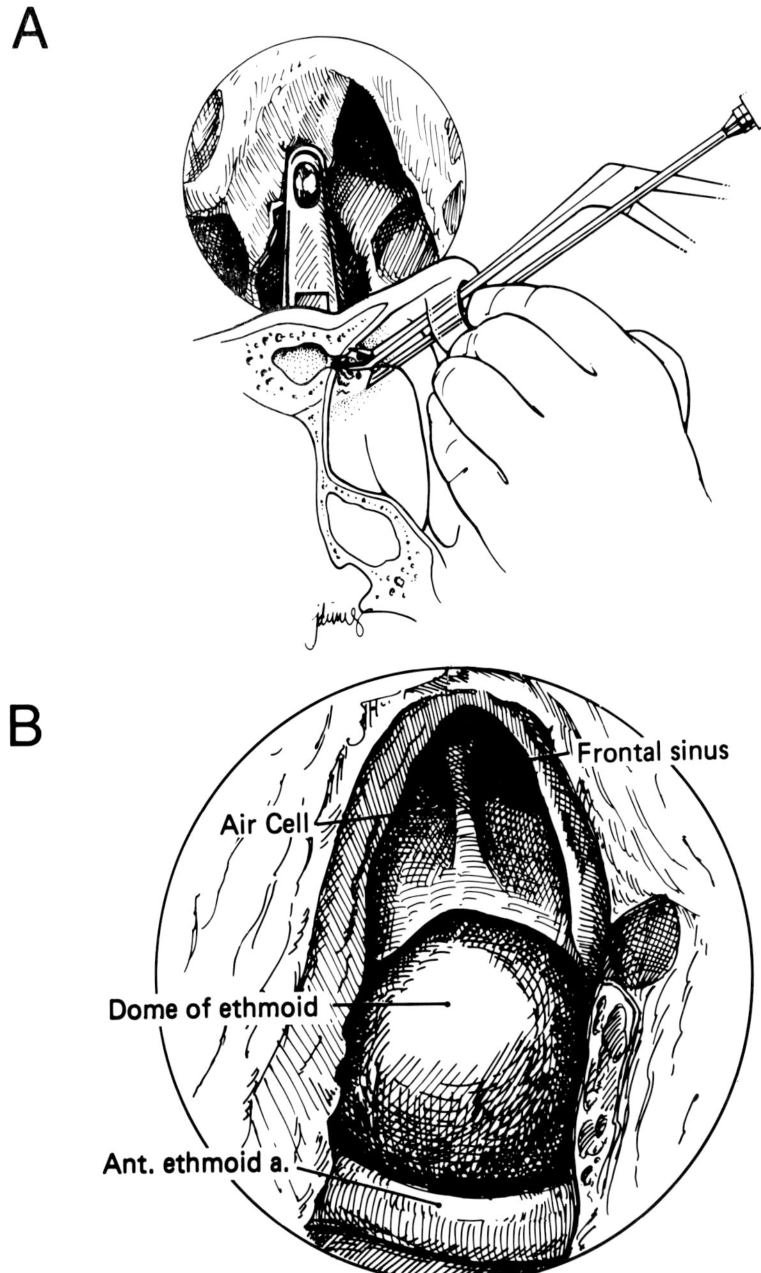

FIG 15–12.
A, after the skull base is identified, the frontal recess area is dissected using up-biting forceps and angled telescopes. **B**, following dissection of the frontal recess, the dome of the ethmoid, internal os of the frontal sinus, and the remnant of an agger nasi cell can be seen. (From Kennedy DW: *Arch Otolaryngol* 1985; 111:643–649. Used by permission.)

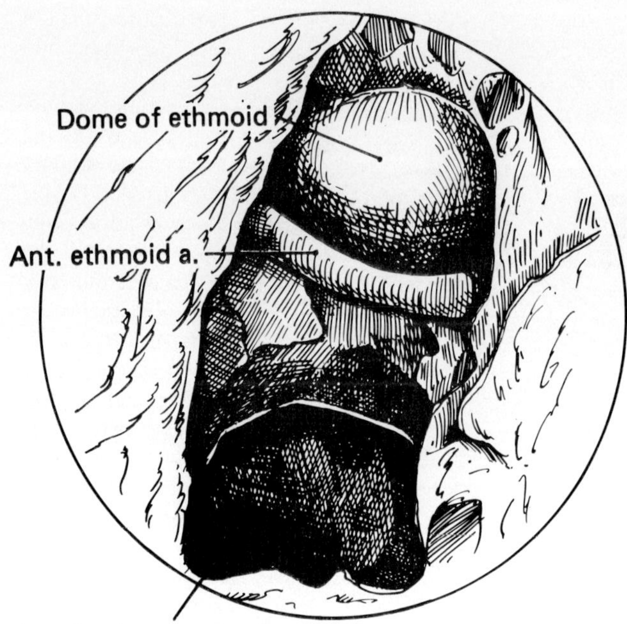

FIG 15–13.
View of the posterior ethmoid after infracture and removal of the ground lamella of the middle turbinate. The ground lamella is always infractured in its inferior aspect after the telescope is partially withdrawn and the position of the instrument reevaluated relative to the middle turbinate. (From Kennedy DW: *Arch Otolaryngol* 1985; 111:643–649. Used by permission.)

and, with curved suctions, from the maxillary and frontal sinus. Crusts and areas of residual mucosal disease or osteitic bone are removed with forceps. Any adhesions are divided, and any infected cells overlooked at the time of the original operation are exenterated. Topical decongestants, saline spray, antibiotics, and perioperative oral steroids are used as indicated.

COMPLICATIONS

Hemorrhage

The concept of ethmoidectomy being, of necessity, a procedure frequently associated with a lot of bleeding is erroneous. It is also a dangerous concept, inasmuch as even a small amount of blood can severely impair visualization within the narrow confines of the nose. Performing an ethmoidectomy without bleeding, however, requires meticulous attention to detail.

Preoperatively, it is important to ensure that acute exacerbations of infection are treated prior to surgery when possible, and in chronically infected patients, it may be possible to reduce inflammation by the use of preoperative antibiotics. Patients with markedly reactive mucosa and patients with diffuse polyposis benefit from the use of oral steroids in the perioperative period, and where the patient is already on oral steroid therapy, it is increased in the preoperative period. When, as is preferable, the operation is performed under local anesthesia, the patient should receive adequate preoperative counseling about what

to expect during surgery. It encourages the patient to feel relaxed and at ease during the operation and decreases the chances that he or she will become agitated and hypertensive.

During surgery itself, it is essential that the surgeon pays meticulous attention to all details of the procedure, much as he or she would when performing a stapedectomy. Thus, care is taken to ensure that maximal vasoconstriction is achieved and that the mucosa of the nose is not unnecessarily traumatized either during the application of anesthesia or during the surgery. The use of suction forceps during endoscopic surgery is helpful in maximizing visualization of the operative field and in reducing the need to alternate forceps with suction. Currently available suction irrigation devices, on the other hand, have proved too traumatic for the functional endoscopic approach, although they are of significant benefit when intranasal ethmoidectomy is performed under endoscopic control (the Wigand technique).

Patients with multiple prior operative procedures, massive polyposis, or acute inflammation are considered at risk for intraoperative bleeding even with good preoperative and intraoperative management. These patients are therefore selected for surgery with the KTP-532 laser. Since, with currently available applicators, the laser is of limited usefulness once bleeding has occurred, the aim here is to identify patients at risk for bleeding prior to the surgery and to use the laser from the outset.

Even with good management, occasional patients will have significant intraoperative bleeding. In this situation, it is often better to apply a temporary packing and return to the site after continuing the surgery at another site. However, if the presence

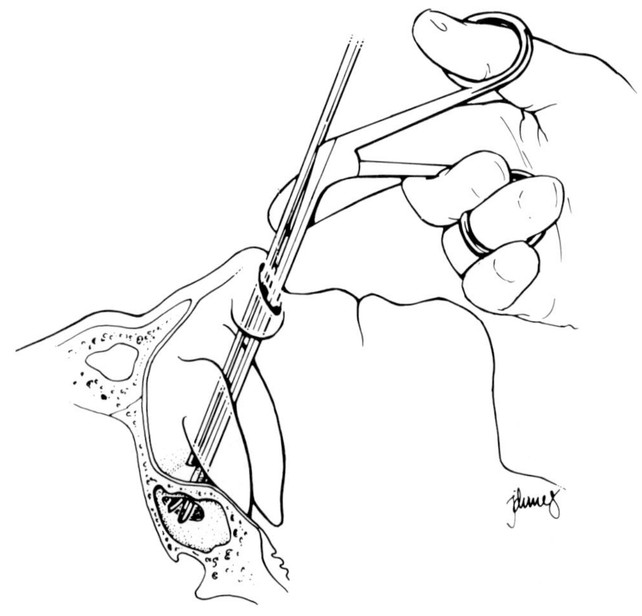

FIG 15–14.
After the bulge of the sphenoid is identified in the posteroinferior aspect of the most posterior ethmoid cell, it may be infractured and entered under endoscopic visualization. (From Kennedy DW: *Arch Otolaryngol* 1985; 111:643–649. Used by permission.)

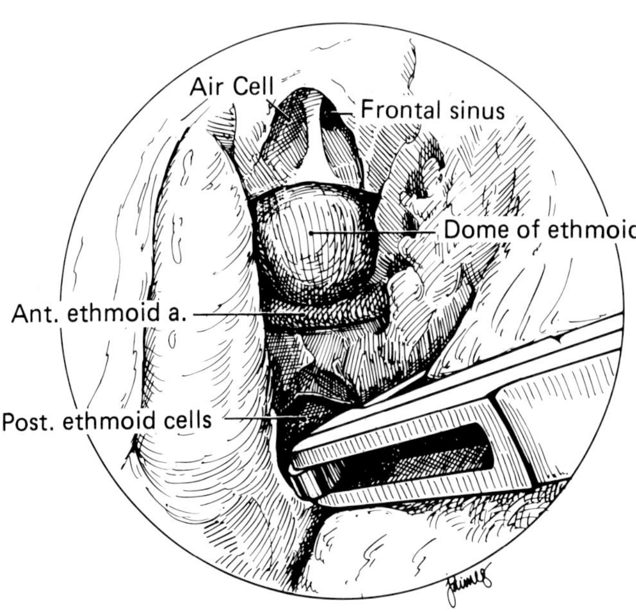

FIG 15–15.
The natural ostium of the maxillary sinus is found at approximately the level of the inferior free boarder of the middle turbinate and, when closed, is surgically opened. After it is opened posteriorly with scissors, it is opened anteriorly with a back-biting forceps. A curette is used to widen it inferiorly and to fold the maxillary sinus mucosa into the nose. (From Kennedy DW: *Arch Otolaryngol* 1985; 111:643–649. Used by permission.)

of bleeding continues to seriously hamper visualization, surgery should be discontinued. The patient can always undergo reoperation if necessary either through the same approach or via an external procedure. It is imperative that intranasal ethmoid procedures are performed under direct visualization if the risk of serious complications is to be minimized.

Arterial bleeding can occur from the anterior or posterior ethmoid arteries or from branches of the sphenopalatine, but significant arterial bleeding is rare with the functional endoscopic approach. The most likely vessel to be encountered is the anterior ethmoid vessel, which usually lies in a bony mesentery adjacent to the inferior portion of the dome of the ethmoid. Bleeding while dissection is performed close to the frontal recess should alert the surgeon that he or she may be approaching branches of this vessel and the adjacent dura. Since the anterior ethmoid nerve also lies in close proximity to the vessel, the sudden onset of pain can also be an important warning sign when the surgery is performed under local anesthesia. Typically, however, the vessel can be easily identified with the 30-degree telescope in cases where frontal recess dissection is required.

Bleeding from the anterior ethmoid artery can usually be stopped by temporary packing of the area. Should this not work, consideration can be given to the use of a bipolar suction cautery or to the placement of microfibrillar collagen. The latter is a very effective hemostatic agent, but any excess should be removed prior to the end of the surgery. In general, the use of oxidized regenerated cellulose is best avoided in the nose,

because when it is left in place, the low pH may cause irritation within the nose, and the material may set into a hard concretion that can be difficult to remove.

The posterior ethmoid vessel is less frequently encountered. It typically lies within the roof of the ethmoid within the posterior ethmoid cells. The arterial branches of the sphenopalatine are also rarely a problem in the functional endoscopic approach. Typically, they may be encountered in two areas with ethmoidectomy: adjacent to the most inferior portion of the basal lamella of the middle turbinate and on the anteroinferior aspect of the sphenoid rostrum. These are areas that are usually not violated during functional endoscopic ethmoidectomy.

The primary concern with ethmoidal artery bleeding is the possibility that the vessel may retract into the orbit and lead to a rapidly expanding intraorbital hematoma. The eyes are always left undraped with this procedure and should be frequently checked. Globe protrusion may occur rapidly from intraorbital bleeding. In this situation, megadose IV steroids are given along with an osmotic diuretic. These measures help to provide time to prepare for external ethmoidectomy and orbital decompression. If the globe protrusion is very rapid, a lateral canthotomy may also be a helpful temporizing step. Ophthalmologic consultation may be sought if immediately available. However, if immediate consultation cannot be obtained the surgeon should proceed with surgical decompression.

Cerebrospinal Fluid Leak

Intracranial entry typically occurs in the medial aspect of

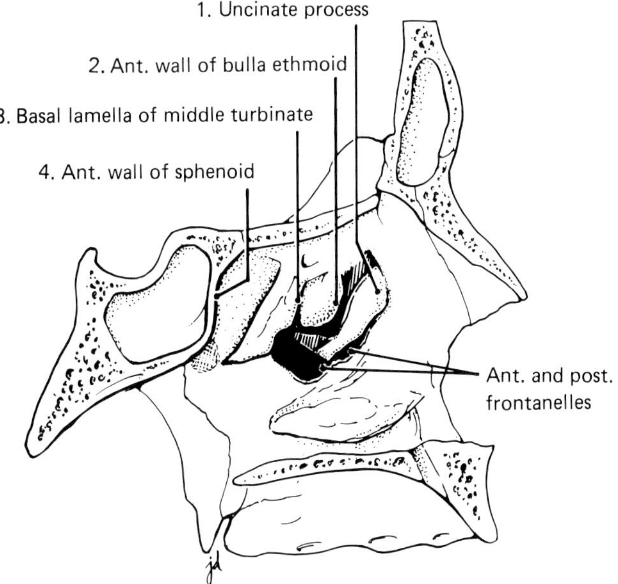

FIG 15–16.
Bony anatomy of the lateral nasal wall demonstrating four bony laminae encountered during endoscopic ethmoidectomy. Numbers indicate surgical order of bony landmarks during approach in a previously unoperated patient. (From Kennedy DW: *Arch Otolaryngol* 1985; 111:643–649. Used by permission.)

the roof of the ethmoid, where the bone is thinner and ma· slope down into the middle turbinate. The roof of the ethmoid may vary from horizontal to steeply downsloping, with up to a 1.7-cm difference between the lateral roof and the cribriform plate. Clearly the latter increases the risk of intracranial entry. The orientation of the roof is best delineated on coronal CT. Care should also be taken to evaluate for bony dehiscences, particularly in the previously operated patient. Dural exposure can also occur congenitally or as a result of chronic disease. During the preoperative endoscopic examination, a nasal polyp that is solitary, is unusually white, pulsates, or occurs in an unusual area (e.g., medial to the middle turbinate) should be considered as a potential meningocele. Aspiration with a small bore needle prior to resection is recommended.

Intraoperatively, the roof of the ethmoid is identified endoscopically and used, along with the medial orbital wall, as a landmark during the surgery. During dissection, the forceps are typically directed laterally so as to avoid the thinner bone of the roof found medially.

The second critical area for intracranial entry lies posteriorly. The sphenoid sinus inevitably lies more inferior and medial than expected, and the most posterior ethmoid cell pneumatizes for a variable extent toward or into the anterior clinoid, superolateral to the sphenoid sinus. If an attempt is made to enter the sphenoid sinus through the most posterior aspect of the last ethmoid cell, the cranial compartment will be breached in the area of the optic nerve.

When a CSF leak is identified intraoperatively, the site should be localized with microscope or endoscope. It is helpful to record the site by performing an intraoperative lateral radiograph with a marker at the site, so as to facilitate reexploration should initial attempts at closure fail. Neurosurgical consultation should be sought, and typically the patient is given broad-spectrum antibiotics that cross the blood-brain barrier. In general, an attempt at closure should be performed during the initial surgery. If for some reason immediate closure is not advisable, no packing is placed on the side of the leak. When the dural opening is minimal and good visualization is possible, intranasal closure with a free mucosal graft and placement of a lumbar drain may be considered. The graft is harvested from the opposite side of the septum and may be secured in place under endoscopic visualization with fibrin glue. Microfibrillar collagen is packed against the graft, and the nose is packed. Larger dehiscences in the ethmoidal roof may be closed with a mucosal flap from the septum or middle turbinate. Exposure, in this instance, is obtained by external ethmoidectomy. Cerebrospinal fluid leaks occurring from the sphenoid sinus are best approached by transseptal exploration. The sinus is packed with fat and fascia, and the anterior wall of the sinus is reconstructed with a free graft of septal bone or cartilage.

Intracranial exploration is reserved for cases where closure from below fails or where intracranial trauma is suspected. In some cases, a transfrontal extradural approach may be helpful in reducing brain retraction. In this case, the frontal sinus is obliterated at the end of the procedure.

All patients who are identified as having CSF leakage should receive an early postoperative CT evaluation to exclude the possibility of intracranial bleeding. Careful monitoring of neurologic status is also performed, even when the leak is stopped immediately.

Performing surgery under endoscopic visualization should reduce the possibility of a CSF leak being missed during surgery. Previously leaks were often not recognized until after the operation. At this time the point of injury is typically uncertain. The first step, therefore, is accurate identification of the leak site. Nasal endoscopy and coronal CT are useful diagnostic first steps. The use of intrathecal radioactive tagged serum albumin and nasal pledgets provides the most sensitive test for the identification of an occult leak but provides little information regarding localization. The combination of intrathecal fluorescein and blue light endoscopy provides a more accurate localization, but the use of intrathecal fluorescein should be undertaken carefully, because seizures and status epilepticus have been reported. A leak may also be visualized with CT using intrathecal injection of a water-soluble contrast agent; however, this requires either a rapid leak or collection within a sinus.

The treatment of CSF leaks that are identified following surgery differs somewhat from those identified intraoperatively. If the leak is minor and the patient is stable, consideration can be given to a period of conservative management. In this situation, the patient is placed at rest with strict instructions to refrain from bending, straining, and engaging in sexual activity. Stool softeners are prescribed as required. The initial attempt at closure with a postoperative leak should also be via an extracranial approach. The method of exposure chosen again depends on site, with an external ethmoidectomy generally the method of choice in an ethmoid leak.

Medial Canthal Ligament Injury

Medial canthal ligament injury is not a risk of intranasal ethmoidectomy. In addition, it appears to be a rare surgical complication even with the external approach. Damage to either the medial canthal ligament or to the trochlea is best avoided by cleanly elevating these structures from the underlying bone with their surrounding periosteum. The periosteal incision is thus made well anterior to the ligament, and care is taken to elevate the ligament atraumatically by staying closely on the bone. Care is also taken not to remove the underlying bone during the surgery. At the end of the surgery, the periosteum should be carefully realigned and closed, and the ligament will reattach to the underlying bone. In revision surgery, elevation of the ligament can be a more difficult problem due to scarring. Greater care is therefore required, and if the periosteum is markedly adherent, it may be advisable to perform the surgery by working around rather than elevating the medial canthal ligament.

Repair of a preexistent medial canthal ligament injury involves reattachment to stable bone. The repair is typically achieved using a wire or nonabsorbable suture. If the bone in the ipsilateral side is mobile or absent, the suture is placed through to the opposite side. It is important to ensure that the two ligaments are at the same vertical height and at the same level in the anteroposterior plane.

Optic Nerve Injury

Loss of vision may occur from direct trauma to the optic nerve or chiasm or from bleeding into the orbit or around the optic nerve. In the external approach, visual loss may occur from overzealous globe retraction. The monopolar cautery has also been implicated but is probably not responsible unless it is used immediately adjacent to the nerve.

Direct trauma to the nerve is most likely to occur while working in the posterior ethmoid in a patient with extensive retro-orbital pneumatization. In these cases the nerve comes to lie in close proximity to the posterolateral ethmoid air cells and occasionally deeply grooves them. In benign disease of the sphenoid sinus, particularly in cases of fungal sinus disease, expansion of the sinus around the nerve can also occur. The keys to avoiding this complication are carefully reviewing the anatomy on the preoperative CT scan and performing the surgery under direct vision. In all intranasal ethmoid surgery, it is imperative to discontinue surgery if persistent bleeding interferes with visualization of the area.

Intraorbital bleeding, either as a result of intraorbital trauma or bleeding from a retracted ethmoidal artery, probably constitutes a more frequent cause of visual loss than direct trauma to the nerve. Similarly, if nasal packing is used in the presence of heavy intranasal bleeding and a dehiscence in the periorbital periosteum, the blood may dissect into the orbit.

Postoperative visual loss, pupillary change, or evidence of orbital bleeding require immediate removal of the packing, neuro-ophthalmologic consultation, and reexploration. Immediate decompression is required if the vision is to be saved. High-dose IV steroid therapy should also be initiated. Ultrasound may be of benefit in identifying an orbital hematoma, but time is the most important factor in this situation. If no orbital hematoma is present, consideration should be given to decompressing the optic nerve.

Enophthalmos Secondary to Periorbital Fat Herniation

I am not aware of enophthalmos as a postsurgical complication from either external or intranasal ethmoidectomy. The creation of enophthalmos would appear to require both the extensive removal of the orbital bone and the creation of large dehiscences in the periorbita. This should therefore be a very rare postsurgical occurrence. However, enophthalmos is a well-known posttraumatic complication and may also occur as a result of severe sinus disease.

The creation of a lasting correction for enophthalmos is difficult. Unless the deformity is severe, it is probably better not to intervene. Where there is a compelling reason to attempt correction, the principle is to correct the bony defect with a free bone graft and to perform a free fat graft to the orbit. However, as a result of the subsequent shrinkage of the fat graft, considerable intraoperative overcorrection is required. At the same time, care must be taken to ensure that intraorbital pressure does not become sufficiently great to compromise vision either intraoperatively or following the surgery when postoperative edema is present. These patients, therefore, require careful ophthalmologic monitoring.

CHAPTER 16

External Sinus Surgery

Approach of

William W. Montgomery, M.D.,

Mack L. Cheney, M.D.,

and

Pamela A. Turner, B.A.

CALDWELL-LUC OPERATION

Indications

The indications for the Caldwell-Luc procedure are (1) intractable infection, (2) failure of resolution of a chronic infection following intranasal antrostomy, (3) polypoid tissue filling the antrum, (4) antrochoanal polyp or cystic disease of the antrum, (5) osteonecrosis, (6) suspicion of maxillary sinus neoplasm, (7) dental cysts, (8) presence of foreign bodies, (9) fractures of the maxilla, and (10) the presence of an oroantral fistula.

Incision

A horizontal incision is made in the gingivobuccal sulcus well above the roots of the teeth (Fig 16–1,A). The incision extends from the level of the lateral incisor to the second molar and through the mucous membrane and periosteum. The periosteum over the canine fossa is then elevated to the level of the infraorbital canal. The infraorbital nerve is identified and carefully preserved (Fig 16–1,B). The best way to avoid injury to this nerve is to positively identify it. An atraumatic method of elevating the periosteum is to place a bit of gauze ahead of a chisel to provide blunt dissection. Gentle retraction throughout the procedure will also reduce the chance for trauma to the infraorbital nerve as well as to the other soft tissues of the cheek. Two retractors are used to elevate the periosteum. They

are placed in a superior medial and superior lateral direction to avoid the infraorbital nerve.

Fenestration of the Canine Fossa

The best way to fenestrate the anterior wall of the antrum is with use of a curette or a rotating bur. If a rotating bur is not available, a square window may be made with a sharp chisel. The four sides of this window are first scored by light tapping to avoid fracture. A sharp gouge is another instrument that may be used to fenestrate the anterior wall. Whichever instrument is employed, a fracture must be avoided, because this may extend to and injure the infraorbital nerve or a tooth root.

The opening in the anterior wall is enlarged with either a burr or Kerrison bone-cutting forceps. Troublesome bleeding may occur from the bone margin, which can be controlled by squeezing tightly with the Kerrison forceps but not hard enough to cut through the bone. It is well to enlarge the sinus opening to a size that will admit the fifth digit. The entire contents of the antrum can then be viewed.

Cysts and benign tumors can be removed with various elevators and forceps, injury to the normal mucosa being avoided. Removal of the entire mucous membrane lining of the antrum is often not necessary. However, when the lining seems irreversibly diseased, it can be easily removed by first elevating it with a curved blunt dissector and then using various elevators,

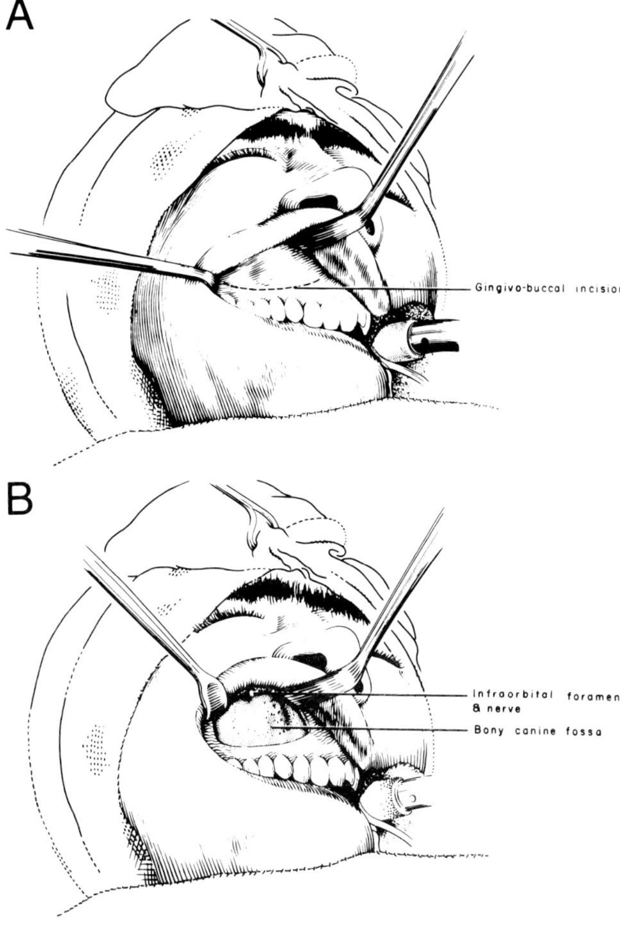

FIG 16–1.
A, the upper lip is retracted superiorly in a direction away from the infraorbital nerve. Stretching of the nerve can cause anesthesia of the upper lip and side of the nose. The endotracheal tube is directed toward the contralateral angle of the mouth. The pharynx is packed both to assist with a closed system of anesthesia and to prevent blood from entering the pharynx. An incision is made about 5 mm above the gum margin. It should be slightly U shaped, especially when the patient wears a maxillary denture. **B,** the periosteum has been elevated superiorly, exposing the bony front face of the maxillary sinus, known as the canine fossa. Again, note that the retraction is in a direction away from the infraorbital nerve, which can be seen as it leaves the infraorbital foramen. Bleeding is controlled by packing with epinephrine-impregnated gauze strips or by cautery. A gauze strip pushed ahead of a chisel assists with the elevation of the periosteum. (From Montgomery WW: *Surgery of the Upper Respiratory System,* vol 1, ed 2. Philadelphia, Lea & Febiger, 1979. Used by permission.)

curettes, and tissue forceps for removal. Dissection in the region of the roof of the antrum must be conducted with care, because the infraorbital nerve may not have a bony covering in this region.

Nasoantral Window

A curved, sharp hemostat is inserted intranasally into the inferior meatus, and by gentle pressure, an opening is made in the anterior aspect of the nasoantral wall. The fenestra is enlarged in an anterior direction with Kerrison forceps and posteriorly with a side-biting forceps. This dissection is much more easily carried out by way of the Caldwell-Luc opening in contrast to the intranasal route. The nasoantral window should be at least 1.5 cm in diameter and should include intranasal mucous membrane, sinus mucosa, and the bony nasoantral wall. Many surgeons hold the opinion that the various mucosal flaps devised for formation of the nasoantral window are not only unnecessary but can, by becoming displaced, close the fenestra.

Before packing, the sinus cavity is carefully inspected for retained sponges. If there is no bleeding, packing is unnecessary. Petrolatum or chlortetracycline (Aureomycin) ointment-impregnated 1-in. iodoform gauze packing may be inserted into the sinus by way of the nasoantral fenestra to control persistent bleeding. The incision in the gingivobuccal sulcus is closed with one or two catgut sutures. Some surgeons prefer not to suture this incision, stating that there is much less postoperative edema if it is not closed.

OROANTRAL FISTULA

Diagnosis

The number of maxillary premolars and molars in intimate contact with the floor of the maxillary sinus is dependent on the size of the sinus. The sinus may be separated from the roots of these teeth by a thin layer of bone, or there may be an absence of bone. On occasion, the roots may extend into the maxillary sinus. There are two predisposing factors to oroantral fistulae: (1) the close proximity of premolar and molar roots to the sinus floor and (2) the presence of either an apical abscess or a maxillary sinusitis with poor drainage at the time of a maxillary molar or premolar extraction. An oroantral fistula may be secondary to compound maxillary fracture, neoplasm of the antrum (especially after radiation therapy), or following a radical antrum operation.

The symptoms of an oroantral fistula, if of recent origin, are blood in the nasal cavity and an escape of air from the fistulous tooth socket. Liquids taken into the mouth may escape through the nostril. If infection is present, it usually is manifested within 1 or 2 days following the extraction of the tooth. Pain over the maxillary sinus and a profuse malodorous nasal discharge are characteristic. The patient complains of foul taste. Purulent discharge can be seen exuding from the extraction site. This discharge may increase when the patient holds his or her nose and increases the intranasal pressure. The patient may have difficulty in developing a negative intraoral pressure such as when drinking through a straw.

The diagnosis is made from the history, signs and symptoms, x-ray films of the sinuses, and probing of the fistulous tract with a small-caliber lacrimal probe.

Indications for Surgical Procedure

The surgical procedure is determined by:

1. The size of the fistula
2. The presence or absence of adjacent teeth
3. Previous unsuccessful attempts for closure
4. Severity of the associated maxillary sinusitis
5. Epithelialization of the fistulous tract

On occasion an oromaxillary fistula may occur following the extraction of a nondiseased tooth. This usually heals rapidly after making local repairs, administering antibiotics, and prohibiting the patient from nose blowing. If a tooth root is broken off during extraction and found to lie within the antrum but submucosally, it is best left alone if there is no infection. If infection is present, antibiotic therapy plus local irrigation may result in resolution of the infection and healing. Otherwise, a more radical procedure is necessary both to remove the foreign body and to close the oroantral fistula.

Repair of Fistula When Teeth Are Present

If the fistula is small and teeth are present, it is closed by using a combination of gingival and palatal incisions adjacent to the teeth (Fig 16–2,A). Antibiotic therapy is instituted several days before the operation. The patient is prepared for operation as outlined for the Caldwell-Luc procedure. The incision is made near the gingival margin. The periosteum is elevated over the anterior wall of the maxillary sinus. The antrum is entered, and a Caldwell-Luc operation is carried out, making certain that a large nasoantral window is fashioned. It is most important to obtain a culture so that sensitivity tests can be performed. All granulation tissue and diseased bone are curetted from both the sinus and oral orifices of the fistula. An incision is made on the palatal side of the alveolar ridge. A counter incision is made over the hard palate; this incision may extend beyond the junction of the hard and soft palate if necessary. The bipedicled flap thus created is elevated so that it may be advanced laterally to obtain tension-free approximation of the flaps. The flaps are securely sutured over the fistula with mattress sutures (Fig 16–2,B). Tha antrum is firmly packed with 1-inch chlortetracycline-ointment-impregnated iodoform gauze.

Procedure in Edentulous Patients

If the fistula is small or of moderate size and there are no teeth present in the adjacent alveolar ridge, a gingivobuccal U flap is used to repair the defect (Fig 16–3,A). The U flap is elevated, and a Caldwell-Luc operation is carried out. The lateral wall of the fistulous tract is completely removed from the alveolar ridge to the antrum. Adjacent bone is also removed laterally so that the U flap may be placed in contact with the entire surface of the trough thus created (Fig 16–3,B). The U flap is then secured in place with no. 3-0 chromic catgut or silk suture material (Fig 16–3,C).

Procedure for Large or Persistent Oroantral Fistula

There are numerous surgical procedures for the correction of a persistent or large oroantral fistula. Probably the simplest and the most successful method is that of providing a posteriorly based palatal flap combined with a buccal flap (Fig 16–4,A). It may be necessary to remove adjacent teeth if they are in close proximity to the fistula. In preparing the palatal flap, one must be cognizant of the location of the greater palatal foramen and artery. The location of the greater palatal foramen is approximately 0.5 cm medial to the last molar. The lateral wall of the fistulous tract is removed in a manner similar to that previously described. A more extensive resection of the alveolar ridge may also be necessary. The palatal flap is then advanced laterally so that it may be sutured to the gingivobuccal flap without tension (Fig 16–4,B).

A connective tissue flap derived from the area above the gingivobuccal flap may be reflected inferiorly into a large oroantral fistula. This is sometimes necessary in conjunction with the palatal and buccal flap to close a very large oroantral fistula.

PARTIAL MAXILLECTOMY

During the past 10 years, we have performed a gradually decreasing number of total maxillectomies along with an increasing number of subtotal maxillectomies combined with postoperative radiation therapy. At the present time, our only indication for a total maxillectomy is extensive disease of the maxillary sinus with involvement of the orbit, alveolar ridge, palatal bones, or pterygoid region. A subtotal maxillectomy, performed by way of a lateral rhinotomy incision or an extended gingivobuccal incision, allows the surgeon to encompass the disease as well as a total maxillectomy in most cases. This, followed by a full course of postoperative radiation therapy, offers our patients an equal chance for cure compared with those patients subjected to a total maxillectomy.

There are a number of reasons for a change from total maxillectomy to subtotal maxillectomy:

1. Our techniques for a partial maxillectomy have improved.

2. Preoperatively, the sites of extension of the disease can be accurately assessed by improved radiographic studies such as polytomography and computed tomography (CT) and magnetic resonance imaging (MRI) scanning.

3. As a result of these improved diagnostic procedures, the surgeon can plan the operation so as to encompass only the diseased segment and its surrounding tissue rather than a large block of tissue that is not diseased. Potential sites for recurrent disease can be accurately designated and reported so that the radiotherapist can concentrate on and include these in the field of radiation therapy.

4. In most cases, the disease can be encompassed as well by the subtotal maxillectomy compared with the total maxillectomy.

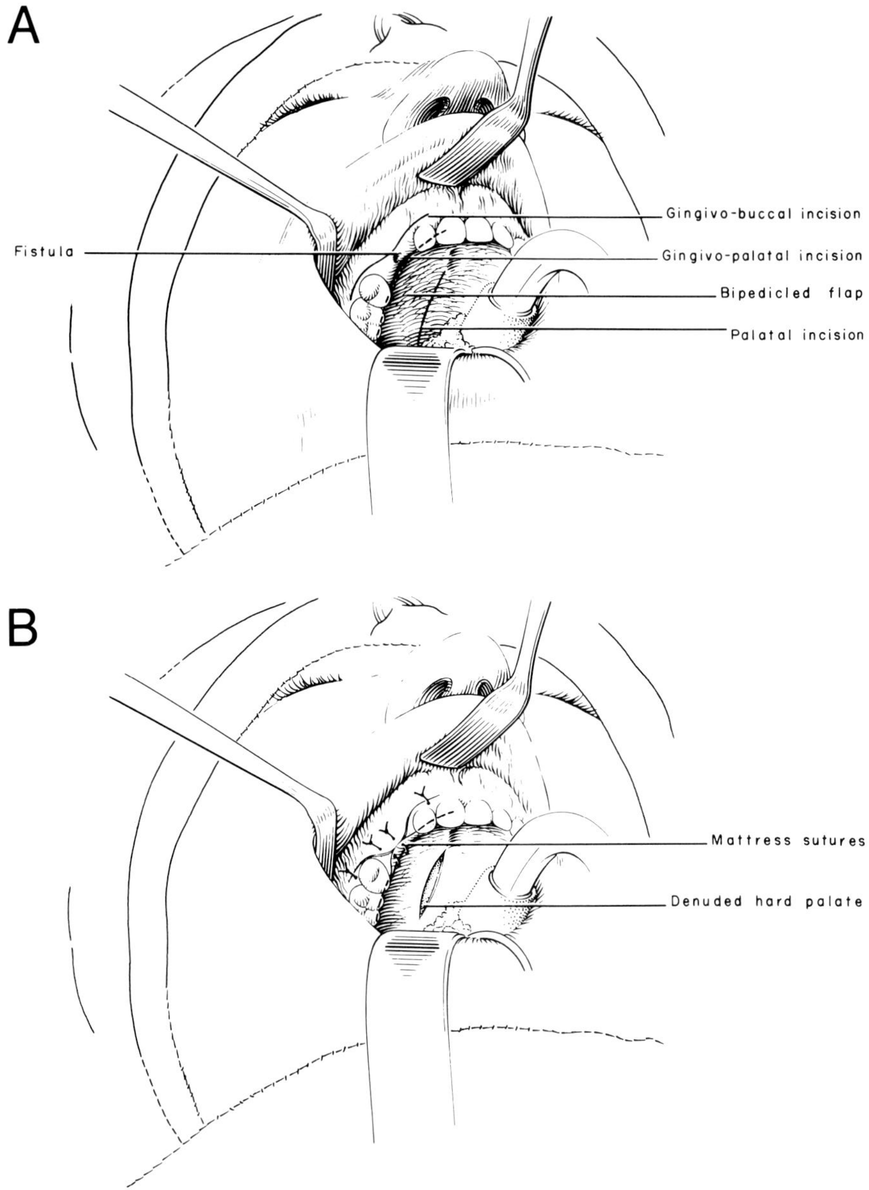

FIG 16–2.
A, the gingivobuccal incision is made just above the gingival margin. The periosteum is elevated over the canine fossa, and a Caldwell-Luc operation is completed. A gingivopalatal incision parallel to the above incision is made just medial to the gingival margin. A third incision begins behind the incisor teeth near the midline and extends posteriorly over the entire length of the hard palate. The mucosa between the latter two incisions is elevated from the hard palate, creating a bipedicled flap. **B,** all diseased bone is removed from the bony fistulous tract. The two flaps are secured over this bony defect with mattress sutures. These flaps can be advanced into position by additional sutures if necessary. A defect over the hard palate is created as the bipedicled flap is advanced in the direction of the fistula. (From Montgomery WW: *Surgery of the Upper Respiratory System.* vol 1, ed 2. Philadelphia, Lea & Febiger, 1979. Used by permission.)

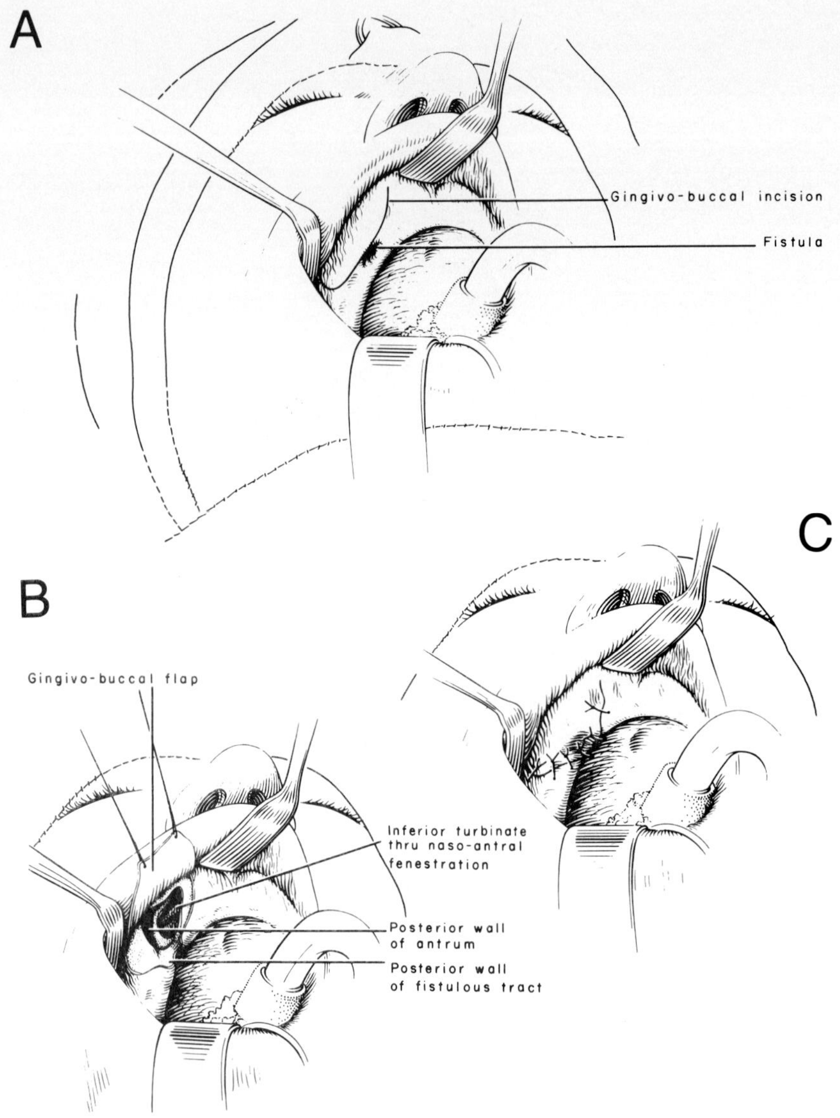

FIG 16–3.
A, a U-shaped gingivobuccal incision is used for a moderate-sized oromaxillary fistula when the patient is edentulous. **B**, the U flap has been elevated and a Caldwell-Luc operation completed. The anterior wall of the bony fistulous tract has been removed. **C**, the U flap has been sutured in place. It makes contact with the posterior wall of the fistulous tract to obliterate and prevent a recurrent tract. (From Montgomery WW: *Surgery of the Upper Respiratory System.* vol 1, ed 2. Philadelphia, Lea & Febiger, 1979. used by permission.)

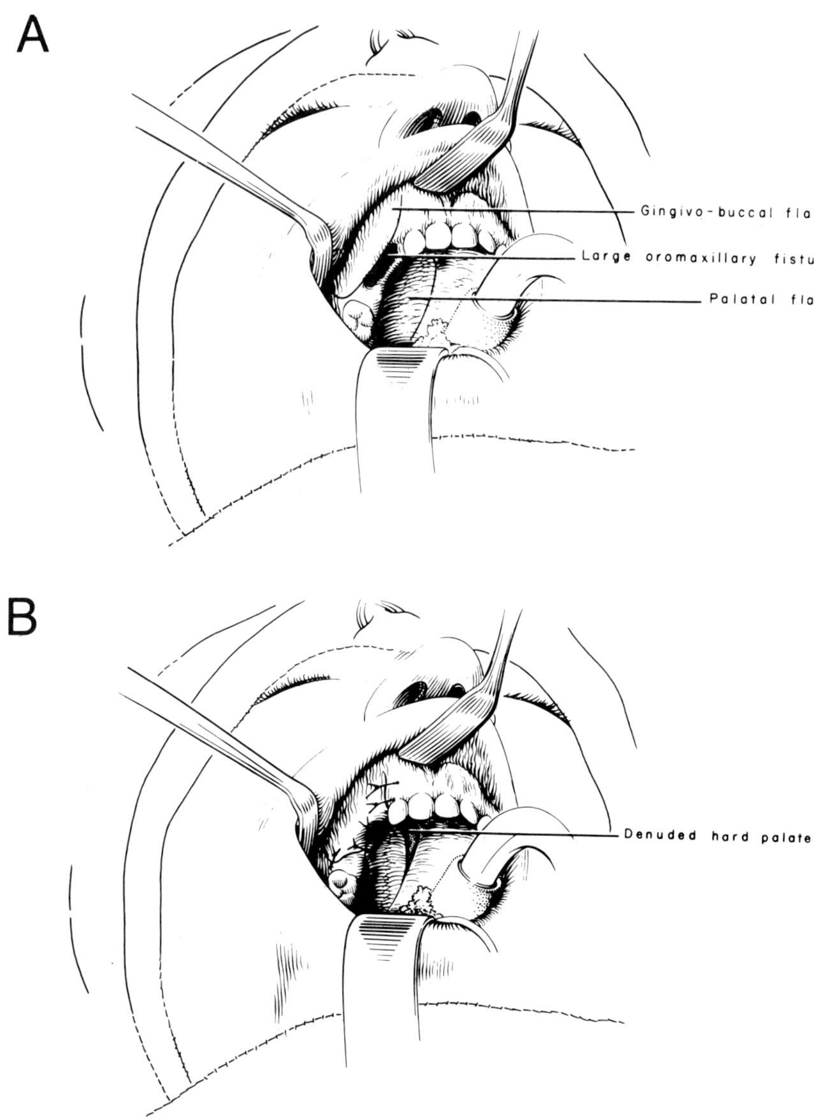

FIG 16–4.
A, combined buccal and palatal flaps are often necessary for repair of a large fistula with adjacent teeth or for repair of persistent fistula. **B,** the palatal flap, which is based posteriorly on the greater palatine vessels, is advanced toward the alveolar ridge, where it is sutured to the buccal flap. (From Montgomery WW: *Surgery of the Upper Respiratory System.* vol 1, ed 2. Philadelphia, Lea & Febiger, 1979. Used by permission.)

5. During recent years, techniques for radiotherapy have improved sufficiently so that the sites for potential recurrence may be treated with a full course of radiation therapy without injury to surrounding structures.

6. The subtotal maxillectomy results in excellent cosmesis compared with the unsightly appearance and facial asymmetry that results from a total maxillectomy.

The obvious disadvantage for this conservative therapy is the difficulty in observing the cavity for recurrent disease and the problem of keeping the cavity free from crusting. These problems have been overcome with the use of straight and angulated fiberoptic scopes for visualization of the cavity along with periodic polytomography. The crusting can be controlled by a lubricating spray such as Spray B (200 mg of camphor, 200 mg of menthol, 0.2 ml of eucalyptol, and petrolatum liquid in sufficient quantity to make 100 mL). Crusting is also controlled by irrigating the cavity with warm saline solution (1 tsp of salt per glass of warm water) or Alkalol solution to which has been added an equal part of hot tap water. The patient thus irrigates with warm, half-strength Alkalol solution.

Nasal irrigations are accomplished by inserting the end of an ulcer or infant enema syringe into the nostril while the patient leans forward, face down, over a sink with the mouth open.

Irrigations are usually commenced 10 days to 2 weeks following surgery when the patient is completely healed. They are continued two or three times daily until crusting becomes minimal. After this, irrigations are carried out several times each week as indicated.

Crusting in a subtotal or total maxillectomy can lead to serious consequences. The accumulation of crusts is a formal invitation for bacterial growth, which, in turn, produces an offensive odor, loss of underlying mucous membrane, and localized osteomyelitis. We have seen a case of metastatic osteomyelitis of the cervical spine resulting from untreated subtotal maxillectomy cavity crusting. Thus, when a patient appears with a much crusted cavity, a culture is taken, the patient is placed on high-dose antibiotic therapy, and irrigations are carried out with sufficient frequency so as to eliminate crusting.

TOTAL MAXILLECTOMY

Maxillectomy is the treatment of choice for a carcinoma confined to the antrum. Unfortunately, these cases are few and far between, because carcinoma in the maxillary sinus usually extends beyond the confines of the sinus to produce signs and symptoms that bring the disease to the attention of the patient.

As a general rule, inferiorly located carcinoma of the maxillary sinus has the best chance for cure. If the lesion has broken through the anterior wall of the sinus, everything under the cutaneous cheek must be removed, and on occasion, the skin of the cheek must be included with the resected specimen. If the carcinoma has broken through the roof of the antrum, the orbital contents must be resected with the maxilla. If the tumor invades the anterior ethmoid cells, the nasal septum and entire

ethmoid labyrinth, including the roof of the labyrinth and the cribriform plate, must be removed. Tumors that extend through the posterior wall of the antrum into the posterior ethmoid cells, sphenoid sinus, or apex of the orbit have a poor prognosis even with preoperative or postoperative radiation therapy. If the carcinoma extends into the frontal sinus, the frontal bone in this area should be resected.

Postoperative radiation therapy is given when posterior extension of the tumor is discovered. In such cases, a radiotherapist can administer the radiation more accurately than would have been possible prior to the operation.

Preoperative Management

Permission for removal of the orbit must be obtained preoperatively in all cases, because an unsuspected extension of disease is not uncommon. The surgeon may choose to begin antibiotic therapy before the operation, especially if the carcinoma is accompanied by secondary infection. Anteroposterior and lateral planograms as well as CT (including coronal sections) of the maxillary sinus are often most helpful in determining the extent of the disease. It is preferable to obtain impressions and a prosthesis before the maxillectomy rather than during the immediate postoperative period. If this is not possible, the impression can be taken following removal of the packing.

Maxillectomy With Orbital Exenteration

The patient is placed on the operating table in the supine position. The head is elevated above the level of the thorax to reduce the venous pressure. Maxillectomy is a difficult, bloody, and high-risk operation. Heavy equipment is necessary.

The anatomic parts to be removed are the orbital contents, the floor and medial wall of the orbit, the malar bone, a portion of the zygomatic arch, the antrum, the ethmoid sinuses, the anterior wall of the sphenoid sinus, the pterygoid plate, the hard palate, and the nasal septum if the ethmoid or nasal cavity is involved with the tumor (Fig 16–5).

Incisions

The eyelids are sewn together with 5-0 silk or polyethylene suture material. The incision begins over the lateral aspect of the nasal dorsum, just above the level of the inner canthus. It is made directly to the bone (Fig 16–6,A). It is extended down over the nasal bone midway between the lateral nasal crease and the dorsum of the nose, around the ala and the nasal labial crease, to the midline under the columella. Cross-hatching of the incision is carried out to ensure a more accurate closure. A vertical midline incision is used to split the upper lip. The upper lip is compressed with a finger and thumb on each side while the lip-splitting incision is made. As pressure is released, the superior labial and lateral nasal branches of the external maxillary artery are easily identified and ligated.

The incisions above and below the eyelid margin are made approximately 2 mm away from the tarsal plates. They rejoin lateral to the external canthus and extend laterally an additional 2 cm. Some surgeons advocate preservation of the lids so that

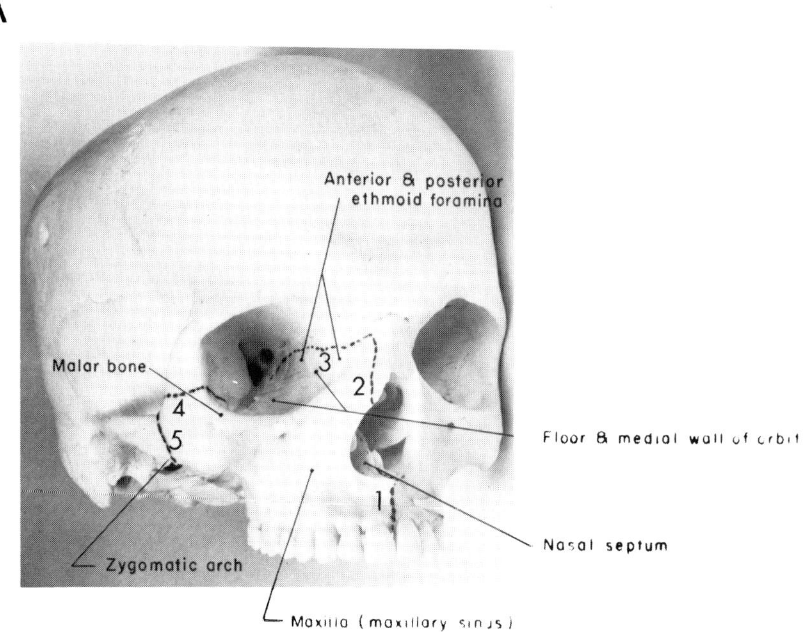

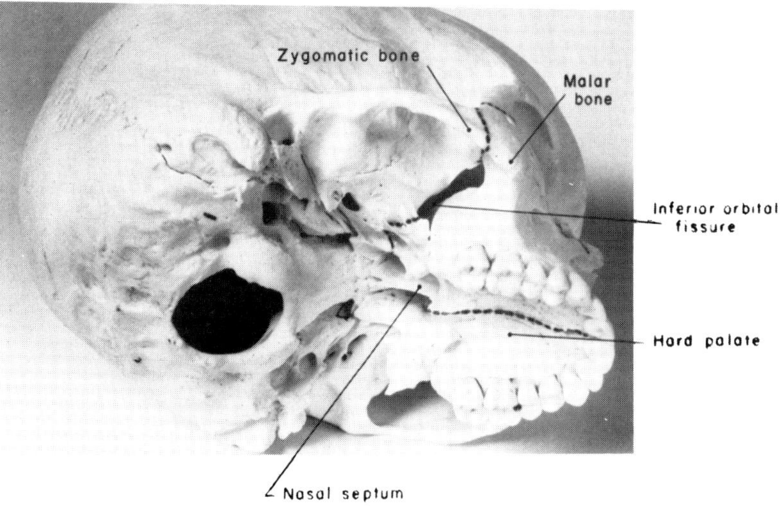

FIG 16–5.

A, the parts to be removed in maxillectomy are floor of the orbit, malar bone, zygomatic arch (medial aspect), ethmoid sinuses and anterior wall of sphenoid, lateral wall of nose with turbinates, hard palate, entire maxillary sinus, and pterygoid plates. Bone incisions are (*1*) anterior alveolar ridge and premaxilla, just to the right of the nasal septum; (*2*) between the nasal bone and ascending process of the maxilla to the level of the nasal process of the frontal bone; (*3*) along the superior aspect of the medial orbital wall, just inferior to the ethmoid foramina and the suture line between the orbital plate of the frontal bone and the lamina papyracea; (*4*) across the malar bone, connecting with the lateral aspect of the inferior orbital fissure; and (*5*) transecting the zygomatic arch medially. **B,** the parts to be removed are malar bone, maxillary sinus, right alveolar ridge, hard palate, nasal septum (if disease is present in the nasal cavity), and pterygoid plates. Bone incisions include malar bone, zygomatic arch, across the base of the pterygoid process (this incision may be made between the posterior wall of the maxilla and the pterygoid plates if the former remains intact and free of tumor invasion), and the hard palate, split in the midline. (From Montgomery WW: *Surgery of the Upper Respiratory System,* vol 1, ed 2. Philadelphia, Lea & Febiger, 1979. Used by permission.)

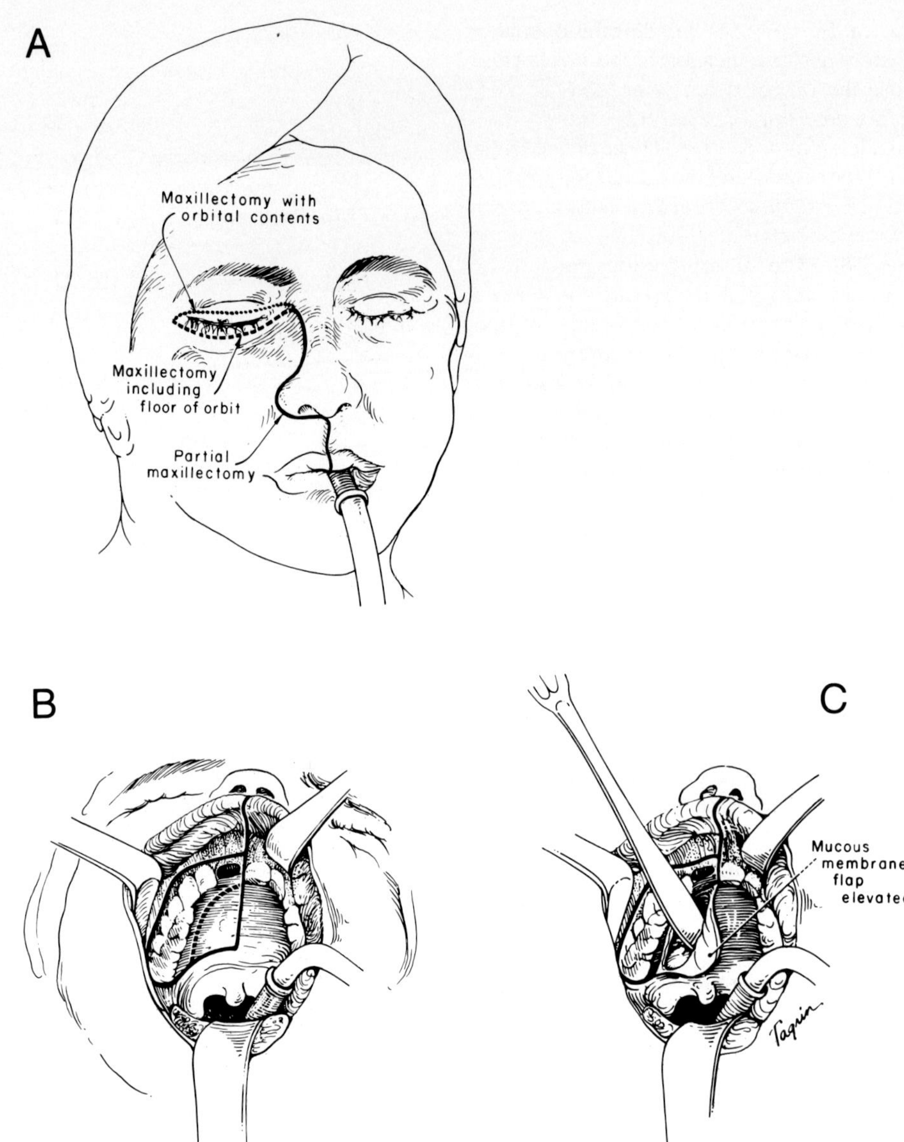

FIG 16–6.
Incisions. *Solid line* indicates partial maxillectomy; *dashed line* indicates maxillectomy, including floor of orbit; *dotted line* indicates maxillectomy with orbital contents. **A,** the incision begins at a point midway between the inner canthus and the nasal dorsum. It extends inferiorly, anterior to the nasofacial crease, until the alar sulcus is reached. It follows the alar sulcus and continues on just below the nasal orifice to the midline. The upper lip is split in the midline. If the floor of the orbit is to be included, the incision must be extended laterally within 4 mm of the tarsal plate inferiorly. An incision just above the tarsal plate in the upper lid is added if the orbital contents are to be included in the resection. The horizontal incisions above and below the lids are connected just lateral to the external canthus and extended lateralward about 1 cm. **B,** the buccal side of the upper lip is split vertically in the midline. The mucosal incision is continued across the space previously occupied by the right median incisor. The mucous membrane over the hard palate is incised in the midline. At the junction of the soft and hard palate, the incision is directed laterally toward the posterior margin of the alveolar ridge. The mucous membrane in the gingivobuccal sulcus is incised along the entire length of the alveolar ridge rather than in the gingivopalatal sulcus. **C,** the mucous membrane is being elevated away from the hard palate. It is unwise to preserve this tissue when the floor of the antrum is invaded by tumor. (From Montgomery WW: *Surgery of the Upper Respiratory System,* vol 1, ed 2. Philadelphia, Lea & Febiger, 1979. Used by permission.)

a prosthesis may be worn. The cosmesis attending this operation is not entirely satisfactory and preservation of the lids is often not advisable, because the orbital defect is needed for long-term inspection and the detection of recurrent disease.

An incision is made along the entire length of the gingivobuccal sulcus and posteriorly around the maxillary tuberosity (Fig 16–6,B). If teeth are present, the median incisor on the side of the maxillectomy is removed.

Either of two methods is used to approach the hard palate. If the lesion extends to or involves the hard palate, the mucous membrane over the hard palate must be removed with the specimen. In such cases a midline incision is made from the anterior midline alveolar ridge to the junction of the hard and soft palates. An incision is then made along the posterior rim of the hard palate. This connects with the gingivobuccal incision, which has been extended around the maxillary tuberosity.

If the hard palate is not involved, the mucosal incision is made along the palatal side of the alveolar ridge parallel to the gingivobuccal incision around the posterior aspect of the palate on the side on which the maxillectomy is being performed (Fig 16–6,C).

Elevation of the Facial Flap

The nasal cavity is entered inferiorly after the upper lip has been reflected laterally (Fig 16–7,A). An electrocautery knife is useful here. This incision is extended laterally and then superiorly in the pyriform aperture to a point on the inferior margin of the nasal skeleton at the junction between the nasal bone and the ascending process of the maxilla (Fig 16–7,B). The periosteum is elevated over the nasal bone and ascending process of the maxilla to the level of the nasal process of the frontal bone, and the nose is retracted to the opposite side.

Elevation of the facial flap is continued in a subcutaneous plane. The skin of the lids is elevated superficial to the orbicularis oculi muscle. (On the other hand, if the tumor does not extend to this region, the orbicularis oculi muscle may be preserved with the facial flap to give a better cosmetic result.) The buccinator muscle is preserved with the facial flap. All other facial muscles attached to the anterior wall of the antrum must be transected. The buccinator can be followed easily, because its fibers are continuous with those of the orbicularis oris muscle and run in a posterior direction. The portion of the buccinator muscle that attached to the maxilla is transected. Elevation of the flap is continued posteriorly to the anterior aspect of the zygomatic arch and to the lateral aspect of the malar bone.

Orbit

As has been mentioned, the skin of the upper lid is usually elevated to include the orbicularis oculi muscle unless there is extension of disease into the orbit. The superior orbital rim is identified. The periosteum is incised along the superior orbital rim and also on the medial and lateral orbital rims to the level of the inner and external canthi (Fig 16–8,A). Elevation of the periosteum is begun superiorly, and the contents of the orbit are dissected inferiorly (Fig 16–8,B). The optic nerve and vessels are transected with curved scissors. Troublesome bleeding can be controlled with packing left in place for a short time.

Malar Bone

The inferior orbital fissure is identified. A long, curved hemostat is inserted under the malar bone and up and out through the inferior orbital fissure (Fig 16–9,A). This hemostat is used to grasp one end of a Gigli saw, which is pulled through and used to transect the malar bone (Fig 16–9,B). The malar bone can also be incised with a Stryker saw (Fig 16–9,C). On occasion, it may be necessary to remove the superior and lateral bony walls of the orbit, thus exposing the dura.

Zygomatic Arch

After the anterior attachment of the masseter muscle is detached, the zygomatic arch is transected (Figs 16–10,A and B) with either a Gigli saw or a Stryker saw (Fig 16–10,C).

Hard Palate

The simplest way to transect the hard palate is with a 2-cm osteotome (Fig 16–11,A). The transection may be accomplished by inserting a Gigli saw into the nasal cavity and out at the junction of the hard and soft palates. The saw is grasped by a curved hemostat inserted through the incision at the junction of the hard and soft palates (Fig 16–11,B). When one is sawing, it is necessary to pull slightly toward the opposite side so that the saw will approximate the midline (Fig 16–11,C). Troublesome bleeding may occur from the greater palatine artery, but this can be controlled by packing or by inserting a cautery tip into the greater palatine foramen. The amount of bleeding can be decreased by employing the electrocautery knife on the buccal and nasal sides of the hard palate prior to using the osteotome or Gigli saw.

Ethmoid

The upper nasal cavity is entered by one of two methods. A 1 cm osteotome is placed between the nasal bone and the ascending process of the maxilla. The osteotome is inserted to the level of the nasal process of the frontal bone (Fig 16–12,A). This is approximately at the level of the inner canthus, cribriform plate, roof of the ethmoid labyrinth, anterior and posterior ethmoid arteries, and the suture line between the orbital process of the frontal bone and the lamina papyracea. The exposure also can be accomplished by removing the ascending process of the maxilla with a rongeur (Fig 16–12,B).

The periosteum is elevated laterally, exposing the lacrimal sac and lamina papyracea. The anterior and posterior ethmoid arteries are identified and cauterized. The anterior and posterior ethmoid foramina accurately identify the level of the cribriform plate and roof of the ethmoid sinuses. An osteotome is used to transect the specimen just below the roof of the ethmoid sinuses (Fig 16–13,A). This osteotome is extended posteriorly to the depth of the posterior ethmoid artery (Fig 16–13,B). If the disease involves the ethmoid sinuses, their bony roof and cribriform plate should be removed, thus exposing the dura. In such cases, cerebrospinal fluid (CSF) leakage usually occurs. Repair is made with a split-thickness skin graft or a mucosal flap from the septum. When the ethmoid sinuses are grossly involved, it is also advisable to resect the nasal septum.

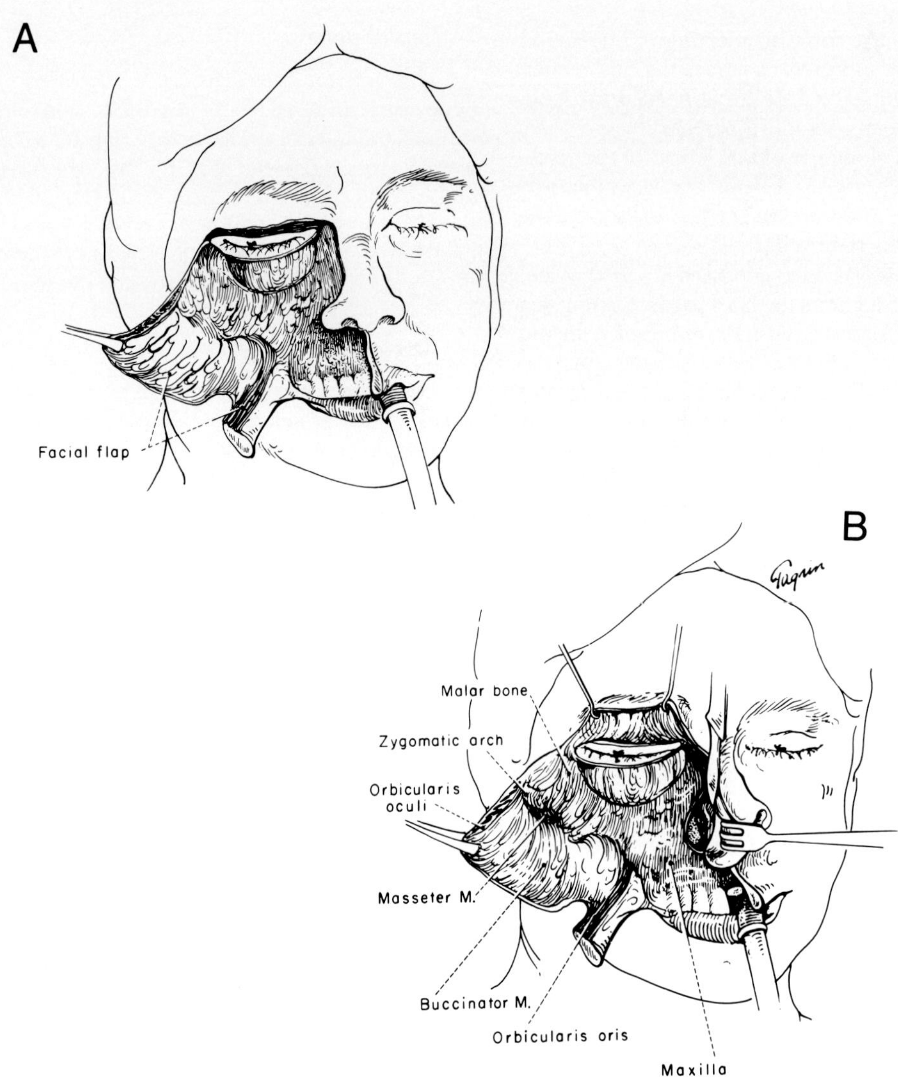

FIG 16–7.
A, the eyelids are sutured, and the facial flap is dissected laterally, exposing the masseter muscle, zygomatic arch, and malar bone. **B,** the nasal cavity is entered laterally. This incision is carried superiorly to the junction of the nasal bone and the ascending process of the maxilla. (From Montgomery WW: *Surgery of the Upper Respiratory System,* vol 1, ed 2. Philadelphia, Lea & Febiger, 1979. Used by permission.)

A

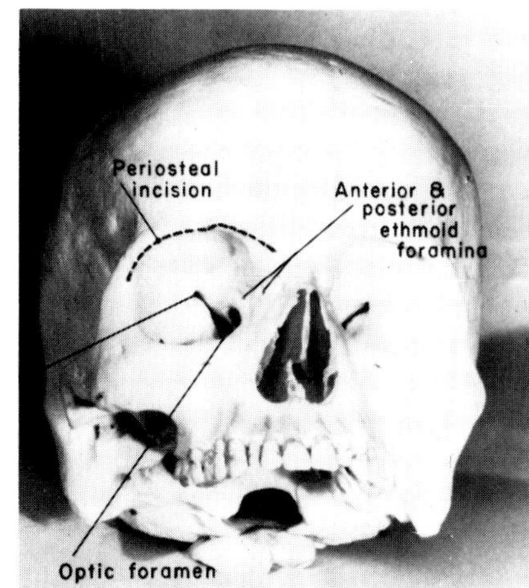

B

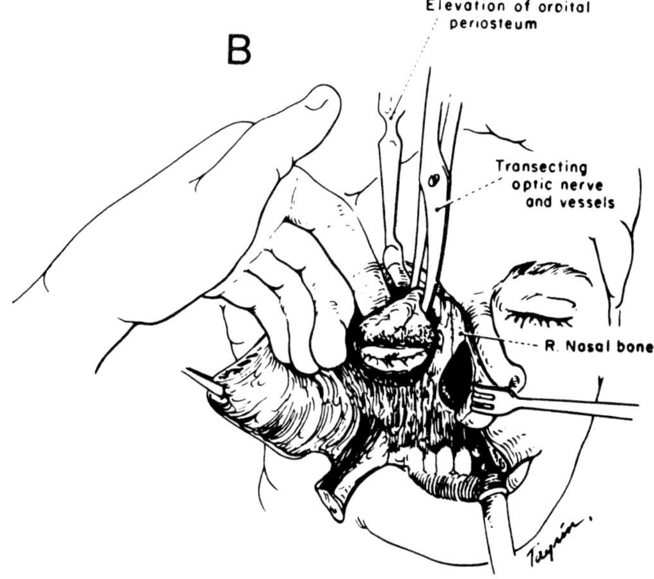

FIG 16–8.
A, the upper lid is dissected and retracted superiorly. The periosteum over the supraorbital rim is incised, as indicated. **B,** the periosteum is elevated from the superior, medial, and lateral walls of the orbit. As the orbital contents are retracted inferiorly with the index finger, a pair of long, curved scissors is inserted, cutting the optic nerve and vessels. The superior orbit is packed tightly with a moist gauze strip to control the bleeding. (From Montgomery WW: *Surgery of the Upper Respiratory System,* vol 1, ed 2. Philadelphia, Lea & Febiger, 1979. Used by permission.)

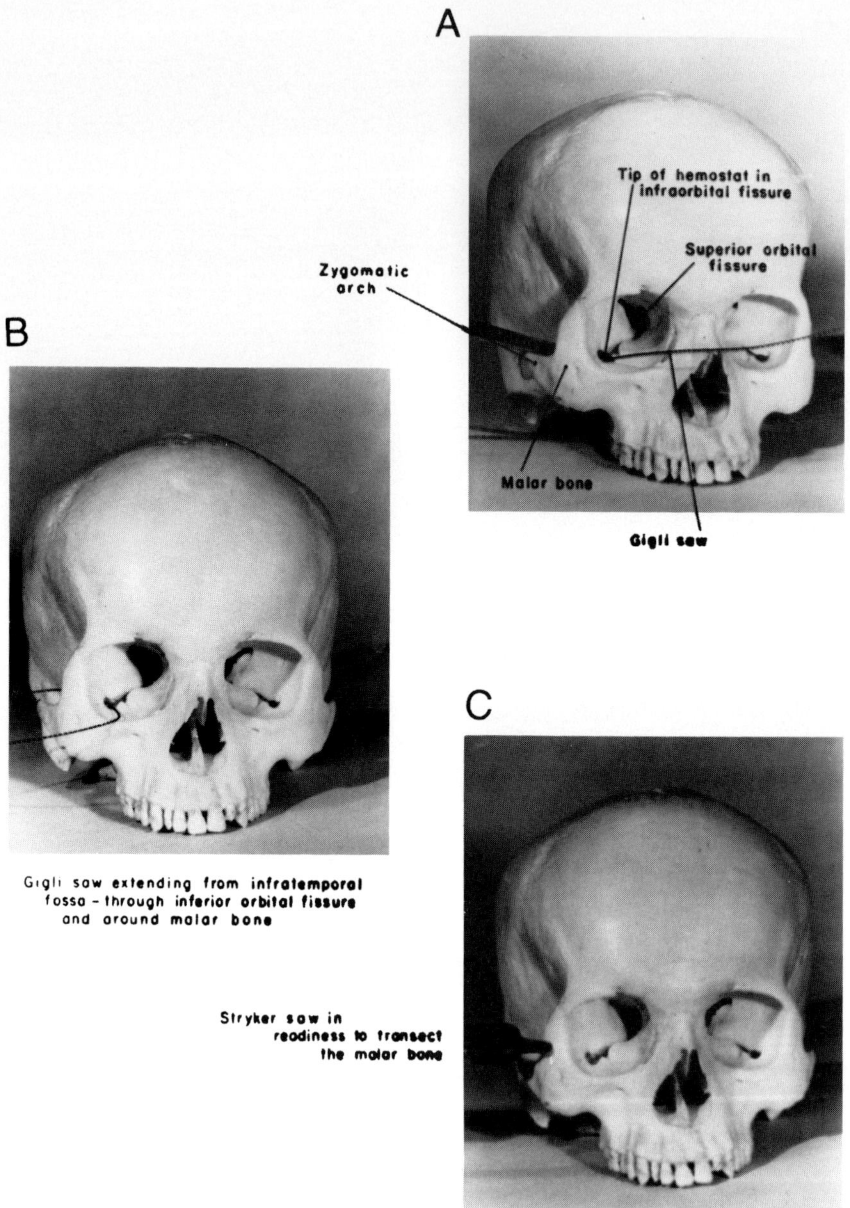

FIG 16–9.
A, the orbital contents are retracted medially, exposing the lateral aspect of the inferior orbital fissure. A curved hemostat is inserted under the malar bone and out the inferior orbital fissure to grasp one end of a Gigli saw. **B,** the malar bone is transected as far superiorly as is possible with the Gigli saw. **C,** a tangential Stryker saw with a sinus blade can be used for this bone incision. (From Montgomery WW: *Surgery of the Upper Respiratory System,* vol 1, ed 2. Philadelphia, Lea & Febiger, 1979. Used by permission.)

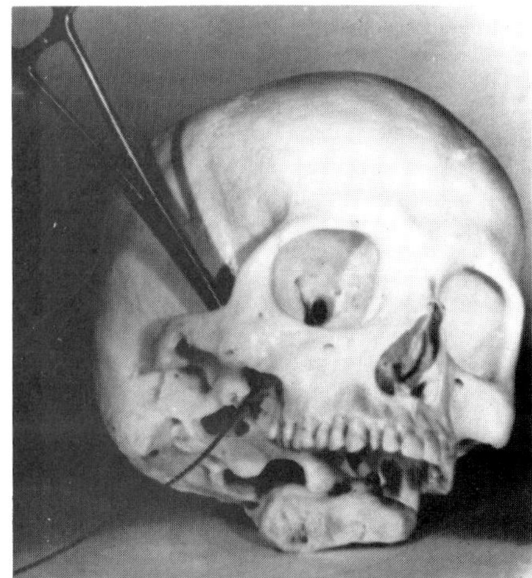

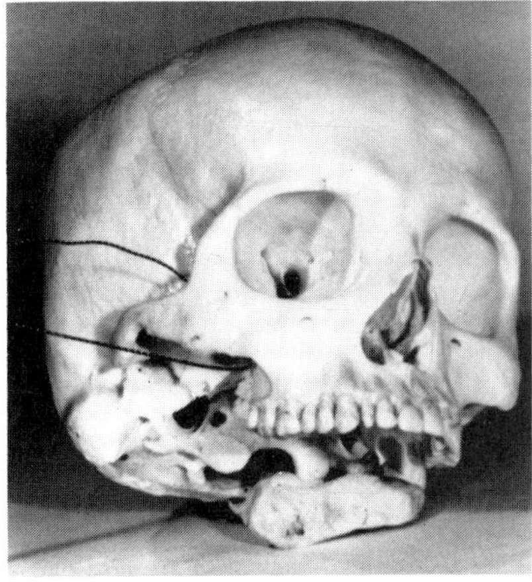

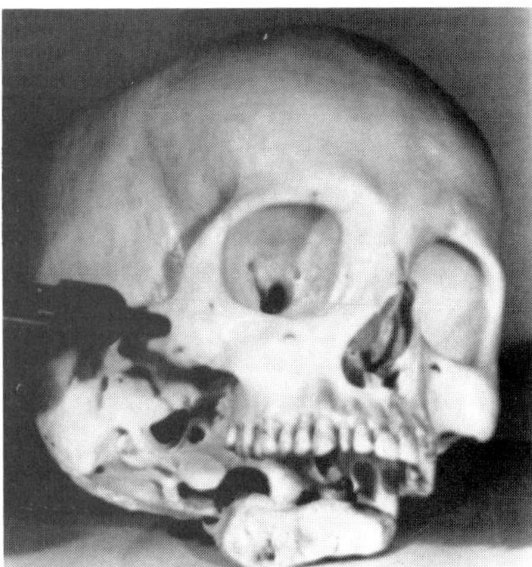

FIG 16–10.
A, a curved hemostat is inserted under the zygomatic arch to grasp one end of a Gigli saw. **B**, the zygomatic arch is transected just lateral to the malar eminence. **C**, a tangential saw can be used to section the zygomatic arch. (From Montgomery WW: *Surgery of the Upper Respiratory System,* vol 1, ed 2. Philadelphia, Lea & Febiger, 1979. Used by permission.)

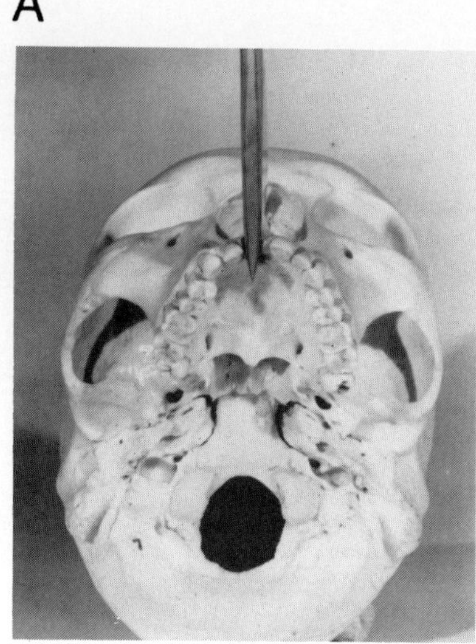

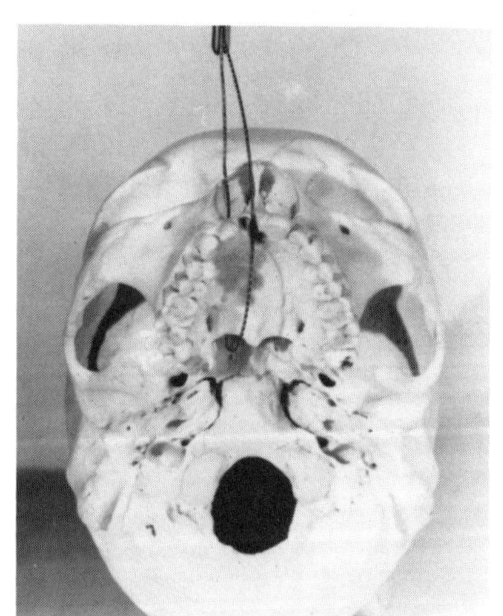

FIG 16–11.
A, the simplest method of sectioning the hard palate is with the use of a wide osteotome. The blade is placed in the midline on the alveolar ridge and just to the right (maxillectomy side) of the nasal septum in the nasal cavity. **B**, the Gigli saw can be used to section the hard palate. A hemostat is inserted into the right nasal cavity for grasping one end of the Gigli saw, which has been inserted in the midline at the posterior margin of the hard palate. **C**, as the hard palate is being sectioned, the Gigli saw is pulled slightly to the left (opposite maxillectomy side). (From Montgomery WW: *Surgery of the Upper Respiratory System,* vol 1, ed 2. Philadelphia, Lea & Febiger, 1979. Used by permission.)

A

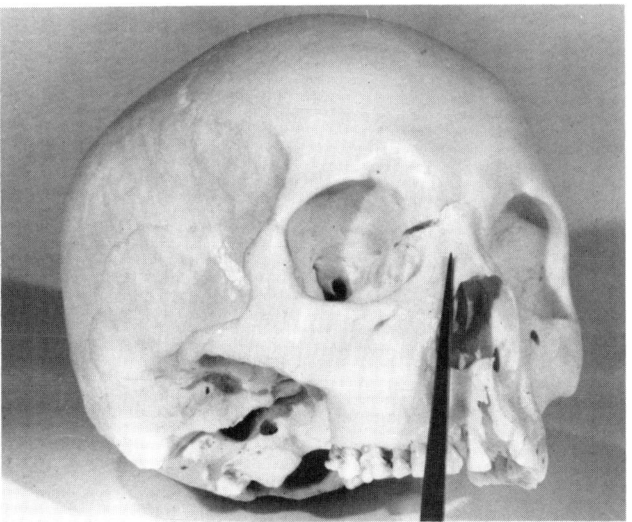

B

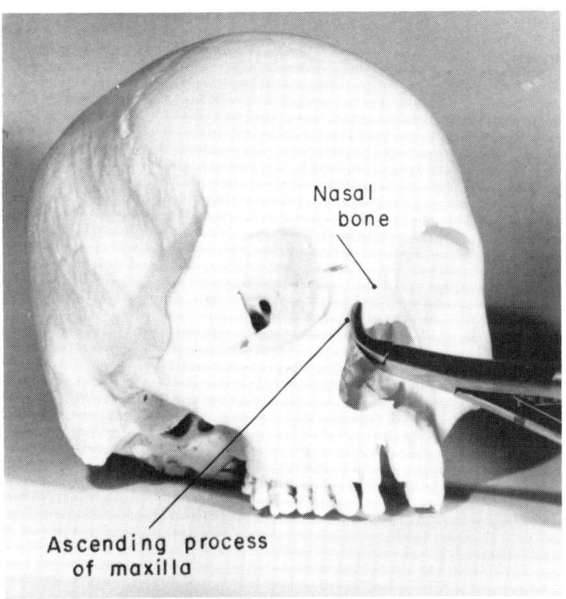

FIG 16–12.
A, the nasal bone is separated from the ascending process of the maxilla by inserting an osteotome between the two. The osteotome is introduced to the level of the nasal process of the frontal bone. **B**, this dissection can also be accomplished by removing a portion of the ascending process of the maxilla adjacent to the nasal bone with a rongeur. (From Montgomery WW: *Surgery of the Upper Respiratory System,* vol 1, ed 2. Philadelphia, Lea & Febiger, 1979. Used by permission.)

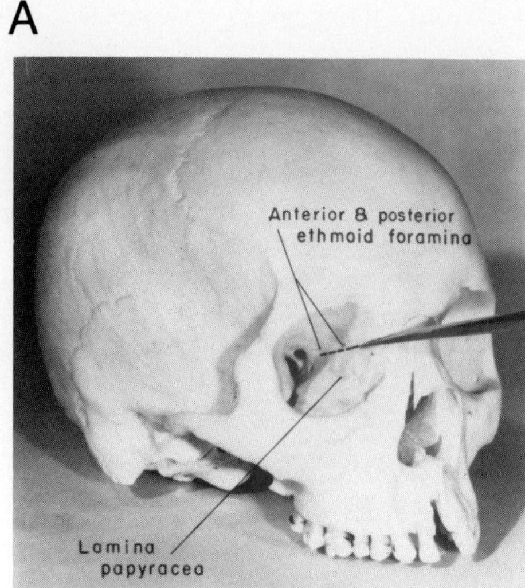

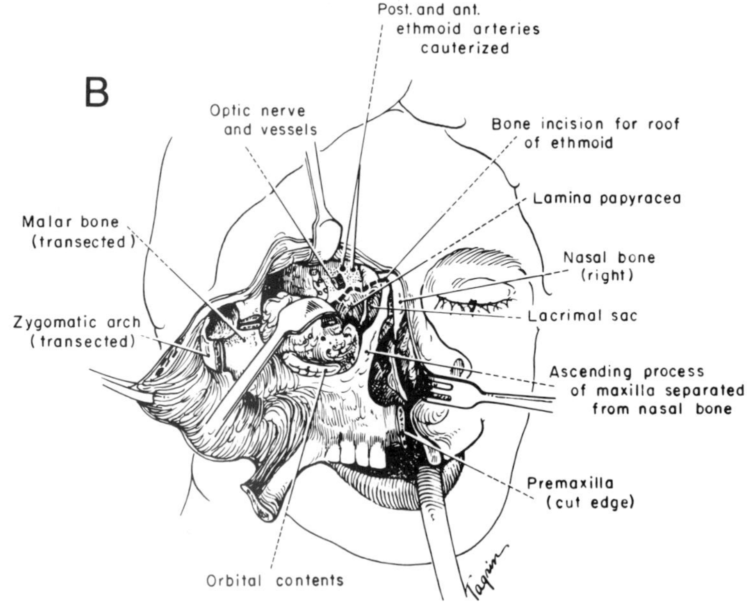

FIG 16–13.
A, the medial wall of the orbit is exposed by retracting the orbital contents downward and laterally. The anterior and posterior ethmoid arteries are cauterized and sectioned. **B,** an osteotome is placed just below the suture line between the orbital process of the frontal bone and the lamina papyracea, using the ethmoid foramina as guides. (From Montgomery WW: *Surgery of the Upper Respiratory System,* vol 1, ed 2. Philadelphia, Lea & Febiger, 1979, Used by permission.)

Posterior Dissection

The masseter muscle is detached from the maxilla. There are two methods to handle the posterior dissection. If the posterior wall of the antrum remains intact, an osteotome is inserted between the maxilla and the pterygoid process (Fig 16–14,A). Most often it is impossible to determine whether or not the posterior wall of the antrum is involved with the tumor, and thus an alternate method must be used. The pterygoid muscles are detached from the medial and lateral pterygoid plates. A large curved osteotome is placed behind the pterygoid plates, and the pterygoid process is transected near its origin from the remainder of the sphenoid bone (Fig 16–14,B). Brisk bleeding from the internal maxillary artery may be encountered in this area.

Specimen Removal (Fig 16–15)

After the pterygoid processes have been freed, the specimen is attached only by the posterior and medial aspect of the bony orbit and the pterygomaxillary fossa. A heavy pair of scissors is placed behind the pterygoid plates and then wherever the specimen remains intact. As soon as the specimen is removed, a large hot pack is inserted into the cavity. Time can now be taken for examination of the specimen to determine the extent of the disease. The packing is removed, and the internal maxillary artery is ligated. The remaining portions of the ethmoid labyrinth, the anterior wall of the sphenoid sinus, and other areas where there could be possible extension of the disease are resected, and the cavity is lined with a split-thickness skin graft (Fig 16–16).

Skin Closure (Fig 16–17)

With the cross-hatchings as a guide, the flap is replaced subcutaneously with 3-0 chromic catgut. Dermal suture material (5-0) is used for the skin closure. A light dressing is placed over the orbit, face, and side of the nose. A nasogastric feeding tube is inserted by way of the nasal cavity opposite the operated side. It remains in place for approximately 4 days or until the patient is able to feed himself or herself properly. If there is any sign of impending respiratory obstruction, or if a radical neck dissection has been carried out with the maxillectomy, a tracheotomy should be performed.

Postoperative Care

The packing is removed between the seventh and 10th postoperative day. An impression for a temporary prosthesis is made at this time if this was not done prior to the operation. Moist cotton packing can be used temporarily to fill the defect. It is changed several times a day, especially after each meal. The cavity should be carefully cleaned each day with hydrogen peroxide solution and irrigated with warm saline solution. Excessive skin that has been grafted is trimmed. A permanent dental prosthesis is made 4 to 6 weeks postoperatively when all healing has taken place.

As a general rule, a dental prosthesis is preferable to a reconstructed palate because it provides for easier inspection of the cavity, and recurrent disease can be identified at an early date. If the mucous membrane and periosteum of the hard palate have been preserved (see Figs 16–5,B and C), the defect in the palate may be eliminated. When the hard palate is reconstructed, the resultant skin-lined cavity, which produces much debris, may result in a crusting and an odor problem. There are three methods for constructing the palate: (1) using a pedicled flap consisting of the entire forehead based on one temporal artery (this is tunneled in through the cheek); (2) using a cervical pedicled skin flap that is pulled up and through the cheek; or (3) swinging the nasal septum, which has been incised anteriorly, superiorly, and posteriorly and hinged inferiorly and laterally to cover the palatal defect.

Maxillectomy With Preservation of the Orbit

A medial and lateral tarsorrhaphy should be performed prior to making the maxillectomy incision. This is done to prevent edema and ectropion of the lower lid postoperatively. The rhinotomy and the upper lip, gingivobuccal, and palatal incisions are made as described previously. The horizontal incision under the eye extends across the lower lid within 2 to 3 cm from the tarsal plates (see Fig 16–5). The lower lid is elevated in a plane above the orbicularis oculi muscle. The flap is elevated, preserving the orbicularis oculi and buccinator muscles. The entire front face of the maxilla, ascending process, inferior orbital rim, zygomatic arch, and malar bone are exposed.

A periosteal incision is made along the inferior orbital rim (Fig 16–18,A). The periosteum is elevated from the floor and lower medial and lateral walls of the orbit. A curved hemostat is inserted under the malar bone, the tip presenting in the inferior orbital fissure (see Fig 16–9) to grasp one end of a Gigli saw, which is used to transect the malar bone. If the floor of the orbit is to be preserved, the orbital periosteum is not elevated from it.

The remainder of the operation is as has been described for maxillectomy with orbital exenteration. The ethmoid is usually transected at a slightly lower level than is shown in Fig 16–13. The remainder of the ethmoid cells are carefully removed after the specimen has been resected.

There are two methods to obtain support for the orbit if the bony floor has been removed:

1. The temporalis muscle is detached from the coronoid process of the mandible. It is slung under the orbital periosteum and sutured in the region of the inner canthus. The temporalis muscle, as well as the remainder of the maxillectomy defect, is covered with a split-thickness skin graft.

2. An alternate, but not quite as effective, method to support the orbit is that of suturing a sling of skin graft under the orbital periosteum (Fig 16–18,B). As the graft becomes attached to the periosteum and contracts, it supplies a good support to the orbit.

It is best not to disturb the tarsorrhaphy incision for several weeks to prevent edema and ectropion of the lower lid. The remainder of the postoperative care is as has been outlined for maxillectomy with orbital exenteration.

A

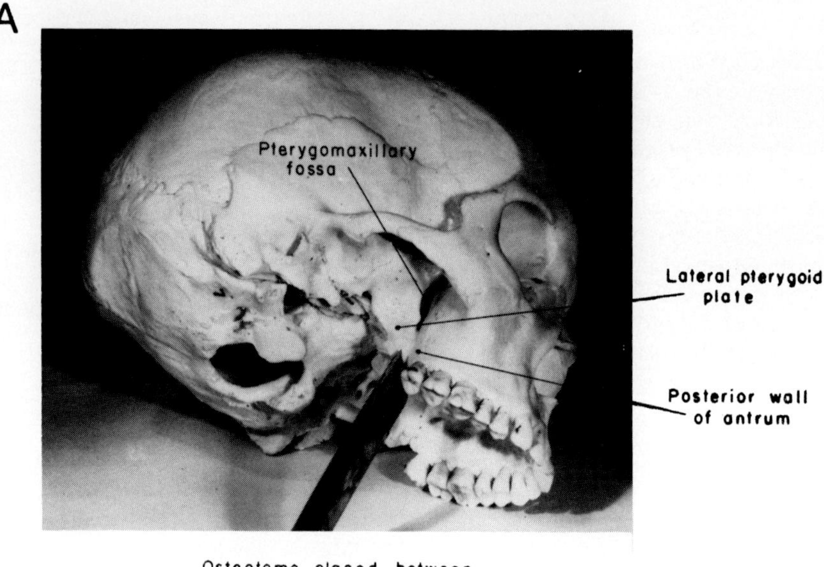

B

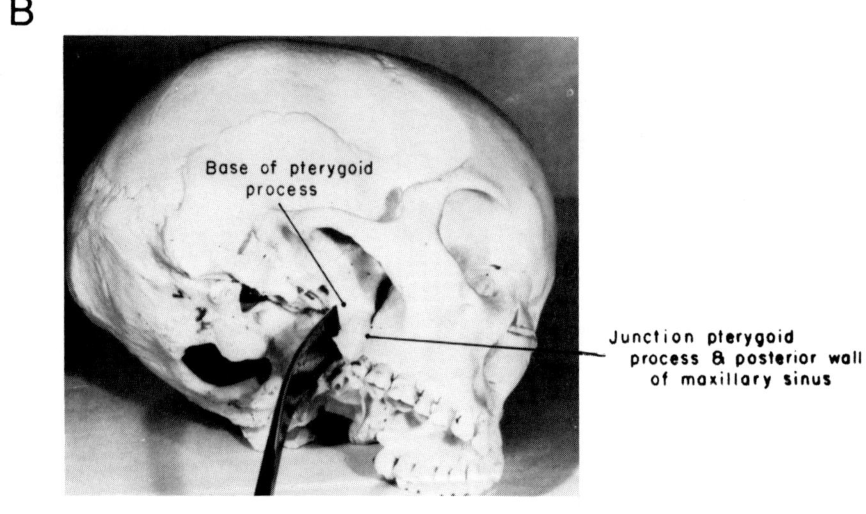

FIG 16–14.
A, if it can be determined preoperatively that the posterior wall of the antrum is intact, the dissection is accomplished between the pterygoid plates and the maxilla. **B,** usually it is necessary to remove the pterygoid plates with the specimen. The external and internal pterygoid muscles are sectioned at their origin. A curved osteotome is inserted behind the pterygoid plates, and the pterygoid process is sectioned at its base. (From Montgomery WW: *Surgery of the Upper Respiratory System,* vol 1, ed 2. Philadelphia, Lea & Febiger, 1979. Used by permission.)

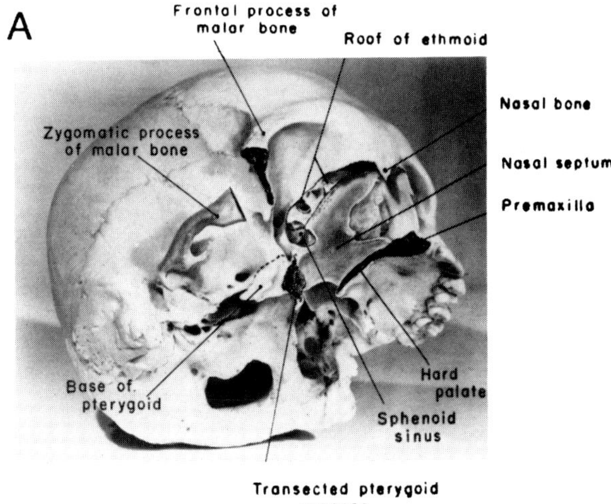

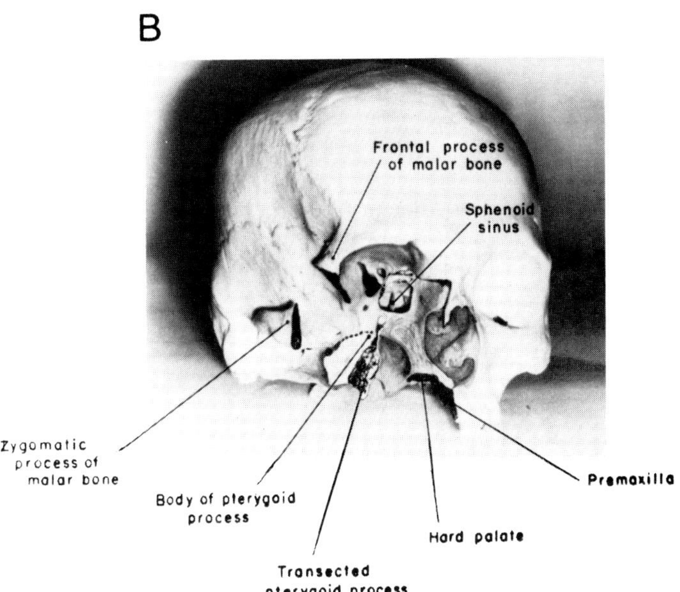

FIG 16–15.
A, the maxillectomy has been completed. The remaining walls of the orbit, the roof of the ethmoid labyrinth, the nasal septum, and sphenoid sinus, and the pterygomaxillary fossa should be clearly delineated. **B**, a frontal view demonstrating the interior of the sphenoid sinus and posterior aspect of the orbit. (From Montgomery WW: *Surgery of the Upper Respiratory System,* vol 1, ed 2. Philadelphia, Lea & Febiger, 1979. Used by permission.)

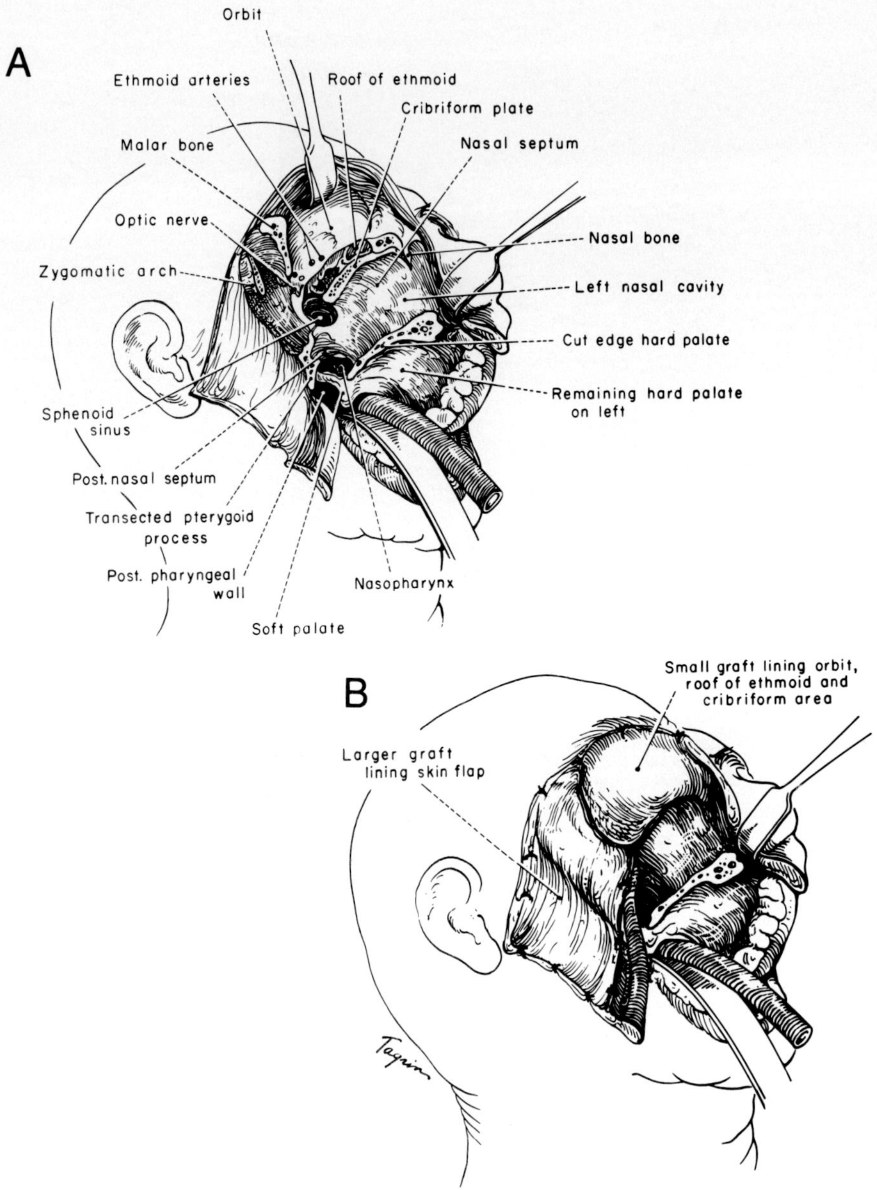

FIG 16–16.
A, a sketch showing the parts mentioned in Figure 16–15 in relation to the surrounding soft tissues. **B,** all areas void of mucous membrane are grafted with split-thickness skin graft obtained from the inner aspect of the thigh. Usually two pieces of graft are used. A smaller piece is used to cover the cribriform area, roof of the ethmoid sinuses, and the orbit. A second piece extends from the front face of the sphenoid sinus, covering the inner aspect of the facial flap. (From Montgomery WW: *Surgery of the Upper Respiratory System,* vol 1, ed 2. Philadelphia, Lea & Febiger, 1979. Used by permission.)

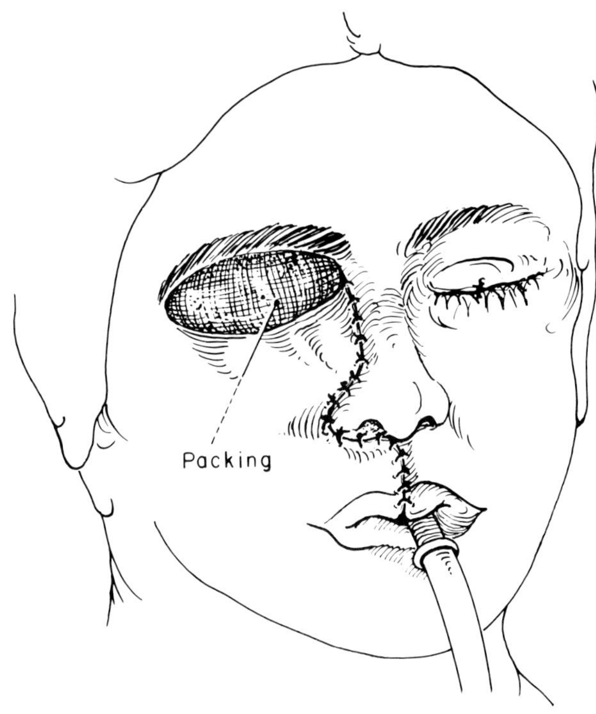

FIG 16–17.
The skin graft is covered with a layer of absorbable gelatin sponge (Gelfoam) to prevent the graft from being pulled away when the packing is removed. The maxillectomy cavity is packed with 1-inch chlortetracycline-impregnated iodoform gauze prior to replacement of the facial flap. The incisions are closed subcutaneously with interrupted 3-0 chromic catgut, and the skin edges are approximated with 5-0 dermal suture material. (From Montgomery WW: *Surgery of the Upper Respiratory System,* vol 1, ed 2. Philadelphia, Lea & Febiger, 1979. Used by permission.)

EXTERNAL SURGERY OF THE FRONTAL SINUS

Indications

Chronic Frontal Sinusitis

Chronic frontal sinusitis that does not respond to medical therapy or conservative surgical therapy or that is complicated by persistent pain, nasal discharge, intracranial extension, bone necrosis, orbital complications, mucocele, or pyocele is an indication for surgical intervention. The osteoplastic frontal sinus operation is the procedure most frequently employed for chronic frontal sinus disease. In the past, the frontoethmoidectomy (Lynch) procedure was popular; however, many patients remained symptomatic after this operation and often required further surgery. The anterior osteoplastic adipose obliteration operation offers several advantages over the frontoethmoidectomy approach:

1. It permits complete and direct visualization of the frontal sinus.
2. It allows visualization and management of the nasofrontal communication.

3. It is not disfiguring, because the anatomic boundaries remain intact.
4. It allows management of the posterior table of the frontal sinus and dura problems.
5. It permits complete removal of the mucous membrane and inner cortical lining of the frontal sinus.
6. It allows the sinus to be completely obliterated with an adipose implant.
7. It reduces postoperative care to a minimum.

Benign or Malignant Tumors

The unilateral osteoplastic frontal sinus operation can be used on occasion with benign tumor such as osteoma. Removal of an osteoma using the frontoethmoidectomy approach can be very deforming. Also, evidence obtained from animal studies and clinical experience strongly emphasizes the necessity of removing both the mucosal and inner cortical lining of the frontal sinus and obliteration with adipose tissue for a successful result.

Malignant tumors of the frontal sinus, which are rare, are most often approached by way of the frontoethmoidectomy procedure because the extent of the disease is undetermined before surgery. The operation is usually followed by radiation therapy.

Trauma of the Frontal Sinus

Depressed and comminuted fractures of the anterior wall of the frontal sinus are best treated by employing the osteoplastic adipose obliteration technique to obtain good cosmesis and avoid sequelae such as mucocele or pyocele.

A fracture of the posterior wall of the frontal sinus (anterior wall of the anterior cranial fossa) may be accompanied by a CSF leak. Surgical intervention is indicated (1) when the leakage is of more than 6 weeks' duration, (2) when the leakage is intermittent, (3) when pneumoencephalus is present, or (4) when there is a history of recurrent meningitis and CSF otorrhea. Defects in the posterior frontal wall are best approached by way of the osteoplastic frontal sinus operation.

Sinocutaneous Fistula

Sinocutaneous fistula from the frontal sinus can extend from the sinus to the skin surface by way of the anterior or inferior walls of the frontal sinus. Occasionally the disease process is directed from the frontal sinus through the ethmoid sinuses before surfacing. Undoubtedly it begins as a localized osteomyelitis. The disease is approached by using the osteoplastic frontal sinus procedure. Intravenous antibiotics must be administered preoperatively and continued postoperatively for 2 weeks, followed by oral antibiotics for 1 month.

Bilateral Osteoplastic Frontal Sinus Operation

Preoperative Preparation

Preoperative radiographs are obtained to determine the extent of the disease. A template outlining the frontal sinuses is fashioned from the Caldwell view. A nasal culture is taken

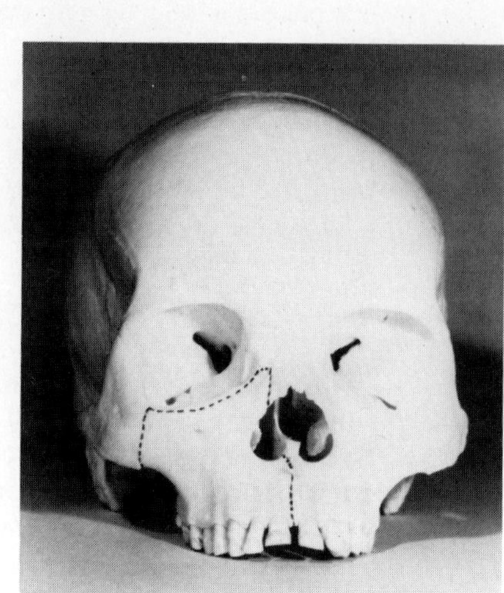

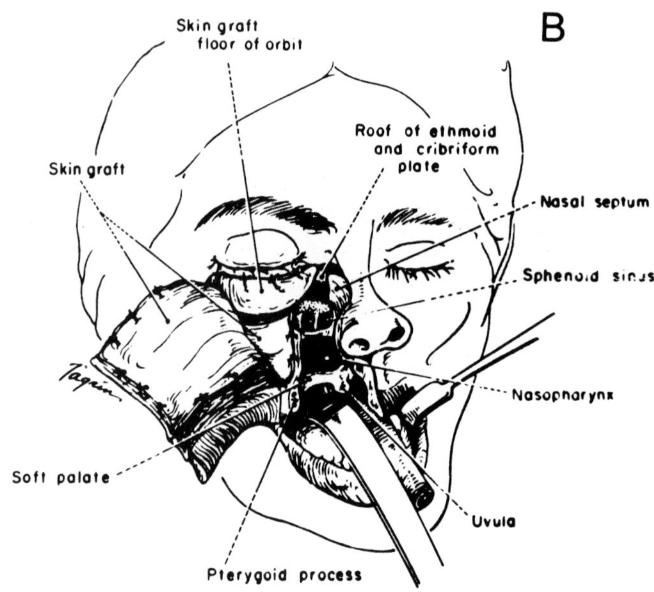

FIG 16–18.
A, periosteal and bone incisions to be used when the bony floor of the orbit is to be preserved. Other bone incisions are similar to those shown in Figure 16–5. **B,** skin grafting is employed to cover either the bony floor of the orbit or the orbital periosteum. In the latter instance, the skin graft, as it contracts, provides support for the orbital contents. A second graft extends from the lateral margin of the front face of the sphenoid sinus laterally, lining the inner aspect of the facial flap. (From Montgomery WW: *Surgery of the Upper Respiratory System,* vol 1, ed 2. Philadelphia, Lea & Febiger, 1979. Used by permission.)

well in advance so that appropriate antibiotic therapy may be initiated before, during, and after surgery. If the coronal incision is to be used, the patient is given a thorough hexachlorophine shampoo the evening before surgery. The abdomen is shaved and prepared so that subcutaneous adipose tissue can be obtained during surgery.

Surgical Technique

Either the eyebrow or coronal incision can be used for the bilateral osteoplastic frontal sinus operation (Fig 16–19). The coronal incision is made approximately 2.5 cm posterior to the anterior hairline. This location is most suitable for female patients but can also be used in some male patients. Hemostatic skin clips facilitate control of bleeding. The bilateral eyebrow incision is made along the entire length of the upper margin of both eyebrows and straight across the nasal process of the frontal bone. The flap is elevated in a plane between the frontalis muscle and the pericranium.

The x-ray template is sterilized and placed over the frontal periosteum. A no. 15 surgical blade is used to incise the periosteum around the outline of the template. A horizontal incision is made in the periosteum over the nasal process of the frontal bone and the supraorbital rims both medially and laterally. Superiorly, a bone incision is made with a Stryker sagittal saw. This incision is made on a bevel to ensure an accurate reapproximation of the osteoplastic flap (Fig 16–20,A).

As the osteoplastic flap is elevated and reflected inferiorly and anteriorly, a fracture invariably occurs just behind the supraorbital rims where the bone is quite thin (Fig 16–20,B). If the interfrontal septum is present and interferes with the elevation of the flap, it is incised by inserting an osteotome from above before the flap is elevated.

The diseased process is visualized and removed along with the mucous membrane of the frontal sinus and superior aspect of the nasofrontal ducts. A rotating cutting bur is used to remove remnants of the mucous membrane and inner cortical lining from within the sinus and the inner aspects of the osteoplastic flap.

Subcutaneous abdominal adipose tissue is obtained by using a left horizontal rectus incision. Subcutaneous catgut sutures eliminate the dead space resulting from the removal. Blood vessels are carefully ligated to prevent hematoma. Closed suction drainage is placed for 24 to 48 hours. It is important to obtain the adipose tissue immediately before its transfer to the frontal sinus. The adipose tissue should not be traumatized by forceps or hemostats. This tissue is fashioned so that it completely fills the frontal sinus cavity and superior aspects of both nasofrontal ducts. The osteoplastic flap is then replaced and secured with multiple periosteal sutures. If there is any doubt as to the stability of the flap, it should be secured with two wire sutures (Fig 16–21).

The coronal incision is repaired as a single layer using 3-0 polyethylene sutures. The double eyebrow incision must be closed in layers with great care using 3-0 and 4-0 chromic catgut sutures for the subcutaneous layers and 6-0 and 7-0 mild chromic suture material for the skin layer. The incision line is supported with adhesive skin strips, and a pressure dressing is placed over

the forehead for 24 to 48 hours. Antibiotics are continued for at least 7 days postoperatively.

Unilateral Osteoplastic Frontal Sinus Operation

The unilateral osteoplastic frontal sinus operation is carried out in much the same manner as the bilateral procedure. The x-ray template of the frontal sinus is prepared from the Caldwell radiograph. The incision is made along the entire length of the upper margin of the eyebrow and is carried through the subcutaneous tissues and the frontalis muscle to the periosteum covering the bone. It is essential not to enter the periosteum, so as to preserve the blood supply to the osteoplastic flap. A plane of cleavage is established between the frontalis muscle and the frontal periosteum. An incision is made in the periosteum around the template, with care not to disturb the periosteum inside or below the incision. The bone incision is made along the outline of the periosteal incision by using a Stryker saw blade designed for this purpose. The flap is elevated and the diseased tissue removed. The mucous membrane of the sinus is removed along with the inner cortical lining, and the sinus is obliterated with fresh adipose tissue.

If a benign tumor such as an osteoma is present, it is

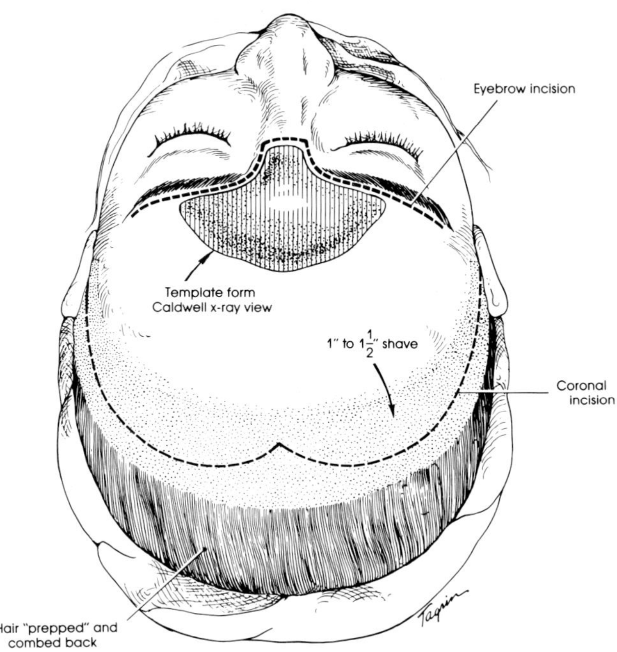

FIG 16–19.
The coronal incision is made approximately 2.5 cm (1 in.) posterior to the anterior hairline. This is most suitable for female patients but can also be used for male patients. The bilateral eyebrow incision is made along the entire length of the upper margin of both eyebrows and straight across the nasal process of the frontal bone. Both flaps are elevated in a plane between the fontalis muscle and the pericranium. A pattern for the periosteal incision is obtained from a Caldwell radiograph. (From Montgomery WW: *Surgery of the Upper Respiratory System*, vol 1, ed 2. Philadelphia, Lea & Febiger, 1979. Used by permission.)

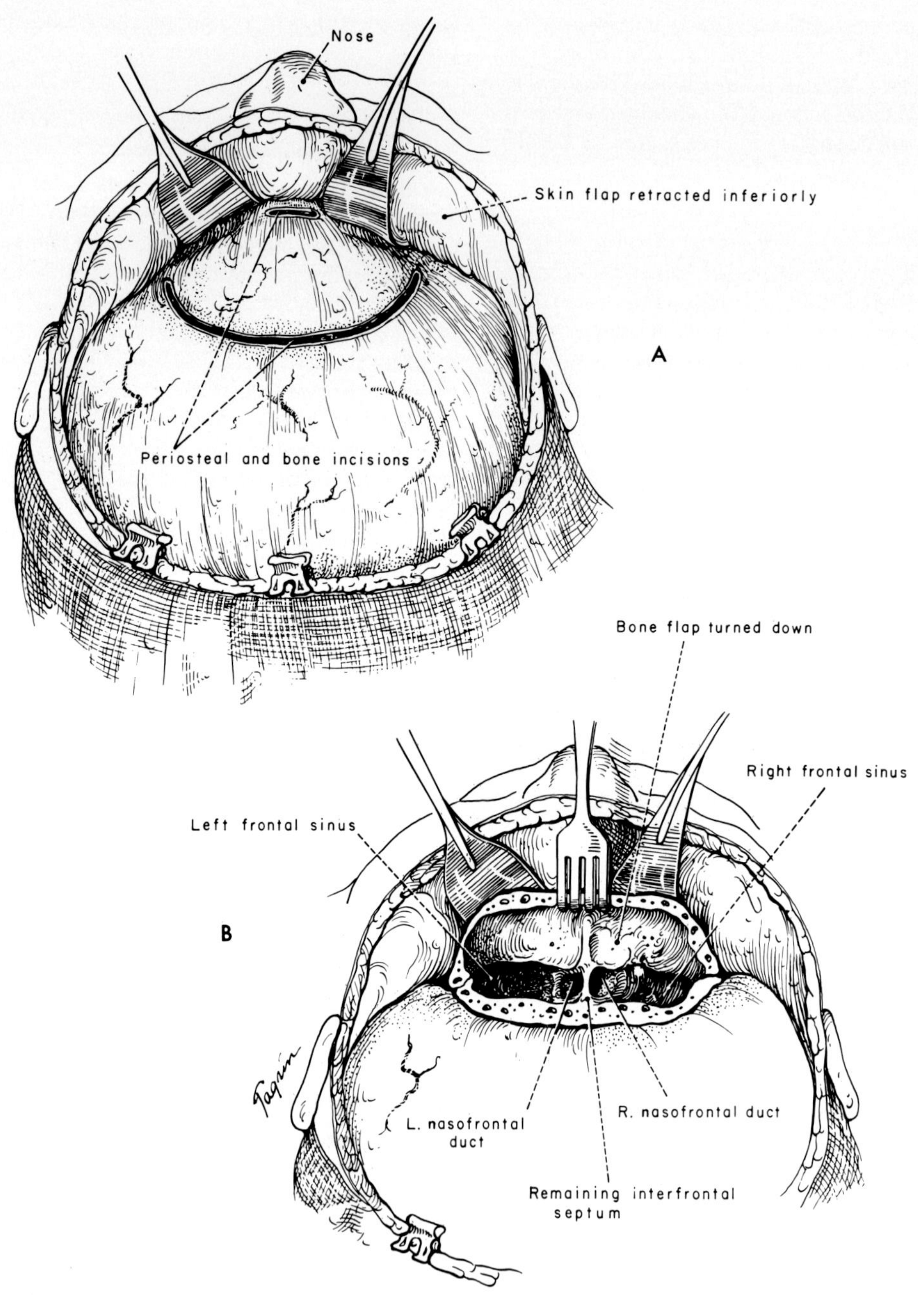

FIG 16–20.
A, the coronal flap has been reflected inferiorly. It is most important that the periosteum and bone incisions include the supraorbital rim medially and laterally on each side. **B,** the osteoplastic flap has been elevated, exposing the contents of both frontal sinuses. (From Montgomery WW: *Surgery of the Upper Respiratory System,* vol 1, ed 2. Philadelphia, Lea & Febiger, 1979. Used by permission.)

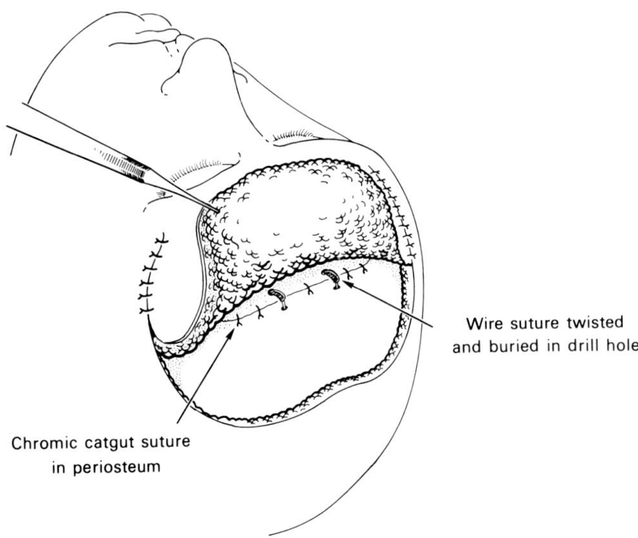

FIG 16–21.
As a general rule, the osteoplastic flap can be tightly secured in place by suturing the periosteum with chromic catgut sutures. If, on the other hand, the periosteum is deficient or defective, or there is any question that the osteoplastic flap might become dislodged and migrate forward, four drill holes should be placed as shown and the wire sutures applied. The twisted ends of these wire sutures are buried in a drill hole, as illustrated. (From Montgomery WW: *Surgery of the Upper Respiratory System,* vol 1, ed 2. Philadelphia, Lea & Febiger, 1979. Used by permission.)

removed and the sinus obliterated with adipose tissue after removal of both the sinus mucosa and inner cortical lining. If the sinus is not obliterated, a mucocele or pyocele may develop.

The osteoplastic flap is returned to its original position, and the periosteum is sutured with 4-0 chromic sutures. The wound is closed with 4-0 chromic catgut sutures subcutaneously and 6-0 mild chromic catgut sutures.

The dressing remains in place 48 hours, and the sutures are removed on the fifth or sixth day. No postoperative care is necessary other than the administration of antibiotics.

Frontoethmoidectomy Operation

The frontoethmoidectomy incision is made along the inferior margin of the eyebrow extending inferiorly halfway between the inner canthus and the nasal dorsum onto the lateral aspect of the nose. It is carried through the skin, subcutaneous tissue, and periosteum. The periosteum is elevated. The anterior and posterior ethmoid arteries are approached carefully and cauterized before being resected. A complete anterior and posterior ethmoidectomy is performed with removal of the middle turbinate. The entire floor of the frontal sinus is resected so that the diseased tissue and mucous membrane can be removed from the sinus. A rubber or plastic tube can be placed between the frontal sinus and nasal cavity by way of the ethmoid labyrinth. If a tube is used, it is left in place for 1 to 3 months after the operation and often requires considerable care. The procedure

is usually followed by radiation therapy when a malignancy is treated.

EXTERNAL ETHMOIDECTOMY

Indications

External ethmoidectomy is indicated for those patients with acute ethmoiditis who do not respond to antibiotic therapy and have redness, swelling, and fluctuation over the ethmoid sinuses, as well as chronic ethmoid infection. Extension of the purulent infection into the orbital cavity with a resultant orbital abscess is also an indication for this operation. Mucocele, pyocele and tumors of the ethmoid must be approached by way of the external route.

With the presence of pain in the region of the ethmoid sinus and a palpable mass in the region of the medial aspect of the orbit or ptosis, mucocele of the ethmoid sinus should be considered in the differential diagnosis. Routine sinus x-ray films will most often confirm this diagnosis.

A mucocele of the ethmoid sinus can be a difficult diagnostic problem. There may be a history of pain, tenderness, and a swelling in the medial aspect of the orbit. If these signs and symptoms are intermittent, they may not be present at the time of examination by the physician. Routine x-ray films of the sinuses can be normal with the presence of a fairly large ethmoidal mucocele. Polytomography of the ethmoid sinus is an essential part of this workup, both to make the diagnosis and to outline the extent of an ethmoidal mucocele. Ultrasonography will demonstrate an orbital mass if the lamina papyracea has been displaced laterally. Computed tomography body scanning will show the presence of an ethmoidal mucocele.

Mucocele of the ethmoid sinus is removed using the external ethmoid operation. The entire ethmoid labyrinth should be resected along with the middle turbinate and its upper extension (medial wall of the ethmoid), otherwise there is a significant chance for recurrence of the mucocele. The external ethmoidectomy also provides the route for external frontal sinus surgery (the Lynch procedure) and an approach to the sphenoid sinus and to the pituitary gland.

Technique

Proper positioning of the patient's head for an external ethmoidectomy is imperative. The plane of the patient's face should be facing and exactly parallel to the ceiling, and the back of the head should rest in a donut-type head support. The patient's entire face, including the eyelids, is prepared using povidone-iodine soap and povidone-iodine solution. The face is scrubbed twice with this soap and each time is rinsed thoroughly using sterile water. Following the last rinse, the skin is dried diligently using sponges. The face is then carefully painted with povidone-iodine solution. After this solution dries, three towels are placed so as to leave both eyes and nose exposed. The towels are stitched together using 3-0 silk suture material on a straight Keith needle. The lids of both eyes are sutured together using 5-0 monofilament polyethylene suture material.

The area to be used for the external ethmoidectomy incision is carefully infiltrated with 1% lidocaine (Xylocaine) with added epinephrine. A half-sheet is applied over the upper portion of the chest such that the long ends cover each side of the table. An A-sheet is used as a second layer to cover the entire patient with the exception of the exposed portion of the face. Several 1/2-inch strips of cottonoid or cotton, impregnated with 4% cocaine solution, are used to pack the entire nasal cavity on the side of surgery. The purpose of this packing is to decongest the nasal mucous membrane and reduce its vascularity. The number of cottonoid, cotton, and gauze strips must be counted before, during, and after surgery.

There should be an interval of at least 10 minutes between the lidocaine-epinephrine infiltration and the skin incision. A slightly curved vertical incision approximately 2 to 3 cm long is made halfway between the inner canthus and the dorsum of the nose (Fig 16–22). Care is taken to make the initial incision through the skin only. Subcutaneous tissues are then carefully dissected layer by layer using a mosquito-type hemostat so that vessels can be identified, divided, and cauterized. Bipolar cautery is preferred to avoid the postoperative subcutaneous thickening that occurs when more than a few catgut ligatures are applied.

The periosteum should be exposed along the entire length of the incision before it is incised. The periosteum is elevated in an anteromedial direction, exposing the ascending process of the maxilla and the suture line between this structure and the nasal bone using a sharp, flat-end periosteal elevator such as is used during mastoidectomy surgery. This same instrument is used to elevate the periosteum in a posterolateral direction until the anterior crest of the lacrimal bone is identified.

Retraction of the incision is necessary at this point. Many self-retaining retractors designed for this purpose are bulky and cumbersome. Excellent retraction can be accomplished by using three no. 00 chromic catgut sutures on a taper needle on each side (Fig 16–23). The needle is introduced in the subcutaneous tissues and then through the margin of the periosteum, which has been elevated. These sutures are weighted by using heavy hemostats and, to protect the eyes, are placed over a folded 4 by 4 in. sponge or eyepad. The hemostats are allowed to hang so that they exert traction.

A more blunt and curve-ended periosteal elevator (e.g., a McKenty or Freer) is used to elevate the periosteum over the anterior lacrimal crest, lacrimal fossa, and posterior lacrimal crest. In so doing, the lacrimal sac, which is in continuity with the orbital periosteum, is carefully dissected laterally. The nasal lacrimal duct is identified so that it will not be injured. The periosteum superior to the lacrimal fossa is elevated by sweeping superiorly with the flap surface of a Ballenger periosteal elevator. This maneuver detaches the medial canthal ligament. The periosteum over the remainder of the medial wall of the orbit is very easily elevated using a Ballenger periosteal elevator aided by a short periorbital retractor.

The anterior and posterior ethmoid arteries are identified. These vessels are cauterized and transected. In so doing, the suture line between the lacrimal bone, lamina papyracea, and the orbital process of the frontal bone is identified. By identifying this suture line, the surgeon learns the level and direction of the roof of the ethmoid and cribriform plate.

The anterior ethmoid cells are located medial to the lacrimal bone and lateral to the upper lateral wall. These cells are entered by way of the lacrimal plate or fossa, depending on which bone is thinner. A mastoid curette is best suited for this dissection. The opening is enlarged sufficiently so that a Kerrison rongeur can be used to remove the entire lacrimal bone and at least a portion of the ascending process of the maxilla. The entire ascending process of the maxilla in this region can be removed without any resulting cosmetic deformity. The membranous and bony anterior ethmoid cells are removed using Brownie or Takahashi forceps and a mastoid curette. The bone medial to the anterior ethmoid cells is carefully elevated from the lateral aspect of the mucous membrane of the superior anterior lateral nasal wall that is anterior to the anterior tip of the middle turbinate. Once the lateral aspect of this mucous membrane is exposed in its entirety, a U-shaped incision is made so as to fashion a posteriorly based mucous membrane flap (Fig 16–24).

The intranasal packing is visualized and removed. The strips are counted so that none remain behind. When this flap is reflected in a posterolateral direction, the mucous membrane of the nasal septum and the anterior tip of the middle turbinate can be visualized. The purpose of this maneuver is to avoid misdirected surgery and injury to the mucous membrane of the nasal septum. The mucosal flap is of no further value at this point and can be resected.

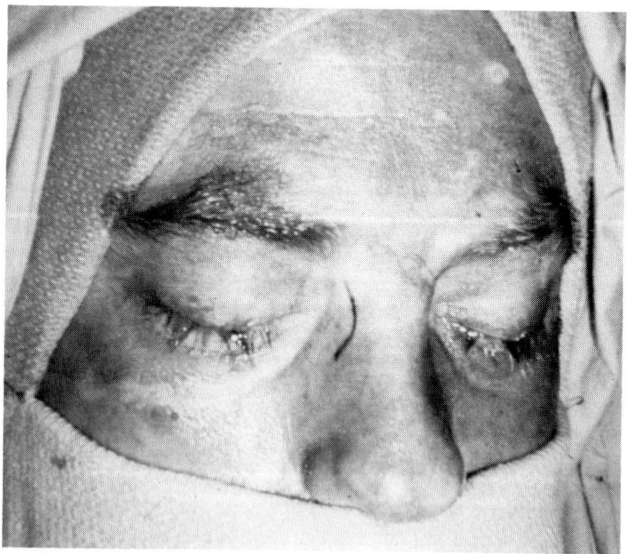

FIG 16–22.
The slightly curved vertical incision is approximately 2 to 3 cm long and placed halfway between the inner canthus and the dorsum of the nose. (From Montgomery WW: *Surgery of the Upper Respiratory System,* vol 1, ed 2. Philadelphia, Lea & Febiger, 1979. Used by permission.)

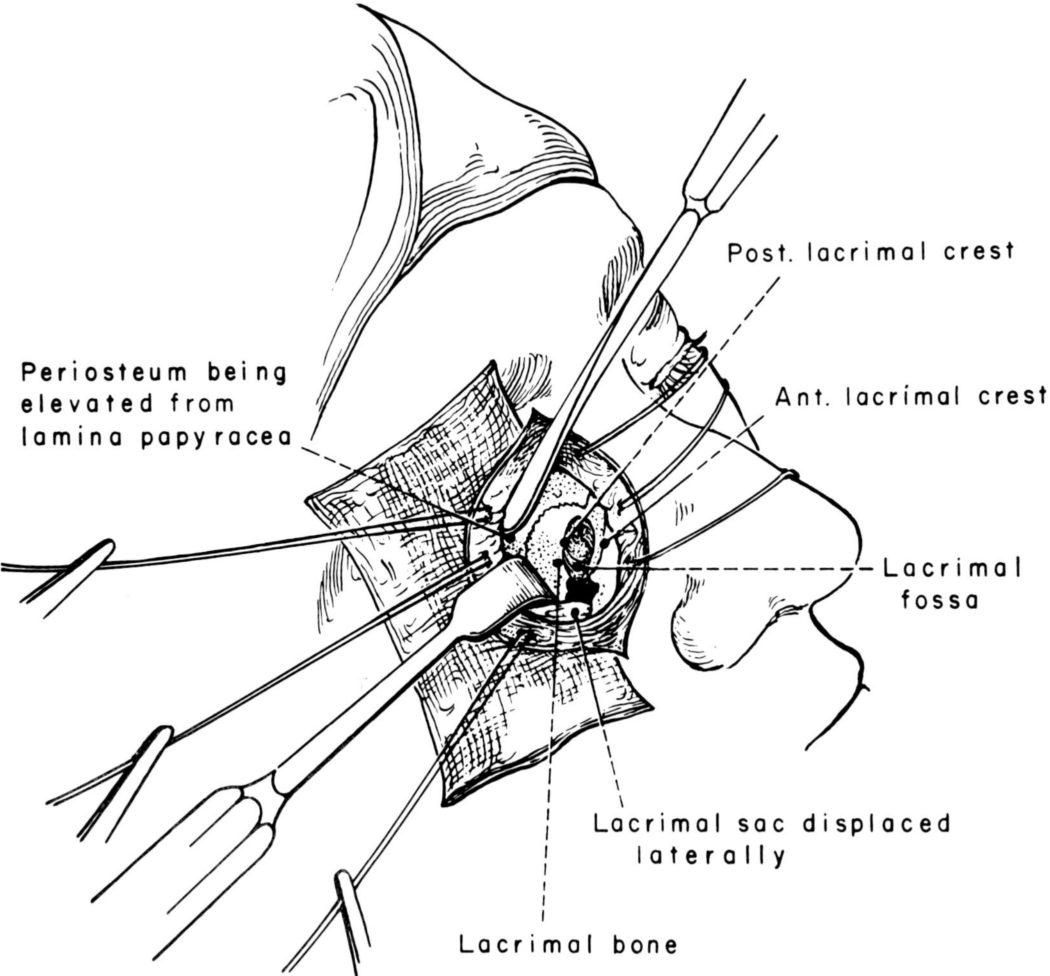

FIG 16–23.
The incision has been carried through the periosteum. Chromic catgut (0-0) sutures are used for retraction. The periosteum and lacrimal sac have been dissected and are retracted laterally. The ascending process of the maxilla, lacrimal fossa, lacrimal bone, and a portion of the lamina papyracea can be seen. (From Montgomery WW: *Surgery of the Upper Respiratory System,* vol 1, ed 2. Philadelphia, Lea & Febiger, 1979. Used by permission.)

At this stage, the middle turbinate and its upper extension, which form the medial wall of the ethmoid labyrinth (Fig 16–25), and the lamina papyracea, which forms the lateral wall of the posterior ethmoid labyrinth, remain intact. Knowing this situation and also having determined the level and direction of the roof of the ethmoid by identifying the ethmoid arteries (this information can be double-checked by examining the lateral view sinus x-ray films), the surgeon can remove the remaining ethmoid cells without fear of misdirected surgery. It is usually necessary to remove approximately one half of the lamina papyracea during this latter dissection. The orbital periosteum is protected during this dissection by use of periorbital retractors of varying lengths.

The anterior tip of the middle turbinate and the entire medial wall of the ethmoid labyrinth are now in view. The upper extension of the attachment of the middle turbinate is cut using turbinate scissors. If these scissors are not available, Mayo scissors can be used. The upper attachment of the middle turbinate is cut to the level of the front face of the sphenoid sinus. If there is any doubt about the position of the front face of the sphenoid, it can be easily identified by palpating the rostrum of the sphenoid bone intranasally with any probelike instrument.

The middle turbinate can be transected posteriorly using a nasal polyp snare or the turbinate scissors. On occasion, it is necessary to remove the turbinate piecemeal. As the turbinate is resected, there is most often rather brisk bleeding from the nasal branches of the sphenopalatine artery. This bleeding is controlled using cautery applied with an insulated suction tip or packing with gauze strips.

At the completion of the ethmoidectomy, the nasal septum, intranasal and ethmoid portions of the anterior face of the sphenoid sinus, the olfactory region, the entire roof of the ethmoid, the ostium of the sphenoid sinus, the communication to the frontal sinus, and the remaining portion of the lamina papyracea should be identified.

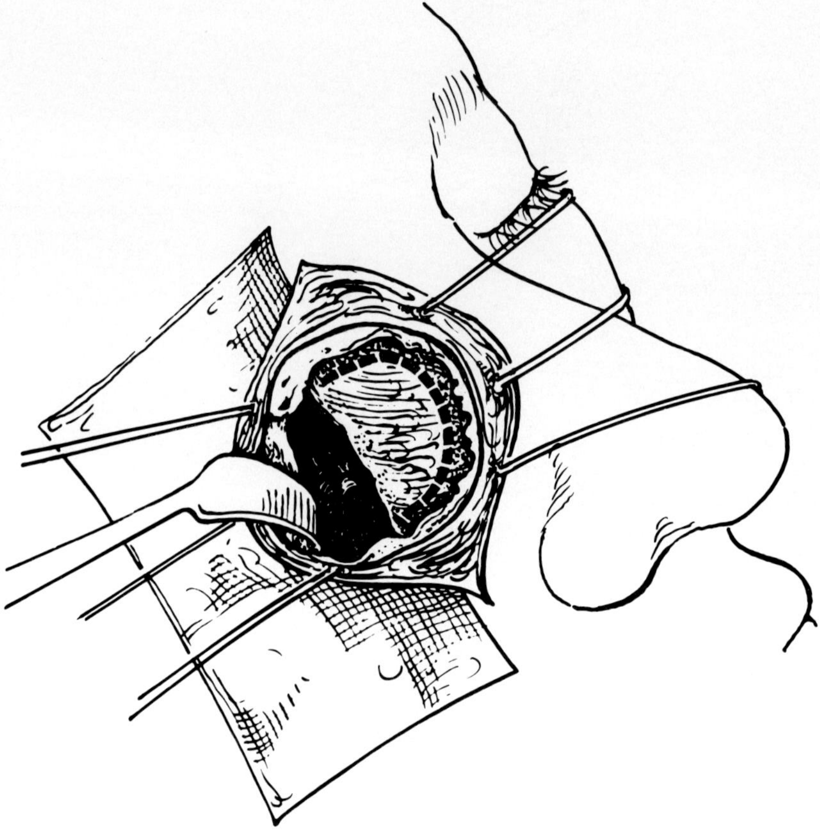

FIG 16–24.
An incision is made in the mucous membrane of the lateral nasal wall as indicated. The posteriorly based flap thus created is reflected laterally, exposing the superior nasal cavity, nasal septum, and anterior tip of the middle turbinate. When these structures have been positively identified, the flap is removed. (From Montgomery WW: *Surgery of the Upper Respiratory System,* vol 1, ed 2. Philadelphia, Lea & Febiger, 1979. Used by permission.)

The entire front face of the sphenoid sinus is resected to determine whether disease exists within the sphenoid sinus.

We believe we get better results by using packing following an ethmoidectomy. One-inch iodoform gauze that has been impregnated with chlortetracycline ointment is quite satisfactory for this packing. The iodoform gauze is introduced into the ethmoidectomy defect by way of the nostril after the roof of the ethmoid has been surfaced with compressed Gelfoam. The upper half of the nasal cavity is also packed with this gauze and is supported by inserting one or two finger cot packs into the lower half of the nasal cavity.

The retraction sutures and those used to approximate the eyelids are removed. A circular piece of compressed Gelfoam is applied over the packing, which can be visualized from the operative field. This layer of Gelfoam prevents the iodoform packing from adhering to the margins of the bony dissection or periosteum. The periosteum is sutured with two or three 4-0 chromic catgut sutures. Subcutaneous sutures are undesirable in this area. The skin is approximated with 5-0 or 6-0 dermal suture.

A moderate-pressure dressing will prevent troublesome postoperative edema and ecchymosis about the eye. A small strip of Telfa gauze is placed over the incision. An eyepad is covered with three or four fluffed 4 by 4 inch gauze sponges. The skin of the forehead and lateral cheek is painted with tincture of benzoin. The dressing is secured in place with three 6-inch strips of 2-inch elastic adhesive.

Postoperatively, the head should remain elevated for at least 24 hours. The finger-cot packing is removed on the first postoperative day, and the dressing is removed on the second. The iodoform packing is removed from the third to fifth postoperative day, depending on the degree of its adherence to the intranasal structures. The patient can usually be discharged from the hospital on the fifth or sixth postoperative day. He or she should be evaluated 2 weeks following discharge from the hospital to detect excessive intranasal crusting or intranasal adhesions. Excessive crusting is treated using a lubricant nasal spray and intranasal irrigation with alcohol solution that is diluted with an equal part of warm water. Intranasal adhesions are disrupted using 4% cocaine solution for topical anesthesia if necessary. An oval-shaped piece of Telfa or silicone sheeting is placed intranasally for approximately 5 days to prevent further synechiae.

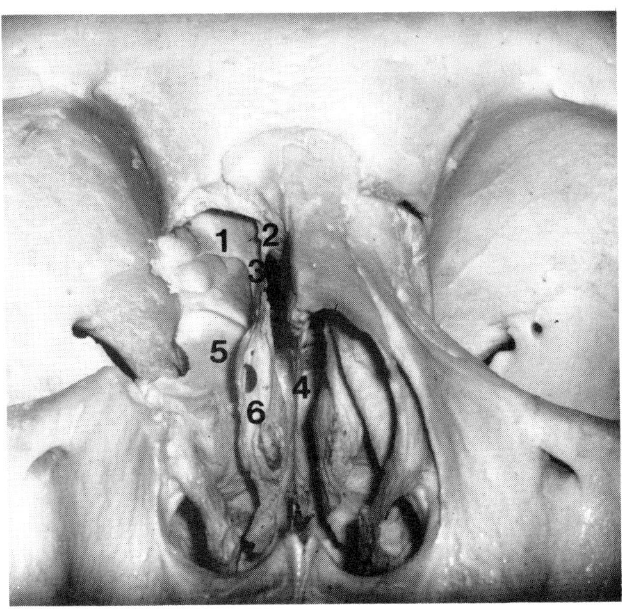

FIG 16–25.
Anterior and posterior ethmoid cells have been removed. The middle turbinate with its upper attachment separates the roof of the ethmoid from the cribriform plate. (*1*) roof of ethmoid, (*2*) cribriform plate, (*3*) upper extension of attachment of middle turbinate, (*4*) nasal septum, (*5*) anterior wall of sphenoid sinus, and (*6*) middle turbinate. (From Montgomery WW: *Surgery of the Upper Respiratory System*, vol 1, ed 2. Philadelphia, Lea & Febiger, 1979. Used by permission.)

REPAIR OF CEREBROSPINAL FLUID RHINORRHEA

A CSF leak is the result of rupture of the arachnoid membrane or herniation of brain through a defect in the protective dura mater and calvarium. The rupture may be small, admitting only herniation or archnoid (meningocele), or large enough to accommodate brain (encephalocele). Flow of CSF through either type of fistula may be a trickle or may be profuse, chronic or intermittent. It usually ceases for a while after an attack of meningitis.

Traumatic and nontraumatic CSF fistulae are limited to basically three areas:

1. The paranasal sinuses (frontal, ethmoid, sphenoid) may have thin walls abutting the anterior and middle cranial fossae. Congenital or traumatic defects may occur in these walls.

2. In the cribriform plate where the olfactory nerve fibers penetrate normal bone, dural defects can be associated with congenital, traumatic bony defects or with tumors.

3. Temporal bone defects may communicate with the middle or posterior cranial fossa.

The CSF leakage is termed rhinorrhea when the source is the paranasal sinuses or cribriform plate otorhinorrhea when the CSF has its origin in the temporal bone and reaches the nose by way of the eustachian tube, and otorrhea when the source is the temporal bone and there is perforation in the tympanic membrane.

Diagnosis

The investigation of a suspected CSF leak must be systematic and thorough, because unless the leakage is profuse and persistent, the detection of its source is difficult. Leakage should be considered in patients who have had severe trauma to the face, especially in the region of the superior aspect of the nasal bone, the forehead, or the temporal bone. A patient who has repeated episodes of meningitis should be thoroughly investigated for CSF rhinorrhea or otorrhea.

A CSF leak is usually unilateral. It may be constant or intermittent. An acceleration of the flow rate with change in position or with straining is rather characteristic. It is important to determine whether the symptoms of leakage are associated with nasal stuffiness or sneezing since the rhinorrhea from vasomotor or allergic rhinitis may be confused with CSF leakage. As a general rule, CSF leakage is unilateral, whereas vasomotor and allergic rhinitis are bilateral. These, however, are not consistent findings.

A salty taste in the throat and frequent swallowing resulting from excessive liquid entering from above are frequent complaints of patients with CSF leakage into the nasopharynx. Leakage occurring in gushes with changes in position suggest emptying of a sinus filled with CSF. On the other hand, CSF otorhinorrhea may occur as a gush when the patient leans forward.

A loss of the sense of smell may indicate a cribriform plate leakage due to fracture or olfactory tumor. A hearing loss or sensation of fluid in the ear may accompany CSF leakage into the middle ear, either directly from the otic capsule or by way of the mastoid. In such cases the findings of fluid or air bubbles behind the tympanic membrane may be apparent.

Visual field examination should be performed because of the frequent association of pituitary tumors with nontraumatic CSF leakage.

Unless contaminated by blood from trauma or by infection, CSF is a clear, colorless liquid with a low specific gravity (1.006), containing no mucus, low levels of protein (<50 mg/dL), and a modest glucose content (50–70 mg/dL). Cerebrospinal fluid will not stiffen a handerchief when dried as do nasal secretions. Nasal secretions may contain glucose as a result of lacrimation and may be "watery" and contain little protein. Testing the fluid with laboratory paper test strips is of little value. In short, a positive diagnosis of CSF leakage cannot be established by chemical analysis. If the nasal discharge can be collected in a test tube, it should be observed for a period of 12 to 24 hours. A sediment will develop in nasal discharge, whereas CSF will remain clear (Fig 16–26).

Routine x-ray films of the skull, sinuses, facial bones, and mastoid may demonstrate the presence of a tumor, fluid, fracture, or air in the cranial cavity (Fig 16–27). X-ray films may demonstrate the air-fluid level in a sinus. To enhance detection of this air-fluid level, the patient remains supine for at least 30 minutes immediately before the x-ray films are taken. Polyto-

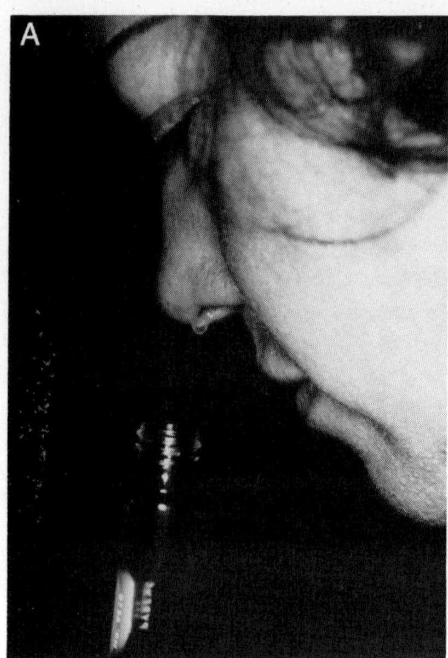
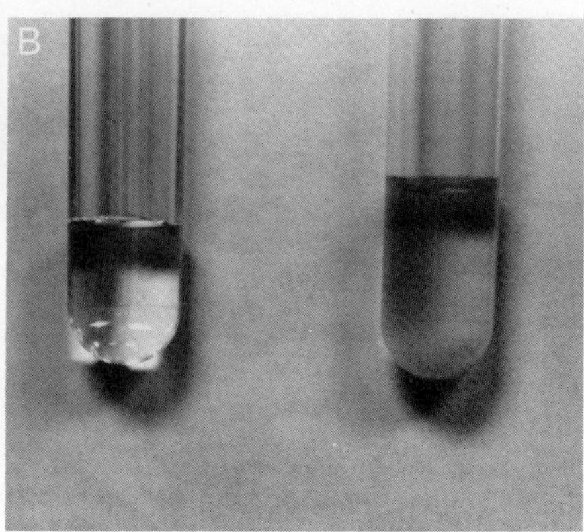

FIG 16–26.
A, patient with CSF rhinorrhea. **B**, the left test tube contains clear spinal fluid and the right cloudy nasal precipitate. Both have been standing for longer than 24 hours. (From Montgomery WW: *Surgery of the Upper Respiratory System,* vol 1, ed 2. Philadelphia, Lea & Febiger, 1979. Used by permission.)

mography and CT scanning are more exact methods for pinpointing the site of the dural defect. The number of positive diagnoses using the various x-ray techniques, however, is disappointing. They may suggest the presence of a small fracture or a defect where there is none. Computerized head scanning should be performed in cases of nontraumatic CSF leakage to detect obstructive hydrocephalus, brain tumor, and other causes of high pressure leaks.

A fairly accurate method of identifying and localizing the source of CSF rhinorrhea or otorrhea is a test consisting of intrathecal injection of fluorescein dye solution. The patient is placed in the sitting position for the first portion of the examination. After examination of the nasal cavities, nasopharynx, pharynx, and ears for the presence of fluid, both nasal cavities are packed with 4% cocaine-impregnated cottonoid strips to shrink the mucous membrane and produce topical anesthesia. The packing is removed after 10 minutes. A separate moist cottonoid strip is inserted into the sphenoethmoidal recess, the region of the olfactory slit and middle meatus, and the anterosuperior nasal cavity.

A lumbar puncture is accomplished, and the spinal fluid pressure is recorded. In patients with a large dural defect, the spinal fluid pressure is often quite low, making a spinal tap in the recumbent position quite difficult. In these cases, the tap is carried out with the patient in the sitting position. Fluorescein (0.5 mL of a 10% solution) diluted with at least 10 mL of spinal fluid is slowly injected intrathecally. In cases in which 10 mL of spinal fluid cannot be obtained because of low spinal fluid pressure, Ringer's or Hartman's solution may be used to dilute the fluorescein dye.

FIG 16–27.
This laminagram demonstrates a defect in the ethmoid-cribriform region and the site of the CSF leakage. The density (*lower arrow*) is an encephalocele, which was resected, and the defect was repaired using a nasoseptal mucosal flap. (From Montgomery WW: *Surgery of the Upper Respiratory System,* vol 1, ed 2. Philadelphia, Lea & Febiger, 1979. Used by permission.)

After the lumbar puncture, the patient is placed in a horizontal supine position. If the leakage has been profuse, the head is elevated. After 10 minutes to 1 hour, depending on the profuseness of the CSF leakage, the cotton strips are carefully removed and labeled according to their intranasal location. The strips are inspected with ultraviolet light in a darkened room for the presence of fluorescein. The presence of dye on the pledget placed in the sphenoethmoidal recess most likely indicates leakage by way of a posterior ethmoidal cell or the sphenoid sinus, or otorhinorrhea. The presence of fluorescein dye on the pledget placed in the olfactory region and middle meatus indicates a leakage by way of the cribriform plate or anterior ethmoidal cells. If the dye is present on the pledget placed in the anterosuperior nasal cavity, the dural defect is most likely behind the posterior wall of the frontal sinus.

In addition to the foregoing technique, the posterior pharyngeal wall is examined for the presence of fluorescein dye with an ultraviolet light source. Both tympanic membranes should also be examined. If fluorescein dye is present in the middle ear, the yellow-green color of the dye will be apparent by ordinary otoscopy.

Reactions to intrathecal fluorescein have been reported. However, I have had no incidence of complication in more than 200 cases in which 0.5 mL of 10% fluorescein is diluted with at least 10 mL of spinal fluid and is slowly injected intrathecally.

Cerebrospinal fluid otorrhea from the mastoid region may be demonstrated by pantopaque study. Proper positioning in serial x-ray films taken over at least 24 hours may be necessary to demonstrate the point of leakage.

Treatment

Early management of posttraumatic CSF rhinorrhea from the cribriform plate, paranasal sinuses, and mastoid is conservative unless the brain is herniated into a sinus or the rhinorrhea is especially profuse. The patient should remain in a semi-sitting position and be instructed to avoid nose blowing, sneezing, and straining. If the leakage is gradually decreasing, surgical intervention can be delayed for 4 to 6 weeks. Prophylactic administration of antibiotics to patients with CSF leakage is common, but as yet there are no controlled studies to demonstrate its proficiency in preventing meningitis. Surgical intervention is indicated in all cases of CSF leakage beyond 6 weeks, because there is a high probability that meningitis, which has a significant mortality rate, will develop. Surgical intervention is indicated in the following instances: (1) 2 weeks after trauma if the leakage is profuse and not decreasing, (2) if the leakage persists more than 6 weeks after the trauma, (3) with any case of recurrence of spinal fluid leakage, (4) when pneumocephalus is present, (5) when there is a history of spinal fluid leakage and meningitis develops.

Frontal Sinus

A dural defect in the posterior wall of the frontal sinus is exposed using the anterior osteoplastic frontal sinus procedure. If the evidence for a dural defect is fairly certain and the patient has been admitted to the hospital for surgery, a fluorescein test should be performed 2 to 4 hours before the scheduled surgery.

The frontal bone is exposed using either the eyebrow or coronal incision. An intrathecal injection of fluorescein dye as already described is repeated before surgery unless performed as a test 4 hours preoperatively. After the osteoplastic flap has been reflected anteriorly and inferiorly and both frontal sinuses have been exposed, the mucous membrane of both sinuses and the interfrontal septum are removed. The fracture or defect in the posterior wall of the frontal sinus is located by the presence of the fluorescein dye (Fig 16–28,A). A linear laceration in the dura can be repaired by suturing; if not, the dural defect can be repaired by using either temporalis or frontalis muscle fascia or frontal pericranium. This tissue should be sufficiently large that it can be tucked between the posterior wall of the frontal sinus and the dura around the periphery of the bony defect. Before the sinus defect is obliterated with adipose tissue, the entire cortical lining of the frontal sinus must be removed with a rotating cutting bur. This procedure ensures complete removal of the mucosal lining of the sinus and adequate blood supply for the adipose implant. Subcutaneous adipose tissue obtained from the lower left quadrant is trimmed and implanted so as to fill the frontal sinus complex completely (Fig 16–28,B). The osteoplastic flap is replaced to its anatomic position and sutured with multiple periosteal sutures. If there is any question of the stability of the osteoplastic flap, it should be secured in place with two wire sutures (Fig 16–28,C).

Cribriform Plate or Roof of Ethmoid

A dural defect above the cribriform plate or roof of ethmoid is by far the most common site of origin for CSF rhinorrhea. These defects are repaired by first performing a complete external ethmoidectomy operation and removing the middle turbinate, then covering the dural defect that has been adequately exposed by using a posteriorly based pedicled mucoperiosteal nasal septal flap (Figs 16–29, A and B). The septal mucosal flap is rotated approximately 90 degrees so as to cover the leakage point and adjacent dura of the olfactory and roof of ethmoid regions (Figs 16–29, C and D). The flap is carefully packed in place with a layer of Gelfoam and then a packing of 1-in. iodoform gauze stripping that has been impregnated with chlortetracycline ointment. A finger cot is inserted into the nasal cavity to prevent inferior displacement of the iodoform gauze packing. After 24 to 48 hours, the finger cot packing is removed. The iodoform gauze packing should remain in place for approximately 14 days.

Sphenoid Sinus

The approach to a dural defect in the region of the sphenoid sinus by the intracranial route is extremely difficult and in some instances impossible because of the anatomic development of this sinus. A complete ethmoidectomy is carried out and a septal mucosal flap is fashioned before the sphenoid sinus is entered, because the mucosa forming the anterior wall of this sinus makes up the base of the flap. It is usually necessary to

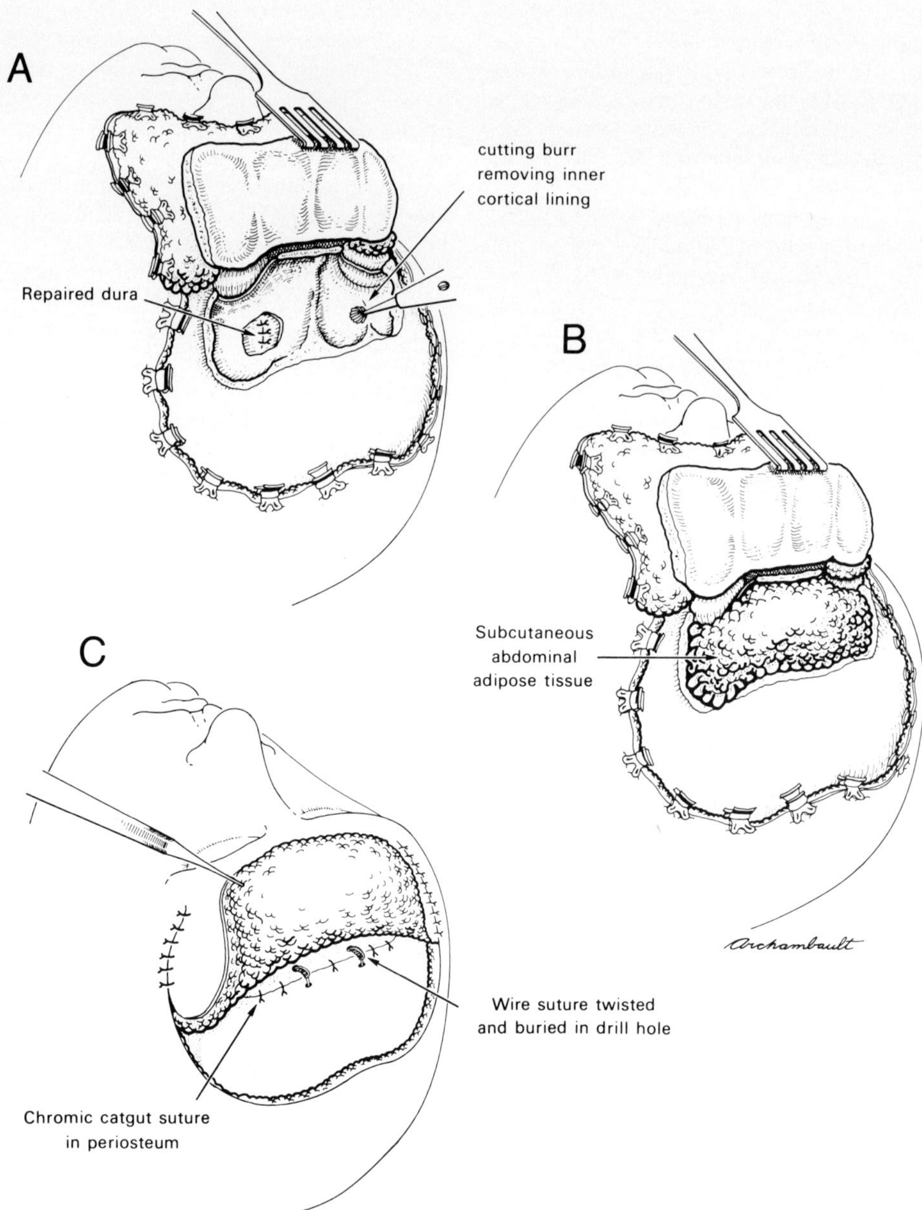

FIG 16–28.
A, reinforcement by fascia is not necessary when linear closure of the dura can be accomplished. It is essential, however, that the mucous membrane and inner cortical lining of the entire frontal sinus complex be removed so that the sinus can be obliterated with adipose tissue. **B**, subcutaneous abdominal adipose tissue has been implanted into the frontal sinuses to create a barrier between the intranasal space and the dura. **C**, as a general rule, the osteoplastic flap can be tightly secured in place by suturing the periosteum with chromic catgut sutures. If, on the other hand, the periosteum is deficient or defective, or if there is any question that the osteoplastic flap might become dislodged and migrate forward, four drill holes should be placed, as shown, and the wire sutures applied. The twisted ends of these wire sutures are buried in a drill hole, as illustrated. (From Montgomery WW: *Surgery of the Upper Respiratory System,* vol 1, ed 2. Philadelphia, Lea & Febiger, 1979. Used by permission.)

remove the intersphenoid septum and a small portion of the posterior nasal septum to provide wide exposure of the sphenoid sinus complex. The mucosal lining of the sphenoid sinus is removed and the mucosal flap placed over the point of leakage. If the dural defect is large, it may be plugged with adipose tissue or fascia before the septal mucosal flap is reflected in place. In cases of recurrent CSF rhinorrhea by way of the sphenoid sinus, it may be necessary to repair the dural defect with fascia and obliterate the entire sphenoid-ethmoidal complex with adipose tissue and cover the anterior sphenoid defect with a septal mucosal flap.

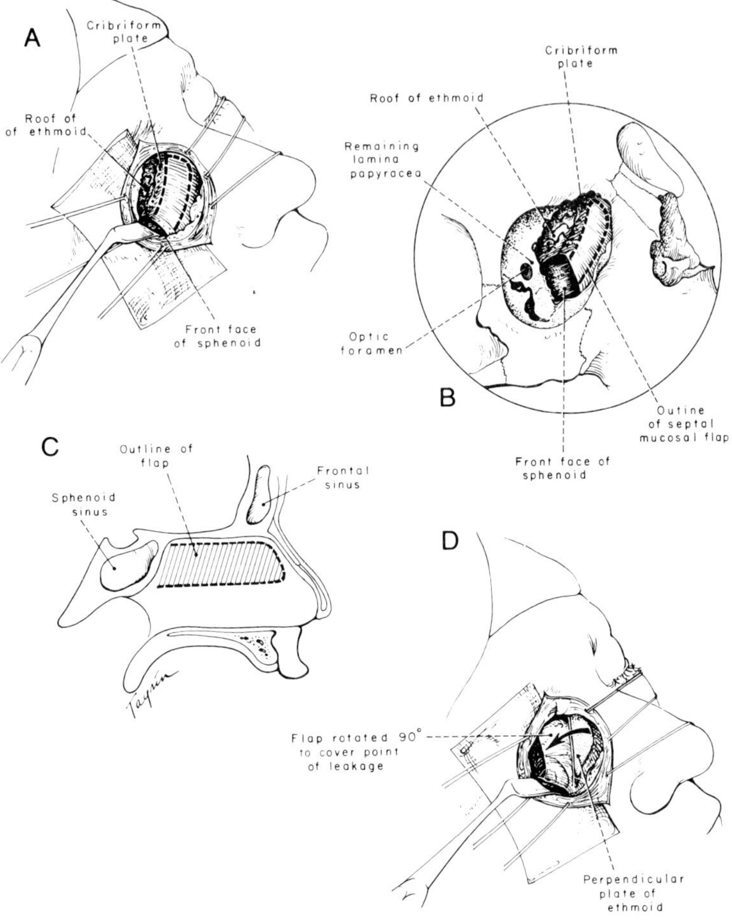

FIG 16–29.
A, the middle turbinate and medial wall of the ethmoid labyrinth have been completely removed. This affords the operator an excellent view of the entire roof of the ethmoid, olfactory slit, front face of the sphenoid, sphenoid ostium, posterior choanae, and the posterior aspect of the laminae papyracea. The outline of the septomucosal flap is shown. The superior incision extends along the anteroposterior dimension of the superior nasal septum at the level of the olfactory slit. The lower incision is parallel to and approximately 1.5 cm inferior to the superior incision. The anterior incision connects the anterior aspects of the above incisions, creating a posteriorly based flap. **B,** the outline of the septomucosal flap, roof of the ethmoid, and cribriform plate are illustrated. A leak in either the cribriform plate or the roof of the ethmoid area can be easily detected. **C,** a midsagittal section, just to the right of the nasal septum, shows the outline of the posteriorly based septal mucosal flap, which is used to repair a CSF leakage by way of the ethmoid labyrinth or cribriform plate. **D,** the septal mucosal flap has been rotated 90 degrees upward to cover both the cribriform plate and roof of the ethmoid. The perpendicular plate of the ethmoid becomes denuded. (From Montgomery WW: *Surgery of the Upper Respiratory System,* vol 1, ed 2. Philadelphia, Lea & Febiger, 1979. Used by permission.)

External Sinus Surgery

Approach of

Frank N. Ritter, M.D.

MAXILLARY SINUS

The maxillary sinus, for an unexplained reason, is more prone to infections and neoplasms than any other group of sinuses. As regard to infections, the surgeon has two well-established technical options—the intranasal antrostomy or the Caldwell-Luc procedure—to employ for a recalcitrant or recurrent maxillary sinus infection.

Intranasal Antrostomy

In general, intranasal antrostomy for its rationale depends on the creation of a window, larger and more inferior in position to that of the natural ostium. This theoretically, then, permits purulent secretions to escape quite readily from the sinus lumen during an infection. In general, I employ it very little for chronic or recurrent maxillary sinus disease. I believe the natural ostium often is not patent but is encroached on by obstruction such as an enlarged ethmoidal bulla, nasal polyps, or infected ethmoid cells that reduce patency of the ostium. The natural ostium should be enlarged surgically.

Technique

This procedure may be performed under a general or a local anesthesia. Regardless of the anesthetic selected, the anterior portion of the inferior meatal area is infiltrated with an anesthetic-vasoconstrictor, such as lidocaine-epinephrine. Unless a patient has hypertension, 1% lidocaine with epinephrine 1:100,000 may be selected. Following anesthesia, the anterior attachment of the inferior turbinate may be severed to gain better access to the meatus. The incision is begun in the mucosa about one half way back and rather superior in the inferior meatus and brought forward for 1.5 cm. The vertical cuts from the top of this incision are made toward the floor of the nose, and the flap is elevated and reflected on the nasal floor. An opening in the meatal bone is made with a punch or chisel and enlarged. It is particularly important to remove sufficient bone to have an opening 1.5 by 1 cm. The edges of the mucosa are electrocoagulated to discourage bleeding. The flap is folded into the sinus lumen and the meatus packed with a Telfa dressing for 24 hours.

Caldwell-Luc Procedure

Although the problem in chronic maxillary sinusitis may be the ostium, there is also a pathologic state of the mucosa. When a pathologic mucosa exists either because of bacterial or fungal organisms, a Caldwell-Luc procedure is indicated, not a nasal antrostomy, in my opinion.

Technique

The operation is usually done under a general anesthetic. I find local anesthesia difficult to render, and if bleeding should be a problem during the surgery, it may be difficult to control with a local anesthetic.

The upper lip is retracted, and the planned area of the incision is infiltrated with an epinephrine-anesthetic solution. I prefer to make an incision with a sharp knife. The soft tissues are elevated from the anterior bony maxilla superiorly until the infraorbital nerve is noted. An opening 1.5 by 1.5 cm is made into the anterior maxillary bony wall. If purulence is encountered, it is cultured for anerobes and aerobes. The cavity is suctioned and irrigated with normal saline, and only diseased mucosa is removed. I then pack the sinus with a strip of gauze moistened with lidocaine-epinephrine mixture for a few minutes. While this is left in the sinus lumen, the intranasal antrostomy in the inferior meatus is made. I believe this is needed to remove the packing postoperatively and to promote ease of irrigation of the antrum later postoperatively.

After the nasal antral window is performed, the natural ostium is inspected and enlarged if needed. The lumen of the sinus is then packed by gauze moistened with bacitracin. This is removed in 24 hours.

Complications

Tooth root injury is rare; I have never encountered it. If it occurs, I would ask for immediate dental consultation when it was recognized. Nasal duct injury is likely nonexistent. Hemorrhage is a possibility during the operative procedure, and tamponade will control it. Postoperatively, I have had a patient with a hemorrhage from the incision in the buccal flap successfully electrocoagulated. Infraorbital injury may occur and does so likely during currettage of the superior wall. Caution and slight force are permitted only to prevent this complication.

EXTERNAL ETHMOIDECTOMY

Indications

The external ethmoidectomy is performed when the patient has ethmoidal disease that has sufficiently distorted intranasal landmarks or is bulky (many nasal polyps) or when the patient has had previous nasal sinus surgery that renders poorly the intranasal landmarks. Even with the most recent vogue of sinus endoscopy, the complication rate regarding the eye and the central nervous system is higher than with external ethmoidectomy.

Technique

The operation is performed with a general anesthetic. A vasoconstrictor anesthetic solution such as lidocaine-epinephrine is infiltrated into the planned area of the incision. A curved incision is mapped with a marking pen around a thumb lightly placed over the eyelids, previously closed by a silk suture. The incision can be staggered to prevent postoperative webbing during healing. Elevation of the periosteum begins anterior to the anterior edge of the lacrimal fossa. The periosteum is more adherent here and the dissection more difficult. The elevation proceeds to just behind the anterior ethmoidal artery. The artery is clipped but not divided, and entry is made into the lamina papyracea at the lacrimal fossa. Directly medially lies the most anterior of the ethmoidal sinus cavities; the agger nasi cells. The lamina papyracea is removed sufficiently to gain visual access to the air cells, usually requiring a 1.5 by 1.5 cm defect in the bone of the lamina papyracea. The ethmoidal cells are removed as needed. The middle turbinate is also removed. Bleeding is controlled by electrocoagulation. Packing is placed to prevent postoperative bleeding, but only lightly, because pressure may encroach on the eye and jeopardize vision. The packing is left in place 24 hours. Postoperative crusting is discouraged by spraying the nose with NaSal, OCEAN, or AYR (over the counter).

Complications

Cerebrospinal fluid leaks are not common, because the anterior ethmoidal artery denotes the level of the cribriform plate. If it occurs and direct suture is not possible, I elevate the dura around the defect and place muscle from the superior part of the incision into the bony defect and then oxidized cellulose (Oxcel) cotton and packing. The patient is kept in the sitting position for 10 days postoperatively. A neurosurgeon should be consulted to see if a malleable subarachnoid needle should be placed in the lumbar region for daily withdrawal of CSF. There is no problem with violation or removal of the cribriform plate if the dura is left intact. However, it should be realized that olfactory filaments penetrate through the cribriform plate, and loss of olfaction may occur if this is done.

Optic nerve injury has no therapy. This nerve is a direct extension of the brain, and violation of it produces irreversible blindness. Ophthalmologic consultation is needed on recognition of it.

Mucocele is a late uncommon complication that can occur as late as even 20 years postoperatively. When it occurs, it must be excised or widely marsupialized and drained into the nasal chamber.

Extraocular injury is not likely when the orbital periosteum is elevated without tearing it. Whenever the periorbitum is torn, it is wise to place a piece of aluminum foil over the periorbitum to prevent further tearing of the rent. The aluminum is removed before the conclusion of the operation. There is no treatment for this condition, but ophthalmologic consultation should be obtained if the muscle is torn.

Orbital abscess may occur, but I have never seen this complication postoperatively from an external ethmoidectomy. Should it occur, it has to be surgically incised, and a drain is left in the lumen of the abscess for several days. After culturing, appropriate antibiotics, and a visual consultation, healing usually occurs.

FRONTAL SINUS SURGERY

Trephination

Trephination is performed for a painful acute sinusitis with retained secretions. Microscopically the mucosa is edematous blocking the sinus ostium. It retains pus in the lumen of the sinus under pressure. When this occurs, trephination is indicated. It can be done either under a local or general anesthesia. The patient should be warned that postoperatively there may be some degree of anesthesia of the skin of the forehead and about the operative site. The incision is placed under the eyebrow, and the fibers of the orbicularis are divided. A small area of the floor of the frontal in its medial aspect near the root of the nose at the glabella is entered with a perforating drill point. A diagnostic radiograph should always be consulted for the anatomy. The opening is enlarged to approximately 4 to 5 mm, and the contents of the sinus are cultured for aerobes and anarobes. The lumen is then irrigated and a small catheter inserted into the lumen. The wound is closed about it, and the catheter is taped to the lateral forehead near the temple.

Postoperatively, the catheter is irrigated daily with the patient in a sitting position until the irrigant passes out the nasal chamber. When this happens, it means patency of the nasal frontal duct. If the disease is not reversed, further surgical drainage is indicated.

Complications

Although I have not seen it, CSF leak may occur when the drill performing the trephine penetrates the dura. If it occurs, the area of the frontal sinus should be explored. Depending on the size of the frontal sinus, a large sinus would permit exploration through the floor of the sinus. A small sinus, however, might require removal of the anterior face of the sinus and the supraorbital rim and exposure of the tear in the dura, and repair by suture or by muscle, Oxycel cotton, and packing are used.

Inability to irrigate via the nasal frontal duct into the nasal chamber would indicate stenosis of the ostium, and the patient has nasal frontal duct closure. This would indicate the need for a second operation, either ablation or osteoplastic flap.

Periorbital infection or hematoma rarely occur postoperatively. Should they develop, wound exploration is indicated. The clot or pus is evacuated, culture is taken, and adequate drainage is performed, and antibiotics are used.

Chronic Frontal Sinusitis

Chronic frontal sinusitis requires surgical intervention. Microscopically there is mucosal disease similar to that in chronic maxillary sinusitis. A procedure consisting of removal of the diseased lining and opening the nasal frontal duct, as performed in the Reidal or Lynch procedure, is done. Since over the years these have not proved to be as therapeutically helpful as desired for a prolonged time, the osteoplastic flap technique has supplanted them. In this procedure, a template of the sinuses is made. The sinus is entered at its superior edge, and the diseased mucosa and periosteum are removed meticulously. The mucosa is then pushed into the nasal frontal duct from the superior direction, and the lumen of the sinus is filled with adipose tissue. This gives rewarding successful results over the long term.

Mucocele

Mucocele occurs because of stenosis of the sinus ostium by infection, polyp, or scar. It is either widely excised or drained into the nose with ablation of the sinus, with later reconstruction of the defect by acrylic cranialplasty or by osteoplastic flap.

Osteoma

Osteomas are osseous lesions within the frontal or ethmoidal sinuses, varying in size. Depending on location, they may produce sinal-osteal occlusion by size or with infection. Therapy is removal of lesion. In practice, I remove frontal sinus osteomas via an anterior osteoplastic flap approach. Since the nasal frontal duct is not jeopardized, usually no ductal work is needed. Recurrence is rare. Postoperative radiographs may still show a shadow of the osteoma on the Caldwell view. However, on lateral view, it will be demonstrated that the lumen is air containing and that the osteoma has been removed.

Osteomyelitis

Osteomyelitis of the frontal bone is rare and usually occurs after swimming or trauma to a preexisting antecedent infected sinus. Allergy is often a component cause. It may be difficult to recognize clinically because the signs are few: tenderness beyond the sinus lumen, persistent leucocytosis, and headache. The radiograph or computed tomogram may disclose loss of the frontal sinus outline or bony intersinus septa. Extensive ablation or osteoplastic flap technique is required.

PART THREE

Head and Neck Surgery

CHAPTER 17

Management of the Primary Site: Oral Cavity

Approach of

Jerome C. Goldstein, M.D.

When one discusses the management of carcinomas of "the tongue," it is extremely important to distinguish between the anterior two thirds of the tongue—the part anterior to the circumvallate papillae—and the base of the tongue—the part posterior to this line. These two parts are embryologically distinct, have different lymphatic drainage, and exhibit different tumor characteristics and behavior. Tumors of the anterior two thirds are usually well differentiated and are detected fairly early in their course. Tumors of the base of the tongue are often poorly differentiated and are difficult to diagnose early. In the patient who presents with pain in the ear yet has a normal-appearing tympanic membrane, symptoms may be due to an infiltrative tumor of the tongue base or other oral site, with infiltrative irritation of sensory nerves V, IX, or X.

The most frequent site of intraoral carcinoma is the tongue (40%). The floor of the mouth is the next most often involved area (15%–20%), then the gum (13%), and then the buccal mucosa (10%), with the remaining sites divided between lips and palate. It is often impossible in advanced lesions to define whether a tumor started in the floor of the mouth and extended to involve the mobile tongue or vice versa. The distinction is unimportant because, regardless of the site of origin, the surgical treatment of large lesions involves en bloc resection, striving for an adequate margin of clinically uninvolved surrounding tissue.

A word must be said about premalignant lesions. The definition of leukoplakia is a white plaque that does not rub off. Histologically, this may represent any of the pathologic premalignancies (parakeratosis, hyperkeratosis, dysplasia of varying degrees), carcinoma in situ, or invasive carcinoma. Such lesions may have carcinoma in one small part with dysplasia in other parts; one cannot predict the histology grossly. Especially beware of erythroplakias (red, velvet-appearing lesions), because in these areas the incidence of carcinoma is even higher. I believe that biopsies should always be performed on both red and white lesions.

SURGERY

Let us consider the determinants of adequate excision once surgery has been decided as the course of action. I believe that frozen sections are mandatory. A close relationship with the involved pathologist is very important; whenever possible, the case should be discussed beforehand, and the pathologist should be alerted to your needs for his or her services in the operating room. The surgeon should be knowledgeable about the histology of the tumor and the different behavior characteristics of, for example, a low-grade mucoepidermoid tumor vs. an adenoid cystic carcinoma, vs. a well-differentiated carcinoma or poorly differentiated squamous tumor. One must reflect on the dimensions of the floor of the mouth and how difficult it may be to get 1 cm or more of clearance around a tumor that widely infiltrates the floor of the mouth. The staging of these lesions is important, and the adept surgeon should know the width of several of his or her fingers and tongue blades. It certainly is far more convenient to insert a finger in a patient's mouth than it is a ruler or tape measure!

One additional fact is important here. The knowledge of reconstructive techniques favors a more aggressive excision of the lesion. One must never compromise an excision for fear of unfavorable defect. If such a mistake is made, one will be quickly impressed with the more severe defect and course of the subsequent recurrent disease. What constitutes adequate surgical resection is a good cuff of normal tissue uninvolved by tumor surrounding a tumor-infiltrated specimen. For well-differentiated encapsulated exophytic (T1) squamous cell carcinoma, a few millimeters of normal tissue will suffice. For a poorly differentiated infiltrative squamous cell carcinoma, one could not be comfortable with this. Faced with an adenoid cystic carcinoma, one would be comforted by seeing that the results of specific neural biopsies in the adjacent nerves were normal and uninvolved with tumor. A very important determinant of likelihood of metastases is the depth of the tumor in the tongue. In my experience, if the depth exceeds 3 mm the metastatic probability significantly increases, and it becomes more important to pay attention to the neck.

RECONSTRUCTION

When possible, the patient should be provided with some mobile tongue remnant for purposes of swallowing and articulation. One must be careful not to bind down the tongue remnant. This is often the mistake of an inexperienced surgeon. Starting with lesions of the mobile portion or anterior two thirds of the tongue, a T1 lesion treated by a wedge excision can be closed primarily. As one progresses to larger lesions, the uninvolved side of the tongue can be advanced and turned on itself, so that the remaining half of the tongue tip can be brought toward the opposite circumvallate line. This will give a smaller, more rounded organ, but it should be functional. A dermal graft may be useful in this reconstruction and will be discussed shortly. If the resection involves a unilateral base of tongue, the defect is best reconstructed by "halving" the anterior two thirds and reflecting posteriorly the mobile tongue on the side of the resected base. The remaining mobile tongue can be closed primarily.

The question arises as to the applicability of a total glossectomy and whether or not the larynx should be included in the specimen. I believe that total glossectomy is warranted in the appropriate patient, and I would not initially sacrifice a larynx not involved with a tumor. The concern here is whether the patient will suffer from aspiration. I still vividly recall the first patient on whom I performed this operation, with the expectation that laryngectomy would soon be necessary because of expected aspiration. I was amazed at how well the patient did, not only with avoiding aspiration but with being able to produce understandable (albeit not normal) speech. The size of a lesion requiring this sort of resection usually requires associated resection of the floor of the mouth. Reconstruction is best accomplished with a pectoralis major flap, with the muscle bulk restoring the floor of the mouth. The patient is best rehabilitated if the mandible can be preserved, but this is an individual decision based on lesion extent. The myocutaneous flap is used to restore the integrity of the floor of the oral cavity, not to reconstruct the tongue. The patient's method of oral feeding will never be normal, but with the help of a knowledgeable speech pathologist and appropriate Gomco-type syringes, nutrition without aspiration should not be a problem.

Regarding tumors involving primarily the floor of the mouth, one must understand the necessity for adequate surgical resection. There are many aphorisms relating to the treatment of cancer, and they all carry the same message: "the first chance for cure is the best chance," and "one cannot play catch up with cancer." Again, there is not much question concerning the T1 lesions. The excisions can either be closed primarily or be left open. If the resection impinges on Wharton's duct, the duct must remain patent intraorally to avoid postoperative swelling of the submandibular gland and the resulting confusion this causes regarding the possibility of metastatic disease. Again, frozen sections are mandatory. Either Wharton's duct must be marsupialized or the gland resected. The larger floor of mouth tumors most commonly leading to this consideration would probably, because of their size, indicate the appropriateness of at least a modified neck dissection with which the gland can be included. This will be discussed later in this chapter.

Dermis as an Intraoral Graft

The histology, characteristics, and techniques of obtaining a dermal graft are well described elsewhere. A brief recapitulation is that this layer of skin contains three epidermal appendages: sweat glands, sebaceous glands, and hair follicles. Dermis contains a full complement of elastic fibers, so that there is no contracture of this graft. The thigh is the preferred donor site. The dermatome is set at 0.012 in., and the first run is taken to raise the epidermis, which is left attached superiorly. The second run at the same thickness setting obtains the dermal graft. The epidermis is then replaced, making the donor site essentially nonpainful and cosmetically acceptable compared with the characteristics of a donor site from a split-thickness skin graft. The dermis in the mouth does not contract because of its full complement of elastic fibers, and the take rate is extraordinarily good. It often rapidly assumes the characteristics of the surrounding mucosa. In fact, in such cases some months later, it is difficult to define as a separate graft. The graft occasionally grows hair. Its take rate intraorally is aided by the use of quilting sutures, described by MacGregor, and by the application of sponge stents secured by through-and-through silk sutures tied over bolsters. I have rarely found the use of such stents necessary.

Clearly the application of the dermal graft is for relatively superficial lesions, the excision of which does not involve a significant part of the muscle diaphragm of the floor of the mouth. If extensive through-and-through resection is necessary, reconstruction is best performed with a flap. A tongue flap may be applicable for small floor of mouth lesions and inferiorly based nasolabial cheek flaps for slightly larger lesions. The pectoralis myocutaneous flap is best for the more extensive floor of mouth lesions. The laterally based MacGregor forehead flap is very useful for intraoral reconstruction but has fallen into some disrepute because of the cosmetic defect it creates. However, the flap should be in the surgeon's armamentarium, and the cosmetic defect can be minimized with delayed skin grafting and in that patient whose hair can be combed down onto the forehead. It is a useful and hardy flap based on the superficial temporal artery. Its viability can be reinforced by beveling the superior flap incision to include the postauricular artery.

Management of the Mandible

There is no controversy concerning the indication for mandibular resection if it is grossly involved by tumor. In such a case, a complete segmental resection is clearly indicated. If the resection approaches the superior condyle, I favor disarticulation of the jaw joint rather than subcondylar resection. Patients undergoing the latter experience annoying jaw joint pain because of pterygoid muscle pull on the small remaining part of the mandible. This is avoided by resection that includes the condylar head. It adds only a moment or two to the operation, and annoying bleeding can be avoided by staying close to the bone during the resection. If the bone is not frankly invaded, I rarely take the mandible except for incontinuity composite resection for tonsil carcinoma. When reconstruction is intended using a pectoralis major flap, removal of the ascending ramus of the mandible facilitates the incontinuity reconstruction, and the bulk of the pectoralis muscle obviates the dead space and cosmetic deformity. For other large lesions of the floor of the mouth approaching but not invading the mandible, in which a neck dissection is to be performed because of palpable nodes, marginal resection of the mandible with inclusion of the periosteum is an adequate operation with little morbidity. If the lesion does not encroach on the mandible, that is, clearly does not approach the periosteum or gingiva, no mandibular resection is necessary, and a pull-through operation should be adequate.

Management of the Neck

There should be no controversy for the neck with palpable nodes. I favor a classic radical neck dissection in such a situation, with the only compromise being preservation of the eleventh nerve in some situations where the patient is a manual laborer or if there is other justification for sparing that nerve and there are no palpable nodes along its course. The modified neck dissection (preservation of the internal jugular vein and sternocleidomastoid muscle) should be reserved for N0 neck with an infiltrative T2 or larger tumor with the expectation that this is a grand biopsy to be followed by radiotherapy if results of sampled nodes are abnormal. The other indication for this grand biopsy is need to enter the neck to resect the submandibular gland, in which case one would do a supraomohyoid operation for purposes of staging. Otherwise, a suprahyoid neck dissection is of no value.

Buccal Carcinoma

Buccal carcinoma, in my experience, is rare. Those cases I have seen are more commonly verrucous carcinoma, which are best treated by wide local excision of the superficial lesion with resurfacing of the defect by a dermal graft. As commented previously, this avoids postsurgical scar contracture. If such contracture is present because of some other surgical treatment, I would favor its excision and repair using a dermal graft. Stenson's duct must be preserved to avoid parotitis. It can usually be easily marsupialized, but if it is left alone, nature favors its fistulization. Carcinoma of the gingivobuccal sulcus is seen in tobacco chewers who hold their tobacco in this area. It is best treated with a composite resection, including treating the man-

dible by the indications previously given for marginal vs. segmental resection.

Conclusion

Reconstruction of the mandible is a significant concern. The fact that no one has a satisfactory answer is attested to by the variety of methods popularized in recent years. The older I get, the more conservative I become, and the more I am impressed with the validity of the aphorism "there is no tissue as good as the original issue." Most large foreign bodies, if followed long enough, extrude or must be removed. This is especially true in the patient who has received significant radiotherapy. You should do everything reasonable to avoid mandibular shift in the patient undergoing a segmental resection. If the patient has teeth, the remaining mandible should be put into occlusion with the maxilla by the application of arch bars at the time of resection. If the patient does not have teeth, one can consider Gunning splints or the insertion of two Steinman pins or Kirscher wires to prevent deviation with the realization that these almost always will subsequently have to be removed. At a later time one can consider mandibular reconstruction using a Vitallium basket, as has been described by multiple authors. In my experience, if one has prevented deviation and reconstructed intraorally with a pectoralis muscle to fill the dead space created by segmental resection, such reconstruction is not necessary.

POSTOPERATIVE RADIOTHERAPY

My indication for postoperative radiation in these lesions is both an unfavorable histology of the tumor and a determination of the adequacy of the surgical resection. Close margins demand radiation therapy. I would routinely irradiate a patient who had an adenoid cystic carcinoma. One can debate whether these tumors are radiosensitive or radiocurable. There is little controversy over the long-term pernicious behavior of adenoid-cystic carcinoma.

A patient with bilateral base of tongue involvement always poses a treatment dilemma. A patient with a T1, T2, or T3 squamous lesion can be treated with external beam radiotherapy and iridium implant, with surgery reserved for clinically abnormal neck nodes. As with other lesions, the cure rate falls with increasing tumor size, and patients with T3 and T4 lesions should be treated with combined surgery and radiation. I have not personally had impressive favorable experiences combining chemotherapy in the treatment plan for these lesions.

Osteoradionecrosis of the mandible is a difficult problem, often associated with poor intraoral hygiene. Obviously, prevention is the best cure, and this will be helped by having oral patients at risk seen by a dentist preoperatively and the best possible status of nutrition and intraoral hygiene attained prior to surgery. If osteoradionecrosis develops, aggressive but conservative therapy is indicated. Hyperbaric oxygen, if available, should be used. Antibiotics, aggressive intraoral hygiene, and pulse steroid therapy (to aid the effectiveness of antibiotics) should be considered. Conservative debridement of exposed bone is usually indicated. Patience on the part of the surgeon and patient is needed.

Management of the Primary Site: Oral Cavity

Approach of

Mark C. Weissler, M.D.

Cancer of the oral cavity was the cause of approximately 21,900 new cancers and about 4,850 cancer deaths[1] in the United States in 1988. The major predisposing factors are tobacco and alcohol abuse. Certainly the most cost-effective means of dealing with these cancers would be through prevention and the elimination of risk factors. It has been estimated that fully 80% of all human cancers are related to life-style.[2] Sites within the oral cavity that can be affected include the tongue, lips, floor of the mouth, alveolar ridges, buccal mucosa, hard palate, and retromolar trigone. Precancerous lesions include leukoplakia and erythroplakia, and precancerous conditions include syphilitic glossitis, Plummer-Vinson syndrome, submucous fibrosis, the erosive form of lichen planus, dyskeratosis congenita, discoid lupus, and chronic hyperplastic candidiasis.

One of the more difficult aspects of the treatment of oral cavity cancers involves the multitude of functions that come together within this limited site. Loss of large portions of the mandible or tongue poses particularly difficult problems. Labial incompetency with drooling, inability to achieve complete dental rehabilitation, leaving patients without dentition and condemned to a life-long soft diet, and articulatory defects resulting from loss of tongue or palate are some of the functional problems encountered. Speech problems may be more difficult to deal with in patients with oral cancers than in many laryngectomy patients, because methods of reconstructing articulators lag behind methods for producing an articulatable tone. If large portions of the tongue base within the oropharynx are involved contiguously, complete resection may add problems of aspiration as well as further articulatory deficits. Local control often can be achieved, only to fail regionally in the neck.

Another problem seen frequently in the oral cavity is that of condemned mucosa, or field change carcinomatosis. In these instances, premalignant or early malignant lesions exist throughout much of the mucosa of the oral cavity. This is a particularly difficult clinical situation since none of the presently available treatment modalities is ideal for the treatment of such lesions. One can hardly remove all of the mucosa from these areas either excisionally or ablatively as with the cryoprobe or laser. Radiotherapy may be effective, but this will burn a valuable bridge should the patient later develop a second more significant cancer, which is often the case. In addition, especially in the young patient, there is a reluctance to use a modality that in itself has known carcinogenic activity. New treatment modalities are needed for the treatment of these patients. Some promising inroads are being made with new treatments such as photodynamic therapy, wherein large surface areas can be treated, theoretically killing off only the abnormal tissues, or with the use of substances such as the retinoids, which may induce differentiation of premalignant tissues.

TONGUE

Squamous cell carcinoma of the tongue is usually seen in tobacco and alcohol abusers. Syphilitic glossitis has been associated with an increased incidence of tongue cancer, though a causal relation has never been shown. Small lesions less than 2 cm in greatest diameter are equally effectively treated by either radiation or surgery, and, therefore, the less morbid therapy is chosen. This usually proves to be simple surgical excision. Radiotherapy requires several weeks of treatment and also burns a valuable bridge should a second primary cancer of the oral cavity develop. A 1 to 2 cm margin usually is considered acceptable, and frozen sections are routinely taken at the time of surgery from remaining tissue in the patient because of the known difficulty of adequately gauging gross margins in the tongue.

Abnormal margins and perineural or vascular invasion are indications for further surgery or postoperative radiotherapy to the primary site. In addition, large invasive lesions are also treated with adjuvant radiotherapy to the primary lesion. Though controversy still surrounds the use of combined surgery and radiotherapy in the treatment of the primary lesion, it is my impression that better local control rates are achieved with advanced cancers.

Fixation, the loss of free mobility in relation to adjacent soft tissues, usually implies direct tumor extension to soft tissue or bone. Evidence of carotid artery or prevertebral muscle involvement is taken as a sign of incurability. Severe trismus most often means pterygoid muscle involvement and is a clue to search diligently for base of skull involvement, often a sign of incurability. The computed tomography (CT) scan, though by no means infallible, may be helpful in suggesting involvement in these areas. When doubt remains, initial surgical exploration of the neck and skull base at the time of operation but prior to committing oneself to resection may help avoid finding oneself in a situation in which total resection is impossible. It is generally assumed that less than total gross surgical cancer removal is not of benefit to the patient.

Bilateral base of tongue involvement does not preclude total surgical removal. Postoperative morbidity, however, will be severe. Some believe that the morbidity precludes total glossectomy as a therapeutic option. This should not be the case. Though attempts at combined external and brachytherapy radiation have yielded good results in some cases, reports are still anecdotal enough not to replace accepted therapy, which consists of combined surgery and radiation. If the supraglottic larynx can be spared, some patients can be rehabilitated by reconstruction with a bulky pectoralis major flap to have somewhat understandable speech without severe aspiration, though they may not tolerate the stress of oral alimentation and may require a gastrostomy. If the supraglottic larynx is removed, aspiration even of the patient's own secretions may make total

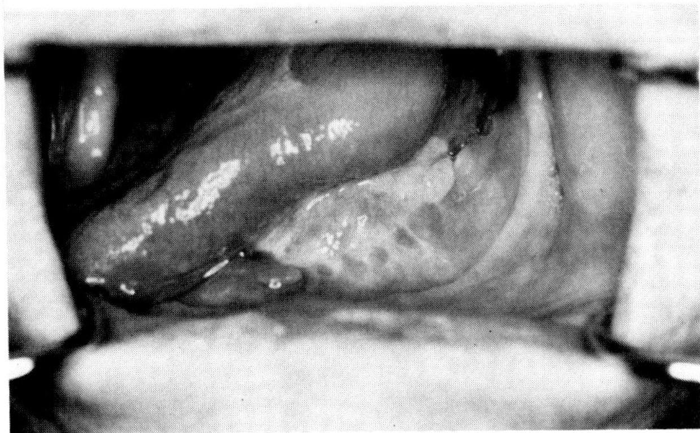

FIG 17–1.
Results obtained with excision and primary split-thickness skin grafting.

laryngectomy necessary. A palatal prosthesis to build up mass may assist these patients with alimentation and speech. All patients considering total glossectomy must be aware of the possible need for immediate (based on surgical findings) or delayed laryngectomy and must be counseled regarding the speech and alimentary morbidity. Ultimately the choice of surgical or some other form of primary therapy must rest with them. Three- to five-year survival will be poor regardless of the method of therapy chosen, but combined surgery and radiation give the best chance of cure and a relatively good chance for locoregional control, which is of great benefit in these cases even if the patient does eventually die from distant metastases.

FLOOR OF MOUTH

Small lesions are excised with 1 to 2 cm margins and skin grafted (Fig 17–1), allowed to granulate, or closed primarily or with local tongue flaps as the case dictates. Tumors adjacent to bone but without radiologic evidence of bone destruction on occlusal dental x-ray films or CT are treated with marginal mandibulectomy removing the inner table of bone. If cortical bone destruction is evident, segmental mandibulectomy with frozen section control of the inferior alveolar canal margins is performed. If there is evidence of invasion to the canal, hemimandibulectomy, including the inferior alveolar canal from lingula to mental foramen, is performed. A variety of reconstructive methods can be used. Defects associated with a marginal mandibulectomy may be closed with a tongue flap, distant flaps, or free flaps, primarily closed or skin grafted depending on the particular situation. Small defects located anteriorly without mandibular loss may be locally excised and Wharton's ducts reimplanted posteriorly with good results. If much of the sublingual gland is disrupted, it should be removed to prevent ranula formation. Larger lesions requiring marginal mandibulectomy or resection of most or all of the submandibular duct are often best treated with a pull-through dissection of the floor of mouth contents along with the mylohyoid muscle and resection of the submandibular gland and contents of the submandibular triangle to achieve complete local tumor removal. Resection of the submandibular triangle contents alone does not constitute adequate prophylactic treatment of the neck for occult metastases. Reconstructive methods should be based on the attainment of optimal functional results with minimal morbidity. With marginal inner table mandibulectomy, closure of the remaining genioglossus, hyoglossus, and mylohyoid muscles to the remaining mandibular arch with absorbable sutures placed through holes drilled in the mandible and covered with a skin graft can give good functional results (Fig 17–2). Distant flaps, such as the pectoralis major flap, heal well and fill soft tissue defects. In some cases, however, these flaps may prove to be excessively bulky and may displace normal remaining tissues, resulting in a large insensate platform that may collect food and saliva (Fig 17–3). With large defects, this is often the only alternative. When placed laterally, segmental mandibular

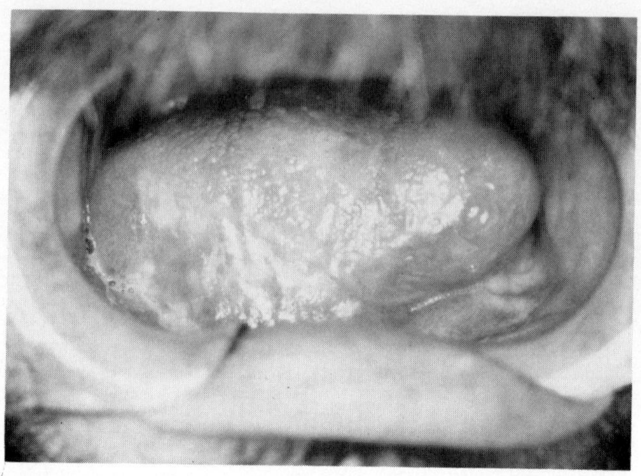

FIG 17–2.
Results obtained after excision of anterior floor of mouth with marginal mandibulectomy of the symphyseal region by pulling remaining genioglossus and geniohyoid muscles up to the remaining mandible and covering with a split-thickness skin graft.

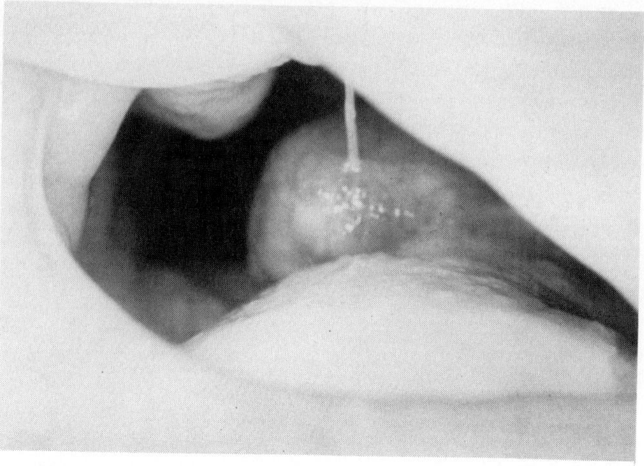

FIG 17–3.
Large insensate platform in anterior floor of mouth following pectoralis major flap reconstruction of large anterior floor of mouth and anterior mobile tongue excision.

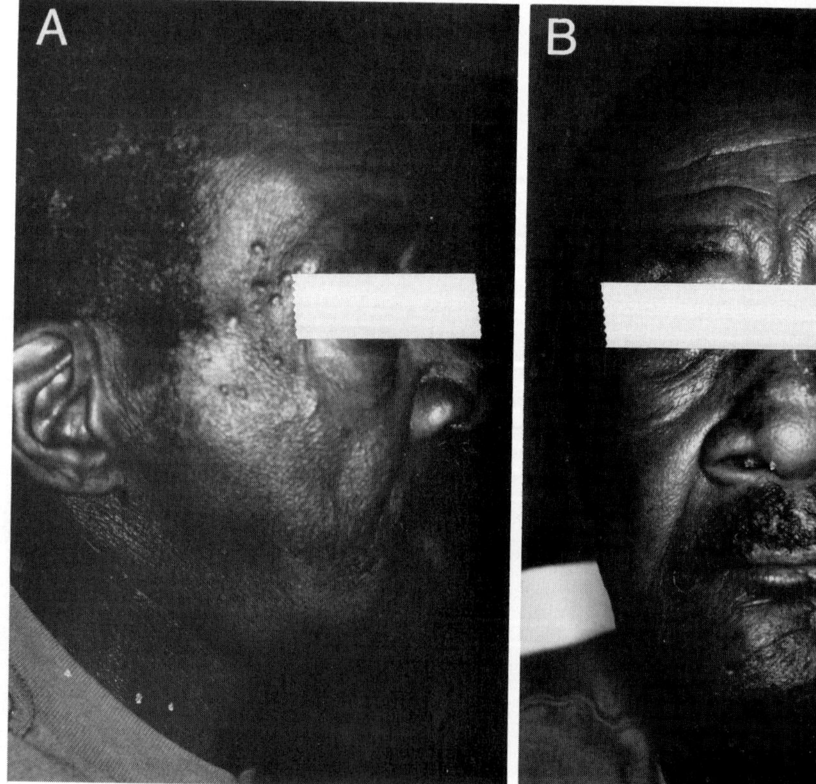

FIG 17–4.
A, lateral view. **B,** Frontal view. Note lack of cosmetic depression or severe mandibular swing following composite resection, including angle of mandible, with pectoralis major flap reconstruction, leaving bone unreconstructed.

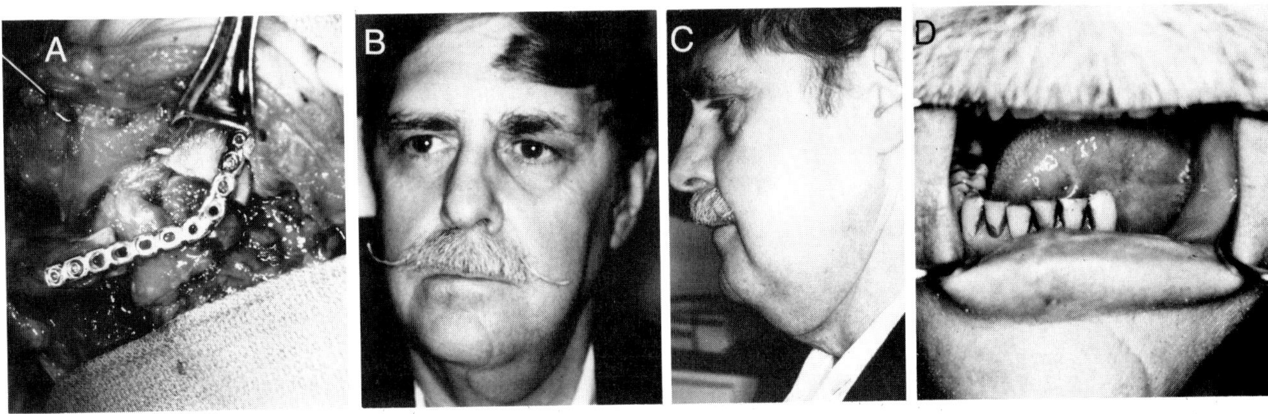

FIG 17–5.
A, surgical defect with bar in place. **B and C,** frontal and lateral views of patient, respectively. **D,** excellent postoperative occlusion. Excellent result obtained after primary reconstruction of a lateral mandibular defect with a metal bar. This case involved a verrucous carcinoma of the alveolar ridge requiring minimal soft tissue resection and no postoperative radiotherapy.

defects can be left unreconstructed, making primary closure easier. Depending on the size of the soft tissue defect, there may be greater or lesser degrees of mandibular drift toward the defect. Patients are often edentulous or will be rendered so in preparation for postoperative radiotherapy, so that a minor degree of mandibular drift may be compensated for in the creation of a denture. There will be a depression at the site of the segmental defect if primary closure is performed. If a distant flap is used to reconstruct the soft tissue defect, the depression is often minimized by the bulk of the pedicle and seems to decrease the amount of postoperative mandibular drift (Fig 17–4). Function is usually quite acceptable.

Lateral segmental defects can be bridged with a metal plate, and, if the plate is fitted prior to mandibulectomy, occlusion of any remaining teeth can be well maintained (Fig 17–5). It may necessitate use of a distant flap where one might otherwise not be necessary, since the plate may prevent collapse of remaining soft tissues. The morbidity of this flap must be taken into consideration when one is making reconstructive decisions. The metal plate can often give good results as either a final reconstruction or intermediary in preparation for later reconstruction. In cases with limited lateral segmental loss, for benign or low-grade neoplasms, or after traumatic segmental loss, it is probably the indicated immediate reconstructive method. However, in the treatment of advanced malignant disease where postoperative radiotherapy will be necessary, there will be an increased incidence of fistulization and exposure that may necessitate secondary procedures or plate removal in some cases (Fig 17–6). The precise effects of the metal plates on postoperative radiotherapy in terms of shielding tissues or causing hot spots of radiation buildup are unknown. The risk/benefit ratio for this form of reconstruction is not well defined. Often the most expedient and functionally acceptable method is to leave the lateral mandibular segmental defect unreconstructed initially. One's concern over reconstructive matters must never dictate over adequate surgical resection.

Segmental defects of the anterior symphyseal mandible are the most difficult to reconstruct. Leaving the defect unreconstructed is generally unacceptable because of the severe functional deficits associated with this "Andy Gump" deformity, including labial incompetence with drooling, poor articulation, inadequate deglutition, and poor cosmesis. In general, the best method of reconstruction is with a vascularized bone graft, either a free flap taken from the iliac bone, scapula, radius, or metatarsal (Fig 17–7) or an osteomyocutaneous flap using either the scapular spine and trapezius muscle or a rib and pectoralis major muscle (Fig 17–8). The bone must be adequately immobilized with either interosseous wires or bone plates. In

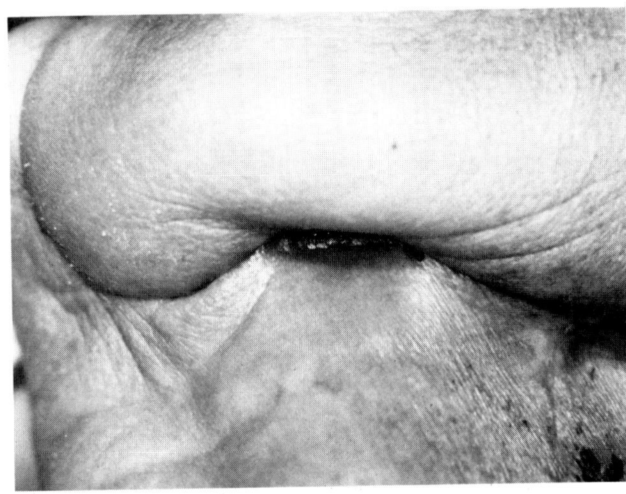

FIG 17–6.
Fistulization at anterior aspect of osteobar reconstruction of lateral mandibular defect.

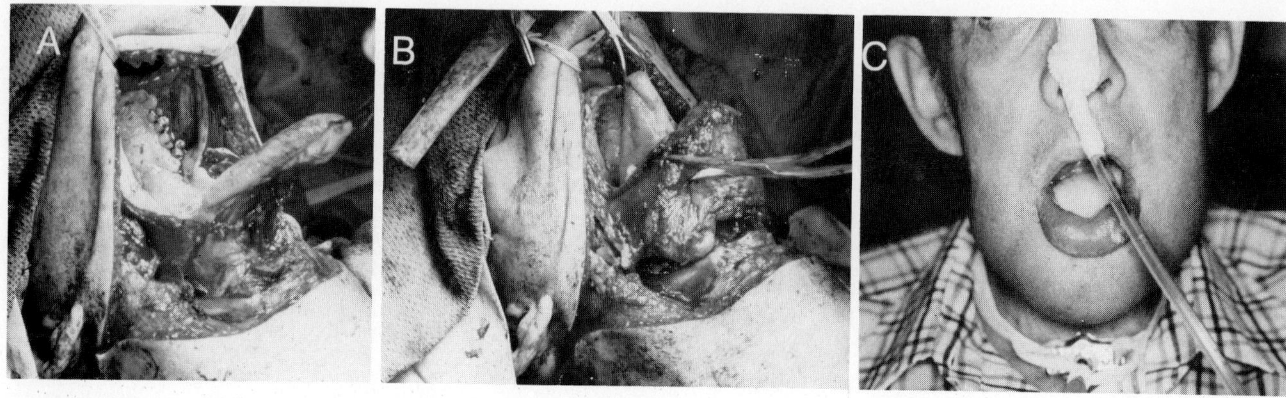

FIG 17–7.
A, surgical defect showing angle-to-angle bony defect. **B,** iliac crest free flap in place. **C,** bulky reconstruction with much soft tissue in floor of mouth. Reconstruction of angle-to-angle mandibular defect along with loss of entire floor of mouth with an iliac crest free flap based on the deep circumflex iliac artery.

these cases, with oral contamination and often a previously irradiated or soon to be irradiated field, free grafts or allogeneic materials such as metal plates will be associated with increased rates of extrusion, exposure, and fistulization. In some cases, however, metal plates may avoid the added morbidity of an osteomyocutaneous or free flap. The use of a myocutaneous flap in association with a plate may improve local healing. Long-term success rates and functional results are unknown. Regardless of the method of reconstruction chosen, it may not be necessary to completely bridge the mandibular defect, especially if the symphyseal defect is combined with a hemimandibulectomy. Acceptable functional results can be obtained by reconstructing to and through the symphysis but leaving the lateral defect on one side unreconstructed (Fig 17–9). The bone can be immobilized with either interosseous wires and an external biphase apparatus or with a compression plate at a single site. Adjuvant radiotherapy to the primary is indicated in the treatment of these advanced lesions.

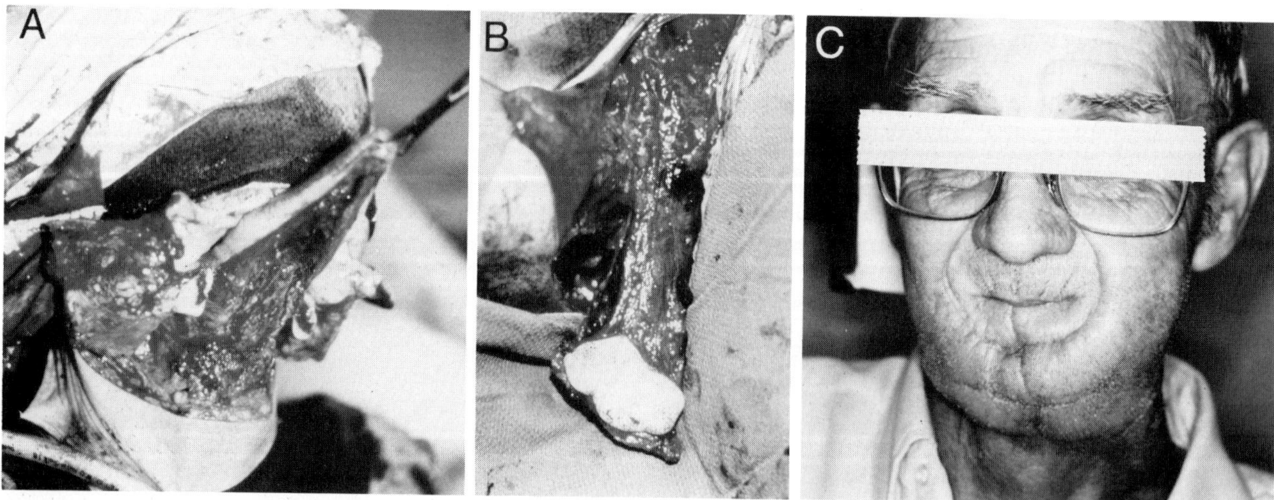

FIG 17–8.
A, surgical defect. **B,** trapezius osteomyocutaneous flap elevated. **C,** final result. Reconstruction of anterior mandibular defect with a trapezius osteomyocutaneous flap. This case also involved loss of most of the lower lip, which was reconstructed with a Karapandzik flap.

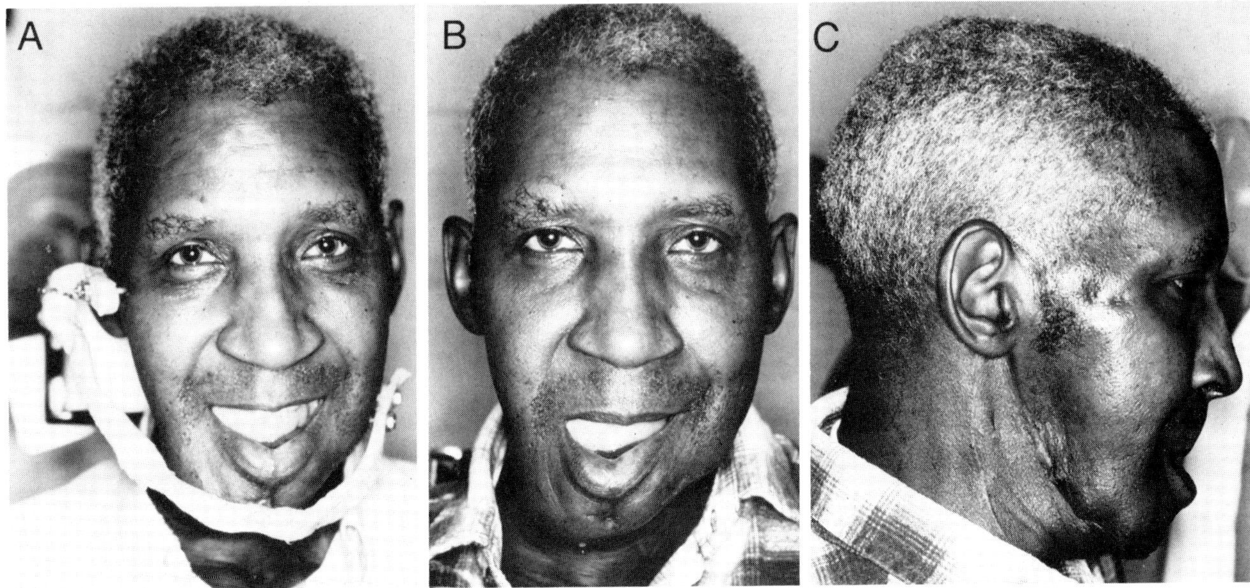

FIG 17–9.
A–C, results of subtotal reconstruction of angle-to-angle mandibular defect with a trapezius osteomyocutaneous flap. The bone was held in place during healing with a hinged external fixation device.

BUCCAL MUCOSA

Small T1 cancers of the buccal mucosa are again best treated by wide local excision. Should the cancer involve the orifice of Stenson's duct, the duct can be ligated with expectations of a limited period of parotid swelling and discomfort. Larger lesions require more complex resections. Because the tissues of the cheek are relatively thin, it is often necessary to perform through-and-through resections. If the lesions approach the subdermal lymphatics, parotid lymph nodes are at risk, and neck treatment whether therapeutic or elective should probably include the intraparotid lymphatics. Small areas of partial-thickness excision almost always can be closed primarily with good functional results. Larger defects can be closed with a superiorly based trapezius myocutaneous flap, or a nape of neck skin flap, the pedicle of which is carried across the midline of the neck posteriorly. The pectoralis major myocutaneous flap also can be used for many of these defects; however, the reach is quite far, and the surgeon must take great care to place the skin paddle at least half overlying the pectoralis muscle (not too far inferiorly on the chest wall) and to bring up the rectus abdominis fascia with the pedicle, otherwise one risks partial- or full-thickness loss of that portion of the skin paddle. Buccal cancers also often encroach on the maxilla or mandible, and in these cases resection of bone is often necessary. Maxillary defects often involve only the infrastructure and are best rehabilitated with a palatal obturator prosthesis. Lesions adjacent to the mandible, without frank destruction on radiologic assessment, can be treated with some form of marginal mandibulectomy removing bone adjacent to the lesion. If bony destruction is clinically evident, segmental mandibulectomy is indicated. When the inferior alveolar canal is involved, it is best to perform a hemimandibulectomy, including the lingula and mental foramen.

ALVEOLAR RIDGE

Cancers of the maxillary and mandibular alveolar ridge are of necessity close to bone. It is safest for all but the most superficial of these lesions to resect some portion of the underlying bone. These lesions, more common than other oral cavity cancers, tend to be misdiagnosed as some form of dental pathology in the dentulous patient, and often tooth extraction has been carried out. In my experience, this is a particularly treacherous situation, since even minimal cancers seem to propagate down the tooth socket toward the marrow space. Frozen sections, so useful in other sites within the oral cavity at the time of excision, are of limited use here because of the bone in the specimen. If bone is excised down to the level of marrow space, frozen section pathology can often be done on this tissue. If there is evidence of such invasion, segmental mandibulectomy should be performed. When the inferior alveolar canal is frankly invaded, hemimandibulectomy from lingula to mental foramen is the preferred method, though lesser segmental resections with frozen section pathology control of the cut ends of the contents of the inferior alveolar canal may be equally effective. What is gained functionally by the lesser segmental resection is minimal and probably does not warrant the increased risk. Issues of mandibular reconstruction are the same as those previously discussed. However, it is most frequently in these cancers that fairly small primaries may leave the patient with segmental mandibular defects with minimal other soft tissue defects, unlike in primary cancers of the tongue or floor of mouth. These patients can expect good long-term primary and regional control and are a group who may not infrequently desire future bony reconstruction. In this case, with plenty of soft tissue to assist with closure, an osteobar may be a good alternative with minimal risk of increasing the likelihood of postoperative fistula, infection, or extrusion. However, most bone-invading lesions will be treated with combined surgery and radiation to the primary site, and the effects of the bars on this therapy currently are poorly understood.

TREATMENT OF THE NECK

For all but T1 lesions of the oral cavity, some form of elective neck treatment is indicated since the incidence of occult metastases is high[3] (Table 17–1). When these lesions approach the midline, bilateral neck treatment is indicated. When clinically abnormal nodes are present in one or both necks, a radical neck dissection on the side or sides of clinical disease, sparing the spinal accessory nerve when the jugulodigastric or spinal accessory nodes are found to be free of disease at the time of dissection, is the currently accepted mode of treatment. If bilateral neck dissections are performed, one internal jugular vein should be preserved, if possible, to prevent a period of severe postoperative lymphedema and venous congestion.

When clinical disease is present in the neck, a dissection that includes all the lymph node-bearing tissue in the anterior and lateral neck is indicated. These dissections may conserve any or all of the spinal accessory nerve, sternocleidomastoid muscle, and internal jugular vein. In unilateral dissections, the spinal accessory nerve is by far the most important of these structures. Its postoperative function will be related to the distance over which it is dissected and stripped of surrounding tissue. In dissections encompassing all the lymphoid tissues of the anterior and lateral neck, the nerve will usually be denuded over 10 to 12 cm and will not function normally immediately postoperatively, though function usually will return to a greater or lesser extent, and the preservation is probably worthwhile.

TABLE 17–1.
Incidence of Nodal Metastases*

		Nodal Metastases	
	N+	N0 Clinically N+ Pathologically	N0 → N+
Floor of mouth	30–50	40–50	20–35
Alveolus	18–52	19	17
Buccal mucosa	9–31	—	16
Oral tongue	34–65	25–54	38–52
Retromolar trigone	39–56	—	10–15

*Adapted from Million RR: The natural history of squamous cell carcinoma, in Cassisi NJ, Million RR (eds): *Management of Head and Neck Cancer: A Multidisciplinary Approach.* Philadelphia, JP Lippincott Co, 1984, p 30.

The role of "partial" neck dissections such as the supraomohyoid, anterior, or posterior neck dissections is unproved in the case with clinically positive nodal metastases, though Jesse et al. have found it adequate for N1 and N2 disease when it is combined with postoperative radiotherapy.[4] Postoperative radiotherapy to the dissected neck or necks is indicated if multiple nodes are found to be involved, if there is evidence of extracapsular spread of tumor, or in cases in which the primary will require radiotherapy.

The clinically normal neck requires prophylactic treatment for lesions greater than T1 in size,[3] though some have suggested that waiting for failure in the neck and treating only at the occurrence of disease is no less beneficial to the patient.[5] The best way to deliver this treatment remains controversial. It is becoming accepted that prophylactic neck irradiation is as effective as prophylactic neck dissection in this setting. Proponents of neck irradiation cite the morbidity of the dissections and argue that in those patients in whom multiple nodes or extracapsular spread are identified, radiation therapy will be given anyway, and the neck dissection will have been unnecessary, since the radiotherapy would have sufficed to treat this amount of disease. Since one never knows whether or not disease actually existed in the prophylactically irradiated neck, this is hard to prove, though it is known that patients with clinically normal necks, even with a high chance of occult disease, seem to do equally well with prophylactic irradiation or surgery to the neck.[6] For midline lesions it may be more expedient for the surgeon, though not necessarily for the patient, to give bilateral prophylactic neck irradiation rather than perform bilateral neck dissections, which may prove a lengthy process. Proponents of prophylactic neck dissection cite the minimal morbidity of a functional or partial neck dissection and the greater morbidity and cost of 4 to 6 weeks of radiotherapy. Functional neck dissections remove all lymph node-bearing tissue from the anterior and lateral compartments of the neck, preserving some combination of the jugular vein, sternocleidomastoid muscle, and, most important, the spinal accessory nerve. Partial neck dissections, such as the supraomohyoid, anterior, or posterior neck dissections, remove nodal tissue only from the most likely involved compartments of the neck. They remain of unproved benefit in this setting.

In addition, proponents of prophylactic neck dissection point out that using radiotherapy at this point may burn a valuable bridge should the patient develop a second primary cancer or a local recurrence. Many patients will have been adequately treated by the single surgical procedure. This is perhaps the most valid argument, because if a patient can be treated by the single modality of surgery, it is much more expedient for the patient and saves a valuable future therapeutic option. This argument is valid only if the primary also can be treated with surgery alone. If the surgeon is unable to get widely clear margins at the primary site, postoperative radiotherapy will be indicated. In such cases, the primary is usually large, with direct extension to the soft tissues of the neck, and combined surgery and radiotherapy to both the primary and neck are the best plan of action.

OSTEORADIONECROSIS

When radiotherapy is planned, a thorough dental examination and appropriate extractions of severely carious teeth or teeth in areas of severe periodontal disease need to be carried out prior to the radiotherapy. During radiotherapy, good oral hygiene and fluoride treatments should be utilized. Osteoradionecrosis, the death and sequestration of bone that usually becomes exposed, is due to devascularization secondary to the effects of the radiation on small blood vessels of bone and its surrounding soft tissues. The bone becomes exposed, and a low-grade indolent infection of sequestered dead bone develops. The underlying problem is the lack of adequate blood supply and not the infection itself. Poor dental care and the presence of severe dental or periodontal disease at the time of radiotherapy are strongly correlated with the development of osteoradionecrosis, which usually affects the mandible and rarely the maxilla. There is conflicting data on whether or not the period of time between tooth extractions and the beginning of radiotherapy is important in preventing osteoradionecrosis,[7] but as a general guideline, at least $1^{1}/_{2}$ to 2 weeks should be aimed for. Extractions may be done preoperatively, during the operation, or postoperatively as is convenient for all concerned. If a midline mandibulotomy has been used, there will be a strip of alveolar mucosa between the floor of mouth incision and the extraction site, which will be very susceptible to necrosis. Two or more weeks between the tooth extraction and the resection should be given for healing. If bone exposure does develop, it should be dealt with conservatively, with minimal sequential debridements in the clinic with a small curette or rongeur. Extensive procedures with much manipulation of the surrounding soft tissues and bone often leads to further devascularization of the area and may only worsen the situation, though in some advanced cases, thorough debridement and bringing in a new blood supply in the form of a vascularized flap may prove necessary. This should be reserved for cases that fail more conservative management. Antibiotics and hyperbaric oxygen treatments also may be helpful, though the hyperbaric oxygen treatments are not universally available and may be quite expensive.

REFERENCES

1. Silverberg E, Lubera JA: Cancer statistics, 1988. *CA* 1988; 38:14–15.
2. Ruddou RW: *Cancer Biology,* ed 2. New York, Oxford University Press, 1987.
3. Teichgraeber JF, Clairmont AA: The incidence of occult metastases for cancer of the oral tongue and floor of the mouth: Treatment rationale. *Head Neck Surg* 1984; 7:15–21.
4. Jesse RH, Ballantyne AJ, Larson D: Radical or modified neck dissection: A therapeutic dilemma. *Am J Surg* 1978; 136:516–519.
5. Vandenbrouck C, Sancho-Garnier H, Chassagne D, et al: Elective versus therapeutic radical neck dissection in epidermoid carcinoma of the oral cavity. Results of a randomized clinical trial. *Cancer* 1980; 46:386–390.
6. Millian RR, Cassisi NJ: *Management of Head and Neck Cancer. A Multidisciplinary Approach.* Philadelphia, JB Lippincott Co, 1984, pp 58–60.
7. Epstein JB, Rea G, et al: Osteonecrosis: Study of the relationship of dental extractions in patients receiving radiotherapy. *Head Neck Surg* 1987; 10:48–54.

CHAPTER 18

Management of the Primary Site: Oropharynx

Approach of

Paul A. Levine, M.D.

TONSIL

Surgical Management

The surgical management of tonsillar carcinomas at the University of Virginia Medical Center is combined with radiation therapy for T3 and T4 lesions to improve survival. Even with combined therapy consisting of 50 Gy preoperatively, the 5-year survival for stage III disease was only 27% and for stage IV was 17% through 1981.[1] More recently, a randomized prospective protocol is in effect that uses mitomycin-fluorouracil and concurrent irradiation to 50 Gy preoperatively to the neck and primary site for stage III and stage IV lesions. This protocol is based on promising initial results of a pilot study performed at this institution.[2]

The T3 and T4 tonsil lesions with metastases in cervical lymph nodes require a composite resection. The resection is performed in conjunction with preoperative or postoperative radiotherapy. Resection of the involved tonsillar region, soft palate, base of tongue, and lateral pharynx is standard, and it is usually combined with a resection of the ascending ramus of the mandible. The reason for resecting this portion of the mandible is tumor invasion of the bone; less valid is resection to facilitate closure. Sparing this segment of the mandible is preferable when possible.

In most clinical situations, x-ray films of the mandible, a computed tomography (CT) scan, magnetic resonance imaging (MRI) scan, or both will not verify invasion of the mandible, and one is sometimes faced with the dilemma of how to proceed. Since there appears to be a natural resistance of the mandibular periosteum to tumor invasion, I usually attempt to preserve mandible, perform an osteotomy, and fix the mandible

with a stainless steel compression plate as part of the reconstruction. This is based on the lateral extension of the disease determined by initial examination and by the findings of the imaging studies. Multiple frozen sections of the lateral margin of soft tissue are obtained at the time of surgery. If there is any question as to the resection adequacy or if the mandibular ramus interferes with the resection, it is removed. The surgical defect is usually reconstructed with a pectoralis major myocutaneous flap, but other myocutaneous or free flaps, or other methods of reconstruction such as split-thickness skin grafts and tongue flaps, can be used.

As mentioned earlier, some surgeons resect the mandibular ramus to facilitate closure. The defect can be closed often without a flap once this is done. Elderly patients with multiple medical problems may require quick, efficient, and oncologically sound procedures. In these cases, the mandibular ramus may be resected, eliminating the need for a flap. Although it is not as cosmetically satisfying, it is functionally acceptable.

Since the technical aspects of the composite resection are basic for the head and neck surgeon, they will not be reviewed, but a few helpful hints are offered. It is simpler to amputate the condyle at its neck when one is performing the mandibulectomy rather than removing the condyle from the glenoid fossa. This prevents excessive bleeding by preserving branches of the internal maxillary artery and the pterygoid veins. Preservation of the condylar head and neck does not interfere with function.

When the surgical plan is to spare the ramus, it is important to decide on the appropriate osteotomy site and the method of fixation. It is my preference to use a dynamic compression plate, and it is important that the plate be bent to conform to the

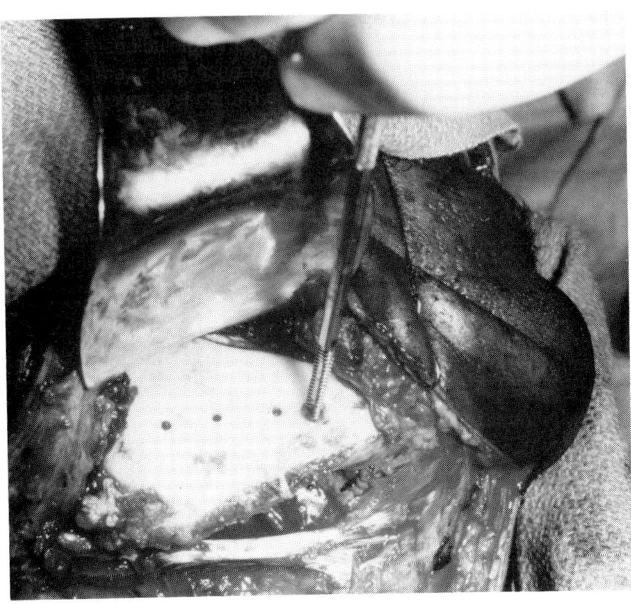

FIG 18–1.
Holes have been drilled, the depth has been measured, and the threads are being tapped prior to the right posterior mandibulotomy and lateral pharyngotomy approach to a recurrent right base of tongue cancer in conjunction with a dissection of the right side of the neck.

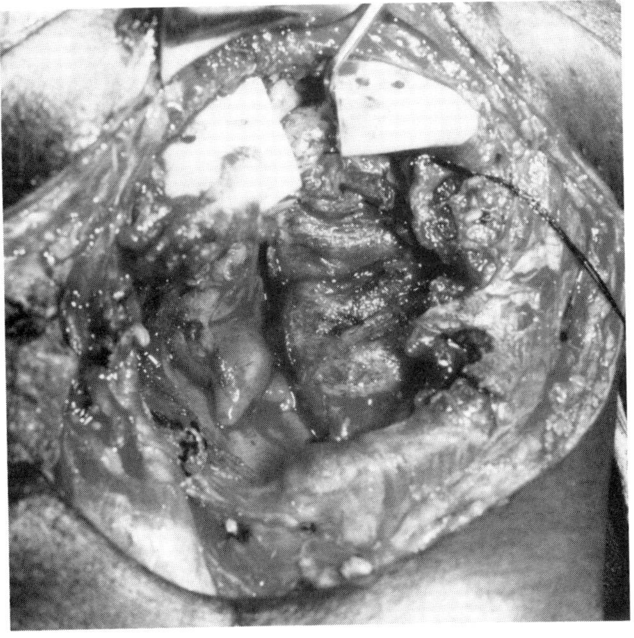

FIG 18–2.
With the mandibulotomy performed, the tumor was resected and a pectoralis major flap used for reconstruction. The muscle pedicle is evident covering the carotid sheath.

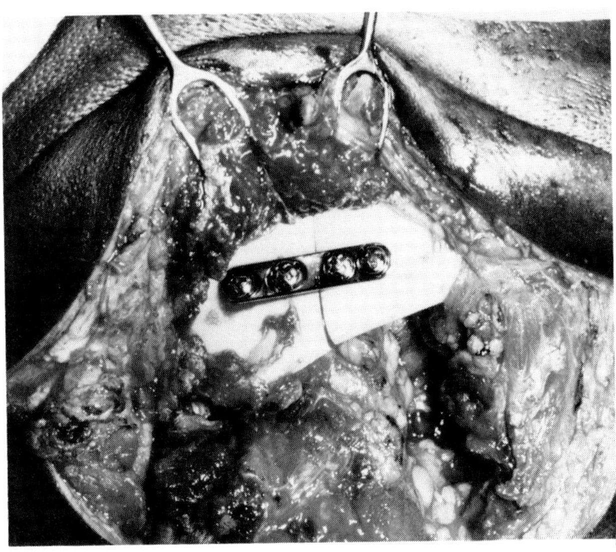

FIG 18–3.
The pectoralis myocutaneous flap is in place, and the mandibulotomy has been immobilized and fixated with a four-hole compression plate.

curvature of the mandible and the holes drilled and tapped prior to performing the osteotomy (Figs 18–1 to 18–4). The mandible will thereby be aligned in the preoperative position, closure will be facilitated, and malocclusion will be avoided. Fixation of the mandible during the reconstructive portion of the operation will take only a few minutes. Other fixation techniques, osteotomies, and osteotomy sites have been advocated,[3, 4] but a vertical osteotomy fixed with a compression plate is my choice.

Radiation Management

Radiation therapy is important in the management of all tonsil cancers, either alone, in combination with surgery, or with chemotherapy. At my institution, irradiation of the primary for cure is the treatment of choice for T1 and T2 tonsil carcinomas and is combined with surgery for T3 and T4 lesions.[1] Those treated for cure receive a radiation dose of 60 to 65 Gy. This dose generally includes prophylactic treatment to both sides of the neck to 50 Gy. Those who received combined therapy receive a dosage of 50 to 55 Gy preoperatively, including both sides of the neck.

Since it is sometimes difficult to differentiate an anterior tonsillar pillar lesion from a tonsil fossa lesion, especially when the tumor reaches the T3 or T4 stage, I treat T1 and T2 anterior tonsillar pillar and tonsil fossa lesions similarly. Both are treated with radiotherapy for cure.

Others have suggested that surgery alone or in combination with radiotherapy is more successful in curing T1 and T2 anterior tonsillar pillar lesions, but their numbers are small.[5] Although there has been a trend to treat small lesions in this region with a combination of external beam and interstitial implantation,[6] my institution has not treated enough patients with this modality to attest to its superiority.

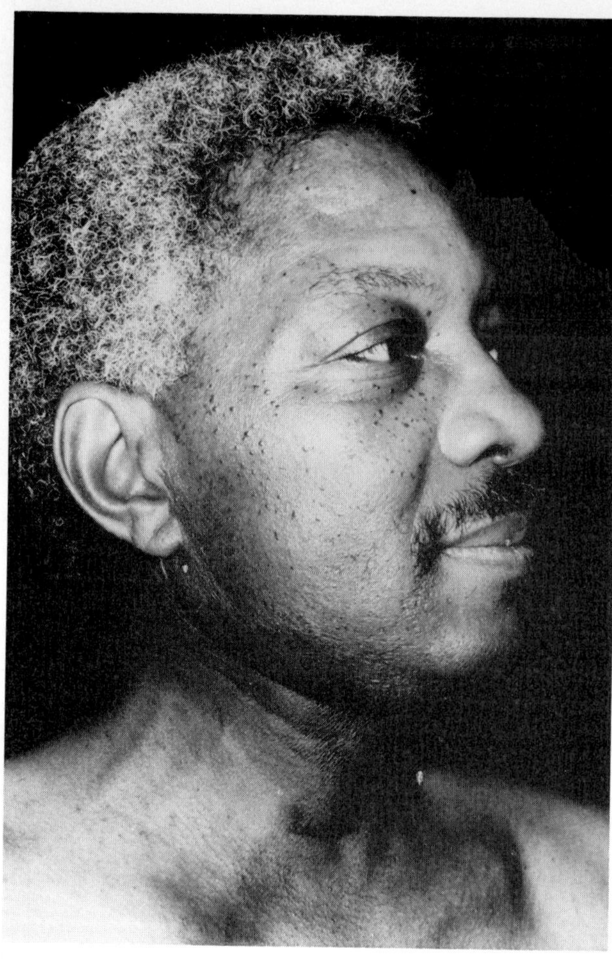

FIG 18–4.
Patient in Figure 18–3, 2 months postoperatively showing excellent mandibular contour. McFee incisions are used for neck exposure.

Neck

My treatment policy for neck disease associated with tonsillar carcinomas is to treat both sides of the neck. If both sides of the neck are N0, they are treated to 50 Gy. If the patient is being treated with a curative dose to the primary, the upper portion of the neck receives a total dosage of 60 Gy. If the neck is N1 or greater, it receives a preoperative dose of 50 Gy, and after a 4- to 6-week rest period, a neck dissection on that side is performed. The type of neck dissection performed is based on the extent of disease, especially in the posterior superior portion of the neck. If the neck nodes have regressed to the point that they are nonpalpable or are mobile and do not involve the spinal accessory or the sternocleidomastoid muscle, a modified neck dissection is performed. Whether or not the sternomastoid muscle or internal jugular vein is spared depends on the judgment and preference of the surgeon. If the node is fixed to deep tissues, or if sparing the spinal accessory nerve is oncologically unwise, a standard radical neck dissection is performed. If the patient presented initially with bilateral cervical metastases, bilateral neck dissections are performed simultaneously. The criteria for sparing the spinal accessory nerve are as stated earlier, but one internal jugular vein is spared on the less involved side, unless this, too, is oncologically unsound. In this case, the neck dissections would be staged with a 3- to 4-week delay between the first and second dissections.

PALATE

Squamous Cell Carcinoma

In general, palatal neoplasms are relatively uncommon. A total of 68 cases of squamous carcinoma of the soft palate were seen over a 20-year period at the University of Virginia,[7] but only 32 cases of hard palate carcinoma were seen at the same institution over a 43-year period.[8] Other institutions have combined their cases to provide data supported by significant numbers.[9] Although soft palate tumors tend to be squamous cell carcinoma, hard palate malignancies are usually minor salivary gland neoplasms. It is important to remember that what may appear to be a hard palate cancer may actually be a maxillary sinus cancer eroding through the sinus floor. High-resolution CT scans can evaluate the extent and location of disease. This is important for pretreatment evaluation of all stage III and IV palatal tumors.

The treatment pattern for these lesions is not as well defined as other head and neck neoplasms because of the paucity of cases within a single institutional experience. The T1 and T2 soft palate squamous cell carcinomas are treated at my institution with radiation therapy for cure, either with external beam alone or external beam plus interstitial implantation of iridium 192 or gold 198. The boost of radiation from 50 Gy of external beam therapy to curative doses of 60 to 65 Gy with interstitial implantation spares the radiation effects of higher doses to the surrounding normal tissue. The T3 and T4 lesions are randomized into our mitomycin-fluorouracil with concurrent irradiation protocol or are treated with preoperative radiotherapy alone, followed by surgery, depending on which arm of the study is chosen by random selection.

Our treatment for hard palate cancers parallels these patterns for soft palate. Our numbers are insufficient to justify arguing for this therapy, and our rationale is based on cures at other sites with combination therapy.

As a rule, I do not reconstruct palatal defects. Surgical prostheses, prepared preoperatively, are placed and modified intraoperatively by the prosthodontist. Although the creation of a satisfactory obturator requires the skills of a competent prosthodontist, and multiple visits are necessary for a final fit, the removal of the obturator allows a complete view of the resected region.

There are a few important basic considerations to remember when one is performing palate surgery. When hard palate lesions are resected, the more teeth that can be spared without sacrificing adequate surgical margins, the better. The teeth supply stability on which the prosthesis can be anchored. The same rule holds true for the alveolar ridge of the edentulous maxilla. When the soft palate is resected, if a 1 cm strip of the posterior edge of the soft palate cannot be maintained after a satisfactory oncologic resection is performed, the small remnant should be excised. A 1 cm or greater rim of soft palate provides enough soft tissue against which the obturator can sit, but less than this provides inadequate tissue and is a hindrance.

Necrotizing Sialometaplasia

The importance of necrotizing sialometaplasia is that it can be mistaken for squamous cell or mucoepidermoid carcinoma. In the original paper by Abrams et al. describing this entity, necrotizing sialometaplasia always involved the mucoperiosteum of the hard palate, primarily in men in the 50- to 60-year-old age group.[10] Since that initial report, a small number of cases in the minor salivary glands or other regions such as soft palate, retromolar trigone, maxillary sinus, and nasal cavity have also been described in the literature.[11] An ulcerated lesion on the hard palate may be necrotizing sialometaplasia, and this differential should be kept in mind. Important features of this lesion histopathologically are that some of the glandular lobules appear to have been infarcted, and the glandular general lobular morphology of the salivary gland tissue is maintained in spite of significant inflammatory and metaplastic changes.[10] The original manuscript states that the lesions were treated by local excision and healed in spite of "positive" or involved margins. Once the diagnosis has been made by incisional biopsy, local treatment or oral irrigations with or without a systemic antibiotic, such as penicillin, is appropriate therapy. This slow-healing lesion will usually heal in 1 month's time. Complete excision of the lesion should be reserved for those with which the pathologist has difficulty diagnosing.

Adenoid Cystic Carcinomas of the Hard Palate

Adenoid cystic carcinoma is a relatively rare neoplasm whose incidence increases as the size of the salivary gland decreases. Its incidence in the nose, sinus, and palate has been reported as high as 41% of all adenoid cystic carcinomas of the head and neck.[12] This tumor has been considered a surgical disease since its recognition, and this basic philosophy has not changed. Contrary to earlier reports,[13] the tumor is radiosensitive, and combined therapy, either preoperative or postoperative radiotherapy, has been used to treat this lesion. Since the palate is amenable to surgical extirpation, the initial therapy is wide local excision with generous, 2 cm surgical margins where possible. Postoperative radiotherapy is suggested because of the propensity of this tumor for perineural invasion. Elkon et al. have shown a decrease in the high local recurrence rate of salivary gland adenoid cystic carcinoma employing postoperative external beam radiotherapy in the range of 50 to 70 Gy.[14] This did not result in increased survival rates, since distant metastases without local recurrence is the rule. Survival rates for this tumor must be measured for 20 years to be significant.

As with adenoid cystic carcinoma in other sites, poor initial prognostic indicators are cranial or sensory nerve involvement at the time of presentation or pathologic evidence of perineural invasion. It follows that those patients with microscopically abnormal margins have a poorer prognosis than those with normal margins.[15] In the Miller-Calcaterra series, all failures occurred

initially at the primary site, with distant metastases following after the recurrence.[15] As with other salivary gland neoplasms, the overall response to chemotherapy at this point in time is poor, though there are some anecdotal cases relating significant tumor shrinkage with chemotherapy.

Postsurgical Velopharyngeal Incompetence

As mentioned in the section on squamous cell carcinoma of the palate, it is not my preference to reconstruct hard or soft palate surgical defects, since the defect provides an excellent access for postoperative observation. When one is performing an appropriate oncologic procedure, it is most difficult to avoid postsurgical velopharyngeal insufficiency, but this is relatively simple to treat if one has access to a well-trained prosthodontist.

The only lesion that will not require either prosthetic or surgical reconstruction following excision are those very rare superficial T1 lesions that can be excised with maintenance of the nasopharyngeal mucosa of the soft palate or the bone or sinonasal mucoperiosteum of hard palate. These defects will heal by secondary intention and require nothing more.

Pharynx–Squamous Cell Carcinoma

A discussion of oropharyngeal lesions confined to the pharyngeal wall is somewhat difficult, due to the paucity of lesions of this area. This is also reflected in the literature in which hypopharyngeal and oropharyngeal lesions are classified together as pharyngeal wall lesions. Marks et al., discussing pharyngeal wall cancer, reported 51 patients treated during a 10-year period, with only 9 lesions in the oropharynx,[16] and an additional 8 years of analysis added only 38 more patients to the series, 20 of these in the oropharynx.[17] With this in mind, the task of providing definitive advice on the best therapy for these tumors is difficult. For this discussion, I will define this region as the region superior to the pharyngoepiglottic fold, posterior to the posterior tonsillar pillar, involving the posterior pharyngeal wall and narrow lateral wall.

When the neoplasms are large (T3 and T4), a decision concerning therapy is not difficult. In most institutions, due to the generally poor prognosis with these tumors, a combined therapeutic approach is used. The standard therapy is surgery and radiotherapy, with radiotherapy given either preoperatively or postoperatively. These patients would qualify for the mitomycin-fluorouracil with concurrent irradiation protocol for advanced head and neck neoplasms at my institution.

A more difficult decision is posed by the smaller lesions (T1 or T2). According to the American Joint Committee on Cancer Staging classification, a T1 lesion is 2 cm or less in greatest diameter, and a T2 lesion is greater than 2 cm but less than 4 cm in its greater diameter. I presently treat T1 oropharyngeal lesions with radiation therapy for cure along with the smaller T2 lesions. For the larger T2 lesions, a more expectant plan is utilized. The patient is treated with a planned preoperative dosage of 50 Gy, and if the tumor has regressed totally with this dosage, the patient is then treated to a curative dose of 60 to 65 Gy. If there has been a less than satisfactory tumoricidal response after the initial 50 Gy, a 4- to 6-week waiting period is followed by a surgical resection.

SURGICAL APPROACHES TO TUMORS

Beyond the transoral approach for small lesions of the oropharynx, the surgical approaches advocated to resect the oropharyngeal wall include the suprahyoid pharyngotomy, the median labiomandibular glossotomy, and the lateral pharyngotomy with or without a partial mandibulectomy or a mandibulotomy. My preference is the lateral pharyngotomy approach for those tumors involving the posterior or lateral oropharyngeal wall with or without involvement of the base of tongue. This approach has been described for many years[18–20] and has been the mainstay of the "commando," or tongue-jaw-neck, procedure.

In those procedures in which the larynx is maintained, a number of points are important. Since swallowing will be altered from a mild to a significant degree, procedures that facilitate deglutition are important for the postoperative recovery. Performing a cricopharyngeal myotomy at the time of the procedure is one of these helpful procedures. In addition, paying careful attention to the superior laryngeal nerve at the time of resection and maintenance of this nerve, if possible, helps prevent postoperative aspiration. In the past, the split-thickness skin graft had been used for reconstruction. Today, the myocutaneous flap and free flaps provide the major methods of head and neck reconstruction. Their great bulk and lack of function interfere with swallowing after surgery.

If the neoplasm extends into the base of tongue or down the posterior hypopharyngeal wall, a decision regarding the larynx must be made. Part of the decision is based on the overall condition of the patient, that is, whether young or healthy or older with chronic obstructive pulmonary disease. More specific anatomic considerations involve the extent of the lesion. If 75% to 80% of the tongue base must be resected for a satisfactory surgical margin, deglutition will be significantly impaired. When the inferior extent of the posterior pharyngeal wall resection extends to the level of the arytenoids, postoperative aspiration is likely. Although it is not often that oropharyngeal lesions necessitate a laryngectomy for oncologic margins, laryngectomy may be necessary to prevent life-threatening aspiration. The decision regarding the larynx is based on these tenets in conjunction with surgical experience and judgment. Finally, if the oropharyngeal lesion involves a majority or all of the hypopharynx, a laryngopharyngectomy with reconstruction should be considered. At the University of Virginia, the preferred method of reconstruction is a gastric interposition.

THE N0 NECK

In general, my approach to the N0 neck is to treat the patient with 50 to 55 Gy. The concept that radiation therapy can control subclinical disease for head and neck squamous cell carcinoma is an accepted one,[21] and this philosophy guides my treatment of N0 necks for squamous cell carcinoma of the pharynx. An important consideration in the treatment of pharyngeal wall cancers is that the retropharyngeal nodes are the primary nodes for metastases, and the cervical nodes are secondary sites.

With this in mind, the retropharyngeal nodes are treated with preoperative radiotherapy that includes the nodes in both sides of the neck.

Occasionally, a neck dissection is performed on an N0 neck in a patient with an oropharyngeal squamous cell carcinoma. When one is faced with a large T3 or T4 lesion that has no clinically palpable disease in the neck, and a flap is needed to reconstruct the pharynx, access and space are needed to rotate the pedicle into position. A neck dissection is performed to provide space for the flap pedicle.

REFERENCES

1. Givens CD, Johns ME, Cantrell RW: Carcinoma of the tonsil: Analysis of 162 cases. *Arch Otolaryngol* 1981; 107:730–734.
2. Kaplan MJ, Hahn SS, Johns ME, et al: Mitomycin and fluorouracil with concomitant radiotherapy in head and neck cancer. *Arch Otolaryngol* 1985; 111:220–222.
3. Spiro RH, Gerold FP, Strong EW: Mandibular "swing" approach for oral and oropharyngeal tumors. *Head Neck Surg* 1981; 3:371–378.
4. McGregor IA, MacDonald DG: Mandibular osteotomy in the physical approach to the oral cavity. *Head Neck Surg* 1983; 5:457–462.
5. Mizono GS, Diaz RF, Fu KK, et al: Carcinoma of the tonsillar regions. *Laryngoscope* 1986; 96:240–244.
6. Puthawala AA, Syed AM, Gates TC: Iridium-192 implants in the treatment of tonsillar region malignancies. *Arch Otolaryngol* 1985; 111:812–815.
7. Chung CK, Constable WC: Squamous cell carcinoma of the soft palate and uvula. *Int J Radiat Oncol Biol Phys* 1979; 5:845–850.
8. Chung CK, Rahman SM, Lim ML, et al: Squamous cell carcinoma of the hard palate. *Int J Radiat Oncol Biol Phys* 1979; 5:191–196.
9. Fee WE, Schoeppel SL, Rubenstein R, et al: Squamous cell carcinoma of the soft palate. *Arch Otolaryngol* 1979; 105:710–718.
10. Abrams AM, Melrose RJ, Howell FV: Necrotizing sialometaplasia. A disease simulating malignancy. *Cancer* 1973; 32:130–135.
11. Maisel RH, Johnston WH, Anderson HA, et al: Necrotizing sialometaplasia involving the nasal cavity. *Laryngoscope* 1977; 87:429–434.
12. Leafstedt SW, Gaeta JF, Sako K, et al: Adenoid cystic carcinoma of major and minor salivary glands. *Am J Surg* 1971; 122:756–762.
13. Foote FW, Frazell EL: Tumors of the major salivary glands, in *Atlas of Tumor Pathology,* section 4, part 2. Washington, DC, Armed Forces Institute of Pathology, 1954.
14. Elkon D, Pope TL, Constable WC: Adenoid cystic carcinoma of the salivary gland. *Arch Otolaryngol* 1980; 106:410–413.
15. Miller RH, Calcaterra TC: Adenoid cystic carcinoma of the nose, paranasal sinuses, and palate. *Arch Otolaryngol* 1980; 106:424–426.
16. Marks JE, Freeman RB, Lee F, et al: Pharyngeal wall cancer: An analysis of treatment results, complications, and pattern of failure. *Int J Radiat Oncol Biol Phys* 1978; 4:587–593.

17. Marks JE, Smith PC, Sessions DG: Pharyngeal wall cancer. A reappraisal after comparison of treatment methods. *Arch Otolaryngol* 1985; 111:79–85.
18. Ogura JH, Watson RK, Jurema AA: Partial pharyngectomy and neck dissection for posterior hypopharyngeal cancer. *Laryngoscope* 1960; 70:1523–1533.
19. Som ML, Silver CE, Carbahal PG: Surgical approaches to the hypopharynx for benign disease. *Ann Otol Rhinol Laryngol* 1966; 83:222–230.
20. Orton HB: Lateral transthyroid pharyngotomy. Trotter's operation for malignant condition of the laryngopharynx. *Arch Otolaryngol* 1930; 12:320–338.
21. Fletcher GH: The role of irradiation in the management of squamous cell carcinomas of the mouth and throat. *Head Neck Surg* 1979; 1:441–457.

Management of the Primary Site: Oropharynx

Approach of

Jack L. Gluckman, M.D.

In spite of multiple advances in diagnostic techniques, the improved capability to resect increasingly advanced cancers and then reconstruct the resultant defect, and new and ever-changing radiation and chemotherapy protocols, the selection of the ideal therapy for the patient with oropharyngeal cancer is as confusing today as it was 25 years ago. The disease is better understood, as are the needs of the patient, and yet this knowledge has not really as yet been translated into improved survival rates. This disappointment should not, however, deter oncologists from using all the powerful new tools that have been placed at their disposal to better help the stricken patient. If, in the end, the only goal that can be accomplished is effective palliation with improved quality of life for the remaining days, this is a laudable accomplishment and worth pursuing. The basic premise of management is to maximize the results of treatment while minimizing the morbidity associated with the treatment.

THERAPEUTIC OPTIONS

Therapeutic options available to the physician are myriad but essentially can be categorized as follows: (1) surgery, (2) radiation, (3) combination surgery and radiotherapy, (4) chemotherapy as an adjunct to surgery and radiation therapy, (5) symptomatic palliative therapy, and (6) no treatment.

Each one of these modalities has its proponents and detractors, but, in the final analysis, because of the absence of any proved definitive approach, the oncologist uses the regimen that he or she feels most comfortable with and that seems best for the individual patient in an individual setting. This treatise reflects, therefore, my philosophy and experience.

FACTORS AFFECTING CHOICE OF THERAPY

Type of Malignancy

Not all growths that develop in the oropharynx are squamous cell carcinoma. A wide variety of benign and malignant tumors may arise from the tissues in this area. In addition, tumors may arise from parapharyngeal structures and present initially within the lumen of the pharynx and mimic primary intrapharyngeal tumors. These obviously need to be differentiated.

Squamous cell carcinoma is the most common malignancy in the oropharynx. Although clinically this cancer appears more aggressive than oral cavity cancer, with a concomitant worse prognosis, this phenomenon is more likely due to the advanced staging at the initial presentation because of late diagnosis. Macroscopically, various types are described: superficial and exophytic, ulcerative and infiltrative, and fungating. The superficial spreading exophytic lesion is found most commonly on the soft palate and faucial arch. These lesions are frequently associated with areas of condemned mucosa and are less aggressive, with a lower incidence of nodal metastases. Ulcerative, infiltrative, and fungating squamous cell carcinomas occur more often in the tonsillar fossa and tongue base and are associated with more aggressive behavior, a higher rate of metastases, and a more ominous prognosis.

Several attempts to correlate histopathologic findings with cure rate and ultimate survival have been made over the years. Squamous cell carcinomas are traditionally graded as well differentiated, moderately differentiated, and poorly differentiated, based on the amount of keratinization, intercellular bridging, and the degree of nuclear pleomorphism. Some authors have noted better prognosis with well-differentiated cancers, however; this has not been a universal experience. The pattern of invasion at the host-tumor interface appears to be the most important prognostic parameter. Carcinomas that invade in small aggregates have a greater propensity to infiltrate blood and lymphatics vessels and have a worse prognosis compared with those that invade with a broad pushing border. In addition, the frequency of mitoses is an important predictor of survival.

Other poor prognostic indicators include tumor size, histologic evidence of nodal metastases, and disease occurring in young patients who are nonsmokers and nondrinkers.

Lymphoepithelioma is a variant of squamous cell carcinoma and represents a poorly differentiated carcinoma with the lymphocytes not actively participating in the malignant transformation. It usually arises from the faucial or lingual tonsils themselves. It behaves somewhat differently from most squamous cell carcinomas in that it has a propensity to early nodal and distant metastases. Histologically, it consists of nests of epithelial cells with lymphocytes scattered between the cells. These tumors are exquisitely sensitive to radiation therapy.

On the other hand, verrucous carcinoma is a very well-differentiated carcinoma, characterized by slow growth and no propensity for local or distant metastases. The treatment of choice for these lesions is surgical excision.

Nonsquamous cell cancers may develop from minor salivary glands in the oropharynx. These should be differentiated from tumors arising in the deep lobe of the parotid presenting in and distorting the oropharynx. Fifty percent to 70% of all minor salivary gland tumors are malignant. Of the malignant tumors, the most common is the adenoid cystic carcinoma, but other malignancies such as the mucoepidermoid carcinoma, adenocarcinoma, acinic cell tumor, small cell tumor, and malignant pleomorphic adenoma all have been described. They usually develop as a painless submucosal mass, gradually increasing in size and rarely become ulcerated. If adenoid cystic carcinoma presents on the palate, the treatment should consist of wide excision usually necessitating an infrastructure maxillectomy. Because of their propensity for perineural spread, great care should be taken to isolate and perform a biopsy on regional nerves (e.g., in the palatine canal) to ensure adequate excision.

Hodgkin's and non-Hodgkin's lymphoma may arise in the tonsil and base of the tongue and should be strongly suspected in a unilateral enlargement of the tonsil, particularly if it is associated with large cervical nodes.

Sarcomas occasionally arise in the oropharynx.

Site of Malignancy

Tonsil

The majority of oropharyngeal cancers arise in the tonsil or tonsillar fossa. As they enlarge, the tumor begins to infiltrate into the surrounding tissues to involve the posterior pharyngeal wall and base of tongue and may extend inferiorly into the hypopharynx. Deep extension can cause fixation to or erosion of the ascending ramus of the mandible or involvement of the medial pterygoid muscle. Parapharyngeal space involvement can result in perineural invasion along cranial nerves with eventual extension to the base of the skull.

Base of the Tongue

Tumors of the base of tongue may arise de novo or may be secondary to spread from regional areas (e.g., tonsil, anterior portion of the tongue, and supraglottic larynx). In any event, these lesions are associated with a poor prognosis because of late diagnosis, difficulty in determining the exact extent of these tumors, and their tendency to early bilateral regional metastases. As the tongue involvement increases, there is spread deeply into the root of the tongue and also into the pre-epiglottic space.

Palatine Arch

Carcinoma of the anterior tonsillar pillar and soft palate usually presents as superficial spreading or exophytic lesions in areas of condemned mucosa, and multicentric cancers are common. Generally, these tumors have a better overall prognosis, but if left untreated, they will extend laterally along the soft palate to involve the lateral pharyngeal walls and the retromolar trigone and assume the more aggressive nature of lesions in this area.

Pharyngeal Wall

Cancer of the posterolateral pharyngeal wall often presents at an advanced stage due to the relative lack of symptoms associated with early lesions. Submucosal spread is not uncommon. Interestingly, the tumors may reach considerable size before invading the prevertebral fascia. This is fortunate, because once they have invaded the prevertebral musculature, the tumor usually is unresectable and probably not curable.

Staging of the Neoplasm

The size and extent of the tumor are most important in deciding the optimal regimen. Smaller, less advanced lesions can be cured by either radiation or surgery, and, therefore, the choice of which approach to use would be entirely dependent on other factors. The large, more advanced tumors, on the other hand, are associated with a poor prognosis regardless of the therapy used. In this situation, although every attempt at cure should be made, one does not want to subject the patient to mutilation and subsequent impaired quality of life in a futile attempt at cure.

To this end, every attempt should be made to delineate the extent of the tumor. A careful head and neck examination is essential. Check for the presence of trismus, limitation of tongue movement, cranial nerve involvement, particularly anesthesia in the distribution of the inferior alveolar nerve, and, of course, for any palpable cervical metastases. A panoramic x-ray view may be helpful in determining mandible involvement. Computed tomography may identify prevertebral muscle or cervical vertebrae erosion and base of skull involvement. Although it also may be helpful in determining the extent of the primary tumor and the presence of enlarged regional nodes, these findings may be misleading and should be correlated with the clinical findings. Magnetic resonance imaging may potentially be better for determining soft tissue invasion.

If suspicion for distant metastases is great, a metastatic workup should be performed; I do chest and abdominal CT scan and a bone scan.

Examination under anesthesia should always be performed to allow (1) more accurate evaluation of the tumor, (2) evaluation for multicentric cancers, and (3) tattooing and multiple deep biopsies. The tumor can then be staged.

Presence of Associated Disease

Head and neck surgery, though complex in nature, in general does not result in a profound disturbance of body metabolism postoperatively. The patient who develops the cancer, however, is frequently poorly nourished and may have significant pulmonary, cardiovascular, and hepatic disease. If severe, they may prevent surgery from being a therapeutic option or may influence the type of surgery proposed (e.g., poor pulmonary reserve necessitating a total laryngectomy in association with glossectomy to prevent aspiration).

Psychologic Attitude of the Patient

The fear of cancer usually outweighs the fear of surgery or radiotherapy. This is, unfortunately, not always the case, and irrational fear may dictate a change in policy. Never force the patient into an option that is not desired.

Attitude of Family and Support System

The family must be involved in the decision-making process. If they fail to live up to their obligations in aiding the patient's rehabilitation and acceptance back into society, the therapy will be judged a failure, no matter how successful it might appear to the oncologist.

Philosophy and Experience of the Oncologist

Each oncologist develops his or her own philosophy of management based on past experience and intuition in dealing with a particular oncologic problem in a particular setting. Until a fail-safe guaranteed "cookbook" cure for cancer is available, a diversity of opinion is to be expected and should, in fact, be encouraged.

Facilities Available

It is a fact of life that many head and neck tumors are managed away from the "ivory tower" of academic institutions, where enormous backup and support systems are in place for the management of these patients. Not every oncologist has access to dedicated nurses, prosthodontists, social workers, speech therapists, and so forth. Perhaps a case can be made for the management of all patients in a controlled centralized environment, but at this moment in time, this is not occurring. The absence of an experienced surgeon, radiotherapist, or chemotherapist, and the absence of support facilities (e.g., intensive care unit) should be taken into consideration when one is making the final decision as to how best to treat the patient.

RADIATION THERAPY

As surgical techniques for ablation and reconstruction have advanced in the past decade, so too have radiotherapeutic techniques. As in surgery, the results of radiation vary according to the skill and experience of the radiotherapist and the facilities at his or her disposal. The results of radiation alone in the treatment of early lesions of the oropharynx are comparable with those obtained from surgery. This usually consists of delivering a dose of 60 to 70 Gy through a shrinking field to the primary lesion and both sides of the neck over the course of 6 to 7 weeks, as indicated. Alternatively, reduced external radiation can be combined with radium implants, thereby boosting the tumor dose. However, implants are difficult to insert in the oropharynx. Likewise submental boosts of external radiation have been used in an attempt to minimize osteoradionecrosis of the mandible. Low-dose rate radiotherapy, as well as twice daily radiation, has been reported as improving local control rates. As the stage of the tumor increases, however, the efficacy of radiotherapy alone declines, and planned combined radiotherapy and surgery appear to offer a better chance for cure.

Radiation alone, therefore, may be used effectively:

1. For small limited cancers.
2. When surgery is not an option because of the absence of an experienced head and neck surgeon or adequate facilities for surgery.
3. When patient is physically or emotionally unable to undergo extensive surgery.
4. If the patient refuses surgery.
5. For palliation in the extremely advanced tumor.

Radiation should not, however, be indiscriminantly used with a view to salvaging the patient with surgery at a later stage if the disease should persist or recur. The success rate with surgical salvage is extremely poor, and the surgery after high-dose curative radiation is associated with a high morbidity.

Radiation itself is not without complications and may be associated with an unpleasant sequelae (e.g., xerostomia, loss of taste, mucosal ulceration, osteoradionecrosis, pharyngeal necrosis with fistula formation, and hemorrhage).

Newer radiation techniques, including the use of hyperthermia, electron beam therapy, and twice daily therapy, all await long-term follow-up so that their precise role can be properly defined.

COMBINATION SURGERY AND RADIATION THERAPY

The concept of combined therapy for advanced cancer is not new; however, only in the past 15 years has it been used on a consistent basis. The rationale for its use is based on the following observations.

The major reason for surgical failure is leaving residual viable tumor cells in the patient. This occurs because of unrecognized peripheral projection of malignant cells, undetected lymphatic or hematogenous metastasis, or the implantation of tumor during the surgery. On the other hand, the major reason for radiation failure is the projection of tumor outside the treatment field or the presence of anoxic cells in the center of the neoplasm remaining untreated. Therefore, theoretically planned combined radiation and surgery should be able to minimize the source of failure in each method.

Although it is strongly suggestive that combined therapy offers the best prognosis for advanced tumors, this remains unresolved, because as yet, no properly controlled trials definitely support this concept.

In addition, it is not yet clear whether preoperative or postoperative radiation should be used. In the 1970s, the use of preoperative radiation usually consisting of 45 to 50 Gy, followed by a 4-week delay to allow the acute radiation reaction to subside before the surgery, was the most popular regimen. The rationale for this approach was that the tumor would be theoretically more radiosensitive if the blood supply would not be compromised by the surgery and also that radiation may seal off the lymphatics, thereby allowing subsequent surgical manipulation without fear of tumor seeding.

In recent years, however, our tendency has been to perform the surgery and to follow it with postoperative radiation. The advantage of this approach is that the operative morbidity is significantly diminished, a slightly higher dose of radiation can be given, and there is less chance of inadequate resection because the margins are more easily identified. A disadvantage exists, however; if a surgical complication should occur, the radiation may be delayed sufficiently to become ineffective. This need not occur, because open wounds may be irradiated without fear of worsening the situation and preventing healing.

Overall, although combined therapy seems to be more effective in advanced tumors, there is little difference in survival rates between patients treated with preoperative vs. postoperative radiation.

ADJUNCT CHEMOTHERAPY

Chemotherapy has been used as a last resort for terminal cancer patients for many years, with its role being palliative in relieving pain and obstructive symptoms. The use of chemotherapeutic agents as an adjunct to both surgery and irradiation in the treatment of head and neck cancer continues to provoke interest. Unfortunately, although many drugs have shown tremendous promise in this role in terms of causing tumor regression, there is no definitive evidence that this therapy has any influence on ultimate long-term prognosis. Whether adjunct chemotherapy will ultimately aid in the control of local disease or prevent tumor dissemination remains, as yet, unanswered. I hope that chemotherapy will one day take its place as part of a multimodality treatment regimen for head and neck cancer.

SURGERY

Historically, it should be appreciated that the reason radiation assumed a dominant role in the treatment of oropharyngeal cancers is because the oropharynx was assumed to be inaccessible to surgical resection. Today, however, a myriad of surgical approaches to lesions of the oropharynx have been described:

1. Intraoral resection
2. Mandible-sparing procedures
    a. Lateral pharyngotomy
    b. Transhyoid pharyngotomy
3. Mandible-splitting procedures
    a. Lateral osteotomy
    b. Midline osteotomy
4. Composite resection (jaw-neck procedure)

Which approach is optimal for a particular cancer is dependent on the site and size of the tumor as well as whether a concomitant lymph node dissection is needed.

Intraoral Resection

Great caution should be exercised before an intraoral resection for cancer of the oropharynx is recommended. It is a very rare lesion, indeed, that is amenable to such an approach. Included in this warning is the inclination to perform a tonsillectomy for squamous cell carcinoma apparently confined to the tonsil. Cancer does not obey normal tissue planes, and this operation can be interpreted at best as a debulking procedure and at worst as opening tissue planes for further spread.

Some lesions may, however, benefit from intraoral resection, and these include:

1. Superficial exophytic lesions, particularly arising from the posterior oropharyngeal wall and soft palate.
2. The "condemned mucosa," with multicentric lesions frequently identified on the soft palate.

The latter may be treated by superficial local excision or ablation of the affected epithelium. The excision can be accomplished using a scalpel, cautery, or carbon dioxide laser with equally good results. The CO_2 laser has some advantages, including improved hemostasis, less edema, and being more precise, but it is not essential for the treatment of these lesions. As always, frozen section control should be performed when these tumors are excised not only from the periphery but from the depth of the resection as well.

After resection, the defect is usually allowed to heal by secondary intention. Occasionally, a nasogastric tube may be needed for a few days to facilitate healing.

Other defects may be closed primarily by mobilizing the surrounding mucosa or using a split skin, which should be quilted into position or, if necessary, stented with a bolster.

Mandible-Sparing Procedures

Lateral Pharyngotomy

Lateral pharyngotomy is an excellent approach to moderately sized lesions on the posterolateral pharyngeal wall, provided they are small enough and inferior enough that adequate access can be attained without disrupting the mandible. Of course, if the lesion is large, the pharyngotomy may be extended superiorly and combined with a lateral mandibular osteotomy to improve access. This technique may be combined with a neck dissection. Key points in the technique are to enter the pharynx by retracting the thyroid ala medially and incising the mucosa of the upper pyriform sinus and extending the incision superiorly. The superior laryngeal nerve must be identified and avoided.

Transhyoid Pharyngotomy

The transhyoid pharyngotomy is an excellent approach to lesions of the lower posterior oropharyngeal wall that are too large or too inferior to remove transorally. Technically, the incision is made over the hyoid bone, flaps are developed, and the body of the hyoid is removed. Care is taken not to damage the superior laryngeal or hypoglossal nerves. The vallecula is entered, and an excellent view of the posterior pharyngeal wall is obtained. After resection, the wound is closed primarily. A temporary tracheostomy is performed, and the procedure can be combined with a neck dissection if indicated. This procedure gives an excellent cosmetic and functional result.

Mandible-Splitting Procedures

If the tumor cannot be readily accessed by working around the mandible, it may be necessary to split the mandible to obtain adequate exposure. After the resection and reconstruction have been completed, the mandible is reapproximated and either wired or plated into position. The osteotomies may be performed in two different sites.

Lateral Osteotomy

Classically known as the Trotter's operation, this technique necessitates a stepped osteotomy of the body of the mandible with the exact site depending on the size and site of the tumor and the state of the patient's dentition. It may be combined with a concomitant neck dissection, and after the mandible has been splayed apart, the tumor is removed in continuity with the neck dissection. After resection, the mandible is approximated using wire or plates.

The ideal indications for this procedure are moderately sized lesions of the tonsil, lateral pharyngeal wall, or base of tongue that are not in close proximity to the mandible or directly invading into the mandible itself. If postoperative radiation is to be given, this type of osteotomy is contraindicated because it will be in the radiation field, and nonunion may result. It would, therefore, be better to perform a midline osteotomy that would be out of the radiation field.

A further, if somewhat minor, sequela of this approach is that the inferior alveolar nerve is transected with resultant anesthesia in its distribution.

Midline Osteotomy

Perhaps a more useful technique for splitting and preserving the mandible is the midline osteotomy. Much discussion exists as to whether the osteotomy should be symphyseal or parasymphyseal or whether it should be straight or stepped. It is my opinion that the actual osteotomy is best performed in a stepped manner just anterior to the mental foramen, ensuring that the inferior alveolar nerve is preserved. The mandible is then swung apart after a release incision is made along the lateral floor of the mouth, leaving an adequate cuff of mucosa on the lingual surface of the alveolar ridge to allow primary closure or flap reconstruction. After the lesion has been excised and reconstructed, the mandible is reapproximated and plated.

This technique is likewise indicated for moderately sized lesions of the oropharynx that do not involve the mandible. It is also an excellent approach to posterior pharyngeal wall and base of tongue cancers.

A variant of this technique is the median translingual pharyngotomy (median labiomandibular glossotomy), which also requires a midline osteotomy. Instead of releasing the mandible along the lateral floor of mouth, however, the tongue is divided down the midline. This is useful as an approach to the posterior pharynx or resection of benign or low-grade malignancies of the base of the tongue. This approach results in minimal functional deformity but is only rarely indicated.

Composite Resection (Jaw-Neck Procedure)

Composite resection consisting of a neck dissection, together with partial mandibulectomy and incontinuity excision of the oropharyngeal lesion, has been and still is the cornerstone for the management of the advanced cancers of the oropharynx. It is without a doubt the method of choice for extensive cancer, cancer with overt mandible involvement, and in postradiation salvage situations where the exact extent of the tumor is unclear. Although regarded as a very radical procedure, under the most ideal circumstances, it may be associated with a very acceptable cosmetic and functional result.

Details of this procedure are readily available in most surgical atlases, and only the highlights will be presented here.

The incision usually consists of a modified Frazier incision that will allow a radical neck dissection to be performed. The upper horizontal incision permits a degloving approach to the oropharynx or may be extended into a lip-splitting incision to improve access if necessary. This is not, in my experience, routinely necessary.

A standard neck dissection is then performed, with the neck dissection being pedicled on the angle and posterior third of the body of the mandible. It is very important to be sure that the neck dissection is completely free from the carotid system before resection of the primary tumor is attempted. Occasionally in advanced tumors where there is a perception that the tumor has extended out into the upper part of the neck, it is better to perform this dissection, particularly the submandibular triangle, in continuity with the excision of the primary tumor.

Initially, intrapharyngeal mucosal cuts are made to delineate the area to be resected, and a spinal needle is passed from the oral cavity into the neck at the site of the anterior line of excision external to the mandible to determine the site of the anterior osteotomy. The periosteum along the lower aspect of the body of the mandible is incised and carefully elevated, exposing the mandible to be excised. The anterior osteotomy is then performed. The superior or posterior osteotomy can be performed just below the sigmoid notch or the condyle may be divided just below the temporomandibular joint. Occasionally it may be necessary to disarticulate the temporomandibular joint to obtain an adequate margin. If reconstruction of the mandible is being contemplated, it may be advisable to perform a vertical posterior osteotomy just posterior to the entrance of the inferior alveolar canal, leaving a 2 cm wide vertical strut of mandible to which a plate can be attached.

Using a heavy scissors intraorally, the surgeon deepens the mucosal cuts on the soft palate through the nasopharynx, and continues the dissection along the mucosal incisions. The segment of the mandible with the tumor is then splayed outward, exposing the full extent of the tumor, which can now be easily resected from the external approach by following the previously performed mucosal cuts. The pterygoid musculature is divided last because dissection in this area is often accompanied by profuse bleeding. The secret to removal is adequate exposure and an exact three-dimensional concept of the extent of the proposed excision.

At this stage, the cut end of the mandible is rongeured to prevent the sharp edge from eroding through the skin. The defect is then reconstructed. After reconstruction, a dermal skin graft is placed over the carotid artery unless it can be covered by the muscle pedicle of a myocutaneous flap.

In an uncomplicated situation, the postoperative management is relatively simple, with the tracheostomy being removed at 5 days and the nasogastric tube a few days later. There may be difficulty with deglutition and aspiration initially, but the patient quickly learns to overcome these problems. Antibiotics are used prophylactically in the perioperative period.

MANAGEMENT OF CERVICAL METASTASES

Controversy has always and will continue to rage as to how best to treat cervical metastases. What is known, however, is that 55% to 75% of patients with oropharyngeal cancers will have neck metastases at presentation, and approximately 20% will have bilateral metastases. Therefore, the neck should be treated in some manner when all but the smallest and most superficial cancers are managed.

N0 necks can probably be treated as well using radiation or surgery, but in my opinion, necks at stages N1 to N3 should be treated with surgical excision in continuity with the primary tumor where feasible. Postoperative radiation, including both sides of the neck, is usually also given in these advanced cancers. If bilateral metastases are present, simultaneous bilateral neck dissections can be performed, with every attempt being made to preserve the contralateral internal jugular vein.

The type of neck dissection to be performed is also controversial; my inclination is to perform a radical neck dissection with sparing of the accessory nerve only if it can be safely performed without compromising dissection of the upper jugular chain metastases.

RECONSTRUCTION

If there has been any advance in the past decade in the management of head and neck cancer, it has been in the realm of reconstruction. Adequate reconstruction not only is important from the asthetic point of view but also, of course, is vital functionally. Poorly conceived reconstruction will result in significant alteration in speech, mastication, and deglutition. Never, however, should the resection be tailored to fit the preconceived reconstructive plan, because any compromise will result inevitably in recurrent cancer and subsequent death.

Healing by Secondary Intention

Small defects of the soft palate and posterior pharyngeal walls following intraoral resection can comfortably be allowed to heal in by secondary intention, particularly if the area excised is relatively superficial (e.g., mucosa and submucosa). This is frequently preferable to primary closure, especially if advancing the edges of the defect will lead to distortion of the pharynx.

Primary Closure

Almost any defect in the oropharynx can be repaired by primary closure. However, the resultant distortion of the pharynx may be so significant that all the vital functions of the pharynx and, for that matter, oral cavity are compromised. Small superficial and through-and-through defects are, however, quickly and easily managed in this way.

Primary closure used to be the technique of choice following composite resection because of its relative ease and because of the difficulties experienced in using a reliable flap. Indeed, one of the indications given for performing a partial mandibulectomy was not for oncologic reasons but to facilitate this closure.

If performed, it should be a three-layered closure, with the most important suture being at the trifurcation between the soft palate, tongue base, and buccal mucosa. Great care should be exercised to avoid tethering the tongue too high on the lateral pharyngeal wall, because it will result in difficulty with deglutition. Also, the contralateral tonsillolingual fold may be released to allow mobilization of the tongue and minimize the tension on the suture line.

Primary closure following a jaw-neck procedure in this modern day is only rarely performed because of the acknowledged advantages of flap reconstruction.

Free Skin Graft or Dermal Graft

Free skin grafts are extremely useful in closing defects of the posterior pharyngeal wall and may be maintained in position by means of stenting or the quilting technique. The use of a stent in the oropharynx necessitates a temporary tracheostomy, and for this reason, quilting is preferable; however, it does not appear to fix the graft as well as a stent.

Split-thickness graft reconstruction following a through-and-through composite resection has been successfully used. This method utilizes a large redundant pouch of either split-thickness skin or dermal graft that is sutured into the defect with a single layer of absorbable suture. This pouch is then packed with a bolster consisting of polymyxin B sulfate (Polysporin)–impregnated iodoform gauze. This results in a saliva-tight anastomosis and minimal shrinkage. Intermaxillary fixation assists in graft immobilization, thereby improving graft take. Although excellent results have been reported and the technique is certainly quickly and easily performed, a regional flap is probably preferable in the vast majority of cases.

Tongue Flaps

The tongue, because of its size, composition, and situation, is ideal for reconstruction of regional defects, particularly following resection of the base of tongue and lateral pharynx. The advantages of the tongue flap are that (1) it has a rich blood supply that ensures viability even under the most adverse circumstances, and (2) no additional defect is created as is the case if regional flaps are used.

The major disadvantage is that speech and deglutition will be adversely affected to a greater degree than when other forms of reconstruction are used. If it is thought that this may be a major factor in the postoperative rehabilitation of the patient, it is better not to use these flaps.

Numerous tongue flaps are available for reconstruction. The easiest technique for reconstructing the lateral pharynx consists of dividing the tongue longitudinally in the midline and basing the flap laterally on the floor of the mouth. The flap is filleted to increase its surface area and then rotated 180 degrees into the surgical defect and sutured into position. The remaining portion of the tongue is closed on itself. A variation of this technique is the setback technique, which can be used to close base of the tongue defects.

Another alternative is to base the tongue posteromedially, but this is possible only if a minimal amount of tongue has been involved in the resection.

Some controversy exists whether to denervate the tongue flap to decrease its movement and, therefore, its metabolism and, therefore, rendering it more liable to survive. Others believe that the intact nerve supply aids in improving subsequent deglutition. It has been my inclination to denervate the tongue flap where appropriate.

Regional Cutaneous Flaps

The advantage of regional skin flaps is that they enable tension-free reconstruction using viable nonirradiated healthy tissue.

The forehead flap, for many years, was the definitive flap for reconstruction of these defects. It was enormously popular because of its great reliability. The donor site defect, however, was unacceptable cosmetically. Even though hardly used today, some knowledge of this flap is essential because it may still be indicated if no other flap is available.

The versatile deltopectoral flap is an excellent means of reconstructing this defect. It may be used in two ways:

1. As a two-stage procedure whereby the flap is sutured into the defect after inversely tubing its pedicle under the skin flaps. This creates a controlled pharyngostoma that has to be closed as a second stage. It is rarely used today.

2. As a one-stage procedure in which the pedicle is deepithelialized prior to suturing the flap into the defect. This allows the pedicle to be buried within the wound and eliminates the need for a second stage. Great care should be exercised when the pedicle is deepithelialized to avoid compromising the blood supply of the flap.

Myocutaneous Flaps

In the past decade, myocutaneous flaps have gained increasing popularity as the definitive method of reconstruction of defects in the oropharynx. The pectoralis major, trapezius, sternocleidomastoid, and latissimus dorsi flaps all have a role either on their own or combined with bone as an osteomyocutaneous flap if the mandible needs to be reconstructed. Of these flaps, the pectoralis major remains the most popular because of its reliability and ease of harvesting. The sternocleidomastoid is the least useful because of its rather tenuous blood supply as it is increasingly mobilized. In addition, it may well be contraindicated in patients who will require a radical neck dissection for ablation of the tumor. Trapezius myocutaneous flaps are not quite as reliable as the pectoralis major flap and, as the patient requires to be repositioned intraoperatively, is not very convenient.

The advantages of these flaps are that a large defect may be closed, and the bulkiness of the pedicle not only protects the carotid system but also camouflages the cosmetic defect created by the neck dissection and partial mandibulectomy. The bulkiness of the flap initially may be a problem impairing deglutition and even the airway occasionally, but this bulkiness usually settles with time.

Free Flaps With Microvascular Anastomosis

Free flap reconstruction of the oropharynx has always been an attractive concept. The groin flap, dorsalis pedis flap, latissimus dorsi flap, radial forearm flap, and free jejunal graft all have been used with great success. Many of these flaps may be used not only on their own but also combined with underlying bone to provide reconstruction of the mandible if indicated.

The major advantage is the ability to harvest almost limitless amount of tissue that can be used to close almost any defect. The disadvantages are that it is time consuming, it requires a two-team approach with personnel well trained in microvascular technique, and the recipient site must have at least one artery and vein available for use. Although the artery poses no difficulty, the venous component may not be readily available after a radical neck dissection, and a vein graft may become necessary. The popularity of this technique will, therefore, always be limited because of the inconvenience associated with this procedure. Where facilities for this technique do exist, however, it is a most attractive alternate approach to reconstruction.

The free jejunal graft can be used as a patch graft for limited repair of the pharynx or as an intact tube for reconstruction following total laryngopharyngectomy for extensive tumors. The major disadvantage as a patch graft is that hypersecretion from the jejunum results in severe aspiration problems, rendering it inconvenient to use. On the other hand, it is an excellent technique for reconstructing the total laryngopharynx with the ability for it to stretch high up into the nasopharynx and down into the superior mediastinum. At this stage, the radial forearm flap is probably at present the most convenient and reliable free flap for reconstruction of partial oropharyngeal defects.

Reconstruction of the Mandible

Significant controversy exists as to the indications for reconstruction of the posterior aspect of the mandible following composite resection. Although asthetically and functionally it appears reasonable to reconstruct, this is not always necessary provided the soft tissue had been adequately replaced. The methods of reconstructing are multiple, and the ideal method in any one situation would frequently depend on the technique used for soft tissue reconstruction. For example, bone can be incorporated in a free flap (e.g., iliac crest or radial forearm flaps) or in a myocutaneous flap (e.g., rib or scapula). There has recently been a resurgence of interest in using mandible replacement plates. This may well prove to be the easiest and least time-consuming method for posterior mandible replacement.

PALLIATION

The management of the patient who is incurable because of either late presentation or failed therapy is a tremendous challenge to the oncologist. Every effort should be made to alleviate suffering and to allow the patient to spend his or her last days with dignity. The use of irradiation or chemotherapy to obtain tumor shrinkage or to alleviate pain should be considered. Tracheostomy, esophagostomy, or gastrostomy may be indicated. Placement in an institution even for short periods to relieve the burden on the relatives and friends may be necessary. The patient's medication (e.g., analgesics) must be constantly reevaluated to ensure that pain is controlled.

REHABILITATION

For too long, the act of ablating the carcinoma, no matter how radical the procedure, to cure the patient was regarded as the goal of both the oncologist and the patient. In recent years, however, great emphasis has been placed on the total rehabilitation of the patient, the most important factor of which is patient motivation. Without the patient wanting to be rehabilitated, the oncologist and the rehabilitation team are helpless. Total rehabilitation is the function of a team of professionals, with the surgeon playing a lesser but coordinating role. Speech therapists, physical therapists, social workers, occupational therapists, prosthodontists, and nurses, together with the patient's immediate family, all are vital members of this team. A number of factors have to be considered.

Cosmetic Appearance

Since younger patients and more women are being treated for this disease, there is an increasing awareness of the cosmetic appearance after therapy. Although much of the surgery is to some degree mutilating, modern reconstructive modalities have been able to minimize the deformity created. As stated earlier, certainly the surgery should never be compromised in an attempt to minimize the defect created. Scars in the neck can be covered with scarves, and hair may be styled to cover the defect. In men, a beard may be grown.

Speech

Dysarthria is a consequence of oral cavity and oropharyngeal resection, with the degree of tongue removal being the dominant factor in determining the severity of the speech defect. The articulation defect most apparent is in the formation of speech fricatives (e.g., this, that) that require lingual-dental approximation. Prevention by assurance that the tongue is not tethered too high or too low if primary closure is used or by the interposition of flaps or grafts to provide more mobility is the best method of treatment. If a tongue tie does result, however, the problem can be improved by dividing the scar tissue and placing a generous split-thickness skin graft to release the tongue or by using a CO_2 laser for tongue release. A speech therapist is invaluable in aiding these patients postoperatively.

Velopharyngeal incompetence due to removal of much of the soft palate is another cause of dysarthria. Although the soft palate can be replaced intraoperatively with an inert flap, it has been my experience that prosthetic rehabilitation in the postoperative period affords the best relief.

Deglutition

If a large portion of the tongue has been removed and the remaining tongue is tethered, the posterior propulsion of food into the hypopharynx becomes awkward. The bolus has a tendency to be propelled down the side of the surgical defect and often directly into the larynx. This, combined with the anesthesia of the flap-covered portion of the pharynx, results in aspiration problems with all the sequelae of repeated lower respiratory tract infections, feat of eating, and debility. Most patients can be trained to correct this problem by swallowing therapy. Occasionally, a cricopharyngeal myotomy may be necessary as a secondary procedure if the swallowing problem continues. Unfortunately, this has been of only limited value in my experience. Velopharyngeal incompetence with reflux of food through the nose is also a problem, but this is helped by the use of a dental appliance.

Mastication

In patients on whom partial mandibulectomy has been performed, the mandible is frequently deviated by scarring, resulting in interference with mastication.

Prevention is vital, and without a doubt the best prophylactic measure is the judicious use of flap reconstruction to prevent scarring and tethering of the mandibular remnant. In addition, reconstruction of the mandible using bone or plating, particularly if the ipsilateral temporomandibular joint has not been disturbed, will further improve this situation. The use of external splints (e.g., Joe Hall Morris splint) for a number of months postoperatively may be advantageous but, in my experience, has proved usually unnecessary.

Psychosocial Functioning

Too often insufficient attention is devoted to the tremendous psychologic adjustments the patient has to make, with attention zeroing in on his or her physical adjustments. The emotional status of the patient in the postoperative period is important. The patient is frequently depressed, and this depression interferes with motivation for physical rehabilitation. An experienced and understanding nursing, medical, and paramedical staff is, therefore, important in aiding the patient to overcome this problem. If necessary, psychiatric guidance should be sought.

In addition, there may be a change in the relationship with the immediate family driven by fear of being rejected by them. Adequate family counseling is vital. The patient must learn to accept the situation and make the necessary alterations in lifestyle to compensate for the particular disability.

CHAPTER 19

Management of the Primary Site: Larynx and Hypopharynx

Approach of

Carl E. Silver, M.D.

CONSERVATION PROCEDURES

Current surgical treatment of laryngeal cancer has been distinguished by the advent of conservation surgery for adequate tumor excision with preservation of essential laryngeal functions. The anatomic and pathologic basis of such surgery is the tendency of many laryngeal tumors to remain confined within the various fibrocartilaginous compartments of the larynx during early stages of development. Its physiologic basis lies in the fact that most individuals are able to adapt to loss of substantial portions of the larynx while retaining ability to breathe, swallow, and speak. Many techniques of conservation surgery had their origins in the late 19th and early 20th centuries but had to await advances in anesthesiology, antibacterial therapy, and improved comprehension of the natural history of laryngeal carcinoma before becoming clinically useful.

Hajek[1] and Pressman[2] employed dye injection studies to demonstrate anatomic compartmentation of the larynx. Frazier observed the embryologic derivation of supraglottic structures from buccopharyngeal anlage and of glottic and infraglottic structures from pulmonary anlage.[3] Tucker and Smith defined the connective tissue structures that form important compartmental barriers by study of whole organ serial sections in the human fetus.[4] These consist of the laryngeal cartilages and associated fibroelastic tissues, the conus elasticus with its thickened upper rim comprising the vocal ligaments, the anterior commissure (Broyle's) tendon, the ventricular connective tissue, and the quadrangular membrane with its ventricular ligaments. Strong barriers to spread of cancer from one side of the larynx to the other and from supraglottic to glottic regions have been demonstrated by numerous authors.

In conservation surgery, resection is established in either the vertical or horizontal plane according to the location of the tumor; thus, a vertical approach is employed for glottic tumors, whereas supraglottic tumors are resected by horizontal section of the larynx. Because exploration may reveal extension of tumor beyond preoperatively estimated limits, consent for total laryngectomy should be obtained prior to attempted conservation surgery.

Vertical Hemilaryngectomy

Laryngofissure

Laryngofissure, or cordectomy via thyrotomy, is suitable for small carcinomas (T1) confined to the membranous portion of the vocal cord without deep invasion. At the present time, laryngofissure is rarely employed for treatment of laryngeal cancer, because lesions suitable for this procedure are most often treated by radiation therapy, endoscopic laser surgery, or hemilaryngectomy. Occasionally, laryngofissure may be useful for treatment of recurrent or persistent tumor following irradiation, particularly in severely debilitated individuals.

The technique is demonstrated in Figure 19–1. In laryngofissure, as opposed to vertical hemilaryngectomy, resection is confined to mucosal and submucosal tissue; cartilage is not resected in continuity with the tumor. The defect heals by reepithelialization with formation of a functional pseudocord. Voice may be improved by subperichondrial resection of a section of thyroid cartilage to permit better approximation of the pseudocord with its opposite member or by transposition of a bipedicled flap of sternohyoid muscle into the laryngeal interior.[5]

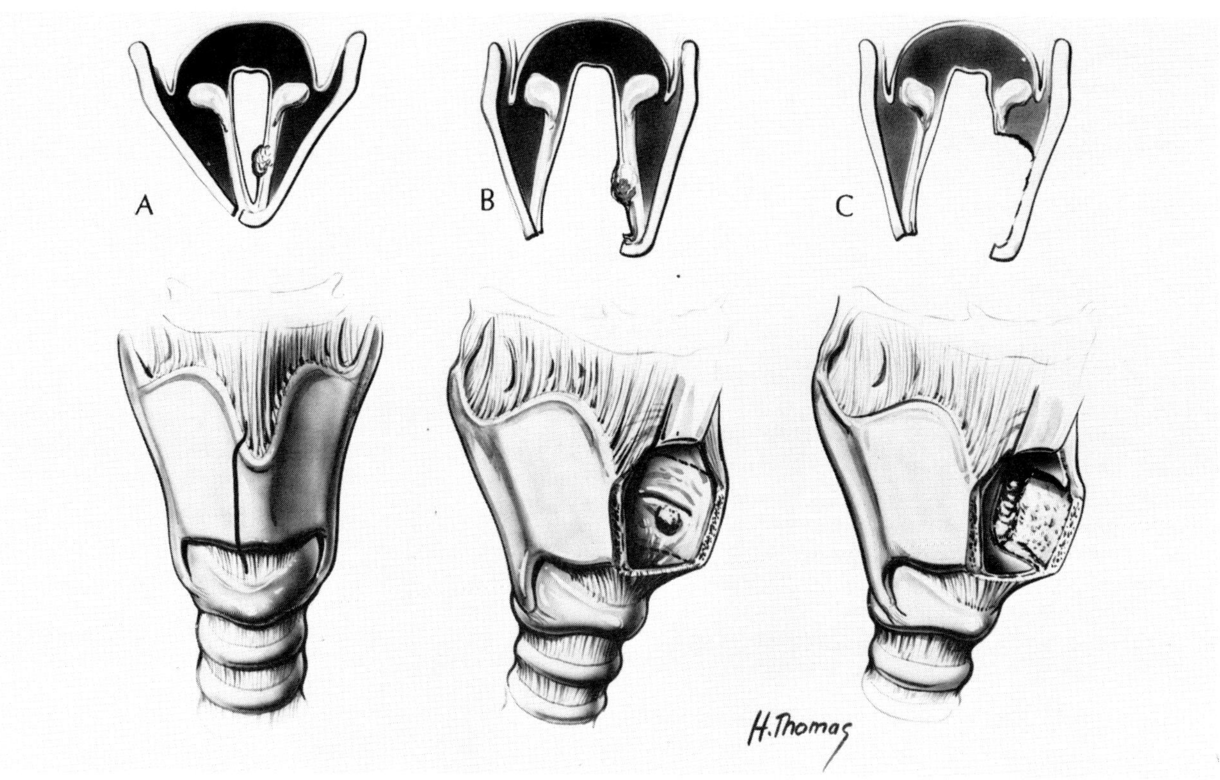

FIG 19–1.
Laryngofissure. **A**, suitable lesion confined to membranous portion of vocal cord. Placement of thyrotomy incision. **B**, endolarynx exposed. Resection outlined. **C**, larynx after completion of resection. The mucosal defect will heal secondarily. (From Silver CE: *Curr Probl Surg* 1977; 14:2–69. Used by permission.)

I always employ tracheostomy as an initial step in laryngofissure and in other open surgical procedures on the larynx. This permits safe, unimpeded access to the larynx and a secure postoperative airway. The tracheostomy is decannulated when the surgical wound has healed and postoperative edema has subsided.

Reported cure rates for laryngofissure performed in the modern era have ranged from 60% to 98%.[6–8] Variation in results has depended, for the most part, on the percentage of radiation failures in the series.

Anterior Frontal Partial Laryngectomy (Anterior Commissure Technique)

Glottic carcinomas tend to progress anteriorly across the commissure onto the contralateral cord. This extension is often superficial and extends only a few millimeters beyond the commissure. Lesions of this sort are amenable to radiation therapy, although if surgical resection is employed, a vertical midline segment of thyroid cartilage should be included. When no more than one third of the contralateral cord has been excised, resurfacing may be accomplished by suture of preserved external perichondrium to the cut margin of the cord. The ipsilateral side is not resurfaced. It will heal by granulation and reepithelialization.

More extensive tumors may cross the anterior commissure and involve significant portions of both vocal cords. Such lesions often extend subglottically or supraglottically in the midline. Because the thyroid cartilage lacks internal perichondrium at the insertion of Broyle's tendon, there is no barrier between tumor and thyroid cartilage at the anterior commissure. Adequate surgical resection of this type of lesion requires removal of a vertical midline segment of thyroid cartilage as well as major portions of both vocal cords. A representative lesion is demonstrated in Figure 19–2,A. The surgical defect following resection may appear formidable, with only posterior commissure mucosa remaining in the endolarynx. Although a variety of reconstructive techniques, including skin grafts, skin flaps, perichondrium, and muscle flaps, have been employed, the simple technique described in 1968 by Som and Silver[9] avoids the need for complex resurfacing procedures by utilizing a temporary midline partition, as developed by McNaught[10] for treatment of laryngeal webs. The partition permits both sides to reepithelialize independently with resultant satisfactory airway and voice.

The technical steps of the procedure are demonstrated in Figure 19–2. Following tracheostomy and exposure of the thyroid cartilage by reflection of the overlying infrahyoid muscles, bilateral thyrotomy incisions are made. Laryngeal soft tissues are separated subperichondrially from each thyroid ala bilaterally as far as the vocal process of arytenoid. The laryngeal lumen is entered anteriorly through the inferior cricothyroid membrane. It is most important to assess accurately the extent of tumor involvement prior to laryngeal entry to avoid compromise of the resection margin. After initial entry, the mucosa is retracted with a small hook as the incision extends posteriorly on the side of lesser involvement. The incision extends vertically at the posterior resection limit immediately anterior to the vocal process. At the superior limit of the posterior vertical incision, the mucosal cut is carried back to the anterior midline as a horizontal incision, traversing the thyrohyoid membrane. At this point, the mobilized portion of the larynx can be retracted forward, affording a panoramic view of the endolarynx and the tumor (Fig 19–2,B). Resection is completed by appropriate circumcision of mucosa and muscle around the tumor. The operation may be extended to include the ipsilateral arytenoid or superior half of anterior cricoid cartilage (or both) to assure a tumor-free margin.

A prosthesis is now inserted to partition the larynx (Fig 19–2,C), and a semirigid silicone rubber keel of the McNaught type may be employed. This type of prosthesis is secured to the thyroid cartilage and requires a second operation in approximately 6 weeks for removal. A soft silicone rubber sheet, secured with sutures through the skin, may be used in place of the rigid prosthesis. The soft partition may be removed endoscopically. I have preferred the semirigid prosthesis because of more secure maintenance of position. The procedure to remove

TABLE 19–1.
Results of Anterior Frontal Partial Laryngectomy

Series	Yr	Stage	Results (%)
Som and Silver[9]	3	T2	26/38 (68)
Kirchner and Som[11]	4	T2	40/58 (69)
Sessions et al.[12]	3	T1–T2	45/61 (74)
Total			111/157 (70)

the prosthesis can be performed easily with local anesthesia.

Reported results of several series of anterior frontal partial laryngectomy are summarized in Table 19–1.[9, 11, 12] Three-year cure in 111 of 157 (70%) cases was reported.

Hemilaryngectomy (Extended Frontolateral Laryngectomy)

The procedure conventionally referred to as "vertical hemilaryngectomy" includes removal of a thyroid ala, arytenoid, and mucosa from aryepiglottic fold to cricothyroid membrane, from anterior commissure to posterior midline. This procedure is indicated for glottic carcinoma with extension posteriorly to involve the vocal process and anterior surface of arytenoid or

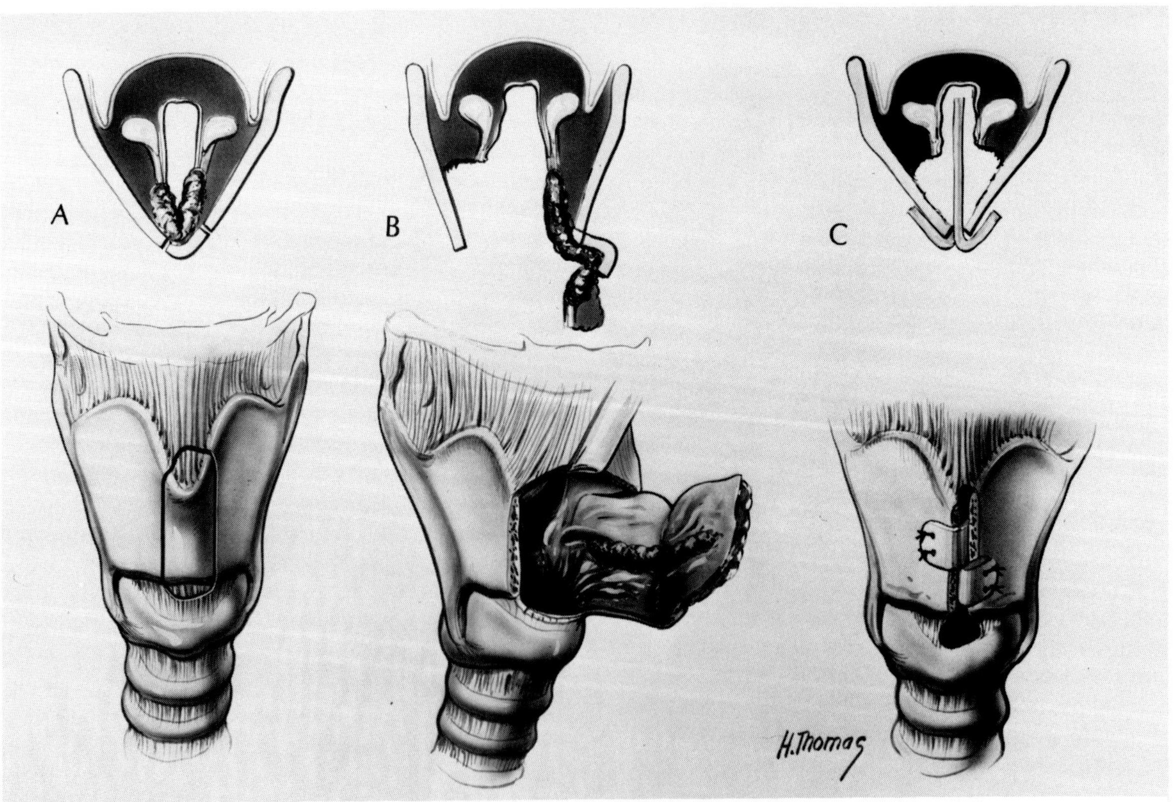

FIG 19–2.
Anterior commissure partial laryngectomy. **A,** suitable lesion involving significant portions of both vocal cords. Placement of bilateral thyrotomy incisions. **B,** larynx is entered on side of lesser involvement posterior to tumor. Appropriate traction exposes the entire mucosal surface to be resected. **C,** placement of "keel" after resection. (From Silver CE: *Curr Probl Surg* 1977; 14:2–69. Used by permission.)

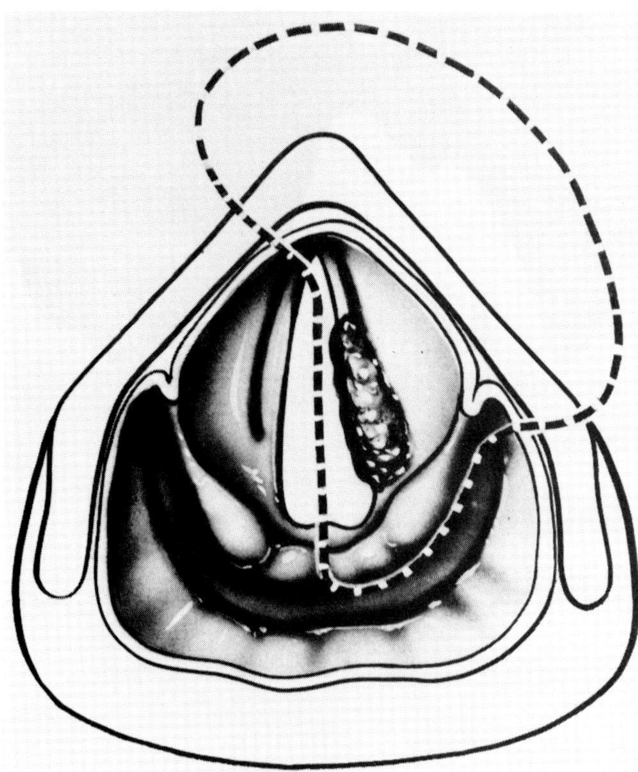

FIG 19–3.
Lesion suitable for vertical hemilaryngectomy with outline of planned resection (From Silver CE: *Surgery for Cancer of the Larynx.* New York, Churchill Livingstone, 1981. Used by permission.)

with involvement of the floor of the ventricle laterally with infiltration of thyroarytenoideus muscle. The procedure may be extended to include resection of various portions of the contralateral vocal cord (extended frontolateral laryngectomy). In such instances, the rules stated earlier for anterior commissure resection apply; if one third or less of the contralateral cord is resected, the laryngeal mucosa of that side may be advanced to the external perichondrium without need of grafts, skin flaps, or prostheses to maintain an adequate laryngeal lumen. If more than one third of the contralateral cord must be resected, various reconstructive measures must be employed to reconstruct the laryngeal framework or mucosal surface.

The most important factors in determining suitability for conventional hemilaryngectomy are degree and location of subglottic extension. Hemilaryngectomy is feasible if subglottic extension does not exceed 8 to 9 mm anteriorly or 5 to 6 mm posteriorly. Limitation of vocal cord mobility, including complete fixation in some cases, does not preclude hemilaryngectomy as long as immobility is not due to subglottic extension beyond the limits mentioned or to invasion of the cricoarytenoid joint. A lesion suitable for vertical hemilaryngectomy is represented in Figure 19–3.

The procedure is commenced by transverse skin incision, elevation of skin flaps, and tracheostomy. The anterior two thirds of thyroid ala is skeletonized by separating thyrohyoid and ster-

nothyroid muscles from the oblique line, leaving inferior constrictor muscle attached posteriorly. Vertical thyrotomy incisions are made anterior to the attachment of inferior constrictor muscle and, on the contralateral side, far enough from the midline to permit adequate resection of the anterior commissure (Fig 19–4,A). After transection of superior laryngeal vessels and nerves, the posterior third of thyroid ala is separated from underlying pyriform sinus mucosa, avulsing the cricothyroid joint to permit retraction of this cartilaginous segment posteriorly.

The laryngeal interior is exposed by retraction of the thyroid alae. Horizontal incisions are made at the level of cricothyroid and thyrohyoid membranes and are continued posteriorly to the midline (Fig 19–4,B). The inferior incision will traverse the level of the cricoid rostrum and cricoarytenoid joint, whereas the superior incision is placed in the aryepiglottic fold as it progresses posteriorly. These are joined in the posterior midline by a vertical incision that will transect the interarytenoideus muscle but not hypopharyngeal mucosa. Proper placement and control of this incision is facilitated by insertion of a finger or instrument into the hypopharynx, pulling the tissue to be incised anteriorly and placing it under moderate tension. With the finger in the pyriform sinus, the cricoarytenoid joint is palpated as it is transected. This maneuver liberates the specimen from its last cartilaginous attachment. The finger remains in the pyriform sinus to protect the mucosa while remaining loose attachments are divided, completing the resection.

At this point (Fig 19–4,C), the specimen has been removed and the pyriform sinus preserved. Reconstruction is commenced by excision of inferior and superior portions of the preserved posterior third of ipsilateral thyroid ala, leaving a central portion of cartilage pedicled on the inferior constrictor muscle that will be used to replace the resected arytenoid, thus reestablishing, at least in part, the vestibule and posterior glottis. The cartilage "flap" is fixed to the cricoid rostrum with polyglactin sutures (Fig 19–4,D), following which, the endolarynx is resurfaced by advancement of hypopharyngeal mucosa, including the preserved pyriform sinus (Fig 19–4,E). The cut edge of aryepiglottic fold should be thinned prior to advancement by removing the remaining cartilaginous and ligamentous material to facilitate mobility of mucosa and avoid creation of an obstructive flap of tissue within the lumen. Suture of hypopharyngeal to subglottic mucosa is carried as far anteriorly as possible, covering the cartilage flap, and resurfacing most of the hemilarynx. Anteriorly the mucosa is sutured to sternohyoid muscle, and the infrahyoid muscles are reapproximated in the midline. Although there is insufficient mucosa for complete resurfacing of the endolarynx, the defect heals without difficulty by secondary intention.

Other methods have been employed for glottic and vestibular reconstruction, including single pedicled sternohyoid muscle[13] and free grafts of fat,[14] muscle,[15] and cartilage.[16] I have found the pedicled cartilage flap, initially developed by Blaugrund and Kurland,[17] to provide the most satisfactory results, because this rigid vascularized flap does not atrophy as do free transplants and pedicled muscle. Although hemilaryngectomy has, in the past, been performed without glottic reconstruction, there is little question in my mind that reconstitution of the vestibule and posterior glottis has reduced the incidence of

TABLE 19–2.
Results of Extended Frontolateral Laryngectomy

Series	Yr	Stage	Results (%)
Ogura et al.[18]	3	T2	45/55 (82)
Som[19]	3	T2	79/104 (74)
Som[19]	3	T3	15/26 (58)
Mohr et al.[20]	5	T2	25/27 (94)
Mohr et al.[20]	5	T3	5/5 (100)

postoperative aspiration and enabled performance of this procedure in a more elderly group of patients than was possible previously.

Results of the effectiveness of vertical hemilaryngectomy for cure of T2 and T3 glottic cancer reported by several authors are summarized in Table 19–2.[18–20] These indicate approximately 81% cure rate for T2 and 58% for T3 carcinoma.

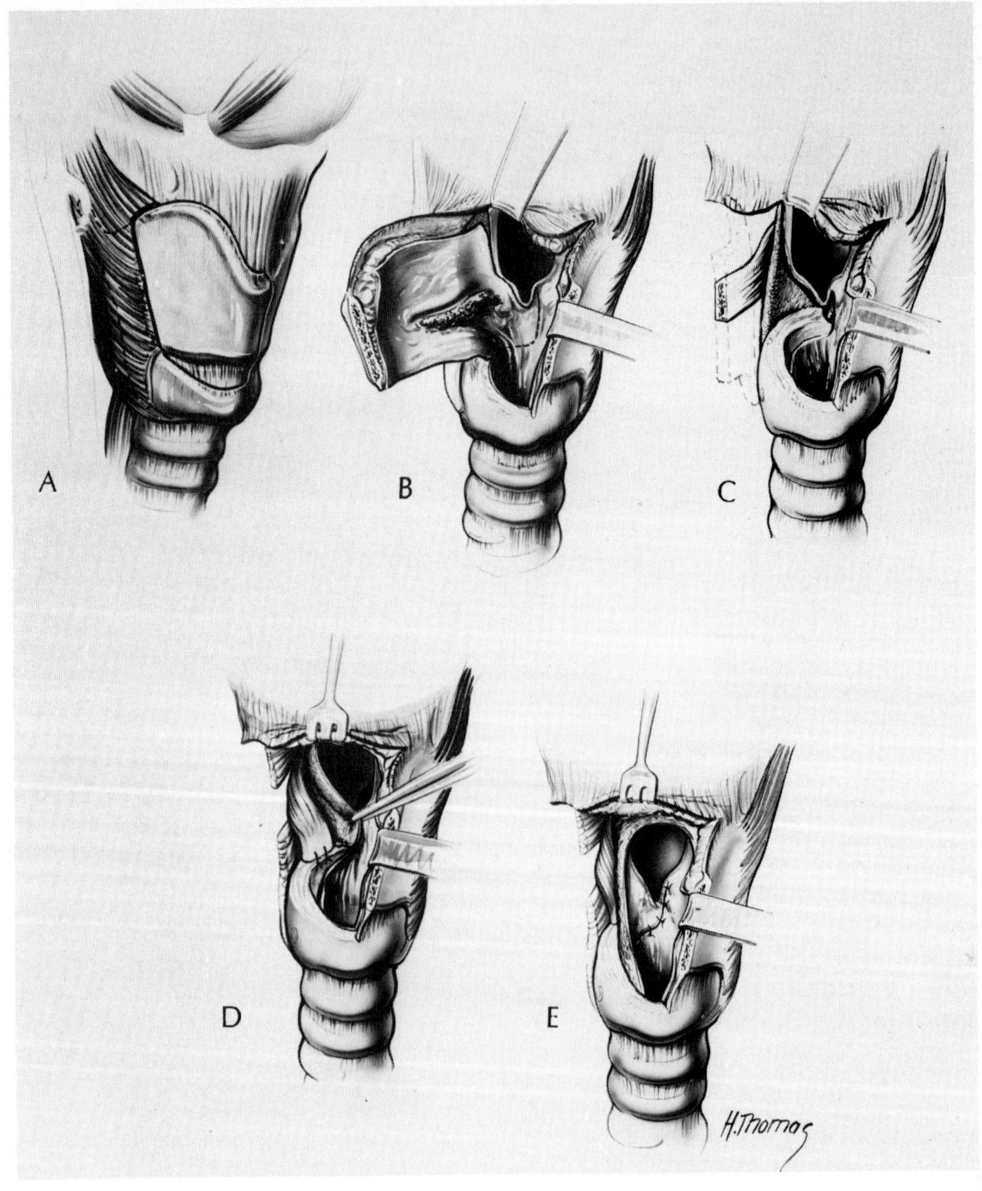

FIG 19–4.
Hemilaryngectomy with cartilage flap. **A**, cartilage cuts. The posterior third of the thyroid ala is skeletonized and is separated from the anterior two thirds. **B**, mucosal incisions. **C**, a block of posterior third of the thyroid ala left attached to perichondrium and inferior constrictor muscle is preserved, whereas the excess cartilage is discarded. **D**, the cartilage flap is rotated into the defect and fixed to the rostrum of the cricoid. **E**, the hypopharyngeal mucosa resurfaces the defect, including the cartilage flap. (From Silver CE: *Curr Probl Surg* 1977; 14:2–69. Used by permission.)

Supraglottic Laryngectomy

Endolaryngeal supraglottic carcinomas usually originate at the junction of epiglottis and false cord. A majority of these lesions are exophytic, well differentiated, and circumscribed, with pushing rather than infiltrating margins. Such tumors rarely extend inferiorly to involve the glottis and rarely invade thyroid cartilage. The preepiglottic space, however, is frequently infiltrated. Involvement is confined above the anterior commissure. As the entire preepiglottic space is removed by supraglottic subtotal laryngectomy, the operation will effectively excise this type of cancer (Fig 19–5). A smaller number of supraglottic carcinomas have infiltrating rather than pushing type of margins. These tumors are usually poorly differentiated, tend to be transglottic, and are rarely amenable to adequate resection by supraglottic laryngectomy.

Supraglottic subtotal laryngectomy is indicated for surgical management of supraglottic carcinomas that do not involve the vocal cord. The procedure may be extended superiorly to include resection of various portions of the hypopharynx and base of the tongue. Only a small margin of uninvolved mucosa is necessary inferiorly because of the barrier to spread of tumor from supraglottic to glottic levels discussed earlier. Even when tumors appear laryngoscopically to extend close to the vocal cord, several millimeters of uninvolved ventricular mucosa are usually found in the resected specimen and constitute an adequate resection margin. Both arytenoid cartilages may be preserved in resecting lesions confined to the laryngeal surface of the epiglottis or anterior part of the false vocal cord, thus preserving vocal cord mobility. For lesions that extend further posteriorly, the ipsilateral arytenoid should be included in the resected specimen. Following this type of resection, the now immobilized vocal cord must be fixed in the midline by suture to the cricoid cartilage to maintain glottic competence.

After incision, elevation of skin flaps, and tracheostomy, the infrahyoid muscles are transected superiorly near their insertions on the hyoid and reflected sufficiently to expose the upper half of the ipsilateral thyroid ala as well as the anterior half of the contralateral ala. Suprahyoid muscles are severed from their attachments to the body and ipsilateral greater cornu of the hyoid bone (Fig 19–6,A). The joint between body and contralateral greater cornu is transected with a small bone cutter. External perichondrium is separated from the ipsilateral and anterior contralateral thyroid alae, creating a flap of tissue that is reflected inferiorly as far as the estimated location of the vocal cord. Thyroid cartilage is transected horizontally at this level and the incision continued obliquely upward to the midpoint of the superior edge of the contralateral thyroid ala. If the valleculae are free of tumor, the hypopharynx is entered in this region by incising the pharyngeal wall superior to the hyoid bone immediately anterior to the epiglottis. This incision is enlarged transversely and the epiglottis secured with a suture and retracted forward into the pharyngotomy (Fig 19–6,B). The mucosal incision is enlarged inferolaterally through the ipsilateral pyriform sinus until both aryepiglottic folds and arytenoids are exposed.

Resection of the supraglottis is now commenced by incising the aryepiglottic folds immediately in front of the arytenoids

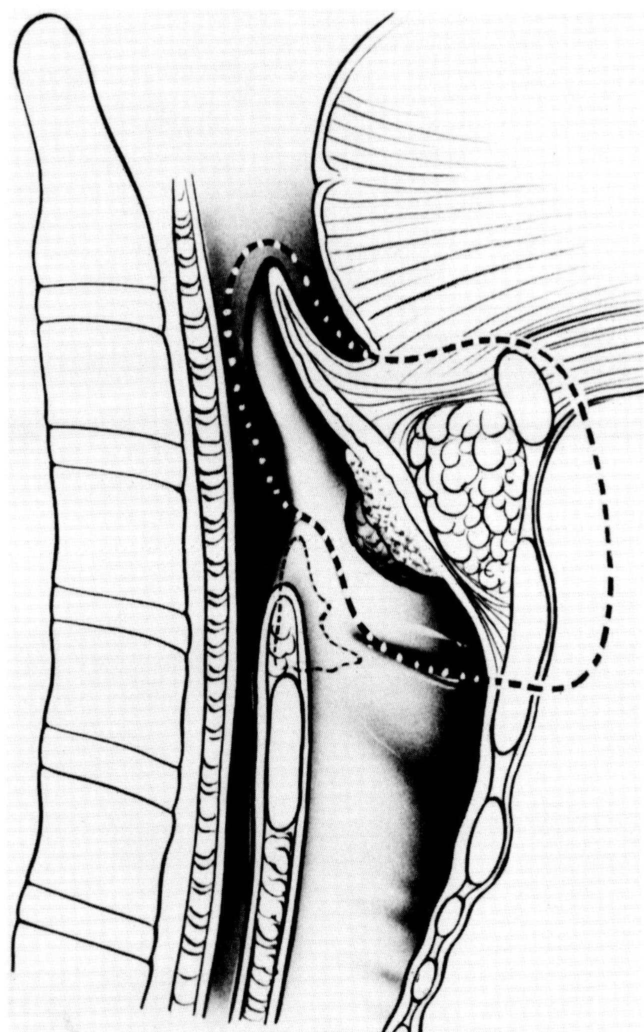

FIG 19–5.
Sagittal view of lesion suitable for supraglottic subtotal laryngectomy with outline of planned resection. (From Silver CE: *Surgery for Cancer of the Larynx.* New York, Churchill Livingstone, 1981. Used by permission.)

(Fig 19–6,C). These incisions are extended inferiorly into the ventricles, then anteriorly, immediately above the vocal cords, to the anterior commissure (Fig 19–6,D). The mucosal incisions are carried through full thickness of the larynx, corresponding externally with the previously placed cartilage cuts. Mucosa superior to the vocal cords should not be preserved even if it is widely free of tumor, because excessive supraglottic mucosa tends to become edematous, producing postoperative glottic obstruction. For small tumors, resection of the supraglottis may commence on either side. For more extensive resections, particularly if arytenoid is included, exposure is facilitated by mobilizing the lesser involved side initially.

Although effectiveness is difficult to measure, I generally perform cricopharyngeal myotomy at the time of supraglottic subtotal laryngectomy immediately after the resected specimen has been removed. This surgical maneuver is easily accomplished at this point, whereas reoperation in cases of persistent cricopharyngeal spasm would be a major undertaking. After insertion of a nasogastric feeding tube, reconstruction is commenced by suturing the cut edges of pyriform sinus and supraglottic mucosa to each other (Fig 19–6,E), reconstructing aryepiglottic folds. The hypopharyngeal defect is closed by direct suture, commencing posteriorly and continuing as far anteriorly as possible. As the region of resected supraglottis is approached, the mucosal edges can no longer be approximated directly. The previously created perichondrial flap is reflected upward and sutured to the cut edge of base of tongue to provide tissue for closure (Fig 19–6,F). Preserved infrahyoid muscles are approximated to cut edges of suprahyoid and inferior constrictor muscles for a second layer of closure.

TABLE 19–3.
Results of Supraglottic Subtotal Laryngectomy

Series	Yr	No. of Patients	No Evidence of Disease (%)
Ogura et al.[21]	3	177	76
Bocca et al.[22]	5	467	75
Som[23]	5	75	68
Burnstein and Calcaterra[24]	2	40	90

Results of treatment of endolaryngeal supraglottic carcinoma by supraglottic subtotal laryngectomy, reported in a number of large series, are summarized in Table 19–3.[21–24] Cure rates achieved by these authors are comparable with those obtained by treatment of similar lesions with total laryngectomy.

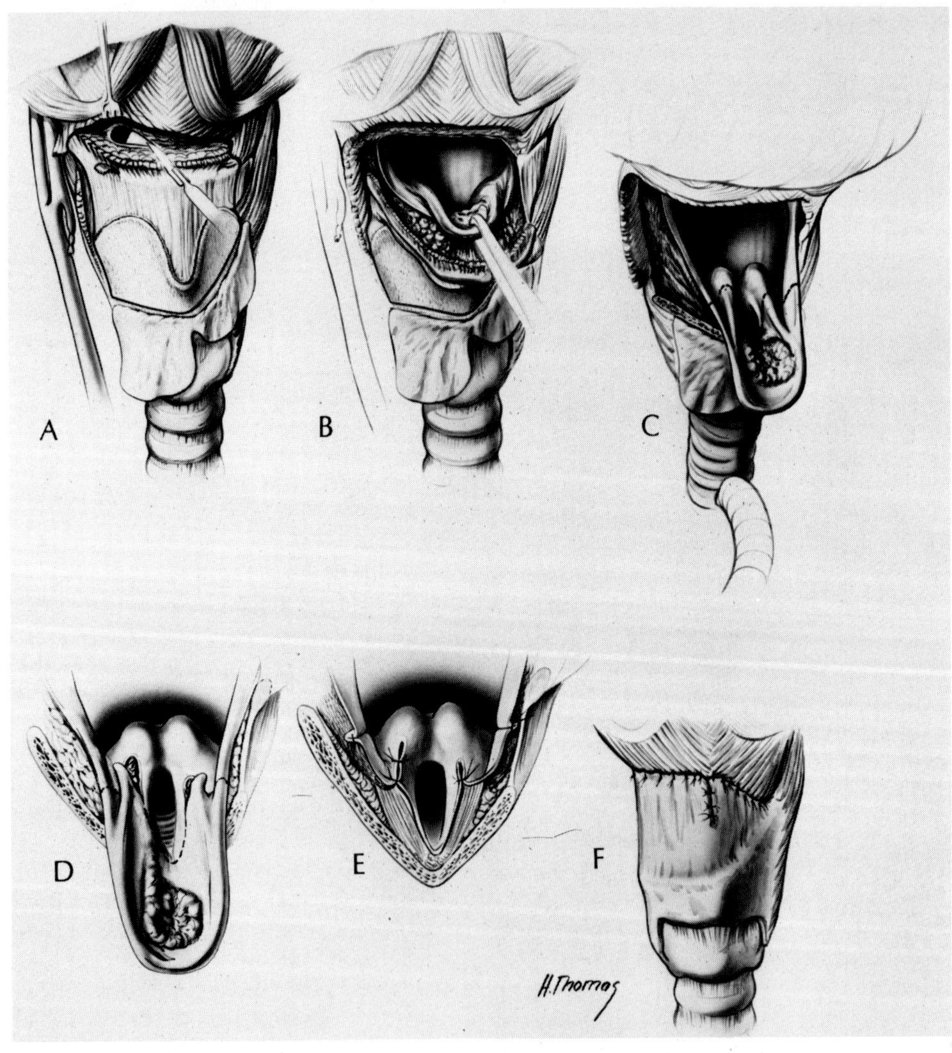

FIG 19–6.
Supraglottic subtotal laryngectomy. **A,** cartilage cuts and perichondrial flap. **B** and **C,** hypopharyngeal entry exposing the epiglottis. **D,** the aryepiglottic folds are incised posterior to the tumor until the ventricles are reached. The resection then proceeds anteriorly through the ventricular mucosa. **E,** closure is commenced by reconstructing aryepiglottic folds. **F,** the perichondrial flap completes the closure anteriorly. (From Silver CE: *Curr Probl Surg* 1977; 14:2–69. Used by permission.)

Extended Conservation Surgery

Various authors have extended the limitations of conventional conservation surgery in series of highly selected cases. Biller and Som employed an oversized thyroid cartilage flap for replacement of cricoid cartilage to facilitate resection of glottic carcinomas with posterior subglottic extension exceeding the limitations discussed earlier.[25] Ogura and Dedo employed an infolded flap of thyroid cartilage for glottic replacement to permit inclusion of the true vocal cord with the supraglottic resection in cases of supraglottic carcinoma extending onto the glottis.[26] Iwai[27] and Friedman et al.[28] have employed long segments of posterior thyroid cartilage for cricoid replacement for functional laryngeal reconstruction after resection of more extensive transglottic carcinomas.

Pearson developed a new concept of conservation surgery by performing a true hemilaryngectomy including cricoid cartilage and perilaryngeal tissues for extensive but unilateral transglottic carcinomas.[29] Although insufficient laryngeal tissue is preserved to maintain an intact airway, a dynamic phonatory shunt is created by preservation of contralateral laryngeal mucosa with an arytenoid cartilage, intrinsic musculature, and the recurrent laryngeal nerve. This permits restoration of a lung-powered voice while preventing aspiration and, in my opinion, has wider applicability in elderly patients as well as for more extensive tumors than operations that attempt to preserve respiratory as well as phonatory and deglutitory function of the larynx. I have found the procedure useful as well for tumors that require extensive hypopharyngeal resection but involve the larynx minimally.

Selection of Patients

Conservation surgery is most often indicated for lesions that, due to local invasiveness or proximity to cartilage, are not readily curable with radiation but are small enough for adequate resection without sacrifice of the entire larynx. Considerable adaptation is required, particularly for recovery of deglutitory function, after removal of large portions of the larynx. Such procedures are usually not suitable for patients with significant chronic respiratory or neurologic problems and should be considered with caution for aged patients who may find adaptation difficult. In some instances, indeed, a patient may lead a more comfortable life following successful total laryngectomy than after a functionally unsatisfactory conservation operation complicated by chronic aspiration of food and saliva. Partial laryngectomy is feasible after irradiation failure, but only for lesions that were amenable to the same resection prior to therapy.[30, 31] The most important consideration is to avoid compromise of a patient's chance for cure by an attempt to preserve laryngeal function with a tumor too large for adequate resection by partial laryngectomy.

Role of Radiation Therapy

Conservation surgery is generally employed for management of relatively early laryngeal cancer. Thus, adjuvant radiation therapy has not been shown to produce significant improvement of cure rates in patients without cervical lymph node metastases. Even the presence of microscopically involved margins in hemilaryngectomy specimens has been questioned as an indication for postoperative radiation therapy.[32] Nevertheless, postoperative radiation therapy is generally employed in cases with inadequate resection margins.

Although elective adjuvant radiation treatment may not be indicated for control of primary tumor in most lesions suitable for conservation surgery, the question of elective postoperative radiation for control of occult lymph node metastases should be considered. Although early glottic carcinomas have a low incidence of cervical metastatic disease,[33] supraglottic carcinomas are often associated with undetected preepiglottic space involvement (thus, apparent T1 lesions may actually be T3) and have a higher incidence of occult lymph node metastases.[34] For this reason, elective modified or complete neck dissection is often performed in association with supraglottic laryngectomy. An alternative to this approach is administration of postoperative irradiation either routinely or if microscopic metastases are found on a staging type of neck dissection. I usually employ the latter approach for supraglottic lesions that are clinically T1 or T2, N0, resecting lymph nodes in the anterior jugular chain, which are the first level of metastases for the supraglottic larynx, and administering postoperative irradiation if microscopically abnormal nodes are found. I usually perform elective complete neck dissection for T3N0 carcinoma and administer bilateral postoperative irradiation if abnormal nodes are found in the specimen. Preoperative computed tomography (CT) of the neck may be helpful in identifying lymph node metastases that are inapparent on physical examination.

MANAGEMENT OF UPPER AIRWAY OBSTRUCTION

Most patients with large laryngeal tumors have some degree of measurable upper airway obstruction,[35] although it may be inapparent clinically in the awake patient. An occasional patient may appear in the emergency room with severe stridor in need of immediate tracheostomy, but most instances of acute upper airway obstruction arise when a patient with laryngeal carcinoma is sedated or when general anesthesia is induced at the time of endoscopic examination of the larynx. The consequences of this situation are most undesirable because of cardiovascular stress to both patient and surgeon and because preoperative tracheostomy is believed to be a predisposing factor in tracheal stomal recurrence.[36, 37]

The best way to deal with this problem is to anticipate it and to avoid oversedating or anesthetizing such patients. It is not necessary to administer general anesthesia to a patient with a large endolaryngeal cancer simply to obtain a biopsy or even to determine the full extent of tumor involvement. Fiberoptic endoscopy and CT of the larynx can, in most cases, afford sufficient information regarding tumor size and extent for staging purposes and treatment planning. A tissue diagnosis may be obtained by fiberoptic endoscopy with topical anesthesia or by the formerly commonly employed technique of biopsy with a curved laryngeal biopsy forceps guided by indirect laryngoscopy. This latter procedure has been in use since the time of Morell Mackenzie but has become a lost art in the era of microlaryngoscopy, fiberoptics, and the laser. I have, nevertheless, found the procedure to be efficacious for obtaining biopsy material from large tumors, particularly supraglottic lesions. Further endoscopic evaluation may be conducted at the time of definitive surgery, after the airway has been controlled by tracheostomy, performed as the initial step in the operation.

Some patients present with high-degree airway obstruction that requires immediate relief. Again, it is desirable to avoid tracheostomy as an independent procedure prior to laryngectomy, if possible. One approach is to perform "emergency" laryngectomy on the basis of a frozen section biopsy. In my opinion, this approach is often impractical and is undesirable with regard to psychologic factors, proper preoperative assessment, and informed consent (a patient struggling to breathe can hardly be expected to adequately evaluate various treatment options). A more desirable approach would be to administer topical anesthesia and intubate the larynx by direct laryngoscopy with a small "laserproof" endotracheal tube. After biopsy, the tumor may be debulked by vaporization with the carbon dioxide laser[38] sufficiently to restore an adequate laryngeal airway.

Endotracheal intubation and laser surgery are, of course, not possible in all cases. Some patients will require tracheostomy, either as an emergency or at the time of laryngectomy. In either case, tracheostomy can be more safely accomplished if the airway is first controlled by endotracheal intubation, relieving the obstruction and permitting orderly performance of the procedure on a well-ventilated patient. Again, topical anesthesia is administered with the patient in a sitting position. If the larynx cannot be intubated with a plastic or rubber endotracheal tube, it is usually possible to pass a small rigid bronchoscope or tracheoscope through the tumor into the unobstructed distal trachea. This instrument can be connected to the anesthesia apparatus and tracheostomy performed under more optimal conditions. Occasionally, tracheostomy or cricothyroidotomy is urgently required without prior control of the airway. In such instances, rapid work and entry into the trachea by the most direct route possible are the main surgical requirements.

An important consideration in tracheostomy performed prior to laryngectomy is placement of the skin and tracheal incisions as high as possible without violating the tumor. Subsequent laryngectomy is greatly facilitated if the tracheotomy site can be circumcised and resected en bloc with the larynx without having to extend the resection into the substernal region. Some large subglottic tumors may present considerable obstacles to control of the airway. Indeed, it is occasionally necessary to force the tracheostomy tube through an obstructing mass of tumor to gain control of the distal airway. If unpreventable, this situation must be managed by adequate resection at the time of laryngectomy, including manubriectomy with thoracotracheostomy[39] and postoperative radiation therapy.

MANAGEMENT OF THE STOMA

Stomal Recurrence

Recurrence of tumor at the tracheostoma is a devastating sequel to total laryngectomy. A number of factors predispose to this condition, including inadequate resection margins, previous tracheostomy, residual disease in paratracheal lymph nodes, and residual disease in unresected thyroid tissue.[36, 37, 40, 41] These conditions are more likely to exist in association with subglottic carcinoma than with other laryngeal tumors. Because elective postoperative irradiation has been shown to reduce the incidence of stomal recurrence in patients with predisposing factors,[42] this adjuvant therapy is recommended for such individuals.

Tracheal stomal recurrence has been classified by Sisson et al. into four types related to location and extent of involvement[43]:

Type I: Localized to superior aspect of stoma; no esophageal involvement

Type II: Localized to superior aspect of stoma with esophageal involvement

Type III: Originating from inferior aspect of stoma and involving superior mediastinum

Type IV: Extension laterally beneath clavicles and into superior mediastinum

Prognosis of stomal recurrence has generally been poor. Treatment by radiation therapy may produce some palliation but rarely results in cure. Wide surgical resection is the only procedure that has produced consistent tumor control, at least in selected cases. Adequate resection includes removal of large amounts of peristomal skin, the manubrium, lymphoareolar contents of the superior mediastinum, trachea, and often pharynx or esophagus. In the past, surgical mortality was unacceptably high due to the frequent occurrence of great vessel rupture after exposure in the mediastinum as a consequence of tracheostomal separation or flap necrosis. Some improvement in mortality was obtained with a two-stage approach developed by Sisson[44] and Sisson et al.[45] More recently, Biller et al. achieved significant reduction in postoperative mortality by use of a pectoralis major myocutaneous flap for single-stage repair after transsternal neck dissection and thoracotracheostomy.[46] Krespi et al. employed gastric transposition for esophageal replacement in association with pectoralis major myocutaneous flap for the Sisson type II stomal recurrence.[47] This combination of procedures has resolved many of the formidable problems associated with resection of this type of lesion.

Gluckman et al. reported results of surgery in 41 patients operated on for stomal recurrence.[48] Overall 2-year survival was only 16% for all patients, but further analysis revealed 45% 5-year survival with type I and II lesions and 9% survival for types III and IV. Thus, acceptable cure rates may be expected in treatment of the less-advanced stomal recurrences. Surgical treatment for type III and IV stomal recurrence, even when feasible, must be considered palliative, and the risk should be evaluated in relation to possible benefit. In many cases, supervoltage radiation therapy, aggressive chemotherapy, or both may produce symptomatic relief and survival comparable to that obtainable by extensive surgery.

Preoperative evaluation should include magnetic resonance imaging (MRI) or CT (or both), contrast esophagography, and endoscopic examination of trachea and esophagus. Evidence of great vessel involvement or free spread of tumor within the mediastinum should be considered contraindications to the procedure.

The following discussion will demonstrate surgical management of a type I stomal recurrence (without esophageal involvement). The technique of gastric transposition for esophageal replacement, as would be employed for a type II recurrence, is discussed later in this chapter. The initial step in the operative procedure is to delineate a wide area of skin to be sacrificed around the stoma (Fig 19–7,A). The superior portion of the incision is extended appropriately to permit exploration of the neck, in particular, the carotid arteries, to determine that these vessels can be separated from the tumor. Pharyngeal or esophageal involvement (or both) and other factors concerning extent and resectability of the tumor should be assessed to the greatest degree possible prior to manubriotomy.

The cutaneous incision is now continued around the delineated area, and the manubrium is transected through the first intercostal space after division of the internal mammary vessels (Figs 19–7,B and C). The costal cartilages of the first ribs are divided, as are the clavicles near the sternoclavicular joints. Appropriate retraction of the now-liberated osteocutaneous island permits access to the mediastinum. The major vessels are identified and skeletonized, reflecting the mass of thymic and lymphoareolar tissue toward the trachea. The left innominate vein is retracted downward for exposure; it may be divided if necessary. The trachea is finally exposed and transected as far inferiorly as necessary, releasing the specimen (Fig 19–7,D).

A pectoralis major myocutaneous flap of appropriate size is created on the chest wall (Fig 19–7,E) and rotated into the defect (Fig 19–7,F). The tracheostoma is created through a small incision placed in the central portion of the flap. The donor site can usually be closed primarily by mobilization of tissues or with a skin graft if necessary.

Stomal Stenosis

The most severe cases of tracheostomal stenosis are caused by separation of the tracheostoma, that is, dehiscence of the cut end of trachea from the skin, in the postoperative period. This particular problem is best prevented by avoidance of excessive tension on the tracheocutaneous suture line. Adequate mobilization of skin flaps and trachea, occasional use of "relaxing" incisions, and manubrial resection in cases of extremely low tracheal transection all are measures that may prevent excessive suture line tension. If tracheostomal separation occurs in the immediate postoperative period, the stoma should be revised immediately, if feasible. Strictures resulting from tracheostomal separation are usually long and difficult to manage either con-

servatively or by corrective surgery. Less severe stomal stenosis may result from hypertrophic scar formation at the mucocutaneous junction of the stoma. This is likely to occur when the tracheostoma has been created directly in the transverse cervical incision rather than a separate small incision in the inferior skin flap. In cases where a previous tracheostomy determines placement of the inferior skin incision and necessitates sacrifice of an ellipse of skin, beveling of the trachea to enlarge its diameter and creation of a vertical incision in the inferior skin flap to accommodate the anterior and lateral walls of the trachea may help minimize stricture formation.

Stomal stenosis may often be managed by the simple expedient of wearing a laryngectomy tube or silicone rubber stent to maintain the lumen after dilation. Initial dilation may be accomplished after application of topical anesthesia with a nasal speculum, followed by insertion of progressively larger metal tracheostomy tubes over a period of days. It is usually possible to insert a tube at least one size larger at each change until a satisfactory diameter (8 to 10 mm) has been attained. In some cases, particularly where stenosis limited to the mucocutaneous junction has occurred in the early postoperative period, the stoma will stabilize at an adequate diameter after a period of several months, permitting decannulation. On the other hand, longer segments of stenosis may resist adequate dilation, and a safe, comfortable airway cannot be maintained with a tube. Some patients may simply object to wearing a tube and desire surgical correction of the microstoma.

The principles of surgical correction of tracheal stomal stenosis are (1) complete excision of the stenotic segment with all scar tissue, (2) reestablishment of the tracheocutaneous junction without tension, and (3) disruption of the straight line of mucocutaneous junction by interdigitation of skin and mucosa with a Z-plasty or other surgical maneuver to accomplish the same purpose. Repair of a long (≥ 1 cm) stenotic segment can present a considerable surgical challenge. After dilation of the lumen and insertion of an endotracheal tube into the distal airway, general anesthesia is induced and a circumferential incision made around the stoma, including all hypertrophic scar tissue. The stenotic segment is now dissected sharply from surrounding tissues until normal trachea is encountered. Dissection proceeds around the trachea until it has been mobilized sufficiently to lift toward the skin. In most cases, surrounding skin from the chest and cervical region may be mobilized sufficiently to reach the trachea without tension. If necessary, a rotation flap can be created for this purpose. Partial manubrial resection may be considered in particularly difficult cases.

Prior to creation of the new tracheostoma, skin and trachea should be incised so as to interdigitate with each other. I prefer a double or single Z-plasty for this purpose. It is fairly simple to create a single Z-plasty on the posterior wall of the stoma. If possible, a second Z-plasty should be placed anteriorly. The resultant stoma will have an adequate diameter and will heal without excessive contraction. If the patient has a tendency to keloid or hypertrophic scar formation, 40 mg of triamcinolone solution should be injected into the skin and mucosal edges at the time of surgery and at weekly and then monthly (for 3 or 4 months) intervals postoperatively.

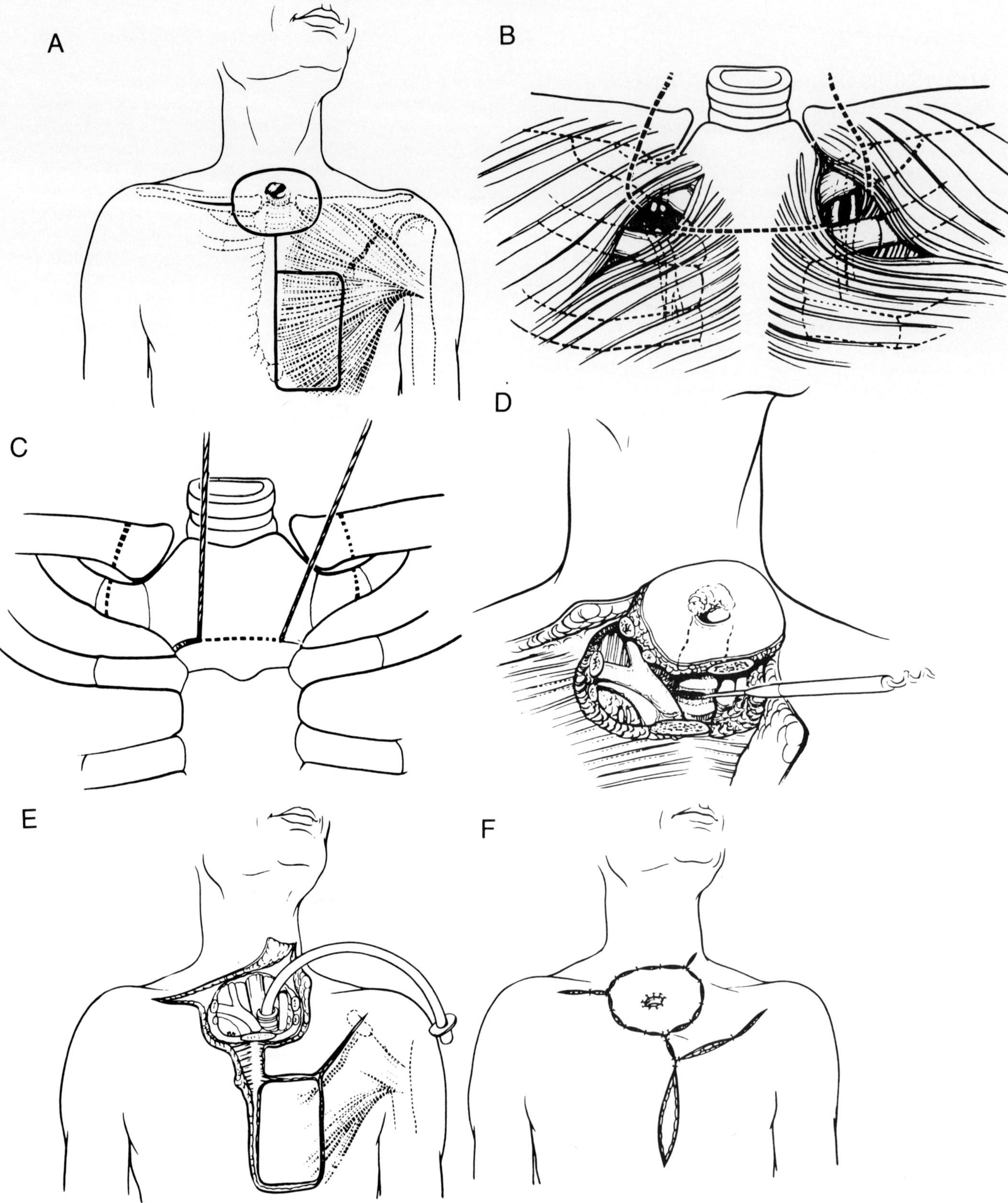

FIG 19–7.
Transsternal neck dissection for stomal recurrence. Repair with pectoralis major myocutaneous flap. **A**, outline of cutaneous incisions. **B** and **C**, outline of bone cuts. **D**, transection of trachea after dissection of superior mediastinum. **E**, pectoralis major myocutaneous flap created. **F**, flap rotated into defect. Thorocotracheostomy created. (From Silver CE: *Surgery for Cancer of the Larynx.* New York, Churchill Livingstone, 1981. Used by permission.)

plane of the strap muscles. The elevation is carried up to the hyoid level and down to the lower margin of the cricoid.

The strap muscles are parted. The angle of the thyroid cartilage, which is the vertical midline strip, often ossified inferiorly, extending from the thyroid notch to the lower border, is exposed. The perichondrium is incised vertically in the midline and elevated laterally for a short distance. If the anterior commissure is well free of the tumor, the thyroid cartilage (only) is cut vertically in the midline with an oscillating saw. Otherwise, the cartilage cut is made 2 to 3 mm to the less involved side. The pertinent anatomy was described by Broyles.[43] The vocal cord ligaments extend forward into the deep surface of the angle of the thyroid cartilage and blend into the fused connective tissues that line the angle from the commissural level to the inferior border of the thyroid cartilage. The anterior connective tissue sweeps downward to continue inferiorly as the cricothyroid ligament. When cancer touches the anterior commissure, allowance has to be made for its possible extension along similar lines. In every case, the entry into the larynx has to be meticulous and well planned.

The anesthesiologist paralyzes the patient to relax the vocal cords. The status of the delphian node in the prelaryngeal fascia over the cricothyroid is noted. A tiny perforating vessel in the cricothyroid ligament, which seems to be a reliable marker for the midline, is cauterized. A short *horizontal* incision made through the ligament enters the subglottis about 5 mm above the upper border of the cricoid. Then a vertical incision is extended upward from the horizontal opening to create an inverted T. An assistant uses skin hooks to lightly retract the two corners of the T. The operator, using a headlight, a scalpel, and a suction tube, continues upward between the cut edges of the thyroid cartilage to complete the "fissure." By observing the tumor from below, one can open the larynx through the anterior commissure or through the uninvolved cord. The object is to achieve adequate clearance of the cancer while producing the minimum disruption of the muscular and tendinous anatomy of the glottic elements on the uninvolved side. To the extent that the uninvolved cord is released from its anterior anchorage, it should be sutured back to two small drill holes in the thyroid ala. If the anterior support and epithelium of the uninvolved cord can be safely and completely preserved, the voice will be remarkably normal after recovery.

The vertical soft tissue opening is extended upward about 1 cm above the true vocal cords, and the retraction hooks now gently separate the cartilage halves as widely as possible. Attention is directed to the side of the larynx that contains the tumor. The lower margin of the specimen is cut in the subglottis with a no. 15 blade. This is the most critical margin after the anterior ones; it should be at least 5 mm from visible tumor. If it is made deep enough, it will cut through the conus elasticus. This permits further retraction of the specimen side by freeing it from the cricoid.

A cleavage plane is opened with a dissector between the inner perichondrium of the involved side's thyroid ala and the external surface of the paraglottic tissues (the neurovascular structures, the thyroarytenoid muscle, and the lateral wall of the laryngeal ventricle). The specimen, which is isolated now, can be elevated forward while the alae are retracted and can be

separated from the supraglottis and the arytenoid with a pair of well-controlled endolaryngeal incisions. The supraglottic one is made through the false cord so that the specimen will include the ventricle. The posterior (arytenoid) one is made through the vocal process with a fine-tipped angle-bladed Panzer scissors. These scissors allow the operator to reach back and transect the posterior attachments of the specimen cleanly without obscuring the view. The cordectomy specimen is thus delivered and can be oriented and submitted to the pathologist. The body of the arytenoid cartilage that remains behind will eventually control a rather credible neocord, which will form in the raw bed of the resection.

Sometimes some not yet cancerous dysplasia is detected on the opposite cord. It should be stripped, and the exposed vocalis muscle should be covered with a posterosuperiorly based mucosal transposition flap, drawn down from the false cord on that same side. Small slivers of soft tissue (surgical margins) should be cut from the edges of the defect to augment the information reported by the pathologist. Throughout this dissection, instruments that touched the specimen (and the surface of the specimen itself) must be treated as tumor contaminated. They are removed from the field, and the wound is irrigated and lightly cauterized while the pathologist is reviewing the frozen sections. The lower epiglottis can be sewn forward to prevent interference with visualization in the postoperative period. The inverted T incision in the cricothyroid membrane should be very accurately repaired with 3 or 4.0 chromic sutures, but no sutures are put through the thyroid alae themselves. The strap muscles are simply approximated over the thyrotomy, and this seems to provide the necessary medialization. No drains are required. The tracheostomy, which is connected to the operative wound just in front of the thyroid isthmus, provides all the wound drainage that is necessary.

Healing after laryngofissure and cordectomy is usually prompt and uneventful. In 3 or 4 days, the tracheostomy tube is removed, and the stoma closes spontaneously. In 10% or 15% of patients, an exuberant granuloma forms at the operative site and may persist for many weeks postoperatively. It usually resolves with time. The extent to which the voice is disturbed on a permanent basis depends on the degree to which it was possible to maintain the anterior commissural attachments and mucosal coverage of the uninvolved cord. If the anterior commissure was slit exactly in the midline and the arytenoid remains present except for the tip of the vocal process, the quality of the voice and even the appearance of the neocord achieved simply with granulation are excellent. Since these patients do not need radiotherapy, appearances gradually stabilize, and repeated follow-up examinations are uncomplicated by chronic edema,[44] cartilage necrosis,[45] or radiodegenerative effects.[46]

Total Laryngectomy

The original "laryngectomies" performed on patients with laryngeal cancer in the late 19th and early 20th century were often partial resections, tailored to the lesion.[47] The principle of separating the airway from the foodway was often subverted by the attempt to preserve some voice. Before long, laryngectomy acquired a reputation for morbidity that quite surpassed the relatively minor difficulties we associate with its more physiologically based counterpart today.[48] Recurrent cancer, intractable aspiration, pneumonia, septicemia, starvation, and death were all common complications, and the technology for long-term tracheostomy care or vocal rehabilitation of the expected aphonia was quite primitive.

Compared with the partial laryngectomies, total laryngectomy achieved a wider resection margin, and it could be taught as a standard anatomic procedure in any medical school. Since it removed the crippled laryngeal remnant that had, in subtotal laryngectomies, connected the foodway to the airway without any sphincteric control, it generated more survivors than any other competitors, and eventually, it acquired a reluctant acceptance that has persisted to modern times.

Most laryngeal cancers unsuitable for cordectomy or laryngofissure came to be considered clear candidates for total laryngectomy. This means all supraglottic, all subglottic, and all T3 and T4 glottic lesions were eligible. After 1922, a few glottic cases escaped excision by responding completely to radiation.[49] And in some centers, limited supraglottic lesions were sometimes removed by transoral epiglottectomy, transhyoid pharyngotomy,[50] or so-called lateral pharyngotomy.[51] On the whole, however, laryngectomy was the centerpiece of primary treatment, and all the failures by radiation or lesser operations also depended on total laryngectomy for salvage. Laryngologists recognized early on that fixation of the vocal cord implied deep invasion by cancer, and this clinical finding became the unquestioned indication for total laryngectomy. The idea that radiation could handle smaller glottic lesions became fashionable, but supraglottic, piriform, and subglottic tumors were rarely considered for anything other than surgery.

By virtue of their delayed effect on the voice, supraglottic tumors usually presented late and so large that a total laryngectomy seemed entirely unavoidable. As for cancers arising in the adjacent hypopharynx, their reputation for aggressive behavior and a miserable prognosis was well recognized, and a total laryngectomy seemed the least one could do in the desperate effort to reduce the mortality. Subglottic tumors were rare, but they often presented in extremis, having escaped detection until their airway obstruction could not be ignored. In such desperate situations, a total laryngectomy was usually advised and accepted.

It should be clearly understood that total laryngectomy was not done because laryngologists were overzealous in ablating cancer or insensitive to the patient's need to speak. It was the knowledge of what befell the patient if he or she tried to preserve the portion of the larynx that was not directly involved. Bitter experience showed this remnant was a liability, not an asset. It could not provide voice because the aspiration and pneumonia killed the speaker. Efforts at voice preservation were thus gradually replaced by the principle of total laryngectomy and separation of the pharynx from trachea. The postoperative course was more predictable, and both cure and recovery from surgery became commonplace events in practice. Ironically, at a time when surgeons were making greater progress in the treatment of laryngeal cancer than in almost any other malignancy, they failed to capture many admirers outside medicine. In the public mind, the loss of the larynx became synonymous with the loss of the voice.[52] So many attempts to avoid this appeared over the next half century that the fundamental simplicity of a total laryngectomy became somewhat overshadowed. Radiotherapy was introduced by Coutard in 1922, but this actually made judgments more difficult and outcomes even more uncertain. Numerous innovative post–total laryngectomy speaking shunt producing operations came and went, but the promise of voice preservation was never quite fulfilled.

Today, total laryngectomy remains an important basic strategy in the treatment of extensive laryngeal cancers. It is also very important after radiation failure for smaller cancers. The true extent of recurrent cancer is often too obscure for a partial laryngectomy, and reconstruction with tissues that have been compromised by radiation is fraught with disappointment.

When a total laryngectomy is indicated, management usually includes the following steps:

1. Pretreatment counseling with a speech pathologist who can discuss rehabilitative strategies while the patient is still able to talk and ask questions.[53]
2. Oral intubation for general anesthesia. If the patient exhibits any stridor preoperatively, a tracheotomy under attended local anesthesia is performed.
3. Direct laryngoscopy, with topographic evaluation, confirmatory biopsies, and final confirmation of the surgical plan.
4. Passage of a nasogastric feeding tube.
5. Creation of a tracheotomy below the thyroid isthmus, with transposition of the anesthetic tubing to this location.
6. Complete neck dissection on the involved side, preserving the accessory nerve[54] but removing all of the fat, fascia, and lymph nodes.
7. Total laryngectomy, partial thyroidectomy, and clearance of the paratracheal nodes.
8. Closure of the defect in the anterior wall of the hypopharynx.
9. Creation of an adequate tracheal stoma.
10. Irrigation of the wound, placement of drains, closure of the neck, and application of the dressing.

After the intubation and laryngoscopy, the technique of laryngectomy is as follows. It is common to site the tracheostomy in the transverse limb of the neck incision, but when the surgeon knows special valving devices will be subsequently fitted to the stoma, a plan to resituate the stoma as a separate wound from the incision is advisable. Otherwise, the crease of the cervical incision notches the stomal margin and interferes with the adhesion or seal of any stomal valvular devices.[55] If a previous tracheotomy was performed, the tracheostomy site should be isolated with an elliptical incision so that it can be included with the surgical specimen.

A complete neck dissection is carried out with the head turned away from the surgeon. The neck dissection provides excellent exposure of the larynx on its more involved side. Since cancer is embolic in lymphatics, not continuous, the neck dissection specimen can be detached before the laryngectomy and sent for histopathologic examination.

The removal of the larynx itself begins with a low transection of both sternohyoid and sternothyroid strap muscles, plus the one remaining omohyoid muscle on the contralateral side. The thyroid lobe on the contralateral side is released from the thyroid isthmus, and its raw edge is oversewn with a running 2.0 chromic catgut suture. The isthmus and ipsilateral lobe of the thyroid, as well as the prelaryngeal fascia and the delphian node, will be removed with the surgical specimen.

The superior and inferior neurovascular bundles on both sides of the specimen are ligated and divided. On the tumor side, these are the superior and inferior thyroid arteries and the superior and recurrent laryngeal nerves. On the contralateral side, the same nerves are divided, but since that thyroid lobe is now reflected from the larynx and preserved, it is the superior laryngeal artery, the inferior laryngeal artery, and the cricothyroid artery that are divided and ligated to isolate the larynx.

The suprahyoid muscles are transected along the upper margin of the hyoid bone, taking care to avoid the hypoglossal nerves and lingual arteries. The larynx is rolled to either side so that the inferior pharyngeal constrictor muscles can be transected all along the posterior border of each thyroid ala. It is also released from its origins on the superior cornua, a bit of the upper margin of the thyroid alae, and the posterolateral surfaces of the cricoid cartilage. The trachea is transected at the tracheotomy site with due consideration for the subglottic–upper tracheal tumor extent. The surgeon will be dividing the lateral walls of the trachea obliquely and aiming for the palpable inferior edge of the posterior cricoid lamina.

The larynx is then removed from below upward. The pharynx is entered through the lateral wall of the contralateral piriform, immediately under the superior cornu of the thyroid cartilage. The removal continues, under strong tension, by carrying the transection of the hypopharyngeal wall across the postcricoid region. From here the surgeon continues up the lateral piriform wall of the involved side. Finally, with the inverted larynx elevated toward the ceiling and the epiglottis everting into the wound, the division across the vallecula is completed. This sequence can be varied to suit the circumstances, of course. If there is a question about the posterior or inferior spread, for example, the operator may enter the vallecula initially and work from top to bottom in the removal.

Stay sutures are placed at the lateral extremities of the pharyngotomy, and the pharynx is repair horizontally or as a very broad T. A vertical closure is undesirable because it gathers the remaining hypopharynx together so as to produce a transverse web. Later, this will impede swallowing. Singer et al. emphasized two refinements of pharyngeal closure that will increase the likelihood of successful vocal rehabilitation.[56] They recommended that the cricopharyngeal fibers of the inferior constrictor muscle, which were transected from their cricoid cartilage insertions by the act of removing the larynx, should not be reunited at the closure. They will only form an encircling band at the cricopharyngeal level, and this might impede release of esophageal air in alaryngeal or tracheoesophageal shunt speech. Myotomy is probably safe because the postcricoid mucosa is strong and redundant enough to repair this portion of the pharyngotomy by itself. They also noted that the crico-

pharyngeal spasm that often complicates puncture and prosthesis vocal rehabilitation techniques can be further averted by a pharyngeal neurectomy. The motor branches of the pharyngeal plexus can be located in the pharyngeal wall medial to the carotid bulb. The operator can confirm their location by taking a few minutes to isolate them and demonstrate their action with a nerve stimulator. If some are divided, reflex spasm of the pharyngoesophageal passage can be reduced.

The operation is concluded with copious irrigation. The drains are positioned so as not to induce a fistula. On the side of the neck dissection, they should not cross the carotid. The tracheotomy is structured very deliberately, each stitch catching the skin with a vertical mattress and the trachea with a simple loop. This induces the skin to slightly overhang the cut tracheal edge. A beveled stoma and prevention of cartilage exposure are important for primary wound healing. Closure of the neck wound should be watertight so the suction drains alone hold the skin flaps down. The anesthesiologist should plan to have the patient breathing spontaneously as soon as the dressing is completed so that positive pressure ventilation will not be required.

A laryngectomy carried out in this manner is safe and relatively rapid. Drains can usually be removed around the third or fourth day, oral feeding commenced on the tenth day, and the patient discharged after complete self-care training in tracheotomy management has been provided. At this time, the plan of approach to the rehabilitation of communication should be clearly established using the collaborative services of the speech pathologist.

Two Additional Strategies

Transoral cordectomy, laryngofissure and cordectomy, and total laryngectomy are the parents of many of today's more contemporary surgical approaches to laryngeal cancer. If two more operations were to be added to these, the group of five procedures we consider basic to the understanding of surgery for laryngeal cancer would be identified. For some medium cancers, a cordectomy was too limited. For others, a total laryngectomy was too much. The fundamental operations that fill the gap between the "too small" glottic operations and the "too big" complete resections of the organ are supraglottic laryngectomy and near-total laryngectomy. Supraglottic laryngectomy accepts two contingencies (temporary aspiration and potentially prolonged dysphagia) to achieve the benefit of voice preservation and the advantage of no need for a permanent stoma. With proper selection, it has replaced total laryngectomy for about one half of all patients presenting with primary supraglottic cancer.

Near-total laryngectomy does not avoid a stoma, but it does allow reliable fistula speech to be developed without prosthetics and without esophageal inflation. It has proved suitable for more than one half of the glottic cases that formerly required a total laryngectomy and relied on esophageal speech or a puncture into the esophagus. It ensures a voice for those supraglottic cases that are oncologically or physiologically unsuitable for the supraglottic operation. It also offers an important advantage (reliable fistula speech) to patients with piriform cancers who would otherwise require a total laryngectomy in concert with their partial pharyngectomy.

The indications, techniques, and expected results of these five laryngeal resections and reconstructions are presented in the belief that each operation exemplifies a fundamentally different idea:

1. Transoral cordectomy exemplifies the concept of complete endoscopic removal.
2. Laryngofissure and cordectomy, the parents of hemilaryngectomy, represent the basic ideas underlying the frontolateral vertical supracricoid resections, which preserve a glottic voice and offer only a minimal risk of swallowing difficulty or airway dysfunction.
3. Supraglottic laryngectomy embodies the basic principles of a horizontal supraventricular partial laryngectomy, again with preservation of voice and minimal risk to the airway. It implies greater swallowing dysfunction, implicit in the loss of the upper laryngeal sphincter mechanism, while trying to preserve an internal airway.
4. Near-total laryngectomy is an en bloc supraglottic laryngectomy, extended hemilaryngectomy, and hemicricoid resection with the creation of fistula voice. The excisional concept is to remove the entire paraglottic space and every structure it touches. This strategy poses a minimal risk to swallowing but for the first time requires acceptance of a permanent tracheal stoma.
5. Total laryngectomy is, of course, a complete resection of the organ (the larynx) but with minimal risk to swallow. Loss of a dependable glottic or fistula voice, so prominent in the public mind, is associated only with this fifth category of surgery; the other four all provide for voice. And today vocal rehabilitation by secondary interventions is feasible. Acceptance of a permanent tracheal stoma is really the only uncompromising requirement of this category.

It deserves emphasis that even though we are talking about the surgery of laryngeal cancer, a strategy for voice preservation or voice production is always included, and swallowing is eventually returned. The majority of laryngeal cancer patients treated by surgery alone will never need a permanent tracheotomy or retreatment for recurrent disease. With a knowledge of the five basic approaches, an appropriate operation can be selected or a modern refinement can be derived for almost every variation of laryngeal cancer that occurs.

The indications for the modern endoscopic technique (e.g., laser cordectomy) are no different than those of transoral cordectomy, and the expected results are the same.

The indications and the safe limits on laryngofissure and cordectomy (the basic vertical operation) have been clarified and extended as the frontolateral and frontoanterior vertical partial laryngectomies and hemilaryngectomy (which is different from "partial vertical" primarily in its entry point, its treatment of the thyroid ala, and its effect on swallow). As the resections in this category have increased in size beyond fissure

and cordectomy, reconstructive strategies have been developed to accompany them to compensate for glottic defects in bulk and lining epithelium.

Supraglottic laryngectomy was originally kept within very strict limits as far as its indications and extent were concerned. It has been successfully expanded laterally to deal with a few piriform lesions (the partial laryngopharyngectomy of Ogura).[57] Numerous other extensions of the supraglottic laryngectomy superiorly and inferiorly have been tried. Currently, clinical experience with the morbidity of these extensions (intractable aspiration) and the alternatives for treatment (near-total laryngectomy) have led to retreat to the original limited form of the operation. In this form, the results of supraglottic laryngectomy are excellent and predictable.

The near-total laryngectomy concept was developed for cancers that fix the vocal cord.[58] The endoscopic resections and the vertical and horizontal conventional partial (conservation) operations *require mobile vocal cords* in most cases. There are a few selected exceptions that allow the larger vertical partial operations, but these are not common, and some surgeons believe they are unsafe except in extremely experienced hands. The near-total laryngectomy includes complete hemispherical resection of the cricoid, which is the lower margin of the paraglottic space. It handles transglottic tumors that are too large for the conventional horizontal operation and piriform carcinomas that are too large for a partial laryngopharyngectomy. It provides reliable tracheopharyngeal fistula voice but for the first time asks the patient to accept a permanent stoma.

Total laryngectomy is the final concept, but cord fixation is not its indication. It is necessary when radiation fails in T3 or T4 glottic cancer, any supraglottic cancer, or any piriform cancer. It is necessary in unirradiated cases where the posterior extent or bilateral ventricular involvement precludes a near-total laryngectomy. Examples are massive bilateral supraglottic cancer with both ventricles involved or hypopharyngeal cancer with extension into the interarytenoid or postcricoid regions. Acceptance of a stoma is mandatory. Voice can be created by air forced up through the pharyngoesophageal segment from the esophagus. This can be impounded to come from an inflated esophagus (esophageal speech), or it can originate in the lungs (after tracheoesophageal puncture and the placement of a prosthetic antiaspiration valve).

The principles and techniques of the three classic procedures have been described. A discussion of the two additional strategies, supraglottic laryngectomy and near-total laryngectomy, will follow.

Supraglottic Laryngectomy

For many years it was recognized that large supraglottic lesions resected by total laryngectomy were often, on closer analysis, confined completely to the supraglottic larynx. The ventricles might be compressed to slits by the bulk of the lesion, but the anterior commissure, vocal cords, arytenoids, and everything below this level were normal. Over the years, Alonso,[59] Som,[60] Bocca et al.,[61] Ogura,[7] and others capitalized on this observation by developing a formal technique for block resection of the supraglottic larynx with preservation of the true glottis and with reconstruction techniques that preserved an airway and allowed the rehabilitation of swallow. Transhyoid pharyngotomy had been employed for epiglottectomy before this time, and the occasional supraglottic tumor had been removed through a lateral pharyngotomy. The oncologic results were never outstanding, however, and only a very small proportion of supraglottic cases were candidates for these earlier operations.

Supraglottic laryngectomy is classified as a true conservation operation because the support of the cricoid is maintained. This is similar to conventional vertical partial laryngectomies, which are also classified as conservation procedures. Circumferential cricoid preservation prevents a permanent tracheostomy from being required.

The selection criteria for this operation are well known now. Supraglottic laryngectomy (horizontal partial laryngectomy) is indicated for squamous cell carcinomas that originate on the epiglottis or the false cords and remain confined to the supraglottic larynx. If their growth pattern is exophytic, the volume may be large, but as long as they do not descend into the glottis or spill out into the pharynx or extend into the base of the tongue, a supraglottic laryngectomy is feasible and usually advisable.

There are two contraindications to supraglottic laryngectomy: oncologic and physiologic. Oncologic contraindications include downward extension to the anterior commissure, posterior spread that would require resection of an entire arytenoid cartilage, forward penetration into the marrow space of the thyroid (ossified) cartilage, upward extension through the valleculae into the base of the tongue, and/or lateral mucosal extension out of the larynx into the surrounding elements of the hypopharynx. Physiologic contraindications are advanced age, failed radiation, and chronic obstructive pulmonary disease for which aspiration would tip the scales toward fatal pulmonary infection.

The technical maneuvers necessary to ensure the restoration of swallowing demand very careful attention to detail and an understanding of the normal physiology of the larynx during deglutition. The normal laryngeal lumen is folded together to resist aspiration during swallow by several related events[62]:

1. Retroversion of the epiglottis into contact with the forward tilting arytenoids.
2. Elevation of the larynx, with compression of the preepiglottic fat pad. This, in turn, displaces the inferior surface of the supraglottic larynx (infrahyoid epiglottis) into the pharyngeal lumen and against the cuneiform and the arytenoid cartilages.
3. Side-to-side approximation of the false cords and ventricular bands.
4. Approximation of opposing true vocal cords and arytenoids.
5. Slight protrusion of the posterior interarytenoid mucosal folds into the interarytenoid space.
6. With elevation of the larynx, telescoping of the intrinsic soft tissues to a more folded lumen-occluding position.

The first three of these six mechanisms are lost in a supraglottic laryngectomy. Compensation requires upward suspension of the remaining laryngeal remnant[63] and the provision of an overhanging tongue base to approximate with the arytenoids. It is obvious that the loss of an arytenoid, paralysis of the vocal cord, or the loss of tension in the vocal cords (e.g., by damaging the anterior commissure) could be potentially fatal flaws in an airway valve already compromised by supraglottic laryngectomy.

The oncologic results of supraglottic laryngectomy are equal to those secured by total laryngectomy for the same lesions.[64, 65] The major threat from a supraglottic carcinoma, having access as it does to the anterior midline prepiglottic space, is bilateral metastases to the neck. A neck dissection is clearly advisable on the side of principle involvement. If this is submitted to histopathologic examination while the supraglottic laryngectomy is in progress, and the analysis shows cancer to be present in any of the resected lymph nodes, the opposite side should be assumed to be highly at risk, and, at the very least, a conservation neck dissection should be performed.[66]

Laryngoscopy and biopsy in supraglottic cancer differ somewhat from those in subglottic procedures. A special laryngoscope that elevates only the tongue base, such as the Lindholm vallecular speculum, may be required.

Visualization of the anterior commissure will be difficult because of the overhanging bulk. The 30 cm 70-degree Mueller subglottic telescope is a valuable device to look around this corner and evaluate the anterior commissure and vocal cords clearly at the time of the direct laryngoscopy.

After the operator confirms that a supraglottic laryngectomy is anatomically appropriate, the operative technique can proceed as follows.

The laryngoscope is withdrawn and a nasogastric tube is inserted. A tracheotomy is performed below the thyroid isthmus, and the anesthetic tubing is switched to this location. A complete neck dissection, sparing the accessory nerve, is performed on the most involved side, even if no cervical metastases are palpable.

The laryngectomy begins with transection of the suprahyoid muscles, taking great care to avoid injury to the 12th nerve. The internal branches of the superior laryngeal nerves are going to be lost in a supraglottic laryngectomy; additional injury to a 12th nerve favors aspiration. The strap muscles should then be transected over the palpable upper margin of the thyroid cartilage on both sides, avoiding the external branch of the superior laryngeal nerve. This incision is deepened through the perichondrium. The perichondrial cut follows the superior margin of the cartilage so the perichondrium (and the strap muscle layer) can be reflected downward off the thyroid alae and angle, almost to the lower margin of the cartilage. A widebladed elevator and gauze help the operator maintain the perichondrial flap (which is rather thin in the midline) as a continuous sheet.

The superior thyroid cornu and the greater horns of the hyoid are freed from their muscular and ligamentous attachments bilaterally, and both the superior laryngeal arteries are divided. The operator should be very careful to note that there is no tumor extending through the thyrohyoid membrane or invading the thyroid cartilage. If the tumor is well enough lateralized, the posterior elements of the internal branch of the superior laryngeal nerve on the side of lesser involvement can be preserved. The anterior branches pass into the specimen.

The horizontal cartilage cut is marked on the thyroid cartilage with surgical ink. The level is critical because it is vital to avoid damaging the anterior commissure. If the attachments of the true cords are destabilized, cord tension will be destroyed and aspiration will almost certainly ensue. The horizontal plane to be marked for the cartilage transection should be no lower than the junction of the upper one third and lower two thirds of the thyroid cartilage at the angle (from notch to lower border), regardless of the sex of the patient. On the ala, the lines extend horizontally backward to intersect the posterior border of the thyroid cartilage at right angles.

The surgeon dons a headlight and makes the cartilage cuts under irrigation with an oscillating saw. The patient is given a paralyzing drug, and the lumen of the pharynx is entered through the valleculae or the piriform on the side of lesser involvement. The tongue base is retracted with a small Deaver (which can be inserted transorally for this purpose or can cross the field in conventional fashion). The hyoid and the epiglottis are grasped with an Allis and rolled forward. The surgeon stands at the head of the table looking down into the supraglottic larynx from above. One scissors blade is inserted across the false cord into the posterior portion of the ventricle. The other scissors blade presses in through the thyroid ala saw cut. With one snip, the false cord is separated from the arytenoid. With two more, directed forward, the junction between the true cord and the ventricle is transected. The transection continues forward, flush with the upper surface of the vocal cords, and is continued horizontally across the midline, below the petiole, and immediately above the anterior commissure. On the second side, the outer scissors blade remains in the saw cut and the inner one in the ventricle. The specimen is continually folded out to improve exposure. The final cuts proceed up across the second ventricular band, false cord, and aryepiglottic fold on the most involved side, right at the attachments of these structures to the arytenoid cartilage.

After the supraglottic specimen is released and delivered to the pathologist, fine slivers of the remaining tissues (surgical margins) should be submitted from any area the surgeon deems important. Biopsy specimens of nearby normal-appearing epithelium sometimes reveal dysplasia, which emphasizes the need to follow-up the surgery with a smoking cessation program.[67]

An intact anterior commissure within a topless thyroid cartilage, two membranous vocal cords, and two partly denuded arytenoids now confront the surgeon. The edges of the piriform mucosa can be tacked forward very minimally with fine chromic sutures, but no attempt should be made to undermine this tissue to advance it. The raw surfaces of the laryngeal interior need not be reepithelized completely, and to deform and denervate the piriform mucosa for this purpose will only delay swallowing.

The principle goal of closure in a supraglottic laryngectomy is to bring the residual larynx up under the tongue base and to maintain it in an elevated (swallowing) position. The sternothyroid muscles, which retract the residual larynx downward, should be taken out of the game by dividing their lower insertions. The preserved thyroid-perichondrial flap, which helps in

the prevention of a supraglottic stenosis and seems to provide a low metabolic demand base for reepithelialization, is sewn to the tongue base along the raw surface of the tongue, not its mucosal edge. To avoid tearing the flap, the operator places multiple sutures while the neck is in extension. These are kept in order, then tied sequentially with the head in flexion. A second layer of closure is achieved by approximating the cut upper ends of the strap muscles to the released lower ends of the suprahyoid muscles. The vertical tensions are reduced further by placing a nonabsorbable mersaline suture through the cricothyroid membrane and sewing it up to the geniohyoid tendons and raphe of the mylohyoid.[63]

Many textbooks advocate asymmetric supraglottic resections and deem it permissible, when necessary, to remove an arytenoid, fillet the upper surface of a vocal cord, or extend the resection out into the piriform sinus. These extensions increase the likelihood of severe swallowing problems postoperatively. Sometimes they also prevent decannulation. I no longer push the supraglottic operation in these directions but prefer the safety and predictability of near-total laryngectomy. It allows a wider excision of neighboring tissues and avoids the swallowing problem. It does commit a patient to a permanent tracheostomy, but it eliminates the need for interoperative conversion of a supraglottic laryngectomy to a total laryngectomy.

The tracheotomy tube and wound restrict the natural upward mobility of the larynx essential to swallowing.[68] Also, the airway leak that continues until the tracheostomy is closed prevents an effective protective cough. It also prevents the "suction pump" action of the lower pharynx during swallow. In the immediate postoperative period, the tracheotomy tube cuff must remain inflated to prevent aspiration. Not until the patient is able to swallow his or her own saliva should the protection of the cuffed tracheotomy tube be forsaken. In the typical case, the tracheotomy tube can be removed around the 7th day, and attempts to swallow pureed food can begin around the 14th (as soon as the tracheotomy is closed). It is not uncommon to send a patient home on supplemental tube feedings after the third week if there is any delay in establishing deglutition. A nasogastric tube can always be removed during a follow-up office visit when progress in swallowing has been demonstrated at home.

Near-Total Laryngectomy

Near-total laryngectomy is a relative late comer to the group of five operations described in this chapter as basic concept procedures. Originally introduced under an anatomic name, "extended hemilaryngectomy,"[69] and subsequently a generic one, "subtotal laryngectomy,"[70] it was erroneously classified with the partial vertical operations for limited glottic cancer. But true partial vertical laryngectomies conserve cricoid integrity and thus do not impose a permanent tracheal stoma. In 1982, the name near-total became attached to this technique because almost the entire larnyx is resected except for a narrow posterolateral strip connecting the trachea and the pharynx, a strip that subsequently becomes the basis of a biologically valved tracheopharyngeal speaking shunt. This strip includes a single arytenoid, preserved from the less involved side.

Compared with a total laryngectomy, the near-total laryngectomy has the advantage of preserving a lung-powered voice. As an ablative procedure, it encompasses the lateralized cord-fixing cancers that are too big for the so-called conventional conservation operations. Like a total laryngectomy, it requires the patient to accept a permanent tracheotomy. Since cordectomies, hemilaryngectomies, and supraglottic laryngectomies do not, they are, of course, preferred when the dimensions of the cancer and the tolerance of the patient permit. They do preserve ipsilateral cricoid and piriform, however, so they are limited as to the extent of the tumor they can address.

The principal indication for a near-total laryngectomy is fixation of one vocal cord by a predominantly unilateral cancer. In addition, the patient has to have an uninvolved laryngeal ventricle on the less involved side. Glottic cancer is only one of the potential candidates for near-total laryngectomy. Other case examples are:

1. Unilateral transglottic carcinomas with cord fixation.
2. Invasive glottic cancer with subglottic spread or cartilage invasion placing it beyond limits of a vertical conservation procedure.
3. Supraglottic cancer with local extension beyond the supraglottis.
4. Cardiopulmonary contraindications too great to tolerate an oncologically adequate supraglottic laryngectomy.[71]
5. Aryepiglottic fold/piriform sinus cancer too large to permit Ogura's conservation partial laryngopharyngectomy.

The voice in a near-total laryngectomy is achieved by the exhalation of air through a primitive tubular tracheopharyngeal shunt. This is fashioned from the laryngeal remnant. Its components can best be described in reference to the anatomic levels of the larynx. The subglottic passage comes from the contralateral subglottic mucosa and conus elasticus, no longer braced open by a ring of residual cricoid cartilage. The glottic portion is partially sphincteric by virtue of its retention of some thyroarytenoid, lateral cricoarytenoid, posterior cricoarytenoid, and cricothyroid muscle. It functions to control aspiration. At the supraglottic level of the shunt, an adynamic entry into the pharynx about 0.5 cm in diameter is maintained with the arytenoid and a small portion of the false cord. This is the portion that appears to vibrate during voice production.

The laryngeal remnant that remains after the ablative portion of a near-total laryngectomy has most of the elements necessary to create a workable vocal shunt except, in some cases, sufficient lining mucosa to provide an adequate shunt diameter, especially at the relatively indistensible glottic level. This requirement is provided by transposing an inferiorly based mucosal flap from the adjacent residual pharynx. This maintains reliability and speed by eliminating the need for skin grafts, distant flaps, or any complex reconstructive technology.

Near-total laryngectomy provides acceptable voice because it meets the following criteria for providing one. It allows voice exhalation to occur at normal or near-normal airway pressures through a shunt from the trachea to the pharynx, which is about

5 mm in diameter or larger. It has a continuous epithelial lining from the trachea to the pharynx, unbroken by any suture line; otherwise it would be subject to stenosis. A neuromuscular valve is incorporated into the shunt to prevent aspiration, just as in a larynx. All that is necessary to produce voice during exhalation is a soft narrow orifice that enters into the pharynx;[72] the laryngectomized patient still has the lips, tongue, palate, motor cortex, and so forth that are needed to articulate the voice into speech.

As with all head and neck oncologic surgery, intraoperative frozen section histopathology has to be expert in near-total laryngectomy. Clinical selection is straightforward in virgin cases. Intraoperative escalation to a total laryngectomy has never proved to be necessary in a personal series of more than 70 patients. Near-total laryngectomy attempts to bloc out one paraglottic space, the contents, the walls, and all the anatomic structures that border on it. Whole organ serial section evidence from the studies of total-laryngectomy specimens seems to indicate that this would be the necessary and sufficient specimen to be removed in most cases of vocal cord fixation by cancer.[73] After radiation failure, definable limits on a tumor and containment within the near-total laryngectomy "block" cannot be ascertained. Therefore, near-total laryngectomy should rarely be employed in radiorecurrent disease.

Voice is a natural result of the deliberate fistula that is formed in a near-total laryngectomy, but to activate it, patients have to learn how to occlude their stoma when they exhale air. No prosthesis is required to hold the shunt open or prevent stenosis, and a near-total laryngectomy does not rely on a prosthesis to prevent aspiration. The dynamics of the shunt itself provides for these features. When a near-total laryngectomy is performed, a voice is obtainable in almost every case. The quality of the voice is good, but it is the reliability of obtaining a voice, not its special quality, that characterizes this operation. The sound does not depend on the ingestion or impounding of air into the esophagus. The near-total laryngectomy shunt enters the pharynx directly. The air does not have to negotiate a passageway up through the resistance of a potentially spastic pharyngoesophageal segment.

The postoperative management of near-total laryngectomy is virtually identical to that of a total laryngectomy. In the first week, patients receive basic wound care. In the second week, they learn self-care of their tracheotomy and lose their nasogastric tube. Fistula speech production does not begin in earnest until around the sixth week, when the tracheostomy is well enough healed to permit valving with a finger. A speech pathologist helps these patients regulate their rate, improve their articulation and phrasing, and valve their stoma more effectively.[74]

The technical sequence of near-total laryngectomy is as follows.[10] For purposes of discussion, we will assume a right transglottic carcinoma that fixes the right vocal cord and invades the paraglottic space (and perhaps the thyroid cartilage) and extends 15 mm subglottically, precluding any safe modification of a conventional hemilaryngectomy. The anterior commissure is involved, as is the right arytenoid, the false cord, and perhaps even the aryepiglottic fold. The vocal cord on the left is slightly involved near the anterior commissure, but it is mobile, and no cancer is present in the left ventricle. The left arytenoid and the interarytenoid area are widely clear of disease.

A careful preliminary laryngoscopy is undertaken. It confirms that the left arytenoid and the left ventricle are free of tumor, and the posterior commissure is clear. The diagnosis is confirmed by frozen section, a tracheotomy is performed below the thyroid isthmus, and a discontinuous neck dissection is performed on the N0 right side of the neck, sparing the right accessory nerve. Now we are ready to address the larynx.

On the side of the major involvement, the right, the strap muscles are cut low over the thyroid gland. The larynx and the right thyroid lobe are turned medially, and the superior and inferior thyroid neurovascular pedicles are divided. The suprahyoid muscles are detached from the right greater horn and body of the hyoid bone. The pharyngeal constrictor is incised all along the posterior border of the thyroid cartilage down to the lower border of the cricoid. To this point, then, on the side of greater involvement, the dissection is exactly the same as that of a total laryngectomy.

Attention is turned to the side of lesser involvement, the left, where the medial edge of the strap muscles is exposed by sharp dissection. The strap muscles are divided at their insertion on the hyoid bone and are reflected back to expose the left thyroid ala and the cricothyroid muscle. The prelaryngeal soft tissues, right strap muscles, and thyroid isthmus will remain with the specimen, and the left lobe of the thyroid is preserved with the patient.

The left cricothyroid muscle is elevated back from the cricoid cartilage and preserved. The hyoid arch is partially resected with a rongeur to remove the anterior end of the left greater horn (the body and right horn will be "specimen"). Similarly, the left thyroid ala is partially resected by cutting out a vertical wedge from its middle third. The apex of the wedge is the cricothyroid triangle below, and the base is the curved upper margin of the ala above. This resection provides a window through which the intralaryngeal soft tissues on the left can be visualized. The amount of thyroid ala removed is roughly the middle third. The anterior third, to which the commissural tendons and the thyroarytenoid muscles are attached, will go with the specimen. The posterior third, which includes the superior cornua, posterior border, and inferior cornua, remains with the patient. It is primarily a pharyngeal structure, on the less involved side, and it is left undisturbed simply to avoid unnecessary dissection. Its removal might disturb the recurrent laryngeal nerve entering behind the cricothyroid joint or the external branch of the superior laryngeal nerve, innervating the cricothyroid muscle. Besides, the thyrohyoid muscle is still attached, and this might help elevate the shunt and reproduce the negative suction pump hypopharyngeal phase of swallow.

The left saccule (that portion of the ventricle that protrudes up over the upper margin of the thyroarytenoid muscle) is opened through its glandular apex. The interior of the ventricle on the left is visually identified. A scissors blade is inserted through this opening, and the dissection proceeds up through the left false cord and then turns horizontally across the vallecula. When the vallecula is transected, the epiglottis and preepiglottic tissues can be turned down and forward (somewhat similar to a supraglottic laryngectomy). From this point on, with

muscle relaxation from the anesthesiologist and good illumination with a headlight, the interior features of the larynx can be properly visualized. The larynx has been entered safely, and the rest of the excision can be conducted with the tumor itself under direct visual control.

Still working on the left (the side of lesser involvement), the surgeon comes down from superiorly and transects the better cord with the scissors, steering clear of any extension of the tumor. Typically, one half to three fourths of the "good" membranous cord is sacrificed. Fortunately, more muscle lies in the posterior half of the glottis than the anterior. Much of the thyroarytenoid muscle sweeps back beyond the vocal process, and no components of the lateral or the posterior cricoarytenoid lie ahead of midcoronal plane. The cricothyroid muscle was preserved in its entirety too, so that all in all, despite considerable sacrifice of the vocal ligament on the less involved side, there is enough muscle left to valve the shunt against aspiration.

Now the line of resection angles down through the anterior arch of the cricoid, curving toward the right in the trachea. It passes around on the right side between the lower border of the cricoid and the first tracheal ring and then rises back up inside the laryngeal midline posteriorly. The posterior incision in the cricoid is made just through the cortex of the cartilage. When this is done and the larynx is elevated forward with a finger inserted into the postcricoid region, a little retraction on the two halves of the subglottic larynx is all it takes to break the postcricoid plate along the score and open out the larynx anteriorly. This provides immaculate exposure of the posterior commissure. The interarytenoid muscle can now be divided on the stretch and any postcricoid (posterior cricoarytenoid) muscular attachments to the specimen can be transected.

The laryngeal specimen and the right thyroid lobe and isthmus are now elevated and divided from their mucosal attachments to the pharynx. As much right hypopharyngeal wall can be included with the specimen as is necessary. Surgical margins are obtained from the patient and delivered to the pathologist independent of the specimen itself. While the frozen sections are studied by the pathologist, the surgeon resects the residual left cricoid support from the laryngeal remnant using nasal subperichondrial elevators. The recurrent laryngeal nerve can be protected from injury by leaving some cricoid in the region of the inferior thyroid cornu. Not enough cricoid would be preserved to prevent the laryngeal remnant from being tubed. The resection of cricoid on the less involved side has nothing to do with cancer. The sole point is to allow uninhibited tubing of the subglottic mucosa.

If enough laryngeal tissue remains to allow the surgeon to form a tube of adequate diameter, the tracheopharyngeal shunt can be reconstructed completely from the laryngeal remnant. If not, a small inferiorly based pennant flap of piriform mucosa is developed from the right pharyngotomy margin. When this is turned down so its base is level with the remaining arytenoid, its mucosa will face the interior of the future shunt. The medial margin of this flap is simply sutured to the (glottic and subglottic) mucosal edge of the laryngeal remnant in the posterior midline. This adds to the width of available shunt mucosa, especially where it is needed, at the level of arytenoid and true cord remnant. A pharyngeal flap added in this way has no contractile powers, so it should probably not be made too large. Otherwise aspiration may ensue.

To determine how much diameter is needed to form an adequate shunt,[75] I measure the caliber of the proposed shunt by tubing it over a 14 F red rubber catheter. The shunt mucosa is folded together anteriorly, and the seam of the tube that results is closed from below upward. A tiny wedge of cartilage sometimes has to be removed from the trachea at the lower apex of the closure line just to get things started. The catheter, which is only a sizing device, is removed. The reflected left cricothyroid muscle is returned and layered onto the shunt to be incorporated into its valve actions. Seam closure is completed up to the level of the corniculate, and the shunt is formed. Only the pharyngotomy remains to be closed. This is done in much the same way as in a total laryngectomy. The shunt itself is already connected with the pharyngeal lumen, since its laryngeal component flows up over the arytenoid and into the pharynx without interruption.

At the conclusion of these internal repairs, the wounds are thoroughly irrigated. The previously reflected left strap muscles are joined back to the suprahyoid muscles. The anterior wall tracheotomy (through the third and fourth rings) is carefully sutured to a stomal opening in the skin. Drainage, closure of the neck flaps, and the arrangement of the dressings are the same as described for total laryngectomy.

Contemporary Extensions of the Five Elementary Operations

There are so many conservation operations for laryngeal cancer that the field seems in hopeless confusion. The reason there are so many operations is that there are so many different diseases. Cancer of the larynx involves different sites, at different stages, in different patients, with and without previous radiation. The differences are important. Undertreatment, driven by the urge to preserve voice, jeopardizes the goal of a cure. Overtreatment in the name of cure may unnecessarily injure the voice. Life is the overriding goal, but the voice has so much to do with our humanity. Individuals who cannot communicate cannot control their environment, carry on their work, or even express their emotions. There are also the issues of swallowing (Can some aspiration be risked?) and breathing (Can a stoma be avoided?). In view of the imperatives of cure, voice, swallow, and airway, no surgeon can long remain satisfied with a limited array of procedures. The "right" operation will be so different from case to case.

On the other hand, there must be some limit on the number of acceptable procedures and some rational basis for selecting them. My premise in this chapter is that if the indications and techniques of a small number of elementary procedures are completely understood, the indications and techniques of their variations and extensions can be readily derived and applied. I have already indicated what I consider to be the five fundamental operations—transoral cordectomy, laryngofissure, supraglottic laryngectomy, near-total laryngectomy, and total laryngectomy. This section presents the rest of the operations as if they were simply extensions of these strategies. These will include laser cordectomy, the vertical and horizontal partial

conservation laryngectomies, near-total laryngopharyngectomy, tracheoesophageal puncture, and laryngopharyngectomy with pharyngeal reconstruction.

Laser cordectomy is, in many ways, a welcome rediscovery of suspension laryngoscopy and transoral cordectomy.[76] The laser offers a new way to cut. The microscope provides precision. In any event, the principles of patient selection and the results of laser cordectomy are the same as those of the classical operation formerly done with the Killian-Lynch suspension system.

Similarly, laryngofissure and cordectomy provide the background of experience from which the vertical partial laryngectomies and hemilaryngectomies for T2 and some T3 glottic carcinomas can evolve. It is not the weakness or strength of one type of vertical conservation operation over another or the school of thought from which one style emerged that determines the best selection. It is an understanding of the extent of the lesion, the requirements of the patient, and the potential of the uninvolved tissues for functional reconstruction. There are no substitutes for a qualified understanding of the meaning of the clinical examination, a thorough knowledge of the techniques of partial laryngeal surgery, and a sophisticated respect for the oncologic and functional limits of each procedure. The contraindication is cancer invasion beyond the point at which a functional reconstruction can be obtained. The reconstruction must produce a valve with the following characteristics:

1. It must close tightly enough to exclude food and fluids from the airway during swallowing.
2. It should approximate lightly enough to permit voice on controlled exhalation.
3. It must open widely and strongly enough to resist collapse (obstruction to airflow) during deep inhalation.

Partial laryngopharyngectomy for selected early piriform cancers[57] is an outgrowth of Ogura's standard supraglottic laryngectomy. To be suitable, an aryepiglottic fold lesion or piriform lesion must show no evidence of (1) piriform apex involvement, (2) vocal cord fixation, or (3) cartilage invasion. It requires, above all, intimate familiarity with the technique of supraglottic laryngectomy and the ability to determine who is a physiologic as well as an oncologic candidate.

The near-total laryngectomy concept has been successfully applied to hypopharyngeal cancer too large for partial laryngopharyngectomy. Near-total laryngopharyngectomy and extended near-total laryngopharyngectomy (in which pharyngeal reconstruction is combined with a near-total laryngopharyngectomy) are valuable concepts whose selection and application become obvious once experience with near-total laryngectomy is gained.

Tracheoesophageal puncture should now be in the repertoire of any laryngologist who deals with cancers. I have already indicated how this technology may influence how the cricopharyngeus is handled and how it may invite a coincidental pharyngeal neurectomy. Finally, I will deal with laryngopharyngectomy, in which major pharyngeal reconstruction technologies are simultaneously applied. In this area, the reconstructive roles of the pectoral myocutaneous flap, free jejunal transplantation, and gastric transpositon (the stomach pull-up) have become clarified in recent years.

Laser Cordectomy

Coherent light from a CO_2 laser source can be used to vaporize tissue in the larynx by linking it to an operating microscope. Marketing brochures trumpet these instruments as "high-precision bloodless light scalpels that offer unparalleled vision and control." The hemostasis and the visualization are excellent with the current generation of instruments. Visual feedback is enhanced by special suction tubes fitted to the laryngoscope, and sometimes to the microforceps, to aspirate the steam and the smoke. The micromanipulator provides no tactile impression of the tissues, but since the cordectomy specimen is usually grasped by a microforceps to prevent destruction of the pathologic specimen, this is not a practical drawback. By adjusting the power (watts) and spot size (square centimeters) and using short sharp pulses instead of a continuous wave, one can dissect a cordectomy specimen with accuracy and at the same time produce a microcauterized base. Special facial protection devices, laser laryngoscopes, and laser-resistant endotracheal tubes are recommended to reduce the risk of injury and of combustion in the oxygen-rich ventilatory atmosphere present in the airway. Jet ventilation avoids an endotracheal tube altogether but is probably less satisfactory from a ventilatory control point of view. The laser works in only a straight line; it does not reach around corners. The surgeon may have to introduce special retractors and protectors to direct and limit the laser's energy to the intended location.

Safety is probably the foremost issue in laser cordectomy, especially eye protection for the treatment team and wet face protection for the patient. A CO_2 laser does add weight to the microscope and expense to the procedure. It also introduces a host of safety regulations into the operating environment, requires special education in laser safety precautions for the operating personnel, and adds a certain amount of set-up time and complexity to an otherwise simple procedure. The "precision" probably comes from the microscope and the micromanipulator, not the laser itself. All in all, it is hard to make the case that laser surgery is a cost-effective improvement over classical transoral cordectomy. On the other hand, it has alerted more surgeons to the possibility of performing a definitive laryngoscopic resection instead of treating their T1 glottic cancer patients with limited biopsy and 6 weeks of radiotherapy. The techniques and the instrumentation will continue to develop, so the full potential of this modality is yet to be realized.

Frontolateral and Frontoanterior Partial Laryngectomy and Laryngoplasty

The anterior commissure is a fixed point and hard to assess clinically as to the depth of invasion. It is a route of spread for invasive glottic cancer into the thyroid cartilage, although the studies of serial sections show that spread up to, but not into, the cartilage is more usual.[3] When glottic cancer involves the anterior commissure but the vocal cords are both mobile, frontolateral and frontoanterior partial laryngectomies offer better control of the disease than does radiation.[77]

Frontolateral partial and frontoanterior partial laryngectomies are simply laryngofissures and cordectomies in which the angle of the thyroid cartilage (the strip that unites the two laminae) is formally included with the specimen. The purpose is to include the anterior commissure and tendon. Frontolateral partial laryngectomy can also include the entire arytenoid cartilage. As in laryngofissure and cordectomy, the petiole, the entire ventricle, ventricular band, and false cord are always included. When the anterior commissure is heavily involved and more extensive bilateral spread is present, the arytenoid is usually free. In this case, the so-called frontoanterior partial laryngectomy is used, taking more cartilage and cord from the less involved side but leaving both arytenoids and any posterior membranous cord tissue that can be spared.

One or other of these vertical partial laryngectomies is indicated in medium to large invasive T1 glottic cancers when radiation is refused, in all cases when the anterior commissure is clearly involved, and where early age mitigates against the use of radiation. It is sometimes permissible in T2 glottic cancers. I never use it for T3 disease; the least operation in cases with cord fixation would be a hemilaryngectomy,[78] to be described in a following section, and more commonly, a near-total laryngectomy would be advised.

When invasive glottic cancer is predominately one sided, the vertical frontolateral partial is appropriate. When an arytenoid is removed or much of the anterior thyroid cartilage ala is lost, soft tissue reconstitution on that side is advisable to avoid a weak breathy voice. Bailey's bipedicled strap muscle/external perichondrium flap provides an excellent method.[79] In the frontoanterior modification, consideration should be given to (1) a temporary glottic keel, (2) bilateral bipedicled strap muscle laryngoplasty flaps, and (3) reconstitution of the anterior defect with a sliding epiglottoplasty.[80]

Lawson and Biller listed the following contraindications to vertical frontolateral partial laryngectomy: (1) greater than one-third involvement of the less involved vocal cord, (2) subglottic extension greater than 10 mm anteriorly or 5 mm posterolaterally, (3) posterior spread beyond the anterior portions of the arytenoid, (4) transglottic extension, (5) thyroid cartilage invasion, and (6) impaired vocal cord mobility (a relative contraindication).[81] These are certainly valuable guides. To them, I would add a seventh, previous radiotherapy.

Frontolateral partial laryngectomy and laryngoplasty is performed as follows. After a preliminary laryngoscopy and a tracheostomy, a transverse skin incision at the lower border of the thyroid cartilage is extended from the medial edge of one sternomastoid muscle to the other. The strap muscles are parted but not elevated, and the delphian node is sampled. The thyroid perichondrium is incised in the midline, partially elevated, and tacked to the medial edges of the strap muscles with fine sutures. The perichondrium from the ala on the involved side is elevated as far back as possible, incised at its attachment, and elevated attached to the undersurface of the strap muscles. A sagittal thyrotomy is made about 3 mm to the less involved side of the midline. A posterior thyrotomy is made on the side of the tumor about 10 mm from the midline. The larynx is entered from below up via the first thyrotomy, like an off-center laryngofissure. The contiguous portions of the thyroid ala, the anterior glottis, the involved true cord, the ventricle and the false cord on that side, plus a portion or all of the involved arytenoid cartilage and its mucosa are removed en bloc. As in laryngofissure and cordectomy, careful note must be taken of the subglottic margin. Preservation of the cricoid ring sets limits on the ability of this operation to deal with subglottic extension. On the other hand, preservation of the cricoid ring guarantees an adequate airway and assures the eventual loss of the temporary tracheotomy.

The reconstructive problem in a vertical frontolateral partial laryngectomy is to provide enough closure to prevent a breathy voice, particularly when the arytenoid has been completely removed. Where the external thyroid perichondrium was tacked to the deep surface of the strap muscles, a bulky muscle-perichondrial flap, pedicled superiorly and inferiorly, is prepared.[79] It is transposed with the residual thyroid ala, and in this position, medial to the ala, it is drawn into the laryngeal defect. The perichondrium is tacked to the cut edges of the endolaryngeal wound with 4.0 chromic sutures. In describing the bipedicled flap technique for a large number of cases, Bailey advocated that the flap should be made as bulky as possible because significant shrinkage is expected.[82] He noted that the perichondrial surface that faces the lumen of the larynx gradually resurfaces with mucosa and provides a satisfactory cushion for phonation.[82]

When the anterior portions of the thyroid cartilage and the contralateral vocal cord are more extensively resected (frontoanterior partial laryngectomy), some means of extending the separation between the two residual halves of the larynx is required. This can be a silicone rubber keel, which is left in place for 4 weeks, under antibiotic coverage, and then removed endoscopically. Alternatively, it might be the epiglottis, advanced downward by releasing the hyoepiglottic ligaments[80] above (Tucker's near-total laryngectomy).[83] If necessary, the epiglottic flap can be cut vertically and folded to deepen the new anterior apex of the glottic chink.[84]

Hemilaryngectomy

Hemilaryngectomy is a more extensive vertical partial laryngectomy than the frontolateral operation. It gives cordal cancer a wider margin by including the thyroid cartilage, but it leads one pyriform sinus into the airway too, so it begins to encroach on the patient's ability to swallow without aspiration. Hemilaryngectomy includes resection of the entire vertical hemilarynx except the hyoid above and the cricoid below. On the side of the tumor, the only element of the thyroid ala that is preserved is a posterior reconstructive strip used to build up the cricoarytenoid region. Hemilaryngectomy is indicated in T2 glottic carcinomas, especially those in which the anterior commissure is involved. Up to one third of the opposite cord may be involved. Subglottic extension should be no more than 10 mm anteriorly and 5 mm posteriorly. In surface extent, the tumors it treats are identical to frontolateral cases. It is when greater depth is suspected or wider margins are desired that hemilaryngectomy is preferred.[85]

Hemilaryngectomy is a useful salvage procedure for early glottic radiation failures, but the specimen excised must encompass all of the tissue in which the cancer was originally present.[86] If this cannot be known because of the patient's transfer from one physician to another, imprecise pretreatment documentation of the original lesion, or interference with the assessment by secondary biopsies or inflammatory events, it should not be tried. Transglottic extension to the supraglottic larynx is a contraindication to hemilaryngectomy. It is also contraindicated in patients with chronic obstructive pulmonary disease who would be intolerant of the aspiration of thin liquids. It probably should not be used in patients more than 70 years old. Near-total laryngectomy can accomplish a higher and lower resection without subjecting the patient to the stress of salivary aspiration, so the justification for extending vertical partial procedures any further than hemilaryngectomy is questionable.

The biopsy should be confined to the center of the lesions, and the border should not be disturbed. The technique originally suggested by Hautant,[87] and described in the modern era by Som and Silver,[88] Mohr et al.,[89] and Biller and colleagues,[90] is as follows.

A transverse incision is deepened through the skin, subcutaneous tissue, and platysma at the level of the lower border of the thyroid cartilage. It extends from the middle of the sternocleidomastoid muscle on the side of the cancer to the anterior border of the sternocleidomastoid muscle on the opposite side. Flaps are elevated to expose the strap muscles and the prelaryngeal fascia from above the hyoid to below the cricoid.

The thyroid cartilage is approached in the manner of the supraglottic laryngectomy. That is, the surgeon transects the strap muscles on the involved side over the upper border of the thyroid cartilage and continues the incision through the perichondrium. The cut edge of the perichondrium is tacked to the cut edge of the muscle. The perichondrial flap is elevated downward to the lower border of the thyroid cartilage. It is released laterally, medially, and inferiorly so that it is completely free and is attached only to the undersurface of the reflected strap muscles.

A vertical saw cut is made in the ala on the side of lesser involvement 3 mm to 1 cm from the midline. The more involved side of the larynx is exposed by rotating the specimen away, and the origin of the inferior constrictor along the posterior external surface of the thyroid ala is exposed. Originally, the entire thyroid cartilage, including the superior and inferior cornu and the posterior strip connecting those two structures, was freed and resected. Nowadays a vertical saw cut is made through the thyroid cartilage just ahead of the origin of the inferior constrictor. The superior cornu, posterior border, and inferior cornu thus remain attached to the muscle for later reconstructive use. Through the thyroid cut, the external surface of the piriform mucosa is mobilized. Then the piriform is entered at the thyrohyoid level.

The resection can now proceed from this pharyngotomy site; the anterior larynx has not yet been opened. A cut is directed horizontally across the aryepiglottic fold above the ventricle and into the infrahyoid epiglottis. Anterior commissure involvement can be assessed with this sequence before it is approached and the principle of entering away from the cancer has been satisfied. The extension proceeds downward across the front of the contralateral ventricular band and into the cartilage cut on the less involved side. It continues down across the true cord on the "good" side, under direct vision, skirting tumor and including in the specimen the anterior commissure and tendon. The view into the laryngeal lumen is excellent at this point. The cut can be continued down to the upper margin of the cricoid, then along its margin horizontally in the subglottis of the involved side, taking care that an adequate resection is achieved. It may also be redirected in the subglottis to include the upper hemicricoid if need be (Biller and Som's extended hemilaryngectomy).[91] The resection continues back to include the entire arytenoid. The final release of the specimen is from the posterior cricoarytenoid and interarytenoid muscle attachments to the muscular process of the arytenoid. Surgical margins are sent separately to the pathologist, and gloves and instruments are changed to prevent cross contamination with any viable tumor cells.

Now the posterior thyroid cartilage remnant can be mobilized, pedicled on the inferior constrictor, and turned down to support the cricoarytenoid defect. This graft is pedicled on the muscle, but to survive, it must also be covered by piriform mucosa from the side of the major resection. The mucosa should be drawn forward to help fashion a partial neocord in the defect and to cover any bare cartilage that remains. The strap muscles and their island of perichondrium can be used to repair the anterior portions of the defect, but of course, in this case, there is no alar cartilage to help medialize the flap.

Mohr et al. reviewed 57 cases in which a hemilaryngectomy, similar to the one described earlier, was applied to a series of T1, T2, and selected T3 glottic cancers.[89] There were only three deaths due to disease, one T1 case (radiation failure) at 11 years and two T2 cases at 4 and 7 years, respectively. Recurrence, when it occurred, tended to be subglottic. Interestingly, the two T2 patients who had recurrences had supraglottic extension of their primary tumors. The authors agreed that this type of extension should be considered transglottic and not amendable to vertical hemilaryngectomy. I would agree; I still have not witnessed any local recurrence when transglottic cancer is treated by near-total laryngectomy.

It is interesting to reflect on what we have learned from frontolateral partial laryngectomy and hemilaryngectomy. Clearly, we see that laryngofissure and cordectomy can be extended, if this is necessary, to control the disease. And the extensions described are tolerable, with the preservation of voice and airway. Aspiration-free swallowing is routine when the aryepiglottic fold and the posterior portion of the arytenoid are retained (frontolateral, frontoanterior). It must be reclaimed by reconstruction when these breakwaters are destroyed (hemilaryngectomy). One can resect the anterior one third of the larynx bilaterally, plus all of one cord, the upper subglottis, the ventricle and the arytenoid, the upper margin of the hemicricoid, and the entire thyroid ala on an involved side. When there is sufficient framework to prevent stenosis, the interior of the larynx can be repaired by granulation, by the reepithelialization of a perichondrial flap attached to muscle, in part by piriform mucosa, and to some extent by the application of a large bipedicled muscle flap. It is clear that a gap will remain in the posterior glottis when reconstruction is overlooked and that the bipedicle muscle flap or other augmentations can partially offset this de-

fect. The pedicled thyroid cartilage reconstructions serve a higher purpose; they are employed principally to prevent aspiration when the resection bares or includes the upper portion of the cricoid cartilage (as well as the arytenoid) posteriorly.

What is not often mentioned in discussions of vertical partial laryngectomies is the fact that a true complete hemilaryngectomy, which would cut the interarytenoid region in the midline and destroy one half of the cricoid, is intolerable. Safe decannulation cannot be accomplished. The remaining single arytenoid is tethered by posterior interarytenoid scarring, so that it can no longer abduct. The airway cannot withstand the negative intra-airway pressure of inspiration because it has lost its cricoid support. Aspiration is also inevitable. With the destruction of the sphincteric capability of so much of the circumference of the larynx and the loss of posterior separation from the foodway normally provided by the arytenoid, the corniculate, the cuneiforms, and the aryepiglottic folds, fluids spill into the larynx. Anteriorly, the ball valve, airway-protecting, occlusive effect of the prelaryngeal fat pad is lost because it can no longer protrude into the laryngeal lumen during deglutition. Finally, a true hemilaryngectomy does not take into account the normal patterns of intralaryngeal cancer spread that have been demonstrated by whole organ serial section techniques.

The term hemilaryngectomy in contemporary parlance refers to a supracricoid and infrahyoid operation. Successful application of the vertical conservation operations that are restricted to this concept has been amply demonstrated for both control of cancer and restitution of breathing, swallowing, and voice. As long as patient selection is rational and the techniques are treated with the respect they deserve, there is no reason why these concepts should not be widely practiced for the benefit of all patients with early and medium glottic carcinomas.

Extended Supraglottic Laryngectomy

Any consideration of the anatomy of the supraglottic "block" reveals that several different potential extensions of supraglottic laryngectomy exist:

1. It could be extended up into the tongue base for vallecular cancer.
2. It could be amplified posteriorly to include an involved arytenoid.
3. It might be enlarged inferiorly to skim off the upper surface of a mobile true cord in a patient with inferior extension by the ventricle.
4. Any of these may be extended laterally to include the piriform sinus on one side when a lateralized supraglottic tumor is primary in the aryepiglottic fold or the upper portion of the piriform.

In fact, there is the occasional patient who develops vallecular cancer for whom a supraglottic laryngectomy extended to include the tongue base is appropriate. The lesion has obliterated the epiglottis and invaded the vallecula. The patient is young, is unirradiated, and has healthy lungs. At least one hypoglossal nerve and a lingual artery can be preserved.

The supraglottic laryngectomy should be performed first

but in a retrograde manner. That is, the surgeon should separate the horizontal saw cuts in the thyroid cartilage and enter the ventricles from below. The site of entry is above the anterior commissure and below the ventricular bands. By working from below upward, the surgeon can elevate the supraglottic specimen, and the tongue base involvement will be exposed by eversion. The portion of the tongue base resected in continuity with the supraglottic specimen should not extend closer than 1 cm to the circumvallate papillae. The lingual artery and the hypoglossal nerve should be identified on the less involved side and be elevated out of harm's way before the tongue base is resected.

A lateral trapezius myocutaneous flap isolated from the bottom of the concurrent neck dissection should be rotated into the defect.[92] Trapezius provides a soft hairless flap based on the transverse cervical vessels, which can be partially folded on itself to simulate the bulk of the tongue base. In closing, every effort should be made to suspend the laryngeal remnant as high up and forward as possible. A neck dissection on the side of lesser involvement can be omitted if results of the first neck dissection are normal. It can be modified if results of the first neck dissection were abnormal and the side of the neck with lesser involvement is N0. Complete simultaneous bilateral comprehensive neck dissections should be performed if bilateral clinical disease is palpable. Steroids will help to diminish the intracranial and facial morbidity of bilateral simultaneous internal jugular vein resection where this proves necessary. The nerves to the mylohyoids and the anterior bellies of the digastrics (the belly often blends into the mylohyoid) should be preserved wherever possible to help elevate the laryngeal remnant.

Most patients with tongue base/vallecular/supraglottic cancer will not meet the criteria for extended supraglottic surgery. When tongue base lesions require supraglottic resections for oncologic reasons, I usually manage the laryngeal excision as a near-total laryngectomy. This can be combined with more extensive myocutaneous flap reconstruction of the tongue base defect, extending, for example, into the tonsillar fossa or up to the oral tongue. The advantage of a near-total laryngectomy is the more extensive ablation (especially of the upper piriform region near the vallecula), the lack of aspiration, and the predictability of a safe airway due to acceptance of a permanent tracheotomy.

Sometimes a supraglottic cancer extends onto the upper surface of the arytenoid or down into the ventricular wall to the plane of the vocal cord. The upper surface of the vocal cord can be filleted obliquely and resected in continuity with a supraglottic laryngectomy. The arytenoid can also be completely resected.[93] When either or both of these extensions are necessary, swallowing will be very difficult for a prolonged period of time, and the voice will be exceedingly breathy. The cord treated this way is partly immobilized and partly lateralized by the scarring that follows.

The indications for arytenoid and partial glottic resections with supraglottic laryngectomy are rare, and the reconstructions are challenging. Preservation of some posterior thyroid ala on the side of greater tumor involvement will allow the development of a local chondro-osseous graft, pedicled on the fibers

of the inferior constrictor, as in extended hemilaryngectomy. After the resection, the flap is sewn to the bare upper edge of the cricoid, to replace lost cordal bulk, as close to the posterior midline as possible. Nearby pharyngeal mucosa must be mobilized to cover this graft; it will do so only posteriorly.

Three-Quarter Laryngectomy

I think the so-called three-quarter laryngectomy, in which a "block" that includes a complete supraglottic specimen plus the standard frontolateral partial vertical or hemilaryngectomy on one side is taken, is a flawed concept. A supraglottic cancer with unilateral transglottic spread should give up the subglottic and cricoid hemisphere on that side, not just the supracricoid tissues.[94] Furthermore, the preservation of the cricoid to avoid a tracheotomy is an invitation to aspiration, and in these cases, aspiration is already a serious probability due to the impairment of both the supraglottic and the glottic sphincters. On the hemilaryngectomized side, the operator is advised to fashion a neocord from a bulky flap of strap muscle and to cover the posterior portions of this with piriform mucosa. On the side with the cord remaining, the anterior commissure portion may be gone, and the surgeon is advised to suture the cord remnant forward to the remaining thyroid cartilage remnant.[95] In practice, the remaining cord ends up bowed and deformed. The reconstructed neocord becomes rigid and foreshortened, and it lies at an inappropriate level. A neoglottis with these deformities simply does not function as an adequate sphincter, and the supraglottic sphincter has, of course, been resected. These patients are bound to aspirate. They cannot be decannulated without great difficulty. Once again, in my view, it would be more appropriate oncologically and for rehabilitative purposes if patients with lesions for which three-quarter laryngectomy was said to be appropriate were treated with a near-total laryngectomy or a near-total laryngopharyngectomy.[71]

In summary, supraglottic laryngectomy is an excellent operation, but its extensions should be restricted to a very few highly selected patients. Supraglottic resections that are kept too small (to be safe) in the extended lesions will rapidly lead to recurrence. On the other hand, rather minimal extensions of the operation, which might be precipitated by the interoperative discovery of a satellite lesion or extended marginal dysplasia, for example, severely escalate the problems of rehabilitation. Of all the operations described in this chapter, extended supraglottic laryngectomies represent the greatest challenge to the patients in terms of pulmonary stress, vocal distortion, and swallowing difficulty. Where the concept of near-total laryngectomy and near-total laryngopharyngectomy is understood and applied, the indication for extended supraglottic laryngectomy becomes rare, and the prospect of escalating from a planned supraglottic laryngectomy to an unwanted total laryngectomy virtually disappears.

Partial Laryngopharyngectomy

Selected aryepiglottic fold lesions and T1 piriform cancers can be successfully treated with a formal supraglottic operation described by Ogura and Mallen as the partial laryngopharyngectomy.[57] It is essentially a supraglottic laryngectomy extended to encompass the piriform fossa of the involved side. The thyroid cartilage cut on the involved side is angled downward on its way toward the posterior border of the thyroid lamina, and the entire piriform down to the apex is included in the specimen. Contraindications are visible piriform apex involvement, local cartilage invasion, or any impairment of movement of the ipsilateral vocal cord.

This procedure extends the rehabilitation period for swallowing, just as any other alteration of the elemental supraglottic operation does, but in 8 or 9 weeks most patients can manage a full diet with care. Piriform cancers are rarely discovered this early, so partial laryngopharyngectomy is an uncommon operation. Any question that one of the classical contraindications is present impels us to advise a near-total laryngopharyngectomy (see later discussion) instead of a partial laryngopharyngectomy. In near-total laryngopharyngectomy the entire hemilarynx (vallecula to trachea) is removed, plus the supraglottic larynx and as much pharyngeal wall as needed. From both the oncologic and rehabilitative points of view, it is a much safer and more predictable procedure. It allows a voice-producing resection for the majority of supraglottic or piriform cancer patients while avoiding the temptation to extend the basic supraglottic operation beyond the excellent predictable functional results it can achieve in the more limited form.

Near-Total Laryngopharyngectomy

Hypopharyngeal cancer is often extensive at presentation. The surgery is usually aggressive, and postoperative radiation is commonly advised. Spread is early, so patients controlled locally and regionally often die of pulmonary metastases. Second primary cancers are common. In many cases, special reconstructions of the pharynx are required.

Voice in this setting is often a secondary consideration for the clinician, but most patients have a near-normal voice when they present for medical advice with piriform carcinoma. One vocal cord is normal, and the other is often normal in shape and restricted only in movement. Such a patient logically resists advice to sacrifice the organ of voice, but this itself escalates the mortality because it delays definitive removal of the cancer. He or she is prone to hunt for second and third opinions, not realizing the compromise.

If patients with piriform carcinoma have a worse prognosis for life than most patients with laryngeal carcinoma, or if they are destined to die of the disease, we are no less obligated to provide voice if we can. The patient's ability to express his or her needs and fears and feelings is paramount during a terminal illness. If they survive, of course a voice is also important, but the prognosis for secondary acquisition of voice after extensive combined treatment for piriform cancer, especially when it includes pharyngeal reconstruction and radiotherapy, is low.

Perhaps fewer patients would be frightened away from the life-saving treatment they need if they were offered a voice-preserving operation. Ogura's and Mallen's partial laryngopharyngectomy for piriform carcinoma is not the answer; it is limited to such small lesions that it can only rarely be employed. A partial pharyngectomy combined with a near-total laryngectomy, however, is a possibility with this operation, because the cord can be fixed, by the cancer, the apex can be involved, and the cartilage can be invaded.[96] Near-total laryngopharyngectomy is an adequate resection for many hypopharyngeal cancers. In 65% of piriform carcinomas in which a total laryngopharyngectomy had been performed, the contralateral hemilarynx was uninvolved on histopathologic examination.

When a near-total laryngectomy was performed for glottic carcinoma, the other side of the larynx was used to make the speaking shunt. But in glottic disease, there was so little larynx left, that the shunt had to be augmented with pharynx. In piriform cancer, there is no pharynx available to augment the shunt. However, more contralateral larynx, such as the entire vocal cord on the uninvolved side, can be preserved. Thus, although we have insufficient pharynx in piriform cases, we can make the shunt entirely with tissue preserved from the larynx.

In a near-total laryngopharyngectomy, a complete hemilarynx, connected to one piriform sinus, is preserved. Therefore, the principle of maintaining a connection between the airway and the foodway is sustained. The intrinsic musculature of the remaining hemilarynx is incorporated into the walls of this construction, and the rigidity imposed by the residual cricoid hemisphere is overcome by submucosal resection. In essence, the shunt is a tubed hemilarynx, reduced to its mucosal, muscular, and neurovascular essentials.

The technique in near-total laryngopharyngectomy is similar to a near-total laryngectomy. The laryngeal and pharyngeal procedures are preceded by a laryngoscopy, a tracheotomy, and a complete neck dissection. The excision resects the involved pharynx with a wide margin plus the epiglottis, preepiglottic space, false cord, ventricle, true cord, subglottis, and cricoid on the involved side. (All of these structures are immediate neighbors of the piriform fossa.) The remaining hemilarynx is tubed after submucosal resection of the cricoid on the less involved side.

At the upper opening of the shunt, a preserved piriform may be all that remains of the pharynx. Any pharyngeal reconstruction that is suited to the patient's needs can be added to this. Therefore, near-total laryngopharyngectomy is not contraindicated by the need for pharyngeal reconstruction. If the cancer involves the piriform, vallecula, and lower tonsillar pole, for example, a pectoral myocutaneous flap might be used. In the case of resection of the lower hypopharynx, where additional tissues might be made up with a jejunal transplant (opened as a patch) or a flap, the concept of a hemilaryngeal vocal shunt can also be sustained.

The terminology to differentiate between cases in which additional reconstruction of the pharynx is required and cases in which the pharynx is repaired primarily are as follows: (1) the term extended near-total laryngopharyngectomy is used to indicate resection extensive enough to require a flap or a graft to repair the pharynx, and (2) the term near-total laryngopharyngectomy is applied to cases in which the pharyngeal defect can be closed primarily. In both situations, the hemilaryngeal unit used to make the vocal shunt is the same.

Vocal rehabilitiation following near-total laryngopharyngectomy duplicates that which follows a near-total laryngectomy. However, two complications that might be encountered deserve special mention. A fistula can form between the seam of the hemilaryngeal vocal shunt and the closure of the hypopharyngeal defect. This causes early massive aspiration. The problem will eventually be identified at a laryngoscopy. It is not necessary to destroy the shunt to correct the aspiration caused by such an H fistula. Just separate the shunt from the pharyngeal closure, and repair the side wall defect in each. Another unusual occurrence is the persistence of a laryngeal ventricle in the wall of the tracheopharyngeal shunt. This acts as a diverticulum that distends with air when the patient tries to phonate. The shunt will seem unable to pass air up from below, whereas on probing from above (at direct laryngoscopy), it will readily admit a dilator. To prevent this problem, one should attempt to destroy the integrity of the ventricle and saccule in the preserved hemilaryngeal remnant at the time of the near-total laryngopharyngectomy[96] itself. If this complication occurs later, the ventricular band maintaining the integrity of the pocket should be divided and the fistula stented for 1 week under antibiotic coverage.

About one half of the patients who present in an otolaryngologist's office with previously untreated piriform sinus cancer are candidates for near-total laryngopharyngectomy. About 80% will accure a voice. If the proper attention is paid to case selection and intraoperative frozen section evaluation of the margins, local recurrence is no more likely than it was with a total laryngectomy. Interarytenoid, postcricoid, or bilateral piriform involvement are contraindications to near-total laryngopharyngectomy or extended near-total laryngopharyngectomy. But the old contraindications to "conservation surgery for hypopharyngeal cancer" that were developed for partial laryngopharyngectomy do not apply when near-total laryngopharyngectomy is the procedure.

Total Laryngectomy and Tracheoesophageal Puncture

Despite modern improvements in early diagnosis, primary irradiation, and conservation surgery, some patients still cannot be cured without a total laryngectomy. The reasons may vary from institution to institution, depending on their surgical or radiotherapeutic bias and patterns of referral. The most common indications for total laryngectomy at Mayo Clinic are (1) T3 or T4 glottic carcinoma recurring in a patient who has failed radiation, (2) supraglottic cancer recurring following failed radiotherapy, (3) subglottic (intracricoid) cancer, (4) hypopharyngeal cancer involving the postcricoid region primarily or spreading to this site from the piriform, and (5) extensive radiorecurrent tongue base cancer.

The restoration of speech after total laryngectomy can often be accomplished by interaction between the laryngectomee and a trained speech pathologist. By learning how to impound air in the esophagus and emit it in a controlled fashion the patient can produce the sound necessary to create voice. A laryngectomee, after all, still has his or her tongue, lips, teeth, palate, and intellect, so if sound can be produced, speech is sure to follow. Over the years, numerous operations were devised to reestablish a connection between the trachea and the esophagus or pharynx after total laryngectomy. This would answer one of the principal objections to esophageal speech, the limited breath support. Communications between the airway and the esophagus or pharynx were constructed with local skin flaps,[97] regional flaps,[98] postcricoid flaps,[99] and esophageal mucosa.[100] Some procedures were multistaged; others were single. Sometimes a pharyngocutaneous fistula was linked to the stoma with an external prosthetic device that directed pulmonary air into the pharynx and also provided the vibrating reed.[101]

Careful analysis of these cases through the 1970s revealed the following characteristics:

1. Some fistula speakers were a spectacular success, and fistula speech was usually of better quality than esophageal speech in volume, phrasing, inflection, efficient use of the air charge, and lack of injection noises.[102]
2. Some fistula speakers were a dismal failure, because the reconstructed passageway stenosed, and voice could not be produced.[103]
3. There was an unacceptable preponderance of additional surgical morbidity related to:
   A. Aspiration[104]
   B. Stomal complications
   C. The need for second or third stages
   D. The need for extra time in the operating room, to perform the reconstructions
4. In successful cases, the use of a hand to valve the stoma was a drawback. Valves that were applied to the stoma, to close during exhalation for speech, were difficult to control. To decompress cough, they had to permit high pressure blowout. They had to remain in place despite the presence of mucus and the pressure of cough. They had to adhere to the skin around the stoma despite creases, scars, radiodermatitis, and sputum.
5. Although long complicated routes were intended for the shunts that were surgically constructed so they could be valved by the elevation or distortion of swallow, most contracted to a short direct connection between the airway and the foodway. Usually this connection had to be occluded with a prosthesis to prevent aspiration.[102]
6. Some shunts could only be kept patent with an indwelling prosthesis. This had to be solid and tight fitting or at least valved against aspiration of food and fluid if vocal function was to remain.[105]

Aware of these elements in their own work, Singer and Blom simultaneously resolved the problems of stenosis, aspiration, and operative morbidity.[106] They popularized the acceptance of the simplest possible operative procedure, a tracheoesophageal puncture. They kept the puncture open with a silicone rubber prosthesis glued and taped to the peristomal skin to prevent dislodgement. Finally, they incorporated a duckbill valve that prevented aspiration while allowing exhaled air to be directed up into the esophagus when the stoma was occluded. Since that time, there have been numerous refinements of tracheoesophageal valves[107, 108] and improved methods of performing the punctures.[109] But at the present time, the basic concept of establishing post-total laryngectomy speech by puncture and prosthesis techniques has been widely accepted and successfully employed.[110]

Some surgeons perform tracheoesophageal puncture as a primary procedure in association with total laryngectomy.[111] They place the feeding tube in the puncture as a "keeper," and no nasogastric tube is required. Patients who are treated this way hope to acquire earlier speech and avoid the need for a separate puncture operation. I have preferred to perform punctures on a secondary basis. My concern is with the possibility of a higher complication rate and a longer hospital stay. Even though most total laryngectomies in my practice are performed for radiation failure, they usually heal promptly. A primary fistula would result in persistent peristomal contamination during the time I expect primary healing to occur. I prefer the patient to have some time to attempt esophageal speech also. Successful esophageal speakers have no need for a prosthesis, risk no aspiration, and have no need to valve their stoma to talk.

Secondary tracheoesophageal puncture is performed after the laryngectomy patient has healed, learned to manage the stoma, and had a reasonable opportunity to learn esophageal speech. Patients unsatisfied with their esophageal or electromechanical speech are candidates. The puncture itself should be sited about 5 mm below the mucocutaneous junction of the upper margin of the tracheal stoma. The layers that will be perforated are the posterior tracheal wall mucosa, the trachealis muscle, the scar that may lie between the trachea and the esophagus, two layers of esophageal muscle, and the thick esophageal mucosa. These layers are not separated or incised. They are simply parted by a blunt technique. The object is to ensure that the patient will have at least three thin muscular layers to keep the fistula sealed around the prosthesis.

I prefer to place a custom-made curved metal sound, similar in shape to a Yankauer suction tube, into the pharynx under strong sedation and topical oral, pharyngeal, and stomal anesthesia. The blunt tip of the sound tents the posterior tracheal wall mucosa forward at the point of the intended puncture. The surgeon lightly nicks the distended tissues over the sound, and the tip pops through into the stoma. A 14-gauge silicone rubber catheter is attached to the eye in the end of the sound with a silk suture. The sound is then withdrawn to bring the tip of the catheter up into the mouth. The silk is cut and removed, with the sound, leaving the catheter protruding from the mouth. I inflate the catheter balloon with about 3 ml of water and then draw the whole catheter back down into the esophagus until the edge of the slightly inflated balloon is apparent at the stomal perforation site. A malleable 4 F wire urologic mandrin (stylette) is then inserted up into the lumen of the catheter to give some control of the tip. The catheter can now be redirected downward using the mandrin to flip the tip. With gentle pressure on the mandrin, the catheter is advanced to lie in the lumen of the lower esophagus. The mandrin is withdrawn leaving the catheter in place. It is corked and taped securely to the skin, near the stoma, and left in place for 7 days. The catheter can be used for tube feeding initially; then the patient can begin eating by mouth on the fifth day. When it is removed, a 2.0 or 2.2 cm Singer-Blom low-pressure valve (with a thin inner retention flange) can usually be fitted to the puncture site. A properly chosen and fitted prosthesis should provide speech similar to

that achieved when the patient occludes the stoma with no prosthesis in place. The patient must learn how to valve the stoma to speak with the tube and must also be taught the ongoing care of the fistula and of the prosthesis. Meticulous hygiene is essential. *Candida* organisms eventually encrust the valve microscopically and cause valve failure.[112] Previous radiation seems to accelerate this problem. The prosthesis should be removed and cleaned every 5 to 10 days and replaced approximately every 3 months.

Later, some patients can be taught to use their prosthesis hands free by mastering the fitting and maintenance of a stomal valve. This works poorly if the tracheal pressure necessary to produce speech is above 40 cm H_2O. In these instances, the operator should evaluate the patient for cricopharyngeal spasm by infiltrating the region of the pharyngeoesophageal segment with local anesthesia and observing a significant drop in the pressure required to speak. In general, patients who demonstrate notable improvements in pressure and speech with this test should be considered candidates for secondary cricopharyngeal myotomy, pharyngeal neurectomy, or both.[113]

Laryngopharyngectomy and Pharyngeal Reconstruction

Cancer of the hypopharynx often requires a total laryngectomy and an associated partial or complete pharyngectomy. Total laryngectomies are probably more frequent now for cancers that were pharyngeal, not laryngeal, in their origin. Partial pharyngectomies can sometimes be repaired by direct closure. However, postoperative pharyngoesophageal stenosis will occur if insufficient mucosa remains.[114]

The laryngectomy patient who winds up requiring repeated pharyngeal dilation or secondary pharyngeal reconstruction often has a typical story. A tight pharyngeal closure was made in association with a laryngectomy-partial pharyngectomy. The lumen of the pharynx was partially obstructed by the presence of the nasogastric tube. Tension and ischemia caused the suture line to break down and leak saliva into the neck wound around the fifth to the eighth day postoperatively. The soilage elevated some of the neck flap and fistulized out through the skin wound around the ninth or tenth day. Healing was then greatly prolonged because of the need to granulate around the pharyngocutaneous fistula. The fibrous tissue response to the infection and the inflammation or to any additional surgical manipulations was amplified by the greatly prolonged period of active wound repair. A narrowed and indistensible pharyngoesophageal segment ultimately resulted.

With the advent of the deltopectoral flap[115] and later the pectoral myocutaneous flap,[116] head and neck surgeons acquired a relatively reliable means of augmenting an inadequate closure.[117] Description of these procedures is beyond the scope of this chapter, but there is no question that they are part of the surgical planning and execution when a total laryngectomy is associated with a pharyngectomy for extensive hypopharyngeal disease.

The greatest preparation of all is required when the cancer involves the postcricoid region of the larynx. In these situations, a total laryngopharyngectomy will be required. The challenge of the reconstruction will be to reconstitute a totally absent segment of the pharyngoesophageal food passageway. Occasionally, this can be done with a myocutaneous flap, but usually the defect is too low, the pedicle would be too distorted, and the flap is too bulky for this situation.

The most successful strategies for pharyngeal reconstruction after total laryngopharyngectomy[118] are gastric transposition[119] and free jejunal transplantation with microvascular anastomosis.[120]

Gastric transposition is the planned elevation of the stomach fundus up to the oropharynx to repair the gullet at the time of a complete laryngopharyngoesophagectomy. This can be accomplished working through only the abdomen and the neck.[121] The stomach will be passed up through the posterior mediastinum, and the greater curvature will be rolled up to the transected margins of the tongue base and oropharynx. If the preoperative images suggest extrapharyngeal extension, the otolaryngologic surgeon should determine the resectability in the neck through a small collar incision before proceeding with the abdominal portion of the operation. Extensive fixation to the major arteries or the prevertebral fascia by extrapharyngeal disease constitute probable contraindications to even a palliative procedure.

The technique of laryngopharyngoesophagectomy and gastric transposition is managed as follows. Two operative teams are required. Two separate instrument tables are provided at opposite ends of the patient, so that no hands or instruments cross the chest from one team to the other. Intravenous cephalsporins and metronidazole are begun before the first incision. The trachea is transected below the thyroid isthmus, and a wire-spiral anesthetic endotracheal tube is placed in the distal trachea. The larynx and pharynx are transected at the hyoid. The paratracheal nodes and fat are mobilized out of the superior mediastinum by following the common carotids down to their origin. A total thyroidectomy is usually included when large low hypopharyngeal lesions are involved because of the high incidence of thyroid invasion. This will often produce a total parathyroidectomy, so that it is worth trying to identify parathyroid tissue and preserve these glands with their blood supply if this does not compromise the resection.[122] Sometimes a parathyroid gland can be dissected safely off the specimen and transplanted into the volar surface of the forearm, adjacent to a prominent vein.[123] At this point, the specimen (larynx, pharynx, thyroid, and paratracheal fat) is mobilized in the neck, attached only by the cervical esophagus.

In the abdomen, lighted retractors, a headlight, and excellent retraction up through the diaphragmatic hiatus are helpful so that the lower thoracic esophagus can be mobilized under direct vision.[124] First the stomach is mobilized. The vascular arcade supplied by the right gastric and right gastroepiploic arteries must be kept intact over the lesser and greater curvatures. The duodenum is kocherized, and a pyloric drainage procedure is performed. The hiatus is bluntly dilated or incised, and the posterior mediastinum is gradually visualized up to the level of the carina. A vascular stapler can be used to achieve a thoroughly dry esophageal bed. When the esophagus is mobile enough to be slipped up and down in this field without any attachment, the stomach is ready to be delivered. A flap of greater omentum can be transposed on the greater curvature of the stomach to cover the exposed great vessels in the neck.

From above, the esophagus is mobilized from its mediastinal (lateral and posterior) attachments as far as finger exploration will permit. Meticulous sharp dissection is usually required to separate the esophagus from the posterior tracheal wall. The endotracheal tube balloon should be partially deflated during this maneuver. Great care must be taken to avoid a tear in the posterior tracheal wall. This is a formidable intraoperative complication, one that is difficult yet vital to repair. When mobilization is complete, traction on the esophagus above and feeding of the stomach from below allows the greater curvature to be drawn up into the neck. Both surgeons must ensure there is no twisting or kinking. The gastroesophageal junction is divided and sealed with a stapling device in the neck. The greater curvature is advanced as high as possible. The highest point of the greater curvature is then opened and anastomosed to the upper defect in the oropharynx. A two-layer closure is carried out.

Sometimes a long portion of the trachea has to be resected because of involvement of the posterior wall. It can be difficult to bring the trachea forward to fashion a tracheostomy. Rather than mobilize the remaining distal trachea upward, it is usually better to elevate the anterior chest wall skin and rotate it back. Usually this can be accomplished with a large upper anterior chest wall faciocutaneous fan flap. The flap, based on the internal mammary perforators, is rotated up and over the clavicular head and down to meet the trachea. Sometimes it is necessary to remove the head of the clavicle and the upper manubrium to facilitate this so-called tracheal exteriorization.

A feeding jejunostomy is constructed. The nasogastric tube is used to decompress the transposed stomach and monitor the fluid and electrolyte loss that occurs into the stomach during the period of gastrointestinal atonia. Chest tubes are placed in the pleural spaces bilaterally so as not to fall behind the possible hemothorax that often develops. The lungs are already compromised by the addition of the stomach's volume to the chest, and an unseen or unmeasured third space fluid accumulation in the stomach or pleural space will only add to the patient's problems in recovery.

When the esophagus does not need to be removed with these resections, a free jejunal or forearm microvascular transplant can be used to reconstruct the gullet. This offers certain advantages over myocutaneous flaps and specific differences in contrast to the use of stomach. Jejunal grafts and free skin grafts present less bulk under the neck flaps. There is no tension on the pedicle of a transplant, which is not always true of the pectoralis flap (or the transposed stomach). The lining obtained is thin, pliable, hairless, and perhaps ultimately more adaptable to vocal rehabilitation strategies than is the stiffer bulkier wall of the pectoralis flap or the thick highly vascularized and secretory wall of the stomach.

The radial forearm free flap provides thin skin and a satisfactory vascular pedicle.[125] There are legitimate concerns related to donor site morbidity, since the bed exposes the flexor tendons, and there is a longitudinal seam to sew that does not exist with a tubular bowel transplant. However, this is one free flap to keep in mind when the prospect of opening the abdomen is distasteful.

Successful free flap reconstruction of the pharynx has most often been accomplished with jejunum.[126] The mesentery of the jejunum is fanshaped, and the position of the mesenteric vessels is relatively inflexible for a given positioning of the transplant. Vascular anastomoses are usually end to side using carotid and jugular sources. For everything to reach without tension, it may be helpful to save the more mobile transverse cervical artery. This artery runs a high oblique course in the lateral neck and is usually high enough to be brought back into the central visceral compartment at a level midway between the upper and lower resection margins. The venous anastomosis will usually be to an internal jugular, but if bilateral neck dissections are performed, it will be too late to look for a high cervical vein.[127] An external jugular vein can be saved by dissecting it down off the sternomastoid muscle first.

Microvascular anastomosis is usually best done by a separate team. In fact, I prefer two microvascular surgeons. One prepares the blood vessels in the neck while the second obtains the section of jejunum approximately 1 ft below the ligament of Treitz. This is delivered onto the abdominal surface, and the vascular supply is carefully dissected and displayed. The mesenteric arteries cannot be dissected further back toward the main blood supply of the jejunum without injuring branches to the adjacent jejunal segments left behind in the abdomen. It cannot be dissected very far toward the bowel either, because it breaks up into many branches.

When the bowel is anastomosed (antegrade) in the neck, the upper anastomosis is done first to avoid any twisting and turning of the transplant. This is the most difficult anastomosis, and it stabilizes the bowel. The vascular anastomosis is performed next. The veins and arteries are large enough that this might be called a "macro" microvascular anastomosis. There are sometimes two veins that can be anastomosed. When the vascular anastomosis is completed, small bowel peristalsis immediately resumes. The lower esophagus-to-bowel anastomosis is performed last, and then a final recheck of the vascular anastomoses is made. Some surgeons leave an observation window in the neck, so that early bowel necrosis is less likely to go unrecognized. The recognition of severe ischemia within 4 hours might allow an anastomotic revision. Later recognition will fail to save the transplant but will at least allow resection to avoid in situ necrosis, with its threat of aggressive septicemia.

NONSURGICAL TREATMENT

Radiotherapy

Should radiotherapy or surgery be considered the foundation of treatment in laryngeal cancer? Well-informed and well-intentioned physicians continue to disagree on this seemingly fundamental question. Effective surgical treatment of microinvasive laryngeal carcinoma is ideal but possible only with the support of a conscientious frozen section pathologist. In general, surgery is probably prudent only when it is directed by a laryngologist who maintains an up-to-date fund of knowledge regarding the biologic behavior of cancer in the larynx and who is properly trained in the principles and techniques of laryngoscopic cordectomy, laryngofissure, vertical partial laryngec-

tomies, supraglottic laryngectomies, near-total laryngectomies, total laryngectomies, vocal rehabilitation, and the extensions of total laryngectomies.

Radiation is a very competitive option for early cancer where these elements are in short supply. It has an important role as part of a combined treatment program in some larger tumors, although it is important to emphasize that it cannot finesse margins, and the indications for radiotherapy are usually related to the findings in the neck.[128] Radiation is only as good as the therapist, the physicists, and technicians, and the sophistication of the planning and the reliability of the equipment at their disposal. The glottis can move out of the central beam with a swallow. Disease in the anterior commissure or cartilage is just below the skin the therapist is trying to spare.[77] The anatomy of extralaryngeal spread is complicated, and the information for planning is often available from only the clinical notes or the indirect appearances of a biopsy-wounded tumor as it presents in the radiotherapy clinic.

As a policy, where surgery and radiation are both excellent, radiation treatment for invasive laryngeal cancer of all stages leads to a higher failure rate and a greater percentage of retreatments.[129] Unfortunately, depending on compliance with follow-up by the patient and continuity by the observer, a percentage of the failed radiation patients will have progressed substantially by the time of their recurrence and rediscovery.[130] This means that even if cure is achieved by salvage surgery, the morbidity inflicted on the patient will be greater than the original lesion required.[14]

Early laryngeal cancer is highly curable. It is often detected when it is extremely small and when no spread has occurred. It could have been well delineated at the time of the biopsy, and any unexpected extensions could have been discovered then or at the improved exposure afforded by surgery. When a complete excision is feasible without escalating the morbidity much more than the biopsy itself entails, this is certainly the most cost-effective method of management. It is also the one least likely to lead to retreatment, loss of larynx, or death. On the other hand, when the morbidity of surgery is significant (as in a total laryngectomy), one would appreciate the voice-repairing promise of radiotherapy. However, here we are dealing with larger cancers, and it is in just such cases that radiation more frequently fails.[131]

In small lesions, radiation is a low-risk gamble (against cure) for a slightly better voice. Studies show it frequently works, that is, the gambler frequently wins. In large lesions, radiation is a risky gamble (against cure) to retain a voice and avoid a stoma. In this very promise, however, it usually fails. Since the surgery of large laryngeal cancers can now be accompanied or followed up by successful voice restoration in almost every case, an important reason for the traditional advocation of primary radiotherapy in the treatment matrix (i.e., larynx preservation) no longer exists.

The contraindications to radiotherapy are prior high-dose radiotherapy and patient refusal. Relative contraindications are (1) previous low-dose radiotherapy (e.g., for acne), (2) alcoholism, (3) refusal to stop smoking, and (4) age less than 45 years. A serious coincidental medical condition is a common reason for selecting radiotherapy, since the acute mortality of radiation is essentially zero. However, the morbidity must also be factored into the decision. A frail elderly patient often does better with a straightforward operation than a protracted course of radiation. Head and neck surgery does not shut down the gastrointestinal tract like perhaps more familiar abdominal surgery. Difficult bronchopulmonary toilet in a chronic lung patient is well served by a tracheotomy. There is no abdominal or chest incision pain to inhibit respiratory movement after neck surgery. Blood loss is minor, and the blood supply to the tissues expected to heal is usually excellent. Modern antibiotics, begun preoperatively, have greatly reduced the prospect of pseudomonas, staphylococcal, and anaerobic polymicrobial infections.

All in all, the morbidity of radiotherapy has increased with escalating dosages[132] and more intensive fractionation schedules[133] in the attempt to achieve higher cure rates in the larger tumors, whereas in the same period, the safety of surgery has been increased and the morbidity of surgery reduced by the development of the numerous technologies cited.

Chemotherapy

It is well known that large or undifferentiated laryngeal tumors sometimes metastasize beyond the neck, and particularly in the case of hypopharyngeal cancer, locoregional cure is sometimes not enough to preserve the life of the patient. Some chemotherapy trials for squamous cell carcinomas of the head and neck have demonstrated reductions in tumor size for a small proportion of the patients enrolled.[134] The side effects are generally severe. Is there any evidence that patients with a poor prognosis can live longer because of chemotherapy? Is there any evidence that temporary reductions in tumor size, called "responses" in the oncologic literature, convey any benefit to the patient? Can the side effects of chemotherapy be ameliorated in some way so that larger doses would be tolerated? So far, it seems there is no value in shrinking a laryngeal cancer without curing it, at least no more value than would be obtained from an incomplete excision.[135] Unfortunately, no chemotherapeutic studies show an improved cure rate, an increase in survival time, or a prolongation of the time between treatment and the return symptoms in laryngeal carcinoma.

Physicians responsible for the care and management of patients with laryngeal cancer must continually evaluate promising new therapeutic modalities. It has been more than 25 years since the first chemotherapeutic agents were introduced. They have completely changed the face of treatment in hemopoietic tumors and some of the pediatric and adolescent sarcomas, but their impact on solid epithelial tumors in adults has been virtually nil. At the present time, the hope for a "miracle drug" in squamous cell carcinoma of the larynx, which has been so alluring to well-meaning physicians, investigators, and health policy planners, must be admitted to be nowhere on the clinical horizon.

CLASSIFICATION AND SELECTION OF TREATMENT

In a sense, this entire chapter is about the selection of treatment in laryngeal cancer. Let us examine at last the role of the TNM (primary tumor, regional nodes, metastasis) staging system in assisting us with our choices.

The TNM classifications of the International Union Against Cancer and those developed by the American Joint Committee on Cancer Staging and Results Reporting[136] have been widely referenced at laryngologic meetings and are passed on to neo-laryngologists in training programs throughout the world. They have helped to clarify discussions in the context of their original intent, which was to help compare outcomes and treatment results among different medical centers. They have also served to emphasize for student laryngologists the need for precision in describing the primary site, spread, and metastatic status of a new neoplasm. Finally, these systems continue to remind us that the three physical findings they catalogue, the site of origin, the size of the primary, and the presence of metastases, are factors that can be taken into account whenever we council a family in regard to prognosis.

When it comes to treatment selection, however, we are not to be overly persuaded by these classifications. The TNM systems ignore important information, such as the patient's history or the physicians's inventory of resources available for treatment, which also have an important bearing on outcome.

The TNM systems are simplification devices for end-stage reporting. They are not prescriptions for therapy. When it comes to selection of treatment, the physician, not the TNM system, is responsible, and many factors must be considered besides the tumor, the nodes, and the metastases.

If a classification scheme were required to help select treatment, I have listed in Table 19–5 some of the factors that might be included. This classification, lightly referred to in our own practice as the LIDREP-SHAMONT system, is obviously ever changing and always incomplete. Nevertheless, it is helpful in demonstrating why a thoughtful clinician who is faced with the same TNM lesion in two patients will select one plan of management in one case and a somewhat different plan in another.

As for the clinicians who like to introduce the TNM designations into their discussions, consultation records, and operative notes, the difficulties this poses in communications should be acknowledged. Most physicians with whom they will communicate do not remember the specific details for staging all cancers for all sites of the head and neck. (Nor do the users in most cases!) When the TNM system is used to describe a tumor correctly, it is usually necessary to refer to the manual. Perhaps whenever the TNM system is introduced into a discussion of laryngeal carcinoma, the participants should also clarify which TNM system they are using (Table 19–6).[137]

TABLE 19–5.
Partial List of the Clinical Factors Useful in the Selection of Treatment for Laryngeal Carcinoma

	Patient Factors	Physician Factors
L	Life expectancy	Laboratory facilities
	Lung disease	Laser equipment
I	Invasiveness of tumor	Intensive care unit
	Illiteracy	Infection control programs
	Insight	Instrumentation
	Insurance certification	
D	Duration of symptoms	Diagnostic imaging
	Diabetes	Diagnosis-Related Group
	Distance from treatment	policies
	facility	
R	Religious Beliefs	Radiotherapist
	Reliability for follow-up	Resident case
E	Emotional health	Expense
	Expectations	Endurance
	Eyesight	Exposure to infectious disease
P	Previous treatment	Pathologist
	Personal hygiene	Preparation and training
S	Sanity	Speech pathologist
	Sex	Surgical experience
H	Heart	Hospital
	Hypertension	Histology laboratory
A	Alcohol abuse	Assistant
	Ambitions	Anesthesiologist
M	Motivation	Medical consultants
	Mental capacity	Medicolegal implications
	Manual dexterity	
O	Occupation	Office
	Oral hygiene	Operating room
	Obstruction of the airway	Organization
N	Nutrition	Nursing
	Number of primary tumors	
	Neurologic disease	
T	Tobacco abuse	Technical support
	Time available for treatment	Transportation

TABLE 19–6.
TNM Staging Systems

Clinical	TNM
Surgical	sTNM
Pathologic	pTNM
Retreatment	rTNM
Autopsy	aTNM

CONCLUSIONS

No list of the principles of treatment in laryngeal cancer is quite equal to the challenge of the disease. Nevertheless, it is perhaps worth concluding this chapter by listing 20 observations I would like to reemphasize:

1. Cancer of the larynx is a highly curable disease.
2. Cancer of the larynx is not a single disease.
3. Cancer beyond the larynx becomes a highly lethal disease.
4. The initial treatment offers the best opportunity for cure and sometimes the only opportunity for cure.
5. The treatment of laryngeal cancer is neither surgical nor radiotherapeutic. It is selective.
6. Cord mobility does not ensure radiocurability.
7. Cord immobility does not mandate total laryngectomy.
8. The TNM classification system does not dictate the treatment plan.
9. Responsibility for cure rests with the physician who prescribes the first treatment.
10. Direct laryngoscopy and biopsy may be the initial treatment.
11. Some cancers can be cured by transoral resection alone.
12. Laryngofissure, the partial vertical laryngectomies, and hemilaryngectomy are specific important treatment strategies for invasive glottic carcinomas.
13. The supraglottic operation works best if it is limited to the basic supraglottic procedure and is worst when it is extended to adjacent sites.
14. Near-total laryngectomy can provide biologic shunt speech for patients who would otherwise require a total laryngectomy.
15. Except for T1 and T2 glottic carcinomas, the treatment of laryngeal cancer must include a rational plan for the neck.
16. Voice is very important, but life is even more important.
17. A surgical bias in initial treatment selection yields more cures and more voices.
18. A radiotherapeutic bias yields some better voices in early disease and some avoidance of a stoma in more advanced disease. The long-term costs in voices, lives, expense, and retreatment are significant.
19. All surgical treatment plans for laryngeal cancer, even total laryngectomy, include a strategy to regain communication.
20. The association of laryngeal carcinoma and tobacco forces us to recognize that this is a largely preventable disease.

REFERENCES

1. Kirchner J, Som ML: Clinical significance of fixed vocal cord. *Laryngoscope* 1971; 81:1029–1044.
2. Olofsson J, Lord IJ, van Nostrand AWP: Vocal cord fixation in laryngeal carcinoma. *Acta Otolaryngol (Stockh)* 1973; 75:496–510.

3. Tucker GF: Some clinical inferences from the study of serial laryngeal sections. *Laryngoscope* 1973; 73:728–748.

4. Freeland AP: Microfil angiography: A demonstration of the microvascular of the larynx with reference to tumor spread, in Alberti PW, Bryce DP (eds): *Workshops From the Centennial Conference on Laryngeal Cancer.* New York, Appleton-Century-Crofts, 1976, pp 279–295.

5. Pressman JJ: Submucosal compartmentalization of the larynx. *Ann Rhinol Laryngol Otol* 1956; 65:761–771.

6. Pressman JJ, Dowdy A, Libby R: Further studies upon the mucosal compartments and lymphatics of the larynx by injection of dyes and radioisotopes. *Ann Otol Rhinol Laryngol* 1956; 65:963.

7. Ogura JH: Supraglottic subtotal laryngectomy and radical neck dissection for carcinoma of the epiglottis. *Arch Otolaryngol* 1958; 68:710–714.

8. Pearson BW: Laryngeal microcirculation and pathways of cancer spread. *Laryngoscope* 1975; 85:700–713.

9. Mittal B, Marks JE, Ogura JH: Transglottic carcinoma. *Cancer* 1984; 53:151–616.

10. Pearson BW: Near-total laryngectomy, in Silver CE (ed): *Atlas of Head and Neck Surgery.* New York, Churchill Livingstone, 1986, pp 234–251.

11. Harrison DFN: Laryngectomy for subglottic lesions. *Laryngoscopes* 1975; 85:1208–1210.

12. Mancuso AA, Cacaterra TC, Hanafee WN: Computed tomography of the larynx. *Radiologic Clin North Am* 1978; 16:195–208.

13. Castelijns JA, Gerritsen GJ, Kaiser MC, et al: MRI of normal or cancerous laryngeal cartilages: Histopathologic correlation. *Laryngoscope* 1987; 97:1085–1093.

14. Berger G, van Nostrand AWP, Harwood A, et al: Failure analysis of T1 glottic carcinoma treated with radical radiotherapy for cure and surgery in reserve in Chretien PB, Johns ME, Shedd DP, et al (eds): *Head and Neck Cancer.* Philadelphia, BC Decker, 1985, pp 195–196.

15. DeSanto LW, Pearson BW: Initial treatment of laryngeal cancer: Principles of selection. *Minn Med* 1981; 64:691–698.

16. Lillie JC, DeSanto LW: Transoral surgery of early cordal carcinoma. *Trans Am Acad Ophthalmol Otolaryngol* 1973; 77:92–96.

17. Saltzstein SL, Nahum AM: Frozen section diagnosis: Accuracy and errors, uses and abuses. *Laryngoscope* 1973; 83:1128–1143.

18. Bauer WC, Lesinski SG, Ogura JH: The significance of positive margins in hemilaryngectomy specimens. *Laryngoscope* 1975; 85:1–13.

19. Lambert PR, Ward PH, Berci G: Pseudosarcoma of the larynx: A comprehensive analysis. *Arch Otolaryngol* 1980; 106:700–708.

20. Lane N: Pseudosarcoma (polypoid sarcoma-like masses) associated with squamous cell carcinoma of the mouth, fauces and larynx. *Cancer* 1957; 10:19–41.

21. Goellner JR, Devine KD, Weiland LH: Pseudosarcoma of the larynx. *Am J Clin Pathol* 1973; 59:312–326.

22. Ryan RE, DeSanto LW, Devine KD, et al: Verrucous carcinoma of the larynx. *Laryngoscope* 1977; 87:1989–1994.

23. Biller HF, Bergman JA: Verrucous carcinoma of the larynx. *Laryngoscope* 1975; 85:1698–1700.

24. Burns HP, van Nostrand AWP, Bryce DP: Verrucous carcinoma of the larynx. Management of radiotherapy and surgery. *Ann Otol* 1976; 85:538.

25. Ferlito A, Recher G: Ackerman's tumor (Verrucous carcinoma) of the larynx: A clinicopathologic study of 77 cases. *Cancer* 1980; 46:1617–1630.

26. Gnepp DR, Ferlito A, Hyams V: Primary anaplastic small cell (oat cell) carcinoma of the larynx. Review of the literature and report of 18 cases. *Cancer* 1983; 51:1731–1745.

27. Coates HL, McDonald TJ, Devine KD, et al: Granular cell tumors of the larynx. *Ann Otol* 1976; 85:504–507.

28. Whicker JH, Neele HB, Weiland LH, et al: Adenocarcinoma of the larynx. *Ann Otol* 1974; 83:487–490.

29. Olofsson J, van Nostrand AW: Adenoid cystic carcinoma of the larynx: A report of four cases and a review of the literature. *Cancer* 1977; 40:1307–1313.

30. Wetmore RF, Tronzo RD, Lane RJ, et al: Nonfunctional paraganglioma of the larynx: Clinical and pathological considerations. *Cancer* 1981; 48:2717–2723.

31. Neel HB, Unni KK: Cartilaginous tumors of the larynx: A series of 33 patients. *Otolaryngol Head Neck Surg* 1982; 90:201–207.

32. Cantrell RW, Reibel JF, Jahrsdoerfer RA, et al: Conservative surgical treatment of chondrosarcoma of the larynx. *Ann Otol* 1980; 89:567–571.

33. Ryan RE, Pearson BW, Weiland LH: Laryngeal amyloidosis. *Trans Am Acad Ophthalmol Otolaryngol* 1977; 8:872–877.

34. McCune MA, Rogers RS, Roberts GD: Laryngeal presentation of blastomycosis. *Int J Dermatol* 1980; 19:263.

35. Bailey CM, Windle-Taylor PC: Tuberculous laryngitis: Series of 37 patients. *Laryngoscope* 1981; 91:93.

36. Kaur S: Respiratory system involvement in leprosy. *Int J Lepr Other Mycobact Dis* 1979; 47:18.

37. Batsakis J, Luna MA, Byers R: Metastases to the larynx. *Head Neck Surg* 1985; 7:458–460.

38. Bauer WC: Concomitant carcinoma in situ and invasive carcinoma of the larynx, in Alberti PW, Bryce DP (eds): *Centennial Conference on Laryngeal Carcinoma.* New York, Appleton-Century-Crofts, 1975, pp 127–134.

39. Doyle PJ, Flores A, Douglas GS: Carcinoma in situ of the larynx. *Laryngoscope* 1977; 86:310.

40. Daly JF, Kwok FN: Laryngofissure and cordectomy. *Laryngoscope* 1975; 85:1290–1297.

41. Neel HB, Devine KD, DeSanto LW: Laryngofissure and cordectomy for early cordal carcinoma: Outcome in 182 patients. *Otolaryngol Head Neck Surg* 1980; 88:79–84.

42. Dickens WJ, Cassissi NJ, Million RR, et al: Treatment of early vocal cord carcinoma: A comparison of apples and apples. *Laryngoscope* 1983; 93:216–219.

43. Broyles EN: The anterior commissure tendon. *Ann Otol Rhinol Laryngol* 1943; 52:342.

44. Fu KK, Woodhouse RJ, Quivey JM, et al: The significance of laryngeal edema following radiotherapy of carcinoma of the vocal cord. *Cancer* 1982; 49:655–658.

45. Litton WB: Preservation of a radionecrotic larynx by excision of thyroid cartilage with flap coverage. *Laryngoscope* 1978; 88:1947–1949.

46. Bird RJ, Bryce DP: Long-term effects of heavy irradiation to the neck. *J Otolaryngol* 1980; 9:18–23.

47. Rosenberg PJ: Total laryngectomy and cancer of the larynx. A historical review. *Arch Otolaryngol* 1971; 94:313–316.

48. Schwartz A, Devine K: Some historical notes about the first laryngectomies. *Laryngoscope* 1959; 69:194–200.

49. Coutard M: Roentgen therapy of epitheliomas of the ton-

sillar region hypopharynx and larynx from 1920 to 1926. *Am J Roentgenol Radium Ther* 1932; 28:313–331.

50. Orton HB: Lateral transhyoid pharyngotomy. *Arch Otolaryngol* 1930; 12:320.

51. Trotter W: A method of lateral pharyngotomy for the exposure of large growths in the epilaryngeal region. *J Laryngol Otol* 1920; 35:289.

52. McNeil BJ, Weichselbaum R, Pauker SG: Speech and survival: Tradeoffs between quality and quantity of life in laryngeal cancer. *N Engl J Med* 1981; 305:982–987.

53. Keith R, Shane HC, Coates HLC, et al: Looking forward...A guide book for the laryngectomies. New York, Thieme, 1984.

54. Weitz JW, Weitz SL, McElhinney AJ: A technique for preservation of spinal accessory nerve function in radical neck dissection. *Head Neck Surg* 1982; 5:75–78.

55. Blom ED, Singer MI, Hamaker RC: Tracheostoma valve for post laryngectomy voice rehabilitation. *Ann Otol Rhinol Laryngol* 1987; 91:576.

56. Singer MI, Blom ED, Hamaker RC: Pharyngeal plexus neurectomy for alaryngeal speech rehabilitation. *Laryngoscope* 1986; 96:50–53.

57. Ogura JH, Mallen RW: Partial laryngopharyngectomy for supraglottic and pharyngeal carcinoma. *Trans Am Acad Ophthalmol Otolaryngol* 1965; 69:832.

58. Robbins KT, Michaels L: A study of whole organ cancerous larynges to determine resectability by conservation surgery. *Head Neck Surg* 1984; 7:2–7.

59. Alonso JM: Conservative surgery of cancer of the larynx. *Trans Am Acad Ophthalmol Otolaryngol* 1947; 51:633.

60. Som ML: Conservation surgery for carcinoma of the supraglottis. *J Laryngol Otol* 1970; 84:655–678.

61. Bocca E, Pignataro O, Mosciaro O: Supraglottic surgery of the larynx. *Ann Otol Rhinol Laryngol* 1968; 77:1005.

62. Fink RB, Demarest RJ: Laryngeal biomechanics. Cambridge, Mass, Harvard University Press, 1978, pp 97–112.

63. Goode R: Laryngeal suspension in head and neck surgery. *Laryngoscope* 1976; 86:349.

64. Coates HL, DeSanto LW, DeVine KD, et al: Carcinoma of the supraglottic larynx. A review of 221 cases. *Arch Otolaryngol* 1976; 102:686.

65. Bocca E, Pignataro O, Oldini C: Supraglottic laryngectomy: 30 years of experience. *Ann Otol Rhinol Laryngol* 1983; 92:14–18.

66. Bocca E, Pignataro O, Oldini C, et al: Functional neck dissection: An evaluation and review of 843 cases. *Laryngoscope* 1984; 94:942–945.

67. Auerbach O, Hammond EC, Garfinkel L: Histologic changes in the larynx in relation to smoking habits. *Cancer* 1970; 25:92.

68. Flores TC, Wood BG, Koegel L, et al: Factors in successful deglutition following supraglottic laryngeal surgery. *Ann Otol Rhinol Laryngol* 1982; 92:579–583.

69. Pearson BW, Woods RD, Hartman DE: Extended hemilaryngectomy for T3 glottic carcinoma with preservation of speech and swallowing. *Laryngoscope* 1980; 90:1950–1961.

70. Pearson BW: Subtotal laryngectomy. *Laryngoscope* 1981; 91:1904–1911.

71. DeSanto LW, Pearson BW, Olsen KD: Utility of near-total laryngectomy for supraglottic pharyngeal base of tongue and other cancers. *Ann Otol Rhinol Laryngol* 1989; 98:2–7.

72. Gutman MR: Tracheohypopharyngeal fistulization (a new procedure for speech production in the laryngectomized patient). *Trans Am Laryngol Rhinol Otol Soc* 1935; 41:219–226.

73. Robbins KT, Michael MD: Feasibility of subtotal laryngectomy based on whole-organ examination. *Arch Otolaryngol* 1985; 111:356–360.

74. Barton D, DeSanto L, Pearson BW, Keith R: An endostomal tracheostomy tube for leakproof retention of the Blom-Singer stomal valve. *Otolaryngol Head Neck Surg* 1988; 99:38–41.

75. Woods RW, Pearson BW: Alaryngeal speech and the development of an internal tracheopharyngeal fistula. *Otolaryngol Head Neck Surg* 1980; 88:64–73.

76. Vaughan CW, Strong MS, Jako GJ: Laryngeal carcinoma: Transoral treatment utilizing the CO_2 laser. *Am J Surg* 1978; 136:490.

77. Kirchner JA: Cancer at the anterior commissure of the larynx. Results with radiotherapy. *Arch Otolaryngol* 1970; 91:524–525.

78. Lesinski SG, Bauer WC, Ogura JH: Hemilaryngectomy for T3 (fixed cord) epidermoid carcinoma of the larynx. *Laryngoscope* 1976; 86:1563.

79. Bailey BJ: Partial laryngectomy and laryngoplasty: A technique and review. *Trans Am Acad Ophthalmol Otolaryngol* 1966; 70:559.

80. Sedláček, K: Reconstructive anterior and lateral laryngectomy using the epiglottis as a pedunculated graft. *Cesk Otolaryngol* 1965; 14:328–334.

81. Lawson W, Biller HF: Cancer of the Larynx, in Sven JY, Myers EN (eds): *Cancer of the Head and Neck.* New York, Churchill Livingstone, 1981, p 470.

82. Bailey BJ: Glottic reconstruction after hemilaryngectomy: Bipedicle muscle flap laryngoplasty. *Laryngoscope* 1975; 85:960.

83. Tucker HM, Wood BG, Levine H, et al: Glottic reconstruction after near-total laryngectomy. *Laryngoscope* 1979; 89:609.

84. Kambič VZ, Radsel Z, Smid L: Laryngeal reconstruction with epiglottis after vertical hemilaryngectomy. *J Laryngol* 1976; 90:467–473.

85. Biller HF, Lawson W: Partial laryngectomy for vocal cord cancer with marked limitation or fixation of the vocal cord. *Laryngoscope* 1986; 96:61–64.

86. Biller HF, Barnhill FR Jr, Ogura JH, et al: Hemilaryngectomy following radiation failure for carcinoma of the vocal cords. *Laryngoscope* 1970; 80:249.

87. Hautant A: Ma technique de l'hemilaryngectomie, ses resultats. *L'oto-rhino-laryngol Int* 1930; 5:217–224.

88. Som ML, Silver CE: The anterior commissure technique of partial laryngectomy. *Arch Otolaryngol* 1968; 87:138–145.

89. Mohr RM, Quenelle DJ, Shumrick DA: Vertico-fronto-lateral laryngectomy (hemilaryngectomy). *Arch Otolaryngol* 1983; 109:384–395.

90. Biller H, Ogura J, Pratt L: Hemilaryngectomy for T2 glottic cancers. *Arch Otolaryngol* 1971; 93:238.

91. Biller HF, Som ML: Vertical partial laryngectomy for glottic carcinoma with posterior subglottic extension. *Ann Otol Rhinol Laryngol* 1977; 86:715.

92. Demergasso F, Piazza MV: Trapezius myocutaneous flap in reconstructive surgery for head and neck cancer: An original technique. *Am J Surg* 1979; 138:533.

93. Ogura JH, Thawley SE: Glottic competence following removal of arytenoid in partial laryngopharyngectomy and subtotal supraglottic laryngectomy. *Laryngoscope* 1978; 88:528–529.

94. van Nostrand AWP, Brodarec I: Laryngeal carcinoma—modifications in surgical technique based on our understanding of tumor growth characteristics. *J Otolaryngol* 1982; 11:186.

95. Ogura J: Personal experience with three-quarter laryngectomy. *Tumori* 1974; 60:527–529.

96. Dumich PS, Pearson BW, Weiland LH: Suitability of near-total laryngopharyngectomy in piriform carcinoma. *Arch Otolaryngol* 1984; 110:664–669.

97. Asai R: Laryngoplasty after total laryngectomy. *Arch Otolaryngol* 1972; 95:114–119.

98. McGrail JS, Oldfield DL: One stage operation for vocal rehabilitation at laryngectomy. *Trans Am Acad Ophthalmol Otolaryngol* 1971; 75:510.

99. Staffieri M: Funktionelle Totale Laryngektomie, Chirurgische Technik, Indikation und Resultate Einer Eigenen Technik 3ur Glottiplastik mit Wiederhestellung der Stimme. *Monatsschr Ohrenheilk* 1972; 106:388.

100. Calcaterra TC: Tracheo-esophageal shunt for speech rehabilitation after total laryngectomy. *Can J Otolaryngol* 1975; 4:568.

101. Taub S, Berguer LH: Air bypass voice prosthesis for vocal rehabilitation of laryngectomees. *Am J Surg* 1973; 125:748.

102. Amatsu M, Kinishi M, Jamir JC: Evaluation of speech of laryngectomees after the Amatsu tracheoesophageal shunt operation. *Laryngoscope* 1984; 94:696–701.

103. Tiwari RM, Snow GB, Lecluse FLE, et al: Observations on surgical rehabilitation of the voice after laryngectomy with Stafflierir's method. *J Laryngol* 1982; 96:241–250.

104. Leipzig B: Neoglottic reconstruction following total laryngectomy: A reappraisal. *Ann Otol Rhinol Laryngol* 1980; 89:534–537.

105. McConnel FM, Teichgraeber J: Neoglottis reconstruction following total laryngectomy: The Emory experience. *Otolaryngol Head Neck Surg* 1982; 90:569–575.

106. Singer MI, Blom ED: An endoscopic technique for restoration of voice after laryngectomy. *Ann Otol Rhinol Laryngol* 1980; 89:529–533.

107. Panje WR: Prosthetic vocal rehabilitation following laryngectomy. The voice button. *Ann Otol Rhinol Laryngol* 1981; 90:116–120.

108. Nijdam HF, Annyas AA, Schutte HK, et al: A new prosthesis for voice rehabilitation after laryngectomy. *Arch Otolaryngol* 1982; 237:27–33.

109. Maniglia A: Newer technique of tracheoesophageal fistula for vocal rehabilitation after total laryngectomy. *Laryngoscope* 1985; 95:1064–1066.

110. Wetmore SJ, Krueger K, Wesson K, Blessing ML: Long-term results of the Blom-Singer speech rehabilitation procedure. *Arch Otolaryngol* 1985; 111:106–109.

111. Hamaker RC, Singer MI, Blom ED, et al: Primary voice restoration at laryngectomy. *Arch Otolaryngol* 1985; 11:182–186.

112. Mahiew HF, et al: Deterioration of voice prosthesis caused by fungal vegetations [letter]. *Arch Otolaryngol* 1985; 111:356–360.

113. Singer MI, Blom ED, Hamaker RC: Pharyngeal plexus neurectomy for alaryngeal speech rehabilitation. *Laryngoscope* 1986; 96:50–53.

114. Kaplan JN, Dobie RA, Cummings CW: The incidence of hypopharyngeal stenosis after surgery for laryngeal cancer. *Otolaryngol Head Neck Surg* 1981; 89:956–959.

115. Bakamjian VY: Total reconstruction of the pharynx with a medially based deltopectoral skin flap. *NY State J Med* 1968; 68:2771.

116. Ariyan S: The pectoralis major myocutaneous flap: A versatile flap for reconstruction in the head and neck. *Plast Reconstr Surg* 1979; 63:73.

117. Ramadan MF, Stell PM: Reconstruction after pharyngolaryngoesophagectomy using delto-pectoral flaps. *Clin Otolaryngol* 1979; 4:5.

118. Missoten FEM: Historical review of pharyngo-oesophageal reconstruction after resection for carcinoma of pharynx and cervical oesophagus. *Clin Otolaryngol* 1983; 8:345–362.

119. Lam KH, Wong J, Lim ST, et al: Surgical treatment of carcinoma of the hypopharynx and cervical esophagus. *Ann Acad Med Singapore* 1980; 9:317–322.

120. Hester TR, McConnel FM, Nahai F, et al: Reconstruction of cervical esophagus, hypopharynx and oral cavity using free jejunal transfer. *Am J Surg* 1980; 140:487–491.

121. Harrison DFN: Surgical management of hypopharyngeal cancer. Particular reference to the gastric 'pull-up' operation. *Arch Otolaryngol* 1979; 105:149.

122. Lore JM Jr, Pruet CW: Retrieval of the parathyroid glands during thyroidectomy. *Head Neck Surg* 1983; 6:610–612.

123. Freeman JL, Brondbo K, Shaw HJ, et al: Parathyroid gland transplantation after total thyroidectomy with pharyngolaryngoesophagectomy. *Head Neck Surg* 1983; 6:610–612.

124. Silver CE: Gastric pull-up operation for replacement of the cervical portion of the esophagus. *Surg Gynecol Obstet* 1976; 142:243.

125. Delaere PR, Boeckx WD, Ostyn F, et al: Hypopharyngeal stenosis and fistulas. Use of the radial forearm flap. *Arch Otolaryngol Head Neck Surg* 1988; 114:1326–1329.

126. Gluckman JL, McDonough JJ, McCafferty GJ, et al: Complications associated with free jejunal graft reconstruction of pharynx and cervical esophagus. *Arch Otolaryngol* 1981; 107:476–481.

127. McConnel FM, Hester TR, Nahai F, et al: Free jejunal grafts for reconstruction of pharynx and cervical esophagus. *Arch Otolaryngol* 1981; 107:476–481.

128. DeSanto LW, Beahrs OH, Holt JJ, et al: Neck dissection and combined therapy. Study of effectiveness. *Arch Otolaryngol* 1985; 111:366–370.

129. Hawkins NV: The treatment of glottic carcinoma: An analysis of 800 cases. *Laryngoscope* 1975; 85:1485.

130. Ward PH, Calcaterra TC, Kagan AR: The enigma of postradiation edema and recurrent or residual carcinoma of the larynx. *Laryngoscope* 1975; 85:522–529.

131. DeSanto LW: T3 glottic carcinoma: Options and consequences of the options. *Laryngoscope* 1984; 94:1311–1315.

132. Cheng VST: Schulz MD: Unilateral hypoglossal nerve atrophy as a late complication of radiation therapy of head and neck carcinoma. A report of four cases and a review of the literature on peripheral and cranial nerve damages after radiation therapy. *Cancer* 1975; 35:1537–1544.

133. Wang CC, Blitzer PH, Suit HD: Twice-a-day radiation therapy for cancer of the head and neck. *Cancer* 1985; 55:2100–2104.

134. Creagan ET, Ingle JN, Schutt AJ, et al: A phase II study of

cis-diaminodichloroplatinum and 5-fluorouracil in advanced upper aerodigestive neoplasms. *Head Neck Surg* 1984; 6:1020–1023.

135. Wolf GT: An overview of preoperative chemotherapy: Where do we go from here? *Am J Otolaryngol* 1984; 5:77–79.

136. American Joint Committee for Cancer Staging and End Results Reporting: *Manual for Staging of Cancer.* Chicago, AJCC, 1977.

137. Chandler JR: Staging of cancer of the larynx, in Chretien PB, Johns ME, Shedd DP, et al (eds): *Head and Neck Cancer.* Philadelphia, BC Decker, 1985, pp 97–99.

CHAPTER 20

Management of the Primary Site: Salivary Glands

Approach of

Michael E. Johns, M.D.

PAROTID GLAND SURGERY

Sacrifice of the Facial Nerve

When does the surgeon sacrifice the facial nerve? This decision is not always easy, because the results are debilitating to the patient. The results of reconstruction, although gratifying insofar as being an improvement over total facial paralysis, are humbling compared with the outcome of embryogenesis and neuromuscular development. Almost always the decision to sacrifice the facial nerve is in the context of an adjacent parotid malignancy. Some surgeons always sacrifice the facial nerve if there is a malignant tumor in the parotid gland. I am selective in my action. Clearly, in cases where malignant tumor encompasses the nerve, it must be sacrificed with clear margins. If the patient presents with a parotid mass and facial weakness or paralysis, one can assume the parotid mass is malignant and that the facial nerve is involved and must be sacrificed. If the nerve had been preserved during the first surgery or grafted during the first surgery, the surgical procedure will of necessity encompass the nerve, because only wide resection of a recurrent malignant salivary gland tumor will offer a chance for cure. When a patient presents with a large tumor in the deep lobe and it is malignant by its behavior or by fine-needle aspiration (FNA), the patient should be prepared for sacrifice of the facial nerve, because adequate resection with free margins will require a wide resection, and the anatomic location of the deep lobe will necessitate inclusion of the nerve in that resection.

The difficult decision comes when the mass is small (<4 cm) and in the tail of the parotid gland. A superficial parotidectomy is carried out, and this accomplishes the removal of the tumor with adequate surgical margins confirmed by pa-

thology. The problem arises when the final pathology results are returned as malignant, usually 3 to 5 days later. There are many surgeons who will return this patient to the operating room and perform a wide resection with sacrifice of the facial nerve. I, however, believe that if the tumor is small (T1 or T2) and low grade (mucoepidermoid or acinic cell carcinoma) and I am satisfied with the pathologic margins, no further treatment is necessary. If the pathology is one of the high-grade malignancies and it is T2 or smaller, the patient is offered postoperative radiation therapy or a wide resection and radiation therapy. The radiation is used to manage any microscopic residual, and thus the facial nerve is left intact. In some instances, the tumor is adjacent to the nerve but separable from it without difficulty. In these cases, I will rely on radiation therapy to manage the microscopic residual. If, however, the mass is densely adherent to the facial nerve and yet I was able to preserve the nerve, I would recommend returning the patient to the operating room for a wide resection and a nerve graft.

Occasionally a patient presents who has had multiple attempts at irradication of a benign pleomorphic adenoma and multiple recurrences. In these cases, nerve sacrifice must be considered. This is because the recurrences are usually multiple, and scarring obscures the dissection and the nerve. Usually the only chance to eradicate the disease (which may undergo malignant degeneration if left unchecked) will require a wide resection, including all or selected branches of the facial nerve.

In every case of a suspected malignancy, the patient must be adequately prepared for the outcome of the facial nerve sacrifice and have a realistic expectation of the potential of the reconstructive procedure. In some cases the patient will take the option to not have the nerve sacrificed, but the surgeon must always respect the patient's opinion.

The reason for my selectively saving the nerve in these situations involving parotid malignancies is based on the accumulating experience that surgery and radiation when used wisely results in an excellent local regional control. The more significant problem that leads to death is the high predominance of distant metastasis. The adenoid cystic carcinoma is a good example of this in that it seems to be controllable locally with combined treatment, but its distant metastasis rate of approximately 40% is so high that the ultimate outcome does not seem to justify the added morbidity of facial paralysis.

When one sacrifices the facial nerve for malignancy during parotid surgery, the surgeon must be prepared for immediate reconstruction of the nerve. This is best accomplished by interposition nerve grafting. An interposition graft must be placed when loss of nerve length is significantly great to preclude approximation by mobilization. The choice of a donor nerve or grafting is based on its size and the extent of functional loss. A large-diameter nerve will become revascularized more slowly than a smaller one. If vascularization is too slow, the graft may undergo fibrosis and degenerate. The length of the graft is not as important because revascularization occurs segmentally and not longitudinally. The most frequently used donor sites of facial nerve grafting are the greater auricular nerve and the sural nerve.

The great auricular nerve is most frequently used. It can be harvested from the same side of the facial nerve resection, or, if there is a question of malignant disease involving the nerve, the contralateral great auricular nerve can be used. The great auricular nerve (C2-3) is a sensory branch of the cervical plexus. It courses over the sternocleidomastoid muscle ascending obliquely toward the auricle and angle of the mandible. Here it divides into three branches, the mastoid, auricular, and facial branches, to supply sensation to the skin and subcutaneous tissues over the parotid gland, angle of the mandible, and lower portion of the pinna. Permanent anesthesia of these areas results when it is used as a graft. It can be identified topographically by drawing an imaginary line between the mastoid tip and angle of the mandible and then drawing a perpendicular line from the midpoint of the line. The greater auricular nerve is on the perpendicular line. If the contralateral nerve is used, a horizontal incision 3 to 4 cm long will allow adequate exposure to mobilize the nerve at the posterior border of the sternocleidomastoid muscle where it has a single trunk. The nerve can then be found superiorly and anteriorly until it branches. Generally there will be two branches that further subdivide. The great auricular nerve has two or three fascicles and is of the same diameter as the facial nerve. However, when the epineurium is resected, the fascicles of the great auricular nerve are frequently smaller than the diameter of the facial nerve, and it is often necessary that a second graft be approximated to the main trunk. The branch of the great auricular nerve can then be approximated to the various distal branches of the facial nerve.

The sural nerve is a valuable donor nerve when multiple grafts or particularly long grafts are needed, as in cross facial nerve grafting or facial rerouting. Up to 35 cm of the sural nerve can be harvested. The sural nerve is generally composed of two to four fascicles and is thin and long. Its absence results in a minimal functional defect. The sural nerve is formed by the junction of the medial sural cutaneous nerve and the perineal nerve between the two heads of the gastrocnemius muscle. It is at this point that the medial sural cutaneous nerve pierces the defect and is joined by the perineal communicating branch of the lateral sural cutaneous nerve to form the sural nerve. The sural nerve descends in close proximity to the lesser saphenous vein to the level of the lateral malleolus and branches on to the side of the foot. This supplies cutaneous sensation to the side and back of the distal third of the leg, the ankle, and the heel. It has separate branches on the side of the foot. This nerve can be reached through a transverse incision just behind the lateral malleolus and stair step incisions used to dissect it. Perhaps less traumatic is a vertical incision that extends along the course of the nerve that does not require as much pulling and tugging on the nerve in the harvesting process. Once the nerve is removed, it can be divided into segments slightly longer than the facial nerve defect to be bridged.

The graft should be handled with the same care given to the facial nerve. It should be longer than the nerve gap to allow for graft contraction and to minimize tension. The graft should be preserved in a balanced salt solution while awaiting placement. The ends of it must be prepared with a careful microsurgical technique, stripping epinerium away 5 mm from the end to be grafted to the main trunk. Sutures of 10-0 nylon placed through the perineurium will allow careful approximation of the graft to the nerve fascicles. Tension is avoided in an effort to minimize connective tissue proliferation. The distal neurorrhaphy is accomplished using 10-0 nylon, but no epineurium is dissected in this epineural repair. This is because the peripheral fibers are so fine that attempts to dissect the epineurium seem to be more injurious than leaving the epineurium intact distally.

The time required for optimal facial function to occur following neurorrhaphy or interposition grafting depends on the distance from which regeneration has occurred prior to reaching its muscular end organ. It is commonly accepted that repairs from the pes anserinus distally generally require approximately 4 months, and repairs in the mastoid segment require 5 months. It is my experience, however, that continued regeneration occurs up to 1 to $1\frac{1}{2}$ years after the neurorrhaphy.

Facial Nerve Injury

The key to prevention of facial nerve injury during parotidectomy hinges on a knowledge of the anatomy of the nerve and the surgical approach to the exposure of the main trunk of the nerve as it leaves the stylomastoid canal or secondary approaches to identifying primary branches for retrograde dissection to the main trunk. Prevention of injuries to the facial nerve hinges on a thorough knowledge of the anatomy of the region. The use of microscopes, loops, and nerve stimulators does not supplant this most essential piece of knowledge. It is beyond the scope of this chapter to give the full surgical approach to the parotid gland, and I would refer you to other articles or atlases. I would, however, like to emphasize some technical aspects that help to minimize facial nerve injury. Adequate exposure is fairly important, and the incision should be placed as cosmetically as possible in the preauricular crease. I prefer to hide the incision behind the tragus and then place it behind the lobule in a soft curve and back down anteriorly into the neck. Greater anterior exposure of the parotid and anterior face can be gained by placing a horizontal extension at the top of the preauricular incision into the sideburn or temporal hairline and by extending the cervical incision anteriorly. The face should be draped so that the eyes, nose, and mouth are exposed. I use a plastic drape positioned away from where my incision is made but over the rest of the face. This will allow the face to be visualized through the plastic drape. An epinephrine solution (1:100,000) injected along the incision line and around the tragus decreases capillary bleeding. Good hemostasis always provides a dry field and improves exposure.

The facial nerve can be identified in one of four ways. These include finding the main trunk by using the tragal pointer or tympanomastoid suture as anatomic guides, identifying the marginal mandibular nerve as it crosses superficial to the posterior facial veins, identifying the parotid duct anteriorly over the masseter muscle and locating the buccal branch that accompanies it, or finding the nerve in the mastoid bone and then following it out through the stylomastoid foramen. In most instances the surgeon must be prepared to use any one or several of the approaches. In most routine cases, I prefer to use the tympanomastoid suture line because it is a constant landmark and the stylomastoid canal can always be located approximately 6 to 8 mm below the inferior border of the tympanomastoid suture line. In recurrent tumors where considerable scarring will be expected around the facial nerve in the retromandibular area, I prefer to begin the case by finding the nerve in the mastoid bone and decompressing it along its entire length until it leaves the stylomastoid canal. In the heavily scarred surgical bed, use of loops or the microscope is a valuable adjunct in recurrent tumor cases. The importance of adequate exposure, especially elevation of the tail of the parotid gland from the underlying musculature, cannot be overemphasized. Wide exposure will prevent "working in a hole" and allow good visualization of all pertinent landmarks required for rapid identification of the main trunk. A nerve stimulator may be used for confirmation of the nerve but should be used sparingly to avoid neural fatigue. I use it only in unusual situations. Once the nerve trunk is identified, the individual branches are followed peripherally, and the tumor with the parotid tissue is removed from the nerve.

When the dissection has been completed, the nerve trunk should be stimulated to be certain that all branches are functioning normally. If any portion of the nerve is not stimulating, careful inspection of the branch using the microscope (if necessary) is imperative.

Another tip to help minimize the chance of paralysis of the marginal mandibular branch is to avoid dissecting and ligating the posterior facial vein. In a superficial parotidectomy, one must remember that the marginal mandibular nerve crosses over this vein and that the vein will not be resected with the tumor mass. Therefore, ligation would only increase the venous

congestion of the gland and, therefore, capillary oozing. In addition, the marginal mandibular nerve runs in immediate proximity of that nerve and can be ligated inadvertently. In the final step in completion of the case prior to closure of the flap, the nerve should be carefully visualized as it leaves the stylomastoid canal and followed out to the periphery. Each branch should be inspected to be sure that it is intact. If it is intact to visualization and to electrical stimulation at 1 mamp but the patient has weakness or paralysis in the immediate postoperative period, the surgeon can feel secure in the knowledge that reexploration will not offer additional benefit to the patient but, rather, that the nerve has undergone a first- or second-degree injury and will recover with sufficient time. The use of steroids to enhance this healing process has been advised by some authors, but there is no evidence to suggest that steroids enhance the facial nerve recovery.

If the careful steps to document the intact presence of the facial nerve have not been carried out and the patient awakes with a facial paralysis, the wound must be explored, preferably within 48 hours of the surgical procedure, to identify the nerve injury and repair it. The technical aspects of the repair have already been discussed. However, I would mention that when the branch of the orbicularis occuli muscle has been either grafted or is severed and reanastomosed that the surgeon could consider a tarsorraphy to prevent corneal drying and ulceration. The use of artificial tears and eye ointments at night are recommended to minimize occular complications.

Frozen Section and Fine-Needle Aspiration Cytology in Parotid Tumors

The application of an FNA technique in salivary gland neoplasms has become increasingly popular in recent years. Although needle biopsy techniques have been discouraged in the past because of the potential for seeding, a thin needle (22-gauge) technique has proved to be very safe and also accurate when managed by an experienced cytopathologist. As the surgeon and the pathologist gain increasing experience, the diagnostic accuracy should continue to improve. For squamous cell carcinoma of the head and neck, the accuracy for FNA is more than 90%. In the area of salivary gland neoplasms, however, the diagnostic accuracy is somewhat less, 60% to 80% in different series. This lower accuracy rate is certainly understandable considering the great diversity of pathology that one encounters in the salivary glands. The results of the aspiration biopsy must be used with caution, particularly if the result does not fit the clinical picture and in view of the moderate level of sensitivity and specificity for this technique in salivary gland tumors. Most important, one must ask whether the utilization of the FNA biopsy will change the way the surgeon manages or approaches the case. Since the majority of these parotid tumors (90%) are less than 3 cm and sit in the tail of the parotid, most of them will be completely removed with a superficial parotidectomy. In the majority of these cases, no diagnostic tests other than a physical examination will alter the ultimate treatment of the patient. However, when the tumor is large, involves the parapharyngeal space, is recurrent or just simply does not quite fit together with the rest of the clinical picture, FNA can be helpful in the decision-making process. I personally do not use it as a routine in the majority of small tumors of the parotid gland.

I must say that the same holds true for the computed tomography (CT) scan. In those majority of cases where FNA will not make a difference in the approach to the parotid tumor, the CT scan also adds very little. The sialogram is almost never used for parotid tumors, but the CT scan with 2 mm cuts can give valuable information in unusual or large tumors. The intravenous (IV) contrast enhancement allows differentiation between masses originating in the deep lobe of the parotid and those originating within the parapharyngeal space.

The use of frozen sections to determine surgical approach is risky. Aggressive surgery should not be based on a frozen section report. The surgeon would regret it if the permanent section diagnosis is changed from malignant to benign, having sacrificed a vital structure! It is better to wait for the permanent section diagnosis and, if it is malignant and the extent of tumor warrants, to return to the operating room and in the next 1 or 2 days complete the operation. Once again, in the majority of cases, the tumor is small, sits in the tail of the parotid gland, and has been completely excised by a superficial parotidectomy. Frozen section will not alter the therapy in any way at all, and frozen section serves only to add to the cost of health care delivery.

In cases of malignant tumors, however, frozen section can be used to determine the adequacy of the margins. This is particularly useful in adenoid cystic carcinomas where nerve margins should be checked when the nerve is resected. The potentiality for perineural invasion is so great, and in addition, skip areas along the nerve can occur. Thus, what appears to be adequate margin around the tumor and nerve involvement should be confirmed by histopathology.

The use of any diagnostic procedure should be based on the fact that the information provided will change what the surgeon will do. Take, for example, a 2 cm tail of the parotid lesion that is painless and mobile, with no evidence of nerve weakness or paralysis (recall this is how 90% of all parotid tumors present). I would contend that CT scans or magnetic resonance imaging (MRI), knowledge of the histopathology in advance by FNA (which is not 100% accurate), or questionable frozen section information during the surgery for this described case will not change the surgeon's approach. The surgeon will inevitably perform a parotidectomy and preserve the facial nerve.

However, in the large parotid mass, mass in the deep lobe or parapharyngeal space, mass with facial nerve weakness at presentation, and when the clinical or surgical picture "does not quite fit," these adjunctive diagnostic procedures can provide useful information.

Frey's Syndrome

Frey's syndrome, also known as gustatory sweating or the auriculotemporal syndrome, consists of sweating or dermal flush in the distribution of the auriculotemporal nerve during the ingestion of food. This phenomenon has often been noted as a sequela of parotid surgery or injury but has also been described after submaxillary surgery,[1] after thoracocervical sympathectomy, and in diabetic autonomic neuropathy.[2]

Estimates of this incidence of Frey's syndrome vary, depending on how rigorously it is searched for. Reports of the occurrence of symptomatic gustatory sweating vary from less than 5% to approximately 25%.[3–6]

Minor's starch-iodine test indicates that the condition is more common than is believed.[7] Some degree of gustatory sweating was reported in 100% of Laage-Hellman's patients,[8] in 36% of Glaister et al.'s patients,[9] in 59% of Spiro and Martin's patients,[10] and in 34% of Gordon and Fiddian's patients.[11] In my experience, among the patients who have this condition, only 10% are aware of it, and even fewer request treatment.

To prevent gustatory sweating following parotidectomy, the surgeon can control at least one variable: the thickness of the skin flap. I have used this in my approach for the past 10 years, and I have not had a single patient request surgical intervention for Frey's syndrome, and only occasionally does a patient mention its presence.

Multiple options are available for the treatment of symptomatic Frey's syndrome; however, none of them is completely satisfactory. In my experience, all of my patients tolerate the symptoms and opt for no treatment.

If treatment is required, strategies can be divided into medical and surgical. The medical treatment is based on the fact that the sympathetic innervation of the sweat gland is cholinergic, not adrenergic; therefore, the use of anticholinergic drugs is indicated. The topical application of 3% scopolamine cream is effective in mild cases. However, because of absorption through the skin, the patient may complain of systemic side effects such as dry mouth and blurred vision. The drug is contraindicated in patients with close-angle glaucoma, gastric outlet obstruction, or bladder neck obstruction. One percent glycopyrrolate cream or lotion is just as effective and has a remarkably low incidence of side effects.[12] Systemic atropine is not as effective, and the problem of dry mouth and blurred vision is intensified. My recommendation for treatment is application of a nonscented antiperspirant to the area involved.

The earliest surgical treatment of Frey's syndrome is credited to Goldwin-Wood,[13] who successfully performed the first three cases of tympanic neurectomy. Since then, this technique has been utilized, providing some relief for the majority of moderately to severely symptomatic patients.[14–17] Long-term results in 13 patients indicate that overall 38.5% were completely relieved of their symptoms, 23% were improved, and in 38.5% the condition remained unchanged.[14]

Rather than nerve section, I would prefer interposition of fascia lata between an elevated skin flap and the gland. Wallis and Gibson[18] and Sessions et al.[15] reported permanent cure in six patients using this technique. Apparently, the number of patients needing this procedure is small. In general, I believe that this complication can be prevented by having as thick a skin flap as possible. To this end I always attempt to raise my parotid facial flaps immediately above the parotid fascia, thus leaving a very thick skin flap. This seems to have diminished the incidence of gustatory sweating in my patients.

Salivary Fistula

Usually salivary fistulae are caused by trauma and are only rarely complications of parotidectomy. If they do occur and persist, periodic aspiration of the accumulated fluid or drainage of the wound is all that is required until spontaneous resolution occurs. Chronic parenchymal fistulae can usually be managed conservatively, unlike chronic ductal fistulae that do not close spontaneously.[19] Antisialagogues may be considered to be useful adjuncts because they temporarily decrease salivary output; however, they may cause distressing side effects.[20, 21]

Since inevitably some parotid tissue persists following parotid surgery, the potential for salivary fistulae is always present. A fistula or sialocele occurs when the flap fails to seal over the remaining parotid tissue, and saliva develops into the flap or drains into the neck. If compressive dressings are used to control the salivary fistula, one must take care to protect the ear to avoid necrosis of the soft tissue surrounding the ear. At this point, I have only rarely had this postoperative complication, and it has always responded to the conservative management approach of aspiration or drainage and a pressure dressing. However, others have described that for fistulae that persist and are leaking for several months or more despite conservative treatment, several options are available. Consideration has been given to secondary surgical closure of small to medium-size fistula tracts, but the rate of success is not high. Low-dose radiation to suppress the remaining actively secreting parotid tissue has been administered, but the doses required are high and may promote carcinogenesis; therefore, I do not recommend them. Tympanic neurectomy has been advocated as the treatment of choice by some. It has been reported that this is the treatment of choice, but to date I have not had to employ any of these surgical options to manage salivary fistulae.

Approach to Deep Lobe Tumors

Most tumors of the parotid gland arise from the lateral lobe, and the incidence of deep lobe tumors does not exceed 11% to 12% in the larger series. Only a small proportion of these patients develop significant retropharyngeal extension. This constitutes a diagnostic and therapeutic challenge among surgeons.

To gain exposure to the deep lobe, a superficial parotidectomy is carried out. Deep lobe tumors generally are defined as those that sit deep to the facial nerve in the parotid bed. When they extend behind the mandible into the parapharyngeal space, they are known as parapharyngeal tumors. For deep lobe tumors, it is generally stated that total parotidectomy should be carried out. This term, strictly speaking, is a misnomer. Removal of all parotid tissue is nearly impossible and usually not necessary in the majority of parotid surgery. The concept of a total parotidectomy is that of removal of the parotid tissue, both medial and lateral to the facial nerve with the accompanying tumor. The particular technique employed may differ depending on the location of the tumor. Once the superficial lobe has been removed, the nerve is exposed and carefully and gently freed up off of the tumor mass. This is accomplished by careful and meticulous dissection of the nerve with sharp pointed scissors and then the use of rubber vascular bands to give gentle retraction on the nerve. Once the nerve is mobilized, the mass is removed by blunt and sharp dissection. Those dumbbell-shaped deep lobe tumors within the isthmus of in front of the stylomandibular ligament or passing posterior to the ligament are called parapharyngeal space tumors. When this situation occurs, further exposure to the portion of the gland medial to the facial nerve is required. To improve this exposure, I approach the parapharyngeal space by excising the submandibular gland and then do a superficial parotidectomy, which allows for identification and protection of the facial nerve. The stylomandibular ligament is then detached from the mandible, thus allowing for anterior dislocation of the mandible to improve access to the parapharyngeal space. This approach suffices for most tumors, which then can be bluntly dissected with the index finger. To date, I have not had to split the mandible to remove a parapharyngeal space tumor. However, if additional exposure is required, anterior mandibular dislocation or a mandibulotomy can be performed at the angle of the mandible space medial to the mandible, and it can then be more completely exposed. Almost all parapharyngeal space tumors can be removed by this technique.

As an alternate approach, a lip-splitting incision with medial mandibulotomy might be considered. After attempting exposure through the neck, the surgeon believes that a lateral mandibulotomy will not allow sufficient additional access, the neck incision is carried through the lip in the anterior midline, and the mandible is transected after a compression plate is bent and shaped to the anterior mandible and four drill holes placed. The incision is carried along the lateral floor of the mouth, avoiding injury to the lingual and hypoglossal nerves and the submandibular contents. As the tongue is pulled medially and the mandible laterally, the incision is carried to the tonsil and pharyngeal regions. With this direct approach to the parapharyngeal space, any mass from the skull base to the lower part of the neck can be removed under direct vision. Although additional cosmetic deformity is encountered through a lip incision, this approach provides direct access to the parapharyngeal space tumors, but usually is not necessary for salivary gland tumors in the parapharyngeal space.

It is apparent, then, that for difficult deep lobe or parapharyngeal space parotid tumors, the surgeon and patient must be prepared for a variety of approaches to ensure complete removal.

Approach to the N0 Neck

It is well accepted and accurately documented that the presence of clinically abnormal nodes alters the prognosis. In the presence of abnormal nodes, surgical management of the neck is indicated. Indications for prophylactic neck dissection, however, are controversial. Many head and neck surgeons might agree that if there is a 25% or greater likelihood of occult metastases, a neck dissection should be done. Others might argue, however, that there is no evidence demonstrating that waiting for occult metastases to become clinically manifest adversely affects the ultimate outcome of the disease process.

It is important to know which of these histologic classes of tumors have a propensity for lymphatic metastasis. At the time of initial presentation, the incidence of cervical metastases is said to be about 13%.[22] The incidence of occult metastases is said to be 16% or less for all parotid cancers except squamous cell carcinoma, in which a 40% incidence of occult metastases is present. I note high-grade mucoepidermoid carcinomas in a superior series had a 60% occult metastases rate.[22]

Occult metastases in acinous cell carcinoma and adenoid cystic carcinoma are rare. In adenoid cystic carcinoma, regional spread occurs by contiguous growth and rarely ever occurs by lymphatic extension.[23] Because of the rare neck metastases in acinous cell carcinoma, earlier proponents of routine neck dissection in acinous cell carcinoma no longer recommend it.[24, 25]

The evidence suggested that in untreated parotid cancers, the incidence of cervical metastasis is very low. More important, occult metastasis is rare in all but squamous cell carcinoma of the parotid. There is no information to suggest that the clinically normal neck is best treated by a prophylactic neck dissection. The use of postoperative irradiation as an adjunct to surgery appears to control occult metastasis.

If we consider the previous discussion, the following philosophy for treatment of the clinically normal neck has evolved. At the time of parotidectomy, the periparotid, upper jugular, and posterior submandibular triangle nodes are inspected. A biopsy is performed on suspect nodes, or they are included in the parotid dissection. Whether further surgery will be carried out or whether postoperative irradiation will be used is then based on the pathology report of the tumor itself and of the nodes sampled. In advanced tumors in which postoperative irradiation is used, I include the neck in the radiation port. The presence of histologically abnormal nodes in the neck is an indication for a neck dissection.

Nonneoplastic Conditions of the Parotid Gland

Sjögren's syndrome can be divided into two types: sicca syndrome and secondary Sjögren's syndrome.

In sicca syndrome, xerostomia and xerophthalmia predominate as a result of diffused exocrine glandular involvement. Salivary gland enlargement is not particularly a hallmark of these patients. They have, however, significant problems with dryness of the eyes and dryness of the mouth and are different genetically than those with secondary Sjögren's syndrome.

Secondary Sjögren's syndrome has a complete triad, that is, xerophthalmia, xerostomia, and an autoimmune disorder. In most cases, this is rheumatoid arthritis. However, in many of the cases, the autoimmune disorder may be lupus erythematosus, scleroderma, polymyositis, or other autoimmune diseases.

Recognition of a benign lymphoepithelial lesion is limited to salivary glands alone, and the pathologic picture is the same as salivary gland changes seen in Sjögren's syndrome.

Diagnosis can generally be confirmed by assessment of xerophthalmia. Xerostomia is not generally quantitatively measured but is more of a qualitative assessment. Flow scanning with technetium 99 can be of some value in showing diminished uptake and can show progression of the disease if there is need for this. Although salivary gland enlargement is perhaps the most frequent reason why otolaryngologists see patients with these disorders. In fact, patients with these diseases as a rule do not as a group have salivary gland enlargement. Only about 30% of all patients with Sjögren's syndrome complain of salivary gland enlargement.

The best diagnostic tool in this disorder is surgical biopsy, and a biopsy is performed most often on the minor salivary glands, generally the salivary gland of the lip. One should carefully evaluate the lower lip to be sure that there is no evidence of recurrent trauma. If this is the case, a simple oral incision can be made in the buccal labial mucosa, and four to five glandular elements should be included in this specimen. It is, indeed, rare that submandibular gland excision is indicated in this disorder. Clearly it would be a last resort in terms of diagnosis. Removing the glands will serve only to further speed and enhance the lack of oral secretions and thus increase the symptoms. The treatment of this disorder generally is the treatment of the entire underlying disease.

Chronic Sialadenitis

Chronic parotitis can be defined as obstructive and nonobstructive. Obstructive parotitis is generally related to trauma that causes strictures of the parotid duct. Sialolithiasis is unusual in the parotid gland. These lesions are best demonstrated by sialography, and it is clearly one area where sialography still plays a useful role. In obstructive sialolithiasis, surgery is generally the treatment of choice for all conditions. Occasionally with the strictured parotid duct, dilation may be successful in the conservative management. However, in most cases, it will not be successful, and surgical excision of the parotid gland is essential. The stones that are within the direct reach of the parotid duct punctum can be managed conservatively; however, the duct rapidly passes over the masseter muscle, and once this occurs, a stone in that portion of the duct is not accessible by the oral route and should be managed by an external approach. The external approach to the parotid gland in obstructive sialadenitis is, in fact, no different from the approaches for parotid tumors I have described.

The second form of chronic sialadenitis is that of chronic nonobstructive sialadenitis. It can occur from a variety of causes. In chronic infectious sialadenitis, the indications for surgery are restricted to those cases that are refractory to medical management over a prolonged period of time. Chronic parotitis frequently can be managed with sialogogues, massage, and antibiotic therapy for the acute episodes. When, however, the problem becomes refractory to this management or the acute episodes become so frequent that they interfere with the patient's function, then excision of the gland is indicated. Again, the surgical approach is not particularly different from that of the superficial parotidectomy already described except that in these cases a total parotidectomy is desirable and removal of as much of the salivary gland tissue beneath the facial nerve as possible is important.

Acute Parotitis

Generally most cases of parotitis are related to penicillin-resistant Staphylococcus or anaerobic infections. Most cases will respond well to antibiotic therapy. If the patient is nontoxic and is reliable, one may take an approach to outpatient management of the infection. However, the patient must be followed carefully and should be seen back within 24 to 48 hours for reevaluation to be certain that the infection is coming under control. In those cases where the patient presents in a toxic condition with elevated temperature, trismus, and erythema, admission to the hospital with intravenous antibiotic therapy is essential. Occasionally the patient will allow the disease to progress to a state where abscess cavities are formed, and although the patient can be brought under some control with antibiotics, the disease does not completely respond to antibiotics. My experience has been rare in that I have generally been able to aspirate these cystic areas repeatedly and bring the infection under control with antibiotics and repeated aspirations. For those cases where the patient remains refractory, my approach is that of surgery and involves incision and drainage. The surgical approach is to raise a parotid flap just as I would for routine parotidectomy and then to use a knife to incise the parotid capsule. The incision should be in the direction of the facial nerve branches. Then a hemostat is inserted through the capsular incision, and the abscessed cavities are opened and drained. Penrose drains should be placed into the drained areas and brought out onto the neck and the facial incision closed loosely. This generally is all that is required to bring these resistant infections under control. Today, however, this is a very rare occurrence, and these infections should generally respond well to antibiotic therapy.

SUBMANDIBULAR GLAND SURGERY

Tumors of the Submandibular Gland

Tumors involving the submandibular gland are usually contained within the gland, and the resection is confined to the gland and the surrounding fat or lymph nodes. If a malignant tumor is invading surrounding tissue, the procedure is expanded to include involved structures with an appropriate tumor-free margin. Structures excised often include the marginal mandibular branch of the facial nerve, hypoglossal and lingual nerves, as well as mandible, tongue, floor of mouth, and skin.

Preoperative evaluation of a submandibular gland tumor, like the parotid, begins with a careful history and examination. As with the parotid, most neoplasms arising within the submandibular gland are asymptomatic. However, if the patient has evidence of neural involvement with loss of marginal mandibular nerve or hypoglossal function and/or loss of sensation and taste, an aggressive malignant disease is probable. Palpation of the mass, both externally and bimanually, aids in localization of the mass. At times, however, one has difficulty differentiating the gland from one or several enlarged lymph nodes overlying the gland. It may also be difficult to differentiate tumors from inflammatory disease, especially if the patient has not had symptoms suggestive of recurrent sialadenitis. Evaluation for reduced salivary flow through the orifice of Wharton's duct and palpation

for ductal stones may support inflammatory gland disease. Discovery of additional adenopathy may indicate nodal spread from a primary gland tumor or may represent nodal spread from a more distant site or lymphoma. Once again, in cases where confusion exists, application of the FNA technique may help solve a dilemma. The gland is quite accessible and easily aspirated. If necessary, the gland may be presented into the neck by placing the finger intraorally and pushing the gland to a more superficial location. Aspiration may help determine whether the mass is within the gland or represents a lymph node and is also useful in differentiating inflammatory from neoplastic disease.

In selected cases, imaging techniques may be helpful, particularly to assess spread beyond the gland. Views of the mandible, including occlusal views, may be obtained when searching for bone erosion. Computed tomography usually does not yield additional information since all surrounding soft tissue spaces can be palpated or visualized without difficulty. The submandibular sialogram is somewhat difficult to perform due to the small ductal orifice. The risk of overinjection and attendant patient discomfort does not justify the routine application of this procedure. For suspected tumors, delineation of the ductal system does not aid in surgical decision making.

Submandibular Gland Excision

The procedure should be performed with the patient under general anesthetic unless the medical status requires local anesthesia. The incision is routinely placed 2 to 3 cm below the inferior border of the mandible and should be hidden in a skin crease if possible. The skin incision may be injected for hemostasis with caution to avoid superior infiltration if an anesthetic is used with the vasoconstricting agent. The anesthesiologist should avoid using paralyzing agents if at all possible. The incision usually measures approximately 5 cm and is carried down through the platysma muscle. The capsule of the gland and surrounding soft tissue should be left intact over the gland when excision is being carried out for suspected neoplasm. Since this technique puts the marginal mandibular nerve at greater risk, the facial vein and artery should be located immediately as close to the gland as possible and, after transection, elevated superiorly to reflect the marginal mandibular nerve from the field. If adenopathy is present over the gland, the marginal mandibular nerve often passes directly over or around these facial nodes, and the surgeon must carefully dissect the nerve from the nodes. The gland and surrounding soft tissue may then be safely dissected from the under surface of the mandible. The inferior border of the gland is elevated from the digastric muscle. The facial artery, if transected superiorly, will again be transected posterolaterally as one nears its origin from the external carotid. The gland is reflected laterally to expose the mylohyoid muscle. As the superficial portion of the gland is dissected from this muscle, the posterolateral border is encountered. A retractor is inserted, and the free edge of the mylohyoid is retracted medially. This maneuver allows exposure of three important structures in the floor of the submandibular triangle: the lingual and hypoglossal nerves and Wharton's duct. With gentle downward traction on the gland, the lingual

TABLE 20–1.
Principles of Management of Salivary Gland Tumors

	Group 1	Group 2	Group 3	Group 4
Tumor type	T1 and T2 low-grade Mucoepidermoid low grade Acinic cell	T1 and T2 high grade Adenocarcinoma Malignant mixed Undifferentiated Squamous cell	T3N0, N+, and any recurrent tumors not in group 4	T4
Parotid gland	Superficial or total parotidectomy Preservation of seventh cranial nerve (CN VII)	Total parotidectomy with preservation of nerve VII Neck dissection for N+ neck only Postoperative radiation	Radical parotidectomy Sacrifice of CN VII with immediate reconstruction Neck dissection for N+ neck only Postoperative irradiation	Radical parotidectomy with resection of skin, mandible, muscles, and mastoid tip as indicated Sacrifice of CN VII with immediate reconstruction Neck dissection for N+ neck only Postoperative irradiation
Submandibular	Submandibular triangle resection	Wide excision of submandibular triangle Preserve nerves unless involved Postoperative irradiation	Radical neck dissection to include CN XII and lingual nerve	Surgery to fit disease extent

nerve is usually noted as a downward curving band with the apex at the midpoint of the gland. This attachment of the lingual nerve to the gland represents the parasympathetic supply to the gland. The duct lies inferior to the lingual nerve and is often surrounded by sublingual glands and may not be well seen initially. The hypoglossal nerve is more inferior yet and is always accompanied by at least one large vein, the ranine vein. The presence of this vein may aid in the identification of the nerve, which often is immediately adjacent or beneath this vessel. Both the nerve and accompanying vein emerge from beneath the digastric muscle and pass anterosuperiorly into the tongue. When all structures are identified, the duct and branch of the lingual nerve to the gland are ligated and transected. The gland and contiguous soft tissue may then be dissected free and removed. A rubber ribbon drain is inserted deep to the platysma and the wound closed in layers.

If a neck dissection is indicated, this procedure is performed in continuity with the gland excision. Tumors may exhibit local invasive behavior, as evidenced by alteration of nerve function, fixation to deep structures, or skin involvement. In these cases, the margin of resection may include the lingual, hypoglossal, or marginal mandibular nerves, floor of the mouth, tongue, mandible, or skin. A careful preoperative evaluation will alert the surgeon to the necessity of extensive surgical procedures in this area and therefore preparation for adequate reconstruction.

Complications of submandibular gland excision are few. The most common postoperative finding is marginal mandibular weakness. This paresis often occurs when the nerve is dissected from underlying adenopathy. Weakness also may occur from persistent traction on the upper flap. Complete return of function is a rule, but it may require several months. Loss of lingual and hypoglossal nerve function is rare unless these nerves are included in the resection.

Histologic grade and clinical staging are the two most important determinants of survival. By combining T classification and histopathologic diagnosis, we have developed a schema for management of malignant salivary gland neoplasms. Four groups are identified for each location. As we pass from group 1 to group 4, increasing severity of disease is matched with progressively more aggressive therapy (Table 20–1).

In group 1, resection of the submandibular triangle is sufficient surgery for the small, low-grade malignancies. A clean plane of dissection between nerves and tumor is usually possible, allowing preservation of these structures. Radiotherapy is not required for malignancies in this group. In group 2 tumors, a wider excision is required for an adequate margin. Nerves are not resected unless they are directly involved with tumor or cannot be cleanly dissected free from the tumor. Postoperative radiation is recommendation.

In group 3 tumors, the lingual and hypoglossal nerves must be sacrificed in most cases, particularly in recurrent tumors. A neck dissection is routinely performed for tumors in this category. Radiotherapy should follow the surgical excision. Surgery for tumors placed in group 4 will be tailored to fit the extent of disease. A marginal or segmental resection of the mandible may be required for these large aggressive carcinomas. Portions of the tongue, floor of mouth, and skin may be included with the tumor and associated nerves. A neck dissection and postoperative radiotherapy are included in the standard management of these tumors. Reconstruction may require transfer of both soft tissue and skeletal elements to reconstitute function and cosmesis.

Sialolithiasis

Proximal Stone

Stones of the submandibular gland are significantly more common than those of the parotid gland. When the stone is proximal near the opening of the submandibular duct, it can be easily managed via an intraoral approach. Generally they can be identified by bimanual palpation of the floor of the mouth. Occasionally I have actually seen them presenting in the punctum of the duct. In these cases, topical anesthesia of the oral mucosa is obtained using your favorite topical anesthestic, either 4% lidocaine (Xylocaine) or topical cocaine. The punctum of the submandibular duct that is involved is identified. The duct is widened with lacrimal dilators, and the lacrimal dilator is passed along the duct until it caputs the stone. This distance can be measured, and clearly if it is within 1.5 cm of the punctum, it should be easily managed by an intraoral approach. The submandibular duct is opened with either a very sharp pointed iris scissors or a knife by cutting along the surface of the lacrimal dilator. This fish mouth opening of the duct will allow the use of either massage or the lacrimal probe to tease the stone anteriorly for easy removal. There is no need to suture the duct closed because it will heal spontaneously. One concern that must be expressed is that if there has been a chronic and long-standing history of recurrent swelling of the submandibular gland, simple removal of the stone will probably not resolve the chronic sialadenitis. In those cases, consideration should be given to excision of the gland and the stone. For the distal stone located near the hilum of the submandibular gland, the intraoral approach will not be successful and will put at risk the lingual nerve and hypoglossal nerve. In these cases, confirmation of the stone's presence can be made by palpation with a lacrimal probe, and the distance can be measured. Confirmation usually is accomplished with radiographic imaging. A submandibular gland resection via the standard approach already described is indicated. This is a conservative resection of the gland with the duct. The duct should be tracked up from the cervical approach as distal as possible to its entrance into the floor of the mouth. It can be ligated and the duct and gland removed. It should be noted that it has been described in the literature that if a ductal stump is left behind, recurrent stones have recurred in the ductal stump.

Neural Injury

Several structures should be identified and protected during surgery of the submandibular compartment. The mandibular branch of the facial nerve, which passes on the undersurface of the platysma superficial to the facial vessels at the mandibular notch, is vulnerable to submandibular incisions along the surface of the gland. Injury to the branch results in partial paralysis of the orbicularis oris muscle. The hypoglossal nerve passes beneath the posterior belly of the digastric muscle along the surface of the hypoglossus muscle. It runs close to the lingual veins and may be injured if obscured by bleeding during surgery. Injury to this nerve leads to ipsilateral paralysis of the tongue. The lingual nerve is located at the uppermost surface of the gland beneath the mandible, and this nerve also may be injured during surgery, resulting in anesthesia of the anterior two thirds of the tongue. The facial artery crosses through the submandibular gland to reach the mandibular notch. It is important to ligate this vessel beneath the posterior belly of the digastric muscle where it leaves the external carotid artery as well as at the mandibular notch. Loss of control of the facial artery can be followed by vigorous bleeding. Persistent ooze from numerous branches of the facial vein may result in hematoma formation. Hemorrhage that occurs within the operative wound during the first few postoperative hours, whether in parotid or submandibular surgery, leads to swelling and extreme pain. In this instance, pressure dressings and wound drain irrigation are not helpful. Instead, the patient should be returned to the operating room and the wound reexplored. Once the vulnerable nerves (facial, hypoglossal, or lingual) are identified and protected, points of bleeding can be located and ligated. The vessels to be looked for in the submandibular compartment have been described previously. The vessels of the parotid area are the external carotid artery and its maxillary and superficial temporal branches, the retromandibular vein (posterior facial), and its tributaries.

First and foremost, it is quite clear that injury to the lingual nerve or hypoglossal nerve should not occur in a submandibular gland resection. I have not yet seen direct injury to the lingual nerve or hypoglossal nerve during resection of the submandibular gland. I believe the technique that I have described allows for adequate identification of these structures, and this is a key to prevention of injury of the nerves. In a routine submandibular gland resection, the hypoglossal nerve, in fact, lies deep to the plane of resection and should not be injured unless the anatomic planes of that nerve are violated or if it is not identified in the submental triangle where it lies in position to the submandibular duct. The lingual nerve is easily preserved as a matter of routine. Once the submandibular gland is mobilized inferiorly, superiorly, and posteriorly, the gland can be retracted inferiorly, and with it, the lingual nerve is drawn down under the mandible and can be easily identified where the submandibular ganglion enters into the submandibular gland itself.

Since at this time I have not had an experience with nerve injury, I can only state that if I were to inadvertently transect either of these nerves, I would simply manage it by repair with a microneural suture as described for the facial nerve. I would point out that the hypoglossal nerve is a pure motor nerve and should, in fact, if reanastomosed properly, provide excellent recovery of 12th nerve motor function on that side. My concern with lingual nerve repair would be centered primarily around neuroma formation and possible paresthesias accompanying the nerve repair. Nevertheless, again I would immediately perform a microneural anastomosis of the severed ends using a good surgical technique.

Sialorrhea

I have had limited experience with the management of sialorrhea. In those limited cases, I have used what I consider to be the best management based on the literature. My approach has centered around bilateral excision of the submandibular glands and then rerouting of the parotid ducts to the tonsillar fossa. This is accomplished by using a buccal flap that encompasses the parotid duct opening and is turned inward. This flap extends from the duct opening to the anterior tonsillar pillar. The goal is to reroute parotid secretions into the tonsillar fossa so that the direction of the flow will be immediately into the oropharynx. My personal experience with this is so limited that I cannot give the reader an adequate idea of the outcome of this approach in a large number of cases, but it seems to have improved the patient with intense sialorrhea. I would refer the reader to the experience of others who have dealt with this problem in a greater number of patients than I have.

REFERENCES

1. Young AG: Unilateral sweating of the submental region after eating (chorda tympani syndrome). *Br Med J* 1956; 2:976–979.
2. Haxton HA: Gustatory sweating. *Brain* 1948; 71:16–25.
3. Singleton GT, Cassisi NJ: Frey's syndrome: Incidence related to skin flap thickness in parotidectomy. *Laryngoscope* 1980; 90:1636–1639.
4. King GD: Complications in the management of surgical disease of the major salivary glands. *Surg Clin North Am* 1968; 3:477–482.
5. Summers GW: Physiologic problems following ablative surgery of the head and neck. *Otol Clin North Am* 1974; 7:217–250.
6. Woods JE, Chong GC, Beahrs OH: Experience with 1,360 parotid tumors. *Am J Surg* 1975; 130:460–462.
7. Minor V: Eines neues verfahren zu der klinischen untersuchung der schweissab-sonderung. *Dtsch Z Nervenheilkunde* 1927; 101:302.
8. Laage-Hellman JE: Gustatory sweating and flushing after conservative parotidectomy. *Acta Otolaryngol (Stockh)* 1957; 48:234–252.
9. Glaister DH, Hearnshaw JR, Heffron PF, et al: The mechanism of postparotidectomy gustatory sweating (the auriculo-temporal syndrome). *Br Med J* 1958; 2:942–946.
10. Spiro RH, Martin H: Gustatory sweating following parotid surgery and radical neck dissection. *Ann Surg* 1967; 165:118–172.
11. Gordon AB, Fiddian RV: Frey's syndrome after parotid surgery. *Am J Surg* 1976; 132:54–58.
12. Hay CL, Novack AJ, Worsham JC: The Frey syndrome: A simple effective treatment. *Otolaryngol Head Neck Surg* 1982; 90:419–425.
13. Goldwin-Wood PH: Tympanic neurectomy. *J Laryngol Otol* 1962; 76:683–693.
14. Parisier SC, Binder WJ, Blitzer A, et al: Evaluation of tympanic neurectomy and chorda tympanectomy for gustatory sweating and benign salivary gland disease. *Ear Nose Throat J* 1978; 57:51–73.
15. Sessions RB, Roark DT, Alford BR: Frey's syndrome: A technical remedy. *Ann Otol Rhinol Laryngol* 1976; 84:734–739.
16. Friedman WH, Pomarico JM: Intratympanic correction of Frey's syndrome. *Arch Surg* 1974; 108:366–368.
17. Smith RO, Hemenway WG, Stevens KM, et al: Jacobson's neurectomy for Frey's syndrome. *Am J Surg* 1970; 120:478–481.
18. Wallis KA, Gibson T: Gustatory sweating following parotidectomy: Correction by a fascia lata graft. *Br J Plast Surg* 1978; 31:68–71.
19. Ananthakrishnan N, Parkash S: Parotid fistulas: A review. *Br J Surg* 1982; 69:641–643.
20. Burch RJ: Spontaneous closure of parotid gland fistulae with the aid of banthine: Report of a case. *Oral Surg* 1953; 6:1191–1194.
21. Cecil AB, Martin GW: Banthine as an adjunct in the treatment of salivary fistulae. *Am J Surg* 1956; 91:421–422.
22. Spiro RH, Huvos AG, Strong EW: Cancer of the parotid gland. *Am J Surg* 1975; 130:452–459.
23. Marsh WL, Allen MS: Adenoid cystic carcinoma: Biologic behavior in 38 patients. *Cancer* 1979; 43:1463–1473.
24. Eneroth CM, Hamberger CA: Principles of treatment of different types of parotid tumors. *Laryngoscope* 1974; 84:1732–1740.
25. Bjorkland A, Eneroth CM: Management of parotid gland neoplasms. *Am J Otolaryngol* 1980; 1:155–167.

Management of the Primary Site: Salivary Glands

Arpproach of

Roger Boles, M.D.

THE PAROTID GLAND

Facial Nerve

Our practice at the University of California at San Francisco (UCSF) has been to preserve the facial nerve whenever possible when it is not grossly or functionally involved by tumor, even with the tumors that are known to propagate along nerves. Our rationale for this is that postoperative radiation therapy in such cases adds the most important additional therapeutic dimension to the cure of such difficult cases and that the minimal additional margin achieved by facial nerve sacrifice does not generate enough enhancement in the overall potential cure rate of these relentless tumors to justify the major functional and cosmetic deficits that such sacrifice creates. Although facial nerve grafting can be expected to compensate for some of these deficits, our experience with such grafts, which are subjected to intensive radiation therapy for the truly malignant tumors as soon after surgery as possible, are not nearly as successful as some other clinical and laboratory reports have suggested, and certainly not as successful as grafts not exposed to high-dose radiation therapy. We use the following criteria for sacrificing the facial nerve during parotidectomy:

1. Malignant tumors have invaded the nerve, causing a preoperative facial paresis or paralysis.

2. Malignant tumors have clearly invaded the nerve or cannot be surgically separated from the nerve even when preoperative facial paresis or paralysis does not exist.

3. Locally aggressive and invasive "benign" tumors cannot be surgically separated from the nerve for complete removal such as certain locally aggressive or invasive pleomorphic adenomas (especially those that have recurred in more aggressive forms than original tumors); rare, locally aggressive and invasive "giant cell tumors" surrounding the nerve; and large cosmetically conspicuous neurogenous tumors of the nerve that involve the less important peripheral branches (frontal and buccal) that can be grafted with fair success.

4. Potentially surgically curable tumor (either malignant or locally aggressive and invasive benign) persists following previous definitive surgery and radiation therapy, and nothing less than a wide-field block resection of the parotid area has a chance for cure.

5. Except for "locally aggressive" and "invasive" recurrent pleomorphic adenomas that are immediately adjacent to or are, in fact, invading the facial nerve, I do not sacrifice the facial nerve for recurrent mixed tumors. For the most part, I consider the excision of most recurrent pleomorphic adenomas "cosmetic surgery" and not as curative treatment, since most recurrent tumors continue to recur. Sacrificing the facial nerve in these cases tends to create more of a cosmetic problem than the tumor itself and, in general, does not lead to longer life for the patient.

Facial Nerve Injury

Intraoperative Recognition.—The main trunk of the facial nerve has a highly consistent and identifiable position as it emerges from the stylomastoid foramen at the base of the skull. This foramen lies immediately posterior to the attachment of the styloid process at the base of the skull and lies directly in the line of the tympanomastoid suture line. These structures are easily identifiable in the majority of parotid surgery cases and reduce greatly the alternative hazards of randomly trying to locate the facial nerve in the posterior part of the parotid gland.

Should the extent of disease at the skull base obviate safe or efficient identification of the main trunk of the nerve at the outset of the procedure, the peripheral branches of the nerve are usually easily identifiable. These branches can be dissected in a retrograde fashion to the pes anserinus. The zygomaticofrontal branches are usually quite superficial in the region of the zygomatic arch, and the buccal branch is usually in close parallel proximity to the parotid duct as it emerges from the front of the gland. The ramus mandibularus usually crosses lateral to the posterior facial vein in the inferior portion of the parotid and can be found by identifying this vein in the upper portion of the neck and following it upward into the gland. In my experience, this latter inferior approach is the most difficult and the most hazardous because of the very small size of this ramus and the risk of damaging it before one finds it.

The most reliable way to avoid injury to the facial nerve is to clearly identify it anatomically early in any parotid procedure and to dissect it anatomically under direct vision throughout the procedure. The operating microscope may be helpful in identifying the nerve when it is obscured by scar tissue in a previously operated, heavily infected, or radiated surgical field.

Intraoperative electrical facial nerve stimulation can be helpful in identifying the facial nerve when there is uncertainty of the anatomic position of the nerve or when it is obscured by tumor or scar tissue. We have recently been experimenting with intraoperative nerve monitoring by recording continuously from electrodes in the facial muscles, as has been successfully reported in acoustic neuroma surgery. Although this appealing technique has been helpful in identifying the nerve in situations of heavy scarring, in general, visual and anatomic identification and dissection of the nerve have been the unsurpassed method for preserving and protecting this structure.

The use of bipolar instead of unipolar cautery for hemostasis in the parotid wound has theoretic potential for lessening thermal injury to the facial nerve.

Intraoperative recognition of facial nerve injury during parotid surgery is most simply and reliably accomplished by direct visualization of anatomic disruption, usually at the immediate time of injury at any point of dissection. Electrical stimulation of the nerve and its branches is an adjunct to confirming anatomic integrity, although it may leave uncertainty in cases of neuropraxia. The facial nerve monitoring technique of electrically recording from facial muscles permits a more quantifiable estimate of intraoperative facial nerve function and permits a much smaller and safer electrical stimulus of the exposed nerve being tested. Almost every recognizable intraoperative anatomic disruption of the main divisions and branches of the facial nerve is corrected by surgical anastomosis or grafting using 8-0 to 10-0 suture material with the operating microscope.

Postoperative Recognition.—Very seldom should postoperative recognition of facial nerve injury come as a surprise to the surgeon if careful intraoperative confirmation of nerve integrity and function has been established. Since many patients have varying degrees of paresis postoperatively despite excellent anatomic integrity of the nerve, the presence of postoperative paresis alone is generally not a very reliable indicator of nerve disruption that needs repair. The only such cases of postoperative recognition of nerve injuries I have had to deal with are those referred by surgeons who were uncertain about injury at the time of surgery and did not check the nerve electrically or who believed the nerve was left perfectly intact as they did the procedure but failed to confirm this anatomically at the end of the operation. Early reoperation of such cases is, of course, the most reliable way to check the integrity of the nerve, to make any surgical corrections before the nerve and field become too heavily scarred, and while electrical excitability of any distal cut branches can still be exploited for help

in anatomic identification. Any reoperation carries the risk of further injury to an already compromised nerve, and the patient should be fully informed of this risk as weighed against the possible benefits of reoperation. The alternative to immediate reoperation would be serial percutaneous electrical testing and, after 2 weeks, electromyography of facial muscles to aid in the clinical decision of whether to reexplore the nerve. Certainly, failure to recover any facial nerve function after 1 year or so in cases in which the main trunk or the primary divisions were thought to be injured is indication to reexplore the nerve and attempt repair, if the patient is willing. Such delayed repairs do not carry the same chances of functional recovery that early repairs do.

Role of Frozen Section and Fine-Needle Aspiration Cytology in Parotid Tumors

Fine-needle aspiration of masses in general in the parotid region has been helpful in my practice. It has been especially helpful to patients in their own understanding and decision making about the management of their parotid problems. In the hands of our cytologists, it has been 85% accurate. It has been especially accurate in identifying lymphomas and Warthin's tumors, both tumors for which we might not elect to proceed with full parotidectomy. It has also been helpful in distinguishing between inflammatory and neoplastic lesions and in demonstrating cysts.

In cases demonstrated to be malignant neoplasms, FNA of incidental lymph nodes in the neck has been occasionally helpful in deciding whether to do a neck dissection along with removal of the primary parotid tumor. When the FNA of the parotid tumor has demonstrated squamous cell carcinoma, a search for another primary focus in the head and neck has been intensified, including, in some instances, "blind" biopsies of suspected primary sites. In general, FNA of parotid tumors has facilitated comprehensive diagnosis and treatment planning by our institutional interdisciplinary head and neck tumor team before the involved parotid region has been surgically disrupted. It has also facilitated, in many instances, a more accurate and better informed preoperative discussion with the patient, particularly with regard to preparing the patient for various intraoperative surgical options in the cases of malignant tumors (e.g., possible facial nerve sacrifice and possible neck dissection in larger more invasive tumors or should metastatic nodes be found intraoperatively in the upper part of the neck that were not palpable preoperatively).

Since the popularization of FNA cytology technique in this country over the past 5 to 10 years, I have not found it necessary to use the frozen section technique nearly so often except to establish whether metastatic disease was present in nearby regional lymph nodes in the surgical field. I do, however, ask for a frozen section reading on any tumor that, in my judgment, requires sacrifice of the facial nerve for resection and where preoperatively there was no clinical facial weakness, even though the FNA had preoperatively suggested a malignant tumor. I ask the cytologist who did the preoperative FNA to participate in this frozen section reading.

Definitive postoperative radiation therapy for parotid tumors in our institution is not determined until after permanent sections of the resected tumor are read and reported by the pathologist. Palliative radiation therapy has been given on the basis of FNA cytology for advanced, inoperable malignant tumors.

Approach to Deep Lobe Tumors

I believe deep lobe parotid tumors are still a rather unsettled issue for which there remains a rather wide range of opinions regarding the clinicopathologic nature of these lesions as well as the therapeutic approaches to them. Better approaches to these tumors are evolving, and the advent of new diagnostic scanning and imaging techniques is supporting these changes with their ability to so elegantly describe the exact size and location of these tumors, as well as their relationships with other important surrounding structures.

Fine-needle aspiration cytology of these tumors, sometimes done under CT control, has also added to our pretreatment information base and has given our interdisciplinary head and neck tumor team, as well as the patient, a sharper perspective of the problem.

One problem with deep lobe parotid tumors is that they tend to be fairly large by the time they are clinically discovered. They are also relatively inaccessible and are in association with important deep structures, particularly the carotid sheath and its contents. By their very location, they are seldom resectable with generous margins. They carry an important differential diagnosis of parapharyngeal space masses, which must be carefully and accurately differentiated before treatment is undertaken.

Most deep lobe tumors in my experience have been benign mixed tumors, which have not recurred despite minimal margins. I have routinely given postoperative radiation therapy for all malignant deep lobe tumors. I have also given radiation therapy for recurrent mixed tumors in which the patients have been considered poor candidates for resection or in which the nature of the tumor has been clinically aggressive and invasive.

Resection of most deep lobe tumors can be satisfactorily and safely achieved through an extended standard parotidectomy approach with initial exposure of the facial nerve, followed by a submandibular approach to the parapharyngeal space with identification and isolation of the great vessels and nerves in this area. Occasionally this simpler approach does not give adequate access to the parapharyngeal space, especially with larger tumors, and the patients should always be asked preoperatively for their consent to permit mandibulotomy as a surgical option in these more difficult cases. Lateral mandibulotomy at the angle of the mandible has served me well for exposing the parapharyngeal space. Anterior mandibulotomy is a more attractive option when postoperative radiation therapy is anticipated for malignant tumors. Preoperative FNA cytology can be helpful in deciding on these mandibulotomy options.

Approach to the N0 Neck

Elective neck dissection has not traditionally been considered a part of the surgical management of parotid malignancies except possibly for the larger tumors and for those that have extended into the upper part of the neck. In these latter instances in which neck dissection is elected, most head and neck surgeons today are tending to modify the operation to some degree to preserve as much function as possible. I have been inclined to follow this surgical practice. In the higher-risk malignant tumors, however, the entire ipsilateral neck is irradiated postoperatively along with the primary. This has seemed to control the neck pretty well. In our experience at UCSF, very few patients failed to have their disease controlled in the neck alone with this approach to management. Almost every patient who has developed uncontrolled disease in the neck has also failed control of the primary site in the parotid.

Frey's Syndrome

Frey's syndrome has not been a common problem in my experience and least of all a problem requiring any sort of remedy. The application of common antiperspirants to the affected area once or twice daily has seemed to satisfy the needs of the few patients I have known who had a particularly troublesome problem with gustatory sweating. I have never performed an operative procedure for this problem, nor have I felt the need to.

Salivary Fistula

In my entire career, I have seen only one persistent salivary fistula that did not subside spontaneously, and it was in a patient who had had parotid surgery 1 year previously in Europe. It was corrected by simple local excision. Because all salivary gland tissue is not entirely removed in most parotid surgery, these wounds tend to be a bit wetter than most and may occasionally accumulate fluid beneath the flaps for 1 to several weeks postoperatively. Simple periodic evacuation of this fluid by needle aspiration or by sterile probing of the wound has always managed this problem satisfactorily until gradual, complete spontaneous resolution occurs.

I do believe that the removal of as much parotid tissue as possible, without jeopardizing the anatomic integrity of the facial nerve, probably reduces the odds of having troublesome postoperative secretion of saliva into the wound. It also widens the margin of resection of the pathologic process and theoretically has the potential for removing possible multiple foci of mixed or other tumors. In my experience, this additional resectional work does not add more than 15 to 20 minutes at most to the primary operative procedure and, in most instances, is worth the effort.

Nonneoplastic Conditions of the Parotid Gland

Sjögren's Syndrome

Sjögren's syndrome is a benign condition that may involve the parotid gland but seldom requires surgical management. Occasionally the parotid gland afflicted with Sjögren's syndrome will enlarge to unsightly proportions, and some patients may wish to have such a gland removed for cosmetic reasons.

Another complication of Sjögren's syndrome of the parotid that occasionally occurs is recurrent or chronic suppurative parotitis as an infected end stage of sialectasis. I believe surgical removal of such glands is better done earlier in the course of such an infectious pattern than later, before abscess formation and fibrosis have had much of a chance to develop and have increased the technical difficulty of a parotid resection. A total parotidectomy is indicated in such end-stage sialectatic suppurative disease, leaving no residual infected pockets of salivary gland tissue behind to continue a suppurative clinical problem. I have not found sialography helpful to me in deciding whether to operate on this condition.

Chronic Sialadenitis

Chronic sialadenitis in children and adolescents is usually quite a different problem from chronic sialadenitis in adults. In children and adolescents, it is seldom due to the obstructive effects of stones and strictures and almost never due to end-stage Sjögren's syndrome. It does seem to be frequently associated with a sialectasis. It tends to differ in behavior from sialadenitis of adults in that it frequently disappears spontaneously following puberty, particularly if the suppuration during childhood and early adolescence is well controlled by antibiotics. Occasionally, such sialadenitis will break from control of antibiotics in childhood and will require total parotidectomy.

Adult chronic sialadenitis, on the contrary, is usually secondary to stones or strictures in the duct or is part of end-stage lymphoepithelial disease. Stones and strictures in the parotid duct are not easily managed by conservative procedures as a rule and, therefore, often require removal of the secondarily infected parotid gland by total parotidectomy. Again, I prefer to resort to parotidectomy in these chronic or frequently recurring parotid infections earlier in their course rather than later after fibrosis and abscess formation have had a chance to develop and to create a much more difficult surgical procedure.

Acute Parotitis Not Responding to Antibiotics

This condition occurs most commonly from dehydration in debilitated patients. It may, of course, develop as already mentioned secondary to stone or stricture or as an acute exascerbation of chronic sialectatic disease, such as in Sjögren's syndrome. In any of these instances, it is important to obtain culture and antibiotic sensitivity studies on any pus expressible from the parotid duct to have the antibiotic coverage of the infection as specific as possible. These antibiotics, of course, should also be given in high doses intravenously along with an aggressive hydration program. When such acute infections fail to respond completely under this aggressive medical therapy, and, indeed, when they begin to become worse instead of better while the patient is on therapy, especially with abscess formation, surgical intervention becomes mandatory. The clinical signs of increasing pain, swelling, and fever are often quite obvious in such cases. More subtle signs are a persistent doughy quality to the swollen parotid with pitting edema, as well as persistent pus from the duct.

Most such infections diffusely involve all parts of the gland.

This necessitates wide exposure of the entire gland through a modified Blair incision and with elevation of a cheek flap as in a standard approach to parotidectomy. Multiple stab wounds throughout the entire parotid can be made with a fine mosquito hemostat, opening the instrument gently in the direction of the facial nerve to minimize injury to the nerve. Several 1/4 or 1/2 in. Penrose drains should then be left throughout the wound for 5 to 7 days and brought out through the loosely closed Blair incision. Any frank pus recovered from this drainage procedure should be submitted for culture and sensitivity studies and antibiotic therapy modified accordingly.

In the case of an unresolved acute infection due to a large stone or as part of a picture of recurring acute infections from either obstructive or nonobstructive disease, total parotidectomy could be elected at this stage of acute infection. In most of such cases, parotidectomy will eventually become necessary, and stopping with only incision and drainage will give fibrosis more of a chance to develop and make subsequent parotidectomy more difficult.

Sialolithiasis

Sialolithiasis in general usually presents as obstructive parotid swelling that is characteristically worse with meals or with salivary stimulation. Most of the time the stones can be seen at the duct orifice in the mouth or palpated in the course of the duct over the masseter muscle. Hilar stones are more difficult to identify, and it is said that only one half of them are radiopaque on standard x-ray films. They all are usually dense enough to be seen by CT scan.

Stones that are in the oral part of the duct can be removed either by manual expression or by surgically opening the duct orifice to release them. Less accessible stones farther back in the duct, particularly in the hilum of the gland, are seldom extractable through the mouth. They usually require parotidectomy with removal of the duct and stone, especially if they are causing too much trouble with secondary obstructive symptoms or infection.

SUBMANDIBULAR GLAND

Neoplastic Conditions

About one half of all submandibular salivary gland tumors are malignant, and malignancies in this gland tend to behave more aggressively than they do in other salivary glands. It is especially important, therefore, that surgical planning for lesions of the submandibular gland, which are potentially malignant, include all of the possible aggressive surgical options that might be required to satisfactorily extirpate the lesions. Whereas for some of the more common disorders of this gland with which malignant tumors can sometimes be confused, such as sialolithiasis and chronic sialadenitis, simple excision of the gland will suffice, such a limited procedure is rarely, if ever, adequate surgery for a malignant tumor of the gland. To plan properly before any surgery of this gland in which there is any diagnostic doubt preoperatively, one can use FNA biopsy to reduce much of the dilemma regarding the most appropriate initial surgical approach and to make it possible to better prepare the patient for all of the surgical options and contingencies. Preoperative diagnostic imaging and scanning have also been very helpful in determining the full size and extent of the lesion in preoperative treatment planning.

As with parotid tumors, the surgical goal in submandibular tumors should be gross total removal of all disease. For smaller benign tumors, it may require only simple excision of the gland. For larger benign tumors and for smaller malignant tumors, it will require at least a suprahyoid neck dissection. For malignant tumors of greater size and extent, particularly those involving the lingual and hypoglossal nerves and other adjacent structures, adequate excision may require a composite resection with sacrifice of involved cranial nerves and with an en bloc neck dissection.

An en block neck dissection should probably always be done in the interest of better surgical margins for larger tumors and for those extending into surrounding tissues, even in the absence of palpable nodes. In such necks, the operation can often be modified to spare function. If results of the preoperative FNA are equivocal, intraoperative frozen section biopsy will usually resolve the issue of how to proceed surgically. Postoperative radiation therapy is given to the entire primary site and to the ipsilateral neck for all malignancies except for the smallest of the low-grade acinar and mucoepidermoid carcinomas. If the adjacent cranial nerves are involved, radiation therapy should encompass the full course of these nerves through the skull base.

Sialolithiasis

Proximal Stone

For orientation, I will define a proximal stone as one that is in the more oral portion of the submandibular duct; that is, more proximal to the surgeon and the mouth than to the more distal salivary gland itself. The distal stone I will define as the stone that is in the more posterior part of the duct, usually in the hilum of the gland itself.

Stones that are in the more anterior or oral portion of the submandibular duct may be removed intraorally under local anesthesia if they are no more than 2 cm back from the duct orifice. The duct can be surgically opened from the duct orifice back to the stone if the stone is within 1 cm or so of the orifice. I usually first pass a lacrimal probe into the duct back to the stone and then incise with a scalpel blade down onto the intraaductal probe. If the stone is more than 1 cm but less than 2 cm posterior to the duct orifice, I usually press the stone upward into the mouth by digital pressure on the submandibular skin and then directly incise down on the uplifted stone and extrude it through the small overlying mucosal incision. This occasionally creates a persistent new salivary fistula posterior to the natural duct orifice that works physiologically as well as the natural duct orifice.

Not infrequently, a number of smaller stones will follow a larger stone. In fact, multiple and recurrent stones, in my experience, tend to be the rule rather than the exception, and I

inform the patients of this to prepare them for possible future such episodes.

Distal Stones

I have made it a general rule not to try to remove intraorally proximal stones that are more than 2 cm posterior to the duct orifice. Beyond 2 cm, the duct is crossed superiorly by the lingual nerve and the lingual artery, and inadvertent injury to these two structures may occur when the duct is incised in the posterior part of the mouth to deliver a stone. To remove these more posterior stones as well as hilar stones, I remove the entire gland and duct through an external submandibular approach.

Some patients elect to keep their stones in situ rather than to have an operation, particularly if they are not too symptomatic and have not been complicated by severe secondary suppurative sialadenitis. I admonish such patients to seek early, aggressive antibiotic therapy for any subsequent severe swelling and discomfort that does not subside spontaneously within 48 hours.

Neural Injury

The problem of lingual nerve injury from intraoral approaches to submandibular duct stones was addressed earlier. Injury to either the lingual or hypoglossal nerves is much less likely when the elective external approach to benign conditions of the gland is used because of proper surgical exposure and direct identification of these structures in the field. In most instances of elective surgical removal of the submandibular gland for benign conditions, the lingual nerve will be encountered and will have to be dissected from the gland and duct. The hypoglossal nerve will usually not have to be exposed.

Should these nerves be inadvertently severed, they should be reapproximated immediately using standard neurorrhaphy techniques. With proper repair, reasonably good function recovery should result, particularly since each of these nerves carries pure sensory and pure motor neurones, respectively, and every bit of neuronal regeneration should result in some functional recovery.

Plunging Ranula

Large mucous and salivary retention cysts of the floor of the mouth that insinuate themselves deeply and extensively throughout the floor of mouth structures are often referred to as plunging ranulas. These may become so large as to displace the tongue and make speaking and eating difficult. They may occasionally become secondarily infected. The exact duct or gland of origin is usually difficult or impossible to establish. Persistence or recurrence following surgical management is common. One very prominent head and neck surgeon once said, "Refer all ranulas to your worst enemy." Simple surgical marsupialization into the mouth is worth an initial try on the basis that if one is going to fail, it might as well be with the simplest, least morbid procedure. Laser may work out to be more efficient for this purpose than more traditional surgical techniques. If a more extensive intraoral excisional attempt is made, one must be very careful not to injure the lingual and hypoglossal nerves or to lose control of the lingual artery. For such large dissections, I prefer the external submandibular approach for better exposure, for more precise control of critical nerves and vessels, and for a more thorough dissection of the region. Even with this, high failure rates can be anticipated, and one may have to resort to periodic local reduction procedures as symptoms demand.

SIALORRHEA

In my entire career, I have encountered sialorrhea as a significant clinical problem only a few times. On the contrary, the opposite problem of too little saliva, for a variety of reasons, with all of its symptoms and sequelae, is one of the most common problems I have seen in my practice.

Sialorrhea can occasionally be a nursing problem in patients with strokes, cerebral palsy, and other neurologic disorders in which deglution or oral competency is impaired. Despite good nursing care in these patients, sialorrhea may create a skin maceration problem of the face that may lead one to consider surgical intervention to reduce the volume of saliva. In such cases, I prefer surgery to medication, since such anticholinergic agents carry so many unwanted and sometimes serious side effects in these patients. I believe the simplest and most efficient procedure to bring the majority of sialorrhea cases under reasonable control is denervation of the submandibular salivary glands by tympantomy and division of the chorda tympani nerves. This technique carries the disadvantage of loss of taste from the anterior two thirds of the tongue, but under the rare circumstances of such surgery, I believe the efficiency and effectiveness of this procedure for resolving the sialorrhea problem outweigh the often unquantifiable problem of dysgeusia in these patients.

Additional denervation of the parotid glands by disruption of the tympanic plexus on the promontory is seldom necessary and does not generally have the permanency of dividing the chorda tympani nerve.

Radiation therapy, in my view, has little or no role in the management of sialorrhea since it usually requires a large dose to significantly diminish salivary production and carries with it significant morbidity and sequelae.

CHAPTER 21

Management of the Primary Site: Thyroid and Parathyroid

Approach of

Alfred D. Katz, M.D.

THYROID

Indications to perform thyroid surgery are hyperthyroidism, huge nodular goiters causing dyspnea or dysphagia, and nodules suspected of being cancerous. Patients with suspect nodules have fine-needle aspiration (FNAs) of their thyroid masses. They are divided into four groups: (1) those patients highly suspected of having malignancy (needle biopsy was 79% correct); (2) those with atypia; (3) patients with needle biopsy results showing follicular adenomas that did not regress while the patient was taking thyroid suppression (in this group follicular neoplasms could not be ruled out); and (4) patients with a history of childhood head and neck irradiation and follicular or colloid nodules that did not regress under thyroid suppression.

Total thyroidectomies are performed on the irradiation group because carcinoma may be found in the contralateral lobe as well as in the ipsilateral lobe. Forty percent of these patients have carcinoma but not necessarily in the dominant nodule.[1,2]

In groups 1, 2, and 3, one lobe of the thyroid is resected. The parathyroids and recurrent laryngeal nerves are identified and preserved. A frozen section of the dominant nodule or another suspicious area is obtained. If the diagnosis is carcinoma or suspected carcinoma, the contralateral thyroid lobe is resected, completing the total thyroidectomy. If the contralateral lobe has discrete nodules or thyroiditis, it is removed even if the primary side is benign.

A total thyroidectomy is performed on well-differentiated thyroid carcinoma. If a subtotal thyroidectomy is performed because the original frozen section is reported as benign but permanent section reveals carcinoma, the patient is returned to the operating room the following day or 2 days later to resect the remaining thyroid tissue, completing a total thyroidectomy. If an occult carcinoma of less than 1 cm is present, reoperation is then not deemed necessary.

If at surgery, metastatic carcinoma to cervical nodes is found, a modified neck dissection is performed. This includes stripping the nodes from the supraclavicular area to the base of the skull. The thyroid incision is enlarged, counterincisions in the upper part of the neck are made so that the dissection can be completed. The sternocleidomastoid muscle, the internal jugular vein, and the submaxillary gland are not resected. A bilateral neck dissection may be performed if necessary. A radical neck dissection is not performed unless the internal jugular vein or muscle is invaded.

For the past 2 years, in a pilot study, I have stripped internal jugular nodal tissue in patients when a diagnosis of thyroid carcinoma is made at surgery and no nodes are palpable. If during dissection, visual or palpable nodes are found, they are not included in this pilot series. The tissue removed includes the internal jugular nodal chain from the supraclavicular area to the carotid artery bifurcation on the involved side. In 19 patients, 8 to 20 nodes were identified on permanent section. Eleven patients had metastatic carcinoma in these nodes. The significance of this can be determined only in an ongoing long-term survival study.

The usual follow-up of patients with well-differentiated thyroid carcinoma is treatment with iodine 131. A 5 mCi ^{131}I baseline scan is performed approximately 6 weeks following surgery. The patient is given liothyronine (Cytomel) for 4 weeks following surgery. This medication is then stopped 2 weeks prior to the dose of ^{131}I. A neck, chest, and body scan is performed 2 to

3 days following the 5 mCi dose. If any functioning thyroid tissue is present, a therapeutic dose of 100 mCi of ^{131}I is then given. This routinely requires 2 days of hospitalization to comply with radiation safety regulations. A posttherapy ^{131}I scan is performed 5 to 7 days later.

Follow-up Intervals

A 1-year follow-up is routinely recommended. However, if there was evidence of extensive disease and or tumor left behind, a 6-month follow-up is recommended. Once there have been two entirely normal follow-up studies at 1-year intervals, a 2-year follow-up is recommended. After two additional follow-ups, periodic checkups at 3-year intervals are recommended.

Thallium 201 is currently being evaluated and compared with ^{131}I imaging and thyroglobulin measurements for following thyroid cancer patients. Thyroglobulin is measured in conjunction with follow-up ^{131}I scans. At the present time, patients are offered a thallium neck and chest scan, which is correlated with the other studies. The thallium scan is performed prior to withdrawal of the thyroid hormone. Iodine 131 studies are performed with the patient off levothyroxine (Synthroid) therapy for 6 weeks and off liothyronine therapy for 2 weeks. A combination of thallium imaging and thyroglobulin in measurement may be substituted for ^{131}I scanning in the future.

Imaging Technique

Following either a 5 mCi dose of ^{131}I, a 3 mCi dose of ^{201}Tl, or a therapeutic dose of ^{131}I, imaging is performed for 15 minutes per view.

All thyroidectomy patients are placed on thyroid suppression after ^{131}I ablation. Levothyroxine or some other synthetic thyroid is given to tolerance. Triiodothyronine (T_3), thyroxine (T_4), and thyroid-stimulating hormone (TSH) levels are followed to determine optimal dosage. Thyroglobulin levels are obtained twice yearly.

Children with well-differentiated thyroid carcinoma are treated like the adults with ^{131}I and thyroid suppression. Patients with medullary carcinoma have total thyroidectomies and nodal dissections if nodes are palpable. Even though the C cells of the thyroid do not concentrate iodine, I still give ^{131}I postoperatively. Calcitonin levels are obtained every 6 months. Radiation is given if there is unresectable residual tumor. The same procedure is used for papillary or follicular carcinoma.

Anaplastic carcinoma is quite rare. Out of 1,265 total thyroidectomies performed, of which there were 439 carcinomas, less than 1% were anaplastic carcinoma. No patients with anaplastic carcinoma lived more than 18 months. In these patients, as much carcinoma was resected as possible with a radical neck dissection, and postoperative radiation was then given. Cisplatin is added with the radiation.

Recurrent Laryngeal Nerve Injury

There is potential danger to the recurrent laryngeal nerves any time the neck and thyroid bed are explored. In surgery, the morbidity documented in the literature ranges from 0.25% to 10% and reveals the extent of danger to the recurrent laryngeal nerve.[3, 4]

The classic anatomic laryngeal pathway fails to outline the many anomalies and the vast variations this nerve follows. Nearly all recurrent laryngeal nerves bifurcate less than 0.5 cm from the cricoid cartilage. Therefore, to have a meaningful statistic as to where the nerves are in danger during surgery, the fixed point in the cricoid cartilage and only nerves bifurcating at a point greater than 0.5 cm from that point are included in this discussion.

In all thyroid or parathyroid surgery, the recurrent laryngeal nerve is visualized along much of its length before any tissue is removed. For the past few years, we have visualized the recurrent laryngeal nerves and measured any bifurcations. We observed 721 recurrent laryngeal nerves in 400 patients, 421 (58%) bifurcated or trifurcated into extralaryngeal of more than 0.5 cm from the cricoid, and 97 patients (24%) who had bilateral recurrent laryngeal nerve bifurcation. Ten patients had trifurcations, seven of which were on the left side. Six patients had direct (nonrecurrent) laryngeal nerves, all on the right side, one of which also had a recurrent laryngeal combination. One direct laryngeal nerve bifurcated. Two patients had recurrent laryngeal nerves on the right side with direct branches from the vagus nerve. These fibers joined the recurrent laryngeal nerve at 6 cm and 13.5 cm from the cricoid. Of the bifurcating nerves, 75% had major division anterior to the cricoid cartilage, 10% were posterior, and 15% were equally divided.[4] These statistics are given to show the variations found and the potential danger to the nerves in the surgical dissection (Figs 21–1 to 21–3).

Since most of the paralyzed cords are in the midline, it is surmised that the smaller posterior division where the nerve and vessels enter the muscle is the portion damaged. Despite careful visualization and dissection with preservation of the recurrent laryngeal nerve in our series, there were 10 paralyzed vocal cords in more than 2,000 thyroid and parathyroid surgeries. This series includes 1,265 total thyroidectomies (Table 21–1). Our incidence of nerve damage, therefore, is about 0.25%. In three patients with huge nodular goiters, the nerves were enveloped by tumor. The nerve endings were cleaned and reanastomosed using 6-0 silk. No motor function ever recurred. In the other seven patients, the branches of the recurrent nerve were visualized and preserved. There were no ties around nearby vessels. Most of these injured nerves were on the right, and therefore, the assumption is that aberrant branches from the vagus to the recurrent, as were found in two patients, were the destroyed elements causing the damage. It is reported in the literature that if a vocal cord is paralyzed, as soon as it is recognized, the nerve area should be reexplored postoperatively. Any ties that may envelope the nerve can be removed.[5] It is far easier to prevent recurrent laryngeal nerve injury than to repair it. If a cord is paralyzed in the midline, there is little loss of quality or strength. If it is in the abducted position, as in two of our patients, injection of Teflon is used. The two patients have had excellent results with good voice return.

Occasionally, patients are seen postoperatively who have dysphagia for an inordinate amount of time. This might be

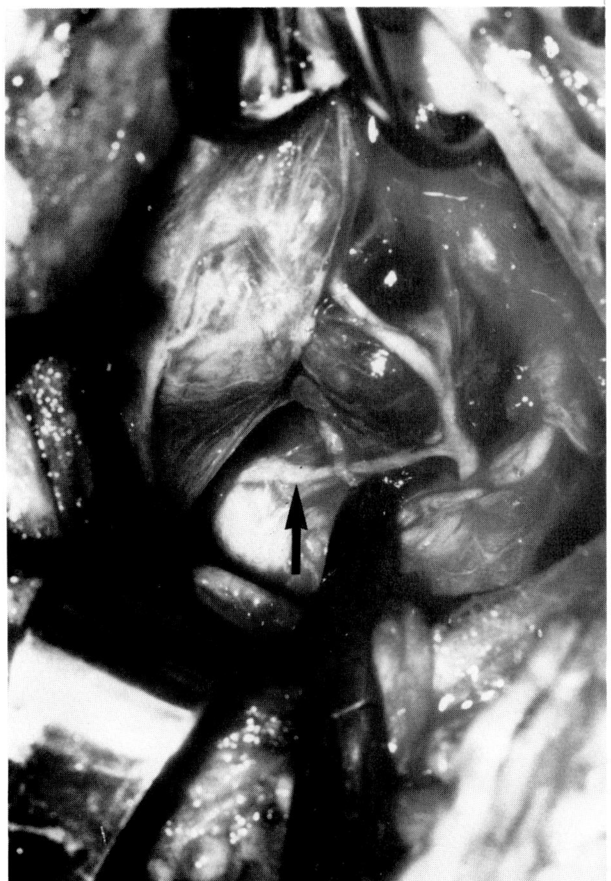

FIG 21–1.
Recurrent laryngeal nerve with the arrow pointing to the branch from the vagus nerve to the recurrent laryngeal nerve 13.5 cm from the cricoid.

explained by damage to the esophageal branches from the recurrent laryngeal nerve. Dissection of recurrent laryngeal nerves have shown a wide variation among patients of the branches to the esophagus. The plexes visualized usually are seen on the left side. The most severe cases of postoperative dysphagia usually involve parathyroid reoperations and not thyroids. During a parathyroid reoperation, the tracheoesophageal groove and esophagus in the retroesophageal area are carefully dissected, looking for parathyroid tumor. The recurrent laryngeal nerves are always identified and are carefully retracted. However, there may be undue tension on the small filament plexes, causing damage.

Management of Devascularized Parathyroid Gland: Parathyroid Autotransplantation

Whenever total thyroidectomy is performed, and no matter how meticulous the surgeon, there are many anatomic pitfalls in parathyroid preservation. Intrathyroid parathyroid glands create the most difficult problems. They must be autotransplanted to be preserved; however, they are identified by the pathologist after he or she carefully sections the specimen, and by then, it is too late to transplant them. Two patients with total thyroidectomies were found to have three intrathyroid parathyroid glands; four patients had two intrathyroid parathyroid glands. About 2% of our patients had intrathyroid parathyroid glands.[6]

The variable and friable blood supply to the parathyroid glands in normocalcemic patients is another difficulty. The inferior thyroid artery is the predominant vascular supply to both the lower and upper parathyroid glands more than 86% of the time.[7] This may explain why viable parathyroid glands at surgery do not function at a later postoperative period. Ligation or dam-

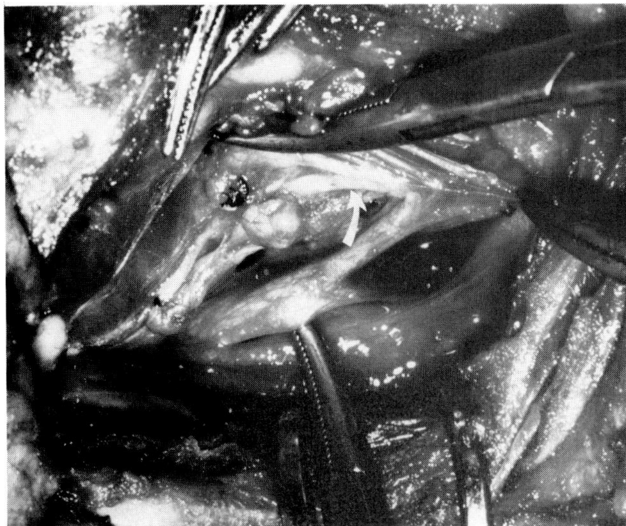

FIG 21–2.
Recurrent laryngeal nerve with the arrow pointing to the bifurcation of the nerve.

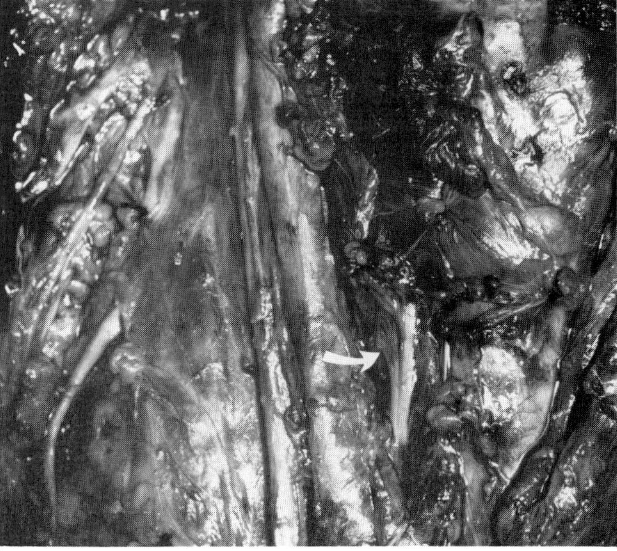

FIG 21–3.
Radical neck dissection and total thyroidectomy. Arrow points to the posterior branch of the recurrent laryngeal nerve (bifurcation 1.5 cm from cricoid).

TABLE 21–1.
1,265 Total Thyroidectomy Patients With 439 Carcinomas
of the Thyroid

	No. of Patients	No. of Carcinomas (%)
Hyperthyroid		
M	25	1
F	139	9
Total	164	10 (6%)
Irradiation		
M	77	30
F	195	75
Total	272	105 (38.6%)
Cold solid thyroid masses		
M	193	93
F	636	231
Total	829	324 (39%)

age to the artery during thyroid surgery may have a latent effect on the glands. Also, one or two viable parathyroid glands may not be sufficient for a patient to have normal calcium levels.

The normal weight of the parathyroid glands may be between 45.6 to 133.6 mg; 88% of normal glands weigh 20 to 49 mg.[7] Bulk tissue, one large normal, or many small parathyroid glands may be necessary for a normocalcemic patient. It should be stressed that when normal, viable parathyroid tissue is in situ, it should be preserved. However, when a hemorrhagic or dusky parathyroid gland is visualized, the capsule should be opened to decompress it to see if there is a viable blood supply. If there is no oozing or visible blood supply, the parathyroid should be removed and transplanted.[8] When a nonviable parathyroid gland is found, it is removed and kept sterile. If the patient preoperatively is known to be normocalcemic, the parathyroid tissue is transplanted into the sternocleidomastoid muscle. Hyperplastic parathyroid tissue should never be transplanted into muscle in the neck. It should be transplanted into the volar surface of the forearm. The tissue is cut into 0.5 to 1 mm size slices, a pocket is made in the muscle fibers, and a hemoclip is placed in the base of each pocket. Two or three slices of parathyroid tissue are placed into the muscle pocket, and the muscle is reapproximated with a figure-of-eight 4-0 silk suture. The hemoclip and the sutures localize the site of the transplant in the event that the transplanted tissue needs to be removed in the future. Several pockets are used for the transplant. If there is any bleeding into the pocket, the tissue is removed, and another pocket is used for transplantation.

Even if normal parathyroid tissue is seen in a patient, I transplant nonviable parathyroid tissue. At present, I have found indications for parathyroid transplantation in about 15% of the patients with a total thyroidectomy. More than 150 patients with total thyroidectomies have had parathyroid autotransplantation. In this group, there are seven cases of permanent hypocalcemia. These cases include huge nodular goiters or invasive malignant lesions. The overall incidence of permanent hypocalcemia is 2% out of the 1,265 total thyroidectomies.

Thyroid Storm

Thyroid storm after thyroidectomy in a hyperthyroid patient can be a severe, life-threatening complication. Clinical findings in patients with thyroid storm include fever, tachycardia, anorexia, nausea, vomiting, abdominal pain, and even cardiac failure. The very anxious patient may have marked agitation, acute psychosis, and confusion and may go into coma.

The treatment of thyroid storm should include propylthiouracil in large doses; 250 mg every 6 hours by nasogastric tube, if necessary, should be given to inhibit extrathyroid production of T_3 as well as thyroidal synthesis of T_4 and T_3. Sodium iodide can be given orally or intravenously to inhibit release of T_4 and T_3 from the thyroid. This is usually given in doses of 500 mg/day. Propranolol in a dose of 0.5 to 1.0 mg/min intravenously for 5 to 10 minutes is the most effective treatment for cardiac and neuromuscular manifestation. This medication lasts for several hours and can be repeated. If marked reductions in pulse are not achieved, larger doses can be given. Twenty to 40 mg of propranolol can be given orally every 4 to 6 hours. Parenteral glucocorticoids are given in large doses as necessary. Hyperpyrexia can be controlled by a cooling blanket. The patient must also be kept well hydrated. Nearly all of our hyperthyroid patients have been well controlled prior to surgery. They were nearly all euthyroid, having taken propylthiouracil or methimazole (Tapezole) and then Lugol's solution in a dose of 10 drops three times daily for the 10 days prior to surgery.

In our series of 164 total thyroidectomies (25 males and 139 females), performed for hyperthyroidism, there was no major episode of thyroid storm. Tachycardia, elevation of blood pressure, and hyperpyrexia, which lasted less than a few hours, were the only symptoms, with no patient having symptoms for longer than 24 to 48 hours.

Hematoma

Our procedure, after the neck flaps have been elevated, is to suture ligate the anterior jugular veins bilaterally, superiorly, and inferiorly. The inferior thyroid artery is ligated with 3-0 silk, but the superior thyroid artery and vein are doubly ligated with 2-0 silk. A 1/4 in. Penrose drain is placed bilaterally paratracheally and brought out between the sternohyoid and sternocleidomastoids and the lateral edges of the incision. The drains are sutured to the skin.

Hematomas requiring reoperation have occurred in six patients. Three of these patients were heparinized dialysis patients who had partial thyroidectomies and total parathyroidectomies. Postoperatively, they had massive bleeding requiring reoperation. They were brought back to surgery, and the bleeding sites were found to be the anterior jugular veins. These cases occurred over 25 years ago. Since then, with our suture ligation of anterior jugular veins, there has been no such bleeding from these sites. Two patients having total thyroidectomies had postoperative bleeding and respiratory distress. At surgery, after evacuation of clots, no bleeding sites were found in either patient, just an ooze. One patient was later found to have a factor 7 clotting defect. The other patient required an emergency tracheostomy, which was removed after 72 hours. Blood transfusions were required in 2 patients during this entire series of 1,265 patients.

Thyroglossal Duct Cyst

A thyroglossal duct cyst is a congenital anomaly resulting from retention of an epithelial tract between the thyroid and the foramen cecum at the floor of the pharynx.[9] The hyoid bone, which forms later during embryologic development, nearly always envelops this tract. Cysts that arise from a persistent thyroglossal duct are usually noticed most frequently in the younger age group but may be symptomatic at any age. The most common presentation is complaint of a pain and swelling in the midline of the neck beneath the hyoid cartilage. An evaluation of this midline mass is the same in all age groups.

A careful history and physical examination, including indirect laryngoscopy, is performed first. Second, as a routine in nearly all cases, thyroid scans are obtained. This was initiated after I recognized the growth of occult lingual thyroids in three children who had their only functioning thyroid tissue removed with their thyroglossal duct cysts. Now, if there is no thyroid in the patient's neck, other than in the cyst, and a lingual thyroid is diagnosed, thyroid medication is started preoperatively. I still suggest a thyroglossal duct cyst be resected, even if ectopic thyroid contained within the cyst is the patient's only thyroid tissue. The cyst is prone to progressive enlargement and to infection. Also, the thyroid tissue in the cyst is frequently insufficient or abnormal for adequate hormonal production. Better control of the patients can be obtained by exogenous thyroid replacement.

Third, and perhaps the most important procedure, is a preoperative FNA biopsy, which greatly aids in the management of the midline cervical masses. With the advent of FNA of all head and neck masses, the techniques and magnitude of head and neck surgery have changed. Two patients originally thought to have thyroglossal duct cysts had midline dermoid tumors diagnosed preoperatively by needle biopsy. These patients had their tumor excised under local anesthesia as outpatients. Needle aspiration is an asset in deciding for or against surgery in patients with an increased operative risk. A 68-year-old man, chronically ill, initially refused surgery for his duct cyst. Needle biopsy diagnosis was carcinoma, and surgery was performed. The diagnosis was papillary carcinoma in a thyroid remnant in a cyst as well as in both lobes of the thyroid. I now have three chronically ill patients with thyroglossal duct cysts who are being followed with serial aspirations.[10]

Surgical Technique

At surgery, with the patient anesthetized and an endotracheal tube in place, a transverse incision is made in the upper portion of the neck. After flaps are elevated and sutured back, the neck mass is dissected up to the hyoid bone. The cyst may then be opened and a frozen section obtained before the hyoid bone is resected. This is done if the needle biopsy is not conclusive or if there is any doubt about the mass being a midline

dermoid.[11] When it is not necessary to resect the hyoid bone, the magnitude of the surgery and subsequent morbidity is greatly reduced. I routinely resect the center of the hyoid bone on all thyroglossal duct cysts and follow the tract, if possible, to the base of the tongue. In resection of more than 85 thyroglossal duct cysts with the center of the hyoid bone resected, there have not been any known recurrences. Three patients who were referred because of a recurrence had not had the center of the hyoid bone excised.

PARATHYROID

Hyperparathyroidism

Primary hyperparathyroidism is not a rare disease. A rapidly increasing number of patients with primary hyperparathyroidism has been reported since the advent of routine determination of serum calcium levels by commonly used automated methods. This is a disease of middle and late life and is found predominantly in women. More than 50% of the patients with hyperparathyroidism are now found without symptoms. However, even in asymptomatic patients, at least one half or more have some clinical problems caused by or worsened by the primary hyperparathyroidism (e.g., urolithiasis, osteoporosis found by routine x-ray or bone density studies, decreased renal function, emotional disorders, peptic ulcer, or pancreatitis). Hypertension is quite common in primary hyperparathyroidism and may be worsened by it.

Surgery is suggested for (1) all symptomatic hyperparathyroid patients, (2) asymptomatic hyperparathyroid patients with clinical problems as outlined, (3) asymptomatic patients with serum calcium levels of 11 mg/dL and parathyroid hormone levels inappropriately high and (4) asymptomatic hyperparathyroid patients who cannot have close continual medical monitoring.

The treatment for primary hyperparathyroidism is surgery and is successful in the first neck exploration in more than 95% to 98% of the cases. In our series of 456 parathyroidectomies in primary hyperparathyroidism, 80% (363 patients) had parathyroid adenomas, and 19% (90 patients) had parathyroid hyperplasia (Fig 21–4). Three patients (two males and one female) had parathyroid carcinoma.

Surgical Technique

A low transverse neck incision is made, and the neck flaps are elevated and sutured to the head drapes. The anterior jugular veins are suture ligated inferiorly and superiorly. The sternohyoid and the sternohyoid muscles are retracted laterally, and the thyroid gland is gently elevated. If at all possible, all four parathyroid glands are identified. However, before any removal of tissue, the two recurrent laryngeal nerves are visualized and dissected from the mediastinum to the cricopharyngeus muscle. If an adenoma or large parathyroid gland is found and removed, a biopsy is done on at least one other parathyroid gland, regardless of size. If this gland is hyperplastic, a biopsy is done on the other two parathyroid glands also. If

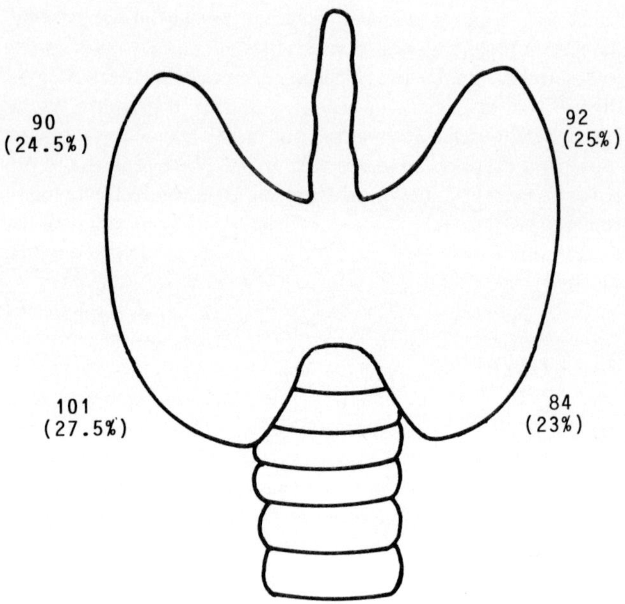

FIG 21–4.
Localization of 367 parathyroid adenomas in 363 patients.

primary parathyroid hyperplasia is diagnosed, three and three-fourths parathyroid glands are removed, and the remaining portion is identified with a hemoclip. During thyroid and parathyroid surgery, hemoclips are only used on parathyroid glands and nowhere else on the neck. Thus, if reoperation is necessary, hemoclips identify the site.

A subtotal or, on a very rare occasion, a total thyroidectomy may be performed if neither normal nor hyperfunctioning parathyroid tissue is found in the neck. Fifteen intrathyroid, parathyroid glands have been located in our series. Since one third of the lower parathyroids may be in the thymus or superior mediastinum, we also explore the mediastinum and thymus bilaterally.[12]

Three of the patients (two men and one woman) had parathyroid carcinoma. Two carcinomas were located in the left lower parathyroid gland area in the superior mediastinum, and one carcinoma was found in the right lower parathyroid gland in the right superior mediastinum. These glands were completely removed without breaking the tumor. The carcinoma was reported only on permanent section. No residual tumor was left, and no surrounding tissue seemed to be invaded by the carcinomas. It has now been 5 years since the elderly woman had surgery, and as yet she has had no symptoms whatsoever. Both men were free of disease for more than 4 years before presenting with invasive, nonresectable carcinoma. One patient died despite radiation and chemotherapy, and the other one is now terminal. Since no further surgery was indicated, because there was no residual disease, no chemotherapy or radiation was indicated in either. In retrospect in reviewing these three cases, we believe that perhaps once a diagnosis of carcinoma is made, and no other tissue can or need be removed, perhaps radiation should be given to this area.

The association between head and neck and chest irradia-

tion and the subsequent appearance of benign and malignant neoplasms in thyroid, salivary, and parathyroid glands has been well documented.[2, 13] In the past 10 years, about 21% of our hyperparathyroid patients who had surgery had a prior history of childhood head and neck irradiation. Of this irradiated group, 79.6% had associated thyroid disease, and ten patients had thyroid carcinomas.

Asymptomatic hyperparathyroidism has also been found at thyroid surgery. Twenty-five asymptomatic patients, 11 with parathyroid adenomas and 14 with parathyroid hyperplasia, were identified at thyroid surgery. This prevented a second or repeat operation in these patients for hyperparathyroidism when the hyperparathyroidism would have become overt in the future. Because of these findings, all patients having thyroid surgery should have calcium and phosphorus levels determined before surgery.

It is important that the surgeon adequately inform the patient preoperatively of the extent of the surgery that might be performed.

Tertiary Parathyroid Hyperplasia

We have performed 81 parathyroidectomies on dialysis patients (40 males and 41 females). In the past, commonplace procedure was the removal of only three parathyroid glands. However, after recurrent parathyroid hyperplasia and the necessity to reoperate on three patients, we started performing total parathyroidectomy on dialysis patients. After performing a total thyroidectomy, we transplant a portion of parathyroid tissue into muscle pockets in the volar surface of the forearm. We use the forearm so that if hyperplastic tissue need be removed, when and if the patients again becomes hypercalcemic, it can be performed under local anesthesia. Ten dialysis patients have had hyperfunctioning parathyroid tissue removed from their forearm, some several times. All of these surgeries were performed under local anesthesia, with the patients having minimal discomfort. Now the accepted procedure in dialysis patients is a total parathyroidectomy.

Scanning Techniques

It is not cost effective to perform localization tests in the primary neck in hyperparathyroid patients. The time and extent of dissection are not appreciably reduced, because the other three parathyroids must be visualized after the adenoma has been localized. In reoperation, localization tests are unquestionably necessary. We have used CT scanning with contrast,[14, 15] selective venous catheterization and parathyroid bioassay,[16, 17] digital subtraction angiography,[18, 19] parathyroid ultrasonography,[20, 21] thermography, thallium 201 and technetium 99 m subtraction scanning,[22, 23] and ^{201}Tl-iodine 123 subtraction scanning.[24] The latter has been most successful. Therefore, [201]Tl-^{123}I subtraction is now the primary localization study performed. Parathyroid imaging is performed immediately following the intravenous (IV) dose of 1 mCi of [201]Tl. Computer subtraction of normal thyroid tissue was performed using 20% increments. Prior to imaging for visualization of normal thyroid tissue, 0.2 mCi of ^{123}I was given orally to the patient. A high-resolution, parallel hole collimator was used with a computer magnification factor of 1.48. Imaging time was 10 minutes for each of two isotopes. Subtraction of normal thyroid significantly improves the detection of parathyroid tumors. In patients with parathyroid adenomas, the sensitivity rate was more than 75%. However, with parathyroid hyperplasia, it was not nearly as successful; only one large parathyroid was found, and the other smaller hyperplastic ones were not.

Hypocalcemia

Postoperatively, the parathyroid patients are monitored every 12 hours for calcium and phosphorus levels. If and when the serum calcium level falls below 8.4 mg/dL (8.4–10.4 mg/dL is normal), oral liquid calcium is started. We use 45 mL of Titralac or Neocalglucon three times daily. When the serum calcium level falls below 8 mg/dL, we start the patient on IV calcium infusion, 5 gm of calcium gluconate in 250 mL of 5% dextrose in water to run over 5 hours. If a second infusion has to be given postoperatively, we start the patient on 0.25 μg of calcitriol (Rocaltrol; 1α,25-dihydroxyvitamin D_3) either once or twice daily. At times it is necessary to use 0.5 μg twice daily along with liquid calcium. We use liquid calcium because, in the postoperative patient who has some dysphagia, it is much more tolerable. We start oral liquid calcium, calcium infusions, and calcitriol at the immediate onset of symptoms, so that patients can be discharged from the hospital sooner in a stable condition. As the patient's serum calcium level rises, we decrease the calcitriol and calcium. Most patients are off vitamin D and calcium therapy in a few weeks to a few months. We do not believe that treating patients before they experience overt tetany slows "return of the parathyroids." It is dangerous to wait the start of calcium until the patient is in carpopedal spasm, hyperventilating, and terrified. We explain to all of our patients that if there is any sign or symptom of tingling in their hands, face, or feet, they should notify the nurses and obtain medication immediately. Surgery is not a contest between the patient and the physician. There has to be complete understanding and cooperation between the physician and the patient.

Reoperation For Hyperparathyroidism in a Previously Explored Neck

In exploration of a neck for hyperparathyroidism that has had previous surgery, the morbidity is at least tenfold, and the success rate is greatly reduced. It is in these scarred and anatomically obliterated planes that localization tests are the most valuable. We have found that ^{201}Tl-^{123}I subtraction tests are the most successful. In our overall series of 537 parathyroidectomies (81 dialysis patients and 456 primary hyperparathyroid patients), 51 patients were identified as having prior head and neck explorations. Thirty patients had parathyroid adenomas, and 10 patients had parathyroid hyperplasia. Eleven patients had prior subtotal or total thyroidectomies, with all of these patients having parathyroid adenomas. No patient in this series had recurrent laryngeal nerve damage after his or her operation.

In reoperation with the distorted anatomic architecture and no normal tissue planes, the thyroid gland may be removed after the recurrent laryngeal nerves are visualized and preserved. When the parathyroid tumor cannot be found in the neck at our initial surgery, and once the diagnosis of hyperparathyroidism is reconfirmed, then and only then, is a mediastinotomy performed. In four of our patients and one referred after initial exploration elsewhere, mediastinotomy was necessary and successful. In 25 referred patients, inexperience or lack of a complete neck exploration with subtotal or total thyroidectomy is the only explanation for initial failure. The need to reoperate in a scarred neck should become less and less as we (1) accrue more knowledge in performing total parathyroidectomies in dialysis patients, (2) remove at least three and three-fourths of the parathyroids in primary parathyroid hyperplasia, (3) have more accurate localization tests at our disposal, and (4) remove the one or two lobes of the thyroid to find intrathyroid parathyroids. Also, in the patients who have prior childhood head and neck irradiation, complete preoperative workup for possible thyroid or parathyroid disease should negate excessive surgery.

REFERENCES

1. Katz AD, Bronson D: Total thyroidectomy. The indications and results of 630 cases. *Am J Surg* 1978; 136:450–454.
2. Katz AD: Thyroid and associated polyglandular neoplasms in patients who received head and neck irradiation during childhood. *Head Neck Surg* 1979; 1:417–422.
3. Foster RS Jr: Morbidity and mortality after thyroidectomy. *Surg Gynecol Obstet* 1978; 146:423–429.
4. Katz AD: Extralaryngeal divisions of the recurrent laryngeal nerve. Report on 400 patients and the 721 nerves measured. *Am J Surg* 1986; 152:406–410.
5. Holl-Allen RTJ: A new approach to the surgical management of paralysis of the laryngeal nerve after thyroidectomy. *Surgery* 1986; 163:543–546.
6. Katz AD: Parathyroid autotransplantation in patients with parathyroid disease and total thyroidectomy. Indications in 117 cases. *Am J Surg* 1981; 142:490–493.
7. Alveryd A: Parathyroid glands in thyroid surgery: Anatomy of the parathyroid glands. *Acta Chir Scand (Suppl)* 1968; 389:9–50.
8. Wells SA, Sturman JA, Boiman RM: Parathyroid transplantation. *World J Surg* 1977; 1:747–756.
9. Moore KL: *The Developing Human. Clinically Oriented Embryology,* ed 2. Philadelphia, WB Saunders Co, 1977, pp 179–180.
10. Katz AD, Hachigian M: Thyroglossal duct cysts: A 30 year experience with emphasis on occurrence in older patients. *Am J Surg* (in press).
11. Katz AD: Midline dermoid tumors of the neck. *Arch Surg* 1974; 109:822–824.
12. Katz AD, Hopp D: Parathyroidectomy. Review of 338 consecutive cases for histology, location, and reoperation. *Am J Surg* 1982; 144:411–415.
13. De Groot LJ, Paloyan E: Thyroid carcinoma and radiation: A Chicago endemic. *JAMA* 1973; 225:487–491.
14. Friedman M, Mafee MF, Shelton VK, et al: Parathyroid localization by computed tomographic scanning. *Otolaryngology* 1983; 109:95–97.

15. Doppman JL, Brennan MF, Koehler JO, et al: Computed tomography for parathyroid localization. *J Comput Assist Tomogr* 1977; 1:30–36.
16. Hsu FSF, Clark OH, Serata TY, et al: Rapid localization of parathyroid tumors by selective venous catheterization and parathyroid hormone bioassay. *Surgery* 1983; 94:873–876.
17. Doppman JL: Parathyroid localization. Arteriography and venous sampling. *Radiol Clin North Am* 1976; 14:163–168.
18. Levy JM, Hessel SJ, Dipple SE, et al: Digital subtraction angiography for location of parathyroid lesions. *Ann Intern Med* 1982; 97:710–712.
19. Esselstyn CB Jr, Buoncore E: The use of digital subtraction angiography and computed tomography scanning in localization of parathyroid adenomas in secondary parathyroid operations: Preliminary observations. *Surgery* 1983; 94:869–872.
20. Reading CC, Charboneau JW, James EM, et al: High-resolution parathyroid sonography. *Am J Radiol* 1982; 139:539–546.
21. Stark DD, Gooding GAW, Moss AA, et al: Parathyroid imaging: Comparison of high-resolution CT and high-resolution sonography. *Am J Radiol* 1983; 141:633–638.
22. Young AE, Gaunt JI, Croft DN, et al: Location of parathyroid adenomas by thallium-201 and technetium-99^m subtraction scanning. *Br Med J (Clin Res)* 1983; 286:1384–1386.
23. Ferlin G, Borsato N, Camerani M, et al: New perspectives in localizing enlarged parathyroid by technetium-thallium substraction scan. *J Nucl Med* 1983; 24:438–441.
24. Brachman MB, Ramanna L, Katz AD, et al: Parathyroid imaging using Ti-201 with I-123 subtraction: Is subtraction necessary [abstract]? *Radiology* 1986; 161:224.

Management of the Primary Site: Thyroid and Parathyroid

Approach of

Dale H. Rice, M.D.

THYROID GLAND

This chapter is written with the assumption that the reader is already familiar with the normal anatomy, physiology, and biochemistry of the thyroid gland, that the workup has progressed to the point that an abnormality of the thyroid has been identified, and that operative intervention is being considered. Both benign and malignant thyroid disease may require thyroidectomy. The most common indications are (1) obstructive symptoms, (2) increased serum calcitonin level, (3) suspicion of malignancy, (4) rapid growth of nodule in euthyroid patient more than 40 years of age, (5) growth of nodule on supression, (6) fine needle aspiration cytology indicating cancer, and (7) psammoma body calcification on CT.

Nonmalignant Disorders

Most nonmalignant thyroid disorders are managed nonoperatively with either antithyroid drugs and ^{131}I if the patient is hyperthyroid or with exogenous replacement if the patient is euthyroid or hypothyroid. Exceptions occur. If the patient has pressure symptoms that fail to respond to drug therapy, the gland is impossibly large, there is strong clinical suspicion of malignancy (e.g., a hard, fixed nodule or lymphadenopathy), or the nodule is substernal, operative intervention is indicated. The extent of the operation indicated depends on the problem. For the unilateral nodule that proves to be benign, lobectomy is sufficient. For Graves' disease or a large multinodular goiter, a total or near-total thyroidectomy should be performed. This choice will be discussed in detail.

Graves' disease presents some special problems.[1] This is the only autoimmune disease leading to glandular hyperfunction. It is characterized by the presence of thyroid-stimulating immunoglobulin (TSI), which probably acts as an anti-TSH receptor antibody. Both autoimmune thyroid diseases show deposition of immunoglobulins (IgG, IgM, IgE) and complement in the thyroid gland,[2,3] but only Graves' disease has TSI. The mechanism of the two common problems associated with Graves' disease, ophthalmopathy and pretibial myxedema, are unknown. Further, since humans are the only animal known to develop autoimmune hyperthyroidism, there is no animal model to study. Ophthalmopathy is present in 20% to 40% and usually develops concomitantly with the hyperthyroidism. Symptoms include pain, increased lacrimation, photophobia, diplopia, and blurring of vision. Signs include proptosis (upper normal level on the exophthalometer is 20 mm in whites and 24 mm in blacks), chemosis, conjunctival injection, and limitation of motion. The disease is characterized by the infiltration of the extraocular muscles and orbital connective tissue with immune cells and mucopolysaccharide. Pretibial myxedema is characterized by mucopolysaccharide deposition in conjunction, with a mononuclear cellular infiltration and degenerative changes in collagen fibrils.

It is critical that the patient with Graves' disease be made euthyroid prior to operation. This is best accomplished with a combination of a thionamide, propranolol, and iodine. The thionamide and propranolol are used initially until the patient is euthyroid. At the time of thyroidectomy, the thionamide and iodine are stopped. The propranolol is tapered over the first postoperative week.

The surgeon must be alert to the possibility of thyroid storm, a rare (in this setting) but dangerous complication. Thyroid storm is defined as severe, life-threatening hyperthyroidism. However, there are no well-established criteria for its diagnosis. The pathophysiology is the same as for hyperthyroidism. It is not caused by a sudden increase in thyroid hormone secretion or mobilization of T_4 or T_3. It is usually precipitated by a major illness such as infection, injury, operation, or parturition. There is usually a history of hyperthyroidism. Findings include fever, tachycardia, abdominal pain, nausea, anorexia, vomiting, pulmonary edema, cardiac failure, and marked anxiety. Both T_3 and T_4 are increased. Treatment consists of inhibiting hormone production, blocking its peripheral action, and providing general supportive measures, which will involve the use of thionamides, propranolol, sodium iodine, and steroids.

Malignant Disorders

Nodular thyroid disease affects approximately 4% of the U.S. population clinically but 15% to 65% in autopsy studies.[4] An appropriate workup must be performed in an attempt to determine the nature of the nodule. The prevalence of thyroid carcinoma in autopsy series ranges from 0.45% to 13%.[5] Historically important data include prior radiation, family history of thyroid or other endocrine neoplasm, rapid growth, symptoms of pressure or hoarseness, age less than 40 years, and sex.

Important physical findings sought are pressure signs, fixation, or lymphadenopathy. Most clinically solitary nodules are the dominant nodule in what is, historically, a multinodular goiter, the presence of which decreases the liability of cancer unless there has been prior radiation. Prior radiation exposure to 2 to 15 Gy increases the risk of benign and malignant neoplasms.[6] Eighty percent to 90% present with an asymptomatic mass in the lower part of the neck. Seventy percent to 80% have a single, palpable nodule. Presence of the mass for many years does not rule out carcinoma.[7]

Seventy percent of thyroid carcinomas are a single cold nodule on scan. However, the scan is of less importance now if the nodule is palpable. Today the most important laboratory test is the FNA cytology. In experienced hands, FNA cytology has an accuracy rate greater than 90%.[8] A cytologic diagnosis of definite malignancy has nearly 100% accuracy (low false positive rate).[9] A definitely benign diagnosis is correct 90% of the time (false negative rate is 5%–10%). Appropriate use of FNA cytology can reduce the number of thyroidectomies by one half without decreasing the number of cancers removed.[10] Other information can help. A finding of punctate calcification on CT suggests papillary carcinoma, whereas TSH, T_3, T_4, and thyroglobulin are of little value in determining the nature of a solitary nodule. The first three merely indicate the state of function of the gland as a whole. Thyroglobulin is a large glycoprotein that acts as a prohormone. Its hydrolosis results in the synthesis of T_4 and T_3. However, it may be increased in hyperthyroidism, subacute thyroiditis, and trauma. Thyroglobulin has significant utility in monitoring patients for recurrence after total thyroidectomy. A change from undetectable or low to high levels indicates recurrent disease.

Computed tomography and radioiodine scans can add information but are more often useful after initial treatment. Preoperative CT will show the size of the thyroid and the presence or absence of substernal extension as well as cervical adenopathy. It is especially useful in the evaluation of cryptogenic neck masses after thyroidectomy.[11] Radioiodine scans are used to check the effectiveness of treatment and to detect recurrences. Recurrences may occur in up to 50% of patients with metastases and 25% of those without metastases and may not become manifest for 5 to 10 years after initial therapy.[12] After treatment, patients should have serial thyroglobulin and radioiodine scans for at least 10 years.

Once the workup has shown that the likely diagnosis is carcinoma, resection is the first line of therapy. Despite this, there is considerable disagreement over the extent of resection that will produce the most benefit with the least morbidity. Several factors account for this. First, complication rates vary from center to center. Second, the natural history of the differentiated thyroid cancers is so long, that a 15- to 20-year follow-up is necessary. Third, the disease is uncommon enough that few institutions or individuals accrue enough patients with long enough follow-up to compare treatments. Fourth, the same cancer may behave differently in different patients. Adverse prognostic signs include moderate to marked angioinvasion, extracapsular spread, and age greater than 40 years for men or 50 years for women. Several studies have found no difference in survival between lobectomy, subtotal thyroidectomy, and total thyroidectomy if the tumor did not breach the capsule.[7] This is despite the fact that up to 38% of cases have multifocal carcinoma involving the opposite lobe, because as many as 90% of these fail to become clinically evident.[13] A similar argument can be made for elective neck dissection. Fifty percent of papillary cancers have at least one abnormal node, but most will not become significant and can be treated when apparent without affecting survival.[14] Further, "node plucking" and formal neck dissection give similar results.[15] Not all agree.[16]

Postoperatively, all differentiated thyroid cancers should be treated with radioiodine. Its efficacy is related to tumor uptake and retention, which occurs in 50% to 80%.[17] Hürthle cell, medullary, and undifferentiated carcinomas rarely concentrate radioiodine. For the differentiated tumors that do concentrate ^{131}I, effective uptake is 0.5% of the dose per gram. The biologic half-life is 4 days. Thus, from a dose of 150 mCi, the tumor will receive a radiation dose of approximately 25 Gy. Objective evidence of a reduction in size occurs in 35%, especially if there are metastases.[18] Further, the evidence that ^{131}I increases life expectancy is limited because of the indolent nature of the disease.[19] However, one study reduced recurrence from 11% to 2.6% with the addition of ^{131}I ablation to resection plus hormonal suppression.[20] Following radioiodine therapy, all carcinomas should be suppressed, preferably with L-thyroxine (T$_4$, Synthroid). Several studies showed a reduced rate of recurrence.[16, 21] The dose should be adjusted to completely suppress TSH.

Papillary Adenocarcinoma

Papillary adenocarcinoma is the most common neoplasm involving the thyroid and accounts for approximately 70%. Peak incidence is in the third and fourth decades. Histologically, the tumor is composed of uniform cuboidal follicular cells arranged in papillae with a fibrovascular stalk. Psammoma bodies—concentrically laminated deposits of calcium—are frequent and nearly pathognomonic. The presenting complaint in 90% is a mass in the neck. The tumor spreads lymphogenously, leading to multiple intrathyroid foci and involvement of cervical nodes. Approximately 45% to 50% will have gross or microscopic adenopathy. However, involved nodes seem to have little influence on prognosis, although recurrences are more common.[14, 15] Angioinvasion and capsular invasion are uncommon.

There is wide divergence of opinion as to the correct amount of thyroid to remove. Some would do a total or near-total thyroidectomy on all papillary carcinomas and cite the following reasons. There is a high incidence of multifocal disease within the gland. Postoperative treatment with radioiodine is easier. It decreases the need for a second procedure. The complication rate (in experienced hands) is small. Others adjust the resection to fit the amount of disease, reserving total or near-total thyroidectomy for those tumors beyond a certain size. One recent recommendation is for lobectomy with a cuff of normal tissue if the lesion is less than 1 cm and entirely intrathyroid. They advise total thyroidectomy for all others.[22] However, since the former condition is uncommon, most patients would undergo a total thyroidectomy. Several studies have found no difference

between lobectomy, subtotal, and total thyroidectomy in eventual outcome.[7] Both approaches give excellent results in experienced hands.

For many years there has been controversy over the management of neck disease. It seems clear now that there is no place for the elective neck dissection. Further, limited nodal resection is as effective as a modified radical or radical neck dissection.[7, 15, 16]

Follicular Carcinoma

Follicular carcinoma accounts for approximately 15% of thyroid malignancies. It is two to three times more common in women, with a peak incidence in the fifth to seventh decades. In contrast to the papillary carcinomas, follicular carcinoma can be difficult to diagnose and usually requires reviewing multiple sections. Thus, the separation cannot be made with FNA cytology or on frozen section. It is probably best to assume follicular lesions are malignant until the permanent sections have been reviewed. The criteria for malignancy include angioinvasion and capsular invasion. Thus, hematogenous spread is more liable to occur than lymphogenous spread. Invasion of the substance of the gland is an adverse sign.[23] The recurrence rate is 5% to 10% with little capsular invasion, but the mortality rises to more than 50% with marked invasion.[24] The best treatment for most patients is total thyroidectomy, followed by ^{131}I ablation, followed by lifelong suppression. Occasionally a well-differentiated thyroid cancer (usually follicular) will undergo anaplastic transformation. This is seen in 25% of anaplastic carcinomas.[25]

Medullary Carcinoma

Medullary carcinoma makes up 4% to 12% of all thyroid carcinomas. It is not a true thyroid carcinoma but arises from the parafollicular of C cells that are of neural crest origin. The male-female incidence is equal. Histologically, the stroma may contain amyloid, and mitoses are common. Both multiple foci and lymph node metastases are common. They may be familial or sporadic. The former is autosomal dominant and may occur in multiple endocrine neoplasia (MEN) type II (medullary carcinoma, bilateral pheochromocytoma, parathyroid adenoma, or hyperplasia) or MEN type III (medullary carcinoma, pheochromocytoma, neuromas). The latter—sporadic—is more common. Diarrhea is a significant symptom in 20% to 30%. This tumor has a convenient biologic marker, the serum calcitonin, which should be obtained routinely for every thyroid nodule. For medullary carcinoma, it is used to follow the patient postoperatively. It is universally agreed that the best treatment is total thyroidectomy. If there is palpable adenopathy, a formal neck dissection should be done. Some would routinely sample the nodes and, if results are abnormal, do a neck dissection. Survival is strongly related to extent of disease. If the thyroidectomy is performed prior to spread, the survival is the same as for controls. If the tumor has spread, the 10-year survival is 42%. Medullary carcinoma generally does not concentrate radioiodine, so ^{131}I has no place in the treatment. Isolated cases of tumors that do concentrate radioiodine have been reported, but they are rare.

Anaplastic Carcinomas

Anaplastic carcinomas account for 10% of thyroid malignancies. The sex distribution is equal, and the peak incidence is in the sixth and seventh decades. This is an unencapsulated, highly invasive, highly malignant tumor. There are several histologic types—giant cell, spindle cell, and small cell. It has recently been recognized that the small cell variant is usually a lymphoma, and this may account for the occasional long-term survivor. Otherwise, long-term survival is rare, with a mean survival of 6 to 8 months. Complete excision should be performed, if possible. Usually it is not. Tracheotomy is often necessary and is best done early. External radiation and chemotherapy are frequently added, but the tumor is usually rapidly fatal.

Complications of Thyroidectomy

Hematoma

As with any operation, hematoma may occur. This is best prevented by good hemostasis. When postoperative bleeding occurs, it is usually from the superior thyroid vessels. Most surgeons routinely drain the operative site and apply a pressure dressing. If a drain is to be used, a suction drain makes more sense than a Penrose, since a Penrose drain may both collapse and kink. Logic aside, many surgeons for many years have used Penrose drains with good success. This may be because a recent prospective study found no difference in hematoma formation between the drained and undrained groups.[26] Likewise, a pressure dressing flies in the face of logic. Bleeding under a pressure dressing would seem to increase the risk of airway compression, but once again, experience does not bear this out, probably because of the rarity of the event. It would seem prudent to use a suction drain and leave the wound uncovered, so that swelling could be noticed early.

Regardless, at the first sign of swelling, the wound should be immediately opened to protect the airway. The patient should be returned to the operating room, the wound explored, the offending vessel ligated, and the incision reclosed.

Recurrent Laryngeal Nerve

Over the years, there have been two philosophies of management of the recurrent laryngeal nerve during thyroidectomy. One was to perform an extracapsular dissection with or without leaving a portion of posterior gland and capsule with little or no effort to identify the nerve. The other was to identify the nerve early in the procedure and keep it visualized throughout the dissection.[27] Since the injury rate is low with either approach, it is clear that the majority of patients could be managed either way. However, early identification of the nerve has more appeal intellectually and seems the surest way to protect the nerve. Maintaining anatomic integrity of the nerve does not guarantee vocal fold function. A normal or near-normal voice postoperatively also does not guarantee normal vocal fold function. The vocal folds should be visualized. Over the years, a number of patients with an (unknown to them) unilateral paralysis have been seen. In every case, the operating surgeons stated it was the first one they had ever had, that they never looked at the vocal folds postoperatively on any patient, and that they identified the nerve and it was intact at the end of the procedure. The nerve can be identified in one of two locations. Most surgeons seem to prefer to find the nerve inferiorly as it enters the neck from the chest. This is usually successful, although there is some variability in the exact location of the nerve, and it is in the lexicon of every surgeon that the nerve has no constant relationship to the inferior thyroid artery. Further, this approach does not account for the rare, nonrecurrent nerve that occurs in 0.3% to 1.0%, usually on the right.[28] The nerve has one constant location at its entrance into the larynx at the cricoarytenoid joint. Many surgeons prefer to identify the nerve at this location and then follow it inferiorly. Both techniques should be in the thyroid surgeon's repertoire. Throughout the procedure, care should be taken to avoid undue traction on the nerve. Although gentle handling of the nerve is the best insurance, nerve function may be assessed with the nerve stimulator. One can either palpate the contraction of the posterior cricoarytenoid muscle or measure fold motion with a pressure-sensitive balloon inserted between the vocal folds. In addition, one can visualize the vocal folds directly at the time of extubation. Should the nerve be transected, accidentally or deliberately, traditional teaching has been that repair is futile, with either no return of function or, at best, some discoordinated motion. Recent evidence, as well as some old literature, showed that repair may be useful in returning enough tone to the vocal fold to yield a normal or near-normal voice[29] despite the absence of purposeful motion.

PARATHYROID GLAND

It is axiomatic that care must be taken to preserve the parathyroid glands. The method of Thompson is effective: ligation of the branches of the inferior thyroid artery on the capsule, medial to the parathyroids with gentle displacement of the glands laterally.[27] Theoretical and clinical experience indicate that a single functioning gland is sufficient. Prudence, however, would dictate that any devascularized gland be minced and implanted into the sternocleidomastoid muscle.

Thyroglossal Duct Cyst

Thyroglossal duct cysts account for approximately 70% of congenital neck anomalies. They occur in the midline, usually at or below the thyroid. The lesion results from failure of obliteration of the duct following thyroid migration from the foramen cecum inferiorly in the 6- to 8-week embryo. Thus, cysts can occur anywhere from the tongue to the thyroid gland. The majority of patients are children or young adults.[30] Cysts average 2 to 4 cm in diameter and are lined by squamous epithelium. Thyroid tissue is not a common finding. However, a preoperative thyroid scan should be performed unless there is clearly palpable thyroid in the normal location. Treatment is excision. It is important to excise the cyst completely as well as the tract up to the foramen cecum. Anatomic studies have demonstrated the intimate association of the tract with the hyoid.[31] The tract passes anterior to the hyoid and hooks under it posteriorly and inferiorly. The tract does not pass through the bone. Regardless, the tract is intimately associated with the hyoid, and a central portion of it and of tongue muscle above must be removed in continuity with the cyst as first advocated by Sistrunk[32] to prevent recurrence.

Hyperparathyroidism

With rare exception, the only functional abnormality that affects the parathyroid glands is hyperparathyroidism. Hypoparathyroidism occurs essentially only as a postoperative phenomenon. Hyperparathyroidism was a rarely diagnosed disease prior to the advent of automated blood chemistry analysis. Now, asymptomatic hyperparathyroidism is probably the most common disease affecting these glands.[33]

The parathyroid gland was discovered by Owen in the Indian rhinoceros in 1862.[34] The function was uncertain until two experiments in the 1890s. In 1892, von Eiselberg performed the first autotransplantation by placing one thyroid lobe with the parathyroids between fascia and peritoneum of cats.[35] The animals did well with removal of the other thyroid lobe and parathyroids but died of tetany with removal of the transplant. Four years later, Vassale and Generali showed that removal of the parathyroid glands alone leads to tetany.[36] In 1908, Halstead demonstrated that less than one autotransplanted gland can prevent tetany.[37] It was not until 1925 that Mandel performed the first parathyroidectomy for primary hyperparathyroidism.[38] One year later, Lahey reported the first autotransplantation in humans.[39]

The diagnosis of primary hyperparathyroidism is best made with an elevated parathyroid hormone level plus the exclusion of other causes of hypercalcemia. The most common other causes are carcinoma with or without skeletal metastases, thiazide therapy, multiple myeloma, sarcoidosis, milk-alkali syndrome, and hypervitaminosis D. Most commonly in this country, the diagnosis is made serendipitously by the finding of hypercalcemia on routine blood chemistries. Of interest, women outnumber men 2 to 1.

The classic symptoms are "bones, stones, and abdominal groans." Skeletal symptoms usually feature osteoporosis, bone cysts, and chondrocalcinosis. The classic x-ray finding was subperiosteal resorption of the radial aspect of the middle phalanges and distal clavicles. The most common site of complications of primary hyperparathyroidism is the urinary tract, usually manifest as calculi or nephrocalcinosis. Abdominal groans were generally caused by ulcer disease or pancreatitis. Many experience nonspecific abdominal discomfort that disappears after successful treatment. Many patients, especially with careful questioning, have neurologic or muscular symptoms, such as somnolence, confusion, weakness, or irritability.

Management

Once the diagnosis of primary hyperparathyroidism is made, the treatment is resection. Seventy percent to 80% of all cases are caused by a solitary adenoma. Localization studies are not mandatory, and some, like selective venous sampling before the first procedure, are probably more troublesome than the information is worth. The CT scan and the Tc–Tl subtraction scan are worthwhile. A normal scan does not rule out an adenoma, but an abnormal scan virtually guarantees it. However, preoperative localization is important only if one believes identification of all four glands is unnecessary once an adenoma is found.[40] Many believe that routine biopsy of the remaining normal glands is mandatory. Others believe that only visual identification is necessary[31, 41] despite the fact this is notoriously inaccurate.[42] This is further complicated by the fact that most pathologists will not commit to hyperplasia or adenoma on frozen section unless there is an unequivocal difference between glands. From a practical standpoint, the incidence of multiple adenomas or synchronous adenoma plus hyperplasia is 1% to 3%,[43] if it even occurs.[44] Further, the only way to absolutely guarantee a second operation will never be needed is to perform an absolute total parathyroidectomy.[45] Few would recommend this for an adenoma.

There is more controversy over the management of hyperplasia. Traditional wisdom is to excise three and one half of the four hyperplastic glands. This is usually successful. Failure resulting in recurrence of hyperparathyroidism may be caused by proliferation of the remaining gland. In the former situation, reexploring the neck is necessary. At that time, one should perform a careful exploration of the superior mediastinum with excision of the thymus. If one discovers only proliferation of the remaining gland, the best procedure is arguable. Many would autotransplant 50 to 75 mg of tissue (normal parathyroid is 30–50 mg) and excise the remainder.[46] In this setting, the average recurrence rate from a compilation of the literature is 17%. Others advocate total parathyroidectomy,[33, 47, 48] followed by permanent medical management or delayed autotransplantation with cryopreserved tissue. If, at the time of the primary resection, the remaining gland is devascularized, it should be transplanted. Whenever parathyroid tissue is transplanted, the site should be marked with a permanent suture and clipped in case future identification is necessary.

Complications

Postoperative hypocalcemia is the most common complication. Following resection of an adenoma, parathyroid hormone levels fall rapidly to less than 1% of the preoperative value, with the nadir between 2 to 4 hours. Recovery generally occurs within 30 hours. The serum calcium level falls more slowly, with the low between 20 to 48 hours and recovery within 60 hours. The patient with symptomatic hypocalcemia should be treated with calcium and calcitriol.

Postoperative vocal cord paralysis occurs in 1% to 2% of primary parathyroid resections and in 6% to 7% of reexplorations. The management is discussed in the section on thyroid.

REFERENCES

1. Makinen T, Wagner G, Opter L, et al: Evidence that the TSH receptor acts as a mitogenic antigen in Graves' disease. *Nature* 1978; 275:314–315.
2. Werner SC, Wegelius O, Fierer JA, et al: Immunoglobulins

(E, M, G) and complement in the connective tissue of the thyroid in Graves' disease. *N Engl J Med* 1972; 287:421–425.

3. Kalderon AE, Bogaars HA: Immune complex deposits in Graves' disease and Hashimoto's thyroiditis. *Am J Med* 1977; 63:729–734.

4. Silverberg SG, Vidone RA: Carcinoma of the thyroid in surgical and postmortum material. Analysis of 300 cases at autopsy and literature review. *Ann Surg* 1966; 164:291–299.

5. Nishiyama RH, Ludwig GK, Thompson NK: The prevalence of small papillary thyroid carcinomas in 100 consecutive necropsies in an American population, in De Groot LJ (ed): *Radiation-Associated Thyroid Carcinoma.* New York, Grune & Stratton, 1977, pp 123–135.

6. Smith RE Jr, Adler RA, Clark P, et al: Thyroid function after mantle irradiation in Hodgkin's disease. *JAMA* 1981; 245:46–49.

7. Friedman M, Deitch R, Grybanakas VT, et al: Thyroid carcinoma. *Otolaryngol Clin North Am* 1986; 19:451–461.

8. Van Herle AJ, Rich P, Ljung BM, et al: The thyroid nodule. *Ann Intern Med* 1982; 96:221–232.

9. Ramacciotti CE, Pretorius HC, Chu EW, et al: Diagnostic accuracy and use of aspiration biopsy in the management of thyroid nodules. *Arch Intern Med* 1984; 144:1169–1173.

10. Miller JM, Kini SR, Hamburger JL: *Needle Biopsy of the Thyroid.* New York, Traeger, 1983.

11. Blum M, Reede DL, Seltzer TF, et al: Computerized axial tomography in the diagnosis and management of thyroid and parathyroid disorders. *Am J Med Sci* 1984; 287:34–39.

12. Krishnamurthy GT, Blahd WH: Radioiodine I-131 therapy in the management of thyroid cancer. *Cancer* 1977; 40:195–202.

13. Tollefsen HR, Shah JP, Huvos AG: Papillary carcinoma of the thyroid: Recurrence in the thyroid gland after initial surgical treatment. *Am J Surg* 1972; 124:468–472.

14. Hutter RVP, Frazell EL, Foote FW: Elective neck dissection: An assessment of its use in the management of papillary thyroid cancer. *CA* 1970; 20:87–93.

15. Beahrs OH, Pasternak B: Cancer of the thyroid gland. *Curr Probl Surg* 1969; Dec:1–38.

16. Mazzaferri EL, Young RL: Papillary thyroid carcinoma: A 10 year follow-up report of the impact of therapy in 576 patients. *Am J Med* 1981; 70:511–518.

17. Pochin EE: Radioiodine therapy of the thyroid cancer. *Semin Nucl Med* 1971; 1:503–515.

18. Benua RS, Cicalle NR, Sonenberg M, et al: The relation of radioiodine dosimetry to results and complications in the treatment of metastatic thyroid cancer. *AJR* 1962; 87:171–182.

19. Beierwalters WH, Nishiyama RH, Thompson NW, et al: Survival time and "cure" in papillary and follicular thyroid carcinoma with distant metastasis: Statistics following University of Michigan therapy. *J Nucl Med* 1982; 23:561–568.

20. Mazzaferri EL, Young RL, Oertel JE, et al: Papillary thyroid carcinoma: The impact of therapy in 576 patients. *Medicine (Baltimore)* 1977; 56:171–196.

21. Crile G Jr: The endocrine dependency of papillary carcinomas of the thyroid, in Smithers D (ed): *Tumors of the Thyroid Gland,* Vol 6: *Monographs on Neoplastic Disease at Various Sites.* Edinburgh, E & S Livingstone, 1970.

22. Gershengorn MC, Robbins J: Thyroid neoplasia, in Green WL (ed): *The Thyroid.* New York, Elsevier North-Holland, 1987.

23. Tubiana M, Schlumberger M, Rougier P, et al: Long term results and prognostic factors in patients with differentiated thyroid cancer. *Cancer* 1985; 55:794–804.

24. Woolner LA, Beahrs OH, Black BM, et al: Thyroid carcinoma: General considerations and follow-up data on 1182 cases, in Young S, Inman DR (eds): *Thyroid Neoplasia.* New York, Academic Press, 1968.

25. Samaan NA, Schultz PN, Haynie TP, et al: Pulmonary metastasis of differentiated thyroid carcinoma: Treatment results in 101 patients. *J Clin Endocrinol Metab* 1985; 60:376–380.

26. Wihlborg O, Bergljung L, Martensen H: To drain or not to drain in thyroid surgery. *Arch Surg* 1988; 123:40–41.

27. Harness JK, Fung L, Thompson NW, et al: Total thyroidectomy: Complications and technique. *World J Surg* 1986; 10:781–786.

28. Wijetlaka SE: Non-recurrent laryngeal nerve. *Br J Surg* 1978; 65:179–181.

29. Crumley R: Nerve transfer versus teflon injection for vocal cord paralysis: Paper presented at the Combined Otolaryngology spring meeting, Palm Beach, Fla, April 27, 1988.

30. Murphy JP, Budd DC: Thyroglossal duct cysts in the elderly. *South Med J* 1977; 70:1247–1248.

31. Ellis PDM, von Nostrand AWP: The applied anatomy of thyroglossal tract remnants. *Laryngoscope* 1977; 87:765–722.

32. Sistrunk WE: The surgical treatment of cysts of the thyroglossal tract. *Ann Surg* 1920; 71:121–122.

33. Saaka MB, Selke FW, Kelly TR: Primary hyperparathyroidism. *Surg Gynecol Obstet* 1988; 166:333–337.

34. Owen R: The anatomy of the India rhinoceros. *Trans Zoological Soc London* 1862; 4:31–58.

35. Von Eiselberg A: Uber erfolgreiche einheilung der Katzenschilddrue in die Banchdecke und Auftreten von Tetanie nach deren Exstirpation. *Wien Klin Wochenschr* 1892; 5:81–85.

36. Vassale G, Generali P: Sur les effects de l'extirpation des glands parathyroidiennes. *Arch Ital Biol* 1896; 26:61–65.

37. Halstead W: Auto and isotransplantation, in dogs, of the parathyroid glandules. *J Exp Med* 1908; 11:175–199.

38. Mandel F: Therapeutischer Versuch bei Ostitis Fibrosa Generaliata Mittels Extirpation cines Epiththelkorperchentumor. *Wien Klin Wochenschr* 1925; 50:1343.

39. Lahey FH: The transplantation of parathyroids in partial thyroidectomy. *Surg Gynecol Obstet* 1926; 42:508–509.

40. Brasier AR, Wang CA, Nussbaum SR: Recovery of parathyroid hormone secretion after parathyroid adenomectomy. *J Clin Endocrinol Metab* 1988; 66:495–500.

41. Duh Q, Arnaud CD, Levin KE, et al: Parathyroid hormone: Before and after parathyroidectomy. *Surgery* 1986; 100:1021–1031.

42. Shaha A: Primary hyperparathyroidism: Changing principles in evaluation and surgical approach. Presented at the Annual Meeting of the American Academy for Otolaryngology Head and Neck Surgery, 1987.

43. Sivula A, Ronni-Sivula H: Natural history of treated primary hyperparathyroidism. *Surg Clin North Am* 1987; 67:329–341.

44. Harnes JK, Ramsburg SR, Nishiyama RH, et al: Multiple adenomas of the parathyroids: Do they exist. *Arch Surg* 1979; 114:468–474.

45. Yagoob M, Ahmad R, Simkin E: Hypocalcemia after parathyroidectomy. *Br Med J (Clin Res)* 1988; 296:1198.

46. McCall AR, Calandra D, Lawrence AM, et al: Parathyroid

autotransplantation in forty-four patients with primary hyperparathyroidism: The role of thallium scanning. *Surgery* 1986; 100:614–620.

47. Saxe AW, Brennan MF: Preoperative parathyroid surgery for primary hyperparathyroidism caused by multiple-gland disease; total parathyroidectomy and transplantation with cryopreserved tissue. *Surgery* 1982; 91:616–621.

48. Billings PJ, Milroy E: Autotransplantation of human parathyroid glands. *Ann R Coll Surg* 1986; 68:11–13.

CHAPTER 22

Oncologic Issues Relating to Neck Dissection

Approach of

Paul H. Ward, M.D., F.A.C.S.

The decision-making process in the approach to the neck containing metastatic tumor varies significantly among surgeons and radiotherapists. The many different methods of managing metastatic squamous cell carcinoma or the probability of metastasis to the neck are based largely on ignorance resulting from the absence of sound data derived from prospective randomized clinical studies.

Most clinicians who perform surgery on a large number of head and neck cases base their decision as to the management of neck metastasis on careful, thorough, clinical assessment of the primary tumor, the patient's general clinical status, and the physical examination. The rapid advancement of diagnostic technology and, more recently, magnetic resonance imaging (MRI) has altered our previous clinical staging. The early (T_1) and delayed (T_2) images have provided considerably more information on the extent of the primary tumor than on the identification of metastatic lymph nodes. It is hoped that with the technology of monoclonal antibody labeling, specific identification of occult nodal metastasis will become a reality.[1] The current state of the art in major medical centers commands imaging as an adjunct to physical examination.[2]

Since it is generally recognized that a 15% to 20% error rate exists in our clinical assessment of nonpalpable neck nodes, the presence of enlarged nodes (> 1 cm) on either computed tomography (CT) or MRI may influence our therapeutic approach to the management of the primary tumor and the potential metastatic disease, if not our clinical staging. I assume that the readers are familiar with the American Cancer Society Joint Commission TNM (primary tumor, regional nodes, metastasis) staging system. This chapter addresses the primary tumor (T) to only a limited extent. The size, location, histologic,

and biologic characteristics of the primary tumor as well as assessment of the patient's immune response and interaction with the tumor are the primary factors determining the management of neck disease.

The presence of a primary tumor that is readily resectable with minimal deformity, morbidity, and the presence of clinically abnormal nodes makes the decision to recommend a surgical resection of the primary tumor and neck disease easy. By contrast, a primary tumor with histologically aggressive behavior located in an area from which resection will cause significant deformity and disability and yet displays no evidence of metastatic disease (even though the probability of metastasis is high) will likely receive radiation to the primary tumor and both sides of the neck with surgery reserved for salvage. In cases with more advanced disease, both in the primary site and in the neck, combined surgery and radiation are recommended even though statistical evidence may be lacking to prove the efficacy of such a radical approach. The essence of a good oncologist (surgeon or radiotherapist) is an experienced clinician who assesses the many variables and individualizes them for each patient.

The following presentation is a relatively rigid cookbook approach to metastatic squamous cell carcinoma of the neck. I expect that the outlined considerations will be modified for each individual patient.

THE N0 NECK

It is a tragedy that controversy still is prevalent over the management of the clinically normal neck. This question could be answered fairly effectively and rapidly with a multiinstitutional, prospective, randomized trial with sufficient numbers and standardization of stratification to provide statistically significant results.[3] The current options are (1) treat the primary tumor alone and observe the neck, (2) treat the primary tumor and neck surgically, (3) treat the primary tumor and side (or sides) of the neck with radiation, and (4) treat the primary tumor surgically and the primary site and sides of the neck with radiation.

My treatment advice to the patient with the N0 neck is similar to that of most major surgical oncologists. That is, either have complete (radical or modified) surgery, including the primary tumor and neck, or have full-course radiation to the primary tumor and one or both sides of the neck. This decision to electively treat the neck is based on the high statistical probability of occult nodal metastasis.[4] The development of unresectable disease in a few anecdotal cases following watchful waiting, even with close follow-up, commends a more aggressive approach with either surgery or radiation.

It is a sad commentary on our scientific efforts that most approaches to the management of the N0 neck are based on empiricism. In all the literature, there is only one prospective randomized trial. A paper from the Institute Gustave Roussy in France published in 1980 is the only study utilizing the prospective randomized approach.[5] They randomized T1N0, T2N0, and T3N0 squamous cell carcinomas of the mobile tongue and floor of the mouth into two groups, either elective neck dissection or watchful waiting with delayed therapeutic neck dissection in reserve. Their 5-year follow-up revealed no difference in the survival of the two groups. This type of study needs to be conducted by others and, if confirmed, should impact heavily on our therapeutic management of the N0 neck in the future.

The N0 neck undoubtedly has led to the popularization of the modified neck technique (the many more conservative varieties of modification of the radical neck are called Bocca and Pignataro).[6] Here again, there is no standardization, no prospective randomized studies on which to base the decision-making process. Nearly all of the retrospective reports are favorable, as would be expected since, even in the worst scenario, if there is no tumor present in a significant percentage of the cases, a good result is a foregone conclusion. There is no doubt that metastatic disease to the neck dramatically decreases the prognosis for 5-year survival.

The reported therapeutic success with elective radiotherapy can be attributed to a "what we don't know won't hurt us" mentality. Snow has so aptly pointed out that "the focus today is not so much on when to treat the neck electively, but rather how best to treat the neck electively."[3] Again, good practice demands, and hopefully will bring forth, some prospective randomized studies to answer these questions. Until these answers are forthcoming, surgery and radiation remain the primary means of treating the clinical normal neck.

THE N1 NECK

The same approach or recommendation for the N1 neck can be taken for the N0 neck, since a significant false positive rate exists for clinical staging, and the retrospective studies can be used to support either surgery or radiation with similar statistical absence of credibility and validity. A surgical approach to any primary tumor with clinically abnormal neck disease is more likely to be advocated. Management of neck disease with surgery over radiation is a matter of personal bias, and valid studies to support this treatment are tenuous at best. There is, however, no place for watchful waiting in the treatment of highly probable metastatic, extracapsular neck disease. Either surgery or radiation or both to both sides of the neck is essential. A merit of surgery is that it allows better postoperative staging of the nodal disease.

I believe there is a place for a modified neck dissection in both N0 and many N1 necks, providing the location of the node is away from, and there are not clustered nodes around, the spinal accessory nerve high in the jugular area. This is an empirical decision and begs for the previously outlined studies. Modified neck dissection in the N0 or N1 neck implies dissection and preservation of the spinal accessory nerve and other structures, such as the sternocleidomastoid muscle and jugular vein. Even with dissection and preservation of the spinal accessory nerve, a 30% to 40% postoperative shoulder morbidity persists.[7] If lesser surgical procedures or radiation prove to provide equal survival results, this will be a significant contribution to the well-being of our patients.

METASTATIC NODAL DISEASE WITH UNKNOWN PRIMARY SITE

Until now, we have been discussing the management of early or statistically highly probable metastatic disease to the lymph nodes. At times, the primary tumor may be large with little or no evidence of metastatic disease; conversely, the primary tumor may be small with large, unilateral or even bilateral metastatic nodes present. In a small percentage of cases (47 of 664 cases of metastatic disease on last review of a 10-year University of California—Los Angeles series), no primary tumor could be found on careful physical examination. After extensive work-up (including a head and neck examination, x-ray studies, and triple endoscopy with biopsies of the nasopharynx, tonsil, base of tongue, and pyriform sinuses), the number of "unknown primary tumors" was reduced to 17. Even over the years of follow-up, only three of the primary tumors became evident and were found at autopsy (maxillary sinus, tongue, and melanoma of the skin).

Fine needle aspirate now assists in the cytologic diagnosis and appears to have no deleterious effects. By contrast, the surgeon poorly trained in head and neck surgery usually yields to the temptation to perform an open biopsy. This does the patient a disservice by making future radical neck dissection with excision of the biopsy site difficult. Intracapsular metastasis is possibly converted to extracapsular disease, and the incisions are invariably in the wrong area to be properly incorporated into the eventual radical neck incision. Actual biopsy should be performed only after the extensive endoscopic "blind biopsy" and MRI or CT scan workup is normal. In these rare instances, an excision biopsy is performed, and if frozen section confirms the presence of squamous cell carcinoma, a modified or conventional radical neck dissection is performed, followed by full-course radiation to both sides of the neck and the entire Waldeyer's ring area.

ADVANCED NODAL DISEASE (N2, N3 AND THEIR SUBCLASSES)

Patients with extensive nodal disease are considered primarily surgical candidates if resectable since the prognosis is poor with all treatment modalities. The election of primary radiation is reserved for those patients with inoperable primary tumors, those refusing surgery, or those who have such advanced extranodal disease that it is attached to the major vessels and en bloc resection is not possible. In these later cases, radiation therapy or protocol chemotherapy and radiotherapy are administered. At the completion of the radiation, the patient is reevaluated, and many are explored beginning by elevation of neck flaps and division of the sternocleidomastoid, omohyoid muscles, and jugular vein. The dissection is carried cephalad, and an attempt is made to form a Conley tunnel by pushing the index finger on the jugular until it is obstructed by metastatic disease or reaches the base of the skull and jugular foramen. If the tumor is adherent to the carotid and no planes exist and the neck is deemed nonresectable, the specimen is replaced in the bed and the wound is closed. If the base of the skull is reached and the carotid artery feels free of tumor, the dissection is continued. I have long passed the phase where resection with or without grafting of the carotid artery in a heavily irradiated bed is deemed worthwhile. The disasters encountered with graft blowouts, hemiparesis, and other complications certainly make it seem like the patient lives longer, but survivors in good health are anecdotal.

In those cases with extensive disease in which surgery was the initial treatment, the current policy is to follow the surgery with full-course radiation to the primary site and both sides of the neck. This latter treatment may be treating only the physician since in only a few primary tumors, (e.g., pyriform sinus carcinomas) is there strong evidence that combined therapy significantly increases the 5-year survival rate.

The management of the opposite side of the neck in patients with extensive unilateral metastasis remains an enigma. Depending on the location of the primary tumor, the opposite side of the N0 neck may or may not be operated on. In midline lesions (i.e., floor of mouth, base of tongue, or epiglottic), one of the modified varieties of neck dissection may be performed for staging purposes. If abnormal nodes are found, the dissection is converted into a radical neck, sometimes with sparing of the spinal accessory nerve. These patients with or without the second neck dissection then receive full-course radiation to their primary site and both sides of the neck through opposing portals.

A question frequently asked concerns the risks of simultaneous bilateral neck dissection. There is little risk except for the additional surgery and time on the operating table when the contralateral jugular vein is saved. When it is possible to save the vein, the neck dissection may not have been needed in the first place. I believe that simultaneous radical neck dissections are of minimal risk provided they are performed rapidly and the operative time remains relatively short (<5–6 hours). The complications in my experiences occur when the surgery is long. Atelectasis, pneumonia, thrombophlebitis, and pulmonary emboli can be attributed to slow surgery and lengthy anesthesia. A teacher of mine once said, "Surgery is like beating a person with a stick. The longer you beat, the more it hurts."

When simultaneous or even staged second neck dissections are performed, a tracheostomy is mandatory. If both jugular veins are taken, rapid onset of laryngeal edema can be an unwelcome seqeula. Management of the cerebral and facial edema is accomplished with corticosteroids and upright posturing of the patient.

CONCLUSION

The last 20 to 30 years have witnessed remarkable advances in our surgical capabilities in the management of head and neck cancer. Our resections have reached spectacular proportions, and the multiple reconstructive flaps and grafts have enhanced the quality of life.

Surgery retains its position as the primary form of therapy for local and regional metastatic diseases. Prospective randomized studies are needed to evaluate the effectiveness of combined therapy (surgery and radiation). When better drugs become available, further protocol studies that include chemotherapy need to be conducted.

REFERENCES

1. Wolf GT: Head and neck tumor immunology, in Veldman JE (ed): *Immunobiology, Histophysiology, Tumor Immunology in Otorhinolaryngology.* Amsterdam, Kugler Publishers, 1987, pp 343–354.
2. Lufkin RB, Hanafee WN: Magnetic resonance imaging of head and neck tumor. *Cancer Metastasis Rev* 1988; 7:19–38.
3. Snow GB: Surgical management. Paper presented at the Second International Conference on Head and Neck Cancer, Boston, August 1988.
4. Byers RM, Wolf PF, Ballantyne AJ: Rationale for elective modified neck dissection. *Head Neck Surg* 1988; 10:160–167.
5. Vandenbrouck C, Sancho-Garnier H, Chassagne D, et al: Elective versus therapeutic radical neck dissection in epidermoid carcinoma of the oral cavity. *Cancer* 1980; 46:386–390.
6. Bocca E, Pignataro O: Conservation technique in radical neck dissection. *Ann Otolaryngol* 1967; 76:975–987.
7. Schuller DE, Caputa M: Surgical management of the N0 neck. Paper presented at the Second International Conference on Head and Neck Cancer, Boston, August 1988.

Oncologic Issues Relating to Neck Dissection

Approach of

Lawrence W. DeSanto, M.D.

NODAL FIXATION

Nodal fixation is associated with a poor prognosis. The word "fixed" is an examiner's interpretation that can mean attachment to structures that can be removed (e.g., the mandible, sternomastoid muscle, external carotid system, skin of the neck, or clavicle) or attachment to structures that cannot be practically removed or that cannot be removed without hazard (e.g., the skull base and common or internal carotid arteries).

Others use the term to describe decreased mobility. This difference in interpretation explains why the frequency of fixation in different series ranges from 5% (in most)[1] to as high as 35%.[2]

The classification systems have had trouble with the concept of fixation, and the current American Joint Committee system has discarded an attempt to classify fixation in favor of recording nodal size.[3] The previous American Joint Committee classification[4] used the designation N2 for fixed, the European Union Internationale Contre Cancer classification uses N3,[5] and the M. D. Anderson system uses N3 for unilateral nodal fixation and N3B for bilateral fixation.[6]

The importance of the distinction between fixed and reduced mobility was demonstrated by Spiro et al.[7] For tumors of the oral cavity and oropharynx, the 5-year cure rate was 40% in patients with a single node of "reduced mobility" but only 13% in those with "fixed" nodes.

Fixation is related to size, because a node is usually quite large before it becomes fixed.[7]

The frequency of fixation varies with tumor site. A multicenter study of larynx cancer in the 1950s and 1960s found fixed nodes in only 14 of 600 patients (2.3%), and only 1 of them survived 5 years (7%), whereas the survival rate with mobile metastatic nodes was 40%.[4] A few years later, the frequency of fixation was reported in other organs. Fixation was observed in 15%, 20%, and more than 30% of patients with primary cancer of the oropharynx, hypopharynx, and nasopharynx, respectively.

The effect on fixation was striking. The 5-year survival rate in patients with unilateral fixed nodes was 7% and in those with bilateral fixation was zero.[8]

Fixation increases with size of the primary tumor. Stell et al. observed that the frequency was 18% with T4 and 3.8% with T1 primary tumors.[1] The difference was highly significant ($P <$ 0.01).

One would like to think that the frequency of nodal fixation has decreased in the intervening 20 to 30 years, and it may have in some places. There are very few data that specifically address the concept of fixation. In the comprehensive report by Stell et al. in 1984, the incidence of large fixed glands was 23% in 1,918 patients seen from 1964 through 1981.[1] The 23% estimate was a clinical judgment. On exploration, some of the large neck masses in the series could be treated with a curative goal, and some were cured. The adjusted estimate of fixation after exploration was about 7%.

This statistic is of interest. It calls into question the whole judgment of fixation and really means that in some patients one cannot be sure a mass is fixed without attempting to remove it. It also raises the issue of definitions of "unresectable" and "incurable." If one assumes that a large mass that cannot be removed is incurable, it would seem that some patients are denied the opportunity for treatment with some probability of cure by a clinical judgment that may not be correct; that is, curability is related to a degree to the skill and determination of the surgeon. This observation also calls into question studies of alternative therapies, such as chemotherapy with or without radiation, in which the criterion for entry is "technical" unresectability or the judgment "inoperable."[9]

On the other hand, not every tumor that is resectable is curable by resection. That issue cannot be predetermined.

The treatment options for a fixed neck mass, regardless of the site in the neck, are limited to four: (1) no treatment, (2) radiation alone, (3) conventional combined therapy with radiation and surgery, and (4) investigative forms of combined therapy with radiation, chemotherapy, and surgery.

No Treatment

The choice between no treatment and palliative treatment with radiation or chemotherapy is difficult. Our society does not easily acknowledge that there are times when its technology is incapable of altering the course of a disease. Sometimes doing nothing could be the right option. When this time occurs can be decided only by the responsible physician alone in a consultation room with the patient and his or her family. An honest discussion of options, consequences, and probabilities with the patient and family at least lets them know that they can choose not to have treatment. Some of the most satisfying letters I have had have come from the families of patients who died of cancer after no treatment was elected. In this situation, a sincere commitment to be available to help with pain relief, feeding problems, and airway management is all the patient really wants from the physician. When the decision not to treat is made, one must be careful about recommendations for diversionary therapies such as tracheotomies. To a patient with clearly incurable head and neck cancer, a tracheostomy is not always a positive addition. One must remember that there is a quality factor in death as well as in life, and some of the things that can be done to a patient may lessen the quality of both life and death. It is really a philosophical issue, but I do not believe it makes a great deal of difference whether I die in April or May. I do care about what those last weeks will be like.

Radiation

The decision to treat a patient with an unequivocally fixed neck mass by radiation alone for palliation is an attractive one. This decision is often made. It must be clear to the patient that the goal of the treatment is to buy time. Making a big neck mass smaller is usually not of any value. The question, then, is how much time one buys with palliative radiation. Stell et al. found that only 3% of untreated patients were alive at 1 year, whereas with radiation about 30% were alive at 1 year.[1] All were dead by 2 years. Fifty percent of those not treated were dead at 6 months, and of those treated by radiation, 70% were still alive at 6 months. These statistics can be interpreted two ways. The most attractive interpretation is that palliative radiation added a few months to the patients' survival. A more realistic interpretation is that the patients who were not treated were into or almost at the final phase of their lives, whereas those who had radiation were a bit healthier and thus lived longer. The radiation was not the reason they lived longer. The interpretation of median survival curves is hazardous without a very clear description of the population involved. The population difference in Stell and associates' large study illustrates this point.[1] The median age of those not treated was 10 years greater than that of those who were (67 compared with 57 years).

There is very little in the literature about radiation to the fixed node. Petrovich et al. noted that of 76 patients with tonsil cancer who had bilateral or fixed nodes treated by radiation alone, none survived for 5 years.[10] Likewise, Saxena and Allt reported that among the 12% of 456 patients with tongue cancer who had fixed nodes treated by radiation alone, nobody was alive at 5 years.[11]

At times, a miraculous response occurs after radiation to a fixed neck mass, and one reconsiders and decides on resection. This is a goal change. The radiation shifts from palliative to preoperative. Stell et al. noted that when this happens, although the survival curve briefly shifts in favor of those who have the combined therapy, by 2 years the curves have converged, with only about 8 of 100 persons alive.[1]

Surgical Treatment

Surgical treatment of the fixed node depends on to what the mass is fixed. Whether fixation is to a structure that can be removed, such as the skin of the neck, the mandible, the skull base, the larynx, or the pharynx, or cannot be removed, such as the internal carotid artery, makes a difference.

The most distressing situation is fixation to the carotid artery. The carotid can be involved in two ways: (1) the mass is fixed only to the external carotid system, or (2) the common or internal carotids are invaded. If only the external system or the external system and the bifurcation are invaded, one can resect the mass by cross-clamping the artery at the bifurcation and above and then closing the arteriotomy with vascular sutures and needles. This can be done safely and without predictable morbidity. When the common or internal carotid arteries are involved, the consequences of resection and grafting are high, and the probability of success is limited. Stroke or death as a consequence is a real risk. Beahrs and Devine did a few carotid resections in the 1960s but abandoned the procedure because the price was unacceptable.[12] Others verified their observations.[1, 13]

There can be a temptation to "peel" tumor off the carotid and finesse what is called "microscopic disease" with postoperative radiation. This approach is almost always followed by early recurrence.[1] Brachytherapy with radioisotope implants may have a place in this situation. Removing all cancer when one can still seems preferable to depending on supplemental treatments. As a rule, if cancer is not removed in toto, it will come back. Debulking is not, in my opinion, a concept worthy of recognition by the committed head and neck oncologic surgeon.

Fixation to the skin of the neck or the mandible is not a hopeless situation. Wide excision of neck skin and partial resection of the mandible when tumor is attached externally can be worthwhile. There are many ways to replace the neck skin, and the old deltopectoral flap is as good as any. When fixation is found on exploration to be direct extension rather than nodal disease, there is usually a chance for bloc excision. I experienced this situation with piriform sinus carcinoma. Tumor had pushed through the constrictor muscles and was palpable in the neck. The mass was close to but not on or into the carotid artery, and resection was possible. A fixed mass by direct extension is possible with supraglottic cancer, but here the mass would be closer to the midline than the usual large metastatic mass. The use of CT scanning in these unusual situations would be prudent.

My experience with CT scanning to determine whether a fixed mass is, in fact, resectable is not extensive. In the few cases in which a decision had to be made about the practicality of exploration, I did not depend on the scan as the final arbitrator. I thought there was too much at stake, and I believe that exploration is the best "test" to determine operability. The routine use of computer imaging in metastatic neck disease does not seem necessary or helpful.

Combined Therapy

The combination of surgery and radiation is an attractive concept. In instances of nodal fixation, radiation before surgery is theoretically better. The theory that radiation can "downstage" a tumor and make seemingly inoperable tumors operable is based on the idea that tumors are "sterilized" from the periphery. The periphery is better oxygenated, and the better the oxygenation, the more radiosensitive the cancer cells, according to the theory. This radiobiologic theory, attractive as it is, breaks down when tested with human cancer. Tumor destruction is not centripetal, and the belief that inoperable cancer can be made operable is wishful thinking.

Very little in the literature supports the concept of combined radiation and surgery for the fixed neck mass. Wang et al. reported that two of seven patients with fixed masses were alive at 3 years after preoperative radiation and neck dissection.[14] Barkley et al. from the M.D. Anderson group found no improvement in survival with combined therapy in patients with unilateral or bilateral fixed nodes.[15]

Combined Therapy With Chemotherapy

The preliminary report on bleomycin-methotrexate and radiation by Fu et al. addressed advanced and "inoperable" cancer but did not reveal whether "inoperable" was based on nodal disease or primary size.[9] The study showed a prolonged relapse-free survival time with combined therapy that could have been related to the drug therapy or to the patient population. There was no difference in survival, however, between radiation alone and radiation plus chemotherapy. One of the objectives of adjuvant chemotherapy is to decrease the frequency of distant metastasis. The study by Fu and associates[9] found a higher incidence of distant metastasis in the group treated with drugs than in the group receiving radiation alone (38% compared with 24%). This observation needs to be followed carefully in patients with advanced disease. We need to start asking critical questions about what our treatments do to the host's own tumor immunity.

Observations

1. Although more than 20% of nodes were thought to be fixed in the largest study to address this specific issue, only 7% were actually fixed;[1] thus, the judgment of fixation is a value one, and when it is in doubt, the neck should be dissected.

2. A survey of the literature suggests that the incidence of death from intercurrent disease between the second and the fifth years is unusually high in patients with fixed neck disease. This finding suggests that the person with cancer who presents with a fixed mass differs in some way from the usual patients with head and neck cancer. That difference needs to be looked at to see if it is a socioeconomic variable or something related to tumor-specific immunity.

3. There are different kinds of carotid artery invasion— some that can be safely treated surgically and others that cannot. Precise definition requires exploration in some patients.

4. Not all fixed masses are nodal disease. Some fixed masses are direct extension of tumor, for example, extension from a piriform sinus cancer. Others are cancer into soft tissue or muscle. These are further reasons to explore the neck when there is doubt. Also, CT scans will help in these instances.

5. Fixed nodes are more common from some sites than from others, possibly because some sites, such as the nasopharynx and piriform sinus, are late in producing symptoms and are more likely to be neglected until obvious signs appear. The frequency of fixation goes up as the tumor stage increases.

Dermal Lymphatic Involvement

Subcutaneous tumor or tumor in the skin is rare. I am unaware of any study that specifically addresses this issue. What this finding means practically is that wide margins of skin need to be resected if the problem is to be managed surgically (i.e., if it is curable). The problem is that tumor can be at a distance from the gross margins of the specimen with skip areas in between. A surgical pathologist skilled in the diagnosis of fresh-frozen sections is essential. What I would do is excise the skin mass in continuity with a neck dissection and submit the specimen to the pathologist. I would then take another margin 360 degrees around the skin defect and ask the pathologist to study that tissue. Management of the skin is essentially the same as that of an invasive basal cell carcinoma with modified Mohs' technique and frozen section control. Relining the neck should not be difficult. The median-based deltopectoral flap or an acromioclavicular flap can resurface almost the entire side of the neck (Fig 22–1).

TREATMENT OPTIONS FOR THE NECK WITH N0 DISEASE

Radiation in the Clinically Normal Neck

The issue of the clinically normal neck is best addressed by answering the question, "Which unnecessary treatment to the truly normal neck is the least harmful — dissection or radiation?" If the neck does not contain metastatic cancer, neither dissection nor radiation helps the patient.

The premise of elective radiation is based on several assumptions that may not be valid. The first assumption is that nonclinical disease is microscopic disease. This is an important issue, because the whole basis of elective radiation is that its effectiveness is related to tumor load and that microscopic tumor is more likely to be cured than gross cancer in nodes. The reality is that disease that cannot be palpated is not necessarily microscopic in size. Nonpalpable disease is often gross cancer after the specimen is exposed. My experience is that at least one third of patients with neck metastasis that cannot be pal-

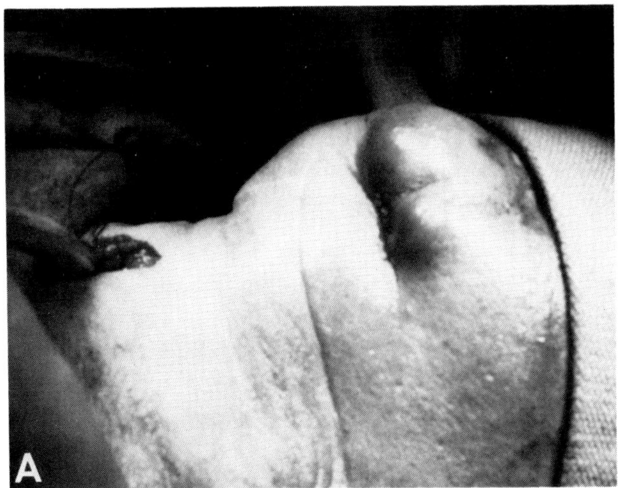

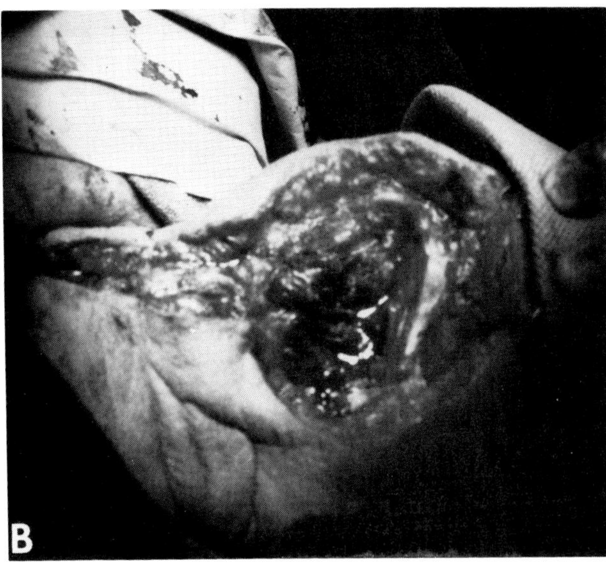

FIG 22–1.
A, dermal metastasis with fixation to mandible. **B,** wide local excision, including rim of mandible.

pated have gross metastasis in the dissected neck specimen.[16, 17] The evolution of the treatment of microscopic disease by radiation is an interesting study in how facts can be stretched from what one knows to be true to what one would like to believe is true.

The idea that radiation could cure microscopic disease began with Cohen in 1968 with an animal experiment (see later discussion of radiation and the neck).[18]

The evidence that microscopic disease is, in fact, cured by 5,000 rad or more to the clinically normal neck is indirect, inferential, conflicting, and confusing about what one can really count on when depending on radiation to control metastatic disease in the clinically normal neck.

One of two random trials of elective treatment to the neck compared elective radiation with delayed neck dissection, and the other compared elective dissection plus radiation in N+ disease with delayed dissection. Although fewer patients in the irradiated group subsequently required neck dissection, the survival rates in both groups were the same. Vandenbrouck et al. treated 75 patients with carcinoma of the tongue by interstitial radiation and 6 weeks later randomized patients to either therapeutic or elective neck dissection or radiation.[19] In the patients with abnormal nodes after dissection, postoperative radiation therapy was added. In the elective dissection group, 19 of 39 (49%) had histologically abnormal nodes. Among the 36 patients in whom dissection was delayed, histologically abnormal nodes eventually developed in 17 (47%) (50% were spared neck treatment). The authors noted extracapsular cancer in 25% of these cases compared with 13% in those with elective dissection, but this difference was not reflected by survival rates. Two patients in whom dissection was delayed could not be treated at the time they were seen with neck disease.

The inferential data on the value of elective neck radiation come from studies that compare neck recurrence rates after elective treatment with the frequency of late neck metastasis after no neck treatment and the frequency of contralateral nodal disease. Also, neck recurrence frequencies when the neck was partially radiated were compared with those after complete neck radiation. Data showed that the neck recurrence rates were less than would be expected in all of these situations when radiation was delivered in proper amounts to the normal neck.[15, 20–27] None of these studies was random, and a variety of tumors and stages were included. Exclusions were numerous. Specifically excluded were patients with uncontrolled primary tumors. Looked at together, the studies demonstrated that the neck recurrence rates were in the 5% range when the primary tumor was controlled. Neck recurrence was less often seen when the whole neck was radiated than when only part was treated. Contralateral nodal disease developed in only about 4% when both sides of the neck were treated but in 24% when the contralateral side was not treated. Unfortunately, none of these studies indicated that elective neck radiation does anything to improve survival. The suggestion that elective neck radiation merely changes the pattern of disease and the cause of death has yet to be studied or refuted.

Elective Neck Dissection

The surgeon's case for elective neck dissection in the clinically normal neck is based on the general belief that the less disease required to be removed, the more effective treatment will be. This belief, too, may not be true. Bocca, an early and vigorous proponent of the elective treatment of the neck, was interested in cancer of the supraglottic larynx and recognized that the main cause of failure in treating this disease was failure in the neck.[28, 29] He made his case for bilateral neck dissection in all instances. Many of the dissections were elective. He cited a 16% attrition in survival between patients who had an elective dissection that was therapeutic (clinically N0 and pathologically N+) and those who had a delayed dissection. Lee and Krause made a similar observation about the benefits of elective surgical treatment of the neck.[30]

Elective neck treatment is criticized because of morbidity and because some patients are necessarily treated but get no oncologic benefit. Morbidity in neck dissection is said to be from 1% to 5%,[31] but this incidence includes the morbidity of treating the primary cancer too. When dissection is compared with elective radiation to the clinically normal neck, there is another issue beyond the effectiveness of one compared with that of the other. When one acknowledges that patients with truly normal neck nodes derive no oncologic benefit and may actually be harmed by the morbidity from the dissection and radiation and that morbidity is related to the immunologic purpose of the nodes, the comparison becomes one of cost vs. benefit. With radiation, there is no specimen, so that no staging or prognostic information is gathered. The dissection is a staging procedure that is, when there is disease, therapeutic. All things considered, this information is worthwhile for planning purposes and peace of mind when the specimen is negative for cancer. The cost of the dissection is extra time and a scar, but no bridges are burned. Radiation is a one-time treatment, and there are long-term consequences.

With this comparison, I believe that the least harm is done with the most benefit (staging) by an elective dissection when it seems appropriate. Elective radiation seems excessive when it is compared with an efficiently executed dissection. I have no regrets if there is no metastasis. If surgery is used for primary treatment and there is a reasonable probability of metastasis in the clinically normal neck, I prefer a staging neck dissection to radiation.

The only reasonable situation for radiation in the clinically normal neck is a primary tumor of low volume that is to be treated with external radiation. Then the neck nodes can be included in the treatment plan. Few data exist on the effectiveness of this approach on survival. Most reports deal with local and regional control.

Modified Neck Dissection

We have taught and performed the most practical modified neck dissection since the early 1960s; that dissection is the Crile operation,[32] with preservation of the spinal accessory nerve when it seems appropriate. The obvious place for this modification is the clinically negative neck, because the dissection is a staging procedure. It is also reasonable to preserve the accessory nerve in some N+ neck dissections if the gross disease is not near the 11th nerve.

Having used a modification of the Crile operation for many years, I find it difficult to understand what all the fuss and confusion are about today surrounding the subject of modified neck dissection. Some of the confusion is semantic. We use the term modified neck dissection for any operation that is not the classic Crile operation. The M. D. Anderson group described a whole series of neck dissections as modified: the suprahyoid dissection, supraomohyoid dissection, the anterior modified dissection, a posterior neck dissection, and so forth.[33] All this means, of course, is that surgeons do as they have always done as they try to fit the operation to the patient's problem.

The prototype modified dissection is the one described by Bocca and Pignataro[34] and Bocca et al.[35] that preserves the 11th nerve, the internal jugular vein, and the sternomastoid muscle.

Bocca evolved the technique because he was convinced that the concept of prophylactic dissection was valuable. He believed that patients had a better chance to get well and stay well if metastatic neck disease was removed while it was occult (nonpalpable) rather than when it became palpable. This belief is intuitive to surgeons, who understandably believe that the less cancer they are called on to remove, the better the outlook. This precept may not be true, because we are now beginning to understand that there is more to curing cancer than removing cells. Bocca was justifiably bothered by the fact that in supraglottic laryngeal cancer, for which bilateral dissections were deemed essential, so many persons incurring the morbidity of losing both accessory nerves were then found to have pathologically negative neck specimens. Bocca never believed, nor do I believe, that sacrifice of the sternomastoid muscle on one or both sides or of both internal jugular veins is a big issue in terms of morbidity.

It seems to me, then, that the modified operation is pertinent only in instances of bilateral dissection. With careful preservation of the accessory nerve in unilateral dissection assumed in the clinically negative neck (N0), the Bocca modified operation is a nice anatomic exercise that really gives very little extra to the patient. There is no value in saving one internal jugular vein. (It is just another vein that is a bit bigger and has a name.) The idea that the cerebral circulation somehow depends on the internal jugular veins is a fallacy. To be sure, there is sometimes impressive facial swelling, and I have observed papilledema after unilateral and bilateral dissection. Nevertheless, it has been known for years that more than 60% of the cerebral drainage is independent of the internal jugular circulation.[32, 36] One can debate the cosmetic value of the sternomastoid muscle. My impression is that when it is preserved, it is denervated and devascularized and shrivels up. The fuss today over modified neck dissection seems to ignore the fact that modified neck dissection has been quietly going on for years.[31, 37]

In bilateral elective neck dissection, there may be some short-term benefits of saving one internal jugular vein along with both accessory nerves. I still wonder if the preserved internal jugular vein stays patent in every patient. I have observed some impressive facial swelling after the Bocca operation. I attempt a Bocca type of modification in patients with supraglottic cancer and some with oropharyngeal cancer (base of tongue, tonsil) when bilateral simultaneous dissection is performed.

I have two concerns about the modified concept today, and neither is with oncologic safety. The first is what I have called the linkage issue, and the second deals with quality.

Bocca was the father of linkage. In necks that turned out to contain cancer, Bocca was concerned, when he started with his modification, that there was an increased risk of neck recurrence when he did something less than the Crile operation. This was at the time when the Halsted concept of "the bloc" was fundamental to oncologic surgery. At least in the upper part of the neck and posterior triangle, the modified operation violated the bloc as it was described by Crile. For that reason, Bocca added postoperative radiation to the treatment of patients who had N+ neck disease. He later looked at his data and, finding that the addition of the radiation did nothing to the neck recurrence rates, abandoned postoperative radiation after neck dissection (an observation that seems to have been ignored in North America).[35]

Jesse and his colleagues did much to institutionalize the linkage of postoperative radiation to modified neck dissection.[38–41] Jesse was impressed by a Memorial Hospital study done in 1969 in which 2,000 rad was delivered preoperatively. The neck recurrence rate compared with that in historical controls decreased from 70% to just 30%. The theory of microscopic disease was then resurrected to justify the shift to postoperative radiation. From this came several decades of connection between modified neck dissection and postoperative radiation, to the point that the two terms almost ran together, like ham and eggs or peanut butter and jelly. There does seem to be a trend to unlink the two. Byers,[33] in 1985, came a great distance from the Jesse attitude when he suggested that postoperative radiation may not be needed in the treatment of the N0 or N1 neck after modified neck dissection. Our two studies of this issue found no stage of neck disease in which the addition of radiation after modified or complete neck dissection made a difference in neck recurrence rates or survival. We believe that a number of patients are incurring an escalation of treatment without benefit, and thus the concern over linkage.

The quality issue involves training and the standards of practice in the community. Cancer surgeons with a large volume of tumor work can mix and match modified operations to the clinical situation without harm. On the other hand, when there are six or more possible modifications in addition to the classic operation to be considered along with the primary ablation, we end up with hundreds of possible combinations that someone responsible must choose from. This variety and the combined therapy conundrum lead to confusion. The resident physician and the community surgeon have little to help them know what is right. This confusion can lead to undertreatment (no dissection) or overtreatment with combined therapy.

The quality of the dissection is another concern. The classic operation with or without preservation of the 11th nerve is a clean and understandable anatomic exercise. It is, in my opinion, a basic infrastructure on which the modifications are built. Unless one has a solid grounding in the basic operation, the modifications become a blur. I doubt this is an overstatement. I have watched for years the confusion in the minds of residents as they struggle to decide what is the right thing to do for neck management. I receive regular telephone calls asking basic questions about neck treatment. The first modification, the preservation of the accessory nerve, can be structured into an understandable list of options. The Bocca operation follows logically. The places of all the others in head and neck oncologic surgery are undefined.

It is naive to think that a modified neck dissection is easier to do than a classic operation. It is more difficult. It is better for patients who undergo neck dissection to have clean and efficient classic operations with or without preservation of the accessory nerve than slow, sloppy modified procedures. The idea that every preserved accessory nerve functions normally is not true either. Preservation and function are two different things. I believe that those who have trained residents will appreciate these observations. Residents must learn that the goal of the operation is to treat cancer and not just to save nerves, veins, or muscles.

To summarize, the modified dissection concept is worthwhile but has become mixed up with peripheral issues. The principal place for the modified operation (not considering the preservation of the 11th nerve) is in bilateral simultaneous dissection. The concept is criticized not because of oncologic concerns but because of the unjustified and at times irrational linkage of the modified operations to combined therapy. My concern is that in our zeal to do modified operations, we are confusing people and diluting the quality of care.

Combined Therapy

No issue involving head and neck cancer evokes more controversy than the place for and value of combined therapy with radiation or chemotherapy or both for head and neck squamous cell carcinoma. The opinions range from "All patients with head and neck cancer require combined therapy" to "None will benefit." The real value of any of the contemporary combined therapy schemes is undecided.

Some of the practical considerations about combined therapy from a patient's perspective are:

1. Any kind of treatment for cancer has problems and complications.
2. If single-modality therapy creates problems, multimodality treatment will create more.
3. Somebody should benefit from any escalation of therapy, and that somebody should be the patient.
4. The benefit to the patient should be an increase in the probability of survival from the treated disease.
5. Changing the mode of death when death occurs from the treatment or the disease is not progress.
6. All combined therapy programs are expensive and logistically inconvenient.

From the physician's perspective, there are other considerations:

1. Most combined therapy schemes are investigative and are best done in protocols with the patient's informed consent.
2. Factors of patient selection can profoundly distort the outcome of clinical trials, so that all studies that use historical controls are suspect without a contemporary comparison group with the same selection biases.
3. Young and sound patients usually live longer and withstand treatment better.
4. All patients reported in statistical studies must be accounted for in the denominators to avoid statistical bias. The discarding of patients who do not complete the program, are lost to follow-up, die from the treatment, or are otherwise ineligible for analysis makes the results for those who complete the program appear better than they really are.

These perspectives apply both to chemotherapy and to

radiation combined therapy schemes, either before or after ablative surgery.

Radiation and the Neck

There is little doubt that in surgically treated head and neck cancer when all the tumor is removed and the margins are confirmed free of cancer, the major cause of failure is uncontrolled metastatic disease. In our most recent analysis of glottic and supraglottic cancer, for example, the frequency of failure at the primary site was less than 2%.[42] The frequency of distant metastasis was less than 10%. Most of those who died did so because of uncontrolled metastasis in the neck. Certain situations are now recognized in which the likelihood of failure to control the disease in the neck is greater, even with a properly executed complete neck dissection. These include the presence of massive and fixed metastatic masses; metastatic tumor that has broken the capsule of a cervical node or extended into the soft tissues, muscle, fascia, or nerves; major skin involvement; and attachment of tumor to parts not usually removed, such as the base of the skull. Another such situation is metastasis to the nodes of the lower part of the neck. Even in the most favorable situation—the neck with no clinical metastasis or only microscopic disease—there are recurrences in the neck, and the rate of recurrence seems to increase as the clinical and pathologic stages of the neck disease increase.

Why even a small focus of cancer in a lymph node so alters prognosis is not known. Possibly a cancer that metastasizes is more aggressive, the host is less resistant, or some combination of both exists.

Because neck dissection alone is now and always has been less than satisfactory in controlling neck disease, efforts to add cancer-directed, potentially lethal particles or drugs are understandable. The concept of combining methods, each of which has some potential to destroy or alter in a positive way malignant cells, is logical until one considers their effects on the host as well as on the cancer. The combination most often used is radiation before or after surgery.

Radiation to the neck can be thought of as either prophylactic or adjunctive to neck dissection. The prophylactic concept was discussed earlier in regard to radiation in the clinically normal neck.

Adjunctive radiation can be delivered either before or after neck dissection. A separate radiobiologic theory covers each sequence. Preoperative radiation is based on the theory of oxygenation, that is, the better oxygenated a tumor is, the greater the positive radiobiologic effect and the more effective the treatment will be. A corollary of this theory is that the periphery of a tumor, either primary or metastatic, is better oxygenated, so that tumor destruction is concentric from the periphery in. Thus we have been told that preoperative radiation destroys cancer cells, reduces the size of the tumor burden, and leaves less material for possible spread during dissection designed to remove only the residual, presumed hypoxic central tumor core. Other positive assets claimed for preoperative radiation are (1) its potential to make fixed masses mobile and thus removable and curable and (2) an option with smaller masses to do a more functional dissection in which a structure, such as the accessory

nerve or sternomastoid muscle, is preserved without any increase in risk.

Unfortunately, radiation before definitive surgery, most believe, creates new problems, such as delayed primary healing, added hospital time, large skin sloughs, blown out carotid arteries, and pharyngeal fistulization. At one time, the proponents of preoperative radiation went so far as to say that if radiation was required after surgery, it was in error, because it really should have been given before.[43] When some data were available and studies of specimens had been reported, the concept of preoperative radiation was finished: there was no increase in cure rates, the sterilization of tumors was not concentric, and the neck recurrence rates were not decreased. Several decades of human misery were required to redirect efforts. Postoperative radiation was an old idea resurrected as a new direction.

Postoperative radiation is based on another theory, that of microscopic disease. The idea here is that cancer cells that remain at the periphery of a surgical site or in the depths of a dissected neck will be sterilized by a dose of postoperative radiation less than that lethal to normal tissue. This idea is not comfortably received by all radiation therapists because it is contrary to the oxygenation concept. Also, it violates the surgeon's general belief that cancer left in patients after resection, either at the margins of the primary tumor or within the neck, is rarely controlled by radiation. That is, positive margins of cancer left on a structure not removed, such as a carotid artery, cannot be predictably finessed by postoperative radiation even if the disease is microscopic.

Some of the hopes for postoperative radiation are that it will provide (1) a decrease in recurrence in the clinically negative neck with radiation alone (this may be the contralateral side of the neck or the undissected ipsilateral neck), (2) a decrease in recurrence in the dissected side of the neck, and (3) the opportunity to do a more conservative resection that removes all "gross disease" but may leave microscopic cancer at the margins and on arteries or nerves. This concept of gross total removal suggests to the oncologic surgeon that, as Fletcher[44] stated, "There is no benefit to be derived from trying to remove all microscopic disease, which cannot be done in all patients anyway. The increase in radicalism of the surgical procedure might be counterproductive by increasing the delay for the start of irradiation."

With a lesser operation, it is said that "diminished surgical manipulation provides less opportunity for throwing tumor cells into the blood stream" and that "there is less scar tissue and, therefore, less possibility of hypoxia of the tumor cells left behind. When surgery is conservative, the quality of life is better" and, of course, complications are fewer.[44]

All of these benefits are theoretical and mostly unrealistic. Nobody has ever quantitated the amount of manipulation in the various neck dissections, found out whether cells go into the bloodstream in different ways, or determined whether scarring is different or makes a difference. The idea that a modified operation to the neck or a conservation operation to the primary tumor is easier and quicker is naive. Most conservation neck and primary operations are technically more difficult and take longer than the classic dissection and require more manipulation. There is not one bit of substantive evidence that more patients get well. There is a real concern that none of these benefits is being experienced by patients. The linkage of the type of operation to combined therapy is, in my opinion, a leap of fancy that defies human reason. There are no data to verify that combining a conservative neck operation with postoperative radiation has any benefit to patients in terms of cure or length of survival.[16, 45–48] Moreover, the concept of removing only gross disease leads to the debulking idea, which permits one to leave behind cancer so long as it is microscopic and cannot be seen with the eye, and then clean it up with postoperative radiation. This is a dangerous idea.

The concept of microscopic disease itself is flimsy, because in the clinical reality, microscopic and nonpalpable are used interchangeably. The experienced head and neck surgeon knows that it is not uncommon to find gross nodal metastatic disease in necks that contain nothing palpable. A microscopic focus of cancer can be up to several millimeters in diameter and contain 10^6 to 10^8 cancer cells. The death of a cancer cell is a random event and is not intrinsic to being irradiated. The cell must be hit by the radiation particle in a critical place. It takes the same amount of radiation to decrease the cell population from 10^7 to 10^6 cells as it does to go from 100 to 10 cells. The mathematical probabilities of predictable control of even microscopic disease are not all that promising.

The evolution of the concept of microscopic disease from a radiobiologic experiment to a clinical assumed truth is a study in how we can take what we would like to believe to be true and evolve it into truth. The experiment cited is that of Cohen, who, in 1968, reported a simple dose survival curve of an experimental mouse adenocarcinoma.[18] With incremental increases in radiation amount delivered to microscopic foci of these experimental tumors, more cancer cells appeared to die, and at radiation amounts greater than 5,000 rad, about 90% appeared dead or incapable of reproducing. Nothing was said in this experiment about persons, squamous cell carcinoma, postoperative radiation, or human survival. We have changed that 90% figure in our meetings and conferences from "theoretically 90% of microscopic cancer will be destroyed," to "90% of microscopic cancer will be destroyed," to "90% of neck recurrences will be prevented," and finally to "90% of people will get well." None of these statements except the initial one of Cohen and the theoretical conjecture has any basis in established data. All are unsubstantiated and probably not true.

In analyzing the available studies on the effectiveness of combined therapy with postoperative radiation, one can find a retrospective study to support any bias one would like supported. As a generalization, if the series is small,[49] the number of exclusions is large, or historical controls are used for comparison, the likelihood is great that postoperative radiation will be found to have a positive benefit in decreasing recurrence rates in the neck.[47] No valid study that I am aware of has claimed an impact of increased survival with the contemporary combined therapy schemes.

Nevertheless, postoperative radiation has become the reality in head and neck oncologic practice to the extent that it is looked on as the community standard to an almost quasilegal degree. To paraphrase Winston Churchill, never have so many been treated so much for so little.

Combined Therapy in Practice

The Mayo Clinic practice is an integrated group practice because multidisciplinary consultation is available to every patient. The ultimate treatment decisions are made after appropriate studies and consultations have been obtained. The treatment decisions are made between the patient and the single consultant responsible for that patient. Tumor boards as a decision-making body have never been popular, because committees cannot assume individual responsibility. Within the institution are several services that treat head and neck cancer. Within a given service, several individuals have a special interest and experience with patients who have head and neck cancer. Treatment protocols for the more common tumors have not been used, with the exception of chemotherapy protocols for patients with advanced and disseminated cancer.

Several principles are shared among the consultants, since all believe that the first treatment should be the one most likely to succeed in solving the patient's tumor problem. To that end, there has been little enthusiasm for a "radical radiation with surgery for salvage" approach to any stage or type of squamous cell cancer. All believe that the control of tumor margins in surgically treated cancer depends on the use and expertise of a surgical pathologist present in the operating area and skilled in the preparation and interpretation of fresh-frozen sections. All believe that the person who recommends the initial treatment retains a responsibility until the patient is declared cured and released or dies. Each consultant shares a well-organized and dedicated follow-up system that assures nearly universal follow-up and statistical analysis, and few patients are lost to follow-up.

Beyond these shared aspects of practice is the freedom for diversity, and this leads to a somewhat random approach to specific issues such as combined therapy. At any one time, one or more consultants may have been enthusiastic toward multimodality therapy, and their patients would be more likely to have received postoperative radiation in more recent years or preoperative radiation in the 1960s and early 1970s than would patients with the same disease at the same stage who were seen by consultants who had less enthusiasm for combined therapy.

This randomness allowed for the comparison of effectiveness of both preoperative and postoperative radiation as supplements to neck dissection in a large group of patients with head and neck cancer. We compared the effectiveness of combined therapy with that of neck dissection alone in two studies.[16, 17] The first addressed primarily preoperative radiation and the later postoperative radiation, and the combined series in 1985 was the largest study to date of radiation on the effectiveness of neck treatment. We were unable to find any stage of neck disease in which neck recurrences were fewer or survival was better with either preoperative or postoperative radiation than with neck dissection alone when contemporary treatment plans and radiation dosages were used.

A sophisticated statistical study used a case-pair method in which patients were matched by all the variables, such as age, sex, primary site and stage, control of the primary lesion, pathologic stage of neck disease, and even date of surgery, that would be applied to a randomized prospective study. The only difference was that one patient received postoperative radiation and the other in the pair did not. Even with this type of analysis, we could not verify that the addition of radiation after neck dissection decreased the frequency of neck recurrences or decreased the probability of death from cancer.

We were careful not to state that radiation after neck dissection was of no value. Rather, we stated that using the data we had and using the statistical methods we used, we simply could not find an instance when radiation plus dissection was superior to dissection alone. These conclusions should not be too surprising. There is no substantive study in the literature that has claimed improved survival (the only worthy goal of combined therapy). A few have claimed fewer neck recurrences in the combined group as a whole or in specific subgroups (patients with extranodal spread of cancer).[33, 47, 50]

A specific question must be answered: What are my indications for either preoperative or postoperative radiation therapy to the neck?

Preoperative Radiation

Preoperative radiation is rarely used, and when it is, it is selected more as a triage technique than a cure-directed treatment. What this means is that some patients have insurmountable neck disease or at least neck disease in which the size of fixation of the neck mass causes one to believe intuitively that neck dissection with a curative goal is unlikely (Fig 22–2). An ablative procedure in these patients is usually the substitution of hope for reality. In that situation, radiation to high, yet preoperative, dosage buys some time to reconsider the surgery option. Usually something intervenes, such as a change in the chest radiograph, a cranial nerve palsy that indicates skull base involvement, or death. Infrequently, the neck mass marvelously resolves, and if no other contraindications come along, a definitive procedure can be considered. Even with a miraculous response to the preoperative radiation, these patients are rarely cured. This is a somewhat cynical attitude toward preoperative radiation, but the human occurrence is real.

Postoperative Radiation

With all the evidence against any curative value of combined therapy that includes postoperative radiation, the answer to the aforementioned question should be "I never use postoperative radiation!" That would not be true. I do not often use postoperative radiation. I do know when the prospects for neck dissection alone are not very good. Big nodes, multiple nodes, low neck nodes, and neck masses peeled off through a subadventitial plane of the carotid artery are all serious conditions, and I discuss them with the patient and the family. I try to be honest in my skepticism toward some magical additional step that will make a difference. I scrupulously avoid promising more than I believe can be delivered by avoiding such statements as, "We need to add postoperative radiation *just to be sure.*" I am convinced that if given a chance, patients understand our humanity and realize that we do not have all the answers and that not everybody we treat will be cured by what we do. Some patients faced with the reality of their disease elect to receive postoperative radiation. Others, when given a choice, prefer to live their lives in another way. No patient or family has come back with criticisms because of this approach. This is not very scientific, but neither is an approach that intuitively believes that in spite of all the data to the contrary, more is necessarily better.

Chemotherapy

The possibilities of chemotherapy are threefold: (1) induction (neoadjuvant) before standard treatment, (2) administration concomitant with radiation therapy, and (3) administration after standard treatment.

Simultaneous drug and radiation therapy has been shown to be extremely toxic at the local level without real gains in survival. Much more experimental work in animals is needed before more experiments are undertaken in humans.

Two randomized studies are in progress to determine the effect of chemotherapy after standard therapy, one in the United States and the other in France.[51] Both are in patients who have histologic metastatic nodal disease with extracapsular spread. In the French study, with more than 100 patients assessed in each arm of the study (with and without chemotherapy), no benefit has been shown from the adjuvant treatment.

Chemotherapy in an adjuvant induction sequence is the current focus in combined therapy. Without question, tumor response rates with the current combinations are impressive, because they approach or exceed those of breast cancer and approach those of lymphoma.[52] The problem is that we really do not know what the response means in terms of survival increments. The effectiveness of induction (upfront) chemotherapy in randomized trials has been strikingly disappointing. In a number of randomized clinical trials with 50 or more

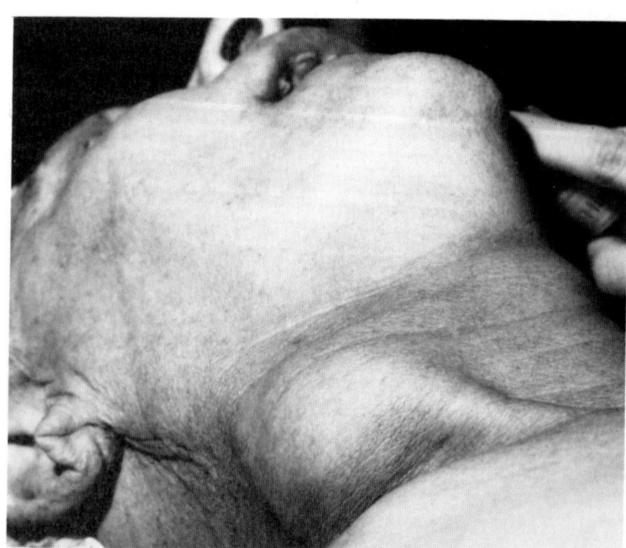

FIG 22–2.
Fixed node to carotid artery in lower part of neck. Successful resection is unlikely.

patients, sequential therapy followed by conventional local-regional therapy has been compared with conventional local-regional therapy alone. Of nine studies summarized by Tannock and Browman, only two using intraarterial chemotherapy showed improved survival in the experimental arm, and two others showed a "trend" toward improvement in patients randomized to receive chemotherapy.[53] The other trials, including the large National Cancer Institute trial, which evaluated a single dose of a large amount of cisplatin and bleomycin given by infusion before surgery with and without radiation, showed a similar survival in both arms. Other studies have preliminary data or too few patients. There have been no striking reports that deviate in their differences from those that can be expected due to random fluctuations about a null effect.

It is clear from the clinical oncology literature that chemotherapeutic combinations with conventional therapy must be conducted as part of a protocol. The protocols must be statistically valid and have contemporary controls. Chemotherapy combined with surgery or radiation is, today, experimental, and the patients who get involved must be so advised. In the community, the use of chemotherapeutic combinations with surgery or radiation cannot be passed off on patients as acceptable clinical practice. To do so would, in my opinion, be unconscionable.

The goals of the chemotherapeutic trials are fairly well understood. The trials must study whether (1) primary and nodal tumor regression will lead to better local and regional control, (2) initially unresectable tumors (Who decides this?) will be reduced in size to permit effective surgical removal (i.e., Can tumors be downstaged?), (3) a patient population can be identified for whom surgical resection can be eliminated or a more conservative procedure can be done (again, downstaging), (4) chemotherapy will eliminate micrometastasis and in the process reduce the risk of systemic metastasis, and (5) more patients will be cured than are now cured with single-modality therapy.

One of the problems the head and neck surgeon has with the current thinking about chemotherapy by the clinical oncologist is that some of the latter's premises are different from the ones the surgical oncologist and, to a lesser degree, the radiation oncologist work with. The clinical oncologist believes, on the basis of autopsy studies, that 30% to 50% of patients with head and neck cancer who die of their disease have clinical or occult distant metastasis.[54] This generalization, which may not be true or, if true, is iatrogenic, implies that head and neck cancer is a systemic disease relatively early. The surgeon's perspective is quite different. The oncologic problems are uncontrolled regional disease and, to a lesser degree, local control. In no head and neck primary cancers that I treat does the incidence of distant metastasis in all stages throughout all phases of treatment come anywhere near that 30% figure. Ten percent distant metastasis is about the highest we have reported.[43, 55] Crile, in his monumental description of en bloc neck dissection in the first decade of the century, cited a study of more than 4,000 cancers of the head and neck treated at that time in which at all stages of the disease and at death the distant metastasis rate was less than 5%.[32] The striking incidence of distant metastasis reported in contemporary studies either reflects a change

in the natural history of the disease or is the result of differences in therapy from Crile's time.

The attempts to redefine head and neck cancer as a systemic disease in the early stages are either wrong or self-serving. One must ask whether the treatment, either through alteration of tumor resistance in the host or through delays caused by sequential therapy, is responsible for the high incidence of distant metastasis. We tend to look at the tumor and our treatment somewhat separately from the host of the tumor, and we seldom ask what our treatment is doing to the host and his or her relationship to the tumor.

The second problem is that clinical oncologists are enamored with response rates of the tumor to the chemicals, and implied is their belief that response rate or degree is somehow related to the goal of curing the patient's disease.

A complete response implies a total disappearance of disease; partial response is more than 50% reduction in the sum of the products of the longest perpendicular diameters of the most clearly measurable lesions. The definition of a complete response seems obvious. The validity of a complete response is directly proportional to the enthusiasm of the investigator. A defined complete response, especially malignant adenopathy, would undoubtedly not be so if measured by CT or MRI. The definition of a partial response also seems unassailable on casual review, but few authors clarify the distinction between a 50% reduction in the sum of the diameters of all measurable disease and a 50% reduction in the single most measurable lesion. Moreover, if most abnormalities decrease by 50% but one increases in size, most investigators would call this a partial response. Aside from these procedural gymnastics, the clinical reality is that most head and neck lesions are not precisely measurable, and all lesions do not have discrete perpendicular margins. Observer bias cannot be ignored. An experienced colleague of mine summarized all the statistical jargon by stating, "There is undoubtedly an inverse correlation between objective response rates and the number of photographs per publication. The higher the number of photographs, the lower the response rate." As Gertrude Stein said, "A difference to be different must make a difference." The equating of response with a service to patients is a giant leap that has never been verified in a controlled study.[54]

Another problem is the interpretation of survival curves by tumor response. Oncologists like to believe that "responders live longer than nonresponders"[56, 57] and that the treatment (chemotherapy) causes longer survival. The reality is that the divergence of survival curves in favor of one treatment over the other reflects a number of interacting factors that may be completely independent of the treatment. The "nonresponders" may be a prognostically unfavorable group in which chemotherapy could accelerate their death and thus artificially enhance the clinical course of those responding. The "responders" may have an advantage regardless of chemotherapy because of more favorable factors, such as overall physical health, minimal weight loss, or the site of disease. Another dubious statistical technique is the comparison of median survival duration without considering the contours of the survival distribution.

Factors of patient selection can profoundly distort the outcome of clinical trials. Young and sound patients without previous treatment will obviously have a better outcome from a specific treatment than old, sickly, and previously treated patients. Patients with progressive disease after an initial chemotherapeutic trial, radiation, or surgery are less likely to respond to further treatment.

My impressions on reviewing the chemotherapy literature on induction programs are as follows:

1. Some squamous cell carcinomas respond dramatically to most of the drugs used today.

2. It is unlikely that current chemotherapy will do what is so greatly needed, that is, get rid of bulk disease. It takes a tremendous amount of chemotherapy to destroy the primary tumor and N2 or N3 disease, but these are the patients who have the greatest need for something better.

3. The duration of response, when it occurs, is short, and one cannot call on chemotherapy to do again what it did the first time. Tumor resistance to the drugs comes on quickly.

4. Patients who have a complete response tend to do better with conventional therapy than those who do not have a good response, although the response and the patient's subsequent course may not be related.

5. Tumor response is not centripetal, so that the idea that chemotherapy as we know it today will downstage tumors or permit more "conservative" operations is unlikely.

6. The induction programs delay the delivery of standard local modalities, and this delay can compromise patient management. The development of drug-resistant clones of tumor is undoubtedly accelerated by induction chemotherapy, especially in patients with bulk disease. Chemotherapy may alter the cause of death because of this effect, and this alteration may be the reason we are seeing reports of distant metastasis rates in the 30% to 50% range.[52]

7. Some patients who experience a complete response paradoxically have a new problem, because they are tempted to refuse surgery or radiation. Weaver et al.[58] observed that 17 of 61 patients (including 13 who had "complete" response) refused planned surgery.

8. Many studies have shown that chemotherapy shrinks tumors. Data are lacking to indicate that shrinking of tumors has much impact on survival. It may well be that induction of adjunctive therapy produces both a benefit and a harm through different mechanisms. The net result is no change in survival.

These generalizations apply to both single-agent and multiagent drug regimens. In all the randomized cooperative studies that analyze multidrug programs, no persuasive data endorse combinations over single drugs. When any of the important variables are compared—objective regression rates, time to progression, and overall survival—no combination has been consistently superior to single-agent regimens.

Randomized trials of the various chemotherapeutic schemes should continue. Ad hoc chemotherapy outside investigative trials is inappropriate. The passing off of chemotherapy as standard practice is dishonest in light of what we know today. The control arm in randomized trials should be conventional surgery or radiation but not both. There is enough statistical con-

fusion without creating triple combined therapy schemes—to say nothing about the cost of such programs. The only place for single-arm studies is to test the feasibility of a randomized study. Reports of promising single-arm studies without controls should no longer be accepted by the editorial boards of peer-reviewed journals.

REFERENCES

1. Stell PM, Dalby JE, Singh SD, et al: The fixed cervical lymph node. *Cancer* 1984; 53:336–341.
2. Snow GB, Annyas AA, Van Slooten EA, et al: Prognostic factors of neck node metastasis. *Clin Otolaryngol* 1982; 7:185–192.
3. Beahrs OH, Myers MH: *Manual for Staging of Cancer,* ed 2. Philadelphia, JB Lippincott Co, 1983.
4. Smith RR, Caulk RM, Russell WO, et al: End results in 600 laryngeal cancers using the American Joint Committee's proposed method of stage classification and end results reporting. *Surg Gynecol Obstet* 1961; 113:435–444.
5. Harmer MH (ed): *TMN Classification of Malignant Tumours,* ed 3. Geneva, International Union Against Cancer, 1978.
6. Lindberg R: Distribution of cervical lymph node metastases from squamous cell carcinoma of the upper respiratory and digestive tracts. *Cancer* 1972; 29:1446–1449.
7. Spiro RH, Alfonso AE, Farr HW, et al: Cervical node metastasis from epidermoid carcinoma of the oral cavity and oropharynx: A critical assessment of current staging. *Am J Surg* 1974; 128:562–567.
8. Smith RR, Frazell EL, Caulk R, et al: The American Joint Committee's proposed method of stage classification and end-result reporting applied to 1,320 pharynx cancers. *Cancer* 1963; 16:1505–1520.
9. Fu KK, Phillips TL, Silverberg IJ, et al: Combined radiotherapy and chemotherapy with bleomycin and methotrexate for advanced inoperable head and neck cancer: Update of a Northern California Oncology Group randomized trial. *J Clin Oncol* 1987; 5:1410–1418.
10. Petrovich Z, Kuisk H, Jose L, et al: Advanced carcinoma of the tonsil: Treatment results. *Acta Radiol (Oncol)* 1980; 19:425–431.
11. Saxena VS, Allt WEC: Cancer of the tongue. *J Can Assoc Radiol* 1967; 18:274–277.
12. Beahrs OH, Devine KD: Personal communciation, 1977.
13. Conley JJ: Carotid artery surgery in the treatment of tumors of the neck. *Arch Otolaryngol* 1957; 65:437–446.
14. Wang CC, Schulz MD, Miller D: Combined radiation therapy and surgery for carcinoma of the supraglottis and pyriform sinus. *Am J Surg* 1972; 124:551–554.
15. Barkley HT Jr, Fletcher GH, Jesse RH, et al: Management of cervical lymph node metastases in squamous cell carcinoma of the tonsillar fossa, base of tongue, supraglottic larynx, and hypopharynx. *Am J Surg* 1972; 124:462–467.
16. DeSanto LW, Beahrs OH, Holt JJ, et al: Neck dissection and combined therapy: Study of effectiveness. *Arch Otolaryngol* 1985; 111:366–370.
17. DeSanto LW, Holt JJ, Beahrs OH, et al: Neck dissection: Is it worthwhile? *Laryngoscope* 1982; 92:502–509.

18. Cohen L: Theoretical "iso-survival" formulae for fractionated radiation therapy. *Br J Radiol* 1968; 41:522–528.

19. Vandenbrouck C, Sancho-Garnier H, Chassagne D, et al: Elective versus therapeutic radical neck dissection in epidermoid carcinoma of the oral cavity: Results of a randomized clinical trial. *Cancer* 1980; 46:386–390.

20. Bataini JP, Ennuyer A, Poncet P, et al: Treatment of supraglottic cancer by radical high dose radiotherapy. *Cancer* 1974; 33:1253–1262.

21. Million RR: Elective neck irradiation for T_xN_0 squamous carcinoma of the oral tongue and floor of mouth. *Cancer* 1974; 34:149–155.

22. Goffinet DR, Gilbert EH, Weller SA, et al: Irradiation of clinically uninvolved cervical lymph nodes. *Can J Otolaryngol* 1975; 4:927–933.

23. Mendenhall WM, Million RR, Cassisi NJ: Elective neck irradiation in squamous-cell carcinoma of the head and neck. *Head Neck Surg* 1980; 3:15–20.

24. Horiuchi J, Adachi T: Some considerations on radiation therapy of tongue cancer. *Cancer* 1971; 28:335–339.

25. Rabuzzi DD, Chung CT, Sagerman RH: Prophylactic neck irradiation. *Arch Otolaryngol* 1980; 106:454–455.

26. Decroix Y, Ghossein NA: Experience of the Curie Institute in treatment of cancer of the mobile tongue: II. Management of the neck nodes. *Cancer* 1981; 47:503–508.

27. Meoz RT, Fletcher GH, Lindberg RD: Anatomical coverage in elective irradiation of the neck for squamous cell carcinoma of the oral tongue. *Int J Radiat Oncol Biol Phys* 1982; 8:1881–1885.

28. Bocca E: Critical analysis of the techniques and value of neck dissection. *Nuovo Arch Ital Otol Rhinol Laryngol* 1976; 4:151–158.

29. Bocca E, Calearo C, De Vincentiis I, et al: Occult metastases in cancer of the larynx and their relationship to clinical and histological aspects of the primary tumor: A four-year multicentric research. *Laryngoscope* 1984; 94:1086–1090.

30. Lee JG, Krause CJ: Radical neck dissection: Elective, therapeutic, and secondary. *Arch Otolaryngol* 1975; 101:656–659.

31. Beahrs OH, Barber KW Jr: The value of radical dissection of structures of the neck in the management of carcinoma of the lip, mouth, and larynx. *Arch Surg* 1962; 85:49–55.

32. Crile G: Excision of cancer of the head and neck: With special reference to the plan of dissection based on one hundred and thirty-two operations. *JAMA* 1906; 47:1780–1786.

33. Byers RM: Modified neck dissection: A study of 967 cases from 1970 to 1980. *Am J Surg* 1985; 150:414–421.

34. Bocca E, Pignataro O: A conservation technique in radical neck dissection. *Ann Otol Rhinol Laryngol* 1967; 76:975–987.

35. Bocca E, Pignataro O, Oldini C, et al: Functional neck dissection: An evaluation and review of 843 cases. *Laryngoscope* 1984; 94:942–945.

36. Batson OV: Anatomical problems concerned in the study of cerebral blood flow. *Fed Proc* 1944; 3:139–144.

37. Ward GE, Robben JO: A composite operation for radical neck dissection and removal of cancer of the mouth. *Cancer* 1951; 4:98–109.

38. Jesse RH, Lindberg RD: The efficacy of combining radiation therapy with a surgical procedure in patients with cervical metastasis from squamous cancer of the oropharynx and hypopharynx. *Cancer* 1975; 35:1163–1166.

39. Jesse RH, Fletcher GH: Treatment of the neck in patients with squamous cell carcinoma of the head and neck. *Cancer* 1977; 39:868–872.

40. Jesse RH, Ballantyne AJ, Larson D: Radical or modified neck dissection: A therapeutic dilemma. *Am J Surg* 1978; 136:516–519.

41. Jesse RH: Modified neck dissection with and without radiation, in Kagan AR, Miles JW (eds): *Head and Neck Oncology: Controversies in Cancer Treatment*. Boston, GK Hall Medical Publishers, 1981, pp 247–254.

42. DeSanto LW: Cancer of the supraglottic larynx: A review of 260 patients. *Otolaryngol Head Neck Surg* 1985; 93:705–711.

43. Lindberg RD, Jesse RH, Fletcher GH: Radiotherapy—Before or After Surgery?, in *Neoplasia of Head and Neck*. Chicago, Year Book Medical Publishers, 1974, pp 47–58.

44. Fletcher GH: Subclinical disease. *Cancer* 1984; 53:1274–1284.

45. Schuller D: Management of the N0 neck, in Chretien PB, Shedd D, et al (eds): *Head & Neck Cancer: Proceedings of the First International Conference*. St. Louis, CV Mosby Co, 1985, vol 1.

46. Snow JB Jr, Gelber RD, Kramer S, et al: Evaluation of randomized preoperative and postoperative radiation therapy for supraglottic carcinoma: Preliminary report. *Ann Otol Rhinol Laryngol* 1978; 87:686–691.

47. Vikram B, Strong EW, Shah JP, et al: Failure in the neck following multimodality treatment for advanced head and neck cancer. *Head Neck Surg* 1984; 6:724–729.

48. Arriagada R, Eschwege F, Cachin Y, et al: The value of combining radiotherapy with surgery in the treatment of hypopharyngeal and laryngeal cancers. *Cancer* 1983; 51:1819–1825.

49. Pearlman NW, Johnson FB, Kennaugh RC: Modified radical neck dissection and postoperative radiotherapy in squamous cell head and neck cancer. *Am J Surg* 1985; 150:488–490.

50. Johnson JT, Barnes EL, Myers EN, et al: The extracapsular spread of tumors in cervical node metastasis. *Arch Otolaryngol* 1981; 107:725–729.

51. Snow GB: Personal communication, 1987.

52. Ervin TJ, Clark JR, Weichselbaum RR, et al: An analysis of induction and adjuvant chemotherapy in the multidisciplinary treatment of squamous-cell carcinoma of the head and neck. *J Clin Oncol* 1987; 5:10–20.

53. Tannock IF, Browman G: Lack of evidence for a role of chemotherapy in the routine management of locally advanced head and neck cancer. *J Clin Oncol* 1986; 4:1121–1126.

54. Clark JR: Induction chemotherapy for advanced head and neck cancer. *Adv Oncol* 1987; 3:23–29.

55. Carpenter RJ III, DeSanto LW, Devine KD, et al: Cancer of the hypopharynx: Analysis of treatment and results in 162 patients. *Arch Otolaryngol* 1976; 102:716–721.

56. Anderson JR, Cain KC, Gelber RD: Analysis of survival by tumor response. *J Clin Oncol* 1983; 1:710–719.

57. Tannock I, Murphy K: Reflections on medical oncology: An appeal for better clinical trials and improved reporting of their results. *J Clin Oncol* 1983; 1:66–70.

58. Weaver A, Flemming S, Kish J, et al: Cis-platinum and 5-fluorouracil as induction therapy for advanced head and neck cancer. *Am J Surg* 1982; 144:445–448.

Vascular and Neural Issues Relating to Neck Dissection

Approach of

Robert H. Miller, M.D.

CAROTID ARTERY

Bradycardia and Hypotension (Carotid Sinus Reflex)

The carotid sinus is a collection of complicated nerve endings located in the wall of the carotid bulb, a swelling at the lower end of the internal carotid artery or the upper end of the common carotid artery. The nerve endings may also be situated in the wall of the internal carotid artery superior to the bulb. The sinus is characterized by an abundance of elastic tissue and numerous nerve endings with little associated muscle. It is a pressure receptor innervated by the glossopharyngeal nerve and should not be confused with the carotid body, a chemoreceptor. Stimulation of the carotid sinus by mechanical manipulation produces bradycardia and a reduction in blood pressure.

A certain degree of carotid artery manipulation during the course of a neck dissection is unavoidable, although it should be manipulated as little as possible not only to avoid stimulating the carotid sinus but also to avoid dislocating atherosclerotic plaques, which could lead to a cerebrovascular accident (CVA). However, should the carotid sinus be stimulated, the anesthesiologist will note bradycardia and a reduction in blood pressure. It is important for the surgeon to notify the anesthesiologist when the area of the carotid bulb is being dissected or manipulated so that he or she will be attuned to the potential cardiovascular changes that might take place and inform the surgeon of such changes. Lidocaine 1% injected into the adventitia surrounding the carotid bulb and internal carotid artery with a 25-gauge needle will block the transmission through the nerve to the carotid sinus and eliminate the reflex. I do not routinely inject this area unless cardiovascular changes occur or if it ap-

pears that a great deal of manipulation of the carotid bulb will be required.

Intraoperative Injury

The key to preventing an intraoperative injury to the carotid artery is careful dissection in the proper plane using careful, atraumatic technique. I begin the dissection of the carotid artery in the supraclavicular area. After identifying the internal jugular vein and vagus nerve, I carefully strip the specimen from the carotid in a plane just superficial to the adventitia. When it is necessary to use scissors to free the specimen from the carotid, it is important to open the scissors and spread with the blades parallel to the carotid in such a way that one of the blades is not pushed into the vessel.

As the dissection approaches the carotid bulb, one must be cognizant of the branches of the external carotid artery and ligate them with a 2–0 silk ligature when it is necessary to sacrifice a branch. Some surgeons prefer to place a suture ligature to reduce the chance of the ligature becoming dislodged. The facial branch is usually ligated during the dissection of the submandibular triangle. The facial artery is an excellent vessel to use when reconstruction with a free flap is planned, so it is important to leave as long a proximal branch as possible.

Should an injury to the carotid artery occur, massive bleeding will ensue. The first step is to apply digital pressure to the bleeding site. Blind clamping should be avoided since there are a number of vital structures (e.g., the vagus nerve) in the area, and one may actually increase the size of the rent during a frantic attempt to clamp the bleeding site. Once the bleeding has been controlled, the carotid artery should be dissected both superiorly and inferiorly to the tear and encircled with plastic vascular loops. When the bleeding has been controlled with the vascular loops, the site of injury can be examined. It may be possible to apply an angled vascular clamp tangentially so that some flow can continue through the vessel during the repair, for which I use interrupted 6–0 Proline sutures. Some surgeons use a shunt to permit flow during the repair; however, its use is controversial, and it may take longer to find and place a shunt than to proceed directly with the repair. If possible, the repair should be made in a transverse direction so as to minimize the narrowing of the lumen. If a portion of the wall is missing and primary repair would lead to stenosis, a vein patch should be used. Nonautogenous material (Goretex grafts) should be avoided, particularly if the pharynx has been entered and the wound is contaminated. It is important to include the intima in the repair since a pseudoaneurysm may result if it is not closed properly. Just prior to the placement of the last stitch, the vessel should be allowed to back-bleed so that all air is removed and an air embolism is avoided.

An injury at the thoracic inlet is particularly troublesome because of the extra exposure that is needed to repair the injury. In addition, the vessels in this area are fragile, and the repair is technically difficult. Blind clamping of the bleeding site should be avoided, and digital pressure will usually temporize the situation. It may be necessary to remove a segment of the clavicle to gain exposure of the injury. This can be accomplished quickly and safely by carefully dissecting around the clavicle and dividing it with a Gigli saw. Unless the surgeon has a great deal of experience in this area, intraoperative consultation with a vascular surgeon would be advisable.

An injury of the internal carotid artery at the skull base can be particularly bothersome because of the limited exposure of this area. After obtaining digital control of the bleeding, the surgeon should obtain proximal control of the carotid artery. Additional exposure of the skull base can be obtained quite rapidly by performing a lateral mandibulotomy.[1] The surgeon can then view the carotid foramen and, if possible, obtain distal control of the internal carotid artery. The repair can be performed with a 6–0 Proline suture. If the surgeon cannot obtain distal control and back-bleeding makes the repair impossible, the vessel should be ligated proximally and the carotid foramen packed with absorbable gelatin sponge (Gelfoam) and muscle.

Postoperative Blowout

One of the keys to preventing a postoperative blowout is to use careful technique in handling not only the carotid artery but also all of the soft tissue of the neck. It is important to prevent desiccation of the carotid by placing a moistened sponge over the carotid when one has completed the neck dissection and is working on another area. The flaps should be handled gently and closed properly without excess tension. Most neck dissection incisions involve a trifurcation, which is the most common area of wound breakdown. Therefore, the trifurcation should not be placed over the carotid artery. Suction drains should be placed so that they do not cross the carotid.

The patient who has received preoperative radiation ther-apy is at particular risk for carotid blowout. Some surgeons save the sternocleidomastoid muscle and suture it over the carotid artery. I have had good success with the use of dermal grafts in radiated patients. The dermal graft has the advantage that if a wound breakdown should occur, the area of exposure will epithelialize without the need for a graft or flap.[2] If the pharynx is entered, salivary fistula are not uncommon, which further endangers the carotid artery. Therefore, many surgeons will create a controlled pharyngostoma to divert saliva away from the carotid. Once healing of the flaps has occurred, the fistula can be closed using fresh tissue. When resection of a large part of the pharynx or oral cavity requires reconstruction with a flap, the pedicle of the flap can be used to cover the carotid.

In the immediate postoperative period, prompt attention to accumulations of blood, serum, or saliva under the flaps will reduce the degree of wound breakdown and subsequent carotid exposure. Hematomas and seromas should be drained immediately, and fistulae should be treated aggressively with pressure dressings and diversion away from the carotid.

Small amounts of bright red bleeding from an open neck wound (sentinel bleeding) should alert the surgeon to the possibility of an impending carotid blowout. This is the appropriate time to make plans should a blowout become imminent or occur. If the patient is terminal and has very poor quality of life, the surgeon should discuss the situation with the patient and his or her family. It may be desirable to write a "do not resuscitate" order so that further suffering of the patient and family is avoided. This will also avoid placing the family and medical personnel in the uncomfortable situation of making a moral decision in an emergency.

If a blowout occurs and it is elected to pursue an aggressive course of therapy, digital pressure is applied to the bleeding point and the patient taken to the operating room. Proximal and distal control is obtained, and the carotid is doubly ligated with a 0 silk suture ligature. Repair with grafts or prosthetic materials should not be attempted since the area is contaminated and success is unlikely.

Intraoperative Cerebrovascular Accident

An intraoperative CVA can be a devastating complication and usually results from the dislocation of an atherosclerotic plaque during dissection. There are frequently no symptoms during the operation, and its occurrence is not detected until the patient is in the recovery room or the intensive care unit. The key to avoiding this complication is careful, atraumatic dissection around the carotid artery. Although it apparently has not been used during a neck dissection, intraoperative electro-encephalographic (EEG) monitoring has been used successfully during other types of surgery. If it is known that a patient is at particular risk for a CVA, EEG monitoring may be of value.[3]

Once it is diagnosed postoperatively, there is not much that can be done for the stroke, particularly if the deficits are fixed. If the deficits fluctuate, the patient may benefit from anticoagulation with heparin, although this may cause wound complications such as hematoma formation. Each case must be managed weighing the benefits and risks of this form of therapy.

INTERNAL JUGULAR VEIN

Venous bleeding in the neck frequently does not carry with it the same degree of urgency one has for brisk arterial bleeding. However, an injury to the internal jugular vein can be an extremely dangerous and life-threatening problem not only from exsanguination but also from other problems such as air embolism, which can be even more difficult to control.

Injury at Thoracic Inlet

Of all the locations of internal jugular vein injury, the thoracic inlet is probably the most dangerous. Identification of the vein and careful dissection are the keys to preventing an injury. Like the digastric muscle in the upper part of the neck, the omohyoid muscle is an important landmark in the lower part of the neck. After removal of the sternal and clavicular insertions of the sternocleidomastoid muscle, the posterior belly of the omohyoid muscle is identified and the scapular insertion avulsed. The omohyoid is then carefully dissected toward its hyoid insertion (which is the medial limit of a standard, isolated neck dissection). As the omohyoid is elevated in the supraclavicular area, the internal jugular vein is exposed and identified.

If the vein is to be sacrificed, it is carefully skeletonized medially and laterally, making sure to be in the same plane (just superficial to the adventitia) on both sides. Any branches are ligated with 2–0 silk sutures. A right-angle clamp is passed posteriorly around the vessel, making sure that the vagus nerve is not included in the tissue around the vein. Silk sutures (2–0) are passed around the vein and tied 1 to 2 cm apart. The area between the sutures is doubly ligated with 2–0 silk suture ligatures, and the vein is divided between the suture ligatures.

If the internal jugular vein is to be preserved, the dissection around the vein is carried out in a plane just superficial to the adventitia using sharp and blunt dissection. One should use care when dissecting with clamp or scissors so that the spreading motion of the instrument is such that the blades do not push into the wall of the vein. Usually the dissection goes very easily by carefully stripping the specimen off the vein.

If an injury occurs, it is usually associated with profuse, dark red bleeding. If there is any doubt, the anesthesiologist should be asked to apply positive ventilatory pressure, which will increase venous bleeding. Although the bleeding may be quite impressive, there is the subtle danger of an air embolism, which may go unnoticed until too late. Therefore, whenever an injury occurs to the internal jugular vein, digital pressure should be applied immediately. The anesthesiologist should be informed of the possibility of an air embolism and the head brought to at least a horizontal if not a Trendelenburg position. The injury can then be repaired with 6–0 Proline suture or the vein ligated, depending on the situation, after obtaining proximal and distal control. As with an injury of the internal carotid artery in this area, removal of the clavicle may be necessary to obtain adequate exposure. The venous structures in the thoracic inlet area are very fragile, and repair is difficult.

Injury at Skull Base

Injury of the internal jugular vein at the skull base is not quite as dangerous as an injury at the thoracic inlet. Injury to the internal jugular vein can occur as the vein is being skeletonized for ligation, if it is to be removed, or as tissue at the skull base is being removed. One can also injure the vein as one dissects the spinal accessory nerve in this area since the nerve may pass anterior, posterior, or actually penetrate the vein at the base of the skull.[4]

Since the internal jugular vein usually has been identified prior to the dissection of the skull base area, careful attention to the vein will help avoid injury. However, should the vein be injured, hemostasis can be obtained by digital compression. Blind clamping should be avoided because of the close proximity of the last four cranial nerves and the internal carotid artery. As with injury in the thoracic inlet area, one must ensure that air does not enter the vein. Proximal control is usually not a problem, but distal compression can be difficult. A Kittner type of dissector can be used to compress the vein as it exits from the jugular foramen. Once the bleeding is controlled, the vein can be repaired or transected and ligated. If the vein has been completely transected and the distal stump has retracted into the jugular foramen so that a ligature cannot be applied, a muscle flap from one of the local muscles can be fashioned to fit into the jugular foramen and held in place with sutures and absorbable sponges.

Bilateral Sacrifice: Staged Neck Dissection

Prior to the development of the modified neck dissection and preservation of the internal jugular vein, bilateral sacrifice of the internal jugular vein was not uncommon. Unfortunately, a number of complications arose from the simultaneous sacrifice of both internal jugular veins. In addition to the marked facial swelling associated with this procedure, cerebral edema is not uncommon and may lead to complications such as blindness and death. In an attempt to avoid these complications, surgeons would stage the neck procedures for those patients who required bilateral internal jugular vein sacrifice.

Now that head and neck surgeons have gained experience with internal jugular vein preservation, it is unusual that both veins must be sacrificed simultaneously. However, if both veins are removed, it is desirable to delay the second procedure approximately 6 weeks to allow time for collateral circulation to develop. Osmotic diuretics and steroids may be helpful in avoiding cerebral edema, which can be quite severe despite the delay.

Air Embolism

Air embolism is the result of introduction of air into the vascular system usually through a hole in the internal jugular vein or one of its major tributaries. Some surgeons will position the patient for head and neck surgery with the head elevated so that there is less venous pressure and bleeding. However, this position places the neck higher than the heart and may create negative pressure in the venous system of the head and neck so that if there is an injury to the internal jugular vein, air can actually be drawn into the vascular system. If the patient is behind in fluids, this may also aggravate this tendency.

The first step to take if injury to the vein occurs is to seal the hole with a finger, even if there is no bleeding. The patient should be placed in a horizontal or a Trendelenburg position to decrease the negative pressure in the vein. If there is concern that a significant amount of air entered the vascular system, the patient should be placed in a left lateral decubitus position so that the air bubble will remain in the right atrium and not be circulated to the pulmonary vasculature where it may cause severe cardiovascular problems. It may also prove helpful to insert a catheter in the vein and pass it into the right atrium so that air can be aspirated.

CHYLE LEAK

Although a chyle leak does not have the same urgency as a vascular injury, this complication can be quite devastating since it may cause a marked prolongation of the patient's hospitalization in excess of an injury to the carotid artery and certainly the internal jugular vein. As with any complication, prevention is the best form of management. It is important to recognize that although the thoracic duct enters the internal jugular vein on the left, there may be an accessory duct on the right, so that a chyle leak can develop on either side of the neck. The lymphatic ducts appear as diaphanous, bulging structures in the supraclavicular area near the thoracic inlet, although there is a great deal of variation in how far superiorly into the neck they extend. After exiting the thoracic cavity, the thoracic duct passes deep to the carotid sheath in its lateral course to join the venous system at the junction of the internal jugular vein and subclavian artery. It has been suggested that the narrower the thoracic inlet, the higher into the neck the thoracic duct travels.[5]

Intraoperative Recognition

If the thoracic duct is injured, there is usually no immediate indication that something is amiss. Characteristically, there is a slow welling up of clear fluid in the inferior portion of the dissection. Since the patient has not eaten any food for several hours prior to surgery, the amount of fluid is frequently scant and does not have the typical creamy appearance of chyle after a meal. If the surgeon notes a collection of clear fluid in the area of the thoracic duct, all attention should be directed at finding its source, since the best way to manage a chyle leak is to control it at the time of surgery.

A meticulous inspection of the area by careful dabbing with sponges will usually reveal the site of the injury. Having the anesthesiologist increase the intrathoracic pressure by giving the patient long, deep inspirations will increase the leak and help demonstrate its source. If necessary, the patient can be placed in a Trendelenburg position. Once the location of the injury is noted, it should be oversewn with nonabsorbable su-

tures. Since there may be more than one channel to the duct, multiple sutures may be required to achieve an absolutely dry field. The duct itself is very friable and does not hold sutures well, so the sutures should be placed in the surrounding tissues. Rotation of a local muscle flap may also help seal the area.

Postoperative Recognition

A chyle leak may not be recognized immediately postoperatively because the patient is usually maintained on intravenous (IV) fluids so that the gastrointestinal tract is at rest. The small amount of chyle that leaks during this period is very difficult to differentiate from the normal serosanguinous drainage removed by the suction drains. However, when the patient is started on enteral feedings that include long chain triglycerides, a chyle leak will become very evident as the drainage from the suction drains becomes milky in appearance. If the drains have already been removed, the flap will elevate in the supraclavicular area, and aspiration of the subcutaneous fluid will confirm the existence of a chyle leak. If the leak is quite large, the patient may develop a chylothorax with radiographic evidence of fluid in the pleural space. The same milky-appearing material will be recovered by thoracentesis.

The vast majority of chyle leaks can be managed without reexploration of the area.[6] Reduction of thoracic duct flow is a cornerstone of treatment. Chyle production is increased by a diet that contains long chain triglycerides, which are carried through the thoracic duct in chylomicrons and enter the systemic circulation via the thoracic duct. A diet that is rich in medium chain triglycerides will reduce chyle production (and thoracic duct flow) since these substances are carried through the portal system. Therefore, the first step in the management of a chyle leak is to reduce chyle flow by eliminating long chain triglycerides from the feedings and placing the patient on a medium chain triglyceride diet.

Chyle must not be allowed to accumulate under the flap so that the flap can adhere to the underlying tissue and seal any leak. In a very small leak, this can be accomplished by repeated aspirations. In the case of a larger leak, insertion of a suction drain in the supraclavicular area, taking care not to injure the great vessels or other structures, will provide an egress for the chyle. Pressure dressings are helpful in maintaining contact between the flap and the muscle bed.

Most chyle fistulae managed with this conservative approach will stop within 1 week. If there appears to be no improvement in the leak within 1 week, surgical exploration may be indicated, but it is usually difficult to identify and ligate the offending duct. The use of muscle flaps to help seal the leak may be of value.

NERVE INJURY

Nerve injury is usually not a life-threatening problem, but it certainly can have a significant effect on the physiologic and psychologic function of the patient marring the otherwise successful treatment of a malignancy. A thorough knowledge of the anatomy of the nerves of the neck is probably the most important key to prevent injury during neck dissection. It is also essential that the surgeon inform the anesthesiologist that a nerve stimulator will be used during the surgery and that the patient should not be given any long-acting paralyzing agents that might affect the response of nerves to stimulation. If a nerve injury is recognized at the time of surgery, the surgeon must decide whether the nerve should be repaired and by what means. This varies depending on the size and function of the nerve as well as other factors.

Many factors affect the results of a nerve repair. The nerves should have sharply incised ends that will reduce the chance of neuroma development at the anastomotic site. There should be no tension on the anastomosis. Although a better result usually follows end-to-end anastomosis, if the transacted nerve does not come together easily, consideration should be given to using a nerve graft, many of which are easily accessible during neck dissection. Monofilament sutures varying from 7–0 to 10–0 are used to repair the nerve. Depending on the size of the nerve to be repaired, no more than three or four epineural sutures are necessary, and in some cases, only one or two sutures can be placed.

Facial Nerve

Ramus Mandibularis

The marginal mandibular nerve is one of the smaller-diameter nerves that are routinely identified and preserved during neck dissection. Although functionally it is not essential, injury of the marginal mandibular nerve will produce an asymmetric smile and drooling from the affected lip. Some patients will have more than one branch of the facial nerve that innervates the lower lip so that injury of the marginal mandibular nerve may not necessarily produce paralysis of this area.

The first step in avoiding injury to the marginal mandibular nerve is during the draping of the patient. The drapes should be placed so that the lower lip is exposed and movement can be seen during surgery. The skin incision should be planned so that the horizontal limb of any Shobinger-type incisions should be made at least two fingerbreadths below the angle of the mandible. Several techniques are used to avoid injury to the nerve during surgery. In the submandibular area, the nerve consistently lies superficial to the facial vein, so that if one divides the facial vein low in the submandibular area and then dissects deep to the vein, the marginal mandibular nerve is avoided. It is important to remember that the nerve may dive deep into the neck so that the vein must be divided very low to ensure avoidance of injury. Another technique is to identify the fascia of the submandibular gland at the inferior margin of the gland. The fascia is then carefully elevated off the gland, and the marginal mandibular nerve, which frequently lies in the fascia, is maintained in the skin flap and preserved. If there is any question about whether the nerve is contained in a piece of tissue that must be cut, the area should be stimulated and the corner of the mouth observed for movement. It should be noted that contraction of the platysma may cause mouth movement, and this must be differentiated from movement caused by stimulation of the marginal mandibular nerve. The use of loops or an operating microscope may also aid in the dissection.

If the nerve is transected, repair is desirable and possible, depending on the location of the injury and the size of the nerve. Good results can be obtained using epineural monofilament sutures if the nerve is large enough to repair. If the injury is quite distal, repair may not be technically feasible and should be aborted if not successful after a reasonable attempt.

If injury to the marginal mandibular nerve is recognized postoperatively, it is probably inadvisable to reexplore the patient since it is unlikely that one will be able to find the two cut ends of the nerve. Furthermore, the paralysis may very well be due to a stretch injury and may recover without any therapy.

Main Trunk

The main trunk of the facial nerve is not usually at great risk during a standard neck dissection. It is possible to injure the nerve while removing the sternocleidomastoid muscle from the mastoid tip; however, this can be avoided by dividing the muscle along an imaginary line drawn from the angle of the mandible to the tip of the mastoid. The posterior belly of the digastric muscle is also an excellent guide to several structures in this area, including the main trunk of the facial nerve. By staying inferior to the digastric muscle, one can avoid the facial nerve trunk. However, if there is any question as to the location of the nerve, the main trunk should be identified. This can be accomplished by either identifying it as it exits the stylomastoid foramen or by tracing the marginal mandibular branch back to the main trunk. If the nerve cannot be found by either of these techniques, it may be necessary to identify it in the mastoid.

If the nerve is injured during surgery, it must be repaired. Very good facial function can be achieved by anastomosis of the main trunk, although varying degrees of synkinesis are not uncommon. However, the results of immediate anastomosis are far superior to any other technique of facial reanimation. If necessary, the greater auricular nerve can be used as a cable graft, but better results are achieved by performing a direct anastomosis.

If the patient is found to have a complete, unilateral facial paralysis immediately postoperatively, a decision must be made as to whether or not to explore the nerve. If the surgeon identified the nerve and believes it is intact, exploration is probably not warranted. However, if the nerve is out completely and the surgeon is not confident that the nerve is intact, reexploration and repair are probably indicated. The patient's overall condition must, of course, be taken into consideration. If the decision to explore the nerve is made, exploration should be carried out within 1 or 2 days so that the distal trunk can be identified using the nerve stimulator.

Hypoglossal Nerve

Unilateral hypoglossal nerve injury can be bothersome, but bilateral injury can be devastating and must be avoided. Fortunately, bilateral injury is exceedingly rare and obviously should not be a concern in performing a unilateral neck dissection. The nerve is quite large and can be identified in a number of ways. It crosses superficial to the carotid arteries, usually just above the bifurcation, and is frequently found as the specimen is being freed from the vessels. Another technique of identifying the nerve is to bluntly dissect through the fascia just deep to the submandibular gland. The nerve usually is located just superior and deep to the digastric muscle running parallel to the latter. In addition, the ansa hypoglossi nerve can be identified as it courses along the surface of the strap muscles and traced back to the hypoglossal nerve.

If the hypoglossal nerve is injured during surgery, it may be worth an attempt to repair as long as the patient's condition allows the little extra time it takes to perform the repair. The nerve is large and repaired easily, but there are no studies to show that repair results in improved tongue function. If unilateral paralysis is noted postoperatively, it is probably not worthwhile exploring the patient and attempting repair.

Lingual Nerve

The lingual nerve can be identified (and potentially injured) quite easily during dissection of the submandibular gland. A very nice way of identifying the nerve is to free the superior and anterior margins of the submandibular gland, place an Army-Navy retractor at the margin of the mylohyoid muscle, and retract it medially. The nerve traveling its curving course is readily visible just deep to the fascia in this area. It is important to identify the nerve so that the small vessel that runs in the parasympathetic pedicle to the gland can be clamped safely without injury to the lingual nerve. In addition, the nerve should be visualized during transection of the submandibular duct.

If the nerve is injured, it should not be repaired, since this may give rise to dysgeusia, not dissimilar to the situation if the chorda tympani is injured or severely traumatized in the middle ear.

Recurrent Laryngeal Nerve

Because of its anatomic location, injury to the recurrent laryngeal nerve is very unusual during an isolated neck dissection. The nerve runs in the tracheoesophageal groove, and if dissection is necessary in this area, the nerve should be identified. One must be very careful to avoid recurrent laryngeal nerve injury if the patient is undergoing supraglottic laryngectomy, because this may preclude performing conservation surgery or at least modify it.

The results of anastomosis of the recurrent laryngeal nerve are, at best, mixed. Because of the complex set of muscles it innervates, repair will probably never produce a normal functioning larynx. However, there may be some merit to anastomosing the two severed ends in that the resultant innervation may provide some tone to the vocal cord and produce a better voice.

If the paralysis is discovered postoperatively, exploration is not warranted. If return of vocal cord function does not occur within 6 to 12 months, medialization of the affected cord with Teflon injection, for example, should be considered.

Phrenic Nerve

The phrenic nerve is identified during the dissection in the lower part of the neck. The nerve is probably easiest to find as it passes in a lateral to medial direction on the anterior surface of the anterior scalene muscle. The fascia overlying the nerve should be preserved during the dissection, so the injury should be avoided if one is in the correct plane. The nerve is probably at greatest risk as one transects the cervical sensory nerves as they traverse the specimen. Care should be taken to divide the sensory nerves well away from the phrenic nerve.

Should the phrenic nerve be injured during surgery, repair can be attempted but will be difficult due to the small size of the nerve. There are no studies to indicate that the repair will be successful. Postoperatively, phrenic nerve injury can be diagnosed on chest x-ray film by noting the elevated hemidiaphragm on the side of the injury. Exploration of the nerve is not warranted, because most patients tolerate unilateral paralysis without significant compromise.

Brachial Plexus

The brachial plexus receives contributions from the lower four cervical nerves and the first thoracic nerve. It passes deep to the anterior scalene muscle and superficial to the middle scalene and then crosses the first rib under the clavicle and wraps around the axillary artery to innervate the upper extremity. The brachial plexus is at most risk when the surgeon is transecting the fat pad in the supraclavicular fossa. Although the planes are usually well defined in this area, this dissection can be quite difficult if the patient has had preoperative radiation therapy. The key to avoiding injury is to identify the plexus prior to clamping and dividing the fat pad.

One way of identifying the plexus is to bluntly dissect down to the phrenic nerve as it crosses the anterior scalene muscle. One can then pass a finger superficial to the fascia overlying the scalene in a lateral direction to the posterior inferior margin of the neck dissection. By elevating the finger, the surgeon should see the brachial plexus deep to the fascia, and the fat pad can be safely divided.

If the brachial plexus is injured during a neck dissection, immediate repair is indicated. Although there is not a great deal of experience in treating injuries that have occurred during neck dissection, most authors recommend repair of other types of brachial plexus injuries if there is functional disability.[7] If the injury is not detected until the postoperative period, consultation with the appropriate service to determine the suitability and timing of repair is indicated.

Spinal Accessory Nerve

Sacrifice of the spinal accessory nerve is part of a standard radical neck dissection. Unfortunately, this produces a dropped shoulder syndrome with limitation of the patient's ability to raise the arm over the head and, perhaps more significantly, chronic pain in the shoulder that can be quite debilitating. However, with the observation that the posterior cervical triangle is infrequently the site of metastases from most head and neck cancers, the classic radical neck dissection can be modified by preserving the spinal accessory nerve in selected cases.[8]

The spinal accessory nerve can be preserved in those cases in which its preservation will not compromise the extirpation of the neck metastases. Virtually all neck dissections for differentiated carcinoma of the thyroid can be modified. Elective neck dissections for clinically normal necks (those without palpable adenopathy) in patients with squamous carcinoma are also suitable for preservation of the spinal accessory nerve. If a metastasis from a squamous carcinoma is present, it should be limited to a single node less than 3 cm not in proximity to the nerve. These patients should receive radiation therapy postoperatively.

The spinal accessory nerve is identified at Erb's point, which is an area along the posterior border of the sternocleidomastoid muscle where the spinal accessory nerve and the greater auricular nerve exit. The greater auricular nerve is identified easily as it crosses the sternocleidomastoid muscle. The spinal accessory nerve can be found within 1 cm superior or inferior to the junction of the posterior border of the sternocleidomastoid muscle and the greater auricular nerve. Once identified, the spinal accessory nerve is traced inferiorly through the posterior triangle to its insertion in the trapezius muscle. Frequently, there are one or two branches to the trapezius as the nerve traverses the posterior triangle, and, if possible, these should be preserved. The nerve can then be traced through the body of the sternocleidomastoid muscle by transecting that part of the muscle superficial to the nerve. This is expedited by retracting the cut margins of the sternocleidomastoid muscle with Allis clamps. The neck dissection is continued in the usual fashion.

If the nerve is cut accidentally during surgery, repair should be considered based on several factors. Although trapezius function is not normal, repairing the injury may reduce postoperative morbidity.[9, 10] If a section of the nerve must be sacrificed for tumor extirpation, a cable graft (usually from the greater auricular nerve) can be performed if time and the patient's condition permits.

Postoperative Neuroma

Postoperative neuromas result from an overgrowth of the axons of an amputated nerve. Although uncommon, they may give rise to a multitude of types of pain ranging from aching to a burning sensation. If large, they may be confused for a possible tumor recurrence, although they are usually small and slow growing. They are most often noted in the subcutaneous tissue and are mobile and well circumscribed. Tinel's sign (a tingling sensation on percussion of the mass) may be elicited. Although not always present, it certainly helps in making the diagnosis.

Treatment consists of careful observation if the patient has no symptoms and there is no concern of a possible recurrence. If the pain is bothersome, phenytoin or carbamazepine can be tried, although one must always consider the possibility of a recurrence. Some investigators have found transcutaneous electrical neural stimulation (TENS) helpful for patients with neuromas in other parts of the body. If TENS is not helpful, excision is usually curative.

REFERENCES

1. Dichtel WJ, Miller RH, Feliciano DV, et al: Lateral mandibulotomy: A technique of exposure for penetrating injuries of the internal carotid artery at the base of the skull. *Laryngoscope* 1984; 85:1140–1144.
2. Corso PF, Gerold FP: Autogenous dermis for protection of the carotid artery and pharyngeal suture lines in radical head and neck surgery. *Surg Gynecol Obstet* 1963; 117:37–40.
3. McFarland HR, Pinkerton JA, Frye D: Continuous electroencephalographic monitoring during carotid endarterectomy. *J Cardiovasc Surg (Torino)* 1988; 29:12–18.
4. Hollinshead WH: *Anatomy for Surgeons: The Head and Neck.* Philadelphia, Harper & Row, Publishers, 1982, p 498.
5. Lissitzyn MS: Ductus thoracicus. *Arch Klin Chir* 1924; 128:215.
6. Lucente FE, Diktaban T, Lawson W, et al: Chyle fistula management. *Otolaryngol Head Neck Surg* 1981; 89:575–578.
7. Stevens JC, Davis DH, McCarty CS: 32 year experience with the surgical treatment of selected brachial plexus lesions with emphasis on its reconstruction. *Surg Neurol* 1983; 19:334–345.
8. Skolnik EM, Yee KF, Friedman M, et al: The posterior triangle in radical neck surgery. *Arch Otolaryngol* 1976; 102:1.
9. Zibordi F, Baiocco F, Bascelli C, et al: Spinal accessory nerve function following neck dissection. *Ann Otol Rhinol Laryngol* 1988; 97:83–86.
10. Saunders JR, Hirata RM, Jaques DA: Considering the spinal accessory nerve in head and neck surgery. *Am J Surg* 1985; 150:491–494.

Vascular and Neural Issues Relating to Neck Dissection

Approach of

Patrick J. Gullane, M.D.

and

Timothy P. O'Dwyer, M.D.

CAROTID ARTERY

Carotid Sinus Reflex

Surgical dissection in and about the carotid bifurcation occasionally results in carotid sinus reflex stimulation with bradycardia and hypotension. When this occurs, manipulation is immediately terminated until the patient's cardiovascular status returns to normal. If bradycardia and hypotension persist, 0.5 mL of 1% lidocaine solution is injected into the adventitial wall in the region of the bifurcation. This usually results in an immediate reversal of the reflex. Failure of this local treatment to correct the problem requires the systemic administration of atropine.

Intraoperative Injury of the Carotid Artery

Intraoperative injury to the carotid artery during a neck dissection is uncommon. However, in certain circumstances the risk is significantly increased, especially in patients who have had prior irradiation or previous surgery and in those with tumor adherent to the carotid wall. If at the time of surgery tumor is found adherent to the vessel wall, proximal and distal control is obtained, allowing immediate repair in the event of an inadvertent injury. In most circumstances, a subadventitial dissection permits the removal of tumor without entering the lumen. However, when tumor is found to have breached the vessel wall, its sacrifice with primary repair remains controversial. When a localized area of invasion is found, sacrifice of the vessel with repair using a saphenous vein graft is employed. A Pruitt Inhara shunt provides carotid perfusion during its repair. In the majority of patients, vessel involvement is so extensive that any attempt at sacrifice and repair is not warranted due to the poor prognosis and potential complications.

Postoperative Blowout

Although its occurrence is rare, blowout is one of the most feared postoperative complications, with an incidence of between 3% and 7% of all neck dissections.[1,2] Contributing factors include prior irradiation, the development of a fistula, or persistent disease in the region of the carotid artery.

The usual sequence of events prior to a carotid blowout is the development of a wound infection, necrosis of the overlying skin (Fig 23–1), and an associated fistula. Should the surgical resection of disease about the carotid necessitate removal of the adventitial layer, a significant reduction in vessel wall perfusion occurs. Further compromise occurs in patients who have had prior irradiation. Subsequent fistula formation with local infection may result in a slow dissolution of the vessel wall (Fig 23–2). In this situation, a warning from a sentinel bleed may occur prior to rupture. The recognition of this sign is vital, and immediate intervention is imperative. Unfortunately, imminent rupture is not often apparent, and emergency ligation of the carotid following rupture has a much higher incidence of neurologic sequelae and death than elective ligation.[2,3]

The immediate management of a blowout should include digital compression of the vessel with placement of the patient in the supine position. If a tracheotomy tube is in place, its immediate inflation to prevent aspiration of blood is imperative. Additional IV lines should be inserted so that volume replacement with fluids and blood is instigated, thereby preventing cerebral anoxia. Once the patient's condition is stabilized, he or she is transferred to the operating room for vessel ligation. Maintenance of digital compression is continued until the isolated bleed is controlled with appropriate clamping. The vessel wall is dissected to a region of healthy tissue prior to its ligation with multiple heavy transfixion sutures of 0 silk. In the postoperative period, the patient is observed for evidence of a pos-

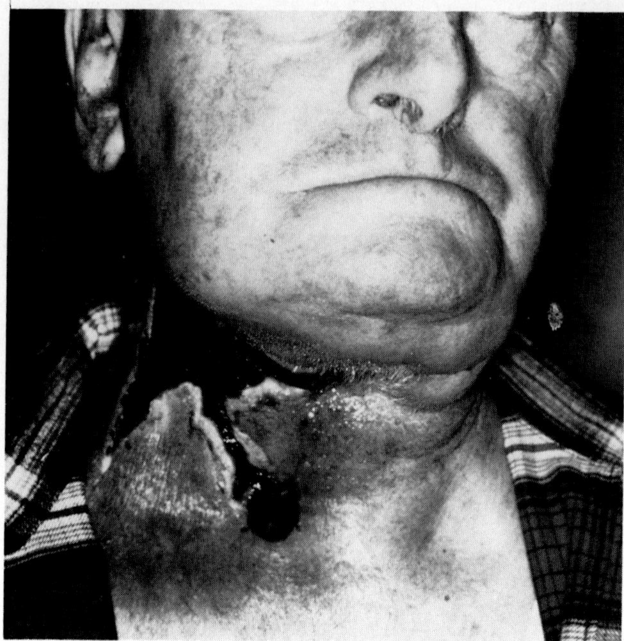

FIG 23–1.
Skin necrosis following neck dissection.

sible neurologic deficit. The potential complications include hemiplegia or monoplegia, aphasia, dysphasia, dysarthria, and occasionally progressive cerebral hypoxia and brain swelling culminating in death.

A number of factors have helped significantly reduce the incidence of this dreaded complication over the past decade. These include improved irradiation techniques and knowledge of the vascular supply to cervical skin with appropriate planning of skin incisions. The more liberal use of myocutaneous flaps with vessel protection from the muscle pedicle and the prophylactic use of antibiotics,[4,5] particularly metronidazole (Flagyl), have also contributed.

Intraoperative Cerebrovascular Accident

Surprisingly, this complication is a rare occurrence since this procedure is performed on an elderly population with significant atherosclerotic disease. Predisposing factors that may result in this potential complication include manipulation of the artery with possible displacement of a plaque, carotid sinus stimulation with bradycardia, and hypotension or unrecognized excessive blood loss with associated hypotension.

Methods of prevention include gentle manipulation of the vessel at the time of surgery and the maintenance of intravascular volume both with fluids and blood. Frequently, intraoperative CVA goes unrecognized.

INTERNAL JUGULAR VEIN

Injury at the Thoracic Inlet

Injury to the internal jugular vein at the thoracic inlet is uncommon. To avoid such injury, one must carefully identify the vessel where it drains into subclavian vein. Disease in the lower part of the neck greatly increases the risk of injury. Once the sternal and clavicular heads of the sternomastoid muscle are detached approximately 1 cm above the clavicle, the carotid sheath is identified beneath the clavicular head. In this location, care must be exercised not to avulse one of the tributaries, which enter the vein medially, or tear the vein when freeing it posteriorly.

If inadvertent opening into the vein occurs, digital pressure is applied and the anesthesiologist is informed. The patient is placed in the Trendelenburg position to minimize the risk of air embolus. In the event of a small localized tear, the vessel is repaired with 6–0 vascular proline. A more major tear is treated with appropriate cross clamping, ties, and suture ligatures, with the preservation of local vascular and neural structures.

Injury at the Skull Base

Disruption of the internal jugular vein in the region of the upper part of the neck, although uncommon, can on occasion be difficult to control. To locate the vein, the operator detaches the sternomastoid muscle from its insertion and transects the tail of the parotid gland. The posterior belly of the digastric muscle is then identified and retracted superiorly. This provides exposure of the internal jugular vein and permits identification of the hypoglossal nerve anteriorly, the vagus nerve posteriorly, and the spinal accessory nerve posterolaterally.

Again, management of an inadvertent tear includes digital pressure and identification of the site and extent of the tear, with either repair or cross clamping with ligation. Occasionally, control of the bleeding is not accessible to ligation, and repair

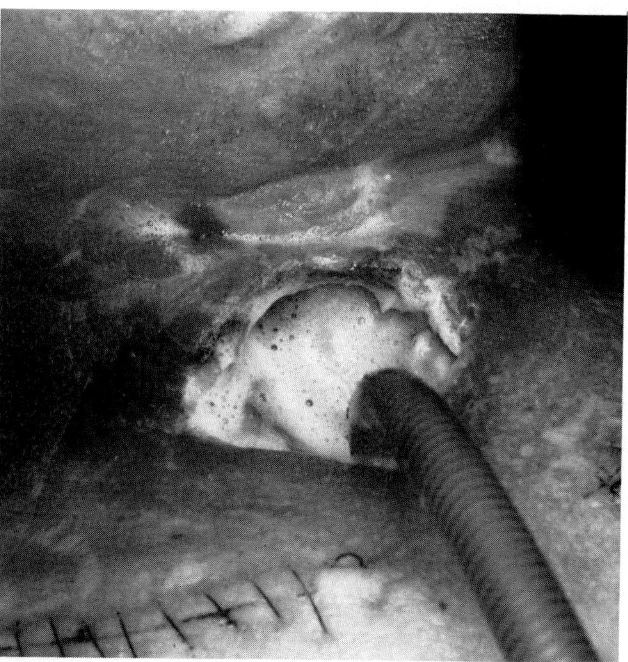

FIG 23–2.
Pharyngocutaneous fistula with skin necrosis and infection. Carotid artery exposed deep in the wound.

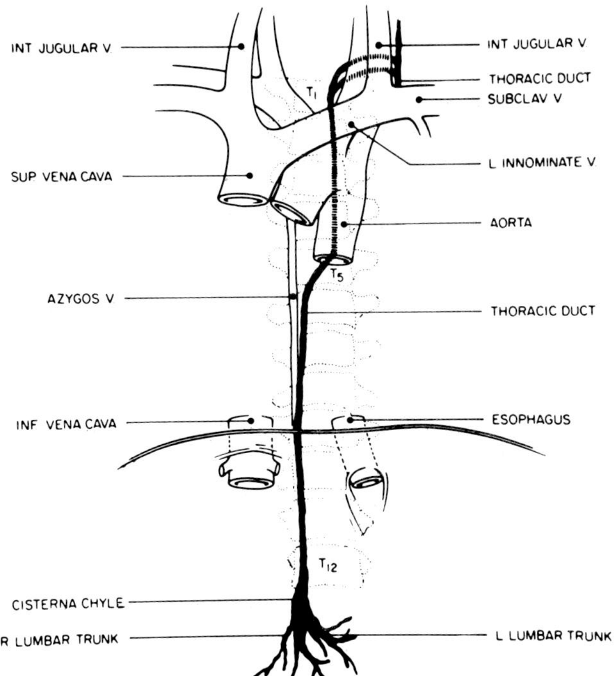

FIG 23–3.
Anatomic relationships of the thoracic duct.

and is treated with tamponade using either oxidized cellulose (Surgicel) or muscle plugs. Rarely is surgical exposure of the sigmoid sinus and jugular bulb necessary to control bleeding from this site.

Bilateral Internal Jugular Vein Sacrifice

The risk of complications following bilateral radical neck dissections are significant. In general, I attempt to preserve one internal jugular vein unless the neoplastic process precludes this. The resulting complications of bilateral radical neck dissections include significant facial edema, upper airway obstruction, and increased venous pressure with associated elevated intracranial pressure. Appropriate preventive measures to avoid these potential complications include a tracheotomy, elevation of the patient's head, maintenance of fluid balance, and the prophylactic use of dexamethasone (60 mg daily in four doses tapered over 5 days). A lumbar drain or ventriculoperitoneal shunt is rarely used except in the extreme case where cerebral edema has resulted in the progressive neurologic deficit.

The potential risk of serious complications is minimized if the previous regime is adhered to and outweighs the advantages of performing the procedure on a staged basis.

Air Embolus

Although uncommon, air embolus is a potentially fatal complication of neck dissection.[6,7] In general, a pressure gradient exists between the internal jugular vein and the heart. This gradient increases with elevation of the head. Inadvertent transection of the internal jugular vein in the neck predisposes the

patient to an air embolus. When greater than 50 mL of air enters the ventricle, acute insufficient right ventricular outflow occurs, resulting in a functional obstruction with cardiovascular collapse. Should this occur, the patient is immediately placed in a Trendelenburg and left lateral decubitus position. Vasopressors and 100% oxygen are administered with closed cardiac massage performed until circulation is restored. If these measures fail to restore the cardiovascular circulation, aspiration of air from the ventricle with a large-bore (14-gauge) needle may be required.

Prevention of this potential, though very uncommon, complication is achieved by placing the patient in the Trendelenburg position in the event of a major venous tear.

CHYLOUS LEAK

Chylous fistula is a rare but serious complication of neck dissection, with a reported incidence of 1% to 2%.[8,9] The majority of fistulae occur on the left side, with up to 25% on the right side.[10] Knowledge of the anatomy of the lymphatic channels in the lower part of the neck is the most important factor in prevention of injury to the duct. The thoracic duct enters the neck and runs anterior to the left subclavian and vertebral arteries, phrenic nerve, and along the medial border of the scalenius anterior muscle. Classically, the duct terminates on entering the left internal jugular vein at its junction with the left subclavian (Fig 23–3).

Recognition of the normal anatomy and its variations is crucial to the prevention of a fistula. Greenfield and Gottlieb found that 89.4% of thoracic ducts ended as a single channel, 6.6% ended as two, and 4% ended as three terminal branches in 75 neck dissections studied.[11]

The majority of injuries to the thoracic duct that occur during neck dissection are recognized intraoperatively. The appearance of a clear or milky fluid in the supraclavicular fossa or a greasy film on the surgeon's glove should alert the operator to the possibility of a chylous leak. In these circumstances, one must painstakingly search for the duct and ligate it. Placement of the patient in the Trendelenberg position with the application of positive pressure ventilation frequently assists in locating the site of the injured duct by increasing the flow of chyle. Once the site of injury is identified, the duct is either simply ligated or occasionally oversewn.

A chylous leak in the postoperative period manifests itself in a variety of different ways, including increased drainage from the Hemovacs, which, in the early phase, may be clear but may have a more milky creamy appearance as the fat content of the patient's diet increases. With time, the overlying skin becomes erythematous, resulting from the irritative effect of the alkaline chyle. Confirmation of a leak is obtained by measuring the specific gravity and fat content of the drainage. If the specific gravity of the effusion is greater than 1.012 with a fat content more than 3%, confirmation of a leak is established.

Immediate management includes maintenance of a closed drainage (Hemovac) system, analysis of electrolyte and protein levels, and the discontinuation of food by mouth. Nasogastric feeding is commensed 24 hours later with the use of a medium chain triglyceride such as Vivonex or Portagen. This fat-free supplement maintains the patient's nutritional status while reducing the volume of chyle produced. If despite this early treatment the drainage continues to increase to a volume greater than 500 mL/day, serious consideration should be given to early open exploration and identification and ligation of the duct. Reexploration of the neck in such circumstances is usually difficult, and a combination of oversewing the duct with the topical application of tetracycline powder is usually successful.

NERVE INJURIES

Ramus Mandibularis and Main Trunk of Nerve VII

The marginal mandibular branch of the facial nerve courses horizontally parallel to the ramus of the mandible between the platysma and superficial layer of the deep cervical fascia. Its caudal limit is variable and during a routine neck dissection can be damaged easily. Selective identification of this nerve is rarely performed unless the ablation of disease high in the submandibular triangle places it at risk. Inadvertent injury to the nerve during this procedure is usually unrecognized. Prevention of injury is achieved by dissecting deep to the superficial fascial layer over the submandibular gland, identifying and ligating the facial artery and vein, thereby displacing the nerve superiorly and the judicious of bipolar rather than monopolar cautery. If the nerve is inadvertently severed, an end-to-end anastomosis is performed.

Injury to the main trunk of the facial nerve is extremely uncommon following neck dissection. Inadvertent injury may occur in circumstances where the normal anatomy is distorted or where advanced disease has invaded the parotid. In the event of nerve transection, primary neurorrhaphy is performed.

Phrenic Nerve and Brachial Plexus

Injury to the phrenic nerve and brachial plexus during a routine neck dissection is extremely uncommon. Anatomically, the phrenic nerve lies along the scalenus anterior muscle, whereas the brachial plexus lies over the scalenus medius and exits the neck between the scalenus medius and posterior on its course caudally into the axilla.

Dissection in the posterior triangle and supraclavicular fossa includes the removal of fat, transection of the omohyoid, and identification of the scalene muscles. In the event of an inadvertent transection of either the phrenic nerve or brachial plexus, primary neurorrhaphy with the use of the operating microscope and 9–0 Ethilon results in a greater than 70% return of function.

Prevention of injury is achieved by having a thorough knowledge of the anatomy of the area with meticulous dissection.

Lingual and Hypoglossal Nerves

Surgical dissection of the submandibular triangle places the lingual and hypoglossal nerves at risk. The potential risks of injury to the lingual nerve are increased in patients who have had previous irradiation or chronic sialadenitis. As the submandibular gland is dissected free, the lingual nerve becomes visible on its cephalic surface and is maintained in the neck by its attachment to the submandibular ganglion. An inadvertent crush injury or transection occasionally results when this attachment is being released. Should transection occur, a primary nerve repair is performed. A permanent injury to the nerve results in significant loss of sensation over the anterior two thirds of the tongue, which, on occasion, can be quite troublesome to the patient.

The hypoglossal nerve is vulnerable to injury as it hooks around the occipital artery and passes over the external carotid artery 3 to 5 cm above the carotid bifurcation. In its transverse course, the nerve lies deep to the digastric muscle surrounded by multiple veins, which, when disturbed, may bleed profusely. Control of such hemorrhage with cautery or ligation increases the risk of injury to the nerve. If disease involves the nerve, necessitating its sacrifice, an interposition cable graft is not routinely employed. However, if the nerve is inadvertently transected, primary repair is performed.

Vagus Nerve

The vagus nerve is most commonly injured at the time of ligation of the internal jugular vein. Occasionally, tumor may involve the nerve necessitating its sacrifice. The morbidity associated with such injury depends on its level of transection. High vagal injuries above the nodus ganglion frequently result in severe dysphagia and aspiration. Routine primary nerve repair following its transection is not performed. Alternatively, immediate vocal cord augmentation is performed, which helps improve the patients tracheobronchial toilet and eliminates aspiration in the early postoperative period.

Spinal Accessory Nerve

The accessory nerve exits the skull base at the jugular foramen and runs laterally posterior to the internal jugular vein. The nerve then descends obliquely, passing medial to the styloid process, stylohyoid, and posterior belly of the digastric muscle. When it reaches the upper end of the sternomastoid muscle, it pierces its deep surface and emerges along the posterior border of this muscle at the junction of its upper and middle third (Erb's point). The nerve courses across the posterior triangle, where it receives branches from the cervical plexus (C2–3) and finally enter the trapezius muscle 3 to 5 cm above the clavicle.

Injury to the nerve may occur with inadvertent deep elevation of the posterior cervical flap. Other situations that put the nerve at risk include tenting of the nerve in the posterior triangle (Fig 23–4) and during a modified neck dissection where the sternomastoid muscle is transected. During a routine functional neck dissection, the nerve can also be injured when stripping the fascia from the undersurface of the sternomastoid muscle. If the nerve is transected, primary neurorrhaphy of the nerve ends alone or with a cable graft should be considered. Continual controversy regarding the functional results of such repair still exists.

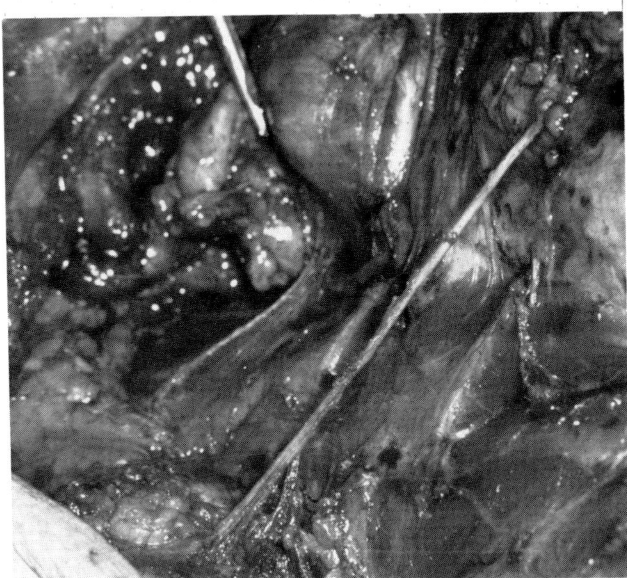

FIG 23–4.
Tenting of the spinal accessory nerve in the posterior triangle.

Prophylactic neck dissection is now performed more commonly with the increased awareness that control of disease within the regional lymph nodes is vital to survival. However, the nerve is always sacrificed in the presence of regional lymphadenopathy along the spinal accessory chain, in the posterior triangle, or with extensive disease in the upper deep cervical region.

Sacrifice of the nerve usually results in postoperative shoulder discomfort and pain. However, these symptoms may also be seen even when the nerve has been preserved. A prospective study by Leipzig et al. showed that spinal accessory nerve dysfunction occurred in 60% of patients following radical neck dissection, in 50% of patients following modified neck dissection, and in 30% of patients following functional neck dissection.[12]

The role of nerve grafting after sacrifice of the accessory nerve during routine neck dissecton is controversial; however, favorable results have been reported in 50% to 100% of cases using the great auricular nerve.[13,14] I do not routinely employ this technique.

Postoperative Neuroma Formation

Neuroma formation resulting from neck dissection is extremely common, but only a minority of these patients have significant complaints. Symptoms of pain aggravated by pressure or palpation usually develop 6 months to 1 year following surgery. The most frequent sites of neuroma formation include the posterior triangle, along the transected cervical roots, the site of spinal accessory nerve transection, and in the terminal sensory roots of the infra-auricular region. Management includes the avoidance of triggering factors such as pressure from tight clothing. In a minority of patients, the topical application of phenol may be used but is of temporary benefit. A more successful treatment is isolating the neuroma with its resection, and burying the stump in the surrounding muscle, and resurfacing the area using either a local or pedicled muscle flap.

REFERENCES

1. Heller KS, Strong EW: Carotid arterial hemorrhage after radical head and neck surgery. *Am J Surg* 1979; 138:607–610.
2. Shumrick DA: Carotid artery rupture. *Laryngoscope* 1973; 83:1051–1061.
3. Moore O, Baker HW: Carotid ligation in surgery of the head and neck. *Cancer* 1955; 8:712–726.
4. Camitz PS, Biggers WP, Fisher NK: Avoidance of early complications following radical neck dissection. *Laryngoscope* 1979; 89:1553–1563.
5. Johnson JT, Yu VL, Myers EN, et al: Efficacy of two third-generation cephalosporins in prophylaxis for head and neck surgery. *Arch Otolaryngol* 1984; 110:224–227.
6. Erickson JA, Gottlieb JD, Sweet RB: Closed chest cardiac message in the treatment of venous air embolism. *N Engl J Med* 1964; 270:1353–1354.
7. Longnecker CG: Venous air embolism during operations on the head and neck. Report of a case. *Plast Reconstr Surg* 1965; 36:619–621.
8. Fitz-Hugh GS, Cowgill R: Chylous fistula. *Arch Otolaryngol* 1970; 91:543–547.
9. Lucente FE, Dicktaban T, Lawson W, et al: Chylous fistula management. *Otolaryngol Head Neck Surg* 1981; 89:575–578.
10. Crumley RL, Smith JD: Post operative chylous fistula prevention and management. *Laryngoscope* 1976; 86:804–813.
11. Greenfield J, Gottlieb MI: Variations in the terminal portion of the human thoracic duct. *Arch Surg* 1956; 73:955–959.
12. Leipzig B, Suen JY, English JL, et al: Function evaluation of the spinal accessory nerve after neck dissection. *Am J Surg* 1983; 146:526–530.
13. Ballantyne AJ, Guinn GA: Reduction of shoulder disability after neck dissection. *Am J Surg* 1966; 112:662–665.
14. Anderson R, Flowers RS: Free grafts of the spinal accessory nerve during radical neck dissection. *Am J Surg* 1969; 118:796–799.

Infectious Issues Relating to Neck Dissection

Approach of

Jonas T. Johnson, M.D.

This chapter will discuss several selected infectious issues involving the neck. Wound infection, its prevention, and management will be presented first, following which parotitis and septic thrombophlebitis of the internal jugular vein will be presented and discussed.

WOUND INFECTION

Postoperative wound infection is an important cause of surgical morbidity. In one study, it was estimated that the development of a postoperative wound infection following major head and neck surgery increased hospitalization by 14 days and cost greater than $10,000 (1985) in direct hospital charges.[1] This figure, of course, does not address suffering or lost income.

The first and most important issue in discussing wound infection must be prevention. The surgeon should consider a successful outcome as the appropriate conclusion to a carefully planned and well carried out surgical procedure. Success, however, requires preoperative preparation, intraoperative skill, and postoperative care.

Preoperatively, the patient must be brought into optimal condition. Clearly, great variability exists between individuals in terms of intrinsic surgical risks. However, every attempt must be made to correct metabolic abnormalities, stabilize chronic diseases, and initiate appropriate nutritional support. The head and neck surgeon should give special attention to the reestablishment of good oral hygiene to prevent dental sepsis from compromising normal wound healing. Nutritional abnormalities must be recognized and corrected preoperatively. Bulky, painful, and sometimes obstructing tumors of the upper aero-

digestive tract are frequently associated with dysphagia, aspiration, and resultant malnutrition. Taken in context with the frequent history of alcoholism and poor diet, this situation mandates preoperative correction whenever possible.

Intraoperatively, the tenants of good surgical care must be followed. This calls for gentle handling of tissue, debridement of necrotic and foreign body material, copious irrigation of the wound, and absolute hemostasis.

It has been clearly established that procedures contaminated by oropharyngeal secretions may be accompanied by a high risk of postoperative wound infection when antibiotic prophylaxis is omitted.[2–6] In a study of patients undergoing major contaminated head and neck procedures in which a cervical incision was used to remove a tumor of the upper aerodigestive tract, Becker and Parell report an 87% incidence of postoperative wound infection among patients randomized to receive no antibiotic prophylaxis.[7] Other placebo-controlled clinical trials have reported excessive infection rates in patients randomized to no antibiotic therapy (Table 24–1). The variability of risk probably reflects methodologic differences in terms of the characteristics of the population studied, drugs used, and the definition of wound infection; nonetheless, the conclusion that antimicrobial prophylaxis is mandatory seems justified.

Saliva harbors about 10^8 organisms/cm^3.[8] This includes both aerobic gram-positive cocci and anaerobic bacteria. However, anaerobes are approximately 10 times more numerous than aerobes. Gram-negative aerobic rods are rarely part of the normal oral flora. These bacteria may be observed on skin, colonizing preexistent tracheostomy wounds,[9] and occasionally on the gingiva following radiation therapy.[10]

Cultures of material obtained from patients with postop-

TABLE 24–1.
Head and Neck Infections Developed in Patients Receiving Perioperative Placebo

Author	No. of Patients Studied	Infection Rate (%)
Piccart et al.[2]	12	24
Dor and Klastersky[3]	50	36
Seagle et al.[4]	25	48
Eschelman et al.[5]	8	50
Johnson et al.[6]	9	78
Becker and Parell[7]	23	87

TABLE 24–2.
Antibiotics With Reported Efficacy in Prevention of Wound Infection: 1 Day of Administration Only

Antibiotic	No. of Patients	No. of Infections (%)
Cefazolin (500 mg)[13]	21	7 (33)
Cefazolin (1 gm)[4]	25	4 (16)
Cefazolin (1 gm)[7]	32	12 (38)
Cefazolin (2 gm)[14]	59	5 (8.5)
Carbenicillin[2]	72	10 (14)
Moxalactam[15]	16	1 (6.2)
Moxalactam[14]	59	2 (3.4)
Clindamycin[11]	52	2 (3.4)
Clindamycin-gentamicin[13]	29	2 (7)
Clindamycin-gentamicin[11]	52	2 (3.4)
Cefoperazone (2 gm)[6]	39	4 (10)
Cefotaxime (2 gm)[6]	32	3 (9)

erative wound infection frequently demonstrate multiple organisms from a single patient.[2,6,7,11,12] These polymicrobial wound infections characteristically demonstrate both aerobic and anaerobic bacteria.

Published reports have indicated that multiple antimicrobial agents may have efficacy in the prevention of postoperative wound infection (Table 24–2).[2,4,6,7,11,13–15] To date, no comparable study has been undertaken to clearly define the "best" choice antibiotic. Direct comparison of results generated in different studies, especially when done by different investigators, is unreliable. The need for administration of an antibiotic effective in eradicating oral flora is apparent.[11] Toxicity, cost, and ease of administration all are reasonable considerations.

Various studies have indicated that aerobic gram-negative bacteria may be isolated from secretions cultured from head and neck wound infections.[2,6,7,11] These organisms may be only colonizing the wound and do not necessarily represent the etiologic agents. Nevertheless, the need for broad-spectrum antimicrobial prophylaxis with efficacy for gram-negative aerobic bacteria continues to be investigated.

Burke demonstrated that a critical time exists during which the antibiotic must be administered for it to be effective.[16] In an animal experiment, he demonstrated that antimicrobials administered 3 or more hours after contamination are ineffective in preventing subsequent wound infection. This observation has been subsequently corroborated in human studies.[13] It is now generally accepted that effective prophylaxis must be administered prior to bacterial contamination.

The duration of postoperative antimicrobial administration remains somewhat contentious. Many experienced head and neck surgeons favor maintenance of antibiotic prophylaxis for several days postoperatively. Various authors have evaluated the optimal duration for antibiotic administration.[2,13,15,17] However, these studies have failed to show improved efficacy for antimicrobial prophylaxis administered greater than 24 hours postoperatively (Table 24–3). It would appear that patients undergoing routine head and neck surgery do not benefit from more prolonged antibiotic administration. Studies of antibiotic prophylaxis in patients undergoing mandibular reconstruction, free tissue transfers, and cranial base surgery have not, however, been undertaken to date.

At the completion of the procedure, drainage catheters must be placed. After radical neck dissection, I frequently observe from 100 mL to several hundred milliliters of serosanguineous drainage in the 24 hours following surgery. Characteristically, this drainage gradually tapers daily until the drains can be removed when less than 15 mL of accumulation daily is observed. This vast amount of material must be adequately drained to prevent elevation of the cervical skin flap, ischemia of the tissues, and invasion by pathogenic bacteria with resultant wound infection. I recommend that at least two, and sometimes four, continuous positive-pressure suction drains (e.g., Hemovac or Jackson Pratt) be introduced to each side of the neck prior to closure. Suction must be applied before the last sutures are tied to assure that all secretions are properly aspirated and to prevent occlusion to the drains by clotted blood.

Postoperatively, proper wound care may reduce the risk of subsequent wound infection. A properly applied compressive dressing serves to coapt the cervical skin flap to the underlying soft tissue, reducing the risk of hematoma and contributing to immobilization of the soft tissues (Fig 24–1). Some judgment must be used in applying compressive dressings inasmuch as free flaps and pedicle grafts must not have the vascular supply compromised by a compressive dressing. Similarly, cervical

TABLE 24–3.
Comparative Studies Designed to Evaluate Duration of Antibiotic Therapy

Authors	Duration Studied (days)	Drug	Infection Rate (%)
Piccart et al.[2]	1		10/72 (14)
	4	Carbenicillin	7/68 (10)
Fee et al.[15]	1		1/15 (6)
	2	Moxalactam	0/15 (0)
Johnson et al.[13]	1	Clindamycin	2/29 (7)
	5	plus	
		Gentamicin	1/27 (4)
Johnson et al.[17]	1		10/53 (18)
(flap reconstruction)	5	Cefoperazone	14/56 (25)

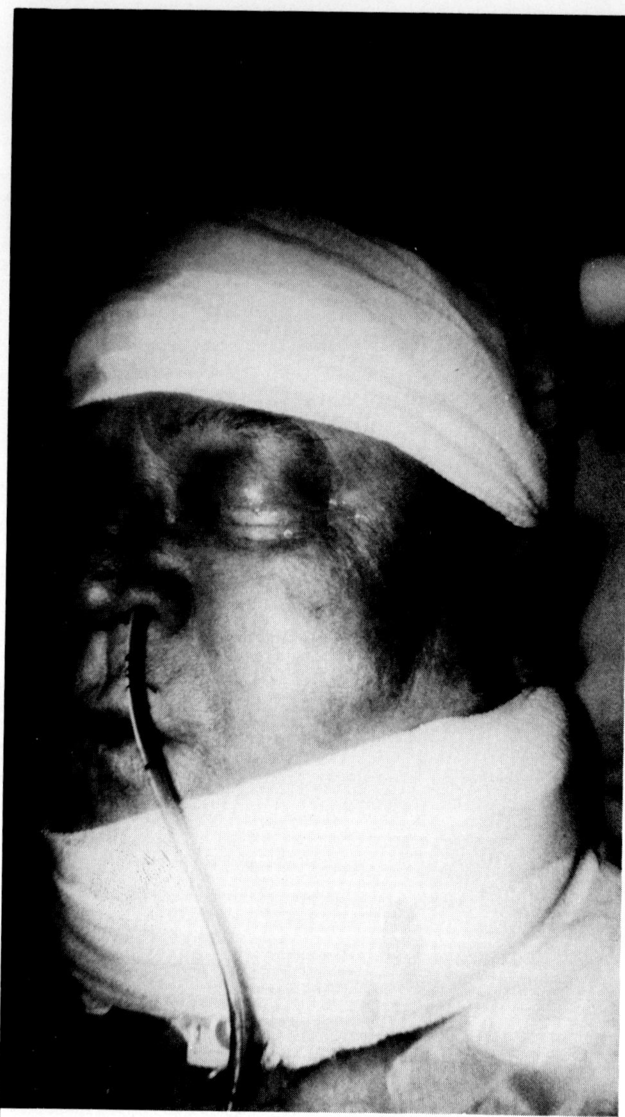

FIG 24–1.
A bulky, compressive dressing assists in immobilizing the patient, reduces cutaneous edema, and serves to coapt the cervical skin flap to the underlying tissues.

dressing is not advocated following bilateral radical neck dissection inasmuch as the dressing may compromise venous drainage, resulting in increased intracranial pressure.

Maintenance of patent cervical drains is critical to postoperative care. Drains should be examined frequently and aspirated every shift by a trained nursing staff to assure that obstruction with clot and debris does not occur. Drain management should be done using sterile technique. If inattention results in occlusion of the drain by clot, subsequent collection in the neck is predictable, with resultant poor wound healing and increased risk for wound infection. Postoperative hematoma is an indication for return to the operating room for clot evacuation and reestablishment of hemostasis.

Diagnosis of hematoma is easily made when sudden swell-

ing of a ballotable cervical mass is observed. Needle aspiration is inadequate to remove clotted blood. Failure to maintain drain patency is the most common cause of hematoma; however, disruption of a ligature occasionally occurs. Johnson et al. have demonstrated that hematoma, properly recognized and evacuated, is rarely the source of major wound sepsis, and the risk is limited to those attendant with a second anesthetic.[18]

Other postoperative conditions that merit special attention include reestablishment of nutritional needs through tube feeding and maintenance of normal metabolic parameters, including hydration, electrolytes, and oxygenation.

Postoperative wound infection may be diagnosed when a purulent subcutaneous collection is recognized or if purulent material is obtained through the Hemovac drains. This represents two distinct circumstances and will be discussed separately.

In most circumstances, when purulence is adequately drained through the Hemovacs, little or no further management is needed. The implication of purulent or mucoid material in the drainage tubes is that salivary material has gained access to the previously closed wound. As long as the material can be adequately drained by the Hemovac, further sequelae are unusual. The cervical suction catheters should be left in place until the drainage stops. Of course, circumstances may develop in which the drainage tubing is actually aspirating salivary material from the pharynx. Under these circumstances, the drainage catheter should be maintained patent until the cervical skin flap has been allowed time to heal to the deep tissues of the neck. This may take 10 to 14 days. At this time, the cervical drainage tube can be advanced, leaving only a small circuitous fistula track that can be reliably expected to close spontaneously by secondary intention. In patients who have received prior radiation therapy, the time elapsed between surgery and removal of the drainage tubes may necessarily be extended to 21 days.

If the purulent collection is not adequately drained by the Hemovac, the cervical skin flap may be elevated with resultant tissue ischemia, necrosis, and wound breakdown. This may result in a mucocutaneous fistula. The wound should be carefully examined daily. A fluid collection may develop if the suction catheters are not draining properly or, conversely, after catheter removal. Surgical drainage should be initiated. A procedure should be planned to divert the draining material away from the great vessels and tracheotomy site. This decreases the risk of vascular erosion and hemorrhage or pneumonia. Compressive dressings are applied, and the patient is treated with parenteral antibiotics and regular dressing changes. Nutritional support is continued through tube feedings.

Small fistulas frequently close spontaneously. However, hospitalization is characteristically prolonged 10 to 14 days.[1] In the face of a patient who has had prior radiation therapy, the resultant perivascular fibrosis may contribute to the development of massive tissue loss and a large mucocutaneous fistula. These defects frequently will not close spontaneously, and secondary surgical procedures must be planned. The literature is replete with suggestions for the management of large mucocutaneous fistulae. Current technology would indicate that the most important considerations include debridement of ischemic and necrotic material, protection of the great vessels and nerves, and replacement with vascularized healthy tissue. Modern microvascular techniques have allowed aggressive management of large fistulae, resulting in improved carotid protection and early return of function.

The creation of planned or "controlled" fistula at the time of surgery has been previously advocated in high-risk patients to allow the surgeon to control the direction of the salivary fistula and facilitate postoperative wound care. Fortunately, improved understanding of surgical nutrition, avoidance of preoperative radiation therapy, and a better understanding of the use of vascularized tissue for reconstruction of major soft tissue defects has made the need for the development of controlled fistulas and planned multistage procedures obsolete. When high-risk patients such as those with malnutrition or prior radiation therapy are encounterd, it is appropriate to delay surgery for appropriate nutritional replacement. Following extirpation, soft tissue defects can be repaired with vascularized tissue employing either pedicle flaps or free tissue transfers using microvascular techniques. This approach obviates the need for control fistulas and multistage procedures. This also facilitates entry into adjuvant therapy programs when indicated.

PAROTITIS

Acute suppurative parotitis is a disease that has been characterized as occurring chiefly in dehydrated postoperative patients. The pathogenic organism is almost always *Staphylococcus aureus*. The incidence of nosocomial parotitis is reportedly decreased since the underlying pathophysiology became widely acknowledged.

Parotitis most commonly develops in debilitated and dehydrated hospitalized patients with poor oral hygiene. Retrograde spread of bacteria from the oral cavity through the parotid duct is the most common mechanism of infection. The parotid gland is particularly susceptible to bacteria because its serous secretions contain no bacteriostatic mucus as do the submandibular glands. The inflammatory lesion produces an accumulation of cells within the larger ducts. Gradually, however, the smaller ducts and parenchyma are involved as the larger- and medium-sized ducts are destroyed. With parenchymal invasion, microabscesses may develop, which may then coalesce.

Krippaehne et al. retrospectively reviewed 161 cases of acute suppurative parotitis.[19] One hundred thirty-one of these patients had severe or multiple illnesses. Carcinoma was present in 25% of cases, and more than 50% of patients had preexistent major infection elsewhere in the body. These authors note that only one third of the patients were postoperative. In fact, Krippaehne et al. note that one third of their patients with suppurative parotitis were admitted from home or from nursing facilities.[19]

Spratt reported a retrospective study of 178 cases of parotitis identified between 1911 and 1959.[20] His data indicated that the introduction of antibiotics between 1940 and 1950 resulted in the almost complete disappearance of postsurgical parotitis. Thereafter, a resurgence of the disease was noted. Acute suppurative parotitis due to antibiotic-resistant *S. aureus* with an accompanying mortality rate of 31% was noted between 1952

and 1959. Spratt interpreted this as an indication that the widespread use of antibiotic prophylaxis in surgical patients had contributed to the development of superinfection with resistant organisms.[20]

Recognition of parotitis is relatively straightforward. Erythema, tenderness, and swelling characteristically develop around the involved gland. Suppurative debris can almost always be milked from Stenson's duct and submitted for bacteriologic study (Fig 24–2). Therapy should be directed at correction of dehydration and metabolic abnormalities, with institution of antimicrobial therapy and other supportive measures as needed.

Radiation therapy has been suggested as an alternative for acute suppurative parotitis. Treatment characteristically consisted of 50 to 150 rad daily from a 250 kV source to a total dose of approximately 600 rad.[20] Spratt points out that this dose of radiation is nonlethal to *Staphylococcus*.[20] In addition, it is unlikely that this dose of radiation would result in significant reduction of parotid secretions. It should be pointed out that most reports are poorly controlled inasmuch as most patients received antibiotics and surgical drainage in conjunction with the radiation therapy.[21, 22] The relationship between radiation therapy and resolution of acute suppurative parotitis is conjectural at best.

Surgical therapy may be required in patients who develop abscess of the parotid gland. Characteristically, microabscesses may coalesce to development of multilocular glandular abscesses. Surgical therapy should be directed at achieving complete drainage of all loculations with preservation of facial nerve function. This requires development of a cervical skin flap, following which, the infected gland can be explored with a blunt instrument directed in the direction of the branches of the facial nerve.

Yonkers et al. retrospectively reviewed the records of 11 patients with parotitis observed between 1948 and 1971.[23] All

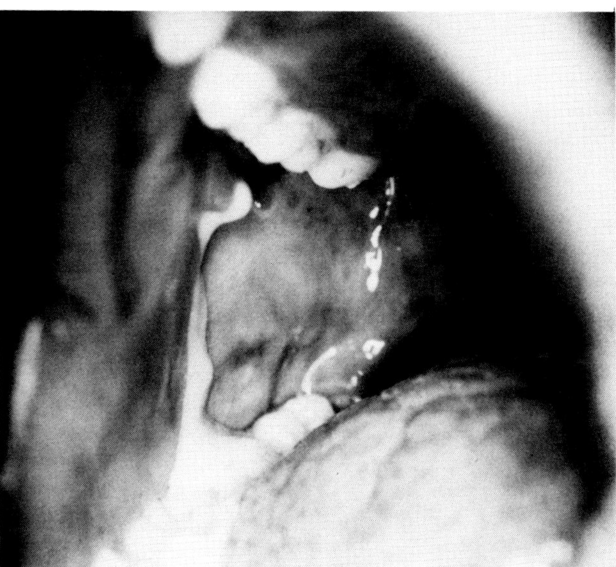

FIG 24–2.
This patient with acute suppurative paratitis demonstrates free flow of purulent saliva from Stenson's duct.

patients were observed between 6 and 107 days postoperatively. The disease manifested itself as an erythematous swollen tender parotid with leukocytosis and fever. *Staphylococcus aureus* was recovered from every patient. Therapy included correction of dehydration and metabolic abnormalities, oral care, warm compresses, and antibiotics. Radiation was employed in two cases (225 and 378 rad). A single death occurred in this series. They consider the irresponsible use of perioperative antibiotics an important causative factor in the development of parotitis.[23]

More recent reports indicate that nosocomial parotitis may be associated with various other bacteria. Pruett and Simmons report enteric gram-negative bacilli as the primary pathogen.[24] These included *Pseudomonas aeruginosa, Klebsiella oxytoca, Enterobacter* species, and *Proteus mirabilis.*

Fainstein et al. documented two patients with nosocomial *Hemophilus influenzae* as the sole isolate in patients with acute suppurative parotitis.[25] In both cases, the disease was bilateral.

Acute suppurative parotitis is a disease of chronically debilitated patients with associated dehydration and poor oral hygiene. Clearly, the incidence of this entity is reduced; however, hospice, nursing home, and occasional hospitalized patients will be encountered. Management should be directed at identification of causative organisms, correction of dehydration and metabolic abnormalities, and institution of appropriate antimicrobial therapy. The patient should be observed carefully. If abscess and suppurative complications should develop, surgical therapy may be indicated.

SEPTIC THROMBOPHLEBITIS OF THE INTERNAL JUGULAR VEIN

Septic thrombophlebitis of the internal jugular vein is a well-recognized complication of deep neck infection when the inflammatory process involves the contents of the carotid sheath. Abscess originating in either the retropharyngeal or, more commonly, the parapharyngeal space may spread to involve the carotid sheath. As the inflammatory process progresses, a combination of venous stasis, perhaps due to compression, and the inflammation itself may result in thrombophlebitis. Untreated, portions of infected clot may result in septic emboli to the pulmonary vascular tree.

Septic thrombophlebitis of the internal jugular vein is an unusual complication of deep neck infection. Recognition requires an adequate index of suspicion. Persistence of a spiking febrile course in a patient who has received appropriate antibiotic therapy and adequate surgical drainage should alert the surgeon to the possibility of septic emboli. Other physical findings that should lead to the suspicion of jugular vein thrombosis include facial plethora, engorged facial vessels, and choked optic discs. The Tobey-Ayer test has been described to identify patients with thrombosis of the internal jugular vein. Lumbar puncture is required so that cerebral spinal fluid (CSF) pressure can be maintained as the jugular veins are sequentially occluded by digital pressure. Compression on the involved side should give no change, but compression of the contralateral (noninvolved) jugular should cause increased CSF pressure.[26] More

modern techniques to assist in making the diagnosis include computed tomography (CT) scan, magnetic resonance imaging (MRI), and contrast vascular studies.

Treatment of jugular venous thrombosis with associated septic emboli has included antibiotic therapy and surgical exploration with ligation of the infecting vein. Attempts at more conservative therapy with intravenous (IV) antibiotics and anticoagulation may be frustrated by septic emboli and serious systemic complications.

More recently, a growing population of patients with thrombophlebitis of the internal jugular vein has been identified. Self-administration of intravenous narcotics by drug abusers may result in thrombophlebitis. In my experience, these patients do not always have abscess formation, and septic emboli has not been observed. I speculate that many of the agents used by intravenous drug abusers produce severe phlebitis with resultant thrombosis without abscess formation. Successful therapy has been accomplished employing intravenous antibiotics. Careful assessment with various imaging techniques is necessary to rule out development of abscess that would, of necessity, be an indication for surgical incision and drainage.

REFERENCES

1. Mandell-Brown M, Johnson JT, Wagner RL: Cost effectiveness of prophylactic antibiotics in head and neck surgery. *Otolaryngol Head Neck Surg* 1984; 92:520–523.
2. Piccart M, Dor P, Klastersky J: Antimicrobial prophylaxis of infections in head and neck cancer surgery. *Scand J Infect Dis Suppl* 1983; 39:92–96.
3. Dor P, Klastersky J: Prophylactic antibiotics in oral, pharyngeal and laryngeal surgery for cancer: A double blind study. *Laryngoscope* 1973; 83:1992–1998.
4. Seagle MB, Duberstein LE, Gross CW, et al: Efficacy of cefazolin as a prophylactic antibiotic in head and neck surgery. *Otolaryngol Head Neck Surg* 1978; 86:568–572.
5. Eschelman LT, Schleuning AJ II, Brummett RE: Prophylactic antibiotics in otolaryngologic surgery: A double blind study. *Trans Am Acad Ophthalmol Otolaryngol* 1971; 75:387–394.
6. Johnson JT, Yu VL, Myers EN, et al: Efficacy of two third-generation cephalosporins in prophylaxis for head and neck surgery. *Arch Otolaryngol Head Neck Surg* 1984; 110:224–227.
7. Becker GD, Parell GJ: Cefazolin prophylaxis in head and neck cancer surgery. *Ann Otol Rhinol Laryngol* 1979; 88:183–186.
8. Bartlett JG, Sherwood LG: Anaerobic infections of the head and neck. *Otolaryngol Clin North Am* 1976; 9:655–678.
9. Niederman MS, Ferranti RD, Zeigler A, et al: Respiratory infection complicating long-term tracheostomy: The implication of persistent gram-negative tracheobronchial colonization. *Chest* 1984; 85:39–44.
10. Brown LR, Dreizen S, Daly TE, et al: Interrelations of oral microorganisms, immunoglobulins, and dental caries following radiotherapy. *J Dent Res* 1978; 57:882–893.
12. Johnson JT, Yu VL, Myers EN, et al: An assessment of need for gram-negative bacterial coverage in antibiotic prophy-

laxis for oncological head and neck surgery. *J Infect Dis* 1987; 155:331–333.

12. Rubin J, Johnson JT, Wagner RL, et al: Bacteriologic analysis of wound infection following major head and neck surgery. *Arch Otolaryngol Head Neck Surg* 1988; 114:969–972.

13. Johnson JT, Myers EN, Thearle PB, et al: Antimicrobial prophylaxis for contaminated head and neck surgery. *Laryngoscope* 1984; 94:46–51.

14. Johnson JT, Myers EN, Yu VL, et al: Cefazolin vs moxalactam? A double blind randomized trial of cephalosporins in head and neck surgery. *Arch Otolaryngol Head Neck Surg* 1986; 112:151–153.

15. Fee WR Jr, Glenn M, Handen C, et al: One day vs two days of prophylactic antibiotics in patients undergoing major head and neck surgery. *Laryngoscope* 1984; 94:612–614.

16. Burke JF: The effective period of preventive antibiotic action in experimental incisions and dermal lesions. *Surgery* 1961; 50:161–168.

17. Johnson JT, Schuller DE, Gluckman JL, et al: Antibiotic prophylaxis in high risk head and neck surgery: One day vs five day therapy. *Otolaryngol Head Neck Surg* 1986; 95:554–557.

18. Johnson JT, Cummings CW: Hematoma after head and neck surgery—a major complication? *Otolaryngol Head Neck Surg* 1978; 86:171–175.

19. Krippaehne WW, Hunt TK, Dunphy JE: Acute suppurative parotitis: A study of 161 cases. *Ann Surg* 1962; 156:251–257.

20. Spratt JS Jr: The etiology and therapy of acute pyogenic parotitis. *Surg Gynecol Obstet* 1961; 112:391–405.

21. Robinson JR: Surgical parotitis, a vanishing disease. *Surgery* 1955; 38:703–707.

22. Gilchrist RK, McAndrew JR: Surgical parotitis. *Arch Surg* 1958; 76:863–867.

23. Yonkers AJ, Krous HF, Yarington CT Jr: Surgical parotitis. *Laryngoscope* 1972; 82:1239–1247.

24. Pruett TL, Simmons RL: Nosocomial gram-negative bacillary parotitis. *JAMA* 1984; 251:252–253.

25. Fainstein V, Musher DM, Young EJ: Acute bilateral suppurative parotitis due to *Haemophilus influenzae. Arch Intern Med* 1979; 139:712–713.

26. Rabuzzi DD, Johnson JT: Diagnosis and management of deep neck infections, in *Self-Instructional Package.* American Academy of Otolaryngology–Head and Neck Surgery, 1976.

Infectious Issues Relating to Neck Dissection

Approach of

David E. Schuller, M.D.

WOUND INFECTION

Wound infections continue to be a major challenge to all head and neck surgeons. The development of newer antimicrobial therapy has had a positive impact on the frequency of such infections. But wound infections continue to be a common occurrence following neck dissection, especially when the pharynx has been entered during the same surgical procedure. Numerous variables and their impact on the frequency of wound infection have been studied. Nutritional status, prior irradiation, stage of disease, and entrance into the pharynx all have been analyzed to determine their impact on the frequency of wound infections. As the operative time and surgical complexity increase, so do the chances of wound infection.[1] But it is important not to lose sight of the single most important variable causing infection, which has been well established by Davidson and co-workers,[2] and that is the presence of bacteria in the surgical wound. Davidson et al. determined that 10^5 bacteria per milliliter was needed to develop a wound infection. This concentration is exceeded in many head and neck procedures. When the pharynx or oral cavity is entered during a neck dissection, it is inevitable that salivary contact with the neck tissues occurs. The bacterial concentration of aerobic organisms is 10^7 per milliliter and 10^8 anaerobes per molliter. This information readily explains the overall complication rate of 50.8% in a group of 788 patients undergoing a radical neck dissection reported by McGuirt et al.[3] This surprisingly high figure includes both medical and surgical complications. Medical complications actually occur in 28% of this series, but major surgical complications, including death, carotid artery rupture, and fistula formation occurred in 16.2%. This information is intended to convince the reader that wound infections following head and neck surgery are common and can have catastrophic consequences. Therefore, it is important to discuss not only means of treating such infections but also how they may be prevented.

Prepping the operative site is an important first step in preventing wound infection. Several effective antimicrobial prep solutions are now available. I currently am using a providone-iodine (Betadine) solution with 70% alcohol. I have not routinely prepped the mucosal surfaces of the upper aerodigestive tract prior to an operation in which entrance into the oral cavity or pharynx is anticipated. The rationale for not prepping this surface is because of the numerous potential areas that will still remain unsterilized, such as the paranasal sinuses. It is, however, important for the surgeon to determine that no chronic sinus infections or dental infections are present preoperatively. These should be resolved prior to any major ablative cancer resection if it does not cause an undue delay in the surgery. It is important to recognize that some prep solutions have the potential to cause either a first-degree or second-degree burn of the skin if they contact the skin for a protracted period of time. If the surgeon does not guard against this by removing any residual prep solution from skin surfaces where there has been runoff of the prep solution, the contact over an extended operative procedure is sufficient to cause a burn. Generous rinsing after prepping the skin and then drying with sterile towels to remove any residual solution and also protection of skin surface area that is in contact with the operating table will minimize the chance of this occurrence. It is also important that the surgeon try to anticipate any unexpected needs for tissue transfer during the planned surgery and to prepare that surface area accordingly. For example, a surgeon may preoperatively anticipate that primary closure may be possible following resection of a particular neoplasm of the pharynx, but submucosal extension may produce a defect larger than anticipated and make flap reconstruction necessary. Surgeons should anticipate this with the original preparation by including the chest area and the thigh in the prepping and draping in case a flap or skin graft is required. This surgical planning decreases the chance of breaking sterile technique by having to prepare another area intraoperatively.

Another important preventive consideration is adhering to sound surgical techniques. This approach means that tissue is handled gently to minimize any chances of necrosis that could eventually become a nidus for postoperative wound infection.

In addition to gentle handling, it is important to keep the tissues moist and to maintain optimal hemostasis. It is also essential to determine that the thoracic duct or other lymphatic channels have not been transsected during the neck dissection. Chyle fistulas can create an impressive amount of inflammation and eventual tissue necrosis in addition to causing hypoproteinemia if the volume of lymphatic flow from the fistula is substantial. It is important to specifically assess the possibility of lymphatic leakage following completion of every neck dissection. The chances of detecting such a fistula are increased by asking the anesthesiologists to vigorously ventilate the patient's lungs for a short period of time to increase the intrathoracic pressure, which will increase the lymphatic drainage. It has been my experience that intravenous fluorescein used to assess flap viability will transform the normally colorless lymph fluid to a greenish fluid and facilitate detection. This approach can be used if the surgeon either suspects a lymphatic leakage intraoperatively or is having difficulty in identifying the location of the leakage.

There are other considerations relative to surgical technique, but if one just remembers that the basic underlying factor responsible for developing wound infection involves a critical concentration of bacteria, certain preventive steps become obvious. In addition to the previously mentioned approaches that increase the chance for tissue necrosis, it is important to keep the tissues moist throughout the procedure and to use aggressive irrigation to remove any clots or to detach tissue fragments from the wound prior to closure. Aggressive irrigation also acts to dilute the concentration of bacteria and possibly has a direct osmotic killing effect on certain bacteria.

The use of antibiotics to prevent wound infections has been clarified in the past 10 years. Although antimicrobial therapy has improved, the optimal antibiotic has yet to be developed. There is a greater appreciation of when the timing of antibiotic administration is beneficial, however, and also what represents the optimal delivery of antibiotics used prophylactically. There appears to be general agreement that prophylactic antibiotics are probably not necessary for head and neck surgical procedures that do not include opening the pharynx or oral cavity. The only time I use prophylactic antibiotics is when saliva bathes the tissues of the neck as a result of resection of an oral or pharyngeal malignancy. The literature abounds with reports evaluating a variety of prophylactic antibiotic regimens,[4–8] but Johnson and his co-workers have done a series of prospective double-blind antibiotic trials that have helped clarify this issue.[9, 10] Most authors have identified that the infection involves both gram-positive and gram-negative bacteria, as well as aerobic and anaerobic organisms. Anaerobic bacteria constitute as much as 42% of the pathogens isolated. It therefore becomes imperative that the prophylactic antibiotic has activity against this broad spectrum of organisms. It is also important that a prophylactic antibiotic be safe and that there is minimal chance of secondary infections following the use of such antibiotics. These previously mentioned studies have demonstrated that there is no increased benefit for prolonged postoperative antibiotic usage vs. a regimen that includes receiving intravenous antibiotics 1 to 2 hours preoperatively and continuing them for

1 day postoperatively. Cefaperazone used with this perioperative regimen is an effective prophylactic antibiotic.

In spite of vigorous preventative measures, the head and neck surgeon can (personally) anticipate encountering wound infections. Prompt and aggressive treatment are the hallmarks of proper management. To begin treatment early, the clinician must be able to recognize a developing wound infection early in its course. A neck wound that heals uneventfully can be characterized by a series of observations. The suture line will be erythematous but not moist. The neck flaps are adherent to the underlying tissue, and they are not edematous and have normal skin color. The wound drainage tubes in the early postoperative period will drain fresh blood, which will become darker and eventually change to just a serous type of drainage. The quantity of the wound drainage will decrease over a period of 3 to 4 days postoperatively. There will be little, if any, tenderness to palpation of the neck flaps.

In contrast, the flaps of a neck wound developing an infection will start to develop the usual signs of inflammation, especially edema and erythema. This can occur at any time during the postoperative period, but it is rare to see these early signs before the third or fourth postoperative day unless there is a major divergence that occurs either with wound healing or with an undetected deviation of normal surgical technique. The natural course of an infection will include progressively severe edema and erythema of the neck flaps and alteration in the wound catheter drainage. Both the quantity and quality of the drainage will change. Rather than decreasing in quantity, the wound catheter drainage will increase. The character of the drainage fluid will change to a more cloudy color. It may even approximate the appearance of frank pus, and it may have a mucoid component consistent with salivary drainage if a fistula has developed. In addition to these physical stigmata, the patients will often become febrile and develop a leukocytosis with a shift in the differential count, indicating inflammation. The temperature is usually elevated only mildly from 38.4°C to 38.9°C. It is only if an actual abscess develops that the potential exists for higher temperatures. If the infection progresses after removal of the drainage catheters, there will be progressive development of mucopurulent or just purulent fluid underneath the neck flaps, which will elevate and separate them from the underlying tissues of the neck. This accumulation of fluid will continue until it produces a breakdown usually at a point along the suture line, with spontaneous drainage of fluid. Hopefully the wound infection will have been recognized in earlier stages of what has just been described, and intervention will reverse the situation.

Treatment of a wound infection is dependent on the stage of its development. This discussion involves the treatment of a wound infection independent of a salivary fistula. Wound infections caused by pharyngeal or orocutaneous fistulae will be discussed later in this chapter.

If the infection is early and there is erythema and edema of the suture line and neck flaps with no drainage or fluctuance, IV broad-spectrum antibiotics are instituted in the absence of any material to culture to obtain specific information regarding the infecting microorganism. The cephalosporin, especially cefaperazone, provide effective broad-spectrum coverage because the infections are usually polymicrobial. If there is any fluctuance underneath the neck flaps, aspiration of the fluid with an 18-gauge needle performed with aseptic technique is a useful means of obtaining fluid for culture and sensitivity. This is intended purely as a diagnostic and not a therapeutic approach. Both aerobic and anaerobic cultures should be taken. If there is any drainage from the suture line, once again, it should be retrieved for culture and sensitivity.

Any amount of fluid collection underneath the neck flaps needs to be drained. It is usually best not to drain this by removing some of the skin sutures or by opening a portion of the suture line that has recently had the sutures removed. The concern is that drainage through the suture line may prompt a greater separation of the suture line than what is needed and produce a wound dehiscence. I prefer to drain a wound through a separate stab incision performed under sterile conditions. Often local anesthetics are not necessary, because the previous transection of the roots of the cervical sensory plexus at the time of the original operation produces anesthesia. If it is possible to place the incision in such a fashion so that the underlying fluid will drain away from rather than over the carotid artery system, it becomes a less dangerous situation. After the wound is drained, it is irrigated with copious amounts of antibacterial solution, such as povidone-iodine. If there is any evidence of necrotic tissue within the wound, it is debrided. The wound is treated with multiple antibacterial solution irrigations, followed by packing. It is not unusual to prescribe these irrigations to occur every 2 hours while the patient is awake. Broad-spectrum antibiotic therapy is instituted at the time of the incision and drainage. Antibiotics are subsequently adjusted according to information obtained with the cultures.

The primary concern with any neck wound infection is an assessment of its potential danger to the carotid artery system. If pus is not draining over the carotid artery and the carotid artery is not exposed, the wound will usually heal uneventfully without the need for additional surgery. If the wound causes necrosis of portions of the overlying neck flaps with exposure of the carotid artery, it becomes mandatory to protect the carotid artery by transferring tissue to cover it. The intent of such a tissue transfer is to protect the carotid artery and not to close an open wound created by necrosis of the overlying neck flaps. The carotid artery can be covered with either a regional skin flap, a musculocutaneous flap, or possibly even a muscle flap.

WOUND CATHETER MANAGEMENT

Wound catheters provide the opportunity to drain fluids from the surgical area, reducing the possibility of any fluid accumulation that may separate neck flaps from the deep tissues. They provide an effective means of facilitating contact of neck flaps with the deep tissues without resorting to large circumferential and uncomfortable pressure dressings. A variety of catheter systems are available. I currently prefer to use the Blake drainage catheters, which have multiple longitudinal grooves around the circumference. They provide an effective means of draining fluid from the wound with minimal chance of the drain being blocked by a fragment of tissue or blood clot. Although many catheters are now made of a soft silicone rubber (Silastic) plastic material, they still cause pressure necrosis of the wall of the carotid artery if they are placed over the carotid artery. It is important to precisely control the position of the wound catheters. They should not course over the carotid artery, and I also prefer to place one of the drainage tubes near the suture line of a pharyngeal closure but not adjacent to the suture line. My concern is that a catheter adjacent to a pharyngeal suture line may facilitate fistula formation by drawing saliva through the suture line. The wound catheters are sutured with absorbable suture material to the deep tissues of the neck in positions that meet these criteria. It is important that the exit point of the wound catheters not be placed indiscriminately in a location that might destroy or weaken an area of skin that has a flap in the future. The neck flaps need to be sutured so that there is an airtight closure with the subcutaneous suture line. It is essential to achieve the airtight closure, because this will optimize the drainage capability of the wound catheters and will prevent the possibility of introducing bacteria via the site of an air leak along the suture line. A pursestring suture is used to tighten the skin around the catheter at its exit point. Two catheters are usually used in a standard neck dissection: one is located posterior to the carotid artery system and usually exits the inferior posterolateral neck skin, and the second is placed anterior to the carotid artery system and drains this region in addition to the submental and submandibular areas exiting either lateral to or superior to a tracheotomy site if tracheotomy has been performed.

It is imperative to monitor wound catheters closely. The primary consideration is to determine that the catheters are draining. The surgeon needs to determine that the neck flaps are flat and adherent to the underlying tissues. The catheters should be checked to assure continuing patency. If there is any question, a large-volume (50-mL) syringe should be attached to the end of the wound catheter and negative pressure applied to determine patency or to dislodge a blocked catheter. I do not advocate injecting air through the catheter to dislodge a plugged drain tube for fear of introducing infection. If negative pressure does not release an obstruction, forceful injection of a small amount of sterile saline can be used, followed by reconnecting the catheter to the negative suction. The criteria for removing the drains are based on the type of surgery in addition to the quantity and quality of fluid from the catheters. The surgeon should be able to assess at the time of surgery whether more or less than the usual wound drainage can be anticipated. This is a function of the magnitude of the surgery and the patient's overall health. For example, a neck dissection as an isolated procedure in an otherwise healthy middle-aged person would usually have considerably less wound drainage than a neck dissection performed in association with a composite resection and flap reconstruction in an elderly debilitated person. It is important to remove the drains as soon as possible to minimize the chances of infection by way of bacteria gaining access along the catheter tracts. The surgeon needs to assess not only the volume of the drainage but also the characteristics of the drainage fluid. If the drainage fluid has progressively decreased so that it is less than 30 mL in an 8-hour shift and is clear to amber, these are the quantity and character of the fluid

that indicate an uneventful postoperative course and usually represent the time when removal is appropriate. If there is an increase in the volume of the fluid or any divergence of its characteristics, the removal needs to be delayed.

If there is evidence of a wound infection noted by the catheter drainage, the catheters can be used to help manage the infection. If the infection has occurred in the absence of any pharyngeal contamination via fistula, the catheters can act as a drainage mechanism for the infected fluid. They can also be used as a means of instilling wound irrigant into the site of the infection. If there is an associated fistula, the catheters can still be used to help drain the wound, but it is best to stop the active negative pressure and to use them as a passive drainage system. This can be achieved by cutting the drains beyond the skin exit point and using them as a passive system for drainage and also wound irrigations.

I do not usually administer antibiotics as a prophylactic measure associated with wound catheter placement. Prophylactic antibiotics are based solely on whether or not the pharynx has been entered and not on wound catheters. Antibiotics are currently being used in a perioperative setting encompassed by 1 to 2 hours preoperatively and 1 day postoperatively; therefore, it is not uncommon for catheters to be present without any antibiotic therapy.

FISTULA

Orocutaneous or Pharyngocutaneous

Spontaneous Fistula

The development of a spontaneous orocutaneous or pharyngocutaneous fistula potentially can be a life-threatening complication. The bacteria within the saliva can produce an infection of the neck tissues, including the wall of the carotid artery. Progression of the infection can produce tissue necrosis with the possibility of developing an exsanguinating carotid rupture. The most important component of prophylaxis centers on meticulous technique in not only the handling of the tissues but also the closure of the pharyngeal opening. When the pharyngeal closure is being done primarily, it is imperative that the suturing technique produces approximation of the submucosa layer, which can form granulation tissue and heal. Approximation of the mucosal surfaces will produce no healing and result in a fistula. The Connell-type suture technique, which inverts the mucosal edge and approximates the submucosal tissues, is an example of an appropriate stitch that will create a watertight closure. It is important to recognize that the suture is intended to only approximate the tissues to provide the optimal environment for healing. Sutures should not be tightened so severely that it produces necrosis of the tissue contained within the suture. Such necrosis, albeit small, can produce enough of a defect to permit salivary drainage onto the neck tissues. If the pharyngeal or oropharyngeal closure involves flap insertion, I prefer to use a musculocutaneous flap that permits one-stage reconstruction. I find the pectoralis musculocutaneous flap is the most versatile and dependable. When the skin island of a musculocutaneous flap is being sutured to seal a pharyngeal defect, the suture material is 3–0 coated Vicryl placed so that it everts the mucosal edge to the skin edge. However, the suture includes a portion of the underlying subcutaneous fat and muscle of the flap. The stitches are placed at a distance that will result in complete approximation of the mucosa to the skin edges circumferentially. The surgeon should be cautioned not to place too many sutures that might cause necrosis of either the skin or the mucosa and facilitate the development of a fistula. The muscle pedicle of the flap is sutured to the underlying tissue to support it so that it does not pull on the pharyngeal closure.

In the case of primary closure of pharyngeal or oral defects, it is advisable to approximate adjacent musculature over the initial closure in a multilayered fashion. After the defect has been closed, the neck wound is irrigated with copious amounts of saline in an effort to decrease the concentration of bacteria introduced by the previously patent pharyngeal defect. As mentioned earlier, my preference is not to place the wound catheters adjacent to the pharyngeal suture line for fear of enhancing the drainage of saliva between the sutures because of the negative pressure from the catheters.

Proper management of a spontaneous fistula is a function of prompt recognition. A fistula will rarely cause any distinctive symptoms, but the clinician can usually detect the early development of a fistula by inspection of the neck flaps. They will start to become erythematous and edematous, which usually become evident between 7 and 10 days postoperatively. The patient's temperature curve will become elevated at this time, and he or she will run a low-grade fever with a temperature of 38.4°C to 38.9°C, in addition to sometimes developing a leukocytosis with a shift of the differential count. These physical findings will occur prior to the appreciation of any fluctuance created by the undermining of neck flaps by saliva draining through a separation in the pharyngeal closure. It is at this time that treatment should begin. Treatment is comprised of two components: (1) instituting intravenous antibiotics to cover the infection of the soft tissues of the neck created by the bacteria within the saliva and (2) providing drainage of the saliva in an optimal fashion. Once again, antibiotic therapy is initially directed at the broad spectrum of microbes usually involved with such an infection until more specific information is obtained from cultures taken when the wound was drained. Drainage of the wound is done even in the absence of palpable fluctuance or other appreciation of fluid accumulation. The wound is drained through a stab incision in the neck skin in a position such that the saliva is directed away from the carotid artery.

Primary intent of any fistula treatment is to protect the carotid artery system. After the skin incision is made, a Penrose drain is inserted into the wound directed toward the presumed location of the fistula. The Penrose drain is sutured into position and is used as a drainage site in addition to a means of irrigating the wound every 2 hours with an antimicrobial solution, usually povidone-iodine. The patient is maintained on nasogastric feedings with no oral feedings until the fistula is completely healed. When it is suspected that the fistula has healed, it is evaluated by having the patient drink a glass of grape juice by mouth to determine the presence of any purple liquid at the Penrose drain site.

If the fistula is wide enough that it is associated with a large amount of salivary drainage, an additional catheter is placed along the Penrose drain tract and put on continuous negative suction to facilitate management of the wound and also to prevent the large amount of saliva from undermining surrounding neck skin flaps that may already be sealed to the underlying tissues. This continuous suction is maintained until the size of the fistula decreases to the point that there is no longer a high output.

It has previously been demonstrated that patients undergoing flap reconstruction have a greater incidence of wound infection.[11] Another factor that needs to be considered is the impact of radiation therapy. In the United States, currently the popular technique of combined therapy is surgery and postoperative radiation therapy as a means of avoiding the potential for delayed wound healing that previously occurred when radiation was administered preoperatively. It has become apparent that there is an optimal time of tumor radiosensitivity postoperatively, and this interval has been determined to be 4 to 6 weeks after surgery. Meeting this time requirement can sometimes be a challenge if a fistula has developed postoperatively and is not closed by the time to start radiation therapy. Does radiation therapy cause an unhealed fistula to enlarge? Does radiation therapy permanently prevent a fistula from healing? These are just a couple of questions that currently stress the surgeon facing this clinical dilemma. However, I believe that these fistulae will eventually heal even while the patient is receiving radiation therapy. There may be a time delay, but they still seem to heal. This impression has recently been supported by review of a series of patients from the University of Florida who received radiation therapy with unhealed surgical wounds.[12] This approach has to be modified based on the surgeon's assessment of the wound. If there is exposure or near exposure of the carotid artery, additional surgery to protect the artery as described earlier in this chapter is recommended.

Controlled Fistula

A controlled fistula used to be commonly employed in conjunction with regional skin flaps when used for pharyngeal or oral reconstructions. This would require a second operation to detach the flap and completely close the defect. Such fistulae were especially useful in patients who had large tumors and were debilitated by other medical conditions, poor nutrition, or other factors. This intentional exit route for saliva theoretically increases the chances of the remaining wound healing without infection and disruption with carotid artery exposure. Controlled fistulae have become less frequently used since the advent of the musculocutaneous flaps. It is still possible to develop controlled fistulae with a musculocutaneous flap. I do not frequently employ controlled fistulae. The basis for my approach rests with continued enthusiasm for the capabilities of the musculocutaneous flaps. They appear to have such a rich blood supply that they often seem to enhance the healing capabilities of a surgically created wound even in a debilitated patient. When I do make the determination that a controlled fistula is in the best interest of the patient, I still prefer one of the regional skin flaps, especially the deltopectoral flap. The thickness and pliability of the tissue lends itself to the development of an effective salivary drainage pathway more so than the skin island of a musculocutaneous flap. It is important to reemphasize, however, that I have not routinely used controlled fistulae since the advent of the musculocutaneous flap. The only clinical situation where it is routinely used is in the case of a large pharyngeal lesion with the neck skin involvement that requires dual flaps for pharyngeal reconstruction and neck skin resurfacing. If the mediastinum has been entered or if the patient is in a poor nutritional state or otherwise debilitated, the deltopectoral flap is used for the pharyngeal reconstruction, provided a controlled fistula and a pectoralis musculocutaneous flap is simultaneously used for the neck skin resurfacing.

PAROTITIS

Parotitis used to be a common postoperative complication when it was not recognized how important it was to maintain proper hydration of the operative patient. The subsequent perioperative dehydration resulted in inspissation of the parotid salivary secretions and obstruction of the parotid duct. The stagnant saliva would become inspissated, and the parotid duct would act as a conduit for oral microflora to then infect the gland. This had the potential of being a life-threatening clinical situation. The frequency of parotitis markedly decreased with the recognition of the importance of fluid hydration. However, it has been reported that parotitis has been increasing with the emergence of certain patient populations. The immunocompromised patient following previous organ transplantation represents a person more likely to develop perioperative parotitis. Patients with other immunocompromised states, such as acquired immune deficiency syndrome, also represent another group more susceptible to parotitis than others. This has not manifested itself in a dramatic increase in my experience with this clinical condition.

The signs and symptoms of parotitis involve a painful swelling overlying one or both of the parotid glands. The pain and swelling are increased with gustatory stimulation either with smelling a fragrant odor or eating. Inspection of the parotid duct orifice reveals that it is erythematous and edematous. Compression of the involved gland will produce an inspissated purulent secretion from the orifice. Treatment of this condition involves fluid hydration in addition to intravenous antibacterial therapy. Some of the infected fluid from the parotid duct is obtained to be sent for culture and sensitivity. *Staphylococcus* is most frequently the offending organism, and antibacterial therapy should include an antistaphlococcal agent until culture results are available. If there is no clinical improvement in 2 to 3 days, the impression is that an abscess may have developed. A parotid abscess usually is not clinically detected by the appreciation of fluctuance because of the numerous septatations within the gland. Lack of clinical improvement with hydration and IV antibiotics usually results in a surgical approach to the gland via a modified Blair incision and development of the usual parotid skin flap. Numerous incisions are made through the fascia overlying the parotid gland, and the gland is then gently

probed with blunt dissection using a curved hemostat to identify and drain the abscess. There is obvious risk to the facial nerve with such an approach, and the surgeon needs to approach this matter carefully. The parotid flap is left open so that the area can be irrigated routinely with an antibacterial solution.

CONCLUSIONS

Infections following neck dissection continue to be a commonly encountered clinical situation for the otolaryngologist-head and neck surgeon. I have attempted to emphasize preventive measures, because the compulsive pursuit of these matters can certainly decrease the frequency of this complication. However, one needs to realize that the proper execution of preventive measures will not guarantee total avoidance of a wound infection. It is at this time that recognition of the clinical situation is so important in the development of an appropriately aggressive management program. The recent antibiotic trials cited earlier in this chapter have given us useful information in not only those antibiotics that are the most effective components but also in the identification of the surgical situation that is most likely to be the setting for the development of a wound infection. The combination of appropriate antimicrobial therapy in addition to local wound care usually results in prompt resolution of the infection without disastrous consequences.

REFERENCES

1. Everts EC: Surgical complications, in Cummings CW, Fredrickson JM, Harker LA, et al (eds): *Otolaryngology—Head and Neck Surgery.* St Louis, CV Mosby Co, 1986, pp 1411–1428.
2. Davidson AG, Clark C, Smith G: Postoperative wound infection: A computer analysis. *Br J Surg* 1971; 58:333–337.
3. McGuirt WF, McCabe BF, Krause CJ: Complications of radical neck dissection: A survey of 788 patients. *Head Neck Surg* 1979; 1:481–487.
4. Eschelman LT, Schleuning AJ, Brummett RE: Prophylactic antibiotics in otolaryngologic surgery: A double blind study. *Trans Am Acad Ophthalmol Otolaryngol* 1971; 75:387–394.
5. Dor P, Klastersky J: Prophylactic antibiotics in oral, pharyngeal, and laryngeal surgery for cancer (a double blind study). *Laryngoscope* 1973; 83:1992–1998.
6. Seagle MB, Duberstein LE, Gross CW, et al: Efficacy of cephazolin as a prophylactic antibiotic in head and neck surgery. *Otolaryngology* 1978; 86:568–572.
7. Becker GD, Parell GJ: Cefazolin prophylaxis in head and neck cancer surgery. *Ann Otol Rhinol Laryngol* 1979; 88:183–186.
8. Goode RL, Abramson N, Fee WE, et al: Effects of prophylactic antibiotics in radical head and neck surgery. *Laryngoscope* 1979; 89: 601–608.
9. Johnson JT, Yu VL, Myers EN, et al: Efficacy of two third-generation cephalosporins in prophylaxis for head and neck surgery. *Arch Otolaryngol* 1984; 110:224–227.

10. Johnson JT, Schuller DE, Silver F, et al: Antibiotic prophylaxis in high-risk head and neck surgery: One-day vs. five-day therapy. *Otolaryngol Head Neck Surg* 1986; 95:554–557.

11. Johnson JT, Myers EN, Thearle PB, et al: Antimicrobial prophylaxis for contaminated head and neck surgery. *Laryngoscope* 1984; 94:46–51.

12. Isaacs JH, Cassisi NJ, Thompson WB, et al: Postoperative radiation therapy of open head and neck wounds. *Laryngoscope* 1987; 97:267–270.

CHAPTER 25

Head and Neck Reconstruction

Approach of

William R. Panje, M.D.

and

Michael R. Morris, M.D.

MANDIBULAR RECONSTRUCTION

General Principles

The impact that reestablishing mandibular continuity has on cosmesis, function, and overall patient well-being underscores the necessity for head and neck surgeons to be well versed in the many reconstructive options. Although there are many methods suitable to replace the jaw, certain principles must be followed if the surgeon is to obtain a successful reconstruction.

Immediate vs. delayed jaw reconstruction following cancer ablation is always a debated issue, especially when the different disciplines of otolaryngology–head and neck surgery, general plastic surgery, maxillofacial surgery, and oral surgery approach the problem of mandible replacement. Replacing part of a missing jaw in a young trauma patient is quite different from doing the same procedure in an older cancer patient. The technique that might work in the young patient may be disastrous in the older cancer patient.

When one is dealing with oncologic resections, especially in an irradiated field or following chemotherapy, the preferred method is to wait on any reconstruction until final pathology confirms complete irradication of the cancer. Once the cancer has been irradicated, the reconstructive head and neck surgeon will select that particular technique most suitable to that particular patient based on basic principles of mandible replacement.

The basic principles of mandible reconstruction were developed primarily for nonvascularized autologous bone replacement of the jaw. Since the bone graft must undergo resorption and substitution, strict adherence to an aseptic en-vironment is mandatory. For this reason, the nonvascularized bone graft must be placed where there is no chance of contamination of the bone graft. To avoid a malunion and to reduce the chance of osteomyelitis, one must attach and stabilize the bone graft such that there is no movement during the healing phase. If there has been soft tissue excision such as following the removal of an oral cavity cancer, soft tissue must be replaced before a bone graft is used. Once adequate soft tissue has been replaced and there is complete healing of the wound, the bone graft can be placed into the jaw region. This delay avoids the intraoral graft extrusion commonly seen with primary repair. Extrusion occurs secondary to erosion produced by pressure from soft tissue placed too tight over the bone graft. Finally, the use of closed suction drainage and liberal use of prophylactic antibiotics are also very helpful in assuring a successful grafting of the jaw.

The development of vascularized bone graft techniques to restore segments of the jaw have been a great impetus to immediate reconstruction of the jaw. Since the vascularized bone graft brings its own blood supply to the area of reconstruction, the same problems are not encountered if contamination should occur. Thus, the bone graft can be used at the time that the oral cavity is open into the wound bed. Soft tissue should be replaced similarly to that required for autologous bone graft placement, but this also can be done at the time of the closure of the oral cavity since composite grafts can be moved on their own vascular supply. Vascularized bone grafts, however, need to be rigidly fixed to the recipient mandible and stabilized for at least four weeks until bone healing occurs. The use of suction drainage and antibiotics is also important to assure success.

The muscles of mastication provide a very powerful force that will cause severe distortion of the jaw following loss of mandibular continuity. Mandibular drift can be particularly aggravated when there is composite loss of oral cavity and jaw tissues without replacement. If there is loss of jaw, soft tissue, or both, there should be proper stabilization of the mandibular remnants with either rigid metal plating, biphase or intermaxillary fixation. An exception to this is when the ramus and partial body defect accompany a composite ablation. This defect is often managed with only soft tissue replacement, usually in the form of a musculocutaneous flap. Mandibular drift has not been problematic in these patients if adequate tissue bulk is used and the jaw is temporarily stabilized for 6 to 12 weeks. This is usually done with intermaxillary fixation, an internal metal splinting device, or an external Joe Hall Morris biphase. The mandibular condyle should also be removed in a composite resection. Osteoradionecrosis of a retained condyle can cause wound breakdown and concern of cancer recurrence. The articular disc is preserved in situ if possible since it can be incorporated into a reconstructive effort.

Preserving the mandibular arch with a marginal resection should always be done if oncologically feasible.[1,2] Although the inner cortex is quite resistant to tumor invasion, any question of bone involvement negates a marginal excision.

The resection of the body or anterior segment of the mandible usually requires reconstruction. This defect produces a significant cosmetic and functional deficiency to the patient. Bone is the ideal material to permanently restore the jaw. Autologous bone is the overall best bone to use. The superiority of autologous bone is because of improved survival of grafted osteocytes, more rapid vascularization, and higher potential to induce osteoneogenesis.[3,4] With the uncertainty of frozen section margins, a contaminated surgical field, and a relatively limited supply of autologus donor sites, it is rarely prudent to reconstruct an oncologic defect with primarily nonvascularized autologous bone.[5,6] If the surgeon is unable to wait for final pathology for margin confirmation, a compromise must be made. The best choice seems to be the use of a local or regional flap (if necessary) to fill any soft tissue defect and metal plating to stabilize the mandibular remnants. This will allow a well-planned, staged reconstruction with a much higher success rate and a better served patient.

Maximizing success with mandibular metal plating requires some attention to detail. A minimum of three-screw fixation is required on each fragment plated. If possible, plates are always adjusted or set before any bony resection. Titanium (Ti) or vitallium (cobalt-chromium alloy) are preferred because of their excellent tissue compatibility and suitable rigidity and because they are nonferromagnetic. Stainless steel, however, is of limited usefulness. Any drilling that is done before screw placement must be done at extremely slow speeds (25–50 rpm) with copious cold saline irrigation. The screw holes must then be tapped before placement of the screw. We have found this of paramount importance if the metal plate is to stay in for the long term.

The use of extracorporally treated autologous mandibular segments (autoclaved, irradiated, frozen) has been extensively studied, but long-term results in restoring the jaw are consist-ently disappointing.[7–12] These segments seemed best suited as templates for alternative reconstructive techniques.

Homograft mandibles have been advocated in reconstructing extensive mandibular defects.[13] The contour and size that the homograft jaw affords as a near exact replacement of the lost mandible's anatomy are probably its biggest advantage. It is not reliable enough in the irradiated compositely resected case to be used alone. To encourage homograft mandible success as well as improve osseous healing, one must complete absolute separation of the oral cavity from the jaw wound bed usually with a soft tissue flap such as musculocutaneous flap. Likewise, if the patient has been irradiated or the surgeon believes the wound bed is incapacitated, the patient should probably have at least 10 to 15 courses of hyperbaric oxygen prior to the implantation of the homograft jaw. Autologous bone (both cancellous and cortical) should be incorporated into the homograft in the form of plating or plugs. The homograft mandible therefore serves as a tray for the autologous bone just as a Dacron or Ti mesh tray would. An alternative method is to implant the homograft into the lower abdominal wall in close proximity to the epigastric vessels. If autologous marrow is implanted into the homograft jaw, osteoneogenesis can often be demonstrated by bone scan several weeks later, at which time the graft can be removed as a compound microvascularized free flap based on the epigastric vessels and transplanted to the jaw area. This, of course, is a quite complicated and sophisticated way of approaching jaw reconstruction and would be indicated in only highly selected cases.

Autologous free grafts of bone are frequently successful when used in mandibular reconstruction.[14–18] The two preferred sites for harvesting bone include the anterior-middle iliac crest and the calvarium. Both cortical and cancellous bone can be easily harvested from the ilium with a minimum of morbidity. A metal or reinforced fabricated tray such as Dacron is then used as a template, allowing the donor bone to fill the defect. The calvarium also provides an excellent source of bone[19,20] for replacing limited mandibular defects (6–8 cm). No tray is necessary when a calvarial bone graft is used. A full-thickness graft of calvarium can be taken with attached pericranium harvested from the parietal region with essentially no patient morbidity. The segment is quite sturdy and excellently suited for mandibular body reconstruction. Rib has been advocated by some authors as an autologous source,[21] but it is definitely inferior to iliac or calvarial bone.

Several of the commonly used musculocutaneous flaps have been combined with a bony element as a means of mandibular reconstruction. These composite flaps offer the potential for immediate reconstruction of jaw defects with vascularized soft and hard tissues. The sternocleidomastoid-clavicle,[22–24] pectoral-rib,[25–27] and latissimus dorsi–rib/myo-osseous flaps are mentioned only to indicate that these areas of the body can act as donor tissues for jaw reconstruction. Because of their variability for successful bone replacement of the jaw and potential for significant patient morbidity, we have favored other body sites for obtaining vascularized tissues for restoring composite oral cavity tissue losses.

The temporal myo-osseous flap has been used with success[17];

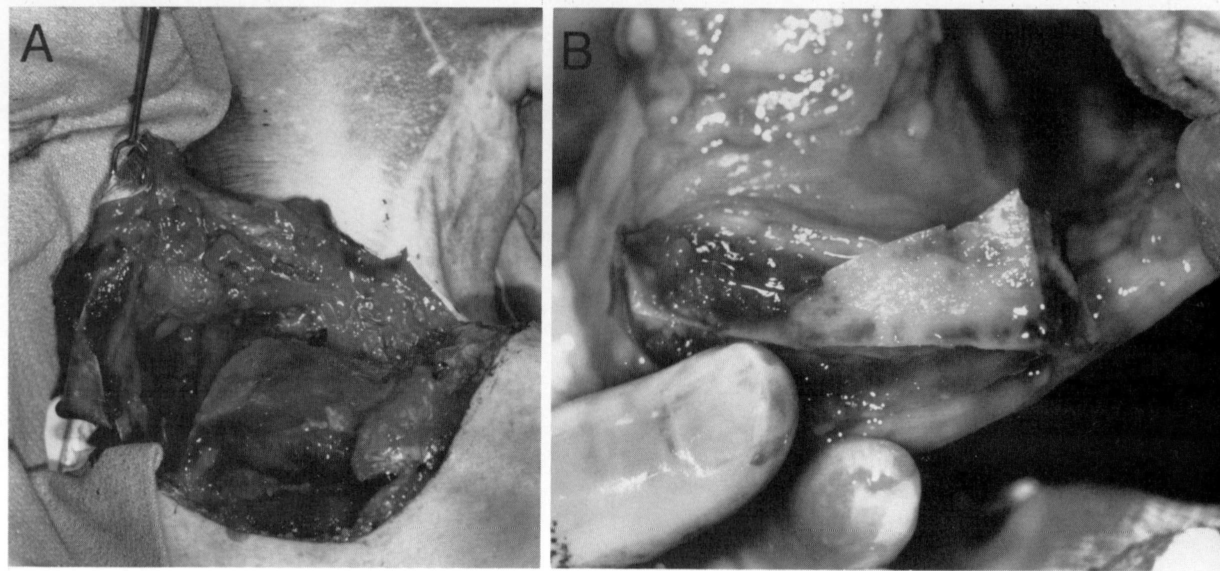

FIG 25–1.
A, trapezius osteomusculocutaneous flap being dissected. **B,** closeup of scapular spine available for mandibular reconstruction.

however, its application is quite limited. A portion of parietal bone is elevated in continuity with the anterior segment of the temporal muscle and overlying pericranium and can be tunneled through the infratemporal fossa for reconstruction of small lateral jaw defects. This compound vascularized flap is probably more versatile and easier to place when used as a free myo-osseous flap. In any case, this flap will certainly provide the operator with a major technical challenge.

The latissimus dorsi–iliac flap has been used with limited success.[28–30] The poor vascularity provided to the ilium by the latissimus dorsi myofacial attachment makes the bone behave like a free autograft. This should be understood and planned for by the reconstructing surgeon.

The trapezius osteomusculocutaneous flap has been demonstrated to be a superior regional compound flap for mandibular reconstruction (Fig 25–1).[31–34] The more dominant role of the periosteal blood supply to the scapular spine[35] (as with all flat bones) enhances this flap's survival and subsequent incorporation into the mandible. The drawbacks of using this flap are its relatively limited supply of bone and potential for patient morbidity. The acromion must be preserved to allow appropriate function of the shoulder girdle.[31, 32] This permits transfer of only the posteromedial scapular spine. In the adult male, this segment measures about 12 by 2.5 cm, obviously limiting the amount of mandible that can be replaced. An additional 1 to 2 cm of bone can sometimes be obtained by bivalving the spine attachment over the acromion; however, this is useful for only a better overlap of the mandibular remnants at reconstruction.[32] This flap should generally be avoided if the accessory nerve must be sacrificed solely for its use. It should be understood that trapezius function can at times be preserved despite the use of this flap.

The advent and application of free osseous flaps for mandibular reconstruction have added a new dimension for con-

sideration in jaw replacement. By providing vascularized bone, they share many of the advantages of regional compound flaps. Like other jaw reconstruction techniques, this highly sophisticated method of transplanting vascularized bone has many potential drawbacks. The free osseous compound flap operation for jaw reconstruction generally takes more than 8 to 16 hours and will invariably require subsequent revision operations for optimum function and cosmetic improvement. The microvascular expertise required is magnified by the consistent need for interposition vein grafting to achieve satisfactory and successful placement of the jaw. These demands translate into a delayed reconstruction or use of multiple surgical specialty teams in managing the head and neck cancer patient. We tend to favor delaying jaw reconstruction to avoid the excessive operating time needed for simultaneous ablation and reconstruction with free flaps. The two preferred sites for free osseous flaps of bone include the iliac crest and the scapula.[36–41] Free rib flaps have been described but are not recommended because of patient morbidity and reconstructive inferiority of rib.[42, 43] Metatarsal osteocutaneous flaps have been used with success[37]; however, they are technically difficult to perform and have reportedly carried a significant donor site morbidity.

The free compound groin flap employs anterior iliac crest with overlying skin and represents an extension of the versatile free groin flap. The free flap is pedicled on either the superficial circumflex iliac, the lateral femoral circumflex, the deep iliac, or the epigastric vessels.[36, 44] Appropriate recipient vessels are located and prepared in the neck, and the mandibular defect is adequately exposed. The flap is then freed and transferred. Fixation to the mandibular remnants precedes any anastomotic effort. The tubercle on the anterolateral ilium seems to form a natural chin,[45] so an attempt is made to use it as such. Immobilization has been problematic, but the placement of Steinmann pins and basket wiring seems to provide an easy and reliable method.[37] The surgeon must be cautioned about using mandibular plating since vascular pedicle compromise can occur.

The scapula has also been used as a source for a free bone flap.[38–41] Like the compound groin flap, it provides excellent vessel diameter for anastamosis and relatively limited patient morbidity. The donor site is hidden and is usually in a non-hair-bearing area. The circumflex scapular artery is the main blood supply and with careful dissection can provide a pedicled length of up to 10 cm.[46] Patient positioning is sometimes cumbersome, requiring a semilateral decubitus position with the arm abducted and prepped free. The lateral border of the scapula provides bone enough to reconstruct defects up about 10 to 14 cm.[38–41] The need for adequate recipient vessels and the problems with bone stabilization are similar to those encountered with the free compound groin flap, but donor morbidity is significantly less.[41] The skin portion of the flap has a separate pedicle, allowing relatively independent positioning compared with the groin flap.[38–41]

Specific Situations

The reconstruction of the various mandibular defects following cancer ablation requires the surgeon to understand the many principles and techniques previously discussed to best serve the patient. Rebuilding the anterior mandibular arch is probably the most difficult task confronting the head and neck reconstructive surgeon. The loss of this segment produces a most significant cosmetic and oral functional loss of patients and therefore requires reconstitution. The use of any nonvascularized bone for reconstruction requires excellent graft bed vascularity, stable immobilization, and an aseptic environment for success.[32] If compound regional or free flaps and only vascularized bone are used, stable immobilization is essential for success. These vascularized flaps can tolerate limited oral contamination without undergoing necrosis[32, 36] and gain strength (stress and strain characteristics) at a substantially greater rate than nonvascularized tissue.[47, 48] Vascularized bone also permits dental prosthetic restoration since it tolerates weight bearing similar to the mandible it replaced.[49, 50] This tissue is thus preferred if the patient's particularities allow its use.

The adult mandible measures about 17 cm from posterior edge of angle to angle, so options for reconstruction of the anterior arch are dependent on the amount and type of the defect present. If a patient has a denervated trapezius from previous therapy, the trapezius osseomusculocutaneous flap provides up to 10 cm of bone ideal for recontouring the anterior arch.[32] Transcutaneous wires and biphase stabilization are usually adequate for preventing migration of the bone. With gaps of more than 10 cm or in a patient without a denervated trapezius, other considerations are necessary. Free flaps can be used if the surgeon has the requisite technical expertise and the patient is an appropriate candidate. This would provide vascularized bone with all the inherent advantages already discussed. Alternatively, an autologous graft can be employed. However, because of its lack of vascularity, the graft can be used only when oral contamination is not present and sufficient soft tissue has been used to repair the cancer-ablated site. In this situation, a tray (e.g., Ti, Dacron mesh, or homograph mandible) is preferred as the template and the iliac crest as the donor bone. Cancellous-cortical bone should be densely packed into the tray. The tray acts as a template while providing rigid internal fixation of the mandibular remnants.

Mandibular body defects are somewhat easier to manage than anterior segmental defects. Rigid metal mandibular plates used to stabilize a lateral jaw defect often provide long-term adequate form and function for patients. The trapezius scapular spine flap again provides an excellent option for reconstruction with vascularized bone. The temporal myo-osseous flap is a more technically difficult alternative for small (6–8 cm) defects.[19] Free flaps offer the same advantages but suffer the same drawbacks previously discussed. If nonvascularized autologous grafts are used, the full-thickness calvarial flap with attached periosteum is preferred. Internal plate fixation with Ti miniplates provides a reliable and sturdy reconstruction. Using the miniplate system, although not as rigid as the larger metal plates, is preferred because it may be left in situ permanently. Iliac crest bone with Ti mesh template or internal metal plating is a second choice.

Larger near-total or total defects require very deliberate planning and technical competence to obtain workable results. The use of homograft mandible is warranted in this situation if regional and free composite flaps cannot provide enough bone to span the defect. The homograft bone is used as a tray augmented with an autologous bone usually taken from the iliac crest. It can also be implanted in the abdominal wall in proximity to the epigastric vessels and later harvested as a free flap. The patient must understand that the requisite time needed for osteoneogenesis to occur prolongs the reconstructive effort. Placement of the homograft mandible in situ is always done as a staged procedure when the surgeon is assured that adequate soft tissue replacement of oral cavity is present and that there is no communication between the oral cavity and the mandibular bed. Internal metal plating with a full metal jaw and condyle and a musculocutaneous flap has also been used with good success. Although the patient demonstrates excellent contouring in the lower half of the face, the mandible cannot tolerate weight bearing of a denture or chewing of solid foods.

Osteoradionecrosis of the mandible following aggressive radiation therapy is often the cause for acquired mandibular defects. This is mentioned only to stress the need for early diagnosis and aggressive treatment of this condition. The use of hyperbaric oxygen therapy, prolonged antibiotics, and judicial operative debridement are essential. The omentum has been used with great success as a free flap to salvage remaining viable mandible.[51] Following debridement, the omentum is transplanted into the neck and circumferentially wrapped around the remaining bone. Often the mandibular arch can be preserved, making subsequent reconstruction much simpler. Musculocutaneous flaps have been used for mandibular salvage in osteoradionecrosis as well.

Dental prosthetic rehabilitation following mandibular reconstruction is often considered important only by the patient. Experience with osseointegrated implants is rapidly expanding and warrants consideration in replacing dentition in the reconstructed jaw.[49, 50] Placement of the implants is always done in a delayed setting after demonstration of bone integration. Penetration of the implants through a mucosal surface is preferred to avoid the chronic drainage and infection often encountered with transcutaneous implantation within the mouth. This technology has in a few cases dramatically improved prosthetic rehabilitation.

MUSCULOCUTANEOUS FLAPS

The vast array of reconstructive options available to the head and neck surgeon today contrasts sharply with that of 20 years ago. The advent of the musculocutaneous flap added significantly to the reconstructive potential available in managing head and neck defects. Basic principles of surgery dictate that the prudent surgeon employ the optimal method for reconstruction based on the patient's occupation, cosmetic concerns, general expectations, and health. This is coupled with the physical qualities of the defect and the nature of the disease process to formulate the best operative plan. Reconstruction is, thus, not a question of whether to use a free flap, a musculocutaneous flap, or a skin graft but of selecting the simplest and best method to achieve a desired result in a particular patient.[52]

Greater Pectoral Flap

The greater pectoral, or pectoralis major, musculocutaneous (PM) flap is certainly the workhorse and probably represents the most familiar flap to present-day reconstructive surgeons. The anatomy is well described and must be understood to properly complete PM flap reconstruction.[53-55]

The PM muscle has primarily two portions. The anterior or clavicular lamina originates from the manubrium and clavicle and acts to draw the humerus forward and medially. The posterior or sternal lamina arises from the sternum, sixth and seventh ribs, and adjacent costal cartilages and is a humeral adductor. An abdominal part arising from the external oblique aponeurosis has also been described and blends with the sternal portion. The two heads of the PM join at their humeral insertion to form the rounded anterior axillary fold. Medial to this insertion, the two laminae can easily be separated. It is through this gap that the thoracoacromial artery (TA) consistently pierces the clavipectoral fascia medial to the tendon of the smaller pectoral, or pectoralis minor (PMn), muscle.[53, 55]

The TA arises from the second part of the axillary artery under the superior edge of the PMn muscle. Once it enters the clavipectoral fascia, it divides into several branches. The pectoral branch is the dominant blood supply to the PM flap. The lateral thoracic artery (LTA) also arises off of the axillary artery along the lateral border of the PMn muscle to supply the PM flap. The LTA also forms the major lateral blood supply to the female breast.[53] A minor contribution to the PM flap from the superior thoracic artery has also been described. In about one third of patients, a major cutaneous axial vessel running from a lateral cephalad to caudal direction arises from either the TA or the LTA. Once the TA and LTA pierce the clavipectoral fascia, they do not give off any branches to the PMn muscle, providing an

excellent and bloodless plane of dissection between the two pectoral muscles.[53-55]

Technique

The technique employed in creating the PM flap depends on the physical qualities desired in the reconstructive plan. The obvious limitations of the flap include excessive thickness or bulkiness, breast distortion, and the presence of hair-bearing tissue in the oral cavity.[56]

If an island type of musculocutaneous flap is desired, its dimensions are carefully diagrammed on the patient's chest wall. By extending the cutaneous portion of the flap outside of the underlying PM muscle, one can obtain additional tissue (Fig 25–2). This skin is randomly supplied and thus not as dependable as that overlying the muscle; however, the thin pliable sternal skin is quite useful in hypopharyngeal and esophageal reconstruction.[57, 58] Random skin overlying the xyphoid and rectus abdominis is sometimes needed to reach the nasopharynx or tongue.[59] The cutaneous portion of the flap is circumferentially incised down to the pectoral fascia with care to bevel the cuts outward from the skin edge. This increases the amount of subcutaneous tissue relative to the skin, hopefully providing more perforators for improved perfusion.[57] Tacking stitches are placed to avoid shearing the skin and subcutaneous tissue from the muscle. The incision is continued from the island superiorly and laterally to join the lateral margin of a deltopectoral skin flap (DP flap). This preserves the option of a DP flap if it is ever needed. The lateral margin of the PM muscle is located, and the avascular plane separating it from the PMn muscle is bluntly developed. This usually allows palpation or even visualization of the vascular supply. The inferior and medial margin of the flap is then quickly developed with care to incise the PM muscle lateral to the takeoff of the internal mammary perforators so as to maintain perfusion to the DP skin. By mobilizing the musculocutaneous flap inferiorly and medially, one can create enough arc to rotate it into the neck. The physical qualities of the defect then dictate the surgeon's next step.

Lifted Flaps That Will Not Reach

Several options to increase the arc of rotation of the PM flap are available. The first step generally is to detach the sternal portion of the PM muscle from its humeral insertion lateral to the TA pedicle.[54, 55] This usually necessitates ligating the LTA but allows isolation of the TA pedicle deep to the clavicular portion of the PM muscle. The pedicle can then be tunneled deep to or turned over the remaining clavicular portion, adding 4 to 5 cm of rotation of the arc.[55] Some clavicular fibers are preserved, if at all possible, to lessen the donor morbidity to the patient.[60]

If the flap still does not reach the recipient site, it can be brought close to the vascular pedicle by positioning the patient's head toward the donor site. Two large sutures are placed from chin to shoulder or chest wall to act as a splint to reinforce the patient position. These sutures should exhibit no tension after proper positioning.[32]

Occasionally a pedicle is externalized to increase its arc (Fig 25–3).[52] Great care is needed postoperatively to avoid des-

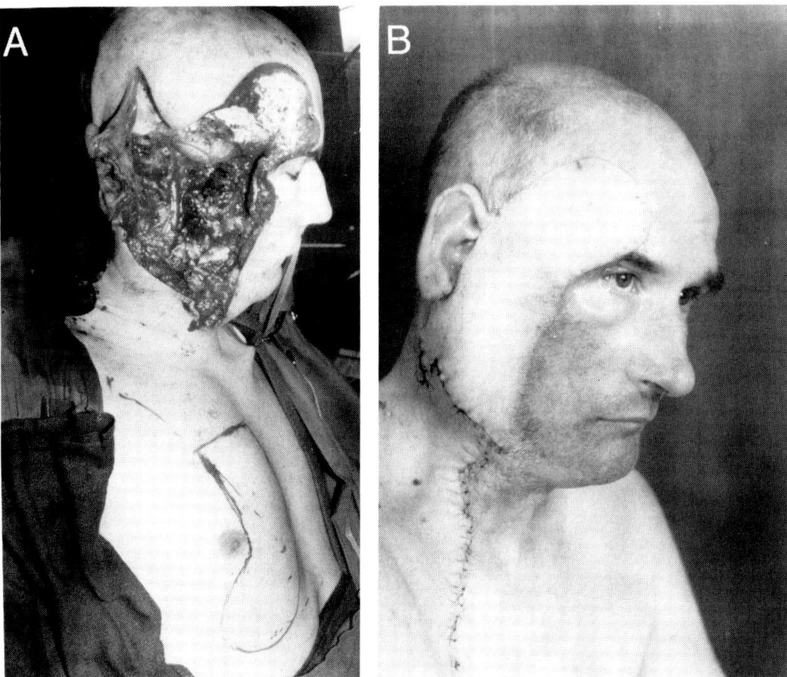

FIG 25–2.
A, random abdominal skin included with greater pectoral flap to increase arc of utilization. **B,** extended greater pectoral flap in place.

sication and pedicle injury. This is accomplished by leaving muscle, fat, and fascia attached to the pedicle (i.e., not skeletonizing) and wrapping the exposed portions with bacitracin-soaked, Adaptic gauze. Bacitracin is used liberally and frequently (six times daily) for the first week postoperatively. The flap is allowed to heal in place for 2 to 3 weeks, at which time flap training is initiated. Occlusive clamping is started for 10 minutes four times daily. The cutaneous portion of the flap is carefully watched during initial clamping to ensure capillary refill changes from a proximal to distal flow. If the flap becomes blue or pale with occlusion, clamping is discontinued and postponed for 1 to 2 days. Once the flap tolerates the 10-minute ischemic period four times daily, the clamp time is progressively increased. The pedicle can be safely divided once 8 to 10 hours/day of ischemic time is well tolerated.[61]

The last option for increasing arc of the rotation for a PM flap is to detach its TA pedicle and create a free flap. This obviously entails microvascular expertise, and the donor site morbidity must be weighed heavily with the many other free flaps available to the reconstructive surgeon.

Separating the clavicle has not been found to be of any benefit to increase the arc of rotation of a PM flap. It does cause significant patient morbidity and thus is not recommended.

Finally, any nerve within the pedicle should be separated to avoid its inadvertent constriction of the vascular pedicle following flap rotation.[56]

Intraoperative Injury to the Vascular Pedicle

Pedicle injury can be either reversible or irreversible. Vascular spasm occasionally occurs, causing concern for flap via-

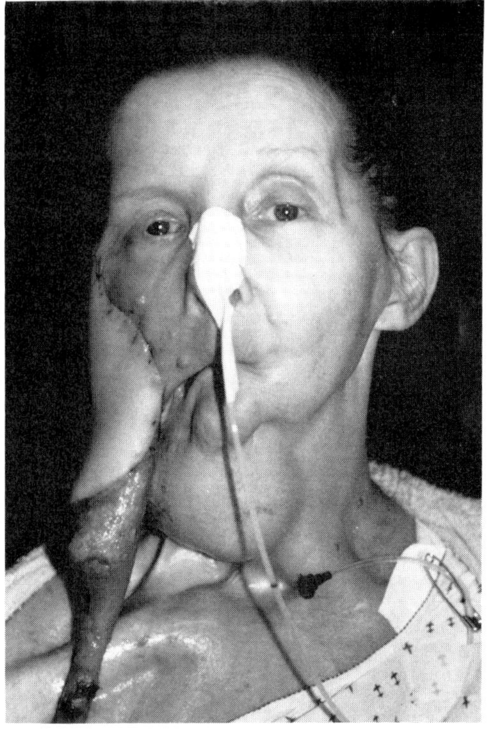

FIG 25–3.
Example of externalization of flap pedicle to increase axis of utilization.

bility. This spasm generally subsides following 10 to 20 minutes of not handling the flap.

Injury to the artery or vein generally negates use of the musculocutaneous flap for reconstructive purposes. An arterial injury may be reanastamosed if feasible; however, it would be preferred to separate the whole pedicle and use it as a free flap. Once again, the patient morbidity must be considered. With obvious injury to the vascular pedicle, the flap is never replaced in its original position as a composite graft. The pedicled muscle is removed, and what PM muscle is left on the chest wall is loosely reapproximated. The skin from the PM flap can be used as a split-thickness skin graft (STSG) to cover the donor defect, or the defect may be closed primarily.

Epidermolysis

Skin loss does not always equate with flap failure. The musculocutaneous skin component of the flap can be tested by simply pricking it with an 18-gauge needle. Alternatively, 10% fluorescein dye (5 mL/50 kg) can be injected intravenously and the skin examined with Wood's lamp.[62] Fluorescence should be seen about 20 minutes after injection. This test is limited by equipment in that unless a microfluorometer is used, it can be performed only at 12- to 24-hour intervals. If no blood flow to the skin is demonstrated, the subcutaneous tissue and skin are debrided promptly. If left untreated, this tissue will become infected and contribute to necrosis of the underlying muscle. Bleeding will be obvious in the denuded muscle if adequate flap perfusion is present. If an external surface is involved, a STSG is applied. Often the excised skin suffices as the STSG. An internal surface is generally left to granulate.

Trapezius Flap

An understanding of the unique advantages of the trapezius musculocutaneous flap over the PM flap allows the reconstructive surgeon to more appropriately manage a defect.[63–66] The relative lack of subcutaneous tissue overlying the trapezius muscle reduces the bulk of the flap. Also, if random skin from the deltoral region is included, a significant amount of pliable, unirradiated, and very reliable tissue is available. This skin is cosmetically superior for resurfacing face and neck defects (Fig 25–4) and can be easily tubed for hypopharyngeal or esophageal reconstruction.[64, 65] The reliability of including the scapular spine as an osseomusculocutaneous flap adds to its reconstructive potential. These advantages must be weighed against the consequence of losing trapezius function, a deformity well known to head and neck surgeons. Once again, the anatomy of the area is paramount to understanding the many options available.

The trapezius muscle has its origin at the occipital bone, ligamentum nuchae, and spinal processes of C1-T12. It is broad, triangular, and flat, inserting into the posterior border of the scapular spine.[63, 66] The function of the muscle can be understood by analyzing the deformity secondary to denervation. First there is absence of the tonic elevation of the shoulder girdle with loss of superior adduction of the scapula. The initial upward rotation of the scapula with arm raising is also lost.[65]

The vascular anatomy of the trapezius muscle, unfortu-nately, is not as consistent as that of the PM muscle. There are four significant sources of blood supply to the trapezius muscle, which actually contains three distinct musculocutaneous segments.[65] The transverse cervical artery (TCA), dorsal scapular artery (DSA), occipital artery (OA), and perforating branches of the posterior intercostal arteries—paraspinous perforators (PPs)—have varying importance depending on whether a superior, lateral, or extended flap is used. The TCA originates medially from the area of the thyrocervical trunk about 80% of the time. With this medial origin, it consistently passes anterior to the scalene muscles and brachial plexus.[65, 67] The TCA origi-nates from the subclavian artery or dorsal scapular artery about 20% of the time and subsequently travels through or under the cords of the brachial plexus before turning laterally to the undersurface of the trapezius. It then divides into a superficial and deep branch, the superficial branch being the key musculo-cutaneous supply to the lateral trapezius.[63, 66] This superficial branch divides into an ascending branch that anastamoses with the PP and OA and a descending branch that passes along the undersurface of the trapezius between the medial border of the scapula and the spinous processes. This artery supplies the extended trapezius flap the majority of the time, but occasionally it will taper quickly, making the DSA the major supply to the lower trapezius fibers.[65]

The DSA arises from the subclavian artery and passes under the brachial plexus and medial edge of the scapula. The artery than may pass between the levator and lesser rhomboid or

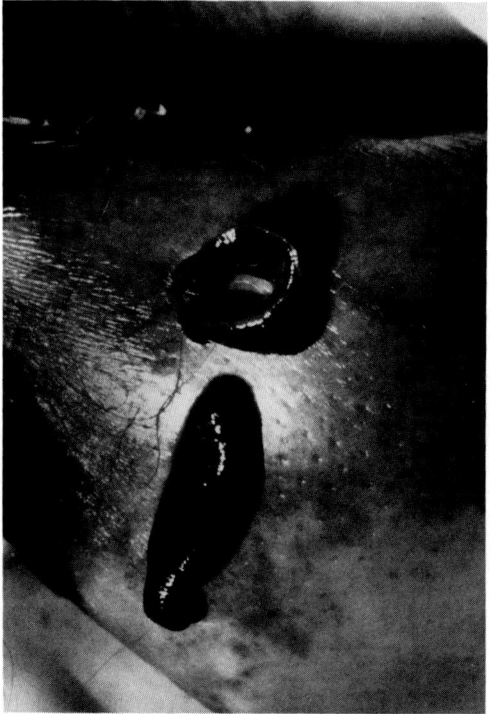

FIG 25–4.
Example of venous congestion of flap being managed with leeches.

inferior to the lesser rhomboid before entering the trapezius.[65]

The PP and OA are not identified during flap elevation, so their anatomy will be omitted. They supply the superior musculocutaneous segment of the trapezius.

The venous anatomy, as always, is quite variable.[67] The transverse cervical vein (TCV) must be present if one is contemplating a lateral or extended trapezius flap. It usually leaves the deep surface of the trapezius and travels adjacent to the TCA for a variable distance. About 75% of the time it will pass deep to and 25% of the time proximal to the omohyoid muscle. It occasionally joins the external jugular vein prior to its insertion into the subclavian vein.[67]

Technique

When one is contemplating use of a trapezius flap, an important consideration is whether the muscle is denervated or if denervation will be required to obtain the desired arc of rotation. It is not recommended to denervate the trapezius muscle for the sake of reconstructing a defect since alternative methods with far less morbidity to the patient are available. Previous oncologic surgery to the neck will often leave questions as to the integrity of the TCA and TCV pedicle. To ascertain whether these vessels are intact requires a neck exploration.[65] Neck incision for a superior or lateral flap must include a vertical limb along the anterior border of the trapezius muscle when it is done in conjunction with a neck dissection. This represents the anterior aspect of the cutaneous portion of the flap.

Superior Trapezius Flap.—This extremely reliable flap can be used regardless of previous neck surgery because its integrity is not adversely affected by separation of either the TCA or OA.[65, 68] In fact, the vascular supply of the PP is more than likely enhanced by previous occlusion of the other vessels. A Mayfield head holder is used to allow easy access to the shoulder and back of the neck as well as patient positioning. The anterior incision is placed along the anterior border of the trapezius muscle. The posterior limb runs inferior and parallel across the back, creating a width of up to 10 cm. At least four PPs should be included in the base of the flap.[65] This obviously makes for a bulky base with a limited arc of rotation, although the ipsilateral neck, lower one third of the face, oropharynx, and floor of mouth can be easily reached. The muscle is separated from its scapular attachments, and the TCA and ascending branch of DSA are ligated unless the needed arc is not hindered by their attachment. This flap is easily and quickly executed and provides excellent coverage for cutaneous defects. The distal skin can be used as an island as well as for internal reconstruction.[65, 68] The donor defect is usually covered with an STSG.

Lateral Trapezius Flap.—The skin paddle is generally centered over the acromion, which should be marked with the patient in an upright position. Up to 40% of the skin can be random, supple deltoid skin.[65] The initial exploration and dissection of the TCA and TCV precede any attempts at flap elevation. The external jugular vein is traced inferiorly, carefully dissecting any posterior or lateral branches. The TCV must be clearly visualized, because its length and axis (i.e., where it joins

the subclavian vein) dictate the arc of utilization of the skin-muscle island. Once the integrity of the TCA and TCV is assured, the distal cutaneous part of the flap is elevated off the deltoid fascia to the scapular spine. Blunt finger dissection at the anterior border of the trapezius muscle deep to the vascular pedicle allows appropriate undermining. The remaining cutaneous portion of the flap is incised down to the trapezius fascia with care to bevel outward as described with the PM flap. Tacking sutures are placed, the muscle is incised, and the flap elevated in a lateral to medial direction.[63–66] The ascending branch of the DSA will be encountered and should be divided as low as possible, providing an option of reanastomosing the artery to the carotid system and improving flap perfusion.[65] The spinal accessory nerve does not need to be divided to use this flap. Because of the supple deltoid skin and good arc of rotation, this flap has use in resurfacing large oral cavity defects and in circumferential pharyngeal reconstruction. The donor site is closed primarily or with an STSG.

Extended Trapezius Flap.—The extended trapezius flap is useful in resurfacing large defects of the face and head in a patient not suited for free flap reconstruction.[65, 69] The patient must be placed in a lateral decubitus or prone position with the upper extremity internally rotated and abducted. This displaces the scapula laterally and provides the space to place the cutaneous paddle between the vertebral column and scapula. The inferior extent of the paddle can be up to 15 cm below the scapular tip if needed.[65, 69] The inferior part of the flap is then incised down to the latissimus laterally and the trapezius medially. The random skin is elevated until the inferior border of the trapezius muscle is encountered. This permits adjustment of the cutaneous paddle to ensure enough skin overlies the trapezius. The upper border of the cutaneous paddle is connected to the neck via a skin incision. The TCA is followed under the trapezius and the descending branch identified. The lower fibers of the muscle are divided around the vascular pedicle, preserving a minimum of 2 cm of muscle on either side. If a prominent DSA supply is present for the inferior trapezius, it must be located under the lesser rhomboid muscle.[65] This situation obviously curtails the flap's arc of rotation; however, the lesser rhomboid may be split on either side of the pedicle to allow some added freedom of rotation.

Once the flap is elevated up to the bifurcation of the TCA, it is rotated over or under the remaining trapezius fibers into the surgical defect. This keeps a functional portion of the trapezius muscle and decreases patient morbidity. The donor site can usually be closed primarily.[65, 69]

Lifted Flap That Will Not Reach

As with the PM flap, positioning the patient to bring the surgical defect closer to the vascular pedicle is a useful first step if flap length is not adequate. Two large sutures are placed from the patient's chin to chest or shoulder to help maintain positioning; however, any tension on the flap requires revision or an alternate plan.[62]

With the superior flap, the inferior incision should cross the posterior midline before turning superiorly to allow added rotation and assure PP perfusion from the ipsilateral side. The random skin portion of the flap can be designed to include up to 10 cm of deltoid skin with good reliability.[65]

Mobilization and anatomy of the TCV generally mandate the arc of rotation of the lateral flap. This vessel can be mobilized down to its (or the external jugular's) insertion into the subclavian vein for added length.[67] Random deltoid skin can be used to increase flap length as well. Up to 40% of the skin paddle can be random with reliable results. The pedicle can be externalized as described for the PM flap.[61] Since this is always a possibility, it is prudent not to skeletonize the vascular pedicle when initially locating it. The same precautions to avoid pedicle dessication and the same scheme for flap training as described for the PM flap are followed.

The extended trapezius flap rarely has a problem with arc of rotation unless a DSA dominant circulation is encountered. The upper trapezius fibers can be split, allowing complete rotation of the vascular pedicle, or it may be converted to a free flap.[65] The vascular pedicle can be externalized as well.

Intraoperative Injury to the Vascular Pedicle

The lateral and extended trapezius flaps must have an intact TCA and TCV pedicle to be used reliably. If no TCV is found on the initial exploration, these flaps cannot be used.[63–67] Injury to these vessels during elevation negates using the tissue as a pedicled myocutaneous flap. With an extended flap, the best alternative would be to convert the tissue to a free flap. Converting a planned lateral flap to a superior flap is always a possibility since the TC pedicle carries no importance to the survivability of the superior flap.[65, 68]

Flap Necrosis

The PM and trapezius myocutaneous flaps are extremely reliable, approaching 90% to 95% success rates.[52] Impending flap necrosis should alert the surgeon that a technical problem is at fault. The operation needs to be honestly evaluated and the patient carefully scrutinized for possible causes of failure. Hematoma, patient positioning, pedicle kinking, or obstruction with circumferential dressings or ties are just a few of the reversible problems encountered. With free flaps, vessel anastomatic failure is always possible. Doppler evaluation is of limited value and should not be exclusively relied on. The flap's capillary refill, temperature, turgor, and color are carefully assessed, and if any suspicion of failure is present, more invasive testing is appropriate. An 18-gauge needle is used to prick the skin, or 10% fluorescein dye is given intraveneously, with either skin bleeding or fluorescence subsequently checked. Cutaneous flaps can survive approximately 8 hours of ischemia before irreversible necrosis occurs.[62] Musculocutaneous flaps, with the higher metabolic requirements of skeletal muscle, can survive only about 4 hours, so immediate postoperative monitoring is critical.[62] The multiple transfers of the patient from operating table to gurney to intensive care unit bed must be supervised to avoid inappropriate tension of the flap's pedicle.

Understanding why flaps fail necessitates a look at fluid mechanics. Poiseville's equation for flow through a rigid cylinder is a useful approximation of blood flow through a musculocutaneous artery.[62] The most critical factor affecting flow is the radius of the vessel since it exponentially affects resistance. Kinking, twisting, or stretching the pedicle would decrease the lumen of the nourishing artery and detrimentally effect flow. Another factor affecting flow is pressure difference between the inflow and outflow of the vessel. The greater the difference, the greater the flow. This probably correlates with increased venous outflow obstruction being detrimental to flap survival (i.e., perfusion). If a flap has a bluish discoloration, the arterial input is exceeding the venous outflow (Fig 25–5).[62] Once again, tension or constriction on the pedicle will adversely affect venous outflow. Hematoma is a common cause of increased pressure, and prevention mandates liberal use of drains whenever pedicled flaps are used. The last significant factor affecting flow is fluid viscosity. Keeping the hemoglobin level in the range of 9 to 10 mg/dL yields better flap survival than if it is increased to 16 to 18 mg/dL. This difference has been proved to significantly affect flap survival in animals.[70]

A theoretical increase in flow resistance involves the elasticity of the donor skin. Once a cutaneous pedicle is incised, the natural elasticity of skin causes shrinkage. This shrinkage inadvertently kinks and impedes the subdermal plexus flow.[71] This increased microcirculatory resistance to flow may explain skin loss with the muscle remaining viable in musculocutaneous flaps. It can be avoided by not using more skin in the reconstruction than was removed during the resection.

Flap failure is not caused by physiologic factors, so the use of such agents as dextran or heparin are best avoided. With appropriate attention to detail, flap necrosis should be quite rare using the techniques herein described.[62]

FREE FLAPS IN THE HEAD AND NECK

With the advent of free flap reconstruction, physiologically similar tissue is available to replace whatever head and neck defect is encountered. Many of the extremely difficult reconstructive problems with musculocutaneous flaps are easily solved with free flaps (Fig 25–6). They provide a 70% to 85% success rate in the head and neck and allow one-stage reconstruction, good wound healing, unirradiated donor tissue, and minimal donor site morbidity.[52] Because of the added operative time, need for microvascular expertise, and additional incisions, free flaps are generally reserved for special indications. A clear understanding of all the available reconstructive options is essential to best rehabilitate a patient's particular problem.

The patient is the first consideration for employing a free flap. Anyone with good vitality is a candidate. This applies to people less than 70 years old with good physical status who are occupationally or socially active. Further limitations on usage would be select cases where function or normality of appearance are better than what is obtainable with regional flap reconstruction.

Free flaps add to the reconstructive potential of head and neck surgeons. The question is not one of using free flap vs. musculocutaneous flap or skin graft but of selecting the simplest

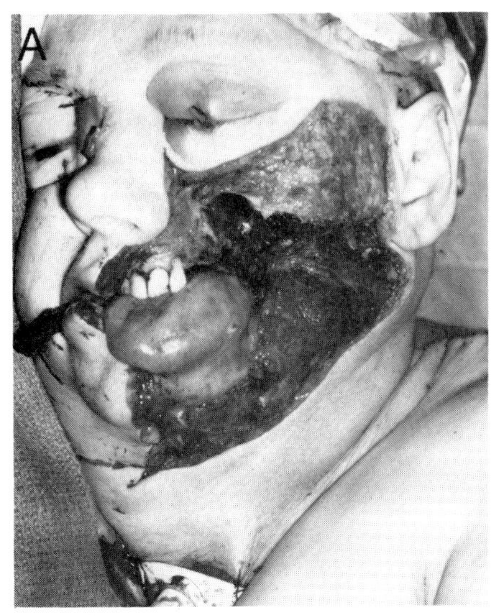
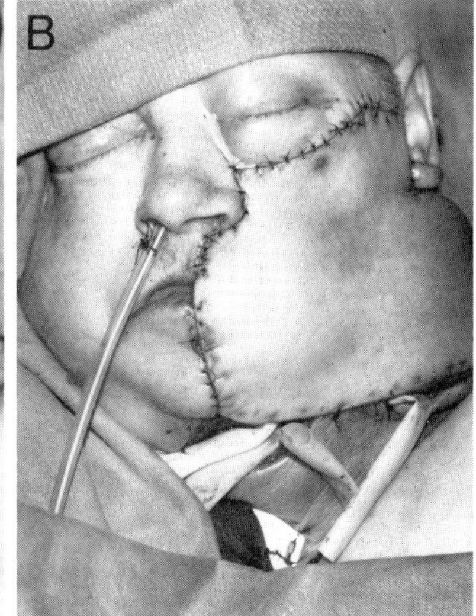
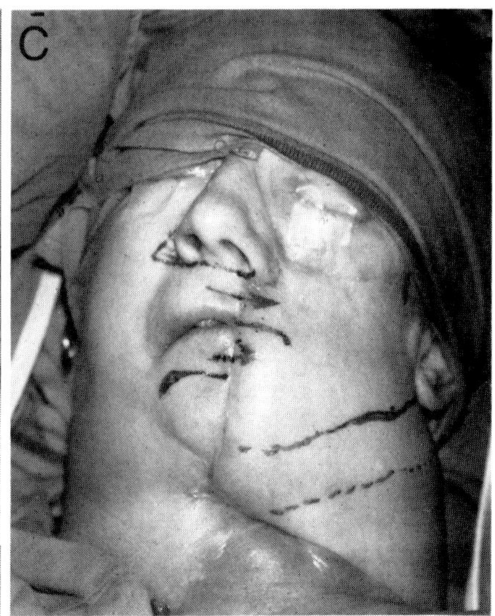
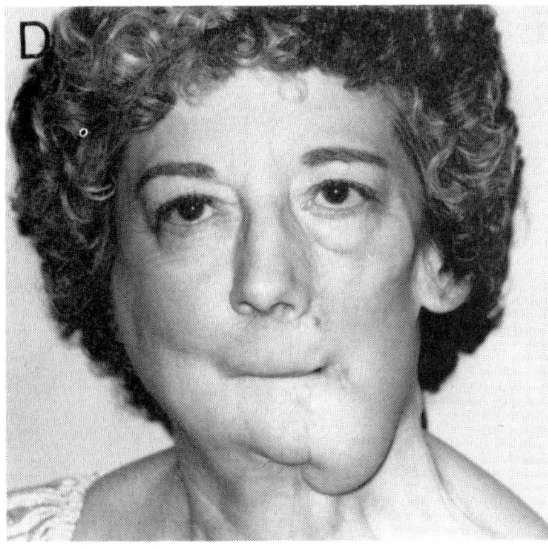

FIG 25–5.
A, large facial defect following ablative surgery. **B,** coverage of facial defect with a trapezius musculocutaneous flap. Notice the excellent color match. **C,** flap revision of trapezius musculocutaneous flap. **D,** patient 1 year after flap revision.

and best method to achieve the desired result in a particular patient.

The free flap is often an axial pattern flap, so the same fluid mechanics described for the musculocutaneous flap apply.[62] Remembering the exponential importance of vessel diameter to vessel resistance makes the accurate control of pedicle tension and position paramount. A pedicle is only minimally skeletonized to afford some protection to inadvertent vessel twisting or kinking.

Recipient vessels are an added requirement to the successful free transfer of tissue. Clinically acceptable vessels are those that appear normal at $\times 16$ magnification with an operating microscope and provide a strong spurt of blood from their cut end.[72]

The superior thyroid artery or lingual artery are ideal recipient vessels even in radiated necks with the resultant fibrosis and scarring. An end-to-side anastamosis to the external carotid artery has also been used with great success. Care should be taken with using the facial artery, because significant atherosclerosis has been occasionally encountered. The venous anastomosis is generally an end to side with the internal or external jugular vein.

Free flaps can tolerate oral contamination as long as a good oral closure is achieved. Previous neck dissection does not preclude their use. Suitable recipient vessels must be identified before harvesting the flap. The Doppler flow meter is frequently helpful in locating arterial vessels.

Systemic anticoagulation is not needed in free flap transfers, and the flap is not perfused. The flap has a relatively low metabolic rate and can undergo relative long periods (hours) of ischemia without sequella.[62] Once the anastomoses are completed, the venous clamp is always released first to prevent congestion. If flow is evident 10 to 15 minutes following clamp removal, a high probability of maintaining patency can be expected.[72] The pedicle is then secured and the transplanted tissue incorporated into the surgical defect.

Skill in microvascular techniques are learned in the animal laboratory. Not until consistent results are obtained with rat vessel anastomosis should a surgeon attempt microvascular surgery on a patient.[73] The extensive experience most head and neck surgeons have with the operating microscope makes the microvascular training a natural extension.

FREE JEJUNAL TRANSFER

In 1959, Seidenberg et al. described the first free jejunal transfer utilizing mechanical methods to join the donor and recipient vessels.[74] The technique was infrequently utilized until the advent of microsurgery in the mid-1970s. Jejunal transfer is now in selected cases the preferred method of reconstructing circumferential pharyngoesophageal defects located above the thoracic inlet.[72] The operation is relatively easy to perform and can be used for defects extending from the nasopharynx to the thoracic inlet. Cervical esophageal carcinomas and other cancers that arise in the esophagus are better managed with a gastric pull-up.[72] The jejunal mucosa is physiologically similar to the pharyngoesophageal mucosa. Unlike a skin flap, the jejunum's surface is moist and supple. The jejunum is a good size match for the pharyngoesophagus, and its vascular supply allows removal of a long pedicled segment (≤20 cm). The inherent peristalsis that aids deglutition somewhat can hinder the development of good esophageal speech. The complication rate is quite low, and early rehabilitation is the rule.[75–78] Split jejunum has been advocated by some to repair oral cavity defects or noncircumferential hypopharyngeal defects. Much thought must be given to the morbidity of an intra-abdominal procedure in light of the various other reconstructive options for this problem. In repair of oral cavity defects, it has been found that the jejunal mucosa often fails to flatten out and can collect food debris, causing severe halitosis.[72]

Technique

While one team of surgeons removes the tumor and pre-

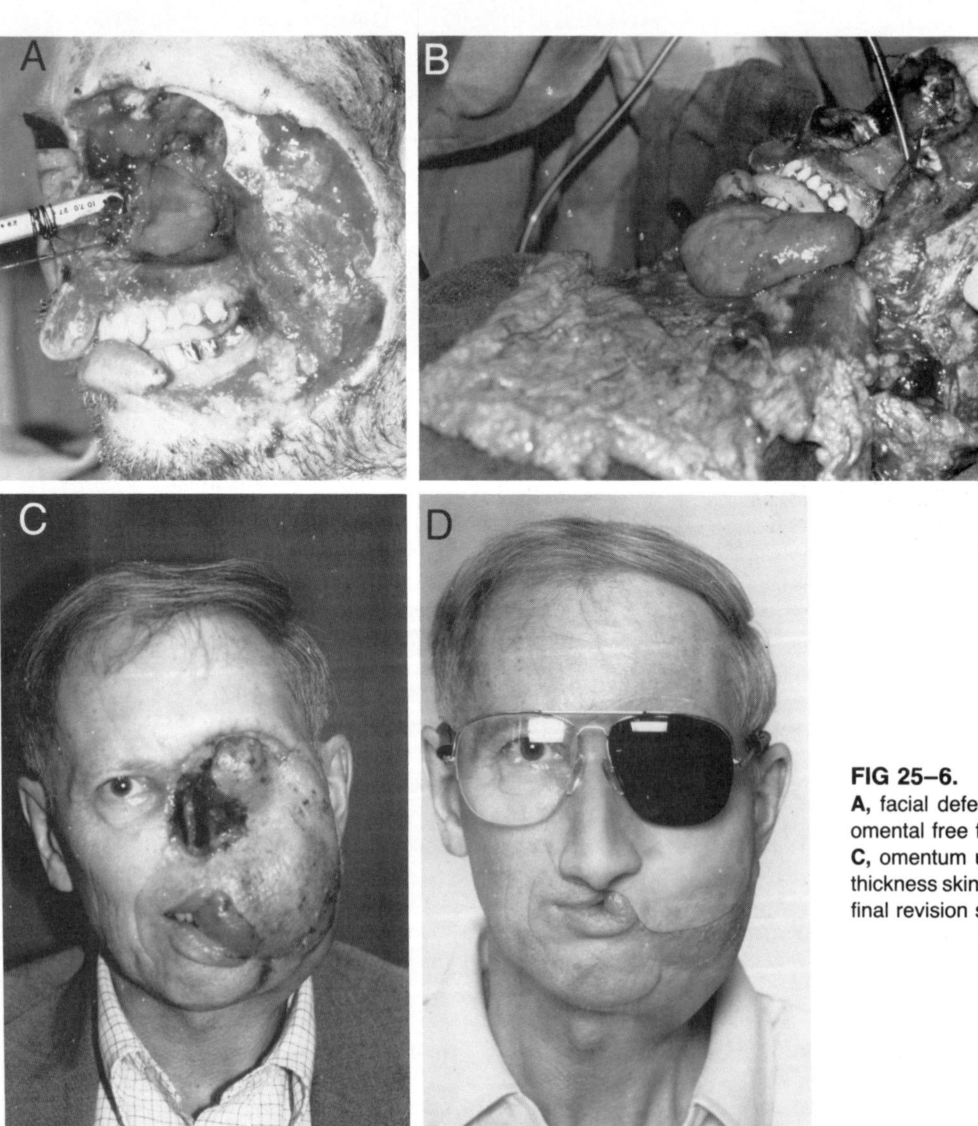

FIG 25–6.
A, facial defect following aggressive removal of angiosarcoma; omental free flap after microvascular anastamosis to neck vessels. **C,** omentum used to reconstruct a cheek and upper lip, with split-thickness skin graft in place. **D,** patient with prosthesis in place before final revision surgery.

pares recipient vessels, a second team harvests the jejunal segment. The area 40 to 60 cm beyond the ligament of Treitz offers a good size match and large, accessible vessels to form a pedicle.[72, 76] Once the donor artery and vein have been isolated, the jejunal segment is divided. Bleeding at the cut ends assures an adequate vascular pedicle. The recipient vessels are then prepared, and when all is completed, the jejunal pedicle is separated and the anastamosis begun. The arterial anastamosis is performed first using the superior thyroid artery or external carotid artery. The venous anastamosis is usually end to side into the external or internal jugular vein. The vein clamps are released first to avoid congestion. Patency is assessed following a 20- to 30-minute observation period and is confirmed by bleeding at the cut end, good color, and normal peristalsis. A two-layer closure is performed distally with care to orient the jejunum in an isoperistalic direction. The esophagus and jejunum are beveled so that they can be anastomosed in an oblong fashion.[72] If more than 10 cm of jejunum is used, an end-to-side anastamosis is performed, with the distal end of the jejunum brought out to the neck skin as a controlled fistula. This also provides a conduit for placing a nasogastric tube to allow decompression. The proximal end of the jejunum is fish-mouthed to open the lumen and provide better pharyngeal approximation. In closing the neck wounds, a window is created by leaving a portion of the serosal surface of the transplanted jejunum externalized.[72] It can be covered with either an STSG or a piece of clear silicone rubber (Silastic), allowing a precise assessment of the jejunum's viability. A tracheostomy is performed if the larynx has not been resected. Drainage is mandatory and passive methods are preferred. Oral intake is started about 10 to 14 days postoperatively; however, if the larynx has been preserved, intake is delayed for 10 to 14 weeks. The larynx should be partially or completely isolated from the digestive tract (i.e., laryngoplasty) if segments of jejunum more than 6 cm are used in the reconstruction. Using longer lengths of jejunum will reduce transit times of food predisposing to aspiration.

Complications

Relatively few problems have been encountered with free jejunal transfer reconstruction of the pharyngoesophageal segment.[75, 78] If a salivary leak occurs, it is managed conservatively and generally heals uneventfully. Stricture occurs much less than with skin flap reconstruction and is usually managed with only dilatation. Beveling the distal end and fish-mouthing the proximal end of the jejunum also minimize stricture formation.

Impending necrosis of the jejunal flap is easily recognized with the window closure technique herein described. The vascular pedicle should be explored and revised if feasible. If the anastamosis is deemed irreparable, several options are available. In an unirradiated patient, the serosa can be removed and the jejunal mucosa used as a free graft over a salivary bypass tube. An irradiated patient should be managed conservatively by making a pharyngostome and an esophagostome and providing carotid protection. A second reconstructive attempt can then be undertaken in 10 to 14 days. Some centers advocate that a second jejunal free flap be immediately attempted if necrosis occurs within the first 24 hours.[79] This places great strain

on both the surgeon and the patient and should be reserved for special circumstances.

Excessive mucous production is expected for the first couple of weeks and may be treated with cimetidine if it is problematic.[72]

FREE SCAPULAR FLAP

The scapular skin provides an ideal source of tissue for microvascular transfer. It is easily dissected with minimum donor site morbidity and provides a large amount of workable tissue. The vascular pedicle is both lengthy and consistently large enough to make installation relatively problem free. The lateral border of the scapula has been incorporated into the flap and allows application to mandibular and midface reconstruction as well. The anatomy of this region allows a three-dimensional versatility to the reconstructive surgeon not afforded by any other donor area.

Anatomy

The subscapular artery (Sa) arises off of the axillary artery and divides into the thoracodorsal (supplying the latissimus dorsi) and the circumflex scapular artery (CSa).[46] The CSa traverses the triangular space and divides into a transverse and descending branch. These combine to supply the skin from the posterior axillary fold to the midline and from the scapular spine to its tip.[40, 41, 46] The descending branch supplies the parascapular and the transverse branch of the scapular skin flap via a rich fascial plexus. This fascial vasculature sends vertical perforating branches up into a subcutaneous plexus. Excess deep subcutaneous tissue and fat can therefore be carefully debulked from the periphery of these flaps, if needed (intraoral resurfacing), by virtue of this fascial circulation.[40, 41, 46] These two flaps can be raised in continuity or as totally separated skin paddles. By having distinct pedicles distal to the vascular supply of the bone in a compound flap, these skin flaps can be moved independently. The three-dimensional flexibility provided by this mobility solves many of the complex reconstructive situations encountered in the head and neck.

The lateral border of the scapula provides the osseous portion of the compound flap. It is supplied by numerous periosteal and muscular branches off the CSa.[38, 41] The lateral scapula provides bone with 1.5 by 3 cm of thickness and 10 to 14 cm of length, depending on the patient's size. If mandibular angle replacement is desired, the medial inferior scapula can be included in the flap, providing an additional 3 to 4 cm of bone.[38, 39, 41]

Two venae comitans generally accompany the named arteries in this area and provide the venous anastamosis for microvascular transfer.[38, 41]

The triangular space previously discussed is a key area for locating the vascular pedicle in this flap. The teres minor arises from the upper two thirds of the lateral scapular edge and forms the upper boundary of this space.[40, 46] The teres major, the inferior boundary, arises from the inferior border of the lateral scapula. Both teres muscles insert onto the humerous but have opposite actions on upper extremity motion.[40] The long head of the triceps forms the lateral margin of the triangular space. Function is always maintained by reattaching all severed muscles to remaining scapula after flap harvesting.

Technique

The reconstructive situation dictates the combination of soft tissue and bone to be used. Preoperative planning is critical, as is proper patient positioning. A Mayfield headrest is standard, and the patient is placed supine but rotated enough to allow access to the midline of the back. Skin paddle design and pertinent anatomy are diagrammed on the patient. Elipses of less than 10 to 12 cm are used to facilitate primary closure.[38, 41] If a single skin paddle is all that is needed, it is generally centered over the transverse branch of the CSa. The skin is then incised and dissected from medially to laterally in the avascular plane of loose areolar tissue just superficial to the infraspinatus fascia. As the lateral scapular border is approached, the triangular space is identified and the vascular pedicle located. The teres major insertion is transected with care to preserve the numerous periosteal branches off the CSa. Pedicle dissection can then be carried back to the Sa or even to the axillary artery if needed. Pedicle length varies on the type of flap employed. If only a cutaneous flap is required, a pedicle of up to 10 cm can be obtained[46]; however, if scapular bone is used, pedicle length averages 6 cm.[38, 41] The thoracodorsal artery is preserved if a latissimus dorsi flap is to be used concomitantly. The CSa ranges from 2 to 3 mm at its axillary artery insertion.[38, 46]

An incision in the infraspinatus is made over the scapula and carried down to the periosteum. The periosteum is elevated just enough to permit osteotomies. Verticle bone cuts on the scapula are next accomplished with an oscillating saw along the junction of the central bone and thicker lateral border bone. Transverse osteotomies are made inferior as needed. Each planned contouring ostectomy requires an additional 1 cm of donor bone.[38, 41] Following mobilization of the bone portion of the compound flap, the defect is reconstituted by reattaching all severed muscles to the remaining scapula.[38, 41] Attention is then turned to the recipient site, where appropriate vessels are located and prepared for anastamosis. The flap is transferred to the neck. Bone fixation is performed before any microvascular suturing. Mandibular contour is created by triangular ostectomies in the donor bone, with care to preserve periosteal attachment.[38, 41] Miniplate stabilization of the donor bone to mandibular remnants has proved adequate, and ostectomies are stabilized with pins.

The microvascular anastamosis is performed in the manner previously described. An interposition graft is often required for the venous anastamosis to provide an unimpeded pedicle.

The donor defect is closed primarily and the shoulder immobilized for 72 to 96 hours. A gradual range of motion rehabilitation is instituted as the patient's recovery permits.

This flap is highly recommended because of its versatility and limited associated morbidity. The amount of available bone limits its use in some situations, but reconstructive surgeons should become familiar with the free scapular flap.

CUTANEOUS THIGH FLAP

Several different cutaneous thigh flaps have been described,[80, 81] attesting to the unique perfusion of extremity skin. It consists of a subdermal plexus and a plexus above the deep fascia connected by vertical perforating vessels. Cutaneous branches of the various muscular arteries end in the deep plexus do not have a typical axial distribution. The shape, location, and pedicle placement of a thigh flap are, therefore, not restricted as in other donor sites.[80] Plexus perfusion also permits a margin for error with limited flap toleration (i.e., survival) of pedicle occlusion and reanastamosis. As a pedicle is traced proximally or distally, muscular branches are ligated, creating a relative hyperperfusion of the cutaneous branch. Flap delineation can then be observed by marking limits of skin flushing[80] to ensure a safe flap design.

Pedicle length and vessel size are generous, averaging 8 to 10 cm and 2 to 4 mm, respectively. Venae comitantes traveling adjacent to the cutaneous artery provide suitable venous outflow for these flaps.[80, 81] Cutaneous nerves are abundant in this area, allowing flap neurotization if desired.

Up to 800 cm² of donor tissue can be harvested on one pedicle from the anterolateral thigh.[80] The donor site is in a hidden area and can be closed either primarily or with an STSG. The available tissue is of relatively uniform thickness and supple enough for external recontouring. Experience with these flaps has confirmed the minimum associated patient morbidity but a consistent need for cosmetic revision with their use.[80]

Anterolateral Thigh Flap

The skin overlying the anterior and lateral surface of the thigh from the level of the greater trocanter to about 3 cm above the patella can be supplied by cutaneous branch off of the descending branch of the lateral femoral circumflex artery.[80] This artery emerges from the deep musculature through a triangle formed by the tensor fasciae latae, vastus lateralis, and rectus femoris. It can be easily traced back to its origin by medially retracting the rectus femoris muscle, producing an 8 cm pedicle with 2 mm vessels. Branches of the anterior femoral cutaneous and lateral femoral cutaneous nerves are within the flap and available for nervous anastamosis.

The patient is placed in the supine position, and the proposed flap is outlined. The area of the vascular pedicle is dissected first on a subfascial plane. Once the cutaneous artery is located, the remainder of the flap can be quickly elevated. The pedicle is traced back to its origin, with care to preserve 1 to 2 cm of surrounding tissue to avoid overskeletonization. No motor nerves need be dissected or severed.

The free flap is then transferred into the head and neck, where a second team has located and prepared recipient vessels. The microvascular anastamosis is completed and the flap observed for 15 to 20 minutes. If perfusion is adequate at this time, the tissue is incorporated into the defect as desired.

Other Thigh Flaps

A posterior flap based on the third perforating branch of the profunda femoris artery has been used with success.[80, 81] Medial thigh flaps based on an innominant branch of the lateral circumflex femoral artery[80] and an innominant branch of the superficial femoral artery[81] have been described as well.

FREE GROIN FLAP

The inguinal area has been used with success as a donor site in free transfer, with up to 500 cm² of relatively hairless tissue.[82] Compound flaps with iliac bone have also been developed, offering the head and neck surgeon another reconstructive option.[36, 37, 44] These flaps involve a hidden donor area and relatively little patient morbidity, but pedicle dissection can be tedious. Another disadvantage with the compound flap is the very bulky cutaneous portion in obese patients. This creates difficulty with flap stabilization after transfer because of gravitational shearing forces. Cosmetic revision surgery is consistently required, and skin color match with facial skin is marginal in whites.[72] These factors, combined with the knowledge that a reconstructive effort employing a compound groin flap takes more than 10 hours, makes proper patient selection paramount. This flap does provide a block of bone averaging up to 10 to 11 by 3 to 4 cm suitably contoured for mandibular reconstruction.[36, 37, 44, 72]

Technique

The free groin flap can be pedicled on either the superficial circumflex iliac artery (SCIa),[36] the lateral femoral circumflex artery,[36] the deep circumflex iliac artery (DCIa),[37, 44, 72] or the epigastric artery.[36] The DCIa appears to be the dominant vessel supplying the iliac bone.[44] This vessel gives rise to a series of musculocutaneous perforators that traverse the external oblique (EO) to supply the skin over the anterior iliac crest. The largest perforator is about 6 to 8 cm lateral to the anterior superior iliac spine (ASIS) and represents the centering point for the skin paddle.[72] The paddle design is generally encompassed in a fusiform incision from the femoral artery to the level of the inferior scapular tip to allow a linear closure. Excess skin can be discarded at a later time. The upper border of the flap is incised first to the level of the EO. The size of the planned skin flap dictates how much EO attachment to the iliac crest must be preserved. Usually 3 to 4 cm of EO is an adequate cuff to maintian good skin perfusion.[44, 72] This incision then curves medially into the inguinal canal with retraction the vascular pedicle can be developed. The DCIa and its accompanying vein are located deep to the posterior wall of the canal. The DCIa is dissected laterally until a large ascending branch is found 1 to 2 cm medial to the ASIS. This represents one of the series of perforating branches but not the dominant vessel supplying the overlying skin. Confusion can be avoided by locating the dominant perforator 6 to 8 cm lateral to the ASIS through the superior incision. This branch can then be dissected medially after the internal oblique (IO) and transversus muscle are incised, with care to preserve a 2 to 3 cm cuff attachment to the iliac crest. This muscular cuff provides accessory nutrient perforator vessels and helps preserve the iliac periosteal attachments. This will improve the blood supply to the bone and subsequent success of the flap.[36]

Transverse fascia is next incised, exposing preperitoneal fat that requires retraction to expose the ilium. The iliac periosteum is finally reached by incising the ilium 1 to 2 cm medial to the transverse-iliac fascial fusion. Attention is then turned to the lower portion of the skin flap. This is incised with care to preserve the SCIa. This vessel is located 1 to 3 cm inferior to and runs roughly parallel to the inguinal ligament. The SCIa can be used as a pedicle for the compound flap if the DCIa vessels are damaged or unsuitable.[36] The tight muscles are detached from the outer iliac crest, preserving a 2 to 3 cm cuff attachment. The inguinal ligament and sartorius muscle are divided, leaving only bony attachments. The lateral femoral cutaneous nerve usually must be sacrificed during DCIa dissection.[37, 44]

A template of the mandibular (or other bone) defect is used to plan the osteotomies. The anteroinferior iliac spine is often included for ascending ramus defects.[37] Osteotomies are performed, at which time final contouring and remodeling of the bone can be accomplished. The inner table can be harvested alone if a particularly thin piece of bone is required.[72]

The recipient vessels and reconstructive site are prepared before pedicle severance. The composite flap is then delivered into the neck and reconstruction begun. Basket wiring and Steinmann pin fixation have proved reliable in stabilizing the bone, which is done prior to any microvascular anastamosis.[36]

Attention to closure is important to prevent donor site morbidity. Iliac fascia and muscle are reapproximated to transverse muscle, and the oblique muscles are sutured to the thigh muscles. The inguinal canal is closed and the ligament reattached to remaining iliac crest. Skin closure is accomplished in a straight line.[44, 72]

The difficulty and duration of this operation should now be apparent and underscore the need for proper preoperative planning and patient selection. It is highly recommended that cadaver dissection be performed before this flap is attempted on a patient. It is a highly reliable technique for obtaining vascularized bone for reconstruction in the head and neck.[36, 37, 44, 72]

If only a cutaneous flap is required, a groin flap based on the SCIa can be designed.[82] The pedicle dissection is less difficult than for the DCIa, which reduces operative time considerably.

REFERENCES

1. Flynn MB, Moore C: Marginal resection of the mandible in the management of squamous cancer of the floor of the mouth. *Am J Surg* 1974; 128:490.
2. Sam ML, Nussbaum M: Marginal resection of the mandible with reconstruction by tongue flap for carcinoma of the floor of the mouth. *Am J Surg* 1971; 121:679.
3. Stringer G: Studies on the revascularization of bone grafts. *J Bone Joint Surg (Br)* 1957; 39:395.
4. Ray RD: Vascularization of bone grafts and implants. *Clin Orthop* 1972; 87:43.

5. DeFries HO, Marble HB, Sell JW: Reconstruction of the mandible. *Arch Otolaryngol* 1971; 93:426.

6. Lawson W, Biller HF: Mandibular reconstruction: Bone graft techniques. *Otolaryngol Head Neck Surg* 1982; 90:589.

7. Hamaker RC: Irradiated autogenous mandibular grafts in primary reconstruction. *Laryngoscope* 1981; 91:1031.

8. Hamaker RC, Singer MI, Shockley WW, et al: Irradiated mandibular autografts. *Cancer* 1983; 52:1017.

9. Cummings CW, Leipzig B: Replacement of tumor-involved mandible by cryosurgically devitalized autograft. *Arch Otolaryngol* 1980; 106:252.

10. Harding RL: Replantation of the mandible in cancer surgery. *Plast Reconstr Surg* 1971; 48:586.

11. Marciani RD, Bowden CM: Reimplantation of freeze-treated mandibular bone. *J Oral Surg* 1975; 33:261.

12. Weaver AW, Smith DB: Frozen autogenous stent graft for immediate reconstruction in oral cancer surgery. *Am J Surg* 1973; 126:505.

13. DeFries HO: Reconstruction of the mandible: Use of combined homologous mandible and autologous bone. *Otolaryngol Head Neck Surg* 1981; 89:694.

14. Giordano A, Brady D, Foster C, et al: Particulate cancellow marrow crib graft reconstruction of mandibular defects. *Laryngoscope* 1980; 90:2027.

15. Schuller DE, Bardach J, Monteith CG, et al: Titanium tray mandibular reconstruction. *Arch Otolaryngol* 1982; 108:174.

16. Schwartz HC: Mandibular reconstruction using the dacron-urethane prosthesis and autogenic cancellous bone: Review of 32 cases. *Plast Reconstr Surg* 1984; 73:387.

17. Albert TW, Smith JD, Everts EC, et al: Dacron mesh tray and cancellous bone in reconstruction of mandibular defects. *Arch Otolaryngol* 1986; 112:53.

18. Baker S: Management of osteoradionecrosis of the mandible with myocutaneous flaps. *J Surg Oncol* 1986; 24:282.

19. Antonyshyn U, Colcleugh RG, et al: The temporalis myoosseous flap: An experimental study. *Plast Reconstr Surg* 1986; 77:406.

20. Tessier P: Autogenous bone grafts taken from the calvarium for facial and cranial applications. *Clin Plast Surg* 1982; 9:531.

21. Ariyan S: The visability of rib grafts transplanted with the periosteal blood supply. *Plast Reconstr Surg* 1980; 65:140.

22. Conley J, Gullane PJ: The sternocleidomastoid muscle flap. *Head Neck Surg* 1980; 2:308.

23. Snyder CC, Bateman JM, et al: Mandibulo-facial restoration with like osteocutaneous flaps. *Plast Reconstr Surg* 1970; 45:14.

24. Hill HL, Brown RG: The sternocleidomastoid flap to restore facial contour in mandibular reconstruction. *Br J Plast Surg* 1978; 31:143.

25. Lem KH, Wei WI, Siu KF: The pectoralis major costomyocutaneous flap for mandibular reconstruction. *Plast Reconstr Surg* 1984; 73:904.

26. Little JW, McCulloch DT, Lyons JR: The lateral pectoral composite flap in one-stage reconstruction of the irradiated mandible. *Plast Reconstr Surg* 1983; 71:26.

27. Maisel RH, Adams GL: Osteomyocutaneous reconstruction of the oral cavity. *Arch Otolaryngol* 1983; 109:731.

28. Sabatier RE, Bakamjian VY: Transaxillary latissimus dorsi flap reconstruction in head and neck cancer. *Am J Surg* 1985; 150:427.

29. Marvyama Y, Urita Y, Ohishi K: Rib–latissimus osteomyocutaneous flap in reconstruction of a mandibular defect. *Br J Plast Surg* 1985; 38:234.

30. Mogi G, Fujiyoshi T, Kurono Y, et al: Latissimus dorsi myocutaneous iliac bone flap for reconstruction of massive defects of mandible and oral basis. *Laryngoscope* 1986; 96:171.

31. Panje WR, Cutting C: Trapezius osteomyocutaneous island flap for reconstruction of the anterior floor of the mouth and mandible. *Head Neck Surg* 1980; 3:66.

32. Panje WR: Mandibular reconstruction with the trapezius osteomusculocutaneous flap. *Arch Otolaryngol* 1985; 111:223.

33. Bern C, O'Hare PM: Case report: Reconstruction of the mandible using the scapular spine pedicled upon trapezius muscle; description of the posterior approach to the transverse cervical vessels. *Br J Plast Surg* 1986; 39:473.

34. Maves MD, Phillippsen LP: Surgical anatomy of the scapular spine in the trapezius-osteomuscular flap. *Arch Otolaryngol* 1986; 112:173.

35. Medgyesi S: Observations on pedicle bone grafts in goats. *Scand J Plast Reconstr Surg* 1973; 7:110.

36. Panje WR: Free compound groin flap reconstruction of anterior mandibular defect. *Arch Otolaryngol* 1981; 107:17.

37. Duncan MJ, Manktelow RT, Zuker RM, et al: Mandibular reconstruction in the radiated patient; the role of osteocutaneous free tissue transfers. *Plast Reconstr Surg* 1985; 76:829.

38. Baker SR, Sullivan MJ: Osteocutaneous free scapular flap for one-stage mandibular reconstruction. *Arch Otolaryngol* 1985; 114:267.

39. Granick MS, Newton D, Hanna DC: Scapular free flap for repair of massive lower facial composite defects. *Head Neck Surg* 1986; 8:436.

40. Barwick WJ, Goodkind DJ, Serafin D: The free scapular flap. *Plast Reconstr Surg* 1982; 69:779.

41. Swartz WM, Banis JC, Newton ED, et al: The osteocutaneous scapular flap for mandibular and maxillary reconstruction. *Plast Reconstr Surg* 1986; 77:530.

42. Serafin D, Riefkohl R, Thomas I, et al: The osteocutaneous scapular flap for mandibular and maxillary reconstruction. *Plast Reconstr Surg* 1980; 66:718.

43. Cuono CB, Ariyan S: Immediate reconstruction of a composite mandibular defect with a regional osteomusculocutaneous flap. *Plast Reconstr Surg* 1980; 65:477.

44. Taylor GI, Townsend P, Corlett R: Superiority of the deep circumflex iliac vessels as the supply for free groin flaps. *Plast Reconstr Surg* 1979; 64:745.

45. Brown RG, Vascomez LD, Jurkrewicz MJ: Reconstruction of the central mandible with a single block of iliac bone. *Br J Plast Surg* 1976; 29:191.

46. dos Santos LF: The vascular anatomy and dissection of the free scapular flap. *Plast Reconstr Surg* 1984; 73:599.

47. Haw CS, O'Brien BM, Kirata T: The microsurgical revascularization of resected segment of tibia in the dog. *J Bone Joint Surg (Br)* 1978; 60:266.

48. Miller JB, Mazur JM: A biomechanical comparison: Vascular and conventional autogenous bone grafts. *Orthop Rev* 1983; 12:49.

49. Vajda TT: Endodonio-prosthetic anchorage and stabilization system for overdentures and fixed bridgework, in *Implantology and Biomaterials in Stomatology*. Tokyo, Ishiyaku Publishing, 1980, pp 199–206.

50. Boyne PJ: Preprosthetic adjunctive surgery in post-cancer rehabilitation, in *Oral Cancer and Jaw Tumors*. Tokyo, Tokyo Professional Postgraduate Services, 1988, pp 244–266.

51. Moran WJ, Panje WR: The free greater omental flap for

treatment of mandibular osteoradionecrosis. *Arch Otolaryngol* 1987; 113:425.

52. Panje WR: Free flaps versus myocutaneous flaps in reconstruction of the head and neck. *Otol Clin* 1982; 15:111.

53. Freeman JL, Walker EP, Wilson JSP, et al: The vascular anatomy of the pectoralis major myocutaneous flap. *Br J Plast Surg* 1981; 34:3.

54. Baek SM, Biller HF, Krespi YP, et al: The pectoralis major myocutaneous island flap for reconstruction of the head and neck. *Head Neck Surg* 1979; 1:293.

55. Wei WI, Lam KH, Wong J: The true pectoralis major myocutaneous island flap; an anatomical study. *Br J Plast Surg* 1984; 37:568.

56. Schuller DE: Limitations of the pectoralis major myocutaneous flap in head and neck reconstruction. *Arch Otolaryngol* 1980; 106:709.

57. Baek SM, Lawson W, Biller HF: An analysis of 133 pectoralis major myocutaneous flaps. *Plast Reconstr Surg* 1982; 69:460.

58. Baek SM, Lawson W, Biller HF: Reconstruction of hypopharynx and cervical esophagus with pectoralis major island myocutaneous flap. *Ann Plast Surg* 1981; 7:19.

59. Sasaki CT, Ariyan S, Spencer D, et al: Pectoralis major myocutaneous reconstruction of the anterior skull base. *Laryngoscope* 1985; 98:162.

60. Morain WD, Glen L, Hutchings JC: The segmental pectoralis major muscle flap: A function-preserving procedure. *Plast Reconstr Surg* 1985; 75:825.

61. Panje WR: A new method for total nasal reconstruction. *Arch Otolaryngol* 1982; 108:156.

62. Panje WR: Musculocutaneous and free flaps, physiology and practical considerations. *Otol Clin* 1984; 17:401.

63. Panje WR: Myocutaneous trapezius flap. *Head Neck Surg* 1980; 2:206.

64. Guillannundegui OM, Larson DL: The lateral trapezius musculocutaneous flap; its use in head and neck reconstruction. *Plast Reconstr Surg* 1981; 67:143.

65. Netterville JL, Panje WR, Maves MD: The trapezius myocutaneous flap. *Arch Otolaryngol* 1987; 113:271.

66. Tucker HM, Sobol SM, Levine H, et al: The transverse cervical trapezius myocutaneous island flap. *Arch Otolaryngol* 1982; 108:194.

67. Goodwin WJ, Rosenberg, GT: Venous drainage of the lateral trapezius musculocutaneous island flap. *Arch Otolaryngol* 1982; 108:411.

68. McCraw JB, Magee WP, Kalvaic, H: Uses of the trapezius and sternocleido mascoid myocutaneous flaps in head and neck reconstruction. *Plast Reconstr Surg* 1979; 63:49.

69. Krespi YP, Baek SM, Surek CL: Flap reconstruction of the upper face: Face flaps versus lower trapezius myocutaneous flap. *Laryngoscope* 1983; 93:485.

70. Earle AS, Fratianne RB, Kiehn CL: The relationship of hematocrit levels to skin flap survival in the dog. *Plast Reconstr Surg* 1974; 54:341.

71. Panje WR, Bardach J: Experimental study on the closure of large defects of the oral cavity using a free island flap with microvascular anastamosis. *Trans Am Acad Ophthalmol Otolaryngol* 1976; 82:434.

72. Panje WR, Moran WJ: *Microsurgical Reconstruction of the Head and Neck.* New York, Georg Thieme, 1989.

73. Panje WR, Krause LJ, Bardach J: Microsurgical techniques in free flap reconstruction. *Laryngoscope* 1977; 87:692.

74. Seidenberg B, Rosenak S, Hurwitt ES, et al: Immediate reconstruction of the cervical esphagus by a revascularized isolated jejunal segment. *Ann Surg* 1959; 142:162.

75. Gluckman JL, McDonough JJ, McCafferty GJ, et al: Complications associated with free jejunal graft reconstructions of the pharyngoesophagus. A multi-institutional experience with 52 cases. *Head Neck Surg* 1985; 7:200.

76. Robinson DW, Macleod A: Microvascular free jejunum transfer. *Br J Plast Surg* 1982; 35:258.

77. Fisher SR, Cole TB, Meyers WC, et al: Pharyngoesophageal reconstruction using free jejunal interposition grafts. *Arch Otolaryngol* 1985; 111:747.

78. Schechter GL, Baker JW, Gilbert DA: Functional evaluation of pharyngoesophageal reconstructive techniques. *Arch Otolaryngol* 1987; 113:40.

79. McConnel FM: Thawley S, Panje WR (eds): *Comprehensive Management of Head and Neck Tumors,* vol 1. Philadelphia, WB Saunders Co, 1987, p 848.

80. Song YG, Chen GZ, Song YL: The free thigh flap: A new free flap concept on the septocutaneous artery. *Br J Plast Surg* 1984; 37:149.

81. Baek SM: Two new cutaneous free flaps: The medial and lateral thigh flaps. *Plast Reconstr Surg* 1983; 71:354.

82. Panje WR, Krause CJ, Bardach J, et al: Reconstruction of intraoral defects with the free groin flap. *Arch Otolaryngol* 1977; 103:78.

Head and Neck Reconstruction

Approach of

John C. Price, M.D.

Numerous disabilities arise from mandibular resection for oral cancer ablation. Airway compromise and swallowing dysfunction are profound, and each may present a threat to life. Crippling of the speech apparatus and communicative ability is variable. Disruption of oral competence and normal mastication alters the diet and seriously limits social functions that center around dining and entertaining. Mandibular shift and muscular imbalance can result in significant pterygoid spasm and temporal mandibular joint pain. The visible deformity presents a very real psychosocial disability in our perfectionistic, cosmetically oriented society; yet most patients fear the cancer more than the disabilities that may arise, and readily enter into therapy. It is the physician's responsibility to design treatments to provide the best chance for cure while simultaneously minimizing resultant disabilities. Mandibular continuity should be maintained if curability is not compromised. Preservation of the mandible is not always possible, and segmental resection is unavoidable.

Mandibular reconstruction is essential if the morbidity of segmental resection is to be reduced. The ideal reconstruction would possess the following characteristics: It would be a primary technique that is highly successful (95%) and accurate in three dimensions, require a short operative time, impose low donor site morbidity, yield long-term retention, and accept a dental prosthesis. Functionally it would provide stabilization of the airway, establish deglutition, improve speech, restore dental occlusion and mastication, and provide satisfactory cosmesis.

No current single technique approaches these stated ideals. Several basic problems invariably inhibit this accomplishment. Adequate oncologic control must not be sacrificed. This frequently produces significant problems in achieving adequate soft tissue coverage of the reconstruction. Requirements for postoperative wound management and observation may interfere with standard techniques for graft fixation or establishment of appropriate dental occlusion. Salivary contamination frequently results in malunion, osteitis, and overt osteomyelitis, with devitalization of bone grafts and high infection rate. The healing power of the soft tissue may be impaired by radiation, diabetes, vascular disease, or malnutrition. The ablative surgery frequently removes considerable musculature, resulting in a-

dynamic tissue in and around the oral cavity. There may be significant tension within flap pedicles, which may compound the effects of gravity. Sensory deficits resulting from the resection, most notable from the mental nerve, deprive the area of kinesthetic and tactile ability.

Special consideration must be given to the fact that almost all patients undergoing segmental mandibular resection for oral malignancy have advanced stage cancer or recurrent disease. As a group they are at risk for a high rate of recurrence. Most will be candidates for combined modality therapy. The reconstruction must therefore provide reliable healing and rapid rehabilitation and permit—and be tolerant of—aggressive irradiation. Very little quality of life is attained if the patient is still recovering from a painful, disabling reconstructive procedure when a recurrence appears. The realization that patients requiring mandibular resection have a 20% or less anticipated 5-year survival may moderate reconstructive plans. The more elaborate the reconstruction the greater the devastation rendered to the patient (and surgeon) by "positive margins" and early postoperative recurrence.

These oncologic considerations influenced the adaptation of the three-dimensional bendable reconstructive plate (3-DBRP) with pedicled myocutaneous flap soft tissue coverage as the major modality for primary mandibular reconstruction. This system provides substantial rehabilitation, is rapid and reliable, produces minimal donor site disability and usually allows rapid healing and early institution of postoperative irradiation. The 3-DBRP may not function as a denture-bearing platform and may ultimately show loosening of screws or metal fatigue. It does, however, allow satisfactory rehabilitation until the problems of the early posttreatment period are resolved. Bone reconstruction may then be considered if indicated because of residual disability.

The reconstructive surgeon must always be motivated and strive for the ideal (perfection) or premorbid function. He or she must also keep foremost in mind the grim realities of cancer management in the oral cavity: (1) biologic consequences of advanced stage malignancy, (2) poor prosthetic and masticatory performance of radiated mandibular bone, either retained or reconstructed, and (3) adynamic nature of soft tissue reconstructions. More pointedly, irradiated bone covered by insensate, nonalveolar, dry soft tissue in a contaminated dry mouth may hold up to prosthetic masticatory loading in only a few lucky circumstances, if at all. Failure to achieve this ultimate step in mandibular restoration should not, however, be the single measure of success. On the contrary, preliminary life quality studies indicate that cosmesis may be the dominant factor in early reentry of the patient into his or her family, social, and work environments. The lack of adequate chewing function seems to become a central focus only in patients in whom all other major functions of the mandible have been retained or restored.

ANTERIOR MANDIBULAR RECONSTRUCTION

Reestablishment of the anterior mandibular arch is the most difficult problem encountered in head and neck reconstructive surgery. Linear, angular, rotational, and loading forces experienced by the bone are complex. Accurate duplication of not only size and shape of the bone but also of strength of bone is important. Soft tissue receives the least support from surrounding musculature in this area. No method of reconstruction approaches the ideal for this defect. The 3-DBRP and pedicled myocutaneous flap provides uncomplicated recovery in 70% of cases. The bar may become exposed in up to 30%, but has successfully been recovered. In other cases the bar ultimately required extraction but provided stability of the mandible through radiation therapy and provided an internal platform for fibrosis and soft tissue contour, persisting even after removal of the prosthesis. The best case for primary reconstruction with microvascular transplantation of bone can be made for defects involving the anterior mandibular arch, although I prefer to reserve this technique for delayed reconstruction and for those patients in which bar exposure is refractory to simple attempts at closure. Pedicled myocutaneous flaps incorporating rib or clavicle simply do not provide bone of adequate quality to hold up to the stress applied to this area. The trapezius myo-osseous flap carries the scapular spine, which is variable in size, shape, and suitability, although it is a well-vascularized bone. It has not, in my experience, held up to the rigors of life as a mandible over 2- or 3-year periods.

Technique

Osteotomy sites are determined by passing the index finger into the lateral posterior floor of the mouth until the radial aspect of the finger contacts tumor adherent to bone. Two centimeters beyond that (usually the width of an index finger) will be the site of the osteotomy (Fig 25–7).

The length of the outer circumference of the lower border of the mandibular segment to be resected is measured and marked with a heavy silk suture (Fig 25–8). Add another 3 cm on either end (total 6 cm) for the mounting section of the bar. A template of the appropriate length is selected and contoured to the mandible. This template is fixed into appropriate position with two plate-holding forceps, and three holes are drilled into

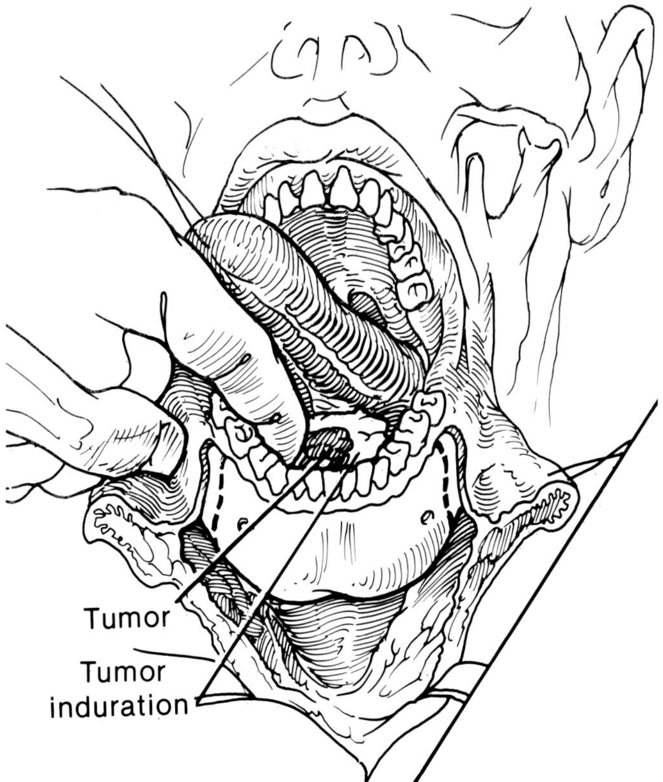

FIG 25–7.
Establishing osteotomy sites. (From Price JC: Management of large anterior floor-of-mouth malignancies with mandibular invasion, in Bailey BJ (ed): *Surgery of the Oral Cavity*. Chicago, Year Book Medical Publishers, 1989, pp 103–115. Used by permission.)

each mandibular segment (Fig 25–9, A). An electric power drill with a 2 mm wire passing bit greatly facilitates this maneuver. Copious irrigation is required to avoid overheating and burnishing the surrounding bone. Each hole must be drilled precisely to be perpendicular to the cortical surface of the mandible and to penetrate cleanly through the lingual cortex. The drill must be positioned carefully in the center of the hole; otherwise, inappropriate contact of the screw with the plate risks stripping of threads from the bone. The depth gauge is inserted into each screw hole, the lingual cortex engaged, the meter set into position firmly against the buccal cortex, and the appropriate length of the screw read from the calibrated scale (Fig 25–9,B). This procedure is repeated for each of the six holes.

Fully threaded screws of proper lengths are selected and arranged in correct order. Machine threads are then established within the bone with the tapping tool (Fig 25–9,C). This tool must be directed perpendicularly to the cortical bone surface so that it will follow the hole drilled previously, and it should pass easily. Encountering significant resistance indicates that the drill hole is incomplete or too small or the tap is placed at an incorrect angle. The tap should be removed promptly and the problem solved before the task is resumed. Failure to pass the tap completely through the lingual cortex may result in out-fracture of the bone as the screws are tightened.

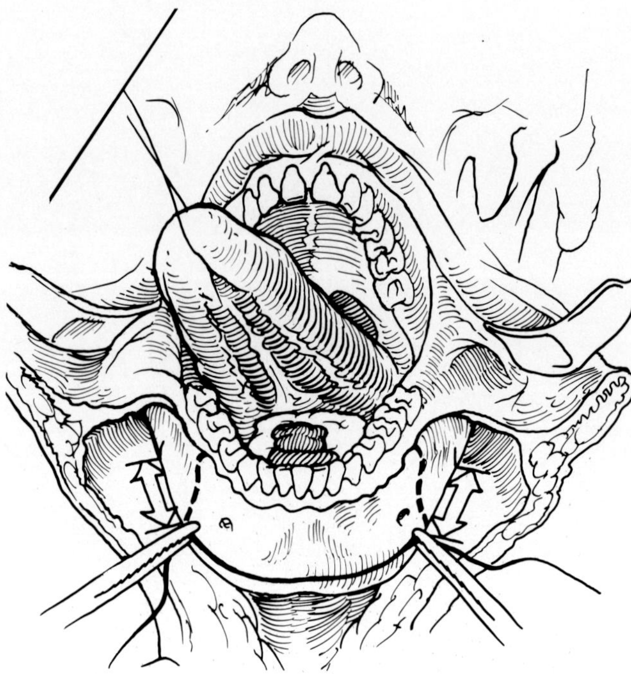

FIG 25–8.
Measuring for width of manibular segments. (From Price JC: Management of large anterior floor-of-mouth malignancies with mandibular invasion, in Bailey BJ (ed): *Surgery of the Oral Cavity.* Chicago, Year Book Medical Publishers, 1989, pp 103–115. Used by permission.)

The template is removed and a corresponding bar bent to the template. A bar 2 cm shorter than the template should be selected and bent to allow reduction in the anterior projection and outer circumference while preserving the angles and relative position of the mounting segments (Fig 25–10). This reduces pressure on the skin of the chin and relieves tension from the intraoral closure. The completed bar is tagged for reference with a suture through the end corresponding to the right side of the patient, then placed on the back table along with the preselected screws.

Bone cuts may be made with numerous devices, including the Gigli saw, large compressed air- or electric-powered oscillating or reciprocating saws, and rotary drills. (Fig 25–11). The new generation of micro saws (either reciprocating or oscillating) are preferred because they produce a much cleaner cut, less loss of bone substance, less overheating of bone, less local soft tissue trauma, and considerable reduction of mechanical energy transferred into the tumor

The mandibular specimen is retracted downward with bone clamps as the tongue is elevated with either towel clips or 0 silk traction sutures. The tumor is carefully inspected and margins marked with electrocautery 2 cm beyond any palpable induration. Tissue transection will generally follow through the floor of the mouth, the mylohyoid, the anterior belly of the digastric, the geniohyoid, the genioglossus, and the intrinsic muscles of the tongue. The specimen is removed and carefully inspected with the pathologist in attendance.

A pectoralis major or latissimus dorsi myocutaneous flap is then designed and deployed into the defect. The posterior (inferior) border is sewn to the posterior oral cavity margin.

The preformed bar is then secured into its permanent position; the screws are tightened only after all have been placed (Fig 25–12). The margins of the transected mandible are smoothed with a rongeur and a power drill to remove threat of perforation of mucosa, transection of sutures by bone, or extrusion of bone spicules. Final closure of the flap to the buccal mucosa is completed.

Closure of the lip begins with placement of a 3-0 polyglycolic acid (PGA) suture deep within the substance of the orbicularis oris muscle at the level of the vermilion border. Note that identical bites of equal position, depth, and width must be taken on both sides (Fig 25–13). This suture is then tied in a secure, nonstrangulating fashion. This is the keystone to accurate reconstruction of the lip, and it must be precise to prevent lip deformity and notching. Inverted sutures are placed in the muscle at each of the four points resulting from the Z-plasty and at each cutaneous mark in the chin and lower lip. Additional sutures are placed as required to achieve an accurate muscular closure. The lip mucosa and vermilion are closed with running interlocking 3-0 PGA. The skin of the lip and chin is closed with running 5-0 nylon. Flat 10 mm Silastic drains are placed in the posterior cervical triangle and along the anterior border of the flap, as previously discussed. These are loosely tacked into position with 3-0 chromic sutures. Next the platysmal layer is closed with interrupted inverted 3-0 PGA sutures until an airtight closure has been obtained. The skin is closed with stainless steel surgical staples. The chest donor site is closed primarily, after placement of two flat 10 mm drains connected to constant negative pressure drainage. Specific instructions are given that nothing should be applied around the neck, including tracheotomy tapes and elastic bands for tracheotomy collars.

LATERAL MANDIBULAR DEFECTS

There are five primary options for management of lateral mandibular defects: primary closure, closure with intraoral skin graft, soft tissue flap closure, 3-DBRP with myocutaneous flap, and primary bone and flap reconstruction. Acceptable, even good results can be attained by any of the first three methods. Each has relative merits and may present a "best choice" in a particular situation. Primary bone grafting without microvascular transfer should not be done. Microvascular osseomyocutaneous flap reconstruction may present an excellent option in selected cases (e.g., full-thickness cheek and mandible and massive defects). Good to excellent results may be achieved by other methods, and extended microvascular repairs may not be the best choice for repair of the conventional "lateral composite" resection.

The 3-DBRP and pectoralis major or latissimus myocutaneous flap technique provides uncomplicated healing in more than 95% of patients. The active soft tissue support of the face, cheek, and neck shield the bar from the adverse effect of a pendulous flap. Suture lines are more reliably directed away

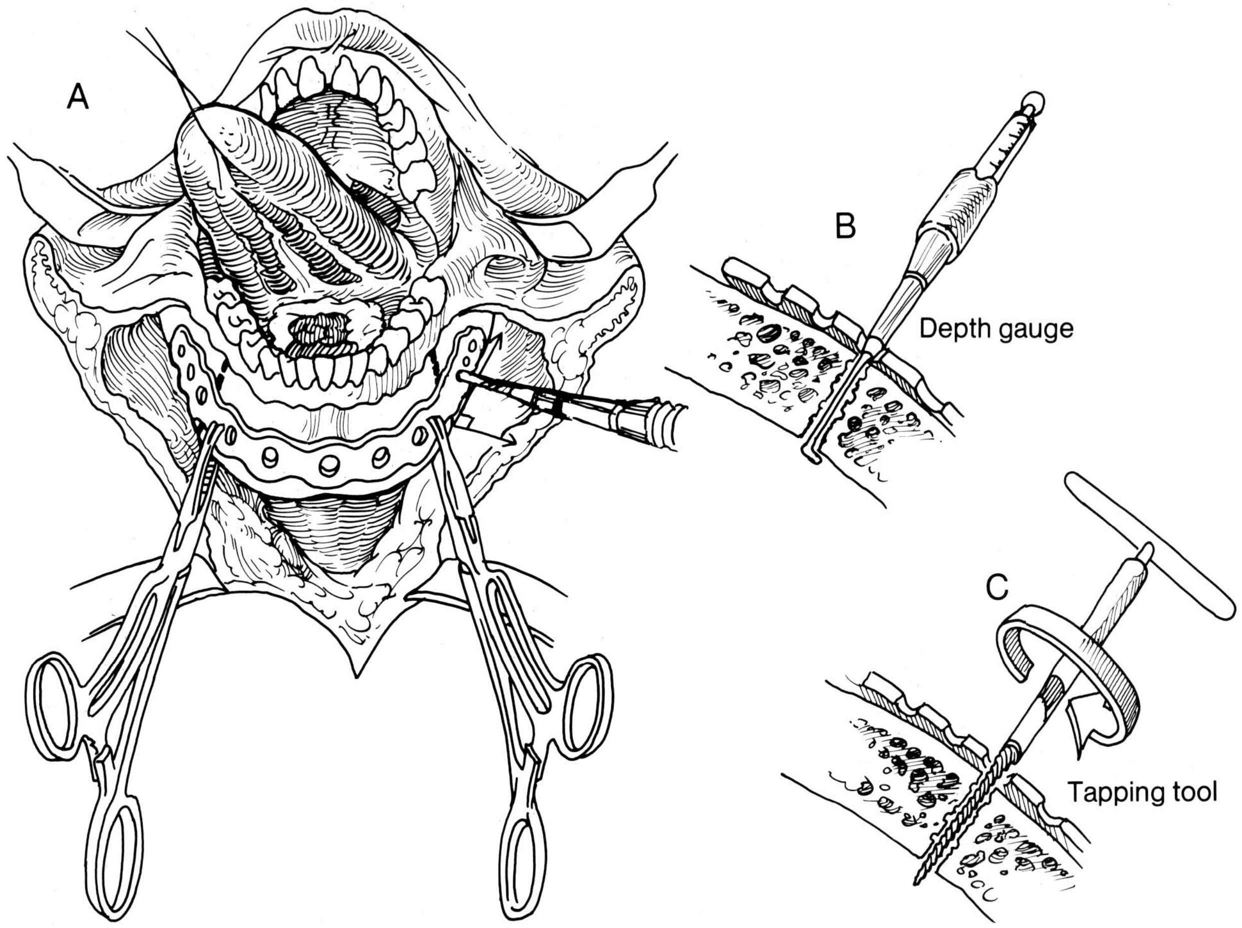

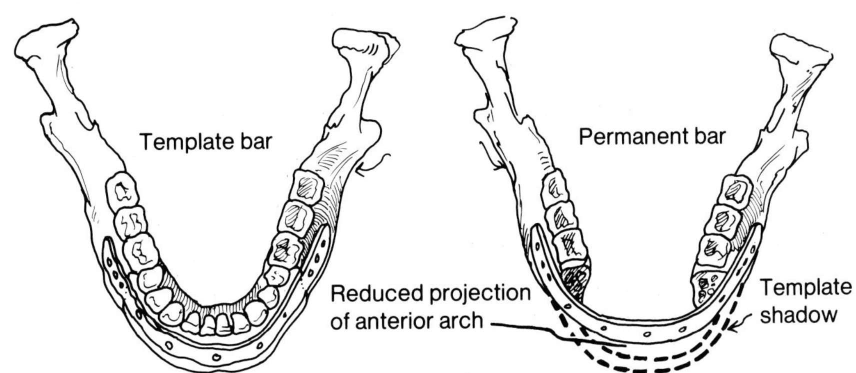

FIG 25–9.
A–C, contouring template and preparing screw holes. (From Price JC: Management of large anterior floor-of-mouth malignancies with mandibular invasion, in Bailey BJ (ed): *Surgery of the Oral Cavity.* Chicago, Year Book Medical Publishers, 1989, pp 103–115. Used by permission.)

FIG 25–10.
Contouring permanent bar. (From Price JC: Management of large anterior floor-of-mouth malignancies with mandibular invasion, in Bailey BJ (ed): *Surgery of the Oral Cavity.* Chicago, Year Book Medical Publishers, 1989, pp 103–115. Used by permission.)

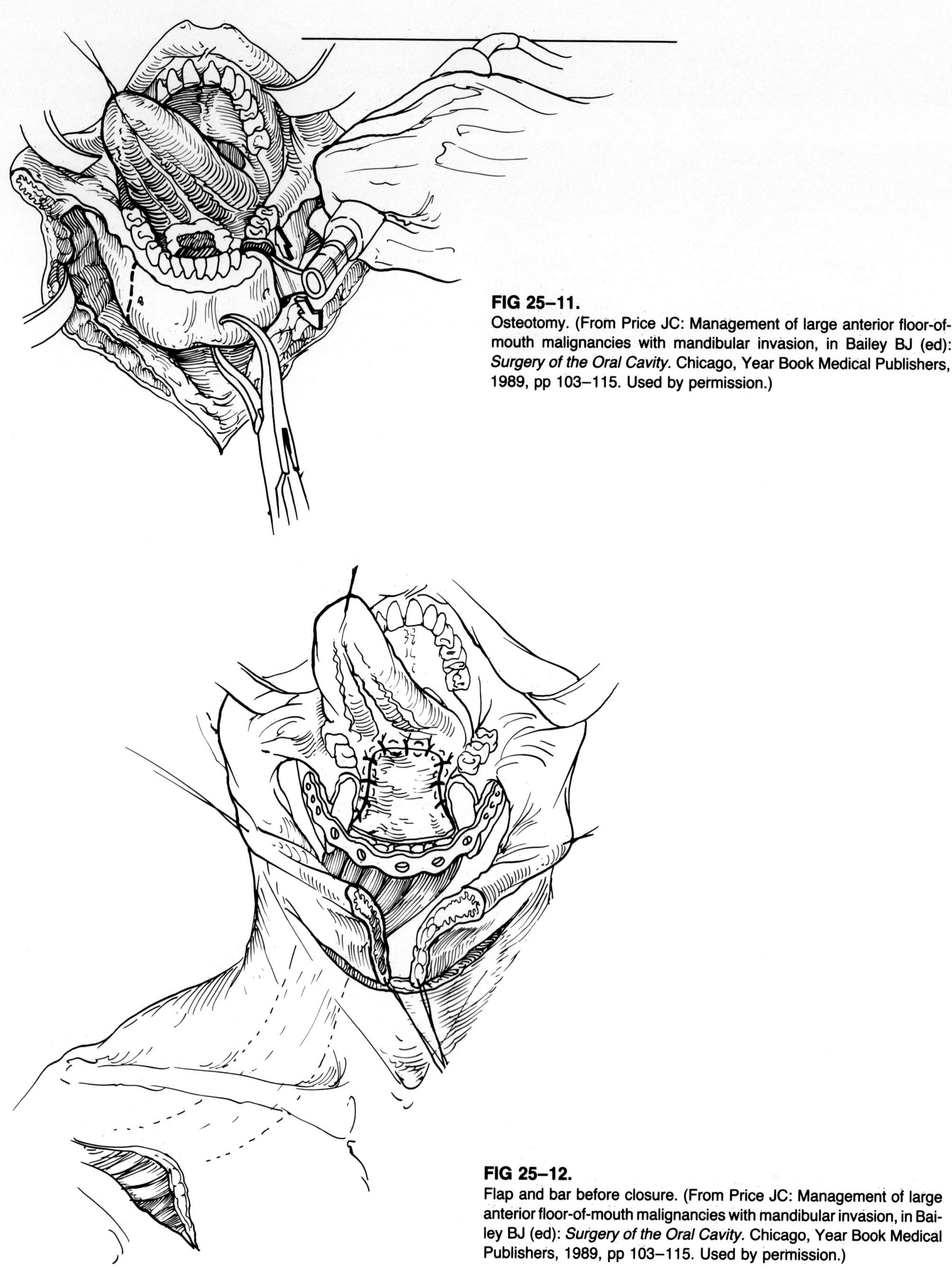

FIG 25–11.
Osteotomy. (From Price JC: Management of large anterior floor-of-mouth malignancies with mandibular invasion, in Bailey BJ (ed): *Surgery of the Oral Cavity*. Chicago, Year Book Medical Publishers, 1989, pp 103–115. Used by permission.)

FIG 25–12.
Flap and bar before closure. (From Price JC: Management of large anterior floor-of-mouth malignancies with mandibular invasion, in Bailey BJ (ed): *Surgery of the Oral Cavity*. Chicago, Year Book Medical Publishers, 1989, pp 103–115. Used by permission.)

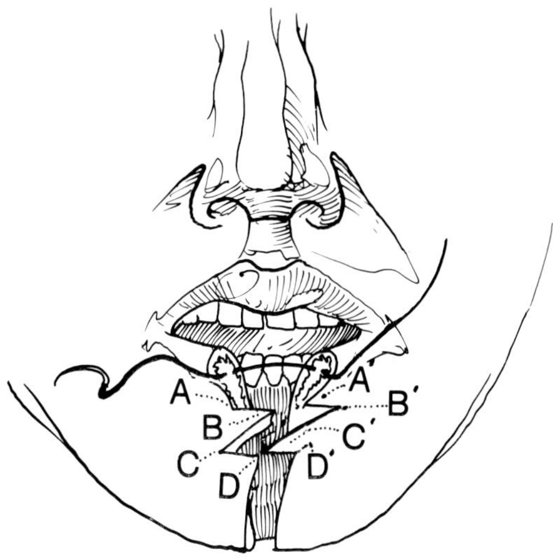

FIG 25–13.
Closure of lip. (From Price JC: Management of large anterior floor-of-mouth malignancies with mandibular invasion, in Bailey BJ (ed): *Surgery of the Oral Cavity*. Chicago, Year Book Medical Publishers, 1989, pp 103–115. Used by permission.)

from intimate contact with the superior surface of the bar. Exposure of the bar has not been a significant problem. Long-term retention of many of these prostheses has allowed development of late complications: loosening of screws, plate fracture from metal fatigue, hematogenous infection, and (rarely) delayed exposure of the plate. These are unusual and account for most of the 5% considered as unsatisfactory results.

The condyle and neck should be preserved whenever possible. The mechanical details of plate bending make accurate alignment of the currently available condylar prostheses difficult. Metal prostheses have been reported to penetrate the condylar fossa and enter the cranial cavity in at least two cases. Both occurred in temporomandibular point surgery, where the muscles of mastication retained their normal attachments. The prostheses used in reconstruction after tumor ablation tend to migrate out of the condylar fossa, and it is unlikely that a similar complication would result when the muscles are removed or completely detached.

TOTAL MANDIBULAR DEFECT

Any mandibular defect resulting from tumor ablation encompassing a condyle to the contralateral mental foramen or beyond may, for practical purposes, be considered a "total" defect. Replacement would require from 20 to 30 cm of bone or even more *after* contouring for accurate replacement. This could be reduced somewhat by "undersizing" the contour of the anterior arch. Bone requirement would still exceed the length of reliable bone available from one adult fibula or iliac donor site. At least two separate bone-carrying microvascular flaps would be required. A squamous cell carcinoma large enough

to require this massive ablation is not a good operative candidate and would be managed in another manner. A massive benign tumor (ameloblastoma) or unusual low-grade carcinoma (e.g., intraosseous mucoepidermoid carcinoma) could present such an opportunity. Alternatives might include primary closure or complete extraoral excision and reconstruction with a custom titanium tray filled with compressed particulate cancellous bone or microvascular bone flap(s) laterally, with the anterior arch spanned by titanium mesh tray and particulate cancellous bone.

PECTORALIS MAJOR MYOCUTANEOUS FLAP

Technique

Flap dimensions are determined by locating the coracoid process of the scapula immediately beneath the inferior margin of the clavicle and marking this spot (Fig 25–14). The first measurement *(I)* is taken from that point directly across the resection bed to the defect margin and represents the distance from the pedicle origin to the base of the skin island. The second measurement *(II)* is taken from the posterior to the anterior defect margins. Determination of the correct position is facilitated by temporarily positioning a paper or cloth template of the defect into the chest. Transverse measurement *(III)* of the defect is taken at its greatest width. The addition of 1 cm or more to the width and length of the skin island deliberately oversizes the flap to allow for proper draping without tension. The shape of the cutaneous paddle should approximate that of the defect. Measurement *I* plus the length of the skin island equals the total length of the flap (Fig 25–15). These measurements will approximate 23 × 8 × 8 cm in most patients. This usually requires little or no random segment along the distal flap margin.

The flap is designed with methylene blue marking pen on the ipsilateral side of the chest, and the skin paddle is sharply released down to the pectoralis major fascia. The surgeon must exercise extreme care to avoid applying shearing forces to the skin island (no traction or countertraction should be applied). After hemostasis is obtained, the dermis of the flap is tacked to the superficial pectoral fascia with 8 or 10 interrupted absorbable 3-0 sutures. Incision is then carried along the lateral margin of the pectoralis major muscle to the apex of the axilla. Skin and soft tissue is sharply elevated from the fascia of the pectoralis major muscle to the deltopectoral groove, clavicle, and lateral border of the sternum. A tunnel, large enough to allow easy passage of the outstretched hand (10cm), is developed underneath the cervical and chest flaps. The surgeon carefully identifies the deltopectoral groove and dissects superiorly the brachiocephalic vein. Blunt dissection is carried down to the underlying pectoralis minor muscle. The index finger is passed inferiorly around the humeral attachment and emerges along the inferior border of the insertion, which is then transected with heavy scissors. The lateral inferior border of the muscle is freed from the underlying pectoralis minor and intercostal muscles and the ribs. The soft tissue between the pectoralis major and minor muscles is carefully elevated and preserved with the flap. The dissection is first developed lateral to medial, then is carried around the inferior border of the flap and vertically 2 cm lateral to the sternal border. Release of the sternal origin of the muscle can be carried out boldly all the way to the clavicle. The muscle is retracted upward, the vascular pedicle identified, and final release of the pedicle completed.

The surgeon next passes the flap through the tunnel and tacks it into position with 3-0 PGA sutures on cutting needles, anchoring the base of the skin island to the center of the defect margin. Horizontal mattress sutures are alternated with simple sutures at 5 mm intervals. This provides the most satisfactory approximation of skin to mucosa. Suturing of the skin is adequate without incorporating underlying muscle. Sutures in the tongue and floor of the mouth must be adequately wide and deep to assure both strength of closure and adequate approximation. Remove the tacking sutures between the skin island

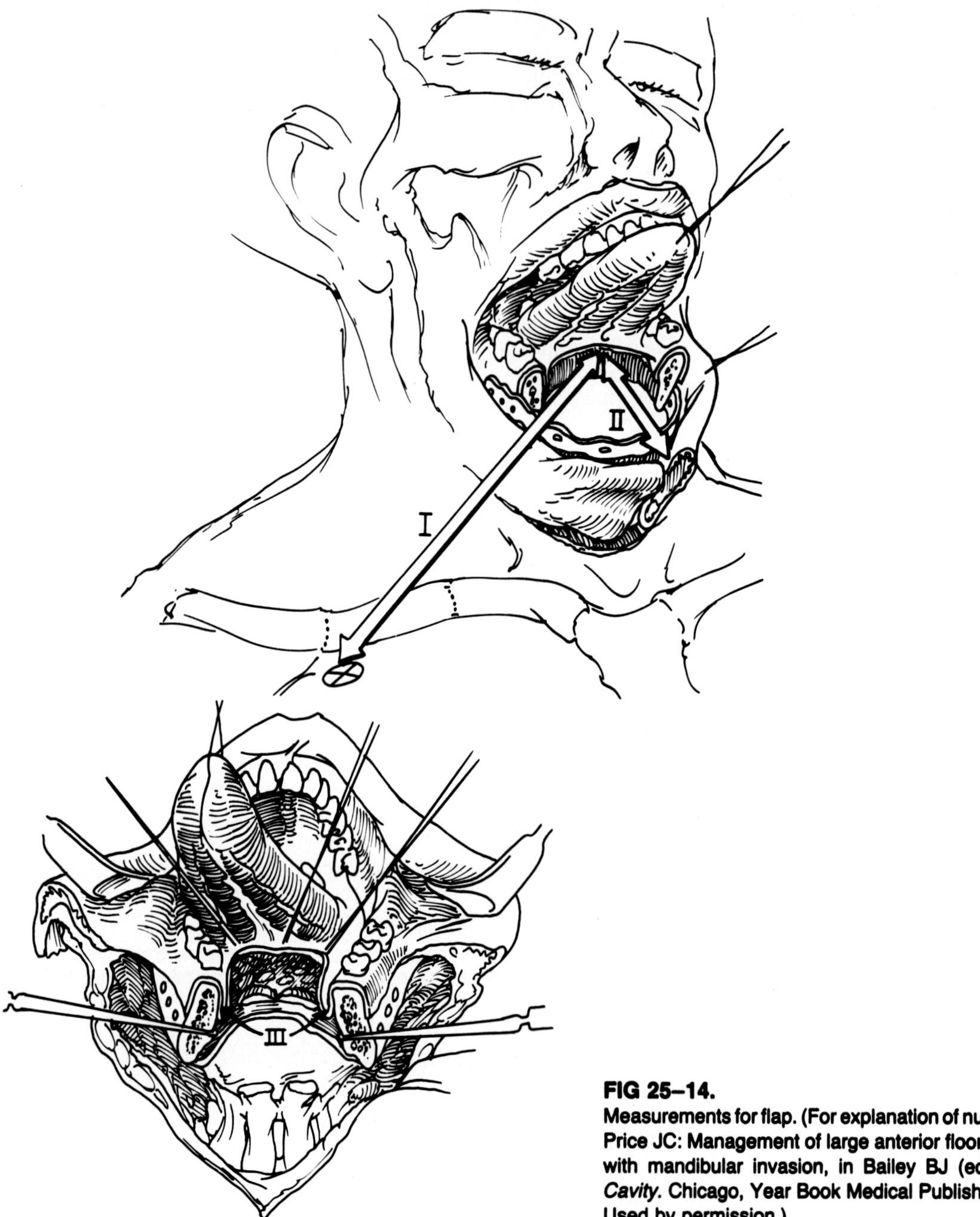

FIG 25–14.
Measurements for flap. (For explanation of numerals, see text.) (From Price JC: Management of large anterior floor-of-mouth malignancies with mandibular invasion, in Bailey BJ (ed): *Surgery of the Oral Cavity.* Chicago, Year Book Medical Publishers, 1989, pp 103–115. Used by permission.)

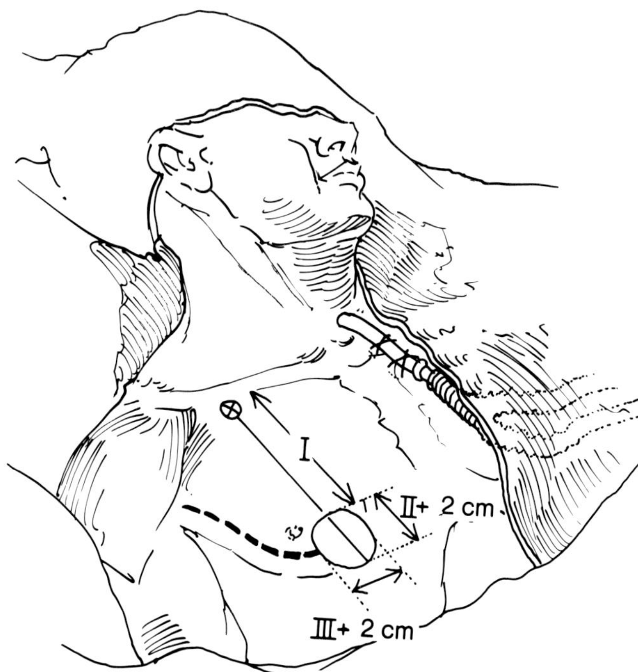

FIG 25–15.
Flap design. (From Price JC: Management of large anterior floor-of-mouth malignancies with mandibular invasion, in Bailey BJ (ed): *Surgery of the Oral Cavity.* Chicago, Year Book Medical Publishers, 1989, pp 103–115. Used by permission.)

and underlying pectoralis fascia as these are replaced by appropriate mucocutaneous sutures; if these sutures are not removed, unacceptable inversion of the suture line may occur. Intraoral defects are closed from back to front. The donor site can usually be closed with minimal tension. Unusually large donor sites may require rotational or advancement flaps or split-thickness skin graft for closure. Two silicone flat suction drains are inserted into the chest wall wound and secured with nylon sutures. A light gauze and antibiotic ointment is placed over the suture line. No ties or constricting bands are allowed around the neck.

Uncertainty of the viability of the vascular supply of the flap may be denoted by (1) pale white coloration of the flap, (2) absence of bleeding from the subdermal vascular plexus, or (3) absence of a "blanch and refill" response. This should stimulate the surgeon to further investigation. Fluorescein (1 ampule in white patients, 2 ampules in darker skinned patients) is administered intravenously and the flap viewed under black light 15 minutes later. Perfusion is indicated by a speckling of yellow-green fluorescence in the skin. A flat, dark blue coloration predicts failure of that section of the flap. A search for any undue tension on the skin island or pedicle is conducted. The muscle pedicle must be free of torsion, kinks, or compression by overlying skin flaps, hematomas, or suction drains. The vascular pedicle itself must be carefully inspected. If there is any suspicion that arterial or vascular injury has occurred, careful microscopic observation is required

Postoperatively the flap should be warm and pinkish. The chest skin normally has a much lighter coloration than that of the neck and face and may confuse the observer. Blanch and refill should be present; if not, the fluorescein test may be conducted at the bedside. A Doppler examination of the flap pedicle may be helpful. Any suspicion of vascular compromise must be followed by careful assessment for tension, compression, constricting bands, and hematoma. Correction of mechanical problems should restore flap circulation. If pallor or cyanosis persists or if epidermolysis develops, medical therapy is directed toward decreasing arteriolar and capillary sludging and platelet adhesiveness, with dexamethasone (Decadron), 8 mg IV every 8 hours for three doses; low molecular weight dextran, 500 ml IV infusion over 8 hours for three doses; and lipoheparin 10,000 Units SC every 8 hours for 3 days. Epidermolysis is likely to progress to demarcation and full-thickness skin loss. No debridement should be attempted until this occurs, however, because some skin survival may be seen and the muscle may remain viable.

A lifted flap that will not reach is to be considered a defect in planning in either flap choice, flap design or flap deployment. If the flap is several centimeters short it should be returned to its donor site and sutured back into position and another flap option selected. If microsurgical capabilities are available and the flap is otherwise viable and of adequate size to repair the defect, transection of the pedicle and transfer to recipient vessels in the neck may be considered. If the flap is only 1 to 3 cm short, enough additional length may be gained by transecting the clavicle immediately above the pedicle, transposing the pedicle underneath the clavicle, and repairing the bone.

Confirmed intraoperative injury to the pedicle of the pectoralis major myocutaneous flap must be dealt with by microsurgical technique. The injured vessel(s) must be freshened back to untraumatized tissue. If sufficient length remains, reanastomosis may be possible. Repair without tension is mandatory; otherwise transfer to recipient vessels in the neck is desirable. An alternative salvage method is sacrifice of the damaged flap and substitution of a trapezius, latissimus, or contralateral pectoralis flap.

REFERENCES

1. Lawson W, Baek SM, Lascalzo LJ, et al: Experience with immediate and delayed mandibular reconstruction. *Laryngoscope* 1982; 92:5–10.
2. Chow JM, Hill JH: Primary mandibular reconstruction using the A-O reconstruction plate. *Laryngoscope* 1986; 96:768–773.
3. Gullane PJ, Holmes H: Mandibular reconstruction: New concepts. *Arch Otolaryngol Head Neck Surg* 1986; 112:714–719.
4. Kellman RM, Gullane PJ: Use of the AO mandibular reconstruction plate for bridging of mandibular defects. *Otolaryngol Clin North Am* 1987; 20:519–533.
5. Papel ID, Price JC, Kashima HK, et al: Compression plates in the treatment of advanced anterior floor of mouth carcinoma. *Laryngoscope* 1986; 96:722–725.

6. DeFries HO, Marble HB, Sell KW: Reconstruction of the mandible: Use of a homograft combined with autogenous bone and marrow. *Arch Otolaryngol* 1971; 93:426.

7. Leipzig B, Cummings CW: The current status of mandibular reconstruction using autogenous frozen mandibular grafts. *Head Neck Surg* 6:922–996.

8. Hamaker RC, Singer MI: Irradiated mandibular autografts update. *Arch Otolaryngol Head Neck Surg* 1986; 112:277–279.

9. Price JC: Management of large anterior floor-of-mouth malignancies with mandibular invasion, in Bailey BJ (ed): *Surgery of the Oral Cavity.* Chicago, Year Book Medical Publishers, 1989, pp 103–115.

10. Price JC, Davis RK: The deltopectoral flap vs. the pectoralis major myocutaneous flap. Which one? *Arch Otolaryngol* 1984; 110:35–40.

11. Ariyan S: The pectoralis major myocutaneous flap: A versatile flap for reconstruction in the head and neck. *Plast Reconstr Surg* 1979; 63:73–81.

12. Baek S, Biller HG, Krespi YP, et al: The pectoralis major myocutaneous island flap for reconstruction of the head and neck. *Head Neck Surg* 1979; 1:293–300.

13. Ariyan S: Further experiences with the pectoralis major myocutaneous flap for the immediate repair of defects from excisions of head and neck cancers. *Plast Reconstr Surg* 1979; 64:605–612.

14. Ariyan S, Cuono C: Myocutaneous flaps for head and neck reconstruction. *Head Neck Surg* 1980; 2:321–345.

CHAPTER 26

Maxillofacial Trauma

Approach of

Robert M. Kellman, M.D.

The assessment and management of maxillofacial trauma patients will often depend on their mode of presentation. Complex and severe injuries often occur in the multiply traumatized patient, typically due to motor vehicle accidents or industrial mishaps. Initial management of these patients frequently entails hemodynamic stabilization and airway access, so that the assessment of facial injuries is often delayed and difficult. Even after we are consulted, necessary radiographic evaluation is often delayed, and we are often told that repair of facial injuries must be delayed until further hemodynamic and neurologic stabilization. This approach has allowed the maxillofacial surgeon to await the resolution of facial edema and has also given us the freedom to plan the surgical repair (and even schedule the surgery) and prepare prostheses, so that it has become an acceptable standard to wait anywhere from 5 to 7 days to as many as 21 to 28 days before proceeding with the major surgical repair. This approach has recently been called into question, and it has been suggested that an earlier and more expeditious repair of facial skeletal injuries will result in less soft tissue injury, scarification, and redraping and may ultimately produce better cosmetic results.[1] Since many of these patients suffer head injuries, we urge our emergency department and neurosurgical colleagues to include the face whenever possible when obtaining the initial computed tomography (CT) of the brain (if, of course, there is any suspicion of facial injury). This at least provides us with an earlier radiologic assessment of the facial skeleton so that we can begin planning our repair immediately. Certainly, if any other service is taking the patient to surgery, we try to take advantage of this opportunity to repair the facial injuries. Otherwise, unless our intervention poses a genuine threat to patient survival, we try to perform our repair as soon as it is feasible.

Some patients present to the emergency room with isolated facial injuries. Rapid and thorough assessment can be performed, and treatment can be planned in a timely and expeditious manner for these patients. A third group of patients includes those who ignore (or due to drunkenness or disinterest fail to recognize) their injuries and then present to the outpatient department with partially healed, malpositioned, or infected fractures. In this group, assessment and treatment generally need to be carried out on a relatively urgent basis, since even a possibly acceptable grace period will have already passed, and infectious complications need to be minimized as much as possible.

The first anatomic area to be addressed in this chapter is the orbital area. As a rule, I obtain an ophthalmology consult for all facial injuries in which there is an apparent potential for globe injury. This includes all zygomaticomaxillary ("tripod") fractures as well as all other injuries involving the periorbital bones.[2] Though the overall rate of ocular injury is relatively low, the result of surgical manipulation of the orbit in the presence of a globe rupture or retinal detachment could be catastrophic, and it therefore behooves the maxillofacial surgeon to have this evaluated before the bony repair (whenever possible). If the ophthalmologist believes that surgical manipulation of the orbit will pose a significant risk to vision, bony repair is delayed until this risk abates, sometimes necessitating a more difficult secondary bony reconstruction. If there is concern about optic nerve compression, it must be evaluated immediately, since any possibility of preventing blindness (if this is even possible) would require immediate decompression (see later discussion).

ORBITAL BLOWOUT FRACTURE

The "pure" orbital blowout fracture occurs when a blunt object (e.g., ball or fist) strikes the orbit in such a way that the energy is fairly diffusely absorbed by a large portion of the orbital rims and contents, so that the rim itself is not fractured but the weaker wall or walls of the orbit give way. It has been suggested that blowout fractures can be the result of trauma to the orbital rim without direct trauma to the orbital contents.[3] Fujino, in fact, demonstrated that a force directed at the inferior orbital rim that is not sufficent to fracture the rim will still transmit enough force to fracture the orbital floor.[3] However, as Converse points out, one still has to postulate a force directed against the orbital contents to explain the phenomenon of entrapment of orbital contents in a fracture, since a crack in the floor produced by trauma to the inferior orbital rim would not force orbital contents into the crack.[4] It is certainly possible that both mechanisms come into play in the production of orbital blowout fractures. Of significant importance here is that since it is most likely that a force directed against the orbital contents plays a role in the occurrence of the blowout fracture, one must always consider the possibility of globe rupture when assessing an orbital blowout fracture. If a minimal injury is missed, the effects of surgical manipulation of the globe when repairing the orbit could prove disastrous. Fortunately, the globe does seem to be somewhat protected and cushioned by the orbital fat and muscles.

Most commonly, the orbital floor is displaced inferiorly into the maxillary sinus. The thin lamina papyracea of the medial wall frequently fractures, but it is less frequently significantly displaced than the floor. The lateral wall may fracture as well, and the superior wall is least likely to fracture without an accompanying rim fracture.[4]

An "impure" blowout fracture occurs when a blowout fracture of the orbital wall is associated with a fracture of the orbital rim. For example, herniation of orbital contents and enophthalmos may be seen in association with a LeFort II fracture, and the enophthalmos may be said to be due to an impure blowout fracture. However, I prefer to reserve the term blowout fracture for the pure blowout fracture (i.e., without associated orbital rim fractures). Other fractures can then be described by the actual injuries that have occurred. When a large defect is produced in one or more of the orbital walls, the orbital contents generally herniate into the defect, thereby allowing the globe to drop posteriorly and most often inferiorly within the orbital cavity. This produces an inferiorly displaced globe and enophthalmos. Enophthalmos occurs because the defect in one or more of the orbital walls increases the orbital volume, thereby allowing the globe to drop back into the orbital cone.[5] When large defects are present, orbital contents will herniate through these defects, thereby further decreasing the amount of tissue supporting the globe in the relatively enlarged orbital cavity, resulting in greater degrees of enophthalmos. Diplopia may be produced due to the change in globe position, though an actual entrapment of orbital tissues is not very likely in a large bony defect. On the other hand, when the defect or crack in an orbital wall is small, any herniating orbital tissue is more likely to remain trapped in the bony defect; thus, a crack or small defect is more likely to produce entrapment. Entrapment most frequently involves the inferior rectus muscle, which can be easily caught in a crack in the orbital floor, and this results in significant limitation of the motion of the involved eye. Of course, other muscles can be affected, and even entrapment of orbital fat can

lead to decreased ocular motility.[6] Diplopia due to impaired motility may also be secondary to neural or direct muscular injury.

With the previous discussion in mind, we can develop an algorithm for the evaluation and treatment of these injuries. The keys to the assessment of orbital blowout fractures are the physical examination and the CT scan. The CT scan should include axials and true coronals (not reconstructions). As previously noted, an ophthalmologic evaluation of a suspected orbital injury is of paramount importance. Evidence of an optic nerve injury should be correlated with high-resolution CT evaluation of the optic canal. Although the benefits of optic nerve decompression remain controversial, it is essential to document the status of vision and follow it carefully. When the patient presents with blindness that occurred acutely, decompression is unlikely to be helpful. However, if severe visual loss develops secondarily, most would recommend treatment with high-dose steroids and would consider decompression if visual loss progressed or failed to improve. When neurosurgical intervention is necessary for other reasons, the optic canal can be safely and easily approached from above via the anterior fossa. When an extracranial approach is indicated, many ophthalmologists favor the lateral orbitotomy approach,[7] whereas otolaryngologists tend to be most comfortable with one of the transethmoid approaches.[8] Note that in the unconscious patient with evidence of optic canal injury on CT scan, the use of visual evoked responses may provide information as to the presence of vision acutely as well as allow for observation of the progress or deterioration of vision.

Once optic nerve and ocular concerns are ruled out or taken care of, we can now deal with the issue of globe displacement, entrapment, and bony reconstruction. As noted earlier, entrapment is generally associated with cracks and smaller fractures. Entrapment can affect muscles in any of the four quadrants (inferior, medial, lateral, and superior), though the inferior rectus is by far the most commonly affected muscle, and the medial rectus is a distant second. In addition to pain on movement of the eye, the patient will complain of diplopia, usually on upward gaze when the inferior rectus is involved and on lateral gaze when the medial rectus is entrapped, though diplopia can be seen in all fields due to voluntary guarding secondary to pain. On examination, limitation of upward gaze suggests inferior rectus entrapment, and limitation of lateral gaze suggests medial rectus involvement. A forced duction test is mandatory, since muscle contusion or neural injury can produce similar findings, but these are clearly not indications for surgical intervention. In the absence of enophthalmos or globe malposition, it is reasonable to wait 5 to 7 days before exploration, since an entrapped muscle may be released as the swelling subsides. However, I believe that waiting beyond this time (as advocated by Putterman[9]) is not recommended, since delayed repairs will likely provide a suboptimal result. When significant enophthalmos is present or the globe is obviously displaced, surgery should be carried out as soon as possible, since delaying surgery offers no benefits but does allow for the buildup of scar tissue, which serves only to make surgery more difficult and may limit the effectiveness as well. The definition of significant enophthalmos is more difficult. Two to 3 mm of difference is often considered clinically significant. I believe that 2 mm is significant if it is associated with a clinically obvious difference when the patient is observed. On the other hand, a measured difference of up to 3 mm will be tolerated if it is not clinically apparent and is not associated with an obvious globe displacement or diplopia. Sometimes minor differences in appearance can be significantly improved by recessing the upper lid, since it is lid position that often exaggerates the appearance of enophthalmos. This should be kept in mind, since unlike orbital reconstruction, there is virtually no risk of causing blindness or worsening diplopia. Enophthalmos of more than 3 mm should probably be repaired. Furthermore, extensive defects such as those involving the entire orbital floor should be repaired as well. Malposition of the globe creates both a cosmetic and a functional defect, frequently resulting in difficulty fusing the images seen by the two eyes. The globe will generally drift in the direction of an extensive bony defect, though the reverse can be seen as well, such as a medially displaced and proptotic globe due to medial and inward displacement of a zygomatic fracture. Finally, when extensive facial fractures that involve the orbit, such as Le Fort II and III fractures and comminuted zygomatic and nasoethmoid fractures are repaired, the orbit should be explored and its bony structure reconstituted after the facial bones are repositioned.

Orbital floor exploration is generally carried out via the subciliary incision using a skin crease 2 to 3 mm below the lid margin.* After the skin is incised, a skin flap is elevated above the orbicularis muscle for a few millimeters in a stepladder fashion, so that during healing the skin is less likely to get pulled down onto the bone by scar tissue. The muscle is then opened, taking care not to penetrate the orbital septum. The periosteum is incised just inferior to the inferior orbital rim, and it is carefully elevated off the orbital floor. The orbital contents are retracted superiorly with orbital retractors or malleable retractors, often walking the retractors over each other to minimize the herniation of orbital contents into the field. The orbital contents are teased out of the maxillary sinus, taking care not to injure the infraorbital nerve, which is particularly vulnerable in the floor of the orbit. (If anesthesia of this nerve is not present preoperatively, the patient should be warned that it may be present postoperatively.) When entrapment is present, it may be necessary to further fracture the orbital floor into the maxillary sinus to release the entrapped tissue. Once this tissue has been released, the floor must be reconstructed so that reentrapment does not take place. For a small crack, a thin piece of silicone rubber (Silastic) sheeting may be adequate; absorbable gelatin film (Gelfilm) or lyophilized dura may be used as well. If autogenous tissue is preferred, a thin piece of bone from the front face of the maxilla may be harvested (particularly if maxillary sinus exposure was necessary to help in the reduction of the orbital tissues), or nasal septal cartilage or bone may be used. Although prolonged antral packing may work when the orbital floor fragments are present and fully reduced, I prefer

repairing and supporting the defect from above. If antral packing is to be used, I would suggest a Foley balloon or tissue expander rather than actual packing. Most important, the antrum should not be packed blindly from below. Larger defects cannot be properly repaired without the placement of a graft. Again, alloplasts are used by many with satisfactory results[10]; however, I prefer autogenous bone. The rib is particularly well suited to orbital reconstruction since split rib can be bent nicely without breaking and will often conform nicely to the desired shape. Split calvarium may be easily accessible, especially when a coronal approach is being used. The best way to repair globe depression or malposition, as well as enophthalmos, is to restore the orbital cavity as closely as possible to its normal anatomic construction.[1] Aichmair and Fries[11] (as cited by Luhr) suggest that volume replacement is an excellent guide to repair, using a 0.5 cc volume of implant for each 1 mm of enophthalmos. The inferior medial wall may be approached through the lower lid incision, but the upper medial wall is best approached through a coronal or an external ethmoidectomy incision. The superior and lateral walls are best approached via a coronal incision, though various brow incisions may be used as well. After placement of any grafts, an intraoperative forced duction test must be performed to make certain that the graft is not interfering with ocular motility. Grafts should be stabilized as rigidly as possible, wired or plated when feasible (e.g., Timesh, as advocated by Manson and Iliff[1]), to prevent migration and resorption. If possible, the periosteum is tacked together. The muscle and skin are laid in position, and a single-layer skin closure is carried out. A Frost stitch (a stitch from the lower lid tarsus taped to the forehead under gentle tension) is placed for 12 to 24 hours. Visual checks are carried out frequently during the first 24 hours.

In summary, the key to the repair of entrapment, globe malposition, enophthalmos and loss of orbital bone is the careful exploration and reconstruction of the bony orbital walls to as near an anatomic shape as possible. It is important to warn the patient that more than one procedure may be necessary to achieve the desired result.

Injuries in this area may be associated with eyelid injuries. In repair of eyelid injuries, several key principles come into play. First is the protection of the cornea. The cornea should not be left unprotected or allowed to dry. The next point is that as much tissue as possible should be saved. Avulsed portions can often be replaced as free grafts, and partially avulsed tissue should be debrided as conservatively as possible. Finally, the repair should be performed to recreate the original anatomic construction as closely as possible. The tarsal plate should be accurately realigned and sutured with a fine, absorbable suture, avoiding penetration of the conjunctiva. (I use the microscope for this.) The lid margin is carefully lined up and sutured prior to repair of the tarsus and skin. The skin is then closed, reapproximating the orbicularis muscle as closely as possible. If there has been conjunctival loss, it should be grafted from another lid or with some oral mucosa. A tarsoconjunctival flap can be advanced when necessary also. Muscle injuries should be approximated as closely as possible as well, since return of motor function is most important. When ptosis results, muscle shortening procedures can be carried out subsequently once

---

*I have had bad luck with the immediate subciliary incision, and the lower lid incision often results in postoperative lower lid edema when carried laterally. A transconjunctival approach can be used in association with a lateral canthotomy.

healing has occurred. Complete eyelid loss presents a potentially devastating problem if corneal protection is not accomplished. Using the tarsus and conjunctiva of the opposing lid, one can sew it to the remaining edge of conjunctiva of the avulsed lid, thereby providing protection for the cornea while the remaining reconstruction is planned. If the avulsed lid is available, it can be grafted into place. Similarly, skin can be borrowed from the remaining eyelids either as grafts or flaps. Finally, a completely lost lower lid can be replaced using a cheek advancement flap. Of note is that when the eyelid is reconstructed, a firm structure should be used to replace the lost tarsal plate. Fascia lata has been used, but cartilage such as nasal septal or lower lateral cartilage provides an excellent source for a graft and is preferred.

Lacerations through the eyelids and medial orbital fractures may injure the lacrimal system and the medial canthal ligament. A canalicular injury is repaired over a stent. A silicone tube is placed through the two portions, and the canaliculus is sutured together under the microscope using very fine suture (usually 10–0). When both the upper and lower canaliculi are injured, the procedure is the same except that the tubing is placed through both canaliculi so that the loop stays in the region of the caruncle and the two ends of the tubing are sutured in the nose. The canaliculi are repaired over the tubing. If the lacrimal sac is injured, a dacryocystorhinostomy is carried out. I prefer an anteroposterior nasal flap sutured to anteroposterior flaps created in the lacrimal sac. This should decrease the likelihood of stenosis of the newly created duct.

Ruptures of the canthal tendons, medial or lateral, must be repaired with permanent suture. The lateral canthal tendon should be reapproximated or wired into the lateral orbit, deep to the lateral orbital rim. Failure to do so will allow it to drop, resulting in an antimongoloid slant to the palpebral fissure, as well as a horizontal shortening. Similarly, the medial canthal ligament should be repaired. If the ends cannot be reapproximated, the ligament should be reattached to the anterior lacrimal crest using transnasal wiring (see later discussion of nasoethmoid complex fractures).

MIDFACE FRACTURES

The approach to midfacial LeFort fractures has evolved greatly during the last 10 to 15 years. The traditional approach using intermaxillary fixation and craniofacial suspension, though still commonplace, is no longer accepted unquestioningly.[12–14] The advent of rigid internal fixation for the repair of facial fractures[15–17] has led to direct interosseous stable fixation of the facial skeleton to the skull, thereby decreasing the dependence on indirect methods like craniofacial suspension. Craniofacial suspension is, indeed, an indirect method of fixation, because it is applied across a distance (from the maxillary arch to either the zygomatic arch or frontal bone) without direct control over the positions of the intervening fragments. Craniofacial suspension wiring has been advocated to prevent the occurrence of facial elongation that can result when intermaxillary fixation is used without fixing the intervening facial skeleton directly to the skull. Mandibular pull can then pull the comminuted mid-

facial bones inferiorly. However, craniofacial suspension wires are often applied blindly, so that in the effort to prevent facial elongation, tightening of these wires can often produce facial foreshortening with overlapping of the comminuted midfacial fragments. Furthermore, the pull on the anterior maxilla is often directed somewhat posteriorly so that inward rotation of the nasal root may occur as well. This rotation can lead to an anterior open bite as well as facial shortening. When the maxillae are rigidly positioned against the zygomas and skull and fixed with rigid fixation devices, neither lengthening nor foreshortening is possible. In addition, advances in craniofacial surgery have been applied in maxillofacial trauma surgery, most notably the wide exposure provided by the coronal incision and the versatility offerd by primary bone grafting with rib and split calvarium. This has led to more direct and accurate repositioning and reconstruction of the facial skeleton after extensive facial injuries.

The most important aspects of LeFort fracture repair are the restoration of the functional portions of the facial skeleton. The orbits have been discussed with regard to globe position and function. Restoration of occlusion is also of critical importance so that masticatory function can be reestablished. Although the use of rigid internal (plate) fixation may often obviate the need for intermaxillary fixation (IMF) during the healing period,[17] IMF must still be used intraoperatively to establish the occlusal relationships. Thus, in repair of any LeFort fractures, IMF is first established with arch bars (or splints, if necessary) before proceeding with direct repair of bony fractures. When mandibular fractures are present also, they are generally repaired after the occlusion has been established, and the LeFort fractures are repaired from the stable to the unstable[14] or, as Champy et al. have described,[18] from the periphery toward the center. This allows for an orderly step-by-step repair of the often comminuted and difficult to align fragments. Once the skeletal position has been reestablished, attention is turned to the reconstruction of the orbital contour (as described earlier).

In a discusion of the approach to LeFort facial fractures, it is easier to start with the most complex LeFort III fractures and work toward the simpler LeFort I fractures. This is similar to the clinical approach of working from the stable periphery (frontal bones) toward the unstable center. Indeed, LeFort III fractures are rarely pure (i.e., with an intact facial skeleton that is completely separated from the skull) but, rather, impure (i.e., complex combinations of LeFort I, II, and III components).[12, 19] Therefore, as one works downward from the frontal bones, sequentially stabilizing the frontal bones to the zygomas, the zygomas to the upper maxillae, and the upper maxillae to the lower occlusal portions, one is stepwise converting a LeFort III to a LeFort II and ultimately to a LeFort I fracture.

With functional occlusion already established, the object now is to reestablish the proper facial shape and contour, both in the anteroposterior and vertical dimensions. This is done by first repairing the buttresses of the facial skeleton.[12, 20] An important determinant of facial height is the vertical ramus of the mandible in its relationship to the skull.[12] Thus, the presence of bilateral subcondylar fractures of the mandible in association with bilateral LeFort III fractures may necessitate the open reduction of at least one, if not both, of the subcondylar fractures.

When the midface is not severely comminuted, it may occasionally be possible to reestablish vertical height without opening the subcondylar fractures by first rigidly repairing the midface and then fixing the mandibular position against the maxilla. With the mandibular rami intact, the midfacial vertical position is established by fixing the vertical dimension from the frontonasal junction down across the pyriform aperture to the anterior dental arch. Posteriorly, fixation is carried out from the front-zygomatic area down across the zygomaticomaxillary area to the posterior dental arch. These bones should be rigidly fixed together using miniplates specifically designed for this purpose (which plating system is used is not as important as the skill and comfort of the surgeon with the particular system). The thick lateral orbital rim in the frontozygomatic region can be solidly fixed with a small compression plate, as can the solid zygomaticomaxillary buttress when it is not too badly shattered. The nasofrontal and pyriform regions are generally adapted together with miniplates without compression. At least two screws should be placed on each side of a fracture line whenever possible. It is also of key importance to establish the anteroposterior position of the zygomas along the zygomatic arches, because failure to properly reestablish this dimension has been a common cause of postreduction facial asymmetry in the past. With the routine use of the coronal flap, direct visualization of the zygomatic arch has made possible the identification and avoidance of this problem. For example, the zygomatic root may be sheared off and overlapping, and it is important to identify this and fix the arch in its proper position. Note that it is often difficult to stabilize the multiple small and mobile facial fragments for rigid repair. It is therefore frequently helpful to first reposition the bone fragments using small wires. Then, once the general position of the facial bones has been reestablished, the more exact and rigid positioning can be carried out with miniplates. The actual plating technique is described elsewhere.[21]

Of paramount importance in obtaining satisfactory results using these techniques is adequate exposure. The bicoronal flap has added greatly to the exposure of the frontal region, frontozygomatic regions, zygomatic bones (including the malar eminences and zygomatic arches), and the nasal root (and nasoethmoid region). The maxillae and zygomaticomaxillary regions right up to the infraorbital rims can be comfortably exposed using the midfacial degloving approach through the sublabial gingivobuccal mucosa. Thus, wide exposure can be obtained, and "blind" repair is no longer necessary. When, for any reason, it is decided not to use rigid fixation, judicious application of craniofacial suspension wires can be effected without risking facial foreshortening as might occur with the blind approach.[19] It is also important to pay attention to the proper repositioning of the soft tissues when extensive elevation is carried out. After use of the coronal exposure to the zygoma, the lateral canthus should be sutured back into position inside the lateral orbital rim with a permanent suture or wire.[22] Similarly, the soft tissues overlying the zygoma should be resuspended superiorly to the temporalis fascia or periosteum using permanent suture material[23]; otherwise, a soft tissue droop is almost always seen after this approach has been used.

After the overall position of the buttresses has been established, thereby reconstituting the facial height and anteroposterior dimensions, smaller fragments can be wired or plated to the larger, more stable segments. Small areas of bone loss can be bridged with plates, so that bony reconstruction may be unnecessary. Larger defects, however, generally require bone grafting. This is particularly important when one or more of the buttresses are severely comminuted. In this situation, bone grafting to reestablish the facial dimensions is of great importance.[24] The use of the coronal approach makes split calvarial bone readily accessible. When an associated skull flap has been elevated by the neurosurgeons, inner table bone is used; otherwise, outer table is harvested.[25] Rib grafts are also easily harvested through a lateral thoracic incision over the seventh, eighth, or ninth ribs. Bone grafts are positioned to both bridge a gap and simultaneously serve as a rigid device linking the bones at either end. These should be rigidly fixed with either a plate or preferably one or two lag screws when possible, because a rigidly fixed bone graft is less likely to undergo extensive resorption. As previously noted, the use of rigid fixation has allowed for decreased use of craniofacial suspension. In an early series of Kellman et al.[17] only 2 of 18 LeFort fractures required craniofacial suspension. Furthermore, 5 of 17 LeFort II and III fractures were treated without any postoperative IMF, and only about one half of the patients had tracheotomies. Moreover, only five of nine patients who had LeFort III fractures in association with mandibular fractures required tracheotomies. Thus, rigid fixation allows for other benefits in addition to the direct advantages of solid bony repair.

Extensive soft tissue loss presents a more difficult problem, since facial skin quality is hard to reproduce. Attention should first be turned to the reconstitution of the underlying skeletal anatomy. Rigid fixation of the remaining bones and bone grafts will decrease the likelihood of infection and increase the probability of obtaining bony union. Soft tissue flaps will be needed if healing is to be anticipated. Either pedicled vascularized flaps or free vascularized flaps can be employed. The deltopectoral flap can provide a large amount of healthy skin, though the color and texture are suboptimal. Vascularized mesentery can provide temporary cover or can serve as a base for skin grafting, as can the temporalis muscle flap. For smaller defects, acute tissue expansion can be employed to allow for closure with neighboring skin.

When a laceration involves Stensen's duct or the facial nerve, it is generally repaired. Stensen's duct is exposed in the wound by cannulating it through the intraoral orifice so that the probe passes into the wound. The proximal end can be located by expressing saliva from it. A tube is then passed through the mouth into both segments of the duct. The duct is repaired with fine suture using the microscope, and the tubing is sutured to the oral mucosa and removed after a few weeks. If repair is not feasible, the proximal duct can be ligated. A facial nerve laceration should be carefully explored and the cut ends carefully approximated using 8–0 to 10–0 nylon under microscopic visualization. Repair is most critical when the branches to the orbicularis oculi are involved. The proximal stumps can be easily identified by performing a facial nerve dissection from the main trunk. Torn distal branches may be difficult to find, but a nerve stimulator may prove helpful. Of course, the more distal the injury, the more difficult it will be to repair it.

Malunited, untreated midface fractures may be quite difficult to repair satisfactorily. Therefore, it is important to try to repair these in a timely fashion whenever possible. Occasionally, neurologic or other bodily injuries will contraindicate the adequate repair of midfacial fractures. In this situation, it is wise to attempt a conservative reduction of the occlusion either as a minor procedure or even at the bedside as early as possible. If the occlusal relationship is reestablished early, the severity of any malunion will likely be minimized, and if nothing else, the functional disability can at least be minimized. Even a patient who is neurologically impaired and in a nursing home will do better if he or she can eat and chew. However, once the malunion has occurred, the treatment selection will depend on the nature of the problem and the patient's needs. An elderly, edentulous or almost edentulous patient may be best served by the creation of an occlusal relationship with modified dentures. When cosmesis and function are both important, mobilization of the fractures by making planned LeFort osteotomies may provide the best results. This requires careful CT evaluation and planning of the osteotomies. When blindness is a particular concern (e.g., an only seeing eye), limited anterior mobilization of the orbital rims can be accomplished. If osteotomies are not desired or seem too aggressive or risky, the facial contour can be improved by the judicious use of bone grafts or alloplastic implants. These may need to be reshaped and replaced more than once before the most desirable result is obtained.

MANDIBULAR FRACTURES

In general, mandibular fractures should be handled conservatively whenever possible. Open reduction should be used when it would appear that closed reduction has a high likelihood of failure or complication or when the patient has a particular need or desire to avoid IMF. However, if open reduction is performed, I believe that rigid fixation provides the best likelihood of healing and the best protection against infection and is therefore the preferred technique when it can be accomplished. Rigid fixation is a demanding and unforgiving technique[26]; thus, it must be carried out properly and meticulously, or it should be avoided and a less rigid fixation technique should be used. Most fractures anterior to the molar teeth can be easily plated via an intraoral approach, though the external approach is technically easier and allows for the use of the specially designed mandibular reduction forceps (Fig 26–1) to assist in fixation and compression. Posterior fractures can be plated intraorally as well, but the technical difficulty becomes much greater the further posterior the fracture. Due to the technical demands of mandibular plating, for optimal results, the external approach is favored for fractures behind the premolars and should be used for anterior fractures as well when technical difficulty is encountered. The specific technical aspects of plate fixation are beyond the scope of this chapter.[21, 26, 27]

Tooth Extraction

Although the issue of whether to extract a tooth in a man-

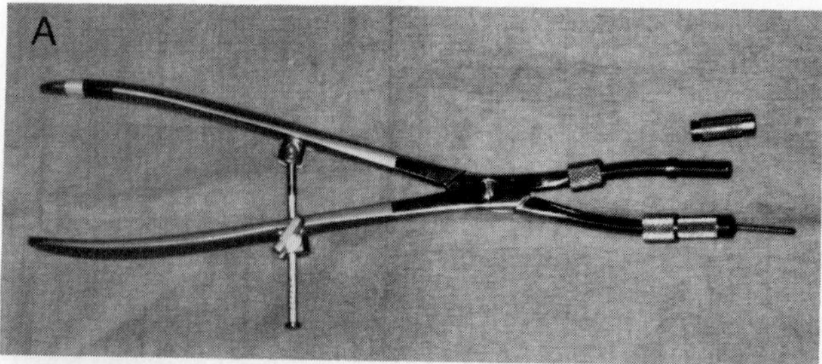
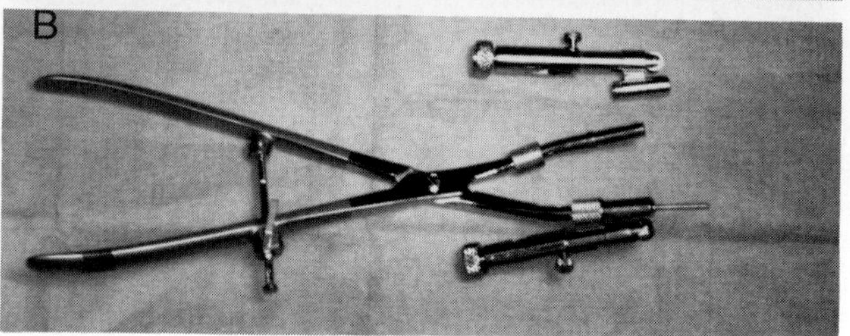

FIG 26–1.
AO mandibular (compression) reduction forceps. **A,** standard mandibular reduction forceps. Two sleeves are screwed into the inferior border of the mandible on either side of the fracture (see Fig 26–2). (One sleeve is seen separately from the forceps in this photograph.) The forceps are then placed into the sleeves and fixed to the sleeves with the cap nuts. The forceps can be used to manipulate the fracture fragments into position and to apply some compression. The compression plate is now applied. **B,** same forceps as in **A,** but the sleeve has rollers attached, which are positioned so that they abut the inferior mandible away from the fracture (relative to the sleeve position, which is close to the fracture). The forceps are then attached to the sleeves as in **A,** and inferior mandibular compression is carried out just as it is in **A.** Since there is no tension band, the alveolar portion of the mandible will be distracted (see Fig 26–2). As the rollers are screwed in, the inferior mandible will be pushed superiorly, thereby compressing the upper portion of the fracture (see Fig 26–4). An eccentric dynamic compression plate can now be applied (see Figs 26–3 and 26–4).

dibular fracture line is still somewhat controversial, more surgeons seem to be in favor of salvaging teeth when possible. In general, the teeth should be considered significant structures, and so they should not be discarded without due consideration. The adage that "any tooth in a mandibular fracture line should be removed" should be stricken from the literature and discarded. Teeth may sometimes provide important alignment when fractures are reduced, particularly in the distal arch. If a distal molar needs to be extracted, I will generally first establish the IMF and plate the fracture. Once the fracture has been satisfactorily stabilized in good position, the tooth can be removed. A tooth in a fracture line should be removed if the root is fractured or if it is already involved in infection. Otherwise, I try to save it. However, I will not reimplant a tooth in a fracture line or save it if it has been totally mobilized. A saved tooth in a fracture line should be removed quickly if any infection develops in it, since, left in place, it will then become a likely source of osteomyelitis.

Comminuted Mandible.

The key to the repair of the comminuted mandible is the establishment of the proper occlusal relationship. Small areas of comminution can then be plated together using compression plates to effect rigid stabilization. When comminution is more extensive, the involved area can be treated as a defect area. This area is bridged with some form of rigid reconstruction plate (a plate designed to bridge mandibular defects as in mandibular reconstruction). Initially all fragments should be maintained to help define the anatomic position of the main segments. A template is used to plan the bending of the plate, making sure that at least four screw holes will overlap the solid bone on either side of the defective (comminuted) area. The plate is then bent to match the shape of the template. Final plate contouring is completed using the mandible itself as the template. Exact bending of the plate with proper conformation to the bone is critical, since minor discrepancies in the plate shape can result in large occlusal discrepancies after fixation to the bone. A plate holder of some type will facilitate plate positioning. The holes are then drilled one at a time, and each screw is placed before the next hole is drilled. At least four screws are used on each side. More can be used. More should be used if the defective area is more than a few centimeters long. If all the pieces are present between larger segments, the smaller comminuted fragments can be compressed between the larger ones to provide greater stability and likelihood of healing. However, if pieces are missing, this is not critical, since the comminuted area is being treated as a defect segment. Once the plate has been stabilized on both sides, the occlusion should be rechecked. If it has been disrupted, the plate should be removed and reapplied. Once satisfactory stabilization has been accomplished, the area of comminution should be evaluated. Small, denuded fragments should be debrided. Larger fragments should be saved, and they should be fixed to the plate if they are unstable and accessible to a screw hole. If they are firmly wedged in place and immobilized, I prefer not to fix devascularized fragments of bone (i.e., bone grafts) to the plate. When necessary, bone grafts can be used to fill in large defects. Cancellous bone from the iliac crest is the preferred choice, providing excellent results in cases of traumatic bone loss. Note that the most important factor in obtaining bony union and protecting against bone infection is rigid stabilization, even in the absence of adequate soft tissue coverage. It is better to properly reposition the bone and fix it rigidly and leave the bone and plate exposed than to foreshorten the mandible to obtain soft tissue coverage.

Condylar-Subcondylar Fracture

The condylar-subcondylar fracture of the mandible provides the area of greatest consternation and controversy in mandibular fractures. It would be impossible to summarize the various opinions, since almost all possibilities have been espoused. It is also unclear whether a good early result will necessarily translate into a good long-term outcome and whether some of the complications (e.g., ankylosis) are due to the treatment or rather to the injury itself.

Generally speaking, I favor a conservative approach to condylar fractures. Early mobilization with minimal intervention should give the best outcome when it works. If the patient comes into a normal occlusion, a soft diet and observation are the rule. Exercises in front of a mirror, including protrusion, side-to-side excursion, and opening in a straight line are practiced at least a few minutes each hour. If opening is limited, exercises (generally with increasing numbers of tongue blades) to increase the excursion are performed. If a malocclusion is present, 7 to 10 days of intermaxillary fixation with elastic traction is attempted. If a malocclusion persists without improvement, open reduction may be considered. Open reduction is also indicated when closed reduction cannot be accomplished (even under anesthesia) and when ramus foreshortening is developing. (Of course, facial paralysis and penetration into the middle fossa would be indications as well, but these are extremely rare occurrences.) Opening a true condylar head (i.e., intracapsular) fracture is frought with risk, and these are usually not amenable to repair. Once opened, treatment may well include condylectomy with or without replacement with an alloplastic prosthesis or an autograft (generally costochondral rib). The subcondylar fracture can usually be approached via a submaxillary incision, though occasionally a facial nerve dissection will be necessary to repair a high subcondylar fracture without injuring the facial nerve. A preauricular incision with dissection onto the zygoma may allow access to a high subcondylar fracture without facial nerve dissection, but rigid fixation via this approach may prove difficult. Once the fracture is exposed, a plate is the preferred method of fixation, though a wire is adequate when a plate cannot be applied for technical reasons. The best way to apply a plate is to pull down gently on the upper fragment and attach the plate (after positioning and bending, of course), and then to align the fragments and screw the plate into the lower fragment. Trauma to the joint should be kept to a minimum. This generally provides excellent short-term results, but whether the long-term outcome is better or worse than after conservative management remains to be seen. Bilateral subcondylar fractures are more likely to require open reduction, at least of one side, since ramus foreshortening and an anterior open bite are much more likely in this situation.

Edentulous Mandibular Fracture

Fractures of the edentulous mandible have always been of concern to maxillofacial trauma surgeons. The absence of teeth, of course, makes it difficult to establish the proper functional relationship between the maxilla and mandible while also eliminating the possible use of arch bars to stabilize the fragments. Furthermore, most edentulous mandibles are atrophic, making stabilization difficult by any means. Since many edentulous mandibles are found in older patients, and since atherosclerotic obstruction occurs early in the inferior alveolar arteries,[28] the blood supply to the fractured fragments is often tenuous, healing is frequently slow, and complications of nonunion and osteomyelitis are all too common.

As a result of frequent treatment failures, intervention for fractures in atrophic edentulous mandibles has become more aggressive. External fixators and primary bone grafts are commonly employed. The advent of mandibular compression plates has improved this situation dramatically. Rigid fixation seems to enhance the healing and protect against infection,[29] and the result is a high rate of primary, bony union even in the most atrophic, pencil-thin mandibles.[30]

I use three different types of compression plates in various combinations depending on the specific circumstances involved. When there is a fair amount of mandibular height remaining, a straight compression plate at the inferior (basal) border of the mandible will result in gapping at the alveolar border (Fig 26–2). An eccentric dynamic compression plate provides compression forces that will compress the alveolar border of the mandible as well as the basal border (Figs 26–3 and 26–4). Anteriorly, where the inferior alveolar nerves are not at risk of being injured, a straight dynamic compression plate can be placed at the midportion of the mandibular height, or, better yet, two plates can be placed so that rotational and torsional forces affecting this area are safely overcome. When there is little mandibular height remaining above the inferior alveolar canals, a straight dynamic compression plate at the basal border may prove adequate. The toughest situation is the thin, atrophic, pencil-thin mandible. This bone is weak and slow to heal. To adequately stabilize a fracture in such a thin area, one must use multiple screws over a lengthier segment, so that the strength of the metal plate can serve to bear the forces and allow the bone underneath to heal. Therefore, at least a six-hole (and preferably a longer) plate should be employed. A reconstruction plate can be used, thereby treating the fractured area as a defect area that is being bridged by the plate. Note that minimal periosteal stripping is performed, and the plate can be safely positioned extraperiostally.

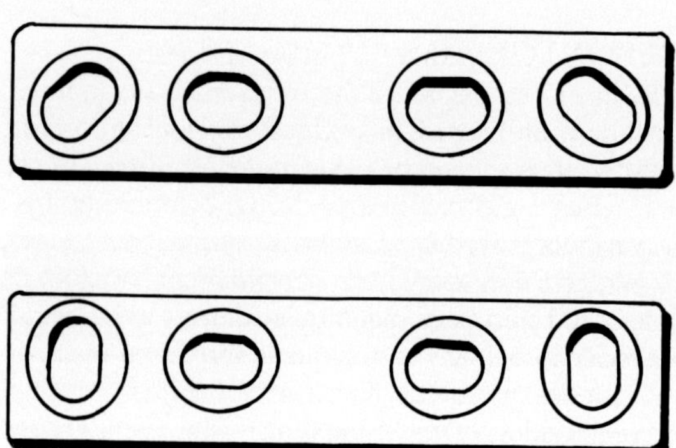

FIG 26–3.
Drawings of AO eccentric dynamic compression plates. Both diagonally directed outer holes and vertically directed outer holes will result in compression of the superior border of the fracture as long as the screws are placed inferiorly in the outer holes (see Fig 26–4). It should also be apparent that the horizontal compression screws must be applied first. Also note that the diagonal holes must point toward the fracture at the superior border of the mandible. If an eccentric dynamic compression plate with more than four holes is used, two horizontal compression screws must be applied, followed by two vertical or diagonal screws, and only then may additional screws be placed. Any other order of placement will defeat the purpose of this plate.

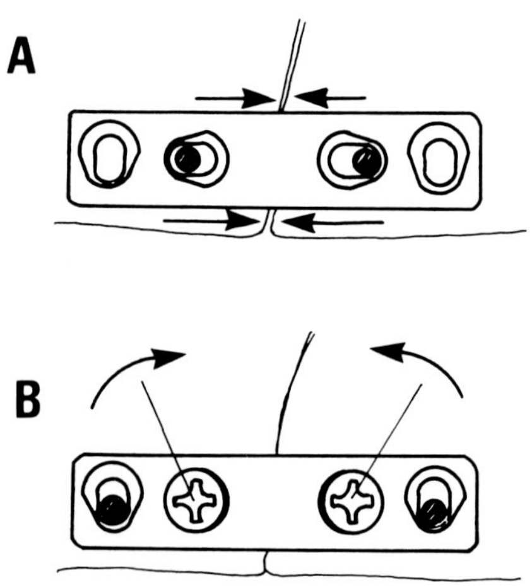

FIG 26–4.
Schematics demonstrating the function of an eccentric dynamic compression plate. **A,** horizontal compression is first applied by placing the screws in the horizontal holes so that they are away from the fracture. As the screws are driven home, interaction between the screw heads and the plate will force the screws to move toward the fracture, thereby compressing the bones together at the fracture line. **B,** placement of the outer screws in the vertical holes so that they are at the inferior portions of the holes forces the screws to move superiorly relative to the plate as the screws are driven home and the screw heads contact the plate. Since there is already a screw in each side of the plate, the bone cannot move straight up; instead, there is rotational movement in a superior direction around the initial screws, which serve as the center of the axis of rotation. The superior borders of the fracture are thereby compressed.

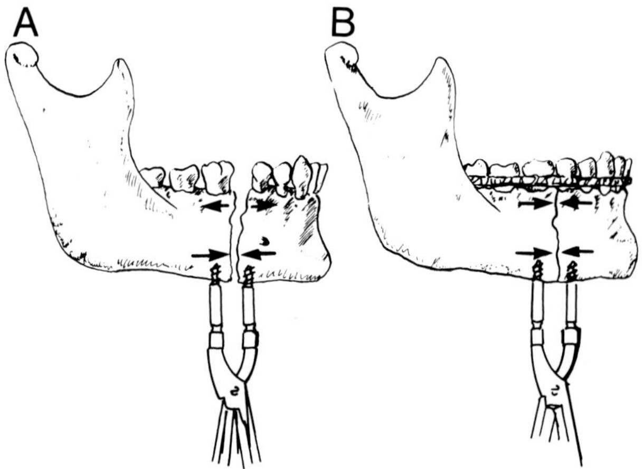

FIG 26–2.
A, compression of the inferior border of the mandible (in this case using an AO mandibular reduction forceps) in the absence of a tension band on the alveolar border will result in gapping at the superior portion of the fracture. **B,** when a tension band has been placed across the alveolar border of the fracture (in this case, an arch bar serves as a tension band), inferior compression now closes (and compresses) the entire fracture. Note that when no tension band can be applied, lateral rollers can be used on the reduction forceps to close the superior portion of the fracture (see Fig 26–1,B).

NASOFRONTOETHMOID FRACTURES

The junctional area of the nasal, frontal, and ethmoid bones is a complex area, and both evaluation and repair of trauma to this area can be difficult and demanding. The nasoethmoid complex fracture is too often underdiagnosed and undertreated. The finding on CT of a fracture through the medial orbit and ethmoid should alert the maxillofacial surgeon to look carefully for the possibility of fractures affecting the position of the medial canthal ligament or ligaments.

Traumatic telecanthus results from the lateral displacement of the medial canthal ligament. This ligament consists of several small slips that interdigitate with the orbicularis oculi muscle and insert on the anterior and posterior lacrimal crests. With direct trauma to this area, the hard nasal bones may telescope inward, displacing the nasal processes of the maxillae laterally and shattering the thinner lacrimal and ethmoid bones. Such fractures are generally comminuted, and the bone fragments attached to the ligaments drift laterally. (Actual disruptions of the ligaments can occur but are far less likely.) This results in lateral and inferior displacement of and rounding of the medial conjunctival sulcus, loss of view of the caruncle, horizontal shortening of the lids, and an increase in the intercanthal distance (between the two medial canthi), so-called telecanthus, or pseudohypertelorism. The laxity and inferior displacement of the lids also result in poor function of the lacrimal collecting system, causing epiphora. If it is left unrepaired, there is significant loss of dorsal height of the nose. As contracture develops, an epicanthal fold usually forms, contributing to the already disturbing cosmetic appearance that this injury creates.

Early diagnosis and repair of this injury is of the utmost importance, since late and secondary repairs are difficult and rarely satisfactory.[10] When a medial canthal detachment is suspected, the examination should include direct palpation of this area. Traction on the lower lid may reveal the laxity and easy distraction of the medial canthal area.[31] Small fragments may be palpable and may move when the medial orbit is palpated, particularly during traction on the lower lid. An instrument should be placed inside the nose, and bimanual palpation of the medial orbit may reveal the lateral displacement of the canthal attachments. Intercanthal and interocular distances should be measured as well.

The key to surgical repair is the refixation of the medial canthal ligament. Proper repair of this injury therefore requires open reduction with direct examination and fixation. Closed reduction using transnasal wiring and lead plates is less likely to provide a satisfactory outcome. After dissection through the skin and subcutaneous tissues, the ligament can be identified by placing a mosquito medially in the conjunctival sac and pushing medially into the wound while carefully dissecting down through the soft tissue. Great care must be taken not to detach the ligament from any remaining bony attachment. Debridement of bone should also be as conservative as possible. A coronal incision is desirable, though local frontoethmoid or open-sky incisions can be used as well. The bony fragments should be repositioned as closely as possible and fixed with wires, plates, or both. The nasofrontal angle and nasal height can be nicely reestablished with small miniplates either from a

solid frontal segment anteriorly onto a solid nasal dorsal segment or from the frontal bones onto each side of the nasal dorsum laterally. However, this will generally not stabilize the fragments holding the medial canthal ligaments, which must therefore be directly wired. The medial canthal ligaments are pulled laterally and inferiorly by their attachments to the orbicularis oculi and lower lid tarsal plate. Repair aims at repositioning the ligament superiorly and posteriorly. The main area of failure is inadequate posterior, medial, and superior positioning of the wire fixation. Due to technical difficulty, it is extremely unlikely that overcorrection will occur; thus, it is important to aim for maximal correction, wiring the ligament superiorly behind the posterior lacrimal crest and pulling medially with transnasal wiring. Wiring itself is technically difficult. Small, thin bony fragments can be difficult to drill, and great care must be taken not to further these fragments. They can also be difficult to drill through in situ, and Manson and Iliff recommend dislocating these fragments laterally and out of the wound to facilitate drilling.[1] Transnasal wiring can be facilitated by drilling holes through the nasal septum, similarly placing them posteriorly and superiorly to aid in the proper positioning of the wires. If the medial canthal ligament has been detached or disrupted, it is critical that a wire passes through the ligament and then attaches it transnasally to the opposite posterior lacrimal crest. Finally, if both medial canthal ligaments have been detached, they must be wired tightly together across the nose. The posterior and superior positioning will be most difficult to maintain in this situation, and bone grafts and plates will facilitate this repair, giving some structural support to help maintain the position of the transnasal wires.

Due to the comminution and telescoping of these fractures, there is often a loss of dorsal nasal height with consequent flattening of the dorsum. This tends to exaggerate any appearance of telecanthus. It is therefore important to graft this area. Minimal flattening can be repaired using otherwise unusable fragments that had been debrided from the medial orbital wall or bone from the nasal septum. Larger defects (particularly when nasal septal support has been lost) require larger grafts, usually calvarium or rib. Primary repair of the nasal dorsum and septum using cantilevered bone grafts will provide better contour as well as better nasal airway function.[32]

Trauma to the nasal area frequently results in septal disruption as well. If the septum is straight, there is adequate septal dorsal support, and there is a good nasal airway bilaterally, then no intervention is required. A mild septal injury such as a dislocation may respond to closed reduction. However, a significant disruption of the septal architecture is best treated via open reduction and immediate septoplasty. The planes will elevate easily due to bleeding into the subperichondrial space. Overlapping fragments can be repositioned, and normal septal contour and even dorsal support can be reestablished. If dorsal support cannot be reestablished, primary bone or cartilage grafting is indicated.

Septal hematomas should always be drained, because failure to do so can lead to avascular necrosis of the septal cartilage or a septal abscess and the later development of a saddle nose. An incision at least 1 cm long is made in the mucoperichondrium. The hematoma is evacuated, and the nose is packed bilaterally for 48 hours. If the hematoma reaccumulates, a vessel loop drain is placed in the cavity, and the nose is repacked for another 48 hours. If this were to fail, I would try to suture the septal space closed with mattress sutures, though I have not had this occur.

The management of frontal sinus injuries, particularly when there is injury to the nasofrontal duct (NFD), remains quite controversial. When the NFD is functioning, frontal sinus infections and mucoceles should not be a problem, and healing of fractures, mucosa, and dura are to be anticipated.[33] However, although obstruction of the duct can be expected to lead to complications, it is not clear how often disruption leads to obstruction. Schultz never obliterates the frontal sinus and claims to have never seen a sinus complication[34]; he carefully reconstructs both the anterior and posterior walls. He did, however, excise the mucosa when there "was marked tearing and displacement of the mucous membrane."[34] Most otolaryngologists recommend obliteration of the frontal sinus either via cranialization (when the posterior wall is fractured)[35] or via osteoplastic obliteration[36,37] when NFD function is at risk of being impaired. I agree with the latter approach and recommend obliteration of the frontal sinuses when NFD disruption is present.

With this in mind, the main question is really when NFD damage is likely so that there is a guide to when to explore the frontal sinuses. May et al. recommended exploration of all frontal sinus fractures,[38] but I do not believe that such an aggressive approach is necessary. When there is gross disruption of the anterior or posterior walls, exploration is indicated for repair of these structures. In a review of 50 patients, Stanley and Becker analyzed the incidence of NFD injury as it related to the fracture pattern.[37] They then suggested guidelines for exploration based on the likelihood of NFD injury. Linear fractures (nondepressed) of the anterior wall without associated nasoethmoid complex or supraorbital rim fractures as well as horizontal linear nondisplaced fractures of the posterior wall were never associated with NFD damage. Similarly, isolated, comminuted anterior wall fractures rarely involved the NFD (1/13th involved the duct). Therefore, if these fractures are seen on CT and are not depressed, no exploration or repair is mandated. If there is a depressed fracture, this should be explored and repaired. On the other hand, vertical fractures of the posterior wall, comminuted fractures of the posterior wall, and fractures associated with nasoethmoid complex or supraorbital rim fractures are highly likely to have associated NFD injuries and should be explored. If at exploration the NFD appears patent, reduction of the fractures should be adequate. If the duct is disrupted, sinus obliteration should be carried out, being extremely careful to eliminate all remnants of frontal sinus mucosa. Fat may be used, but if there is extensive damage to the floor of the sinuses, bone grafts should be placed over a fascial plug to separate the nose and ethmoid from the frontal sinuses. For linear, nondepressed fractures of the posterior wall, the sinus may be explored more conservatively using sinoscopes via a trephination approach. If there is no evidence of NFD injury or cerebrospinal fluid (CSF) leakage, and mucosa does not appear to be trapped in the fracture, no further intervention is warranted. When a disrupted posterior wall can be repaired, an osteoplastic approach is used; if the dura is intact, obliteration should be carried out over the reconstructed or repaired posterior wall. Small dural tears can also be repaired via this approach, though this is more controversial. When this is done, a layer of fascia should be placed over the repaired back wall of the sinus.[39] Finally, when the back wall is severely disrupted, the dura should be explored and repaired through a craniotomy, and the sinus should be obliterated via cranialization. After the back wall remnants are completely removed, great care should be taken to obliterate the communication between the anterior fossa and the nose and sinuses with fascia and bone as needed.

REFERENCES

1. Manson PM, Iliff NT: Orbital fractures. *Facial Plast Surg* 1988; 5:243–259.
2. Miller GR, Tenzel RR: Ocular complications of mid-facial fractures. *Plast Reconstr Surg* 1967; 39:37–42.
3. Fujino R: Experimental "blowout" fracture of the orbit. *Plast Reconstr Surg* 1974; 54:81–82.
4. Converse JM: Orbital fractures, in English GM (ed): *Otolaryngology.* Philadelphia, Harper & Row Publishers, 1977, vol 4, pp 1–22.
5. Converse JM, Smith B: Enophthalmos and diplopia in fractures of the orbital floor. *Br J Plast Surg* 1957; 9:265–274.
6. Korneef L: Current concepts on the management of blowout fractures. *Ann Plast Surg* 1982; 9:185–199.
7. Holt JE, Holt GR: Ocular injuries in craniofacial trauma. *Facial Plast Surg* 1988; 5:237–242.
8. Osguthorpe JD, Sofferman RA: Optic nerve decompression. *Otolaryngol Clin North Am* 1988; 21:155–169.
9. Putterman AM: Late management of blow-out fractures of the orbital floor. *Trans Am Acad Ophthal Otolaryngol* 1977; 83:650–659.
10. Converse JM, Smith B, Wood-Smith D: Malunited fractures of the orbit, in Converse JM (ed): *Reconstructive Plastic Surgery.* Philadelphia, WB Saunders Co, 1977, vol 2, pp 989–1039.
11. Aichmair H, Fries R: Therapie des enophthalmus nach orbitafraktur. *Klin Mbl Augenheilk* 1971; 158:109, as cited by Luhr HG: Midface fractures involving the orbit and blow-out fractures, in Kruger E, Schilli W, Worthington P (eds): *Oral and Maxillofacial Traumatology.* Chicago, Quintessence Publishing Co, 1986, vol 2, pp 197–222.
12. Manson PM, Hoopes JE, Su CT: Structural pillars of the facial skeleton: An approach to the management of LeFort fractures. *Plast Reconstr Surg* 1980; 66:54–61.
13. Sofferman RA, Danielson PA, Quatela V, et al: Retrospective analysis of surgically treated LeFort fractures: Is suspension necessary? *Arch Otolaryngol* 1983; 109:446–448.
14. Kellman RM, Schilli W: Plate fixation of fractures of the mid- and upper face. *Otolaryngol Clin North Am* 1987; 20:559–572.
15. Luhr HG: Compression plate osteosynthesis through the Luhr system, in Kruger E, Schilli W (eds): *Oral and Maxillofacial Traumatology.* Chicago, Quintessence Publishing Co, 1982, vol 1, pp 319–348.
16. Michelet FX, Deymes J, Dessus B: Osteosynthesis with miniaturized screwed plates in maxillofacial surgery. *J Maxillofac Surg* 1973; 1:79–84.

17. Kellman RM, Woo P, Leopold DA: Rigid internal fixation of mid- and upper facial fractures. Paper presented at the Middle Section of the Triological Society, Cleveland, Ohio, January 1987.

18. Champy M, Lodde JP, Muster D, et al: Osteosynthesis using miniaturized screw-on plates in facial and cranial surgery. *Ann Chir Plast Esthet* 1977; 22:261–264.

19. Stanley RB, Toffel PH: The extended access approach for treatment of maxillary fractures. *Facial Plast Surg* 1988; 5:213–219.

20. Stanley RB: Reconstruction of the mid-facial vertical dimension following LeFort fractures. *Arch Otolaryngol* 1984; 110:571–575.

21. Kellman RM: Methods of rigid fixation for facial fractures, in Cummings CW, Frederickson JM, Harker LA, et al (eds): *Otolaryngology—Head and Neck Surgery: Update I.* St Louis, CV Mosby Co, 1989, pp 160–191.

22. Gruss J: Personal communication, 1988.

23. Phillips J: Personal communication, 1988.

24. Gruss J, MacKinnon SE: Complex maxillary fractures: Role of buttress reconstruction and immediate bone grafts. *Plast Reconstr Surg* 1986; 78:9–22.

25. Marentette LJ: Bone grafting techniques in craniofacial trauma. *Facial Plast Surg* 1988; 5:207–212.

26. Kellman RM: Repair of mandibular fractures via compression plating and more traditional techniques: A comparison of results. *Laryngoscope* 1984; 94:1560–1567.

27. Kellman RM (ed): Facial plating. *Otolaryngol Clin North Am* 1987; 20:425–639.

28. Bradley JC: Age changes in the vascular supply of the mandible. *Br Dent J* 1972; 132:142–144.

29. Beckers HL: Treatment of initially infected mandibular fractures with bone plates. *J Oral Surg* 1979; 37:310–313.

30. Levine PA, Goode RL: Treatment of fractures of the edentulous mandible. *Arch Otolaryngol* 1982; 108:167–173.

31. Mathog RH: Post-traumatic telecanthus, in Mathog RH (ed): *Maxillofacial Trauma.* Baltimore, Williams & Wilkins Co, 1984, pp 303–318.

32. Gruss J: Complex nasoethmoid-orbital and midfacial fractures: Role of craniofacial surgical techniques and immediate bone grafting. *Ann Plast Surg* 1986; 17:377–390.

33. Hybels RL, Newman MH: Posterior table fractures of the frontal sinus: I. An experimental study. *Laryngoscope* 1977; 97:171–179.

34. Schultz RC: Frontal sinus and supraorbital fractures from vehicle accidents. *Clin Plast Surg* 1975; 2:93–106.

35. Donald PJ: Frontal sinus ablation by cranialization: Report of 21 cases. *Arch Otolaryngol* 1982; 108:142–146.

36. Montgomery WW: Surgery of the frontal sinus, in Montgomery WW (ed): *Surgery of the Upper Respiratory System,* ed 2. Philadelphia, Lea & Febiger, 1979, vol 1, pp 117–173.

37. Stanley RB, Becker TS: Injuries of the nasofrontal orifices in frontal sinus fractures. *Laryngoscope* 1987; 97:728–731.

38. May M, Ogura JH, Schramm V: Nasofrontal duct in frontal sinus fractures. *Arch Otolaryngol* 1970; 92:534–538.

39. Stanley RB: Management of frontal sinus fractures. *Facial Plast Surg* 1988; 5:231–235.

Maxillofacial Trauma

Approach of

Robert H. Mathog, M.D.

ORBITAL BLOWOUT FRACTURES

Indications for Surgery

Surgery for blowout fractures is indicated when there is (or impending) a dysfunction or deformity that likely can be corrected by an operative procedure. One must weigh the risks, however, and if there is a chance of blindness or complications from the anesthesia, these potential sequelae must be taken into consideration.

All surgery should be planned with ophthalmology. Globe rupture and retinal displacement should be ruled out or corrected prior to repair of orbital blowout fractures. Surgery should not be performed on an only seeing eye. The cardiovascular and central nervous systems should be evaluated and their stability assured prior to any surgical intervention. Timing and comprehensive diagnosis, therefore, become important variables in applying indications to the operative procedure.

Clinical findings that determine if and when a surgeon should operate may vary within and across specialties. Putterman et al. believe that there are few long-term problems following blowout injuries and that surgery should be delayed until there is evidence of incapacitation.[1] This philosophy also is consistent with camouflage or touch-up procedures rather than any major surgical intervention. At the other extreme, one can make a case that it is impossible to rely on signs and symptoms or imaging studies and that exploration becomes an important part of the diagnostic and treatment program. My group takes a middle of the road approach, which individualizes and evaluates each case as to present and future possibilities of functional and cosmetic problems.[2]

Any patient showing acute enophthalmos or hypophthalmos (globe ptosis) is considered a surgical candidate. Usually, the casual observer will note 2 to 3 mm of enophthalmos and 1 to 2 mm of hypophthalmos, and for these reasons, patients with measurements exceeding these degrees of displacement should be encouraged to have a corrective procedure. Quantitative data can be obtained by measuring the projection of the globe from the lateral orbital wall with a ruler or with a Hertel exophthalmometer, but one must be assured that measurements are referred to an orbital rim that is in a normal position. According to my scales of measurement, a 1 to 2 mm difference between sides is classified as mild; 3 to 4 mm is moderate; and 5 to 6 mm is severe. On this basis, I consider patients with a moderate to severe deformity to be excellent candidates for surgery. It should be recognized that initial findings can be misleading, that usual posttraumatic swelling will disappear, and a discrepancy between orbital volume and intraorbital contents will increase with time.

Entrapment is also a strong indication for surgery. Mobility of the eye should be evaluated by asking the patient to look in four quadrants of gaze. The observer should then determine if there are any differences between conjugate movements. The patient should be queried about double images, and the diplopia should be classified according to fields of gaze. I use a grading system in which mild is equivalent to diplopia in one field of gaze, moderate is diplopia in two fields of gaze, and severe is diplopia in three fields of gaze. Prisms and red glass tests also can be used to elicit small differences.[2]

Because dysfunctions of gaze can develop from either injury to one of the nerves or muscles or as a result of entrapment, and because entrapment can be corrected with surgery and neuromuscular injury often cannot, it is important to distinguish between these conditions. Any inability to move the eye should be evaluated by passive forced duction tests, and the degree of restriction should be determined. My method is to apply a topical solution of 4% cocaine or ophthaine to the conjunctiva and wait several minutes for anesthesia. I then grasp the insertion of one of the rectus muscles 5 to 7 mm from the limbus and compare the motility of the globe in any of the desired directions. One side is compared with the other. Any impairment of movement is interpreted as entrapment; normal motility implies a neuromuscular dysfunction. One must also be aware

of diplopia from retinal detachment, but since this is a monocular phenomenon, it can be distinguished by careful questions about the symptom. Ophthalmoplegia secondary to a retrorbital hemorrhage can also limit movement of the globe, but this condition can be diagnosed by proptosis, tension on the globe, and conjunctival inflammation and edema.

As a general rule, I will explore any blowout fracture associated with persistent signs of entrapment or diplopia. Timing, however, is important. In the early period following injury, there can be transient swelling and neuromuscular dysfunction causing diplopia, and only after the acute reaction has disappeared, is it possible to make a clear-cut evaluation. Traumatic diplopia and dysfunction are treated expectantly, but if there is persistent diplopia with motility problems (usually beyond 7 days), I would consider the patient for surgical exploration.

I am also aware of site and size of injury as important considerations. Blowout fractures can occur as small or large defects of one wall, or they can involve several walls separately or together in what may be a junctional injury. The large defects are characterized by expansion of the wall or walls and extravasation of soft tissues from the orbit into the nose or paranasal sinuses. These defects are rarely associated with entrapment, but because of significant discrepancies between orbital volume and intraorbital contents, they often present with acute enophthalmos. Occasionally patients with large defects show no early signs of enophthalmos, and only after time, when the soft tissue swelling subsides, do they exhibit this complication. According to some of our experimental work, 2 to 3 mm of wall displacement will cause problems,[3] and when this degree of wall displacement is observed on CT scan, it is an indication for surgery.

The smaller orbital wall defects are not necessarily benign. These defects can be associated with compression of soft tissues, fat necrosis, and later, loss of tissue volume. If any of these should occur, enophthalmos will gradually appear over several weeks. These patients are also prone to entrapment of a portion of the periorbita and dislocation of orbital septa.[4] In fact, these patients can often end up with a more severe type of entrapment and diplopia. Thus, with regard to the small defects, if there are signs of entrapment, I will explore; otherwise, I will follow the patients for a sufficient time to rule out a late development of enophthalmos.

Since some fractures of the orbital wall can extend to the orbital apex, one must be aware of the possibility of a variety of neural injuries and the potential for correction. One must, however, recognize the safe limits of exploration and not cause or aggravate further neural damage. In general, I explore the orbital floor to the junction of the inferior orbital fissure and infraorbital canal; occasionally I follow a ledge created by the ethmoid cells to its plateau. I also restrict my dissection on the medial wall to an area anterior to the posterior ethmoidal artery. In my experience, fractures that affect the annulus tendineus and the insertion of muscles cannot be corrected. Injury to nerves III, IV, or VI at the superior orbital fissue can occasionally be improved by decompression, but this is still a controversial subject. For those patients with orbital wall fractures and optic nerve injury, there is some optimism, and I will usually administer a course of megadose steroids (100 mg of dexamethasone/day).[5] If vision does not improve in 24 to 48 hours, I will explore the orbital wall fracture and optic canal, and at the time the wall is repaired, I will surgically decompress the optic nerve. In those patients who have a return of vision on steroid therapy, I proceed more cautiously, and in such cases, rather than put mechanical pressure on the orbit, I would delay surgery and relax the indications for exploration.

Operative Techniques

Orbital blowout fractures can involve one or several walls of the orbit. The site and severity of the injury will determine the surgical approach. Often the fracture is impure and associated with other fractures; in such cases, repair is part of more comprehensive surgery.

For orbital surgery, general anesthesia by orotracheal intubation is preferred. The face and upper part of the neck are prepared as sterile fields. Both eyes are left exposed, and a clear drape is used to cover the oral and nasal areas. Markings of incisions are made with a Bonnie blue solution, and the skin and deeper tissues are infiltrated with 1% lidocaine (Xylocaine) containing epinephrine 1:100,000. Vasoconstriction can be achieved in approximately 5 to 7 minutes, and surgery should begin at that time.

For the floor fracture, I use either a high medial lower eyelid or an infraciliary incision (Fig 26–5).[6] The eyelid approach should use a high crease line, and to avoid postoperative edema, it should not extend beyond the middle of a line drawn perpendicular downward from the pupil. Medial extension should be limited so as not to injure the puncta or canaliculus. The incision is then deepened through the orbicularis oculi musculature to the level of the orbital septum. Hemostasis is achieved with fine electrocautery. The muscle is elevated off of the septum, and the septum is followed to the inferior orbital rim.

The infraciliary incision is designed 2 to 3 mm below the cilia, again carefully avoiding damage to the puncta and canaliculus. Through this incision, one then dissects off the attachment of the orbicularis oculi from the tarsal plate. The orbicularis oculi is elevated with the skin in a plane external to the septum to create a skin-muscle flap. This plane is dissected to the orbital rim. If the septum should be entered, the surgeon should return to a more superficial plane. It is not necessary to repair the septal defect.

Both high eyelid and infraciliary approaches provide satisfactory exposure. The direct eyelid incision is easier to accomplish and avoids postoperative eversion or inversion of the eyelid margin, but it also has limited exposure laterally if one desires to repair parts of the malar or maxillary bone. The infraciliary approach, if not done properly, can cause postoperative ectropion and for this reason should be avoided by the novice surgeon. On the other hand, exposure laterally is facilitated by this incision.

Both approaches will bring the surgeon to the inferior orbital rim. With a Senn retractor pulling the eyelid inferiorly and malleable retractor protecting the septum and globe, an incision is made through the orbicularis oculi and zygomaticus muscles as they insert into the anterior wall of the maxilla. This incision allows one to develop a cuff of periosteum that can

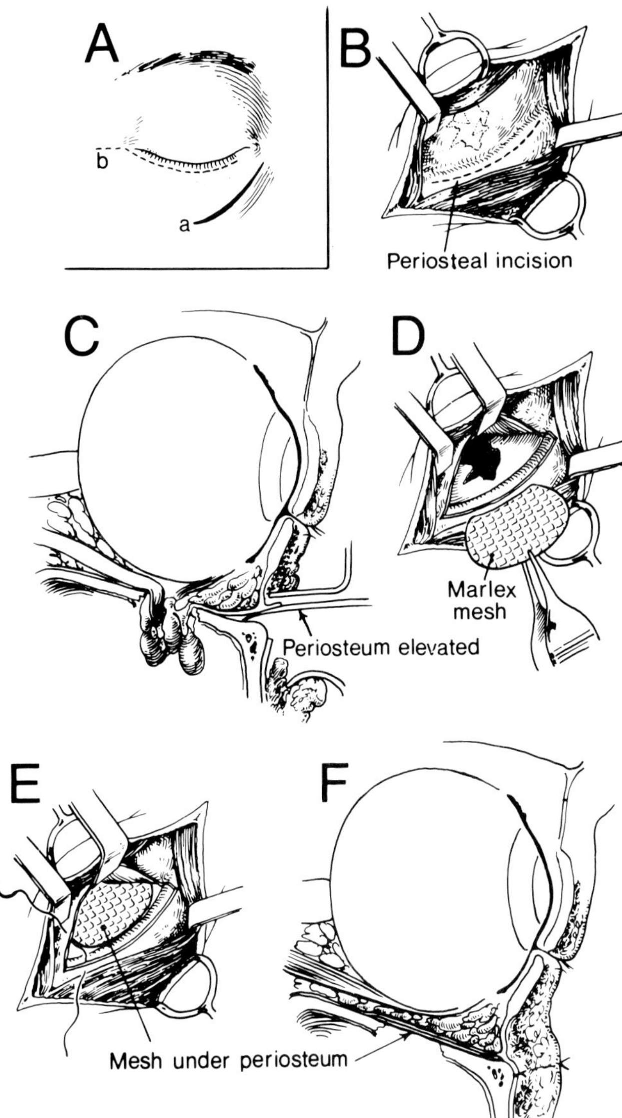

FIG 26–5.

Technique for repair of blowout fracture. **A,** choice of infraciliary (*a*) or high eyelid crease (*b*) incisions. **B,** dissection through orbicularis oculi and periosteum overlying the anterior wall of the maxilla. **C,** elevation of the periosteum and herniated soft tissues. **D,** insertion of Marlex mesh to cover orbital floor defect. **E,** closure of periosteum, **F,** closure of skin with subcuticular nonabsorbable suture. (From Burres S, Cohn A, Mathog RH: *Laryngoscope* 1981; 91:1881–1886. Used by permission.)

then be elevated superiorly across the orbital rim and into the floor of the orbit. Care must be taken to avoid damage to the infraorbital nerve.

With Joseph and Freer elevators, the periosteum is elevated off the floor of the orbit. A surgeon-controlled placement of the table and lighting is essential for adequate visualization of the floor area. The dissection should be directed medially, laterally, and posteriorly to surround and define the entire site of the fracture. All fat should then be elevated from the maxillary sinus with small sharp elevators. Bony trapdoor fragments can then be brought up into position with a small single skin hook. If there is a residual hole or a suggestion of instability, a piece of Marlex mesh is placed over the defect. The Marlex should be cut in such a way that there is a curvature to fit under the rim anteriorly and a notch posteriorly to accommodate the neuromuscular structures. Forced duction tests are then applied to determine the adequacy of the reduction and to assure that there is no entrapment. Closure is accomplished with a single 4–0 chromic catgut suture approximating the periosteum. The skin is closed with a 5–0 nylon running subcuticular suture.

My approach for a medial wall blowout fracture is via a Lynch incision. For this surgery, the incision is made one half the distance between the inner canthus and dorsum of the nose. Hemostasis of the angular vessels is controlled with an electrocautery. The periosteum is elevated off the nasal bones toward the medial orbital wall. The trochlea should be elevated from its attachment and the medial wall dissection continued to the level of the anterior ethmoidal vessel. The surgeon should stay superior to the attachment of the medial canthal ligament. Usually with medial wall blowout fractures, the anatomy of the wall is very much distorted, and it then becomes necessary to identify the posterior ethmoidal vessel or at least to work cautiously beyond a level 25 mm from the orbital rim. Medial wall blowout pathology can vary from a punched-out ethmoidal cell to a comminuted lamina papyracea. After elevation of fat, the bony wall fragments should be gently teased into position and the area lined with a piece of Marlex mesh. Closure is accomplished by several 4–0 chromic catgut sutures approximating the trochlea to the periosteum. The rest of the tissues are closed with subcuticular chromic catgut sutures and the skin with a fine nylon suture. Forced duction tests are performed to assure adequacy of reduction and avoid postoperative entrapment.

Superior and lateral orbital wall fractures are rare and require special techniques.[7] The anteriorly occurring roof fracture can often be explored and repaired through a lateral brow incision, but frequently the fracture extends backward and involves the floor of the frontal sinus and floor of the anterior fossa. When the fracture is confined to the frontal sinus region, a coronal incision and osteoplastic flap can be used for exposure and reduction. For fractures involving the anterior fossa, craniotomy and neurosurgical assistance is necessary. For any of these superior orbital wall fractures, the bone should be elevated into the anatomic position. The orbital rim and frontal bones should be reduced and fixed with wires or plates.

The lateral orbital wall blowout fracture usually occurs deep to the frontal process of the zygoma and involves a fracture of the zygoma and greater wing of the sphenoid. These blowout fractures are often associated with injury to the superior orbital fissure, and if the injury is associated with neuromuscular dysfunction, this may be a reason to reduce any displaced fragments. Extravasation of intraorbital soft tissues rarely occurs because of the pressure from the dura or soft tissues of the infratemporal fossa. Replacement of the lateral wall to the proper position usually will correct entrapment phenomena involving the lateral rectus muscle.

There are many variations of the orbital blowout fractures and the surgeon must be prepared for these differences. Occasionally, part of the floor is severely comminuted and involves the inferior portion of the medial wall. In such a situation, Marlex mesh is not strong enough for support, nor is there enough tissue to compensate for the discrepancy of orbital volume and contents. When this occurs, I prefer to use a separate incision vertically through the parietal scalp and remove one or several pieces of outer cranial plate from this region. Pieces of split cranial bone can then be cantilevered to close over the defect. Severely comminuted medial wall and superior wall injuries can also be treated in a similar fashion.

When the blow out injury also involves the malar bone, the frontal process of the zygoma and the infraorbital rim should also be exposed. Following reduction of the malar fracture, the floor should be examined to determine the size of the defect. If there is a large defect or instability, Marlex mesh can be used for reinforcement of this area.

When a medial orbital blowout fracture involves the optic foramen and is associated with blindness, the procedure should be combined with an optic nerve decompression. In this case I would explore more posteriorly, and using the posterior ethmoidal vessel as a landmark, I would expose the posterior limits of the ethmoidal air cells. The body of the sphenoid is then identified, and the thick bone around the optic canal is removed. A splitting of the sheath, as one would do with a facial nerve decompression, is unnecessary, and damage to the sheath can lead to a significant CSF leak.

With regard to results from early repair of blowout fractures, one must consider the site and severity of damage. Most simple fractures can be repaired with an expectation of normal appearance and function. In my 20-year experience with Marlex mesh, I have had no displacement or infection, and in only one patient was there a complaint of eyelid swelling and pain. The material is incorporated into the periosteum, and, in fact, it is difficult at a later time to remove it by usual surgical techniques.

The procedures, however, have limitations. If the fat is injured or lost, there will be enophthalmos. If there is muscle or nerve injury, there will be diplopia. Injury to the annulus tendineus will also result in neuromuscular problems. Because of all these factors that can affect the results, patients must be followed for at least 1 year to determine the final result. Although all patients are informed about the possibility of loss of vision as a result of the surgery, this should be considered a rare complication.

EYELID AND NASO-ORBITAL TRAUMA

Soft tissue injuries to the eyelid present a challenge to reconstructive surgeon. Poor healing from such injuries can result in a deformity and dysfunction. Patients can thus develop epiphora, retraction, and inadequate closure of the eyelid, corneal exposure, and pain.

When the eyelid is injured, as in a full-thickness laceration, it is important to identify and approximate the different levels of tissue—eyelid skin, orbicularis oculi, tarsal plate and conjunctiva.[8] The conjunctiva is first closed with a fine chromic or Vicryl suture in such a way the knots avoid abrasion of the cornea. The tarsal plate should be brought together with 4–0 chromic catgut sutures. Using the gray line (meibomian orifices) as a landmark, one should then close the eyelid skin. Since the orbicularis oculi is attached to the skin, closure of the skin will effectively repair any muscle injury. Sutures placed through the muscle should be avoided since they can cause a reaction and subsequent postoperative contraction.

Injuries that are associated with avulsion of the eyelid pose unique problems. Small defects can be wedged out and closed directly, whereas larger defects require special reconstructive techniques. Several methods use a switch type of flap where part of one eyelid is used to replace part of another. For details of these techniques, readers are referred to an oculoplastic text. When there is a complete avulsion of the eyelid, the tarsal plate can be reconstructed with nasal or auricular cartilage and the cheek tissues closed over the defect by advancement or rotation flaps.

Injury to the lacrimal collecting system should be recognized and treated as soon as possible. The upper canaliculis may be considered superfluous and need not be repaired, but the lower one is very important, and without its function, there is a good chance that epiphora will develop. One can often evaluate the injury by dilating the puncta with a Bowman probe and passing the probe into the area of the laceration. Using a microscope, one can pass a Silastic catheter through the canaliculus, from one segment to the other, and out through the lacrimal sac. A catheter attached to the Silastic tubing (Guibor tube) can then be passed through the lacrimal sac and out through the nose. As an alternative, one can bring the other end through the upper canaliculis and pass both ends through the nose to be tied as a knot within the nose. With the catheter as a stent, the torn canaliculis can be approximated with 10–0 nylon sutures, How long the catheter should remain in place is debatable, but several weeks are desirable.

Injury to the medial canthal ligament must also be appreciated and treated early.[9] Using a classification dependent on whether there is a simple avulsion or a laceration (type 1), comminution of the bone involving the medial wall of the orbit (type II), or comminution of both orbital walls (type III), I tailor a surgical approach for each condition (Fig 26–6).

Usually repair of the type I injury is through a medial canthal or Lynch incision one half the distance from the caruncle to the dorsum of the nose. After ligation of the angular vessels, the periorbita is elevated off the medial wall of the orbit. The trochlea is detached, and a generous exposure is obtained to demonstrate the medial canthal ligament and the enclosed lacrimal sac. Drill holes are then placed through the superior portion of the posterior lacrimal crest and the ligament secured to these holes with a fine 30-gauge wire. Often this wire suture can be passed through the anterior and posterior parts of medial canthal ligament and the fundus of the sac without damage to the function of the lacrimal collecting system. If there is a need to obtain additional relaxation, a lateral canthotomy through a lateral brow incision should also be performed. Attempts should be made for overcorrection. The soft tissues are then closed in layers. Buttons are avoided since they frequently cause necrosis of the soft tissues.

For the type II injury, my approach is identical, except

another Lynch incision is made on the opposite side of the nose to expose the opposite lacrimal bone. This repair is then carried out by passing a 30-gauge wire on a large curved needle to the opposite side, where the wire is secured to the upper part of the lacrimal crest. A lateral canthotomy is also an important part of the procedure. As with the type I repair, overcorrection for placement of the ligament is desirable.

When there is a type III injury, again the approach is through bilateral Lynch incisions. After adequate exposure, the medial canthal ligaments are secured to each other. For this procedure, it is important to place the wire as high and as posteriorly in the nose as possible, so that the eyelids are drawn up and back against the globes. Failure to do so can result in an epiphora and excessive scleral show.

SURGERY OF MAXILLARY FRACTURES

Introduction of the miniplate has significantly changed the treatment of maxillary fractures. In years past, one would use IMF, circumzygomatic wires, and frontal suspension almost routinely; now many fractures are stabilized by several small miniplates placed in strategic areas for stability and strength.

In preparation for repair of maxillary fractures, I usually wait 7 days until most swelling has disappeared and the sinuses have started to obtain air. Sinus radiographs and CT scans are then obtained, and initial impressions are checked. The Le Fort classification is used for the description of the injury and appropriate planning. The patient is usually anesthetized with a tracheostomy tube, since nasal tubes interfere with any nasal fracture reduction, and oral intubation will preclude accurate fixation and occlusion.

Le Fort I Split Palate and Segmental Fractures

The Le Fort I injury can often be approached conservatively with good results. For such an injury in the patient with teeth, Ivy loops or arch bar fixation is satisfactory. One would think that the mandible would eventually displace the maxilla, but this does not occur, and healing is usually uneventful. If the patient is edentulous, I would prefer plating the inferior portion of the maxillary buttress. If the fracture is associated with comminution of the alveolar ridge, dentures or prefabricated splints, secured by circumzygomatic and circummandibular wires, would be preferred.

Special techniques are necessary for the split palate and segmental fractures. If the palate is fractured and there is a displacement of the lateral portions of the palate, reduction should be carried out with Rowe disimpaction forceps, and the fragments should be stabilized across the midline (Fig 26–7).[10] I still prefer a strong arch bar across the incisors, but if the patient is edentulous, I would stabilize the roof of the mouth and alveolus with dentures or a palatal splint. Any instability can be corrected further by placing bone screws through the plate into the palatine bone on each side of the fracture. The denture additionally can be held to the maxillary arch with circumzygomatic wires and then placed into an occlusal relationship with the lower denture. Hooks or arch bars affixed to

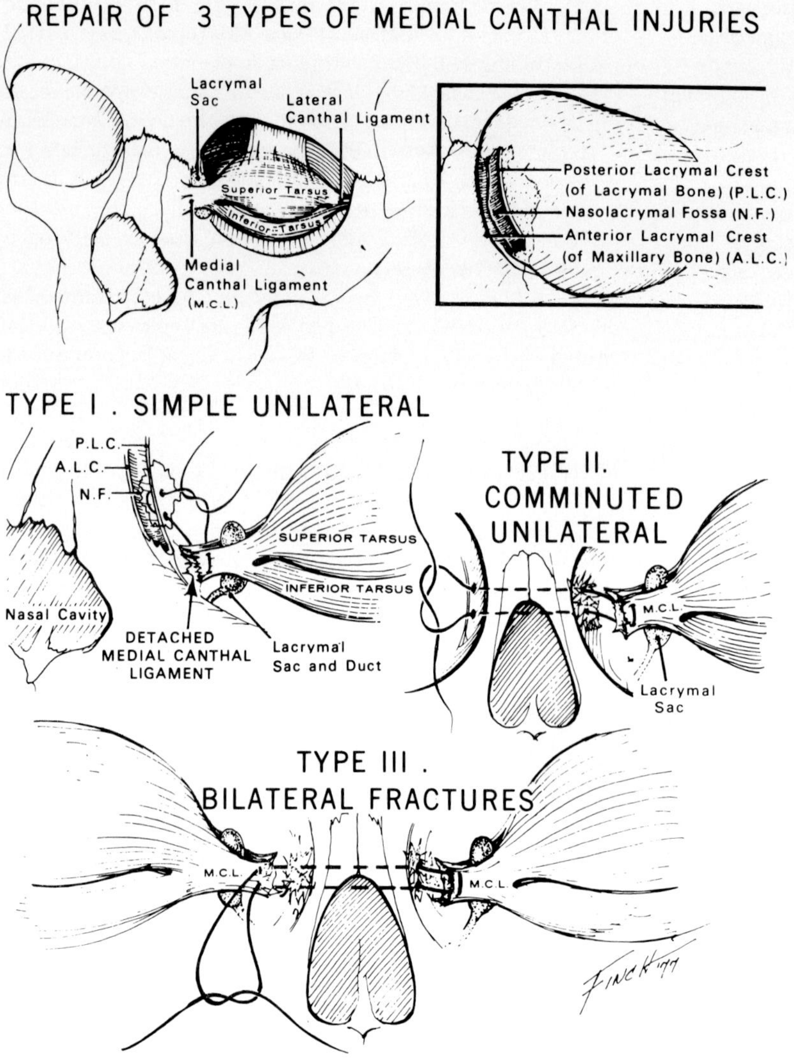

FIG 26–6.
Repair of three types of medial canthal injuries. *Type I:* avulsion or laceration of medial canthal ligament or simple fracture of medial wall of orbit. Repair by attachment of ligament to the superior portion of the posterior lacrimal crest. *Type II:* comminuted fracture of medial orbital wall. Repair by transnasal attachment of fine wire (no. 30) to contralateral lacrimal crest. *Type III:* bilateral comminuted fractures of the medial orbital walls. Repair by transnasal attachment of medial canthal ligaments with fine wire (no. 30). (From Mathog RH, Bauer W: *Arch Otolaryngol* 1979; 105:81–85. Used by permission.)

the dentures can be used for the IMF.

For the repair of segmental fractures, placement of an arch bar over the area of instability is usually sufficient. If the patient is edentulous, dentures fixed to the jaws via circumzygomatic and circummandibular wires with IMF is a satisfactory method. High fractures can be treated with interosseous wires or plates, but if the fractures are near the alveolus, the wire or plate can protrude into the labiobuccal or labiogingival sulcus and become a nuisance in the postoperative period.

Le Fort II Injuries

For the repair of the Le Fort II injury, I usually approach the fracture by sublabial degloving and infraciliary incisions. After adequate reduction usually with Rowe disimpaction forceps, I establish occlusion with two Ivy loops and then use plates or fine wires to stabilize the zygomaticomaxillary buttress. The inferior orbital rim is usually repaired with a 28-gauge wire.

I choose not to plate near the orbital rim since the plates are often palpable and can often be observed after surgery. I also explore the floor of the orbit and treat any fracture in this area.

If the Le Fort II fracture is comminuted, I prefer to plate the larger fragments and hold the smaller fragments into position with fine wires. Usually I find that parts of the zygomaticomaxillary buttress are sufficiently intact for application of the plates. If the comminution extends into the alveolus, dentures and splints with circumzygomatic suspension wires are preferred. Rarely do I use bone grafts to stabilize the areas of comminution.

For the edentulous patient with a Le Fort II fracture, I would reduce the fracture and then approximate the maxillary arch in an occlusal relationship to the mandibular arch. If plating and wiring techniques provide sufficient stability, I will forego any IMF. If, on the other hand, interosseous fixation is unstable, dentures, circumzygomatic wires and IMF would be adjunctive measures.

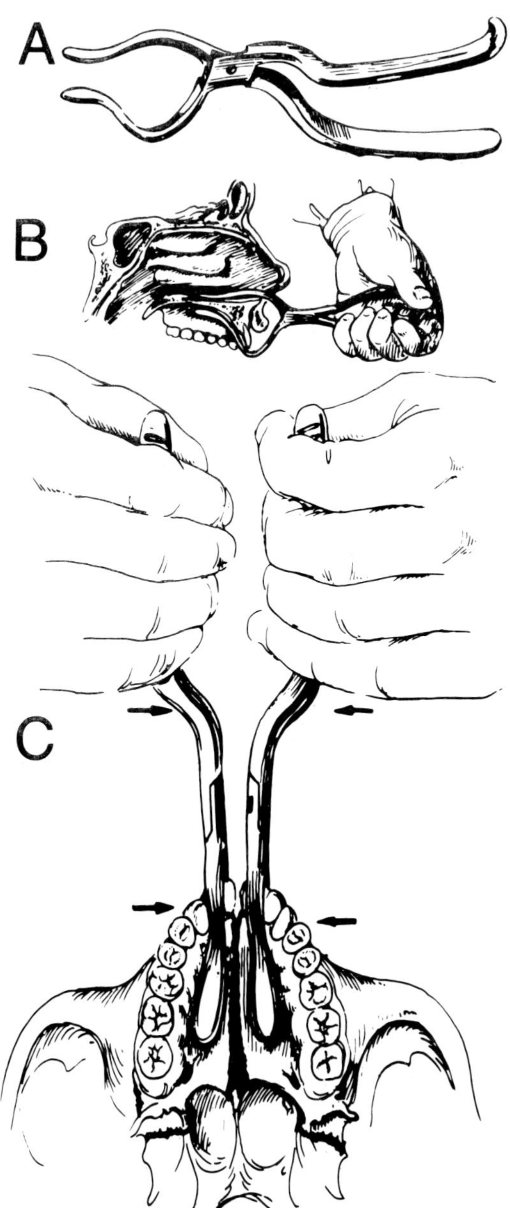

FIG 26–7.
Technique of disimpaction with Rowe's forceps. **A,** Rowe's forceps. **B,** position of forceps for disimpaction. **C,** use of forceps to approximate maxillary fragments in sagittal fracture. (From Converse JM: *Kazanjian and Converse's Surgical Treatment of Facial Injuries,* ed 3. Baltimore, Williams & Wilkins Co, 1974, vol. 1, pp 230–236. Used by permission.)

Le Fort III Fractures

The Le Fort III injuries are probably the most challenging of the facial injuries since they are often complex and can be associated with other maxillofacial bone fractures. According to the classical description of the Le Fort III injury, these fractures cause malar bone instability, and fixation can be obtained only by securing the facial skeleton to the cranium.

Many techniques are available to deal with Le Fort III injury. Preferably, I like to expose as many of the involved facial bones as possible. The degree and site of fracture will determine the approach. If the fractures are extensive and involve the frontal region, a coronal flap approach is desirable. For fractures involving the frontozygomatic suture, one can use the brow incision, and for the nasomaxillary buttress and the zygomaticomaxillary buttress, I prefer the sublabial degloving incision. Fractures of the inferior orbital rim can be managed by infraciliary incisions.

My aim is to reduce the fragments and plate over the buttress. I do not believe that plates are needed everywhere but just in those areas of stress where the bones are naturally thickened. Thus, plates can be placed along the nasomaxillary portion of the maxilla, the frontozygomatic suture lines, and the zygomaticomaxillary buttress. I try to avoid plates near edges (i.e., the orbital rim), however, because they can be palpable or seen through the skin. Displaced small pieces of bone can be either wired directly or, if they are unstable, held in position by periosteal sutures. If the frontal bone is unstable, it may be advantageous to apply a Georgiade halo and maintain the position of the facial prominences with halo supported wires (Fig 26–8).[14] This technique also has the advantage of allowing the surgeon to make adjustments in the position of the facial bones in the postoperative period.

If the patient with the Le Fort III fracture is edentulous, I essentially use the same open procedures that I would apply to the patient with teeth. Occasionally a patient will show instability, retrusion, or lengthening of the face, and if this occurs, dentures or splints with intermaxillary fixation must be considered. However, proper suspension techniques are necessary to avoid overcorrection, compression of the midface, and open bite deformity.

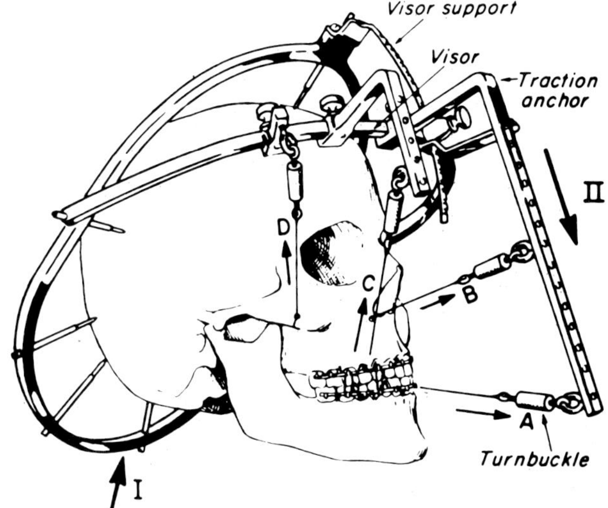

FIG 26–8.
Halo frame used for traction and immobilization of intermediate and high maxillary fractures, especially when fracture involves frontal bone. (From Georgiade N, Nash T: *Plast Reconstr Surg* 1966; 38:142–146. Used by permission.)

MANAGEMENT OF MASSIVE SOFT TISSUE INJURY

Early Treatment

Extensive soft tissue injuries of the face also require special considerations and techniques. Massive loss of tissue usually associated with gunshot wounds and avulsions from industrial accidents present with severe life-threatening problems. The first order of business is to secure an airway and stop bleeding. Second, the patient should be immunized for tetanus and treated appropriately with antibiotics.[12] Once these precautionary measures are accomplished, the damage can be evaluated and repair anticipated.[13]

Wounds should first be cleansed with saline solution and the patient given prophylactic antibiotics (i.e., intravenous penicillin). Vitality of the tissues should be evaluated, and if vitality is questionable, the tissues should be retained. Only "dead" tissues should be debrided.

One of my initial concerns is often the facial nerve. As a general rule, injuries anterior to a line drawn from the lateral canthus to the corner mouth need not be repaired. However, injuries of the nerve proximal to this region should be considered for either anastomosis or grafts. Usually, my approach is via a superficial parotidectomy, and since the superficial lobe of the parotid is often injured, it can be removed and discarded. The course of the nerve can then be followed to the periphery. If the branches are not easily seen, I will use landmarks such as the posterior facial vein to find the mandibular branch or Stensen's duct to find the buccal branch. As many branches as possible should be exposed and should be repaired with anastomotic techniques. Usually I use a 7–0 nylon placed in four quadrants around the nerve. If a section of the nerve is missing, I will obtain a piece of greater auricular nerve as an interposed graft. I do not believe it is desirable to tag ends and come back later, since the best opportunity for repair is as early as possible after the injury.

With regard to a Stensen duct injury near the orifice, it need not be repaired. However, damage close to the parotid will require stenting with a Silastic tube and careful microscopic approximation of the duct wall with fine suture technique. If a portion of the duct is macerated, there is also an option of securing the proximal end to the buccal mucosa, allowing the duct to empty directly into the mouth.

Repair of soft tissue injuries to the face depends on the site and degree of loss. Mucosal lacerations and tears should be closed with heavy 2–0 chromic catgut sutures. Fractures should then be repaired with traditional techniques. If muscles of mastication are torn, the bundles should be brought together and secured with 2–0 or 3–0 chromic catgut mattress sutures.

With regard to skin loss, one should use direct closure or, if not possible, local or regional flaps. When a small area of skin is involved, adjacent skin flaps can be undermined, elevated, and approximated to close the defect. If the area of skin loss is large (i.e., 8–10 cm²), one must consider the use of local tissues such as cheek or neck rotation or regional tissues such as pectoralis major or deltopectoral flaps. Immediate full-thickness coverage is important and should be obtained as soon as possible. If the patient's condition should be unstable, I might consider the need for speed and apply split-thickness grafts. However, these grafts are certain to contract, and they will not establish those optimal conditions that I would like for further reconstruction.

Late Treatment

For the most part, extensive soft tissue injury of the face will result in deformity and dysfunction. Beyond the early phase of treatment, the surgeon is confronted with the problems of scarring, loss of tissues, malunion of bones, and failure of physiologic systems. My approach for surgical rehabilitation is to first reestablish the bony architecture and then to reconstruct the soft tissues. For this to be successful, there must be sufficient soft tissues to cover the bones. If this is not the case, additional soft tissues from adjacent or regional areas must be mobilized to the defect.

For repair of deformed facial bones, I prefer osteotomy and adjunctive bone grafting (iliac crest, split cranium, or rib grafts). Usually I will expose the fracture site, recreate the original fracture lines with osteotomy, and move the bone into a desirable position. Bone grafts are then placed or wired behind the mobilized bone to maintain long-standing stability.[14] If, however, there has been some comminution of fragments or fracture lines extending into the cranium or near the optic nerve, I will choose onlay techniques. For these procedures, I create subperiosteal pockets, carve the bones to appropriate size and shape, and place the grafts into the pockets. Often the grafts will be held securely by closing the periosteum over the graft with 2–0 chromic catgut sutures.

After the bony structures are restored, I usually proceed with the soft tissue reconstruction. Gingivolabial or gingivobuccal sulci are created with split-thickness grafts or Z-plasty techniques. Lip reconstruction is usually performed by advancement or "lip switch" flaps. The nose and perinasal tissues are restored with adjacent rotation and advancement flaps, coupled with rhinoplasty and septoplasty techniques. Oculoplastic methods are used to reconstruct the form and size of the eyelids.

In the final phase of surgical rehabilitation, consideration should be given to revision of scars and dermabrasion.[15] I will revise as many scars as possible at one sitting as long as the revision of one scar will not affect the skin tension of another. I usually use Z-plasty techniques to transpose tissues, change lines, and reduce contraction. The Z-plasty technique is used frequently for scars longer than 2 cm. When the revised scars have matured, I dermabrade that area of the face, often several times, to obtain desirable results.

TREATMENT OF MANDIBLE FRACTURES

Successful treatment of mandibular fractures requires reduction and an accurate stable fixation. These objectives can be achieved by a number of techniques, such as closed reduction and intermaxillary fixation as well as open reduction with interosseous wires, plates or external fixation devices. Adjunctive

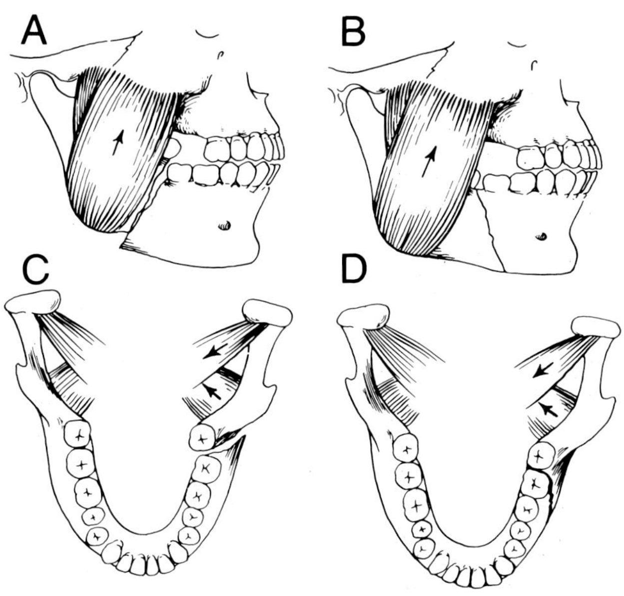

FIG 26–9.
Muscle attachments and forces that affect stability of angle-body fractures. Vertically unstable (**A**) and vertically stable (**B**) as a result of temporal, masseter, and suprahyoid group of muscles. Horizontally unstable (**C**) and horizontally stable (**D**) as a result of pterygoid muscles. (From Stanley RB: Pathogenesis and evaluation of mandibular fractures, in Mathog RH [ed]: *Maxillofacial Trauma.* Baltimore, Williams & Wilkins Co, 1984, pp 136–147. Used by permission.)

methods include the use of splints and stents. What techniques should be used depends on the site and the severity of the injury, age and physical status of the patient, and quality of the dentition.

As to the site of fracture, much will depend on the line of the fracture and whether it is accompanied by other fractures.[16] The attachment of muscles to the mandible in relationship to the line of fracture will determine whether the fracture is unstable or stable (Fig 26–9). Usually fractures that are unstable will require an open technique, whereas fractures that are fairly stable can often be treated with a closed technique. In general, fractures of the parasymphysis and angle are unstable and are better handled by the open methods. Fractures of the body are stable and are more suitable for the closed techniques. Condylar fractures, by tradition, have been successfully treated with one of the closed methods.

It should also be noted that more than one fracture can affect the stability of the segments. For example, there will be a tendency for displacement or rotation if there are two fractures on the same side of the midline. This is often seen with a fracture of the condyle, or angle, in combination with a fracture of the parasymphysis, in which the intervening segment is rotated into the oral cavity (Fig 26–10).[17] Comminution should be a variation of multiple fractures on one side and would also pose similar problems. These types of fractures must be handled by special techniques.

The status of the dentition is also an important part of the decision-making process. Usually when there is an adequate

dentition, closed methods are more easily applied. On the other hand, when the patient is edentulous or has an edentulous segment, an open technique may be necessary for stability.

Other considerations are the age and physical condition of the patient. For the most part, the elderly or debilitated patient does not do well when his or her jaws are closed by intermaxillary fixation. Consequently, open techniques that provide for early postoperative mobility are desirable. However, if the patient is so debilitated that surgery carries excessive risk, a conservative approach may be the better choice.

The Dentulous Mandible

Assuming that the patient has an adequate dentition and is healthy, there is a "cookbook" for the management of the common fractures. For the isolated subcondylar fracture without much displacement, the patient can be treated with soft diet and analgesics. If the fracture affects the bite or causes pain, the fracture is best treated with a variable period of IMF. This can be accomplished with arch bars or Ivy loops for 4 to 6 weeks in adults and 2 to 4 weeks in children. If the fracture is badly displaced or associated with a foreign body, the fracture may need to be explored and treated with open techniques (Fig 26–11).[14] Before this is done, Ivy loops are used to approximate occlusion. I then approach the condyle by a preauricular incision, expose the capsule of the joint, and follow the fibrous tissue to the neck of the condyle. This dissection should put the fracture in direct view, and when this occurs, two small Steinmann pins or Kirschner wires are drilled directly into the

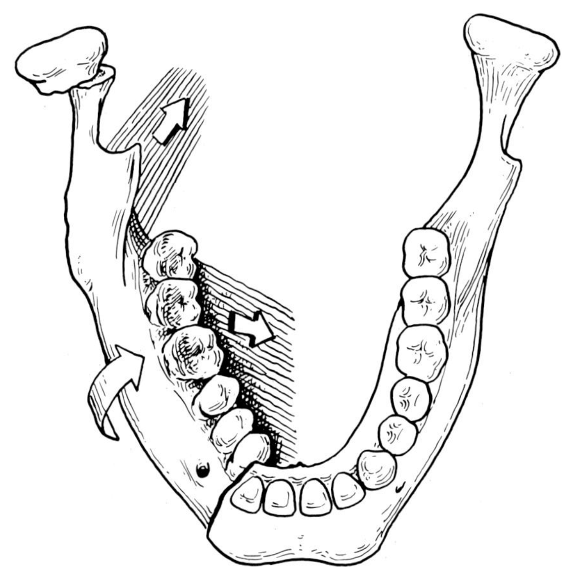

FIG 26–10.
Instability of jaw when more than one fracture occurs on the same side. Note that with ipsilateral subcondylar and parasymphyseal fractures, the hemimandible is pulled and rotated with the forces of the myelohyoid and pterygoid muscles. (From Fernandez J, Mathog RH: *Arch Otol Head Neck Surg* 1987; 113:262–266. Used by permission.)

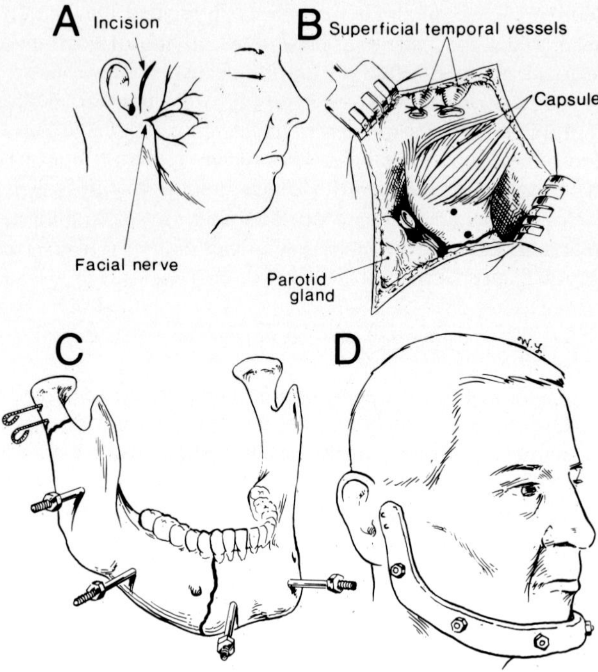

FIG 26–11.
Technique of open fixation of subcondylar fractures. **A,** preauricular incision. **B,** ligation of superficial temporal vessels and exposure of capsule of temporomandibular joint. **C,** pin fixation of mandible and condyle. **D,** application of acrylic bar (biphase technique). (From Fernandez J, Mathog RH: *Arch Otol Head Neck Surg* 1987; 113:262–266. Used by permission.)

neck of the condyle. Two other pins are placed into the ramus or angle of the mandible. The pins are then brought into a position that is consistent with reduction; they are subsequently held in this position with an acrylic bar.

In the treatment of fractures of the angle, which often are characterized by instability, the fracture can be effectively (and traditionally) treated with interosseous wiring and IMF. In recent years however, I have, as an alternative, used compression plates (Fig 26–12).[18] Although there are many types of plates, I have had good experience with the Luhr system. I still set the occlusion temporarily with Ivy loops and then apply the plate to provide an accurate and stable fixation.

Exposure to the angle is usually through a submandibular incision several finger-breadths below the angle of the jaw. I first identify the mandibular branch of the facial nerve as it dips beneath the angle of the mandible and then proceed with the dissection to a deeper level, which will carry us directly to the inferior border of the mandible. If I choose to apply interosseous wires, I usually place the holes for the wires strategically along the sides of the fracture so that the segments are pulled together. A figure-of-eight wire can be applied, but one must be careful that the diagonal of the wire does not enter the fracture. For application of the plate to the angle, I like to secure at least two holes on each side of the fracture. Stripping of periosteum may be considerable, and this is one of the disadvantages of the plate system. In the presence of teeth, an arch

bar can serve as a tension bar. In the absence of a tension bar, however, one must consider using the eccentric dynamic compression plate to achieve a stable fixation.

In a patient with teeth who has a body fracture, IMF alone will be satisfactory. These fractures are usually quite stable and

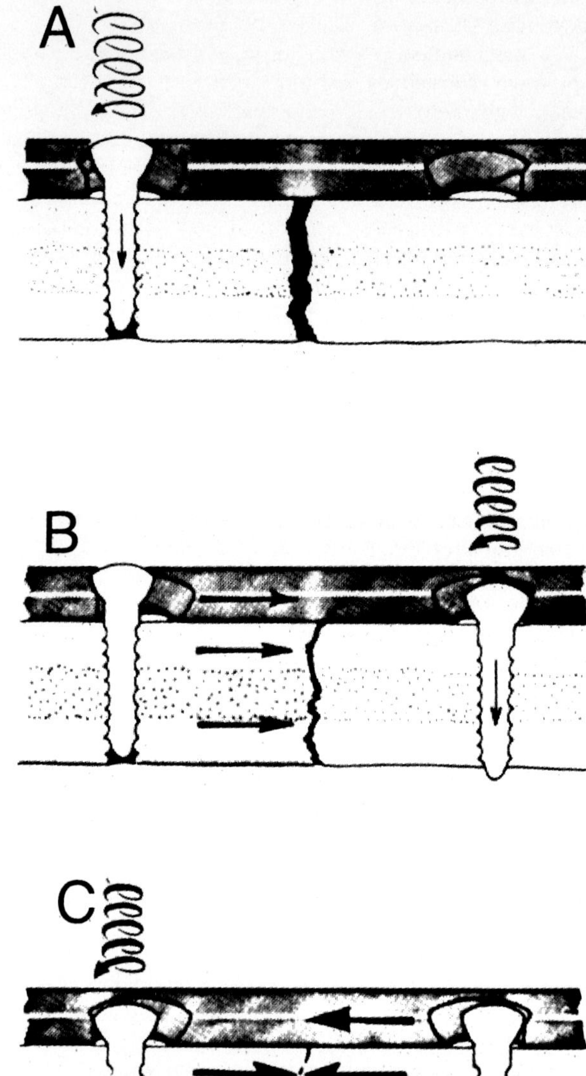

FIG 26–12.
Dynamic compression plate. **A,** the first screw is partly inserted to secure plate. **B,** the second screw is inserted and then tightened to push the fragments together. Eccentricity of the screw hole forces a sliding action so that the bone moves underneath the stationary plate. **C,** the tightening of the first screw advances further the segments to provide a rigid fixation. (From Spiessl B [ed]: *New Concepts in Maxillofacial Bone Surgery.* New York, Springer-Verlag New York, 1976. Used by permission.)

do not require open reduction. If the body fracture is complicated by comminution, or severe displacement, however, it should be opened. My surgical approach would be an incision several centimeters below the lower margin of the jaw. I would then dissect the fascia over the submandibular gland and ligate the facial artery and vein. If the fracture appeared unstable, compression plates could be used. In many cases, a simple 25-gauge wire satisfactorily secures the fracture.

In the treatment of a parasymphaseal fracture, there is often a problem of instability. For these reasons, the fracture is best treated with interosseous wiring and IMF. Plates can be applied, but they are difficult to contour to this "rounded region," and postoperatively the patient may complain of a "feel of the plate through the skin." Occasionally patients complain of pain because the plate tends to interact with the mental nerve. Exposure to the parasymphyseal region is usually through a submental incision. The dissection is fairly safe since one is not near the facial vessels or the mandibular branch of the facial nerve. Still, there is a possibility of injury to the mental branch of the inferior alveolar nerve, and to avoid this complication, one must be aware of its exact anatomic location.

The Edentulous Mandible

Treatment of mandibular fractures in patients without teeth is a serious problem. Stable fixation is difficult to obtain, and if the jaw has become atrophic as a result of edentulation, treatment options are limited. On the other hand, exact occlusal relationships are not required, and minor discrepancies in occlusion can be corrected by modification of a denture.

In considering treatment for an edentulous condylar fracture, one must evaluate the degree of displacement and dysfunction (i.e., trismus, pain, and open bite deformity). If the displacement is minimal and opening and closing functions are near normal, a soft diet and analgesics would probably be adequate therapy. If, however, this is not the case, one would use circummandibular or circumzygomatic attachment of splints or dentures and IMF, or open reduction of the fracture. Usually my open techniques are reserved for bilateral condylar fractures with open bite deformity, displacement of the condylar head out of the glenoid fossa, fracture associated with a foreign body, and fracture associated with an ipsilateral mandibular fracture. I prefer the open method of pinning the fragments with a Kirschner wire and biphase fixation as described earlier.

The angle fracture in the edentulous patient is preferably treated with a compression plate. External fixation via a biphase is used when there is contamination of the wound or multiple (comminuted) ipsilateral fractures. If the patient has dentures, there is a third option of interosseous wires and securing the dentures via circummandible or circumzygomatic wires and IMF.

Body fractures associated with the absence of teeth may pose special problems because of atrophy of the jaw and a poor blood supply to the area. For the treatment of a mandible of normal size, open reduction with internal or external rigid fixation is satisfactory. If the mandible is thin, I would prefer either a closed method (dentures, splints, and intermaxillary fixation) or an immediate onlay bone grafting of the fracture site. In such a case, I would use a split rib and secure it to the mandible with circummandibular wires. Additional fixation with splints or dentures is desirable.

For the edentuous patient with a parasymphyseal fracture, an open technique is the treatment of choice. Such a fracture can be stabilized with interosseous wiring, and additional fixation can be obtained with the IMF via denture or splints. A rigid internal fixation plate is also applicable, but one must be prepared to accurately fit the plate to the curved surface of the mandible. External biphase fixation is technically easier and provides satisfactory stability, but it does have the disadvantage of an outside fixation device and will create small posttreatment scars in the chin region.

Postoperatively, I examine the reduction of mandible fractures by x-ray film and check occlusion and stability of the jaw. Antibiotics are used prophylactically for at least 5 days after surgery.[12] Patients are instructed in the use of a water pick for oral hygiene, and they are seen in the office every 2 weeks in the postoperative period. After removal of the fixation device, the patient bites on a tongue blade and is evaluated for movement of the fragments and pain. If there is a question of healing, fixation can be prolonged for longer periods of time. Usually the patient is seen one or two times later for a final evaluation.

Teeth in the Fracture Line

How to manage teeth in the fracture line is a controversial issue. Unfortunately, the tooth, which is a valuable guide for occlusion and stability, can be a problem and may need to be sacrificed. As a general rule, a tooth that is carious, loose, or in a site of fracture should be considered for removal. Retention may promote bacterial invasion. If the tooth is injured by the fracture in such a way that it is nonviable, it can serve as a foreign body and increase the chance of infection. Fractures to the pulp can also provide a portal of entry for infection into the apical area. Thus, any fracture that is associated with a fracture of the tooth root is suspect, and for this reason, such a tooth should be removed.

There are, however, situations in which it is not easy to determine whether to extract a tooth. This occurs when the fracture runs to the side of the tooth, and removal of the tooth will lead to a bone deficit next to the fracture site. In such an instance, my decision is based on the health of the tooth and the need for the tooth to provide stability to the fixation. For this reason, I will often retain the tooth when the tooth lies in the posterior segment and provides a stop against the maxillary dentition. Also, if the tooth is part of the anterior fragment near the angle and blocks the rotation of the posterior fragment upward, it is best retained. Teeth should also be considered for retention when they are needed to provide a wire loop from one tooth to the other or in the manufacture of a tension bar needed on the alveolar surface of the mandible.

Comminution of the Mandible

Multiple fractures of the mandible pose another set of conditions that require modifications of surgical technique. Many fractures classified as comminution are associated with gunshot

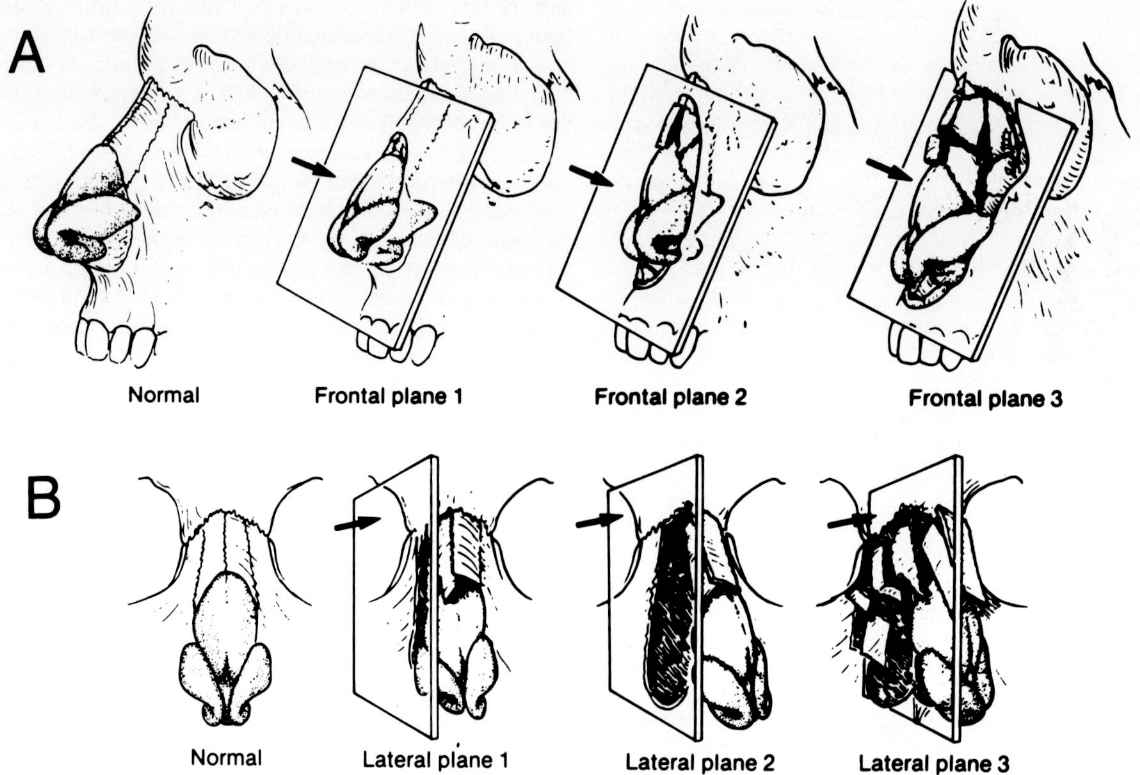

FIG 26–13.
Concept of impact forces and levels (planes of destruction). **A,** with frontal forces, fractures can involve (*1*) nasal tip; (*2*) nasal dorsum, septum, and anterior nasal spine; and (*3*) frontal process of maxilla, lacrimal, and ethmoid bones. **B,** with lateral oblique forces, fractures can involve (*1*) ipsilateral nasal bone; (*2*) contralateral nasal bone and septum; and (*3*) nasal bone, frontal process of maxilla, and lacrimal bone. (From Mathog RH: Acute nasal fractures, in Cummings CW, Fredrickson JM, Harker LA, et al [eds]: *Otolaryngology—Head and Neck Surgery.* St Louis, CV Mosby Co, 1986, pp 628–637. Used by permission.)

wounds, and because of the potential for contamination, these fractures are usually treated in a conservative fashion. For example, in the patient with teeth, IMF may be all that is needed for a successful result. If the patient has dentures, they can be affixed to the maxilla and mandible and then to each other. If there are no dentures and the patient is edentulous, I would prefer to use a biphase technique and span the comminuted segment. I usually avoid a bendable plate since there is a potentially contaminated wound, and I suspect that the plate can act as foreign body and promote infection. Moreover, plating requires stripping of periosteum, which can further devitalize the fragments and predispose toward complications. Interosseous wiring is also avoided since it also requires stripping and provides little, if any, stability.

NASOFRONTOETHMOID FRACTURES

An impact to the midface can affect the nasal bones, the frontal processes of the maxilla, the lacrimal, ethmoid, and frontal bones, the quadrilateral plate of septal cartilage, and the perpendicular plates of the ethmoid and vomer.[19] What bones are injured depends on the direction and force of the blow (Fig

26–13). In severe injuries, many bones may be damaged; there may also be associated cranial injury, CSF leak, and damage to orbital soft tissues.

Nasal Fractures

My preference for the treatment of nasal injuries is to use closed techniques. Exceptions, though, are open wounds or nasal fractures associated with medial maxillary or medial orbital wall fractures in which there is a need for additional surgical exposure. Also, if there is a failure to reduce the fracture by closed techniques, open methods are employed.

A closed reduction of a nasal fracture requires careful anesthetic preparation of the nose. After treatment of the nasal mucosa with 4% cocaine containing 5 drops of epinephrine 1:10,000, I perform a regional block with 2% lidocaine containing epinephrine 1:100,000. The nose is then inspected, and reduction is performed. Usually there is a depressed side opposite to a lateralized side of the nose. In such cases, the depressed side is elevated with a Boies elevator while the opposite side is pushed down with the thumb of the other hand (Fig 26–14). These maneuvers should project and straighten the nose. For the reduction of the septum, I massage the septum supe-

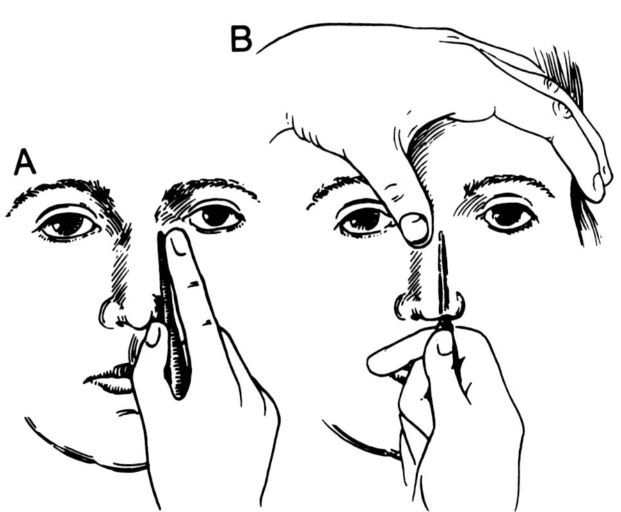

FIG 26–14.
Reduction of nasal fracture. **A,** Boies elevator is placed along the lateral wall of the nose to a point below the nasal frontal angle. Distance to ala is measured with the thumb. **B,** elevator is then placed under the depressed nasal bone, lifting it into position. The opposite thumb carefully exerts downward pressure on the elevated contralateral bone. (From Mathog RH: Acute nasal fractures, in Cummings CW, Fredrickson JM, Harker LA, et al [eds]: *Otolaryngology—Head and Neck Surgery.* St Louis, CV Mosby Co, 1986, pp 628–637. Used by permission.)

riorly with a forceps (i.e., Asche type) and manipulate the caudal part of the septum back on to the maxillary crest. The septum is then held in the midline with light bacitracin gauze packs or tampons. The nasal bones are held in position and protected with tapes and a plaster dressing.

In patients requiring open methods, I prefer to make intercartilaginous incisions, expose the lower portion of the nasal bones, and minipulate the nasal bones into position with needle-nose rongeurs (Fig 26–15). If there is already an incision for a medial canthal or a medial maxillary exposure, these incisions are also used to reduce and fix the nasal fracture. When the fracture involves the larger thicker portions of the pyriform aperture and frontal processes of the maxilla, I try to wire directly the fragments with 28-gauge wire techniques.

If the septal injury requires open reduction, an intermembranous incision is developed alone or in combination with an intercartilaginous incision (i.e., transfixion). As in a septoplasty, a mucosal-perichondrial and periosteal flap is elevated beyond the level of the overriding fracture. The dissection is usually carried out on the same side of the displaced fragment and across the fracture to the opposite side to completely free the posterior fragment. If the fragment cannot be easily manipulated into position, it is trimmed and replaced. Also, it can be held in position by replacing the flaps and applying thin plastic splints to the outside of the flaps. These splints are secured to the columella with 3–0 nylon sutures. If the replaced septum is still unstable, it can be held with a figure-of-eight suture in which the suture is placed between the fragments and then across

each of the fragments. At the conclusion of the procedure, a light packing or splints are applied.

In some cases the patient may develop a septal hematoma. This complication can occur at the time of injury or even after the reduction. A clue to a septal hematoma will be swelling of the nose, pain, and oozing of blood from the nostril. There will also be a noticeable widening of the septum. When I diagnose a septal hematoma, I prefer immediate drainage by incision of the mucosa on one side and removal of the blood by suction. Mucosal flaps are put back into position and held there with a bacitracin gauze packing. The packing should be removed within 24 to 48 hours, and the nose should be inspected again for accumulation of blood clot. Antibiotic coverage is mandatory during and after these manipulations.

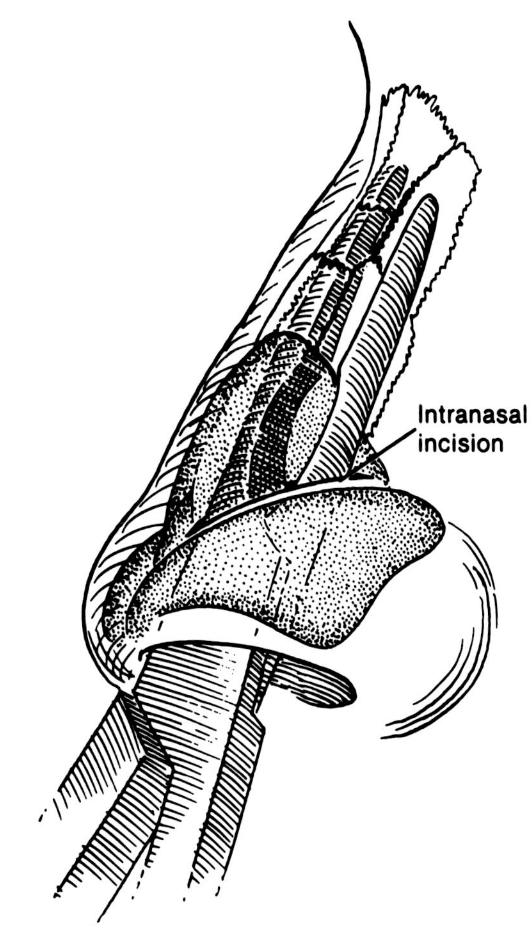

FIG 26–15.
Open reduction and manipulation of nasal bones using Lempert rongeur. After intercartilaginous incision and elevation of dorsal skin, blades of Lempert rongeur are inserted on each side of the depressed nasal bone and used to mobilize the bone for a correct position. (From Mathog RH: Acute nasal fractures, in Cummings CW, Fredrickson JM, Harker LA, et al [eds]: *Otolaryngology—Head and Neck Surgery.* St Louis, CV Mosby Co, 1986, pp 628–637. Used by permission.)

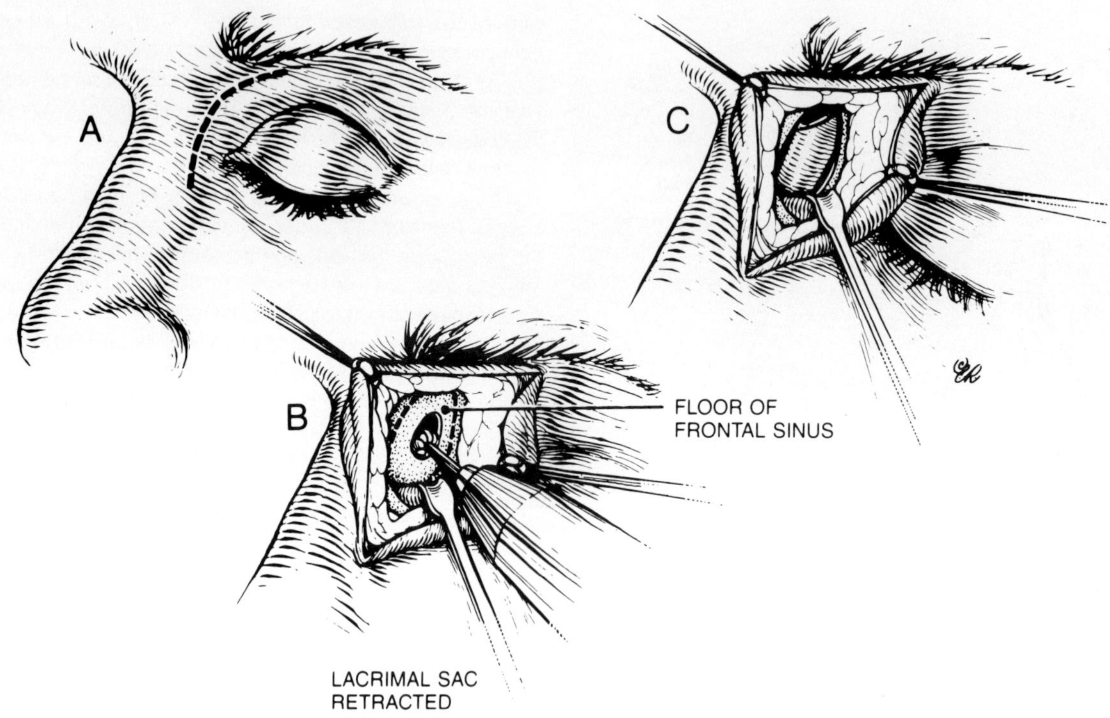

FIG 26–16.
Reduction of frontal sinus fracture and reconstruction of nasofrontal duct with tube technique. **A,** Lynch type of incision. **B,** removal of floor of frontal sinus, portion of frontal process of maxilla, and anterior ethmoid cells with cutting burrs. **C,** exploration of sinus, reduction of fractures, and insertion of large (no. 26 French) Silastic chest tube. (From Owens OT, Mathog RH: Frontal sinus fractures, in Foster CA, Sherman JE [eds]: *Surgery of Facial Bone Fractures.* New York, Churchill Livingstone, 1987, pp 13–23. Used by permission.)

Comminuted nasal bone fractures are usually best treated by a closed technique, but if the bones are so unstable and packing pushes the bones outward, a lead plate method is desirable. In treating such a condition, I manipulate the bones into the appropriate position and lightly pack the nasal cavities. Oval-shaped lead plates are then placed along the side of the nasal bones on top of a thin sheet of Silastic, which is used to protect the skin from the hardness and cutting effect of the plate. Two drill holes are placed through each plate, and with Keith needles, a 28-gauge wire is placed in mattress fashion across the plates and through the nasal pyramid. Good results are often obtained if the plates are placed posteriorly and the pyramid contoured to as narrow a shape as possible. In the postoperative period, there will be swelling, and the plates will tend to widen. The plates should be removed in 7 to 10 days.

Fractures extending into the frontal process of the maxilla and ethmoid and lacrimal bones are often associated with a traumatic telecanthus. These injuries may be handled by Lynch incisions, but if additional exposure is necessary, the incisions can be extended across the glabella angle with an H or I design ("open sky" approach). The management of these injuries is discussed in the section on eyelid trauma.

Frontal Sinus Fractures

Frontal sinus fractures are classified according to site of injury, that is, anterior, posterior, and inferior wall.[20] Usually the anterior wall fractures are caused by a blow to the frontal or brow region and are associated with a laceration or hematoma of the forehead. Depression of the forehead is common, because there is often a displacement of a large fragment or comminution of the bone. Injuries to the posterior wall can occur from severe injury to the anterior wall, but they are usually seen with other cranial fractures. Individuals with posterior wall fractures also have a history of unconsciousness with varying degrees of brain injury and CSF leak. Injury to the inferior wall is often associated with fracture to the posterior wall and superior wall of the orbit. These fractures present also with cranial damage and CSF leaks. In addition, inferior wall fractures have the potential to affect the nasofrontal duct and cause obstruction and later complications of sinusitis. They, moreover, can affect orbital volume and cause enophthalmos or exophthalmos, depending on the direction of displacement of the bones.[7]

Anterior wall fractures can usually be treated by open or semiopen techniques. Sufficient exposure can often be obtained through laceration, but if this is not possible, it may be necessary to create a coronal or inferior brow incision. If one needs only an exploration and a simple manipulation, a Lynch (medial canthal) approach is satisfactory (Fig 26–16). Through these exposures, the anterior wall fracture should be reduced, and if necessary, the fragments should be wired to each other with 28-gauge wires. If there is severe comminution, and wiring or

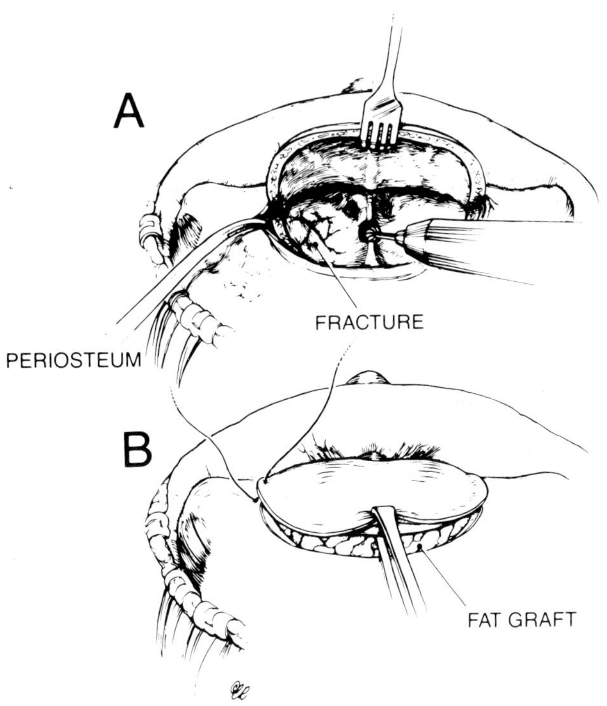

FIG 26–17.
Osteoplastic flap approach to frontal sinus fractures. **A,** elevation of flap via coronal incision and template made from 6 ft Caldwell view. Sinus is explored, fractures are reduced, and dura is repaired, if necessary. For obliteration, the mucosa and intersinus septum are removed. **B,** obliteration of frontal sinus with fat and closure of flap. (From Owens OT, Mathog RH: Frontal sinus fractures, in Foster CA, Sherman JE [eds]: *Surgery of Facial Bone Fractures.* New York, Churchill Livingstone, 1987, pp 13–23. Used by permission.)

plating is not feasable, the fragments can be supported by packing the sinus with a absorbable gelatin sponge (Gelfoam)–soaked antibiotic solution.

For the posterior wall fracture with minimal displacement, exploration without reduction should be satisfactory. In such a case, an inferior frontal sinusotomy (Lynch incision) can be used. However, if there is a displaced fracture of the posterior wall with a suspicion of dural injury, a coronal incision and frontal osteoplastic flap will be necessary (Fig 26–17). In patients with intracranial injury and known CSF leakage, the approach should be planned with a neurosurgeon and provisions taken to perform a frontal craniotomy as well. If on exploration the posterior wall fracture is displaced with a CSF leak, the fragment should be elevated, and the dura should be repaired. If the fracture is comminuted, it is prudent to remove the mucosa from the sinus and obliterate the sinus with abdominal fat. Sometimes the posterior wall of the frontal sinus has to be removed because of severe comminution, but if this type of cranialization is necessary, one must be sure to remove all of the mucosa and obliterate some of the frontal sinus space with a muscle flap or fat (Fig 26–18). One of our popular methods of protecting the anterior fossa and helping to obliterate the sinus is to rotate a temporalis muscle–galea flap into the defect.[21]

Occasionally, I will encounter a condition of posterior wall

sinus fracture that extends beyond direct visualization and precludes a complete removal of the mucosa. In such a situation, I restore the walls as best as possible and reconstruct the NFD with a no. 26 chest tube. As a part of the procedure, the NFD is enlarged with an anterior ethmoidectomy. The chest tube is strategically placed so it does not butt against the dura and yet provides a clear passageway for drainage of blood from the area. In my experience, a CFS leak can occur for several days, but if the fragments are accurately positioned, the leak will stop and healing will take place.

Fractures of the inferior wall of the frontal sinus by definition cause damage to the NFD. Once this type of injury is diagnosed, the duct must be opened and reconstructed, or the sinus must be obliterated. Not to recognize this condition will lead to obstruction, sinusitis, and late developing mucoceles. My preferred management is to remove the mucosa and obliterate the sinus with abdominal fat. Either a coronal or inferior brow incision with an osteoplastic flap provides sufficient exposure. If there is a comminution, and removal of the mucosa is not possible, an ethmoidectomy and chest tube drainage is a reasonable alternative.

Regardless of the type of frontal sinus injury and repair, periodic postoperative evaluations are important. I check the CT scan every 6 months or sooner if there is any pain, drainage, evidence of meningitis, or proptosis. Patients need to be followed for several years before there is assurance of success.

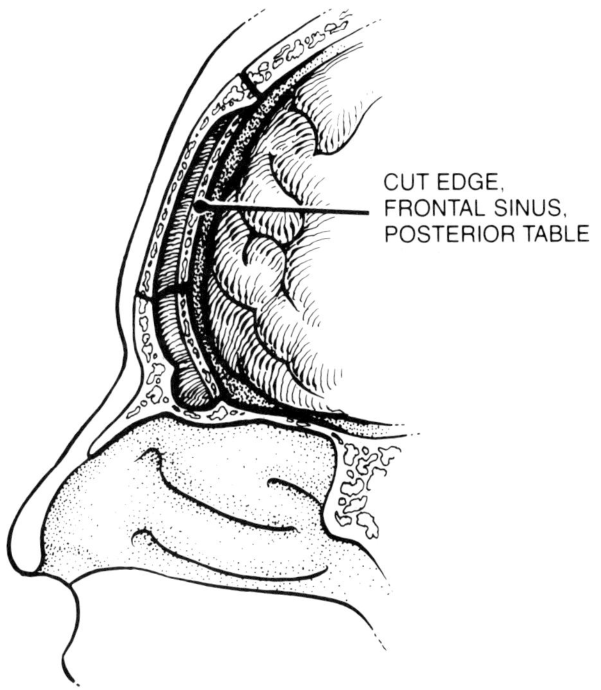

FIG 26–18.
Technique of cranialization after removal of posterior wall of frontal sinus. Some of the space can be filled with free fat or muscle or a vascularized muscle flap. (From Owens OT, Mathog RH: Frontal sinus fractures, in Foster CA, Sherman JE [eds]: *Surgery of Facial Bone Fractures.* New York, Churchill Livingstone, 1987, pp 13–23. Used by permission.)

REFERENCES

1. Putterman AM, Stevens T, Urist MJ: Nonsurgical management of blowout fractures of the orbital floor. *Am J Ophthalmol* 1974; 77:232–238.
2. Nesi F, LiVecchi J, Mathog RH: Blowout fractures of the orbit, in Mathog RH (ed): *Maxillofacial Trauma.* Baltimore, Williams & Wilkins Co, 1984, pp 319–328.
3. Parsons GS, Mathog RH: Orbital wall and volume relationships. *Arch Otolaryngol Head Neck Surg* 1988; 114:743–747.
4. Koorneef L: Current concepts on the management of orbital blow-out fractures. *Ann Plast Surg* 1982; 9:185–200.
5. Ghobrial W, Amstutz S, Mathog RH: Fractures of the sphenoid bone. *Head Neck Surg* 1986; 8:447–455.
6. Burres SA, Cohn AM, Mathog RH: Repair of orbital blowout fractures with Marlex mesh and Gelfilm. *Laryngoscope* 1981; 91:1881–1886.
7. Potter JA, Siddoway JR, Mathog RH: Injuries to the orbital plate of the frontal bone. *Head Neck Surg* 1987; 10:78–84.
8. Letson RD: Ocular injury. *Otolaryngol Clin* 1976; 9:465–476.
9. Mathog RH, Bauer W: Post-traumatic pseudohypertelorism (telecanthus). *Arch Otolaryngol* 1979; 105:81–85.
10. Converse JM: *Kazanjian and Converse's Surgical Treatment of Facial Injuries,* ed 3. Baltimore, Williams & Wilkins Co, 1974, vol 1, pp 230–236.
11. Georgiade N, Nash T: An external cranial fixation apparatus for severe maxillofacial injuries. *Plast Reconstr Surg* 1966; 38:142–146.
12. Mathog RH, Crane LR, Nowak GS: Antimicrobial therapy following head and neck trauma, in Johnson JT (ed): *Antibiotic Therapy in Head and Neck Surgery.* New York, Marcel-Dekker, 1987, pp 31–49.
13. Mathog RH, Nelson RJ, Petrelli A, et al: Self-inflected gun shot wounds to the face. Surgical and psychiatric considerations. *Otolaryngol Head and Neck Surg* 1988; 88:568–574.
14. Mathog RH, Leonard M, Bevis R: Surgical correction of maxillary hypoplasia. *Arch Otolaryngol* 1979; 105:427–439.
15. Mathog RH: Scar revision. *Minn Med* 1974; 57:31–36.
16. Stanley RB: Pathogenesis and evaluation of mandibular fractures, in Mathog RH (ed): *Maxillofacial Trauma.* Baltimore, Williams & Wilkins Co, 1984, pp 136–147.
17. Fernandez J, Mathog RH: Open treatment of condylar fractures with biphase technique. *Head Neck Surg* 1987; 10:78–84.
18. Spiessl B (ed): *New Concepts in Maxillofacial Bone Surgery.* New York, Springer-Verlag New York, 1976.
19. Mathog RH: Acute nasal fractures, in Cummings CW, Fredrickson JM, Harker LA, et al (eds): *Otolaryngology—Head and Neck Surgery.* St Louis, CV Mosby Co, 1986, pp 628–637.
20. Owens OT, Mathog RH: Frontal sinus fractures, in Foster CA, Sherman JE (eds): *Surgery of Facial Bone Fractures.* New York, Churchill Livingstone, 1987, pp 13–23.
21. Arden R, Mathog RH, Thomas LM: Temporalis muscle-galea flap in craniofacial reconstruction. *Laryngoscope* 1987; 97:1336–1342.

CHAPTER 27

Cervical Trauma

Approach of

Nicholas J. Cassisi, D.D.S., M.D.

MANAGEMENT OF BLUNT TRAUMA

Trauma to the upper aerodigestive tract most frequently occurs from automobile accidents. However, recreational vehicles such as dirt bikes, all-terrain vehicles, go-carts, and boats are becoming a leading cause of cervical injuries such as laryngeal fractures and laryngotracheal separation.

The structures of the aerodigestive tract are quite flexible and are afforded some protection by the mandible superiorly, the sternum inferiorly, and the spine posteriorly. However, the spine, because of its rigid nature, can also contribute to laryngeal, tracheal, or esophageal injuries.

In automobile injuries, the cervical region is typically injured by a blow with the steering wheel or dashboard. The speed of the vehicle and the use and type of seat belt determine the extent of injury. Lap-type seat belts can result in trauma to the neck and upper aerodigestive tract as well as to the head and face, depending on the height of the individual, because these are the areas that commonly hit the steering wheel, dash, or windshield. Lap-shoulder type of seat belts can result in trauma to the upper aerodigestive tract, but the injury is much less severe than with lap-type belts.

Complete transection of the trachea is becoming more frequent due to the use of recreational vehicles. Fence wire and clothesline injuries are particularly severe because they are difficult to see and are usually struck when going at a high rate of speed.

Strangulation is another cause of blunt trauma to the upper aerodigestive tract.

Proper management of blunt cervical trauma is dependent on proper workup and diagnosis. Signs and symptoms such as creptius, dyspnea, stridor, dysphagia, hemoptysis, or a flattened thyroid prominence are suggestive of significant upper aerodigestive tract injury (Fig 27–1).

Endoscopy, using the flexible fiberoptic endoscope, is extremely important in the initial evaluation. If the patient is stable, computed tomography (CT) scanning is invaluable for showing laryngeal and cricoid fractures and has replaced other x-ray studies in the workup of the patient with cervical trauma (Fig 27–2).

Immediate Management

Maintaining the airway is the major concern and can be established by either intubation, tracheostomy, or cricothyrotomy. In laryngotracheal injuries, intubation in the emergency room should be attempted only by experienced personnel, since more serious injuries and even death can be caused by an inexperienced person. A false lumen or mucosal tear can be worsened during intubation; therefore, before this procedure is attempted, flexible endoscopy should be performed to determine if either of these conditions is present. If no lumen is seen, immediate tracheostomy or cricothyrotomy should be done. If a cricothyrotomy is performed, a tracheotomy, away from the injury, is done as soon as possible. In a severe upper airway emergency, a temporary measure is to place three to four 14-gauge needles through the cricothyroid membrane until a thyrotomy or tracheostomy can be performed.

MANAGEMENT OF LARYNGEAL FRACTURES

Laryngeal fractures can be classified as supraglottic, lateral glottic, multiple comminuted, and isolated cricoid fractures. In acute supraglottic fractures, there is usually separation between the true and false cords. The thyroid cartilage is displaced superiorly because of the pull of the thyrohyoid muscle, and the arytenoid cartilage is edematous and displaced. Often these

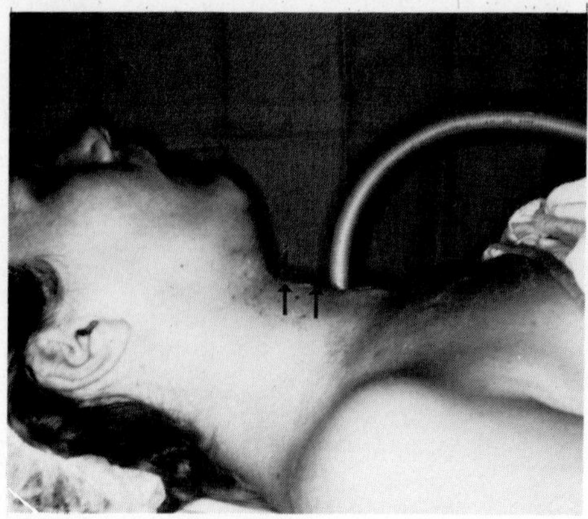

FIG 27–1.
This 25-year-old woman struck her neck on the dashboard. Presenting symptoms were dyspnea, stridor, and crepitus. Note the flattened thyroid eminence (*arrows*). Cricothyrotomy was done initially. Note high level of endotracheal tube.

patients are left with a paralyzed true vocal cord because dislocation of the arytenoid goes unrecognized (Fig 27–3).

In lateral glottic fractures, false passages occur, and cartilage fragments are often visible. In multiple comminuted fractures in which both the hyoid bone and laryngeal cartilage are fractured, the epiglottis and thyroid cartilage are often displaced so that structures under the supraglottic area cannot be seen.[1]

Medical Management

In mild injuries where there is no displacement of the thyroid cartilage and minimal or no mucosal tears, medical management should be the treatment of choice. Often, only a hematoma of the true or false vocal cord is apparent with a minimally fractured thyroid cartilage. Medical management consisting of humidification, antibiotics, racemic epinephrine, and helium and oxygen mixture should be used in these mild injuries. The use of steroids is still controversial, but I tend to use them if they can be started within 1 hour of the injury. I prescribe 100 to 200 mg of hydrocortisone 21-sodium succinate (Solu-Cortef) intravenously every 3 hours for four doses and then taper the dosage over the next 36 hours.

More severe fractures, where there is cartilage displacement or significant mucosal tears, require surgical management (Fig 27–4). Direct laryngoscopy is done prior to all open procedures or laryngeal fractures to assess arytenoid dislocations and to try relocating them onto the cricoid cartilage. However, I have not been too successful in my attempts to do this. Mucosal tears and false passages are also assessed at this time.

When the neck is explored, a horizontal skin incision is used. The strap muscles are retracted, and the larynx is entered through a vertical incision in the midline. If a lateral or supraglottic fracture of the larynx is present, however, the larynx is often best entered through the fracture line. All mucosal tears are carefully approximated using Maxon or chromic suture. Cartilage fractures are reduced and held in position with wire or other nonabsorbable suture material.

In severe cricoid fractures where there has been tissue loss, the hyoid bone is readily available to provide anterior support (Fig 27–5,A). The use of stents is controversial. I tend to limit the use of stents to those situations where because of mucosal loss a split-thickness skin graft is needed (Fig 27–5,B). I will also use a stent if the reduction cannot be maintained by wiring alone. The most commonly used stents are the Montgomery, T tube, or Teflon stents. T tubes, however, should not be used in children, because they may become occluded. I

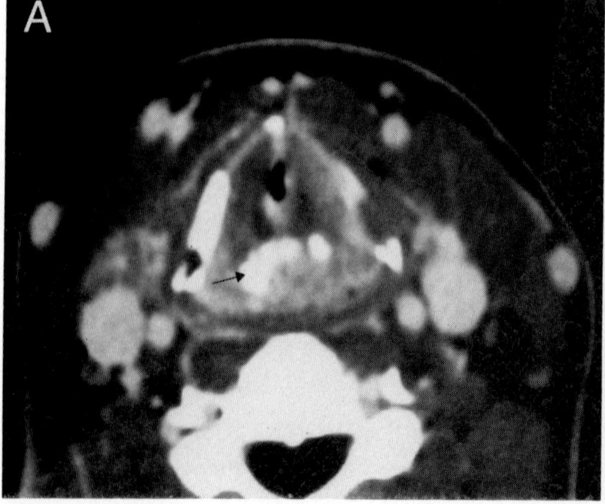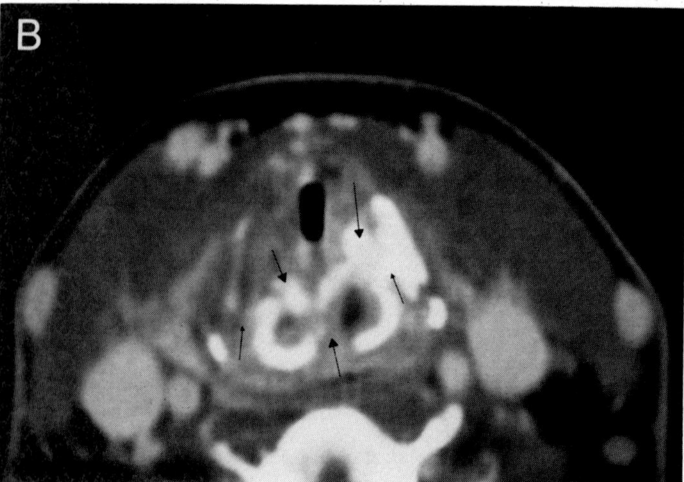

FIG 27–2.
Young boy sustained severe head trauma in motor vehicle accident. This study was done 2 to 3 weeks after trauma when symptoms of glottic dysfunction were first appreciated clinically. **A,** arytenoid dislocation on right (*arrow*); marked glottic and paraglottic edema narrow airway. **B,** comminuted fractures and fragments of cricoid cartilage (*large arrows*). Bilateral disruption of cricothyroid joints (*small arrows*).

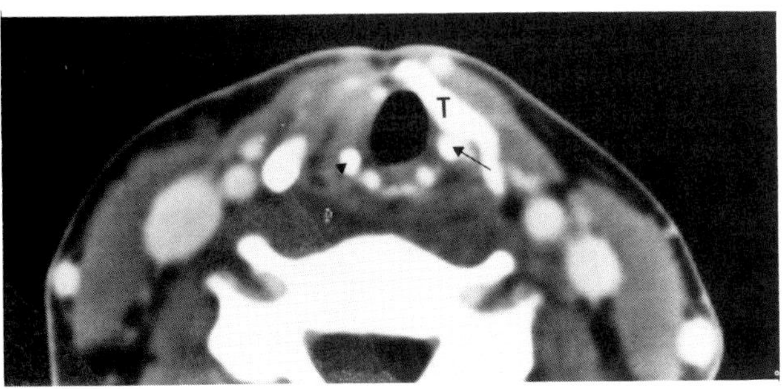

FIG 27–3.
Middle-aged woman presented with chronic progressive glottic dysfunction about 20 years following untreated laryngeal trauma. Section through the midplane of the true vocal cords shows chronically dislocated left arytenoid cartilage (*arrow*); compare this to the normal arytenoid on the right (*arrowhead*). This is probably fibrosed or ankylosed to the deformed thyroid cartilage lamina (*T*).

prefer to remove the stent in 2 to 3 weeks. A tracheostomy is performed whenever a stent is used unless a T tube is placed.

Severe supraglottic injuries, in my experience, are best treated with supraglottic laryngectomy. In the past, when repair was attempted, the resulting scarring has been so severe that a subsequent supraglottic laryngectomy was required to decannulate the patient.

Complete laryngotracheal separation requires end-to-end anastomosis in such a manner so that there is no tension on the suture line. If more than 2 cm of trachea has been resected or lost, I prefer to do a suprahyoid release of the larynx to minimize the tension on the suture line. Advise the patient that he or she may have some initial swallowing difficulties, but these soon resolve. Wire or nonabsorbable suture, such as a 3-0 Vicryl, is placed in the submucosal plane to circumscribe the supporting cartilages. The back wall sutures are placed first, and all sutures are placed before being tied down. The head is flexed, and then all sutures are tied.

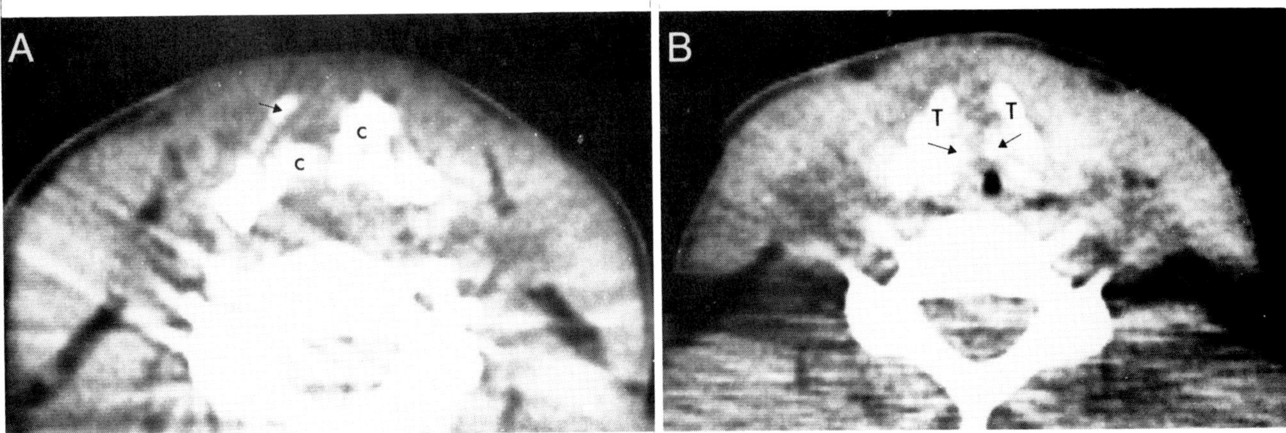

FIG 27–4.
Patient was in a motor vehicle accident and suffered cricotracheal separation. **A,** cricoid cartilage has essentially been released from the trachea and rotated such that the fractured cricoid lamina (*C*) lies in the axial plane of the section (i.e., the cricoid cartilage has rotated 90 degrees). The relationship between the cricoid and thyroid (*arrow*) cartilages is grossly disrupted. **B,** fragments of the fractured cricoid (*arrows*) lie between the thyroid lamina (*T*).

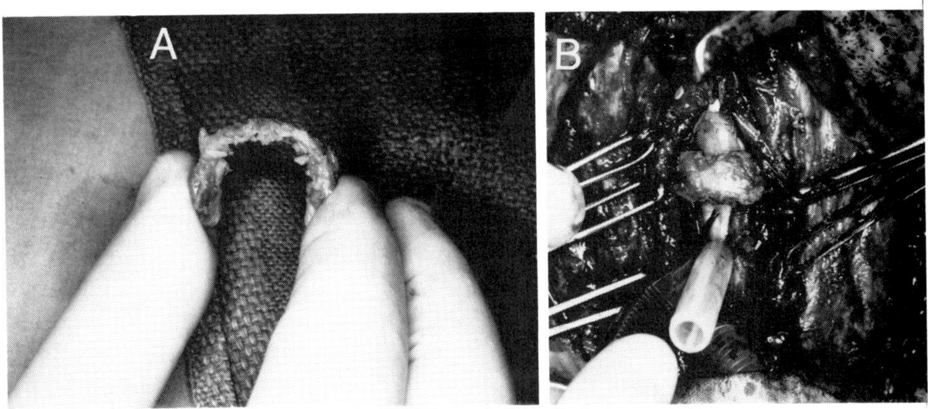

FIG 27–5.
A, hyoid bone used to provide anterior support when the cricoid has been lost. **B,** hyoid is wired in place and the Montgomery T tube placed to hold the skin graft in place. The strap muscles are then closed over the hyoid and the stent.

Because the recurrent laryngeal nerves are often injured in these types of injury, the status of the vocal cord mobility must be evaluated preoperatively. If paralysis is present, the recurrent laryngeal nerves should be identified and examined directly. If they are found to be severed, I have not had success in reanastomosing them. Instead, I perform a tracheostomy well below the suture line of the end-to-end anastomosis and later perform a laser arytenoidectomy. If the vocal cords are mobile, no tracheostomy is performed. The patient is left intubated for 24 hours in the intensive care unit with a suture placed between the chin and the anterior chest wall to remind the patient not to hyperextend the head.

MANAGEMENT OF PENETRATING INJURIES OF THE NECK

Until May et al. published their article in 1976,[2] there was a great deal of debate over whether all penetrating wounds of the neck should be explored. Using their criteria since that time, I have never had an instance where a patient should have been explored and was not. Their criteria for exploration follows.

Indications For Exploration

I. Vascular injury
  A. Absolute indications
    1. Active hemorrhage from neck wound
    2. History of hemorrhage from neck wound with hypotension
    3. Active bleeding from the mouth not accounted for by visible oral injury
    4. Clear or milky, greasy fluid exuding from wound indicating leakage of chyle
    5. Expanding cervical hematoma
    6. Widened superior mediastinum
    7. Compression of airway due to displacement of trachea
    8. Bruit
    9. Absence of pulses in extremities; superficial temporal, facial, or retinal arteries
    10. Progressive central nervous system deficit (due to diminished cerebral circulation or thrombosis of major cervical arteries)
  B. Relative indications: Penetrating object coursing near major vessels (if one or more of the following, explore)
    1. Lateral radiograph shows widening of parapharyngeal space
    2. Radiograph shows injury to transverse process of cervical vertebra (suspect vertebral artery violation)
    3. Abnormal arteriovenogram
  C. Late complications (exploration indicated)
    1. Thrombosis of major cervical vessel
      a. Change of consciousness
      b. Hemiplegia
      c. Aphasia
      d. Blindness
      e. Diminished visual fields
    2. Occult hemorrhage
      a. Expanding cervical mass
      b. Widened superior mediastinum
      c. Supraclavicular fullness
      d. Airway compression
    3. Arteriovenous fistula (confirmed by angiogram–subtraction technique, demonstrates filling and emptying, efferent and afferent flow)
      a. Widened pulse pressure
      b. Tachycardia slowed by vessel compression (Branham's sign)
      c. Continuous bruit with systolic and diastolic component
    4. True aneurysm (confirmed by angiogram–subtraction technique, demonstrates filling and emptying), systolic bruit
    5. Pseudoaneurysm (confirmed by angiogram–subtraction technique, demonstrates filling with delayed emptying), systolic bruit
    6. Vertebral artery injury (confirmed by angiogram–subtraction technique)
      a. Hemorrhage from posterior neck wound, not controlled by common carotid artery compression
      b. Expanding mass in posterior triangle
      c. Fracture of transverse process of cervical vertebra
    7. Injury of subclavian and other vessels of the thoracic outlet (confirmed by angiogram)
      a. Pulseless arm or leg
      b. Hemothorax
      c. Supraclavicular fullness
      d. Widened superior mediastinum
      e. Clear or milky, greasy fluid accumulating in or leaking from wound, indicating violation of the lymphatic channels at the neck base
II. Nervous system injury: relative indications (neurologic signs that may lead to location of possible vascular injury)
  A. Deficit of cervical sympathetic (Horner's syndrome with sweating intact) nerves IX, X, XI, and XII with injury near the jugular foramen (arteriovenography indicated)
  B. Deficit of XIIth and lingual nerves with injury in submandibular space (evaluate facial artery and vein)
  C. Horner's syndrome with injury anywhere along cervical sympathetic trunk.
    1. Injury to only external carotid may result in only anhydrosis on injured side.
    2. Injury to carotid at bifurcation or proximally results in total Horner's syndrome (ptosis, miosis, corneal flare, anhydrosis).
    3. Injury above bifurcation to only internal carotid results in Horner's syndrome with intact sweating on injured side (carotid arteriogram indicated).
  D. Brachial plexus deficit (evaluation of subclavian system, transverse cervical and suprascapular vessels indicated)
  E. Hemiplegia
    1. Contralateral damage of brain by direct injury (may be associated with decreased consciousness, aphasia, and visual changes)
    2. Contralateral damage from interruption of carotid system (may be associated with decreased consciousness, aphasia, and visual changes)

3. Cervical cord injury
F. Diminished visual acuity or constriction of visual fields; carotid or vertebral artery injury
III. Respiratory tract injury
   A. Early signs: relative indications
      1. Crepitus
      2. Dyspnea or stridor
      3. Dysphagia
      4. Dysphonia
      5. Aspiration
      6. Hemoptysis
      7. Hyoid, thyroid, or cricoid cartilages painful to palpation (indicates fracture)
      8. Flattened or deviated thyroid prominence (indicates fracture)
      9. Pain on opening mouth or protruding tongue (suspect fractured hyoid)
     10. Hemopneumothorax
     11. Abnormal endoscopy
     12. Positive dye contrast study
   B. Late signs: absolute indications
      1. Neck infection
      2. Mediastinitis (chest radiograph)
IV. Digestive tract injury
   A. Early signs: relative indications
      1. Crepitus
      2. Dysphagia
      3. Drooling
      4. Positive dye contrast swallow
      5. Abnormal endoscopy results
      6. Pneumomediastinum
   B. Late signs: absolute indications
      1. Neck infection
      2. Mediastinitis (chest radiograph)

Management of Penetrating Esophageal Injuries

Injury to the digestive tract results in crepitus, dysphagia, and often drooling (Fig 27–6). A cineesophagram using a water-soluble dye rather than barium is used to identify the location and extent of the esophageal tear. I do not do flexible or rigid esophagoscopy in penetrating wounds of the esophagus, since it can only worsen the condition and cannot lend any new information.

My philosophy is to explore most penetrating esophageal injuries unless the rent in the esophageal wall is small, as indicated by the extravasated dye in the cineesophagram. In these cases, a nasogastric tube is placed, and the patient receives nothing by mouth and is observed for signs of pain, fever, and abscess formation. Broad-spectrum antibiotics, such as cefazolin (Ancef), 1 gm every 8 hours, and metronidazole (Flagyl), 500 mg intravenously every 6 hours for 10 days, are used. In larger tears of the esophagus from penetrating objects, the esophagus is explored through a horizontal neck incision. The dissection is carried down between the sternocleidomastoid muscle and the carotid sheath. The carotid sheath contents are retracted laterally, and with blunt finger dissection, the area of the esophagus just below the cricopharyngeal muscle is exposed. Care must be taken not to injure the recurrent laryngeal nerve with either the retractor or via the dissection. With this method, the esophagus can be exposed from just below the cricopharyngeal muscle all the way down to the thoracic inlet. Care must be taken, however, not to explore or expose the esophagus any further into the mediastinum than necessary to prevent mediastinitis should a leak occur. When the esophageal tear is encountered, a double-layer closure, whenever possible, is utilized using a continuous inverting mattress suture of 4-0 Maxon for the mucosa and a 4-0 interrupted Maxon for the muscular layer. If the tissues do not approximate well, I use either the mylohyoid muscle or the sternohyoid strap muscle as a patch over the torn area. The neck is copiously irrigated, and a Penrose drain, as well as a nasogastric tube, is placed. I prefer a Penrose drain rather than a Jackson Pratt drain because the latter can draw saliva into the neck and contaminate the area. All patients are placed on antibiotic therapy and given a repeat cineesophagram in 7 days. The drain is not removed until after the repeat study in case a small leak occurs. If a small leak is still present at this time, the nasogastric tube is removed and oral feedings are begun, first with liquids and then with solid foods. The drains are not removed until a tract to the outside is well formed. Using this technique, I have never seen a small leak not close spontaneously. I learned this technique from my general surgeon colleagues in dealing with Zenker's diverticulum and the gastric pull-up operation.

Management of Carotid Artery Injuries

Once the patient has been stabilized in the emergency room and any bleeding or airway difficulties have been controlled, arteriograms are done to evaluate the aortic arch, subclavian, innominate, common, external, and internal carotid and vertebral arteries.

For major vascular injuries, such as carotid artery injuries, I often work with the vascular surgeons. Tears in the common carotid artery are sutured directly whenever necessary, or I use a vein patch graft. Injuries to the external carotid, its branches, or the vertebral artery are ligated, since complications from this procedure are rare. I prefer not to use synthetic graft material because of the possibility of infection, particularly if the wound was contaminated by a knife or gunshot.

Management of Penetrating Laryngotracheal Injuries

Penetrating injuries to the larynx and trachea occur from such objects as bullets, knives, flying glass, and sharp sticks. Because the object is usually sharp or traveling at a high rate of speed, and because it is usually small, there is less likelihood that the cartilage is fractured. Crepitation and subcutaneous emphysema are the most common signs, and airway distress is usually a result of bleeding or mucosal tears. In penetrating wounds caused by a bullet, there is often both an entrance and an exit wound. Indirect laryngoscopy using the flexible endoscope determines if there is vocal cord paralysis, and the status of the airway can be assessed. If there is no significant cartilage injury or mucosal tears, the patient is admitted, placed on antibiotics therapy and humidified oxygen, and observed for 48

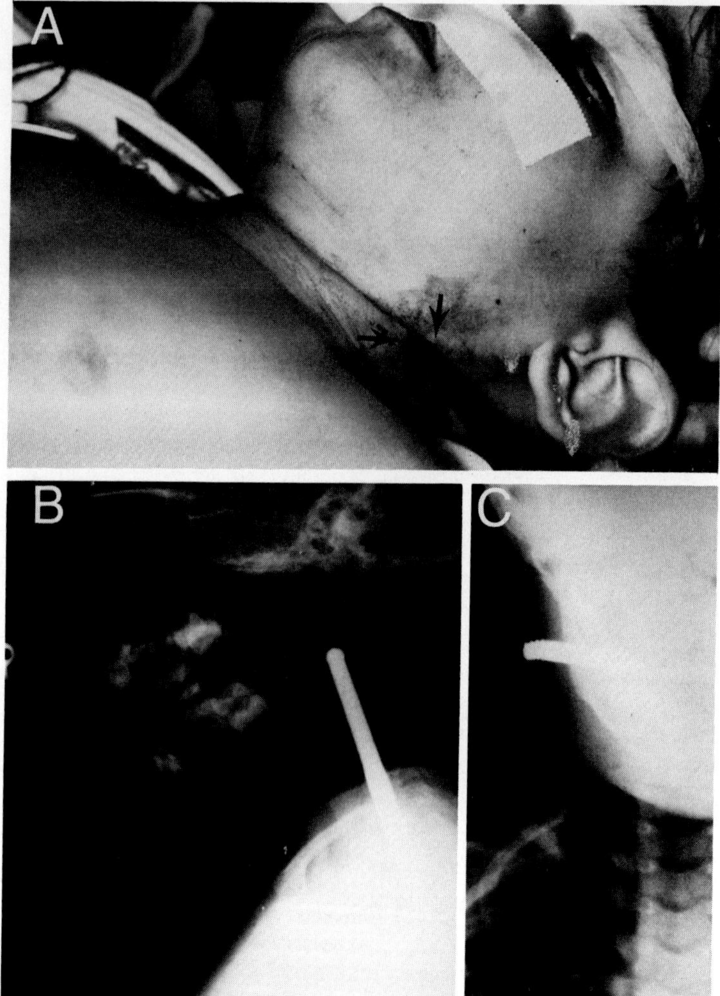

FIG 27–6.
A, 8-year-old fell from a trampoline onto a metal rod. No evidence of vascular or neurologic damage is evident. **B** and **C,** radiographs show the rod passed between the constrictor muscles and the cervical vertebrae. The pharynx was not penetrated. The foreign body was simply removed with no sequela.

to 72 hours. If a significant portion of the larynx has been destroyed, as in a shotgun blast, a tracheostomy is performed. I prefer to pack the wounds open rather than do an immediate repair, since wounds caused by guns with high velocity tend to bring debris, such as clothing, into the area and the possibility of an infection occurring, even with the use of antibiotics, is high. I tend to debride any devascularized cartilage, irrigate the wound, pack the area, and place them on intravenous (IV) antibiotic therapy. I then prefer to do the definitive repair 7 to 10 days later after the possibility of infection has lessened. In reconstruction of the larynx after a gunshot blast, usually both cartilage and soft tissue are lost. I have used a composite graft of nasal septal cartilage with attached nasal mucosa to reconstruct the larynx in two cases, with excellent results. I used a Montgomery stent in both instances, leaving the stent in place for 3 to 4 weeks. If the epiglottis is still intact, it too can be freed of its attachments and brought down to reconstruct the

anterior portion of the larynx, as described by Icambic[3] and Tucker et al.[4]

ELECTRICAL INJURY TO THE HEAD AND NECK

Electrical burns to the mouth classically occur in toddlers less than 2 years of age. Electrical burns occur in two forms: arc and contact. Contact burns occur where an electrical current enters and exits the body and can be lethal if the current passes through the brain or heart. Arc-type electrical burns occur where the arc approximates the tissue and causes heat up to 3,000°C, producing tissue necrosis and coagulation.[5]

Oral Commissure Electrical Injury

Electrical burns of the oral cavity and lips are usually the arc type, because the saliva allows the circuit to be complete within the local area and causes the burning arc to char the tissue. A 110V current can cause a severe burn but is rarely fatal.

Electrical Burns of the Lips

The degree of tissue destruction is extremely difficult to determine in the postburn period. Twelve to 14 days after the injury, the eschar separates. It is at this time that one can distinguish between vital and nonvital tissue. Usually, the amount of tissue destruction is greater than what was expected at the time of the initial evaluation because of progressive tissue necrosis. Because of this, debridement of necrotic tissue and reconstructive attempts should not be done before 2 weeks after the initial injury. There is much controversy in the literature as to when the reconstructive procedures should be done. There are those proponents of immediate reconstruction after 2 weeks, and there are those who believe that it is better to wait longer to allow healing and scar contracture to form before initiating the reconstructive process.[6]

I prefer to begin reconstruction of the burned area after the 2-week period, since no further demarcation occurs after this time, and scar formation and contracture have not begun. I believe it also lessens the sequelae of healing by secondary intention, such as microstomia and increased amounts of scar tissue.

For minor burns, where there is commissure but only a small amount of lip involvement, no surgery is done after the 2-week period, and scar revisions, if necessary, are done at a later date. Moderate acute burns, where the commissure is involved along with more than one sixth of each lip and where there is not a lot of mucosal loss and no involvement of the buccal sulcus, a vestibular flap using the buccal mucosa is used.

For severe burns, where there has been loss of epithelium, muscle, and involvement of the buccal sulcus, the forked tongue flap, as described by Ortiz-Monasterio and Foster,[7] works well. This is a flap using the mucosa and muscle from the lateral and underside of the tongue, splitting it longitudinally and suturing each limb to either the upper or lower lip. After 2 weeks, the pedicle is divided from the tongue. Dehiscence is prevented by placing a heavy suture through the tongue, near the base of the flap, and into the oral commissure.

Another technique that has been reported but that I have not tried is the use of an acrylic obturator, with commissure posts, to prevent constriction or cohesion of the lip and commissure during healing.[8] There are two drawbacks to this: (1) a dentist with this type of experience is necessary; and (2) patient compliance, especially in a young child, may be a problem.

APPROACH TO THERMAL INJURY OF THE HEAD AND NECK

Thermal injury of the head and neck requires that a thorough assessment be made of the upper airway. Endotracheal or nasotracheal intubation is the preferred method of airway maintenance rather than tracheostomy. It has been shown that increased morbidity and mortality result from early tracheos-

tomy. Tracheostomy should be done only if the patient cannot be intubated because of other head and neck injuries or if the patient cannot be weaned from the ventilator.[9]

Eyelid Burns

Full-thickness eyelid injury is best treated with skin grafting. Whenever possible, skin from the contralateral eyelid should be used. However, usually there is not enough tissue to accomplish this, since both sides are often involved. Full-thickness skin grafts for the lower eyelids should be used because of the tendency of ectropion to occur. Such full-thickness skin grafts for the lower eyelids are best obtained from the postauricular or supraclavicular area to provide the best color match. Full-thickness skin grafts to the upper eyelids should be avoided, since the lack of suppleness will prevent adequate function. The best donor site for split-thickness skin grafts for the upper eyelids is the inner aspect of the arm. Adequate amounts of skin graft must be placed over the eyelids to prevent wound contracture.

Nasal Burns

Severe nasal burns result in foreshortening, with retraction of the nasal ala. Delayed reconstruction should be done using local flaps such as nasolabial, midline, or forehead flaps or composite grafts from the ear.

Ear Burns

The ear is involved in about 80% to 90% of burns to the face. Damage occurs because of direct thermal injury or because of subsequent chondritis. The organisms most commonly involved are *Pseudomonas* and *Staphylococcus* species, and the chondritis can occur after epithelialization; therefore, the ear must be closely observed for 5 to 6 weeks. Reconstruction of the helix is accomplished using rib cartilage. For total ear reconstruction, I prefer to have the maxillofacial prosthodontist make a prosthetic ear. Having to glue the prosthetic device on every day is bothersome to the patient, but recent advances in implanting magnets into the bone of the skull and into the prosthesis have minimized this disadvantage.

Neck Burns

Burns to the neck can easily be covered using skin grafts. Neck contractures resulting in distorted facial expression or drawing of the head and skin toward the chest are common; however, I have lined the side of the neck with a deltopectoral flat after a severe radiation burn, with excellent skin and color match.

REFERENCES

1. Cassisi NJ, Isaacs JH: Trauma, in Cummings, Fredrickson, Harker, et al (eds): *Otolaryngology — Head and Neck Surgery*. St Louis, CV Mosby Co, 1986, pp 1943–1964.

2. May M, Tucker HM, Dillard BM: Presenting wounds of the neck in civilians. *Otolaryngol Clin North Am* 1976; 9:361–391.

3. Icambic V: Epiglottoplasty — new technique for laryngeal reconstruction. *Radiol Yugoslavic* 1977; 2(suppl):33–43.

4. Tucker H, Wood B, Levine H, et al: Glottic reconstruction after total laryngectomy. *Laryngoscope* 1979; 89:609–617.

5. Kelley DR: Burns, in Cummings, Fredrickson, Harker, et al (eds): *Otolaryngology — Head and Neck Surgery*. St Louis, CV Mosby Co, 1986, pp 1249–1253.

6. Orgel MG: Electrical burns of the mouth, in Wachtel TL, Frank DH (eds): *Burns of the Head and Neck*. Philadelphia, WB Saunders Co, 1984.

7. Ortez-Monasterio F, Factor R: Early definitive treatment of electric burns of the mouth. *Plast Reconstr Surg* 1980; 65:169.

8. Wood RE, Quinn RM, Forgey JE: Treating electrical burns of the mouth in children. *J Am Dent Assoc* 1978, 97:206.

9. Hammond JS, Ward GC: Burns of the head and neck. *Otolaryngol Clin North Am* 1983; 16:679–695.

Cervical Trauma

Approach of

W. Frederick McGuirt, M.D.

BLUNT NECK TRAUMA

The most common cause of blunt neck trauma has historically been the automobile accident; the nonrestrained driver strikes his or her neck against the steering wheel, or the passenger is thrown into the dashboard with his or her neck extended. The results are laryngocricoid crush and laryngotracheal separation injuries. Although the incidence of automobile accidents as a cause of blunt neck injury is decreasing, and the incidence of personal assault as a cause is increasing, the nature of the injuries and their evaluation and treatment are the same.

The mechanism of injury has been well described by Travis et al.[1] and consists, in its simplest form, of a compression injury of the laryngeal-cricoid complex, which is caught between the inflicting force and the cervical spine. In older men, with their ossified cartilage and marked prominences, multiple fractures of the thyroid lamina occur before the cricoid loading. In younger men and in women, who have less thyroid cartilage depth and a more flexible cartilage, there is earlier sharing of the loading force with the cricoid, and the injury is more often a single paramedian or midline laryngeal fracture alone or with associated cricoid fractures. Cricoid fractures exhibit a sequentially worsening complexity, depending on the force exerted. The cricoid has a slender anterior arch that blends laterally into rigid tubercle buttresses. An initial arch fracture is therefore midline and causes little compromise of the airway lumen. How-

ever, greater force causes secondary fractures of the lateral arch with depression and obstruction of the airway.

Airway Compromise

The problem of airway compromise is what can actually turn blunt cervical trauma into a true emergency vs. an expedited evaluation case. Maintenance of airway integrity must be assured before any tests, evaluations, or treatments are considered. The method of airway control remains controversial. For the person qualified to do a low tracheotomy, it is the preferable method since it effectively bypasses the area of injury and prevents further instrumental injury to preexisting mucosal and cartilaginous injuries within the larynx. On the other hand, for emergency medical crews who are usually the first to see the patient in respiratory extremis and who are more likely to be able to intubate a patient than to perform an expedient tracheostomy, intubation is acceptable. It will probably save more lives than it will lose through completing a partial laryngotracheal separation or producing a false passage into the neck or the mediastinum through mucosal tears and fracture sites. If a patient cannot be intubated, a true emergency cricothyrotomy or tracheotomy must be performed. Obviously the health care provider on the scene must determine the severity of the problem and use his or her capabilities to correct it. There are a few patients who must have emergency intubation (i.e., those

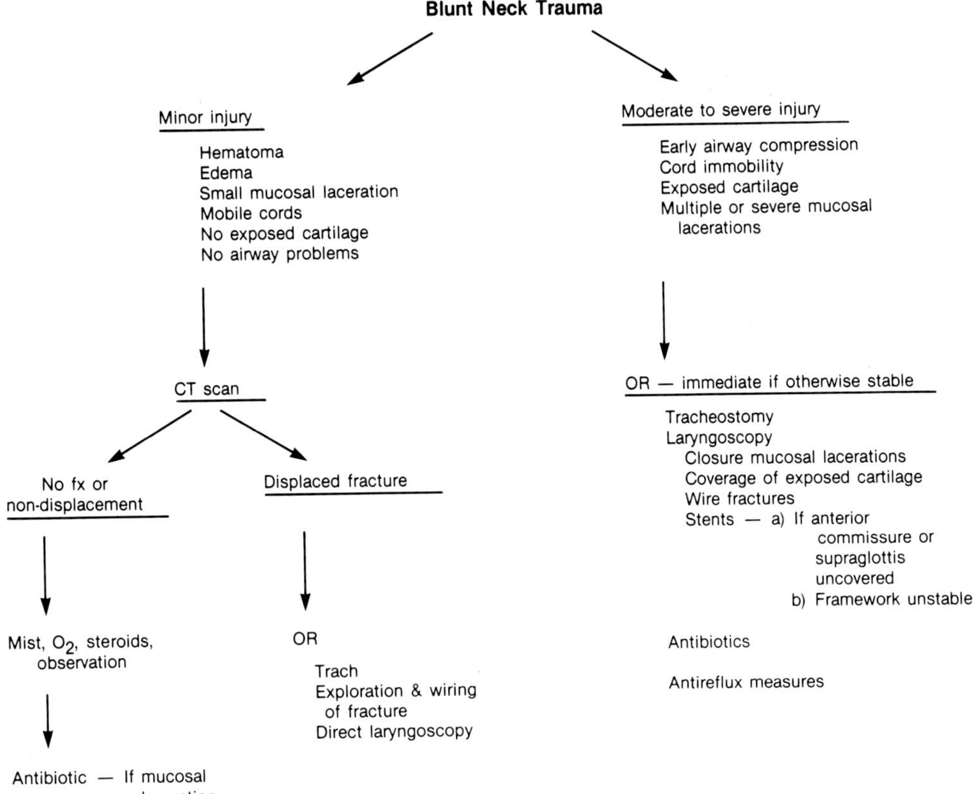

FIG 27–7.
Algorithm for management of blunt neck trauma.

with total occlusions and in extremis) rather than oxygen and mist support during transport to an emergency suite or operating room where the ideal therapy of tracheostomy can be done. For all of these patients, the emergency crew must always assume that the patient has a concomitant injury to the cervical spine, since a blow severe enough to cause this type of airway injury often has associated cervical trauma as well.

Physical Examination

Since the degree of injury is usually proportional to the force of impact, the symptoms generally reflect the magnitude of injury. Occasionally, though, the symptom complex will be minimal in relation to the magnitude of the injury, so a high index of suspicion should be maintained and a thorough examination performed in every patient with blunt cervical injury. Symptoms associated with these injuries include pain, odynophagia, change in voice, hemoptysis, and difficulty in breathing. Minor injuries may be associated with all of these symptoms, but any one of them should alert the physician to the possibility of more major problems.

Once the airway is secured, further evaluation and management can be carried out. Fortunately, few of the patients with blunt neck trauma present with severe airway compromise. Therefore, even in the absence of airway compromise, elicitation of any other of the previous symptoms is presumptive evidence for laryngeal injury and requires a very thorough examination. For the patient with an isolated neck injury or the cooperative patient with multiple trauma, indirect laryngoscopy is mandatory, as is careful palpation of the neck for crepitus, loss of the normal laryngeal cricoid landmarks, subcutaneous emphysema, or crepitant cartilaginous fractures. If indirect laryngoscopy is technically impossible due to anatomic variations, associated injury, or lack of patient cooperation, flexible nasopharyngoscopy should be performed. Evaluation should include identification of hematomas, edema, and cartilaginous injury and assessment of cord mobility, mucosal integrity, and size of the airway lumen.

On the basis of the history and physical examination with laryngoscopy, the patients can generally be placed in one of two groups (Fig 27–7): (1) minimal or mild injury or (2) moderate or severe injury.

Treatment

The group of less-injured patients are those having no presenting airway problems but having hematoma, edema, or both only within the larynx; those having small mucosal lacerations; and those having mobile vocal cords with no exposed cartilage. All of these patients should undergo a CT scan to rule out displaced laryngeal cricoid fractures. Stanley and Hanson[2] as well as Schaefer and Brown[3] have reported late abnormal voice changes, displaced laryngeal cricoid fractures, and delayed edema with airway compromise in patients with only mild to moderate signs and symptoms on presentation. Patients with nondisplaced fractures are treated expectantly with steroids, mist, and observation. If mucosal lacerations are present, antibiotics are added to the regimen since the lesion represents an open fracture bathed by secretions. If the CT scan shows a displaced laryngeal-cricoid fracture, the patient is taken to the operating room, a tracheostomy is established under local anesthesia, and displaced cartilage fractures are reduced and wired to prevent late-occurring problems. With the patient still in the operating room, direct laryngoscopy is performed to search for further endolaryngeal injury. Caution is advised in sending these patients with seemingly less severe blunt neck injuries to the x-ray department unattended. Delayed airway obstruction may occur at any time, and, therefore, these patients must be attended by a health care team member who can recognize such a development and take steps to relieve it.

The second, or moderate to severe injury, group comprises patients who may have one, some, or all of the following: early airway compromise, cord immobility, exposed cartilage, and multiple or severe mucosal lacerations. Computed tomography assessment is not needed for these patients, since it will not influence the method of management, which must be tracheostomy, direct laryngoscopy, and probably open exploration, including median thyrotomy. All exposed cartilage is reduced and covered with mucosa, and all mucosal lacerations are closed primarily with 5-0 or 6-0 chromic sutures. The anterior commissure and cord are positioned with sutures to the midline external perichondrium, and all fractures are reduced and wired.

Stents are used only when the anterior glottic or supraglottic area cannot be covered or when the damage to the cartilage framework requires them for stabilization. Cricoid and anterior glottic stents, such as the Negus silicone rubber (Silastic) stent, are form fitted; a foam-filled finger cot is used for supraglottic areas. Both types of stents should be maintained by two coated, braided wires (cardiac pacer wires) passed transversely and secured on both sides of the neck by Silastic buttons and lead shot. Thus secured, the stents do not rotate but can move with swallowing. As the neck edema decreases, additional lead shot may be attached to the suspension wires to maintain immobility of the stent and prevent mucosal abrasion.

In general, whenever airway integrity can be maintained without stents, stents should not be used, because as confirmed by Leopold,[4] posttreatment voice and airway are better in non-stented larynges. This difference seems particularly significant in the patient with mobile vocal cords and not so significant in the patient with immobile cords. The poorer voice and narrower airway in stented patients are believed to be due to submucosal scarring from chronic irritation by the stent with mucosal debridement.

Stents, if they must be used, should be left in place for no more than 3 weeks. Beyond this period, the degree of scarring increases, and the voice and airway are adversely affected. In all patients with laryngeal injury, and especially in those with stents, an aggressive antireflux regimen should be instituted. In a controlled study, Little et al. have shown stomach acid to produce subglottic scarring and stenosis in the injured larynx.[5]

The development of trauma centers for the more acute care of the injured patient has resulted in better function after cervical trauma and shortened hospitalization for patients with laryngeal cricoid injury from blunt trauma. Complex injuries should be repaired as early as possible, ideally within the first few hours of injury. When mucosal flaps and muscle injury are identified before granulation tissue appears and cartilaginous fractures are reduced before edema develops, the results are a more anatomic repair and a better voice and airway.

Laryngotracheal Separation

Laryngotracheal separation represents an extension of the blunt trauma to the neck and prognostically has a much worse outcome than other degrees of blunt trauma. Patients with such a severe injury are also the patients in whom endotracheal intubation may result in iatrogenic death, which is the main reason why patients with blunt neck trauma and airway compromise should, when possible, have open tracheostomy and exploration. The diagnosis, as well as a relief of airway compromise, is usually accomplished by tracheostomy.

A force sufficient to cause laryngotracheal separation will usually also cause avulsion or compression of the recurrent laryngeal nerve with secondary vocal cord paralysis, which is often bilateral. One should document this injury by direct laryngoscopic examination after the airway is secure. If vocal cord paralysis is seen, the recurrent nerves are not looked for or repaired because:

1. Long-term tracheostomy in these patients is already necessary, and if the nerve is intact, spontaneous functional return may develop within several months.
2. Successful anastomosis with normal function from a disrupted recurrent nerve has not been reported, since the adductor fibers outnumber the abductor fibers 8 to 1, and the resulting adduction theoretically would result in airway occlusion should reinnervation be successful.

Primary laryngotracheal suspension using fine wire with a distal tracheotomy and no stent is my preferred method of acutely managing laryngotracheal separation. Decisions on options for restoration of voice and airway must be made later by the patient based on the end result of the acute trauma.

PENETRATING NECK TRAUMA

Diagnosis and Treatment

The neck contents include many vital structures whose integrity is necessary for survival. These are closely juxtaposed and are quite vulnerable to penetrating injuries. The appropriate diagnosis and management of these injuries are challenging and necessary, as shown by data on combat mortality. From World War II to the Vietnam War era, the mortality from penetrating neck injuries had been reduced from 15% to about 5%, and much of this reduction in mortality was attributed to the policy of exploring surgically any wound that penetrated the platysma.[6] Many surgeons, including myself, believe that this reduced mortality was not so much a result of that policy as it was the result of better technology, which allowed earlier field triage, diagnosis, and definitive therapy. The delay factor in treatment is most important for survival of patients with penetrating neck injury, especially carotid vascular injury. Rubio et al. pointed out the effects that improved carotid vascular techniques have on delaying death from carotid involvement.[7] All surgeons are in agreement that active intervention is necessary in the patient with injury to obvious vital structures; the point of disagreement is whether to explore penetrating neck injuries unless certain criteria are met.

Proponents of selective surgical exploration have pointed out that routine exploration does not obviate the possibility of missed injuries (4%).[8–11] More than one half of routine explorations are normal, and up to one fourth of normal explorations have complications from the surgery. Furthermore, studies on selective exploration have shown that patients with no clinical evidence of an injury do not later prove by special studies or operation to have such an injury, and the average hospital stay of patients undergoing observation approximates only one half that of patients who have surgical exploration with normal findings (1.8 vs. 3.8 days). A further important consideration in this era of cost containment is the saving of operating room charges and time if not all penetrating neck injuries are explored routinely.

Conservative management of patients with penetrating injuries is accepted, safe, and effective in the absence of specific signs and symptoms, as has been pointed out by the large series of selective exploration (1,300 cases, 6.2% mortality) compared with mandatory exploration (1,200 cases, 5% mortality) described by Bivins.[12]

The specific signs and symptoms indicating the need for exploration are present in all patients with significant injury, but in many they may be subtle or delayed. Thus, the clinician must be alert and suspicious and must use repeated clinical examination with appropriate ancillary clinical testing to identify and localize the site and magnitude of a penetrating neck injury to be managed conservatively.

Penetrating trauma can damage the vascular, nervous, respiratory, and digestive systems as it traverses the neck. Specific signs and symptoms referable to injury of these systems must be sought and, when found, are indications for surgery (Table 27–1).

The most obvious indications are those of active hemorrhage, expanding hematoma, pulsatile hematoma, and airway compression or interruption as evidenced by stridor or dyspnea. Less urgent indications for exploration include an altered sensorium that makes clinical evaluation difficult, neurologic paralysis or paresis, bruits, decreased pulses, subcutaneous emphysema, change in voice, hemoptysis, and palpable disruption of the tracheal or laryngeal cartilage. When these present individually or collectively, surgical exploration of the neck is appropriate. One must determine, though, the urgency of the exploration vs. the value in delay for further diagnostic study and planning (Fig 27–8). In the unstable patient, immediate

TABLE 27–1.
Signs and Symptoms of Neck Trauma Indicative of Surgical Therapy

System	Signs and Symptoms
Neurologic	Changing sensorium
	Paresis or paralysis
	Neuropathy
Vascular	Acute hemorrhage
	Expanding hematoma
	Pulsatile hematoma
	Hematoma with airway compression
	Bruit
	Decreased pulse, asymmetric
Respiratory	Respiratory distress
	Crepitus or subcutaneous air
	Dyspnea, stridor
	Hemoptysis
	Disrupted thyroid cartilage
Digestive	Difficult assessment
	Bloody secretions or vomitus

exploration is indicated, but in the stable patient, arteriographic and CT examinations of the neck and spine are in order. Many physicians would also include a contrast study of the upper aerodigestive tract and esophagus. I concur with this for the stable patient who has normal clinical indications and will otherwise be observed. However, in the patient with abnormal findings or symptoms who will need surgical exploration, this test is not necessary, since the same information will be gathered more directly during the operation. Every patient who has the neck explored externally should also have an internal examination of the aerodigestive tract by endoscopic methods, including direct laryngoscopy, pharyngoscopy, tracheoscopy, and esophagoscopy. If possible, a CT scan of the head is also obtained preoperatively in the stable unconscious or neurologically impaired patient to help differentiate cervical vascular damage from blunt head trauma as a cause of the impairment.

When a vascular injury is documented or suspected by the clinical or arteriographic evidence, the area in question must be identified directly, exposed, and treated.[13–17] For damage to the external carotid artery, the vertebral artery, and the external jugular vein, simple ligation is all that is necessary and is without sequelae. Injury to the internal jugular vein, when readily accessible, should be repaired primarily with simple sutures. Injuries involving the common carotid artery, the internal carotid artery, or both, are more serious, are technically difficult to repair, and are fraught with neurologic morbidity. They are best corrected by restoration of vascular continuity and flow by either lateral repair, end-to-end anastomosis, or interpositional grafting. The exceptions to this principle are the patient with a known central, focal ischemic neurologic deficit and the patient who is comatose but has a normal blood pressure. In these instances, the risk of the neurologic deficit worsening from revascularization of an infarct may actually be increased by hemorrhage into the infarcted area. These patients should merely have the carotid artery ligated, as should patients who have primary injury in a technically unrepairable location (e.g., high in the base of the skull). On the other hand, in the acutely injured patient who arrives unconscious and hemodynamically unstable and must be taken to the operating room immediately without benefit of a CT scan or a meaningful clinical and neurologic examination, most would agree that the damaged carotid system should be revascularized. Direct repair or resection and reanastomosis is preferable to grafting in patients with moderate vascular wall trauma, traumatic aneurysms, or arteriovenous fistulae, because graft placement in the neck with a penetrating wound has an increased risk of infection. Only when there is no alternative to restore continuity should grafts be used, and autologous vein grafting is then preferable to grafting with a synthetic material, again due to the risk of infection. Few head and neck surgeons are trained sufficiently in such vascular surgical techniques, and in general they should consult their vascular surgical colleagues for assistance in these cases of major carotid vascular injury.

Penetrating cervical esophageal injuries should be suspected in the patient who is spitting up blood-tinged mucus or has air in the neck. These injuries are easily diagnosed by performing direct endoscopic examination in all patients who are operated on early in their course. Contrast studies in the asymptomatic patient who is initially assigned to the observation group (stable, normal arteriogram, and normal laryngoscopy) will sometimes also show penetrating esophageal injury. Primary repair of mucosal tears or lacerations, placement of a feeding tube for 7 to 10 days, copious irrigation of the area, and placement of a drain tube for 3 to 4 days with broad-spectrum antibiotic coverage for 7 to 10 days are routine components in the management of this problem. When penetrating cervical esophageal injuries are recognized and treated in this manner, sequelae are rare. It is the nonrecognition of these injuries and the failure to treat them that lead to deep neck infection or mediastinitis, both of which can be devastating to the patient.

Penetrating injuries of the larynx and trachea are usually associated with less destruction and disruption than blunt injuries. However, the symptoms and signs of airway compromise—changes in voice, hemoptysis, subcutaneous emphysema, and loss of normally palpable cricoid laryngeal landmarks—are the same for both types of injury, and they should alert the physician to the presence of injuries of the laryngotracheal complex. The definitive diagnosis is made by visualization of the injury. In the cooperative patient not in extremis, it can be done in the emergency suite by indirect mirror or flexible laryngoscopy. In the uncooperative patient, laryngoscopy must be done directly in the operating room. In fact, laryngoscopy should be performed in all patients taken to the operating room for exploration of penetrating neck trauma, regardless of the preoperative findings and especially in any patient having indirect findings suggestive of laryngotracheal injury. The question of tracheostomy vs. endotracheal intubation and the guidelines for repair of laryngotracheal injuries, including the use of stents, covered in the preceding section on blunt cervical trauma are apropos to penetrating trauma.

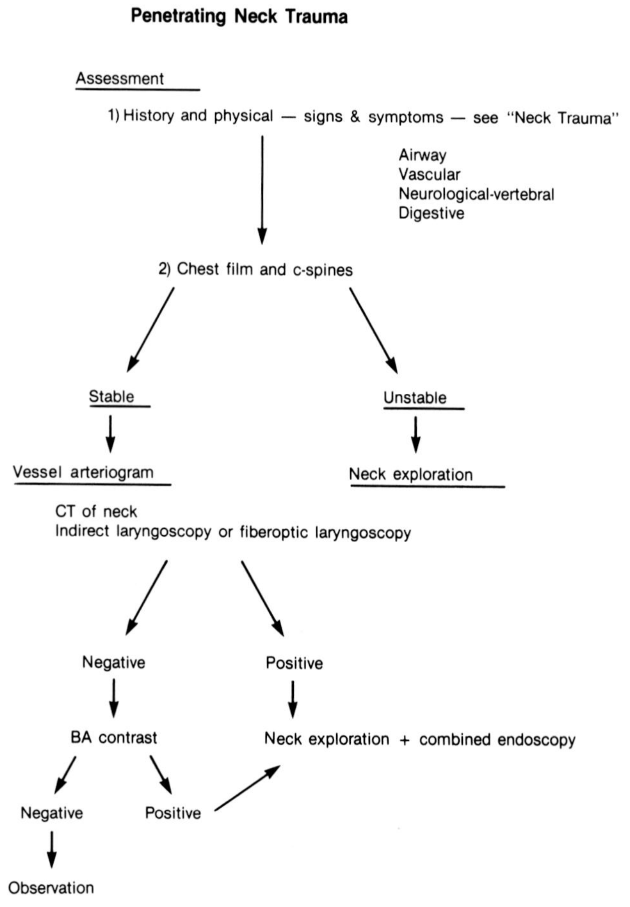

Penetrating Neck Trauma

Assessment

1) History and physical — signs & symptoms — see "Neck Trauma"

Airway
Vascular
Neurological-vertebral
Digestive

2) Chest film and c-spines

Stable → Vessel arteriogram
CT of neck
Indirect laryngoscopy or fiberoptic laryngoscopy

Unstable → Neck exploration

Negative → BA contrast

Positive → Neck exploration + combined endoscopy

BA contrast → Negative → Observation

BA contrast → Positive → Neck exploration + combined endoscopy

FIG 27–8.
Algorithm for management of penetrating neck trauma.

ELECTRICAL INJURY TO THE HEAD AND NECK

Electrical injury to the mouth is essentially an event of young children who chew on a hot electrical cord. The current passes through the tissues in the most direct route where resistance is least, and moist lips have a very low resistance. Low-tension household current is alternating and thus causes tetanic spasms, which increase the difficulty in detaching the child from the cord and augment the insult by prolonging the duration of flow. Once the current enters the body, it traverses along blood vessels and tissue fluids, producing an exothermic reaction to 3,000°C that results in local ischemia and coagulation necrosis. Because of the low resistance and high electrolyte content of saliva, some arc burn is also produced.

Oral Commissure Injuries

The injury produced by electric current is usually much deeper than is immediately apparent. The initial superficial burn is a coal gray or yellow depressed area of full-thickness skin loss with a surrounding hyperemia. After 36 hours, the surrounding tissue becomes red, and the deep tissues become edematous. Tissue necrosis and tissue loss progress over the following week. The eschar sloughs by enzymatic dissolution later than other types of burns unless those burns are complicated by secondary infection. In addition to the soft tissue injuries, devitalization of teeth and changes in the growth of adjacent bone and facial skeleton have been reported.

Electrical injuries of the head and neck usually cause no pain but do cause major functional problems. These problems are due to the loss of lip control, which leads to drooling, and to the inability to masticate efficiently. With careful supervision, oral nutrition can usually be maintained with liquids and vitamins. Although the Louisville experience showed that patients treated with antibiotics had an infection rate no lower than that in patients not treated with antibiotics,[18] all patients at my institution are initially started on penicillin unless they are allergic to it. The principle behind this policy is an attempt to prevent secondary bacterial infection of the burn wound, which is associated with greater tissue loss, faster sloughing with a higher risk of delayed bleeding, and greater cicatricial deformity. The theoretical benefit of the penicillamine by-product on wound healing and contracture is also cited. Topical antimicrobial agents, such as silver sulfadiazine cream and polymyxin B–bacitracin–neomycin ointment, are not used because they are washed off too rapidly by the salivary flow to be effective.

The nature and timing of management of the electrical wound itself are controversial and include operative vs. nonoperative therapy and, if the former, then immediate excision with reconstruction vs. a more conservative delayed approach to debridement. The point of early therapy is to lower the risk of secondary infection, minimize scarring, and prevent interruption of lip growth.[19] However, those opposing early repair report no difference in morbidity or cosmesis by delaying closure,[20] and they believe that less normal tissue is sacrificed with delay, since early debridement must be carried down to obviously normal, bleeding tissue. I agree with this nonsurgical, conservative initial management with delayed reconstructive repair as necessary. Only one third of all cases managed conservatively require late correction of deformity, and only about one fifth require late flaps, Z-plasties, or reconstruction of the commissure.[18] Thus, early excision would submit two thirds or more of the children with this injury to unnecessary surgery. The nonoperative, prolonged use of an intraoral appliance to minimize contracture formation and thus prevent microstomia is quite helpful and is recommended in all patients for 8 to 12 months after injury.[21] It is used continously for the first 6 months except when the patient is eating and is used at night for an additional 6 months. Use of these splints should markedly decrease the number of patients requiring reconstructive surgery.[21] In young patients in whom noncompliance in wearing the splint is foreseen, a fixed appliance cemented to the molars can be used.

The patient being treated conservatively and the parents of a child so treated must be instructed on how to manage lip bleeding from labial artery erosion and slough. This complication is not common, but it does occur.

Despite the best attempts at early management, late deformity may still occur due to treatment failure or to failure of the patient or parents to carry out the follow-up instructions. A contracted, concave commissure with limited excursion and extension of scarring beyond the vermilion border into the lateral perioral skin are the problems most often seen with conservative management (Fig 27–9,A). The method of repair that I prefer for most of these deformities is illustrated in Figure 27–10. This procedure has been more successful in increasing the size of the oral stoma than in restoring true symmetry (Fig 27–9,B). Loss of muscle function laterally sometimes leaves a small gap in mouth closure with attendant drooling.

Arc Injury

The introduction to this section on electrical injuries of the head and neck points out that they are the result of both thermal and arc injuries. Pure arc injury is caused when high-voltage sparks bridge the gap between the energized conductor and the body. The tissues are heated locally to 2,500°C to 3,000°C, and thermal charring burns are superimposed on the deeper coagulative electrical burn. Immediate postinjury excision and primary grafting as appropriate are recommended when the area of injury is limited. Areas of disturbed function or cosmesis will be better served by delay to allow their delineation before definitive therapy. Bone lesions are frequent, despite a very high resistance of bone to electrical current. The extent of skeletal injury is not immediately discernible, and months may pass before sequestration occurs. In skull injuries, removal of the outer table and skin grafting over the granulation bed will speed healing.[22]

THERMAL INJURIES OF THE HEAD AND NECK

It is written that 2 million people in the United States are burned each year, with 300,000 being burned severely enough to require hospitalization.[23] Burns of the head and neck region represent one fourth to one third of all thermal injuries. Concerns of both function and cosmesis enter into the treatment plan for head and neck burns, which can be divided into acute and chronic phases.

Acute Treatment

The acute phase encompasses the time of injury to completion of wound coverage. The initial concern must be the status of the respiratory system.[24] Inhalation of hot air may damage the mucous membrane of the upper airway, causing severe edema and obstruction. True thermal injury to the lung itself is rare except for steam inhalation. What is more common is the inhalation of toxic gases, resulting in a chemical tracheobronchitis, and this type of burn must be suspected in any patient receiving a flame burn within an enclosed space. Singed nasal vibrisi, expectoration of soot, and the presence of lung rales, rhonchi, or wheezes are diagnostic of this problem. A lung scan with xenon will show segmental trapping, with failure of the Xe to clear over 90 seconds. This finding, along with bronchoscopic findings of edema and blisters as well as extramucosal carbon and bronchorrhea, confirms the clincial diagnosis. These two diagnostic tests, Xe scanning and tracheoscopy, should be performed in all patients suspected of having inhal-

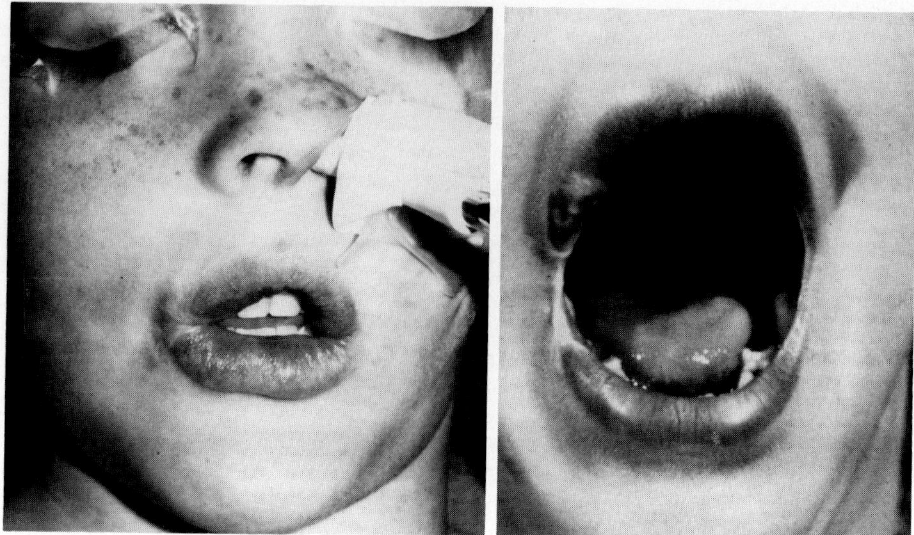

FIG 27–9.
A, scarring beyond vermilion border into lateral perioral skin in child with electrical burn managed conservatively. **B**, postoperative appearance. Size of oral stoma is adequate.

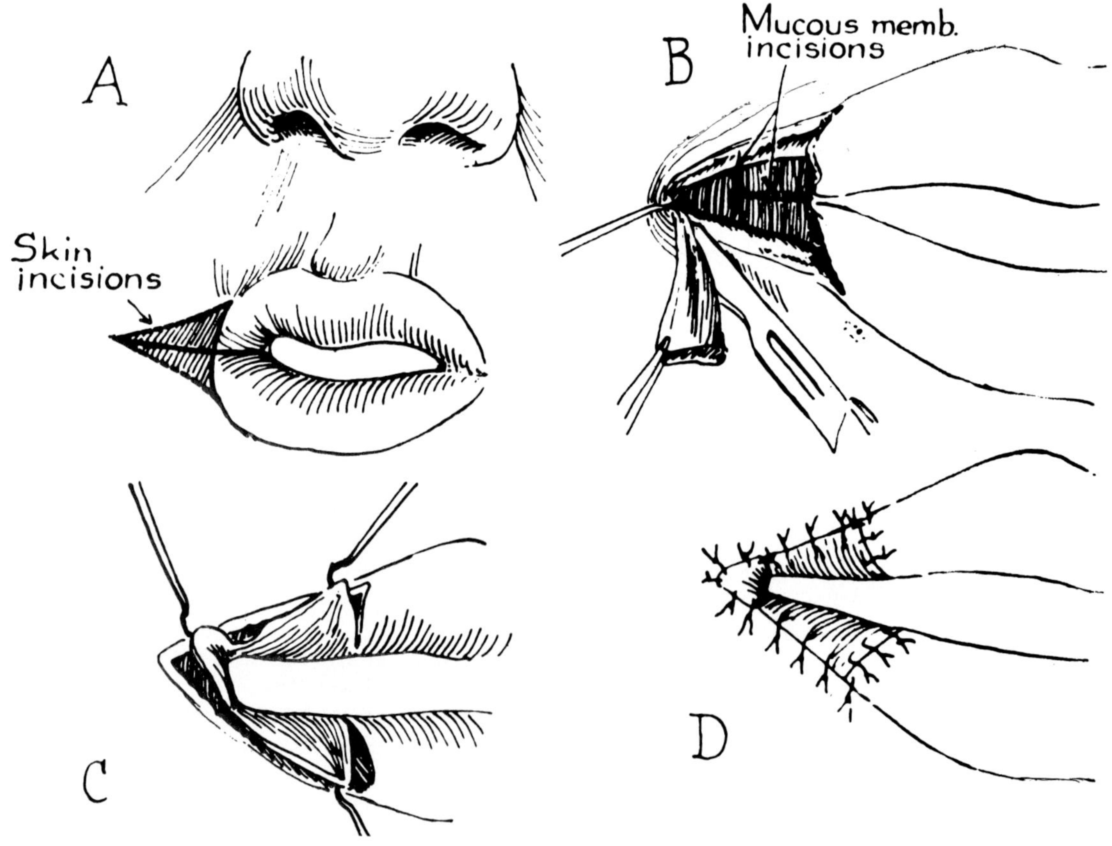

FIG 27–10.
A–D, technique for repair of scarring as seen in Figure 27–9,A. (From Converse JM (ed): *Reconstructive Plastic Surgery,* vol 2: The Head and Neck. Philadelphia, WB Saunders Co, 1964, p 855. Used by permission.)

ational burns. Because a latent period of up to 48 hours may occur before signs of respiratory distress appear, close monitoring of PaO_2 is important. Hypoxemia developing along with clinical signs of respiratory insufficiency such as restlessness, tachypnea, wheezing, retraction, and nasal flaring indicates a need for intubation. Intubation should be done early before edema develops and makes the procedure more difficult. Deep facial burns about the mouth and nose or burns of the pharynx are nearly uniformly associated with upper airway compromise at least and thus should prompt early intubation. This intubation is preferably done through a nasal endotracheal tube when neck burns are present, since, in such instances, placement of tracheostomy tubes has a six times greater incidence of secondary pulmonary infections, which often result in pulmonary sepsis and death.[25] The nasotracheal tube is more easily anchored against dislodgment and causes less patient annoyance than the orotracheal tube. The endotracheal tube with a low-pressure cuff can be left in place for 3 to 4 weeks, by which time wound healing in the neck should be complete. If continued ventilatory support is necessary beyond that time, it can be provided by placement of a tracheostomy tube through a cleaner field with less risk of infection. Usually, except in the most severe burns, it is unnecessary to leave the tube in for more than 3 to 5 days, at which time edema of the upper airway should have subsided. For the patient with anterior neck burns who is likely to require a long-term tracheostomy, early excision of the burn eschar and grafting is indicated so that the tracheostomy can be established through healed, grafted skin.

Again, because of nasal and pharyngeal edema, placement of a nasogastric tube early after presentation is much easier than waiting for signs or symptoms of the intestinal ileus that nearly always occurs. Prolonged enteral feeding, though, which may be important for wound healing and may be dictated by facial and mouth burns, should be given through a small-bore soft nasogastric tube that replaces the large-bore, hard tube initially placed for gastric suctioning.

The outcome and speed of repair will depend primarily on the extent and depth of the burn. I do not advocate primary excision of facial burns except for very small areas that can be closed primarily or with adjacent rotation flaps. Larger burns should first undergo local wound cleansing with a sponge and poloxamer 188, a skin-wound cleanser that does not interfere with wound healing. Blisters are left intact, hair-bearing areas are shaved, tetanus prophylaxis is given, and the head and neck are elevated on a foam donut to avoid pressure contact with compromised skin areas. Parenteral antibiotics and steroids are not used in the acute period.

Superficial burns are treated with moist compresses of saline, which are changed every 6 hours. An alternative is placement of petrolatum-impregnated gauze over the burn and allowing it to form a coagulum that will permit reepithelialization underneath within 10 to 14 days. This latter technique is believed to cause more scarring, and in general I do not recommend it. Deeper wounds with a heavy eschar are treated with topical antibiotics in the form of silver sulfadiazine on the thinner eschars and mafenide acetate (Sulfamylon) on thicker eschars. The former is relatively ineffective against staphylococcal infection and must be closely monitored. It is placed on the burn twice daily after the previous application has been removed. Mafenide acetate, though penetrating deeper into the eschar, is associated with pain on application and occasionally causes acid-base disturbances when it is used on large areas. An open technique is preferred in the application of these topical antibiotics because of the risk of pressure necrosis, especially to the ears, when a closed technique is used. Surgiflex netting easily holds a minimal dressing in place and is often necessary since early facial muscle exercises are recommended and encouraged to decrease underlying scarring and fibrosis.

Enzymatic debridement with a proteolytic drug such as Sutilain's ointment (Travase) can avoid tangential incisions on the face and the loss of viable tissue that might result from such incisions.

When the eschar has been removed, early grafting should be the goal. In facial grafting, one must think in terms of aesthetic appearance, and sometimes it may be better cosmetically to excise some undamaged skin to achieve a uniform regional appearance. In general, full-thickness or thick (0.015 mm) split-thickness skin grafts produce less contracture and should be used whenever possible. Grafts to the face and neck are not meshed but are placed as solid unit sheet grafts held in place by a bolster-stent dressing. Antibiotics such as penicillin are usually given at this stage of treatment. Matching the graft color should be a prime consideration, and skin of the supraclavicular, retroauricular, and scalp areas should be the initial choice when it is available.

Chronic Burn Care

The chronic stage of burn wound care has to do with the management of contraction and hypertrophy. The keys to the management of these problems are exercise, traction, and pressure. In healing, an axiom has been that the position of comfort is also the position of deformity. Therefore, to prevent this deformity, the patient must do active and passive range of motion exercise of all joints several times daily. Splinting is also necessary to maintain proper position. Regions with large amounts of elastic tissue, such as the neck, are especially prone to contractures. Conforming neck splints of Orthoplast or Isopreen are good for immobilizing the neck in the extended position, supporting the mandible, and holding the head correctly during healing. It is important that these splints be fitted on the patient early enough in the burn management period that scar contractures have not started forming. Another device that works well in the prevention of neck contractures and the treatment of neck contractures is the Watusi collar. Periodically, additional rings are placed around the neck to gradually extend it and compress the scarred area.

In wound healing, collagen is formed in a random interwoven manner. This jackstraw arrangement of collagen fibers can be realigned by prolonged pressure. Elastic garments and soft silicone rubber inserts are used for this, as is a clear plastic Uvex mask with pressure fasteners to hold it in place.

Triamcinolone administered by forced-air or small-needle injection is also quite successful in softening and reducing hypertrophic scar. This treatment is repeated every 3 to 4 weeks, with up to 40 mg of triamcinolone being given each time.

Late secondary reconstructive procedures such as hair transplants (as free grafts for eyebrows, a pedicle graft for a mustache, or punch grafts for the scalp) may help to camouflage scar tissue and restore distinctive facial features.

Specialized Areas of Burn

Certain areas must receive special attention when facial burns are being treated. The ear is so exposed that it is involved in nearly 90% of facial burns; chondritis may occur in 25% of these burns. Chondritis requires aggressive debridement, warm compresses, and topical antibiotics such as 0.25% polymyxin B sulfate irrigant applied every 6 hours. It is imperative that a partial-thickness burn of the ear or mastoid area not be converted to a full-thickness burn by pressure necrosis and that a donut head rest be used in all these cases. Partial-thickness burns are treated with topical antibiotics daily as mentioned. Full-thickness burns are treated by removal of the involved skin, application of moist soaks, and positioning of split-thickness skin grafts held in place with stents made of a bolster of mineral oil–impregnated cotton balls maintained with a mastoid-type dressing.

Burns of the lower eyelid are treated by excising the involved skin and grafting a full-thickness skin graft taken from the supraclavicular or postauricular area for its better color match and texture. The upper lid is often best treated by a skin graft from the inner arm since it is a thinner skin than that from the postauricular or supraclavicular region and is more capable of allowing the full motion associated with upper lid activity. A Frost stitch is placed, and bolster stents are used to prevent motion while the graft is healing.

Due to the thickness of the skin on the nose, nasal burns are more commonly partial thickness rather than full thickness. The major disfigurement in nasal burns is loss of the subcutaneous tissue, with secondary scarring of the nasal alae and nasal ectropion and destruction of the cartilaginous framework. A "ram's horn" full-thickness skin graft is used to release this alar ectropion. I have found the use of pedicle flaps to replace most of the nasal surface to be the best way to correct the deformity from cartilage loss along with overlying skin loss in the area of the lower half of the nose.

For the management of thermal burns in and around the mouth, the orthotic appliances described in the section on electrical burns are recommended.

REFERENCES

1. Travis LW, Olson NR, Melvin JW, et al: Static and dynamic impact trauma of the human larynx. *Trans Am Acad Ophthalmol Otolaryngol* 1975; 80:382–390.
2. Stanley RB Jr, Hanson DG: Manual strangulation injuries of the larynx. *Arch Otolaryngol* 1983; 109:344–347.
3. Schaefer SD, Brown OE: Selective application of CT in the management of laryngeal trauma. *Laryngoscope* 1983; 93:1473–1475.
4. Leopold DA: Laryngeal trauma. A historical comparison of treatment methods. *Arch Otolaryngol* 1983; 109:106–111.
5. Little FB, Koufman JA, Kohut RI, et al: Effect of gastric acid on the pathogenesis of subglottic stenosis. *Ann Otol Rhinol Laryngol* 1985; 94:516–519.
6. Obeid FN, Haddad GS, Horst HM, et al: A critical reappraisal of a mandatory exploration policy for penetrating wounds of the neck. *Surg Gynecol Obstet* 1985; 160:517–522.
7. Rubio PA, Reul GJ Jr, Beall AC, et al: Acute carotid artery injury: 25 years' experience. *J Trauma* 1974; 14:967–973.
8. Campbell FC, Robbs JV: Penetrating injuries of the neck: A prospective study of 108 patients. *Br J Surg* 1980; 67:582–586.
9. Rao PM, Bhatti MFK, Gaudino J, et al: Penetrating injuries of the neck: Criteria for exploration. *J Trauma* 1983; 23:47–49.
10. Narrod JA, Moore EE: Selective management of penetrating neck injuries. A prospective study. *Arch Surg* 1984; 119:574–578.
11. Belinkie SA, Russell JC, DaSilva J, et al: Management of penetrating neck injuries. *J Trauma* 1983; 23:235–237.
12. Bivins B: Discussion of Roon AJ, Christensen N: Evaluation and treatment of penetrating cervical injuries. *J Trauma* 1979; 19:391–397.
13. Bradley EL III: Management of penetrating carotid injuries: An alternative approach. *J Trauma* 1973; 13:248–255.
14. Brown MF, Graham JM, Feliciano DV, et al: Carotid artery injuries. *Am J Surg* 1982; 144:748–753.
15. Karlin RM, Marks C: Extracranial carotid artery injury. Current surgical management. *Am J Surg* 1983; 146:225–227.
16. Liekweg WG Jr, Greenfield LJ: Management of penetrating carotid arterial injury. *Ann Surg* 1978; 188:587–592.
17. Thal ER, Snyder WH III, Hays RJ, et al: Management of carotid artery injuries. *Surgery* 1974; 76:955–962.
18. Palin WE Jr, Sadove AM, Jones JE, et al: Oral electrical burns in a pediatric population. *J Oral Med* 1987; 42:17–34.
19. Small A: Early surgery for electrical mouth burns. *AORN J* 1976; 23:126–140.
20. Orgel MG, Brown HC, Woolhouse FM: Electrical burns of the mouth in children: A method for assessing results. *J Trauma* 1975; 15:285–289.
21. Silverglade D, Ruberg RL: Nonsurgical management of burns to the lips and commissures. *Clin Plast Surg* 1986; 13:87–94.
22. Sturim HS: The treatment of electrical injuries. *J Trauma* 1971; 11:959–965.
23. Hammond JS, Ward CG: Burns of the head and neck. *Otolaryngol Clin North Am* 1983; 16:679–695.
24. Edlich RF, Nichter LS, Morgan RF, et al: Burns of the head and neck. *Otolaryngol Clin North Am* 1984; 17:361–388.
25. Eckhauser FE, Billote J, Burke JF, et al: Tracheostomy complicating massive burn injury. A plea for conservatism. *Am J Surg* 1974; 127:418–423.

Facial Plastic and Reconstructive Surgery

CHAPTER 28

Pediatric Issues in Facial Plastic and Reconstructive Surgery

Approach of

J. Richard Casuccio, M.D.

Pediatric facial plastic and reconstructive problems fall into four major areas. The first of these includes facial clefts. The management of velopharyngeal insufficiency is a related but separate topic. Cutaneous vascular anomalies constitute the third major area of interest, and the management of nevi is the fourth area. This chapter will deal with my approach to each of these four areas.

RECONSTRUCTION OF THE UNILATERAL CLEFT LIP NOSE

Many of my colleagues have conceded that the reconstruction of the unilateral cleft lip nose is perhaps the most difficult rhinoplasty that a reconstructive surgeon can be asked to do. It is certainly a challenge for the best trained and most experienced nasal surgeons because the unilateral cleft lip nasal deformity lacks symmetry. In the standard cosmetic rhinoplasty or one done to correct a traumatic deformity, there is an identifiable plane of symmetry, which is completely absent in the harelip patient. This makes the unilateral deformity a three-dimensional nightmare requiring a surgeon with a keen eye and a geometric mind who can define and then correct the problem. Miracles may not be possible and should not be offered, but improvement of nasal symmetry and contour are realistic goals.

Several concessions must be accepted before the cleft lip nose is reconstructed. The first, and most important, is to realize that the deformed nose demonstrates an abnormal anatomy that cannot be made normal. One must accept that the best possible result will be gained not by making the abnormal normal but by establishing some form of symmetry that creates the illusion of normal. Second, a surgeon should not try to solve all the problems at one time. Colloquially expressed, less is best. Time can be a great benefactor in defining both the type and magnitude of the deformity, which will allow the surgeon some flexibility with future reconstructions. Also, it is possible that the patient will grow out of some problems. Therefore, it is advised not to be too rambunctious, particularly in the younger patient. A third concession is that growth is an unknown variable. Since most congenital deformities of the nose are addressed early in life for social reasons, it must be conceded that even the most artistic of repairs can be distorted by the unique growth program of the patient. For this reason, surgical touch-ups are frequently required. Finally, and unfortunately, the mobility of American society interferes with the establishment of a long-term surgeon-patient relationship. Both patient and physician often relocate, requiring that that patient find a new specialist to complete the unfinished labors of a previous surgeon. As a consequence, a patient may be subjected to a multiplicity of surgical philosophies, some of which may contrast, others of which may confuse the patient, leading to frustration and adding to his or her psychologic burden. Consequently, a surgeon who deals with cleft lip and palate patients must be well versed in the various philosophies and techniques described for treatment of this condition.

The most important step in the surgical correction of the unilateral cleft lip nasal deformity is the analysis of the problem. In truth, defining the problem is the initial step of any reconstructive operation, and surgeons should refine their powers of observation so that they are acute and accurate. As Sherlock Holmes said to his friend Dr. Watson as they both examined an old, tattered felt hat, "Watson, you can see everything. You fail, however, to reason from what you see. You are too timid in drawing your inferences."[1] Cleft lip nasal surgeons cannot be timid in their observations; they must be able to see all that is wrong.

The cleft lip nose has a cornucopia of abnormalities that must be broken down into their component parts. These parts will be to a greater or lesser degree depending on the extent of the cleft. There is obvious asymmetry not only between the two sides of the nose but also between both sides of the face. These asymmetries are caused by the lack of skeleton both cartilaginous and bony as a result of the cleft. In lesser clefts, there is a distortion of structures. In total clefts, these supporting structures are absent, and that carries greater implications when the reconstruction is designed. A surgeon must analyze the architecture of the cleft nose defining the nasal skeleton as an engineer might illustrate the framework of a building on a blueprint. There must be a clear picture of what structures are absent, present, and distorted. These problems must be qualified and quantified so that a surgical plan that includes all the little anatomic quirks that must be addressed can evolve. This attention to detail requires that a surgeon also account for all the associated problems that accompany the cleft lip nasal deformity that may have some bearing on future nasal surgery. Such considerations include nasal airway obstruction, dental malocclusion, speech impairment, and hearing difficulties caused by a recurrent otitis media. Nearly all of these patients will need orthodontic treatment and possibly orthognathic surgery, and these considerations must be recognized when one is planning the timing of corrective surgery. It would be ridiculous to embark on a surgical venture that could possibly be undone by some future manipulation. Finally, the social impact of the patient's deformity must be considered. Many decisions regarding the patient's care may have to be addressed in light of the patient's peculiar living circumstances. These patients through no fault of their own have a significant social and psychologic burden, and their treatment should be directed so as to lessen this burden and not to amplify it.

In short, the need for a critical evaluation of all aspects of the cleft lip nasal deformity cannot be overemphasized. Several hours of evaluation may be required, as well as discussions with the patient, parents, and other consultants, before a comprehensive outline is prepared. Photographs should be taken from a variety of angles to assist the surgeon in the preoperative planning. A plaster cast of the face is an extremely valuable tool, allowing the surgeon to find even the most subtle of deformities. The surgeon should not hesitate to review and review the literature and to discuss problem cases with colleagues.

In recent years, the timing of the cleft lip nasal repair has undergone a rethinking. Classically, rhinoplasty was deferred until nasal growth was nearly complete, that is, surgery was done when patients were in their teenage years. Several years ago, a few surgeons began doing tip rhinoplasties in the preschool-aged group, hoping that the growth distortions that typically evolved with age could be avoided. Their results were encouraging. More recently, a good number of plastic surgeons have used that same philosophy as their motivation for performing some minor modifications of the nose at the time of cleft lip repair. Though skeptics question whether such early maneuvers will result in retarded growth rates for the nose, early results seem to support this approach. Establishing some semblance of symmetry at an early age can prevent the gross nasal deformities often seen if surgery is deferred until the child is of school age. I must emphasize, however, that these results are preliminary, and it may take another 5 to 10 years before the final results of early nasal surgery are fully appreciated.

Unless the nose is relatively normal, as it may with incomplete cleft lip deformities, I routinely do some surgical manipulation of the nose at the time of cleft lip repair. I am careful not to disturb the normal side and concentrate my efforts on the lower lateral cartilage on the cleft side. One advantage of the Millard[2–4] cleft lip repair is that it includes a reconstruction of the nasal sill as part of the standard procedure (Fig 28–1). When this technique is used, the ala of the cleft side is rotated in such a way to match the ala on the noncleft side, providing symmetry at the base of the nose. The C flap, which is harvested from the noncleft side of the lip, provides extra tissue that can be inserted into the columella to straighten or lengthen it. It also can be used to provide both bulk and form to the nasal sill. One of the criticisms of this repair is that it creates a buckle along the anterior alar rim when the advancement flap is moved medially. This is particularly true of wider clefts where the lateral flap must be advanced across the midline and positioned in a backcut that is often made under the opposite nostril. Buckling of the nostril results from a relative excess of alar tissue that once bridged the cleft, which is now squeezed into its new position by the tight lip closure. With the ala recontoured into an oval, the lower lateral cartilage bends in such a way as to create a rim that is both lower and longer than on the noncleft side (Fig 28–2). As mentioned earlier, traditionally this deformity has been addressed in later years; however, many surgeons now free the lower lateral cartilage from the overlying and underlying skin at the time of the primary lip repair and move it superiorly to a position immediately adjacent to the opposite lower lateral cartilage. The domes of both lower lateral cartilages are placed side by side and secured to each other with a permanent suture. In many cases the distorting buckle is avoided, and the tip of the nose is more symmetric. The redundant skin usually is rolled into the nostril. Some degree of nasal obstruction is possible, but it is often a positive trade-off when the asthetics are considered.

Recently, Mohler[5] described modification of the Millard cleft lip repair that requires less advancement of the lateral flap (Fig 28–3). Less buckling of the nostril occurs because the advancement flap never crosses the midline. Consequently, this technique allows nasal recontouring with less manipulation of the lower lateral cartilage commonly done in the Millard approach. Time and experience will determine whether the Mohler operation is less disturbing to nasal growth.

As a child approaches school age, cosmetic nasal surgery

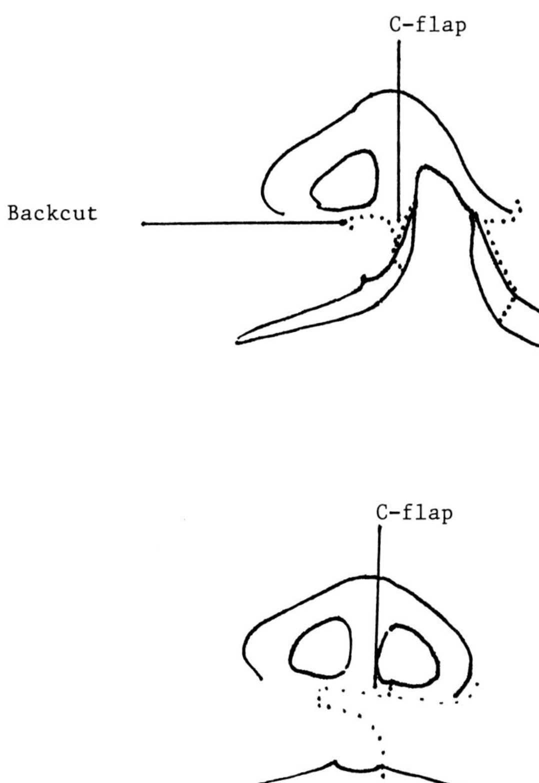

FIG 28–1.
The standard Millard unilateral cleft repair.

often becomes necessary to prevent ridicule by peers. When indicated, the open rhinoplasty is an excellent technical option for the unilateral cleft lip nasal deformity. This operation and its variations, as reviewed by Tebbetts,[6] allow the supporting anatomy to be visualized directly, facilitating the correction. The cartilaginous skeleton can be elevated, rotated, excised, or otherwise modified to bring about nasal symmetry. Soft tissues can be tailored to correct asymmetries of the nostrils and columella. Repositioning of the alas as well as Wehr-type excisions can be included in the operation. In many cases, the open rhinoplasty and a secondary revision of a previous cleft lip repair can be done at the same sitting.

A second operation that has proved very effective in the correction of asymmetries resulting from the unilateral cleft lip deformity is the Dibbell[7] tip rhinoplasty (Fig 28–4). In this operation, the nostril, including a completely mobilized lower lateral cartilage, the nasal sill, and the ala are rotated as a single unit. The dome of the mobilized lower lateral cartilages is positioned next to its normal counterpart and secured there with permanent suture. This operation attempts to refine the tip by rearranging the nostril so that it reflects the shape of the normal side. Skin excess along the anterior nasal tip just inferior to the dome is usually excised in such a way as to reflect the contour of the nostril on the normal side. In addition, there is frequently an excess of skin in the adjacent lip that can be narrowed by the excision of a small triangle. The beauty of this operation is not that it creates nasal symmetry but more the illusion of symmetry. Surgeons often find themselves excising excess tissue from the cleft side when, in fact, these tissues are often deficient. This is done to construct lines and contours that appear normal to our eyes.

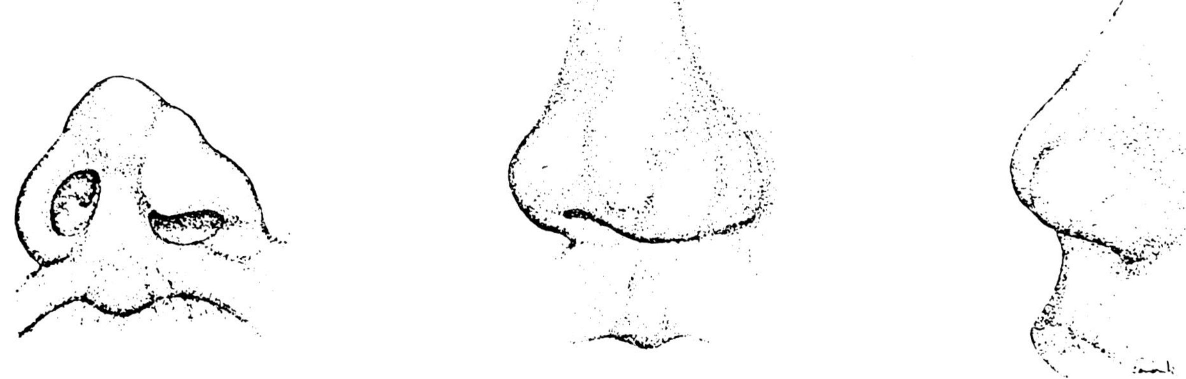

FIG 28–2.
The typical unilateral cleft lip nasal deformity. (From Dibbell DG: *Plast Reconstr Surg* 1982; 69:264. Used by permission.)

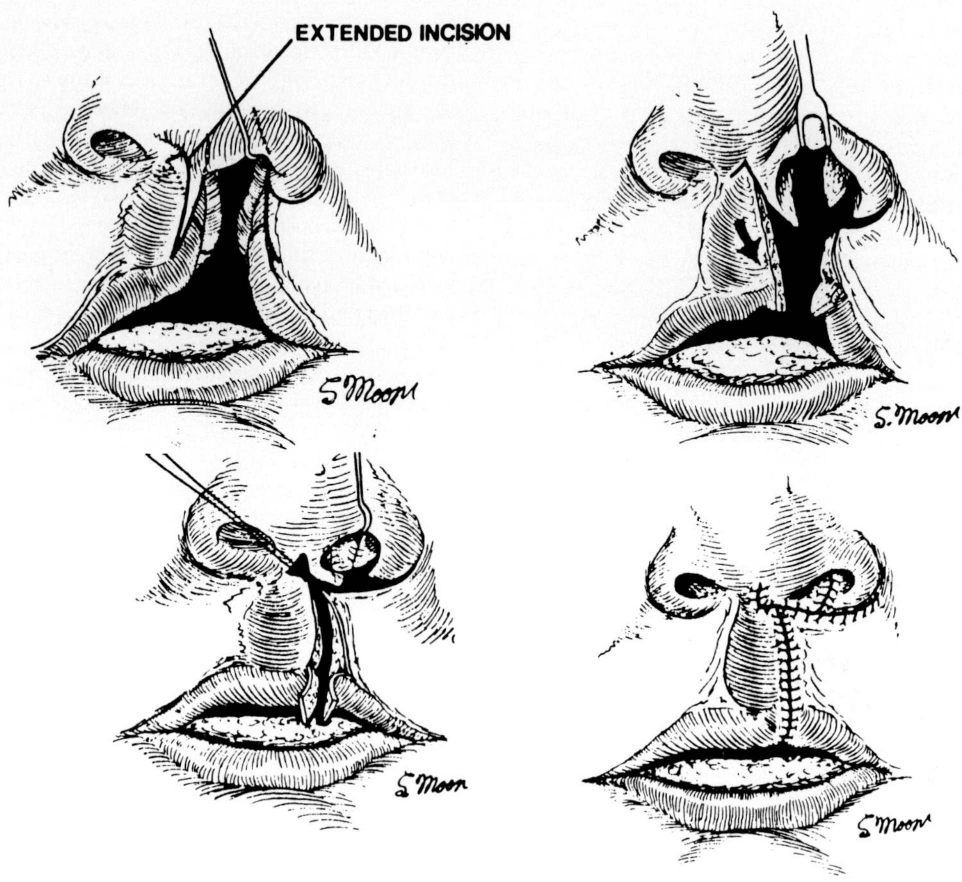

FIG 28–3.
The Mohler modification of the Millard unilateral cleft lip repair. Notice the 90-degree backcut into the nasal columella. (From Mohler LR: *Plast Reconstr Surg* 1987; 80:511. Used by permission.)

Perspective in dealing with the cleft nasal deformities is paramount. These anomalies are never isolated and are accompanied by a host of other congenital and developmental problems that must be addressed. If a patient presents for nasal surgery with a major lip problem, my approach is to correct that problem first, even if it requires redoing the entire lip closure. If, however, the lip deformity is minor, the lip correction and the nasal surgery can be done at the same time. Orthodontic treatment is required in most cases, and I believe this should be well underway before any nasal surgery is attempted. Since palatal expansion is a common orthodontic goal, the base of the nose may be shifted or in some way altered. Therefore, unless the nasal deformity is severe, I believe the nasal surgery should be deferred until the orthodontist is comfortable with the patient's progress. Growing interest in bone grafts of the alveolar clefts in young patients may also alter the timing of a tip rhinoplasty. With the ability to provide skeletal support where it was lacking previously, true nasal symmetry may be a step closer. If such bone grafting is contemplated before the age of 7 years, I believe it is reasonable to postpone nasal surgery until the bone graft is well healed. A final consideration is orthognatic surgery. If either maxillary or mandibular osteotomies are planned, nasal bone osteotomies should be deferred until orthognatic treatment is completed.

A standard rhinoplasty with osteotomies can be offered to those older patients who have widened nasal dorsums, a dorsal hump, or asymmetric nasal bones. Hopefully, by this time tip symmetry has been gained, and the objective of this operation would be the refinement of nasal features. Cartilage and bone grafts can be used to elevate the nasal tip as well as to augment and project the nasal dorsum to give the patient a more mature look. These surgeries can be done either through the usual internal approaches or by the open technique.

The successful reconstruction of the cleft lip nasal deformity requires a dedicated surgeon with a game plan. This plan is based on careful observations of the patient's problem, which includes not only the nose but the other surrounding facial features that may be deformed as well. It is important for the surgeon to maintain an open mind and be willing to change the plan if the patient's physical needs change. Surgical conservatism is to be encouraged so that both the patient and the surgeon are left with future options, particularly with those severe deformities where no single operation is likely to solve the problem. Versatility should be numbered among the virtues of a cleft lip nasal surgeon, who should be aware of all of the technical options and should be able to use them should the situation arise. The surgeon also should know when not to operate. Also among those virtues is a driving compulsiveness that allows one to agonize over the placement of a single suture to gain that optimal result. Finally, but most important, is a sense of compassion for the patient. These children must live with their deformity, suffer ridicule, undergo numerous operations, and yet remain confident in our limited abilities, keeping an open mind to our suggestions for further surgery.

VELOPHARYNGEAL INSUFFICIENCY

Velopharyngeal insufficiency is a long and technical term for those people who "talk through their nose." This hypernasal speech sounds as if words are connected and preceded by an "n" or "gn" sound. Unless they speak slowly, these people are unintelligible and, unfortunately, their speech is interpreted wrongly as being characteristic of an intellectually impaired person. Such speech patterns are seen commonly in the cleft palate patient but may be appreciated in persons with cerebral palsy or heard transiently in some patients after tonsillectomy or adenoidectomy. Velopharyngeal insufficient speech is also expected in those patients who have lost some or all of their palate to tumor or tumor surgery.

Traditionally, the cause of hypernasal speech was thought to be due to the reverberations of sound through an excessively large resonating chamber that could not be adequately sealed off during connected speech. The soft palate and pharyngeal

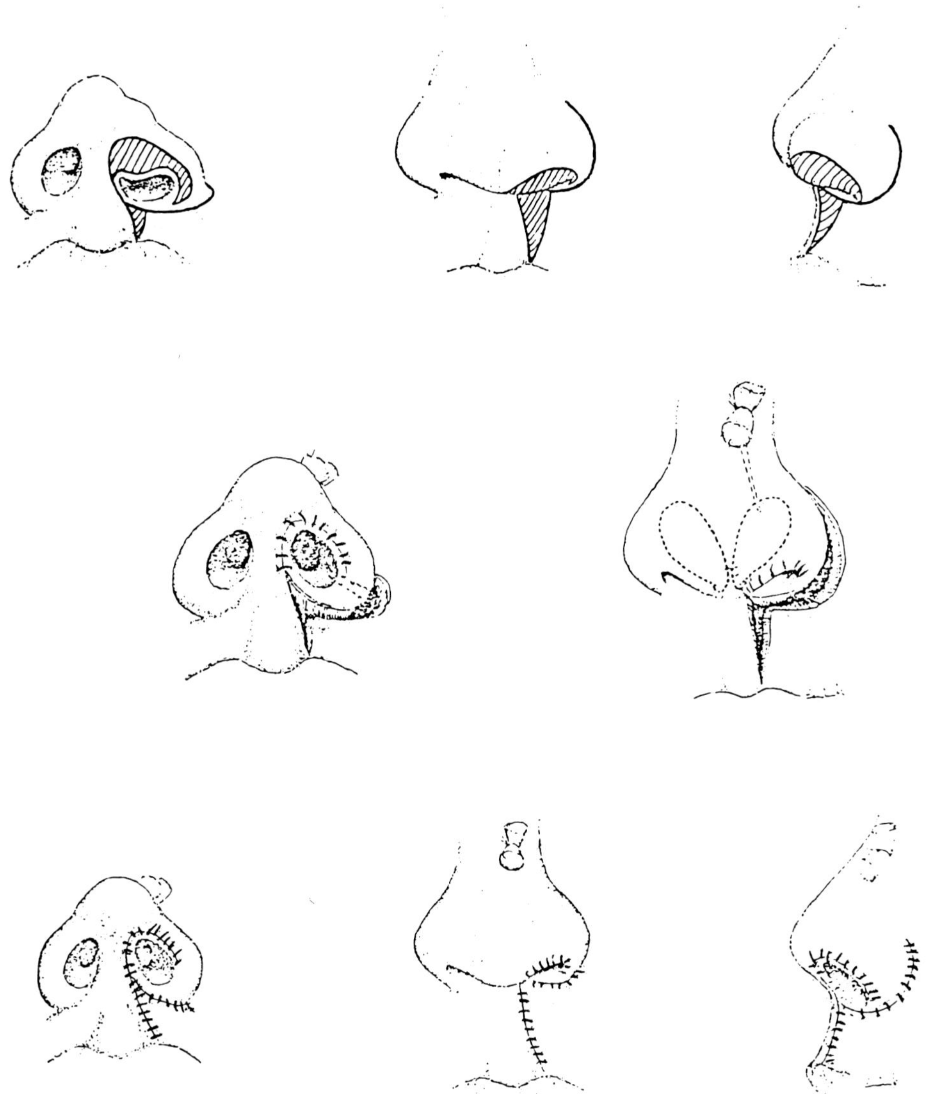

FIG 28–4.
The Dibbell reconstruction of unilateral cleft nasal deformity. (From Dibbell DG: *Plast Reconstr Surg* 1982; 69:264. Used by permission.)

muscles were in some way lax in closing off the nasopharynx, thus the term velopharyngeal insufficiency. Whether this is an anatomic problem or a physiologic one because of improper muscular coordination of the soft palate and pharynx has yet to be determined. Regardless of cause, hypernasal speech is most likely due to the excessive passage of sound through the nasal chamber instead of being diverted through the oral chamber. In severe cases, patients may suffer not only from a speech impediment but also from difficulties with eating. Far from unusual, complaints about nasal regurgitation of foodstuff are heard from embarrassed parents. In milder cases, problems may be limited to an odorous discharge from the nose.

Velopharyngeal insufficiency should be diagnosed, treated, and cured during early childhood. Speech patterns are difficult to change after the age of 9 years and may be impossible to manipulate significantly after the age of 12 years. A common, everyday example of this are those people who are educated in a language during their youth but then learn to speak a second language as an adult. Regardless of how fluently they speak, their diction allows them to be identified as a foreigner. In contrast, many young European children are able to speak several languages each as if they were native to that country. There is a certain plasticity to the nervous system that is lost as we mature. Consequently, if a speech problem exists in a child, the sooner it is recognized the better the chance for the patient to overcome the problem. In the final analysis, this neurologic flexibility may be the key to the successful treatment of velopharyngeal insufficiency, and our alacrity in diagnosis and therapy may be more important than the type of treatment rendered. Our artistic and ingenious operations may be no more than a crutch that helps the individual to a more normal speech pattern.

The best way to evaluate a patient with suspected hypernasality is simply to listen. Physicians should train their ears to the speech patterns of friends and associates as well as their patients. Thus, they can accumulate 20 years of listening experience prior to beginning their training. The specialist should be able to pick up an abnormal speech pattern as easily as an orchestra conductor can detect the one violinist playing out of tune. Although single-word testing is the hallmark for identification of malformed speech patterns, it is probably more informative to listen to the child in casual, playful conversation. We speak not in words but in sentences, and if we are going to evaluate speech, sentences are what we must evaluate. Of course, this takes time. A rapport must be built with patients so that they are as comfortable talking with you as they might be with their parents and peers. To do this effectively may take two to three interviews. The first meeting is merely to become acquainted. Much of this time is spent making the patient and parents comfortable and learning the background of the child and the child's problem. By the second interview, the patient is at ease, talking in his or her usual fashion. I have found that by distracting children with toys and comic books they will jabber freely without shyness or embarrassment. I also take off my white coat and sit on the floor, if necessary. An accurate assessment can then be made.

The expertise of a speech pathologist is essential in the evaluation of children with velophayngeal problems. This is

their life and livelihood, and, in truth, they have more time than the average surgeon for the thorough testing that is necessary. Their advice should be sought before any physical management is attempted. I have found them to be extremely helpful in those difficult cases where the hypernasality is subtle or where there are multiple speech impediments to be distinguished. Written reports are necessary; however, I recommend a direct person-to-person consultation to learn those little nuances about the patient that are often lost in a formal report. The speech pathologist will often consult with the patient's teachers who deal with the child on a daily basis. These educators can be a very valuable source of information regarding the patient's ability to communicate both formally and casually.

I have consciously omitted parental opinion from the diagnostic equation of a child with a speech impediment. I consistently find parents to be of little help to my understanding of their child's speech behavior, and I find this to be both expected and understandable. All parents bear prejudice toward their children, which allows them to ignore many of their problems, particularly the minor ones. By the time the child appears in the physician's office, the parents have been totally acclimated to the child's speech pattern, and they are fully capable of understanding the child when, in fact, no one else can. I have found it to be a common experience that a child and his or her parents will be referred to my office at the direction of the school therapist without the vaguest notion of why the evaluation is needed. In addition, I have been involved in many situations where a child, after 6 to 12 months of intensive speech therapy, shows great improvement according to the parents, but none is found on my testing or that of the speech therapist. In this circumstance, the parents have improved their listening abilities rather than the child improving his or her speaking capability. In contrast, the patient's siblings and peers have been a much greater source of information than the parents. A tragic characteristic of human nature is that children will make fun of their less fortunate colleagues and may even try to mimic the deformity. This is very useful information and should be indicative of the need for expedient therapy before the speech impediment becomes a psychologic problem.

A complete head and neck examination is important to identify any anatomic abnormalities that may impair speech. Repaired or unrepaired cleft palates, submucous clefts, palatal and alveolar fistulae, tongue ties, and dental abnormalities are all considerations. Should that examination be normal, an evaluation of function is in order. Simple techniques include having the patient drink water to demonstrate nasal regurgitation or having the child inflate a balloon to see if air leaks through the nostrils. Placing a mirror under the child's nose as he or she speaks is another way to estimate the amount of air leaking through the nose. The humidified air emanating from the nostrils during connected speech will fog the mirror, and by comparing normal and hypernasal fog patterns, the examiner can get a rough idea of the degree of insufficiency.

Clearly, the best tool in the evaluation of patients with speech impediments, particularly that of velopharyngeal insufficiency, has been the pediatric flexible fiberoptic nasopharyngoscope. This device can be comfortably inserted into the patient's nose to visualize the simultaneous movements of the soft palate and pharynx as they work in tandem to produce speech. Although this sounds technically difficult, it has actually been quite easy to slide a lubricated scope along the floor of the nose to the choana where both the soft palate and the pharynx can be visualized. Earlier in my career I anesthetized these children topically with cocaine; however, in recent examinations no anesthetic has been used. Once inserted, the child is allowed to become comfortable and is then asked to speak, generally repeating what I say. The pattern of palatal and pharyngeal motion can be monitored and characterized in such a way that future therapy, including surgery, can be individualized. I take as much time as needed to make a diagnosis. In some patients, particularly those with mild forms of cerebral palsy, the early part of the examination may be normal; however, as the patient fatigues, problems with speech and motor movement of the pharyngeal structures become evident. On occasion, I have evaluated a patient under general anesthesia. If a child needs ventilation tubes inserted into the eardrums or is undergoing other surgery, I have taken advantage of the anesthetic to insert a fiberoptic scope through the nose and into the nasopharynx, securing it with tape. As the child awakens and begins to call for a parent, a useful examination is accomplished. Thus, the potential for early diagnosis and treatment of the problem-prone child now exists by virtue of recent technology.

Despite the usefulness of the fiberoptic scopes, the cineradiographic studies have not been replaced. Handicapped by producing a two-dimensional image, it nonetheless can render a broader perspective of the motor activity involved with speech by simultaneously demonstrating the coordination among the palate, pharynx, hypopharynx, and tongue. These cine studies also serve as a check on the endoscopic findings, clarifying or rejecting previous assumptions. Lateral and submental vertex views should be obtained.

With all the fancy gimmicks available today, it is possible to lose perspective and see more problems than actually exist. Speech is heard and not seen, and any visual examination must be correlated with the patient's speech pattern and any treatment directed at improving sound rather than anatomy. This point is well made by numerous anecdotal reports by surgeons who have been terribly disappointed in one of their palate repairs only to have the patient speak normally. Conversely, there are those individuals who speak poorly in spite of normal anatomy and function. The key is to consider each patient as unique and to define therapy based on an exhaustive evaluation. Although our understanding of the correlation between speech and anatomy is limited and our therapeutic options are few, treatment by rote is to be discouraged. Perhaps future research using endoscopy and cineradiography with simultaneous audio and video recordings with computer analysis of the findings will define those elusive physical components of speech.

Technology will answer many of our questions in speech pathology, but some can be resolved with simple maneuvers. A frequent diagnostic dilemma occurs in those children who have hypernasal speech following cleft palate closure but who also have an alveolar or palatal fistula. Whether the patient has poor dynamics of the soft palate and pharyngeal wall musculature or is simply leaking air through one of these fistulae is

sometimes difficult to discern. I try to solve this problem by using chewing gum or putty to close off the fistula. The speech evaluations both before and after sealing the open areas are compared. If improvement is noted, surgical closure of the fistula is recommended; otherwise, further speech therapy and perhaps a pharyngoplasty are indicated.

When speech therapy fails to improve hypernasal speech sufficiently, physical management is advised. Although palatal obturators and stimulators are available, most authorities would concur with surgery for the pediatric population. In my practice, I employ both the superiorly based flap as described by Hogan[8] and the Orticochea[9] pharyngoplasty. I cannot say whether either operation has been superior to the other, but rather, in selected cases both flaps have worked well. The superior-based flap creates two lateral ports, both of which should be kept small by making the flap as wide as possible. The mucosal lining on the nasal side of the soft palate should be undermined and rotated distally to cover the exposed muscle of the pharyngeal flap. This will minimize the scar contracture that narrows the flap with time, making the lateral ports larger. I generally use this flap for those patients who demonstrate minimal or no palatal and pharyngeal wall motion with speech. I also use it on those patients who show good lateral wall motion but are unable to seal off the nasopharynx. In contrast, I employ the Orticochea operation when soft palate and pharyngeal wall motion is present but inadequate to form a competent sphincter. This pharyngoplasty constructs a single, central port by rotating the posterior tonsillar pillars with its palatopharyngeus muscle behind the soft palate, securing them to the posterior nasopharyngeal wall. This narrows the inlet to nasal chamber. From my point of view, this operation requires some dynamic activity of the surrounding musculature to make it effective. I have also used it in those cases where there is good elevation of the soft palate and a strong definition of Pasavant's ridge but no evidence of lateral wall motion. To be sure, these indications are arbitrary, and the results to support them lie in the future; however, they are based on findings derived from fiberoptic endoscopy and cineradiography and represent a logical correlation of anatomic and physiologic data gained from a careful and complete examination.

In summary, the essence of velopharyngeal insufficiency lies not in the surgical techniques to correct it but in the long and compulsive approach to its diagnosis. The value of taking time to listen to the patient cannot be minimized, and by maintaining open communications with speech pathologists, parents, teachers, and peers, one will glean beneficial information about the patient's communications skills. A physician should be resourceful when approaching the problem of velopharyngeal insufficiency and should avoid coming to any premature conclusions before a comprehensive evaluation is completed.

CUTANEOUS VASCULAR ANOMALIES

A peculiar personality trait among scientists is trying to establish order and organization where none was before. Thus, many hours of effort have been expended over the ages in what must be the dullest occupation, the classification of everything.

This is often done with a rigid compulsiveness in an attempt to show that nature allowed no loose ends in creation since the time of creation. One gets an eerie feeling when reviewing the variety of classification schemes by which science has regimented nature into artificial categories that make the universe better known but less free. One mistake of nature has consistently baffled scientists in every attempt at classification, stands out due to its lack of conformity, and has character so varied that no one can agree what to call it. These curious quirks of nature are currently known as cutaneous vascular anomalies.

With such interesting and colorful terms as strawberry hemangioma, cavernous hemangioma, cystic hygroma, and port-wine stain, a Victorian novel seems a more likely place to read of them rather than in a text of dermatopathology. Indeed, some of the more notable and tongue-twisting nomenclatures used to describe syndromes with vascular abnormalities are themselves verbal anomalies. For example, such famous syndrome names as Rendu-Osler-Weber, Klippel-Trenaunay, Maffucci, and the blue rubber bleb nevus are more likely to be the brainchild of W. C. Fields than of a notable scientist. In short, the cutaneous vascular anomalies have an image as well as a name problem.

When one is dealing with these lesions, it is best to remember the old adage: Not all hemangiomas are strawberries, and not all strawberries are hemangiomas. Though these lesions may look alike and, in fact, are related histologically, a few important differences must be discerned to determine prognosis and prescribe treatment. The best way to do this is to forget about all the fancy names and cumbersome classification schemes. The goal should be to keep things simple.

The cutaneous vascular anomalies are the most common congenital skin problems of infants and young children. Fortunately, the overwhelming majority are small, require no treatment, and disappear leaving no trace, but this is not always the case. When one of these lesions is recognized, the mission is to decide which lesions can be watched and which will require either medical or surgical therapy. A clear description of the problem and the management options must be presented in a simple and logical way to the parents, many of whom are distraught—blaming themselves for their child's unfortunate blemish. Sadly, many wives' tales about the causes of hemangiomas abound, and these must be dispelled before the physician can win the confidence of all involved and guide them to the proper therapy. This is perhaps the most critical aspect in the treatment of children with vascular anomalies since the most common therapy is no therapy at all. Predictably, the common reaction of parents is to question the judgment of their physician and to seek another opinion or even a quick fix by finding a surgeon willing to operate despite the likelihood that the lesion will spontaneously resolve in time. Therefore, physicians who participate in the evaluation and care of these children should be knowledgeable, conversant, and convincing.

Recent studies[10] suggest that the vascular anomalies may be divided into two broad categories: the hemangiomas and the vascular malformations. This is not an arbitrary separation of terms or even a convenient breakdown of lesions based on obvious clinical differences, but is based on certain cellular characteristics that are noted in the laboratory. The hemangiomas demonstrate an increased rate of endothelial turnover or angiogenesis. Also, during the proliferative stage, an abnormally high count of mast cell may be seen on histologic sections. Finally, harvested capillary endothelial cells will grow easily in tissue culture. In striking contrast, the endothelium from the vascular malformations has a slow turnover rate and grows with difficulty in vitro. The mast cell count is normal. These findings are astute but totally useless in day-to-day clinical practice. Other than the port-wine stains, it is likely that the cutaneous vascular anomalies will appear somewhat similar, particularly in infants; therefore, an approach is needed to properly diagnose and treat these lesions.

The importance of distinguishing these lesions is that the hemangiomas generally disappear and the vascular malformations generally do not. In one situation, it is a matter of waiting for involution, and in the other, it is choosing the right time to begin treatment. This decision is made easier by knowing the natural progression of these lesions. A diagnosis more specific than a cutaneous vascular anomaly may not be possible at the first interview, nor is it important if the child is otherwise healthy. In fact, in some cases it may take 1 year or more of careful and repeated examinations to fully appreciate the problem. Thus, any cutaneous vascular lesion should be judged from the perspective of time.

Hemangiomas are rarely found at the time of birth or, if present, are usually represented by a small pale mark. The vascular lesions, in contrast, are always definable at birth, albeit they may not be classic in appearance. Both lesions will grow as the child grows for much of the first year of life, but the hemangioma will show signs of involution thereafter. Thus, all questionable lesions should be given the benefit of the doubt and observed for as long as possible before the patient is committed to treatment. Of course, lesions that risk the patient's well-being deserve expedient treatment, but in lieu of those few exceptions, the benefits of waiting and watching cannot be overemphasized. Serial photography can be a great aid in the proper and timely care of these children.

The involution of a hemangioma is predictable. The only questions to be answered are how much shrinkage will occur and how quickly will it go. The process commonly begins during the second 6 months of life and may be heralded by a change in color or texture of the lesion. Early on, the hemangioma may grow rapidly, but during the involution phase this growth may arrest or slow to the point where it grows proportionally with the child. During the child's second year, gradual shrinkage of the lesion begins and usually continues for the next 5 to 6 years. Despite many decades of careful observation by researchers and clinicians, none of the characteristics or history of a particular hemangioma predicts the rate and extent of resolution, but complete disappearance can be expected in 50% of children by age 5 years and 70% by age 7 years. After that time a hemangioma may still shrink, but it is unlikely to disappear. In the wake of these lingering lesions, a spongy fibrofatty type of tissue, which at times resembles a hypotrophic scar, is left behind.

Treatment of hemangiomas is reserved for those lesions that threaten the good health of the patient or present a cosmetic concern in school-aged children. Some tumors can be problems more for their location than their bulk. For example, small hemangiomas of the eyelids can cause significant amblyopia and astigmatism. Similarly, a small lesion in the external auditory canal impairs hearing, and airway hemangiomas can be life-threatening. Oral mucosal hemangiomas may impede deglutition. Large hemangiomas may lead to platelet consumption, causing bleeding, congestive heart failure due to blood shunting, and skeletal distortion from compression of an expanding lesion on growing bones. Ulceration with subsequent infection is an uncommon problem with skin lesions. In these circumstances it is still better to wait for involution if the problem can be managed for the short term; however, if the physical development of the child becomes compromised, the treatment should be expedient.

Systemic corticosteroids enjoy popularity at this time as the preferred treatment, particularly if the patient is younger than 6 months of age. The response rate is generally better than 50% in those hemangiomas that are in the proliferative phase. These lesions are seen to involute quite rapidly. Older hemangiomas do not fare as well with this treatment, and the risk of using steroids in young children must be weighed against the clinical situation and the other options for treatment. Hypertension, growth retardation, and rebound growth of the hemangioma are some of the negative considerations with corticosteroid therapy. Interlesional steroid injections, though technically difficult, seem to be an effective mode of treatment yet offer an avenue of safety not afforded with systemic use. Surgery is particularly useful for small lesions that can be excised easily and without a resultant deformity. Small hemangiomas of the ear canal as well as those in concealed areas of the body where primary closure is possible are obvious situations, but excisional therapy can be used when other modalities of treatment have failed or for cosmetic reasons when the resultant deformity is likely to be less than the current deformity. The surgeon needs to have an extensive and versatile repertoire of techniques to afford the patient the best possible result.

Among the other treatment modalities are compression, cryosurgery, sclerosing agents, and the argon laser. Compression of lesions can be of use when one is dealing with large hemangiomas of the extremities but is difficult to apply to other areas of the body. Cryotherapy and sclerosing have been used with limited success and are better used as adjuvants to other forms of treatment. The argon laser holds future promise as a tool that may prevent proliferation of young hemangiomas.

The best approach to the vascular malformations is first to simplify the terminology. Conveniently separated into the low-flow anomalies, including the capillary, lymphatic, and venous malformations, and the high-flow variety, the arteriovenous malformation, this group can now be studied with much less confusion. Words such as lymphangioma, cystic hygroma, cavernous hemangioma, and lymphangiohemangioma are outdated because they are not accurate descriptions of the lesion's histology. They should be retired. A second consideration when one is addressing this family of vascular problems is to concede that there is no ideal treatment prescribed for these lesions. They do not respond to humoral therapy or any other form of medical management, and surgery and other manipulations are often ineffective and technically difficult.

The vascular malformations are present at birth and continue to grow as the individual grows, with an occasional case report of a spontaneous involution. The lesion can grow to be large and grotesque and may become invasive and life-threatening. Treatment options are few and generally limited to surgery, which itself is limited. Once the proper diagnosis is made, the only decisions needed are when to operate and how much to remove.

The capillary malformations or port-wine stains commonly are found in the head and neck, frequently in the distribution of the trigeminal nerve. They are pink in infants but become purpler with age. As the patient enters adulthood, the flat, smooth surface of the discolored skin will become rougher and more irregular. This change in texture is due to the dilation of the vascular channels. Traditionally, camouflage with heavy makeup and tattoos has been used as treatment, but patient and physician satisfaction has been low. Staged surgical excision with skin graft reconstruction exchanges one deformity for another and cannot be recommended. More recently, excision after tissue expansion allows the use of normal head and neck tissues as flaps to replace the pathologic skin. The benefit of this approach is that an unlimited amount of regional tissue can be made available for massive reconstructions with less surgery and, hopefully, less scarring. Though the use of tissue expanders sounds exotic and simple, it is not without its technical problems. Often there is very little usable good skin in continuity with the stain that can be conveniently stretched to cover all the lesion at one operation. Reexpansions of the same expanded skin is frequently done, and the stain is removed in a serial fashion. Technical hassles increase as the expansion approaches an orifice such as the mouth or eyelids. There is very little tissue in these areas on which the advanced flap can be anchored. These flaps have a tendency to retract, causing distortions of the adjacent structures. Perhaps repeated small expansions followed by frequent short advancements are the way to proceed, but this has yet to be demonstrated.

The Ar laser has been a large step forward in the treatment of capillary malformations using light energy to selectively erase the stain. The Ar light coagulates the abnormal capillaries, making the remaining channels smaller, thus preventing further ingress of red blood cells. If the Ar laser is to work adequately, the lesion must be a deep uniform color. Consequently, smooth purple-colored lesions are optimal, but, unfortunately, this type of port-wine stain seldom is found. Young people have the smooth lesions, and older people have the purple ones. Thus, this inherent difficulty in finding the ideal candidate is probably responsible for the irregularities in skin color and texture seen so often postoperatively. In addition, the Ar laser does burn the epidermis and superficial dermis, which may lead to unwanted scarring and pigmentation. Despite these problems, most patients undergoing this treatment achieve improvement and appear to be satisfied with the result. Recent work with the krypton laser suggests that this modality may be more selective for the capillary lesions and less damaging to the adjacent skin.

Lymphatic malformations are found in the head and neck, axilla, and groin most commonly but may be found in any tissue through which lymphatics run. Formerly known as lymphangiomas and cystic hygromas, this group of hamartomas represents a proliferation of lymphatic channels that fail to adequately couple with the venous system. Many such lesions include abnormalities of veins and venules that have been inaccurately but colorfully designated as the lymphangiohemangioma. Despite the confusion of terms, these lesions have an easily recognizable character simulating jelly under a thin skin covering. Besides the unrelenting growth of the lesion that parallels the growth of the patient, soft tissue hypertrophy and skeletal deformities are typical of this family of lesions. In addition, the lymphatic malformations are plagued with recurrent bouts of infection that present as areas of cellulitis or small abscesses. They are easily treated with rest, elevation, and penicillin, but may, on occasion, progress to sepsis.

As with the other vascular anomalies, treatment is conservative. Many of these lesions will arrest and even regress, albeit few, if any, completely disappear. Therefore, surgery is reserved for those aggressive, disfiguring, and functionally impairing lymphatic anomalies. The operation should be well planned, with the goal being to remove all the tumor while avoiding mutilation. Approaches and techniques need to be well thought out so as not to compromise the patient or limit the options for future operations that may be necessary. Computed tomography (CT) is a great aid in measuring the extent of the lesion and planning surgical approaches. Despite one's best efforts, resections are often incomplete, and both patient and surgeon will have to return to the operating theater another day. Regardless, a sufficient bulk can be removed to arrest or even prevent skeletal deformities.

The venous malformations may vary widely in appearance. Ranging from small punctate telangectasias to large, spongy, deeply purple lesions, these anomalies have been given a variety of names, among which is the commonly overused term cavernous hemangioma. These are low-flow entities often seen with other capillary, lymphatic, and arterial anomalies. Blood can be forced from them easily, but, like a sponge, they quickly refill. Frequently, several small, hard nodules can be felt in the lesion. They are phleboliths caused by the sluggish blood flow and, when found, establish the diagnosis of a venous malformation. On occasion these phleboliths may consume platelets and clotting factors, leading to a bleeding diathesis. As with the other vascular malformations, the venous anomalies grow proportionately with the patient but can be seen to expand further if traumatized either accidentally or by subtotal surgery. Unexplained growth may be seen during puberty or may be iatrogenically induced by ill-advised hormone therapy. Treatment is total surgical excision when possible and subtotal excision when necessary. Use of sclerosing agents has aided management by shrinking large lesions as well as limiting the bleeding during surgery.

Arteriovenous malformations are high-flow lesions that may appear anywhere within the body. They may be small and innocuous for years and then suddenly begin to grow and become symptomatic. When they are close to the surface of the skin, they may demonstrate pulsations, thrills, and bruits. The surrounding skin can be warm, and on occasion, port-wine staining may be seen. Although these lesions can distort skeletal anatomy, they are more likely to destroy bone by erosion. Bony overgrowth of arteriovenous malformations is common. The shunting of blood from the arterial to the venous circulation robs adjacent tissues of oxygen and nutrients, and skin necrosis overlying such lesions is a clear indication that blood flow to that area is insufficient. If the shunting becomes excessive, high-output cardiac failure occurs. Small asymptomatic lesions may be watched, but large ones often require medical treatment for cardiac failure and consumptive coagulopathy. Ultimately, surgery is the required treatment to stabilize a life-threatening condition and to relieve a grotesque cosmetic deformity. A total excision is the preferred treatment and is frequently facilitated by preoperative CT and angiography with selective embolization. Feeder vessel ligation, major artery bypass, craniofacial reconstruction, and a variety of plastic and reconstructive techniques frequently come into play when one of these malformations is removed.

In summary, all patients with cutaneous vascular anomalies deserve the benefit of an accurate diagnosis that often does not require exotic testing or transfer of care to a specialist. Careful observation and time are all that are needed in most cases to guide patients and their parents to a successful understanding and resolution of the problem. Treatment of any type should be withheld until a diagnosis is made and then prescribed only when absolutely indicated. When surgery is advisable, it should be as complete as possible, utilizing all the techniques and modalities available to ensure patient safety and to gain an acceptable, aesthetic result.

For completeness, the vascular malformation syndromes are defined:

1. *Sturge-Weber syndrome*—capillary hemangioma (port-wine stain) in the cutaneous distribution of the trigeminal nerve with extension of the vascular abnormality to the brain. Glaucoma, buphthalmos, optic atrophy, and seizures may occur.

2. *Rendu-Osler-Weber syndrome*—also known as hereditary hemorrhagic telangectasia. This syndrome is transmitted as an autosomal dominant trait. It presents in adulthood, and symptoms include nose bleeds, gastrointestinal bleeding, and hematuria. Neurologic symptoms may result from central nervous system bleeding.

3. *Kasabach-Merritt syndrome*—rapid expansion of the vascular malformation with generalized body bruising and bleeding. Disseminated intravascular coagulation results from the consumption of platelets and clotting factors by venous-type malformations usually of the extremities and trunk. Symptoms generally appear in the first year of life and may lead to death. Treatment consists of systemic steroids, surgical excision of the lesion, and arteriographic embolization of the malformation.

4. *Klippel-Trenaunay syndrome*—an irregular and patchy combination of capillary, venous, and lymphatic malformations usually involving a single extremity, generally a leg. Bony overgrowth and growth distortion may occur. Early treatment consists of custom-made elastic stockings.

5. *Maffucci's syndrome*—endochondromas accompanied by vascular malformations. These patients have shortened bones and exostoses of the digits, some of which may progress to chondrosarcomas. Vascular malformations of the internal organs and intracranial tumors may occur.

6. *Von Hippel–Lindau disease*—rare, inherited disorder causing hemangiomas of the retina and cerebellum. Other visceral organs may be involved with cystic angiomas.

7. *Beckwith-Wiedemann syndrome*—a rare combination of port-wine stains of the face and macroglossia. Hypertrophy of the liver, pancreas, and kidneys occurs in addition to hyperinsulinemia and hypoglycemia from the hyperplasia of the pancreatic islets.

8. *Blue rubber bleb nevus syndrome*—vascular malformations of the skin and bowel. The blebs are distinctive and easily compressible. Popping a bleb will express a small amount of blood, which then leaves a wrinkled sac of skin. Bowel lesions may require a segmental resection, and skin lesions can be excised generally subtotally if they become a problem for a patient.

MANAGEMENT OF NEVI

I am frequently asked by my patients and physician colleagues about moles. Specifically, their query is how one distinguishes a mole from a melanoma. It is a germane question considering both the health and medicolegal implications of skin cancer in our sun-soaked culture. I have found that many generalists are uncomfortable with this mole vs. melanoma problem and quickly refer the patient to a specialist, many of whom often are equally confused about the best approach to evaluation and treatment. Making the correct diagnosis without performing too many biopsies is the challenge that confronts physicians as skin cancer begins to reach epidemic proportions.

Two important assumptions need be recognized before one approaches this problem. The first is that Americans are not going to quit going out in the sun. Because of our advice, some may reduce their exposure by limiting their time outdoors, others might apply sunscreen, albeit sparingly, and a few may even wear a hat and shirt occasionally; but to suggest that people give up their seaside vacations, take up bowling instead of golf, or move to cloudy West Virginia instead of sunny Florida will lead them to find another physician, preferably one who enjoys a year-round suntan. (Interestingly, several of my plastic surgery colleagues own or routinely use suntanning beds.) The second consideration is not to underestimate the seriousness of a melanoma. These cancers have the potential to kill, maim, and disable if the diagnosis is missed or if the tumor is treated inadequately. These tumors should be approached with the same diligence and completeness a physician uses when performing a direct laryngoscopy for a head and neck lesion or reading an electrocardiogram of a patient with chest pain.

Although a discussion of skin cancer includes basal cell cancer, squamous cell cancer, and melanoma, the diagnostic dilemma focuses on the melanoma. With a variety of presentations and patterns, this deadly tumor seems camouflaged when surrounded by skin bearing a multiplicity of pigmented lesions, the overwhelming majority of which are benign. Melanoma will strike 1 in every 150 Americans over a lifetime, accounting for about 20,000 cases annually. Of these, 5,000 can expect to die of their disease. A more sobering statistic is that melanoma was diagnosed in 1 out of 300 persons in 1975 and since then has risen at a rate that would predict an incidence of 1 in 100 by 2000.[11] This makes melanoma the fastest increasing cancer second only to lung cancer and implies that 10% of all primary practitioners now have an annual opportunity to diagnose a melanoma if they can recognize it. Therefore, it is imperative, considering the fatal implications of this disease, that all physicians be able to distinguish a mole from a melanoma.

Much of the confusion surrounding melanoma comes from the terminology that has a histologic orientation but is of little, if any, practical use to the clinician. Correlating such terms as dysplastic nevus, junctional nevus, compound nevus, lentigo maligna, and amelanotic melanoma with a dark spot on the skin is mind boggling. This is not to suggest that the terminology be changed or dropped; rather, it should be ignored as a matter of practicality. Instead, pigmented lesions of the skin should be approached as either moles or melanomas, letting pathologists worry about the proper names. The question should not be what is it but, rather, whether it warrants a biopsy. This is the only question to be answered at the initial examination.

Several years ago the American Cancer Society published its ABCD approach to the diagnosis of suspect pigmented skin lesions, which, when correlated with a patient history, greatly simplifies the examination. Any "mole" can be evaluated according to the following scheme:

A—*a*symmetry
B—irregular *b*orders
C—variable *c*olor
D—*d*iameter greater than 6 mm

Certainly, any mole with all four characteristics merits biopsy at the earliest convenient opportunity; however, if not all the criteria are met, the patient history plays an important role. The key question is that of any noticeable change in the lesion. Although the changes frequently mentioned in the literature include changes in color, size, shape, surface texture, surface elevation, surrounding skin (i.e., appearance of satellite lesions), and sensation (i.e., pain or itching), this endless alliteration serves to confuse rather than help when taken in the context of day-to-day clinical practice. More simply, any change of any mole bearing any of the ABCD features deserves biopsy or, at the very least, careful observation. In addition, any suspicious lesion in a person with a family history of melanoma warrants early biopsy. In contrast, any mole that is small, round, regular, and uniform in color with no history of change may be allowed to live with the patient.

Perhaps somewhere in this country medical students are taught the techniques of a careful skin examination, but more likely, the students are given some cursory instruction, which, in many cases, leads to a cursory examination. In light of the near epidemic increase in skin cancer in our society, this deficiency in medical education must change. An examination of the skin should be done in a deliberate and organized fashion similar to a cardiac or neurologic evaluation, and all that is required is a good light source, a magnifying lens, a ruler, and a naked patient. The examination should start at the head with a complete going-over of the scalp and progress to the neck, back, buttocks, legs, and feet, after which the anterior body surface is studied. The upper extremities as well as perineal, scleral, and mucosal surfaces should be viewed. Any interesting lesions should be magnified, measured, and palpated. If a lesion is to be observed over time, it should be described and recorded on a body map; however, a photograph of the lesion makes a quicker and clearer record. Two exposures are generally necessary, the first being a photograph of the body part of interest (e.g., a hand, the back) and the second being a close-up of the lesion with a ruler beside it. This technique should afford maximum protection for those borderline lesions for which a period of observation may be practical.

When a pigmented lesion merits biopsy, a complete excision is the preferred treatment. If this cannot be done without inflicting a functional or aesthetic deformity, a simple incisional or punch biopsy in the most suspicious area can be done. Photographs are tremendously helpful in this situation to pinpoint further changes should the initial biopsy miss a cancer. Electrodesiccation and electrocoagulation are not to be used prior to the histologic analysis of the lesion.

The treatment of the congenital nevus sparks controversy among experts. There is uniform agreement that nevi that are present at birth and are greater than 20 cm in diameter possess a sixfold increase in the incidence of melanoma; however, there is no consensus of the risk incurred for those congenital nevi that are less than 20 cm. Although it is safe to recommend removal of all such lesions, it is not always practical for functional and cosmetic reasons. The best approach is to establish a photographic record of the lesion while examining the patient every 6 months through the early years. The parents must also be educated as to the possible changes that may occur so that there is no delay in diagnosis should the lesion turn suspicious. If changes occur, the lesion is removed, but if the nevus remains stable, it can be watched indefinitely. Commonly, the parents will request excision to eliminate the risk of cancer in the child or they and perhaps the young patient may seek surgery for cosmetic reasons. If the lesion is small or in an area that lends itself to simple plastic surgical techniques, surgery can be done when the patient is old enough to participate in his or her care, usually around the age of six years. The removal of a large congenital nevus or even a moderately sized one requires a grand plan that often includes multiple surgeries employing a variety of plastic surgical approaches. This plan must emphasize functional and physical aesthetics so as to improve the situation rather than to replace one deformity with another. Initial surgeries must be done with future operations in mind so as not to limit other technical possibilities. Recent work with tissue expanders has been exciting and offers tremendous promise to these patients.

In summary, the approach to nevi should be simple and logical. Although some would argue that this approach will increase the number of biopsies done, the justification lies in the number of people who will benefit from the early diagnosis of a melanoma.

REFERENCES

1. Doyle AC: The adventure of the blue carbuncle, in Baring-Gould WS (ed): *The Annotated Sherlock Holmes.* New York, Clarkson N Potter, 1967.
2. Millard DR Jr: *Cleft Craft—The Evolution of Its Surgery,* vol I: *The Unilateral Deformity.* Boston, Little, Brown & Co, 1976.
3. Millard DR Jr: *Cleft Craft—The Evolution of Its Surgery,* vol III: *Alveolar and Palatal Deformities.* Boston, Little, Brown & Co, 1980.
4. Millard DR Jr: *Cleft Craft—The Evolution of Its Surgery,* vol III: *Alveolar and Palatal Deformities.* Boston, Little, Brown & Co, 1980.
5. Mohler LR: Unilateral cleft lip repair. *Plast Reconstr Surg* 1987; 80:511.
6. Tebbetts JB: Cleft Lip. II: Secondary Deformities. *Select Read Plast Surg* 1985; 3:17–22.
7. Dibbell DG: Cleft lip nasal reconstruction: Correcting the classic unilateral defect. *Plast Reconstr Surg* 1982; 69:264.
8. Hogan VM: A biased approach to the treatment of velopharyngeal incompetence. *Clin Plast Surg* 1975; 2:319.
9. Orticochea M: Construction of a dynamic muscle sphincter in cleft palates. *Plast Reconstr Surg* 1968; 41:323.
10. Mullikan JB, Young AE: *Vascular Birthmarks, Hemangiomas and Malformations.* Philadelphia, WB Saunders Co, 1988.
11. Friedman RJ, Rigel DS, et al: *Early Detection of Malignant Melanoma.* New York, American Cancer Society, 1985, p 4.

SUGGESTED READINGS

Bardach J, Salyer K: *Surgical Techniques in Cleft Lip and Palate.* Chicago, Year Book Medical Publishers, 1987.

Friedman RJ, Rigel DS, Kopf AW: Early detection of malignant melanoma: The role of physician examination and self-examination of the skin. *CA* 1985; 35:130–151.

Mulliken JB: Cutaneous vascular anomalies of children. Handout given at the Plastic and Reconstructive Surgery Board Review Course. Northwestern University School of Medicine, Chicago, December 1986.

O'Brien JC: Skin tumors II: Melanoma. *Select Read Plast Surg* 1986.

Rohrich RJ, Spicer TE: Hemangiomas and vascular malformations/lymphedema. *Select Read Plast Surg* 1986; 4(8).

Shprintzen RJ, McCall GN, Skolnick ML: The effect of pharyngeal flap surgery on the movement of the lateral pharyngeal walls. *Plast Reconstr Surg* 1980; 66:570.

Pediatric Issues in Facial Plastic and Reconstructive Surgery

Approach of

Nigel R. T. Pashley, M.B., B.S., F.R.C.S.(C), F.A.A.P.

DERMATOLOGIC LESIONS

Hemangiomas

Congenital hemangiomas may be present at birth or may erupt within the first year of life. Clinically they are either compressible, which implies a cavernous component, or firmer, which implies a more capillary arrangement. A pure form of either is possible, and a mixed type also exists.

The degree of cutaneous involvement varies extensively, and many different sites of occurrence are possible, including the cutaneous facial areas, the tip of the nose, and the major salivary glands. Clearly the challenge is to decide whether surgical intervention is needed and, if so, when?

It is the general approach by parents that they would like their child restored to near normality as soon as possible with no apparent residual deformity or scar. If a surgical attack is contemplated at all, although it may be possible to provide such a result, it would be foolhardy to imply guarantee. A period of observation (watchful benign neglect) is always justifiable, therefore.[1] In general, hemangiomas do not grow explosively, and measurements and photographs are always worthwhile at the first visit. Clear instructions are given at that time that if more enlargement or increasing deformity is noted, the parents should promptly return for a reassessment of this approach.

In the young infant with an enlarging mass, a rapid taper of oral corticosteroids has often been advised and in some cases may have prompted some degree of involution in hemangiomas. No controlled trials have ever satisfactorily determined their efficacy; however, a 7-day course may help and carries little risk of side effects. Thereafter, periodic (about every 3 months) visits with repeat photographs, if needed, should occur (Fig 28–5).

Overall, hemangiomas present at birth stand a roughly 50% chance of involution up until the age of 2 years, provided expansive growth is not occurring. It is prudent if the offending lesion is not growing to wait unless extenuating circumstances such as a pedunculated hemangioma on the lip or the isolated hemangioma on the tip of the tongue is present, in which case a simple prompt excision will take care of the problem.

If the lesion is not changed by the end of the second year or if it starts to expand, removal before the mass becomes more unmanageable is warranted regardless of the age of the patient.

Operative Technique

Isolated discrete small hemangiomas may be simply excised and the defect closed without deformity.

Pure capillary lesions with cutaneous involvement are best treated by Ar laser bursts, which essentially scar the capillary component. Repeated treatments may be needed to avoid a large area of tissue damage.

Hemangiomata that deform by mass effect or by their infiltrative nature in subcutaneous areas will need surgical excision. The approach is dictated by the location; for example, the tip of the nose is approached by an external rhinoplasty and the parotid by formal parotidectomy with facial nerve dissection. When the mass is removed, care needs to be taken of the skin overlying the mass, which may be directly infiltrated or may have a tenuous blood supply (in particular, venous drainage). Excision of skin at the margin of the approach is usual because the skin overlying the lesion is often atrophic and excessive once the mass is gone (Fig 28–6). Where appropriate, suction drains without an overlying dressing provide the best bedding of one's flap with a lessened risk of seroma.

In the parotid area, the surgeon needs to be aware both in hemangiomas and lymphangiomas that these lesions will deform and alter the position of the nerve branches. As the lesion grows, it may compress normal tissue to the point that the medial parotid lobe, for example, may be present to only a rudimentary extent, or occasionally one finds that the pes anserinus has been tractioned or pulled down to an abnormally low level by an apparent mass. By using standard dissection with a facial nerve stimulator and no traction on nerve branches during dissection, one can perform these often tedious and bloody excisions without facial nerve injury (Fig 28–7).

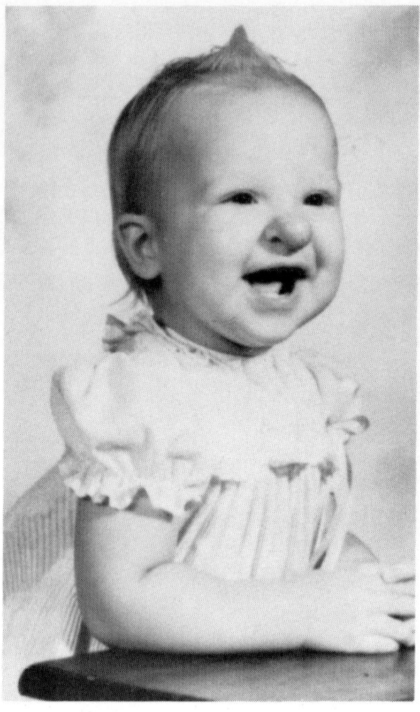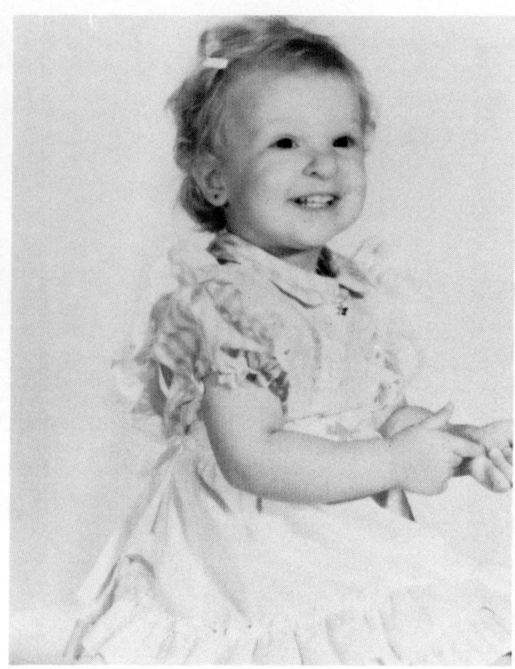

FIG 28–5.
One-year-old girl with a progressively enlarging hemangioma of the nasal tip extending to the vestibular skin (*left*). She was initially followed for 6 months, and the mass was removed at age 15 months. Postoperative view at age 2 years 3 months (*right*). The child won a beauty pageant at age 3 years.

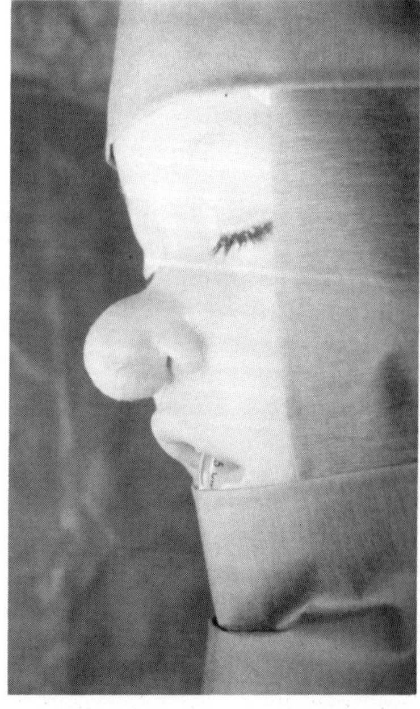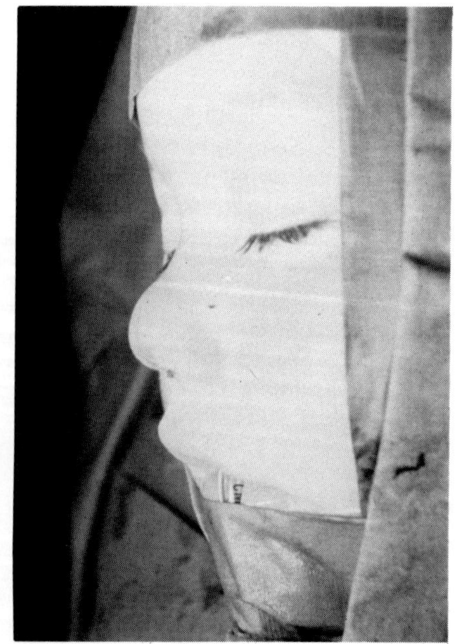

FIG 28–6.
Intraoperative view of a large hemangioma of the nasal tip in a 2-year-old. It required extensive skin resection to successfully close the defect. An external rhinoplastic approach places the resection margins in a hidden area under the nose and within the vestibule.

The original surgeon has the best opportunity for complete excision, and unless the surgeon is performing these procedures on a regular basis in small children, it is better to solicit the help of someone who is.

It is wise for the surgeon to remember that hemangiomas like lymphangiomas may extend through tissue planes, and where cervical involvement or extension into the floor of mouth exists, the airway may be threatened, particularly after excision when edema occurs in a hidden portion of the mass or in adjacent areas.

Hemangiomas of the subglottis occur with another hemangioma in 50% of children. A child with stridor or muffled cry who has a hemangioma in evidence elsewhere in the body must be assumed until proved otherwise to also have one in the subglottis, which may require management first.

Cystic Hygroma and Lymphangioma

Lymphangiomas occur more frequently in children, are more diffuse, may be massive and more deforming, and tend less toward spontaneous involution than hemangiomas. There is more of a tendency toward delayed presentation, no mass being noted at birth but a mass being noticed some months later, except in the truly massive hygromas. Very large hygromas of the head and neck are truly massive, very deforming, in particular, altering bony growth of the maxilla and mandible and invariably threatening the airway. Palatal, tongue, and floor of mouth extension is common, and a long-term tracheostomy quite likely is required.[2]

The general rules applied to a hemangioma also apply to lymphangiomas (wait unless the deformity is threatening or rapidly enlarging).

Operative Management

Excision of lymphangiomas, because of their more diffuse nature, requires some modification. In general principle, opening of the fluid-containing cysts may be all that is required, although the desire is excision without sacrifice of vital structures such as nerves (facial, in particular).

Caution in massive hygromas is certainly the key word, because the facial nerve is displaced in three dimensions by the mass, and the tissue of a cyst wall, once opened, is very similar in consistency and appearance to the nerve itself. I prefer magnification by loupes or the microscope in the infant or child together with the use of a facial nerve stimulator in the appropriate regions.

Where neck extension exists, an excision equivalent to a modified radical neck dissection is used, preserving the sternocleidomastoid muscle and the internal jugular vein but resecting en bloc lymphatics that are the source.

Intralaryngeal hygroma is best treated by laser excision or incision of the cysts, and this may be required over several treatments. Although excisional methods for tongue and floor of mouth are still in vogue, the scar resulting from a large hygroma is truly crippling to the tongue and floor of mouth of a child, and one is limited by the major salivary gland ducts as to the extent of possible resection. Far better is to use cryo-therapy in hygromas. A repetitive freeze and thaw in four to five cycles to each affected area works by freeze-fracturing the cysts that contain lymphlike fluid and preserves muscles and normal cells, which are far more thermally resistant than the hygromatous tissue.

A simple, cheap, effective probe can be made from a Teflon rod[3] with a solid brass or copper end, which is immersed in liquid nitrogen until isothermic and then directly applied to the tissue until the entire area is treated. The limitation of this type of therapy is the volume of tissue to be treated, otherwise wider application in other areas of the body might be possible.

Where the hygroma creates bony facial deformity, later mandibular or maxillary osteotomies, once the second dentition is present, may be required, with coordination with a craniofacial team or surgeon. These massive hygromas have a tendency to have areas of hemangiomatous histology and, where mucosal surfaces are involved, may intermittently bleed. Topical cryotherapy will control this but is palliative until some sort of involution occurs.

Following excision, suction drains without pressure dressings are mandatory in cystic hygromas and one needs to warn parents that commonly another area will bulge into prominence within a short time of a "successful" excision. As the hygroma communicates with (abnormal) lymph channels, it is not uncommon for another unsuspected area to arise often temporarily until lymph drainage from the operative site is established.

Nevi

Hairy Nevus

Pigmented hairy nevi are markedly deforming unsightly lesions in children and may have a potential for more aggressive malignant transformation if left in place. Practically, most hairy nevi in the head and neck occur on the scalp and are best managed by excision, which in most cases, to avoid deformity, requires a serial staged excision, gradually allowing primary closure and removal without grafting. On the neck, either application of a skin graft, which is less cosmetically acceptable, or a bilobed rotational flap closure can usually be achieved. Wide margins are not required and will, indeed, create more problems for closure.

CLEFT DEFORMITIES

Cleft Lip

Preferred Techniques

In a child with a unilateral cleft of the lip, whether complete or incomplete, the repair technique regarded as an industry standard is a rotational advancement (Millard's repair). This type of repair embraces the basis of any repair, which is transferring tissue from the lateral side of the cleft and inserting it in the medial (columella) side that is deficient. The advantage of a Millard-type repair is a great deal of flexibility in transferring tissue with little disposal of tissue, and in particular, an integral correction of some of the nasal deformity, especially the ala base and the columella.[4]

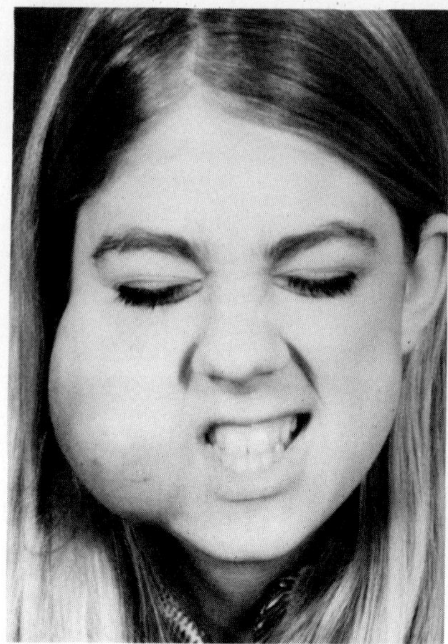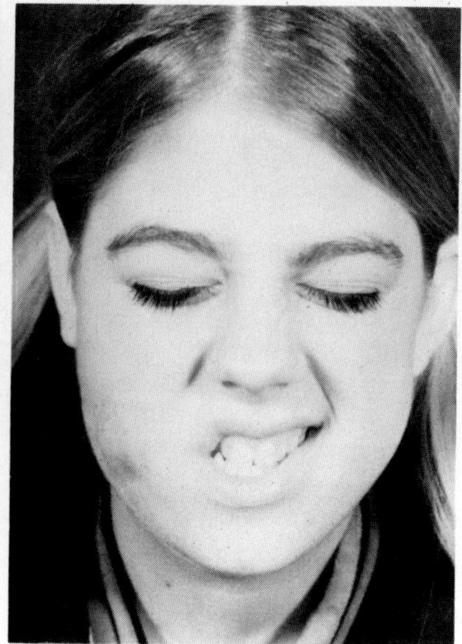

FIG 28–7.
Preoperative and postoperative view of a massive hemangioma of the parotid and cheek in facial animation. There is no change in premorbid facial nerve function following resection, which required parotidectomy with facial nerve dissection.

The nasal deformity is always present no matter how minor (incomplete) the cleft, in addition to which, tissue along the margins of a cleft lip has a growth potential and therefore should never be discarded. Other techniques (triangular or rectangular flaps) tend to waste more tissue, which increases tension within the repair and leads to a secondary deformity.

With any cleft, however, it is important that the surgeon and the parents start with modest realistic aims. The more severe or wide a cleft, the less likely a perfectly normal appearance (see discussion of wide bilateral clefts).

Bilaterally cleft lips can be repaired by a doubled unilateral technique, but there is a substantial risk of compromising the repair to preserve blood supply of the prolabium and vice versa. Most surgeons repairing bilateral complete clefts use a modification of a simple straight line closure along the cleft margins, which saves tissue (the prolabium is often hypoplastic and will, over time, enlarge) and provides two vertical scars along the lines of the philtral columns (a desirable orientation on a lip since horizontal scars tend to catch the light).

Difficulties can be anticipated in wide bilateral clefts where the premaxilla projects markedly. The past practice of early premaxillary setback, which creates a wholly (more) unstable premaxilla, can only be condemned. Staged (one side at a time) closure of a wide bilateral cleft lip is more conservative and physiologic in creating lip pressure that will gradually bring a premaxilla into an arch relationship with the maxilla alveoli laterally.

Lip adhesion has been used, but the creation of a secure adhesion requires tissue sacrifice, and later resection of what is often an unsightly scar creates more tissue loss long term.

The timing of any lip repair has undergone philosophic changes in recent years. With increased safety of pediatric an-aesthesia offered by children's hospitals with qualified pediatric anaesthesiologists and improvements in pediatric and neonatal preparation, we realize that the old rule of waiting until the child weighed 4.5 kg and was at least 10 weeks old was really instituted to provide a healthy child who was in positive nitrogen balance and who could heal an electively performed surgical incision.

Increasingly the trend is toward an early repair within the first or second week of life, provided no other health problems exist; a lip repair is elective even though feeding is more difficult until the repair is complete.

Cleft Palate

Although there has been a modest trend toward repairing clefts of the palate earlier, when a complete cleft is present, early banding of the palate by scars (before the primary teeth are starting to come into occlusion) leads to restricted maxillary development later. Like lip surgery, palatal surgery is elective. About 1 year of age is a common age for palatoplasty to be performed.

The vogue for soft palate repair early (staphylorrhaphy), followed later by a repair of the palate, has for the most part been abandoned as providing little additional benefit over waiting until a definitive repair can be undertaken. Prosthetic splinting of the palate to provide better sucking has been shown to help bring palatal (bony) shelves into better alignment, and for wide palatal clefts with very vertical shelves, this is a useful device.

The technique with better healing and lengthening of the palate potentially is a V-Y pushback (so-called Wardill-Kilner-Peet technique) rather than the older and technically less challenging Von Langenbeck repair, which really failed to adjust the misalignment of the soft palate muscles (the levator sling of the palate).

Also, there is a sensible trend away from primary incorporation of a pharyngeal flap into the cleft repair at the time of primary palatoplasty. Placement of a flap at the time of palatal repair seems to doom the palatal repair or, at the very least, draw into question the adequacy of one's technique and also ensures a fixed static palate rather than a mobile (desired) one. Under exceptional circumstances (extreme palatal cleft usually due to a prior resection, for example, of a teratoma), a flap is inserted early after palate resection to reconstitute function.

Velopharyngeal Incompetence

Incompetence of the velum occurs (1) as a result of clefting of the palate, (2) as a result of palatal paresis in primary neurologic diseases or in acquired bulbar paresis due to cerebral palsy, and (3) as a result of neurapraxia or premorbid anatomic deficiencies as occur or are brought to light by the injudicious removal of an adenoid.

A clinical impression of incompetence can be confirmed by phonation, during which the nose is pinched closed or during which a cold mirror is held at the nostril documenting air escape during phonation. Flexible nasopharyngoscopy can be tolerated as young as 4 years (less than this age with only the most cooperative patients) and, of course, is better tolerated in the older child as a confirmatory endoscopic measure.

A confirmatory phonating cephalometric cinefluorogram in the anteroposterior and lateral plane simultaneously is certainly a superior way to judge movement and provides a measure of lateral pillar movement, which is important for the operative surgeon to judge the size of lateral ports that will be created to provide the nasal airway.

In my experience, because the adenoid may enlarge with restricted mucus flow (stasis), one is asking for a series of obstructed noses post pharyngeal flap unless one removes the adenoid first. Normally, a minimum of 2 weeks is required for healing of the adenoid bed prior to flap insertion. This, of course, creates worse velopharyngeal incompetence, which the parents need to understand.

Occasionally in a submucous cleft, one finds massive superior enlargement of the adenoid, which contacts the nasal surface of the palate and provides "palatal cutoff," which on more than one occasion has resulted in improvement of motion to near competence by simple removal of the adenoid. This normally leads to a recommendation for resumption of speech therapy, which should, incidentally, always precede pharyngeal flap.

Teflon injection, insertion of cartilage, or the plication of muscle in the area of Passavant's ridge has been used in incomplete palates with less than 0.5 cm of velopharyngeal gap. The long-term results in growing children are inferior to those in young adults, possibly due to growth and development.

Pharyngeal flap surgery is a nondynamic admission in the case of a cleft or failure to create a moving palate (sometimes a physical impossibility) and so should take its place as a court of last resort.

A period of at least attempted intensive speech therapy is certainly worthwhile in all except defined neuropathies, and even then some improvement can occur through improved function in the compensatory areas of the lateral (tonsillar) pillars.

Once one reaches a point of no progress or of frustration in speech therapy, a surgical attempt at improving the competence of the velum can be attempted.

For this reason, it would be unusual to embark on a pharyngeal flap in a child younger than 3 years, before which speech patterns may not be established well enough for meaningful therapy.

Operative Management

The operative management is simply the creation of a full-thickness muscular and mucosal flap from the posterior pharynx, which fits best when made square and is less likely to compromise the posterior oropharyngeal airway when superiorly based. In addition, a superiorly based flap places the ports on each side at a much more easily adjusted position where the bare (muscular) surface of the flap can be covered by advancement of the thicker palatal muscle and mucosal layer over the muscle of the flap.

The flap must be stretched out to fill the palatal gap created by the fish mouthing of the palate by creating a deep enough pocket (at least 1 cm deep) and a wide enough pocket (starts and ends at the anterior tonsillar pillar on each side). The best way to extend the flap is to exit one's sutures (usually 3-0 or 4-0 chromic) at the junction of the hard and soft palate on the oral side at five strategically and evenly spaced points with a Dingman gag unless basket weaving of chromic sutures is the surgeon's forte.

Before the flap is sutured into the palate, two endotracheal tubes cut so that their curvature follows the floor of the nose and with openings beveled to face downward (which would provide an opening on the ventral surface of the pharynx) are introduced per nasum.

The size of these tubes is based purely on nostril size and the potential mobility of the lateral (palatopharyngeal) pillars. Restricting the nasopharyngeal port to a smaller size than the nostril guarantees the feeling of nasal obstruction to the child. Creating a port so large that the child cannot possibly achieve competence guarantees a poor (incompetent) result. A certain amount of nasal obstruction usually evidenced by nocturnal snoring is almost desirable at the outset, and the parents need to be warned of this.

Placing the sutures through the tip of the flap in vertical mattress fashion first protects oneself from crossing sutures, which is fairly easy to do. The needle fixed end is then held within the gag toward the surgeon, who is seated at the head, and the free end of the suture is held above on the retaining Dingman springs. By alternatively driving the fixed needle end, then taking a free (herniotomy or Keith) needle on the free suture end and passing this adjacent but separately, one can tie the sutures along the palatal surface sequentially without tangling. (Any other order is acceptable so long as the surgeon does not break a suture, cross a suture, or cut off the blood supply by overtightening sutures.)

The defect left in the posterior pharynx should be closed by approximation, catching the prevertebral fascia centrally to obliterate dead space. Care is needed superiorly near the flap or the ports on each side to avoid cutting off the blood supply or compromising the nasal port.

The nasal tubes can be left in place until removed either by the patient or the surgeon the next morning. Fixing the tubes together with a safety pin ensures protection from aspiration. This is a painful operation for the child, and 2 days in the hospital is certainly normal.

In general, an improvement is noted straightaway, although there is no doubt that speech therapy will be required after a pharyngeal flap to readjust for a different set of oropharyngeal circumstances regarding speech.

In the child who has a cleft palate as a result of Pierre Robin anomalad, the surgeon needs to be aware that edema in the flap or in the tongue or palate compromises the airway, and there have been tragedies when this has not been recognized. Some intensive monitoring of the airway and oxygenation may be required without oversedation.

Secondary Nasal Deformity of a Cleft Lip

The term secondary is a misnomer; the deformity is present as a part of the original cleft, although it remains after cleft lip repair (to a certain degree), and should. It is folly to attempt correction of the entire nasal deformity in an infant and dooms the nasal cartilage (lower lateral and lateral crus of the lower lateral, in particular) to a deformity from which it will not recover if this is attempted.

The nasal deformity has to be understood in its entirety and extent before one can attempt a staged reconstruction. Integrated with this are some surgical limitations that have to be superimposed above the actual deformity. If one sacrifices the following basic principles, too extensive a dissection too early is occurring, and a poor long-term result will likely occur.

Overzealous extension of dissection is the anathema; it creates scar that fails to grow with the child and leads to a secondary restriction of growth or a secondary deformity. The two areas of importance are the face of the maxilla, in particular, lateral to the alar base, and the area superficial and intranasal over and under the lower lateral cartilage, which is itself deformed during development when a cleft exists.

In a bilateral cleft, there is no normal side for reference, and in superficial observance the deformity is less. Indeed, deformities in general are more apparent when one-sided; the eye of the observer is drawn by side-to-side contrasts.

As a corollary, a general rule is that the nostril should under no circumstances be narrowed by any surgical approach. Vestibular stenosis (the result) is notoriously difficult to correct, and the very idea that a scar in the vestibule will correct with time is unfounded.

The deformity starts with an understanding of the base, the maxilla. On the cleft side the maxilla is smaller due to the cleft arising, in all probability, from a failure of arrival or delay of arrival of the reinforcing mesoderm that will form bone or muscle.

The base of the ala is displaced in three directions: laterally, inferiorly, and medially. To a large extent, the first two are correctable during the primary lip repair. The last is correctable only by augmentation (usually later, if needed at all) by placement of a graft of cartilage under the ala base (Fig 28–8).

Secondarily, over time a deviation of the anterior caudal septum occurs toward the cleft side, and later without ala base correction, the nasal bone itself is drawn down and across toward the cleft side. The latter two deformities can be altered by an early correction of the lower nasal deformity but can be hastened by the creation of scar across the maxilla and lower lateral cartilage.

The columella on the medial side of the cleft is short (correction, again during the primary repair, is partially possible), and the remaining deformity is confined to the lower lateral cartilage and its adherent skin. The dome of the nose is lower, the lateral crus is drawn out over an increased distance with the ala base, and this draws the vestibular skin into a more horizontal naris with prolapse downward, perhaps best described as producing a horizontal S-shaped orientation to the naris. The lateral crus is physically wider and longer and thinner with less support and rigidity.

Operative Management

Although attempts to correct the nasal deformity are clearly indicated at the time of primary lip repair, each time a surgical attack is mounted more scar is created, which limits growth, and the law of diminishing returns starts to apply. Because the cartilage of the lower lateral is the primary source of the problem, operations limited to the skin without correction of the excessive thinning and prolongation of the lower lateral cartilage will not achieve as desirable a result as an approach directly aimed at correcting this deformity, such as an external rhinoplasty. This approach provides a one-stage complete correction, in particular, with suturing of the exposed domes of the lower lateral cartilages together at an equal height and the luxury of complete lateral crus exposure with, if necessary, augmentation of the lateral crus to provide more support. Vestibular skin prolapse may still be a problem, but an offset Z-plasty with transfixion suturing after an external rhinoplasty will often correct the problem in two stages.

The external approach can be used as early as 5 years without risk of injury to the cartilage, particularly if magnification is used and one avoids injury to the medial crus during the dissection of the nasal skin upward and over the domes. This is a convenient age before serious schooling or school disruption occurs.

In the older child with a preexistent deformity, a staged approach, including as a last stage the external correction of the lower lateral nasal deformity, is best. If possible, the base is corrected first, the septum is straightened, the ala base is corrected, and then the lower third of the nose is tackled. A lip revision is best timed with the external rhinoplasty so that columella lengthening can be achieved simultaneously if needed.

Later, if the lip scars are prominent or irregular, dermabrasion may be used, or an excisional reclosure once growth is complete may be contemplated. In general, the inclusion of an orthodontist in one's planning or review by a team will help

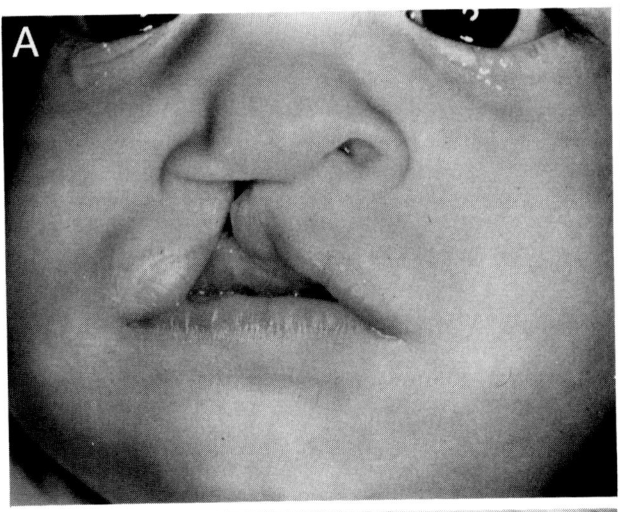

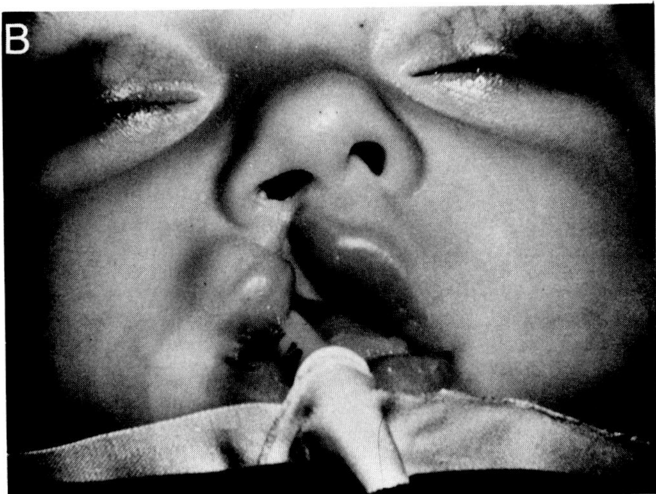

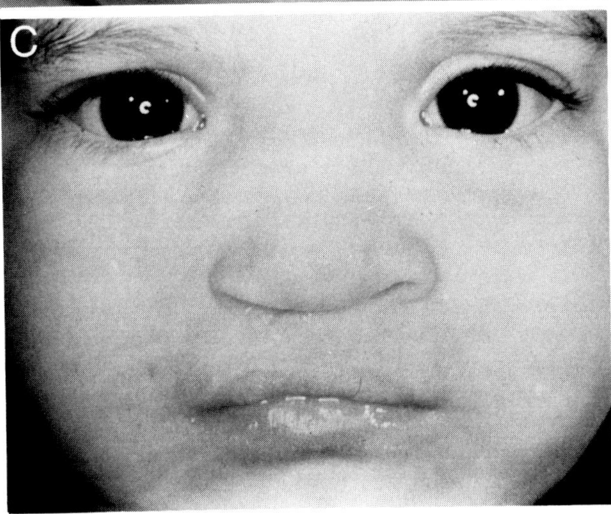

FIG 28–8.
A cleft of the lip (**A**), even a minor one (**B**) has the same nasal deformity, which is partially corrected by the lip repair (**C**) but will likely still require an external rhinoplastic correction later.

minimize the number and frequency of surgical attacks on a limited area and help minimize a certain inevitable deformity, which, in a wide cleft, may have to be accepted.

REFERENCES

1. Batsakis JG: Vasoformative tumors, in *Tumors of the Head and Neck.* Baltimore, Williams & Wilkins Co, 1979, pp 293–296.
2. Batsakis JG: Vasoformative tumors, in *Tumors of the Head and Neck.* Baltimore, Williams & Wilkins Co, 1979, pp 301–304.
3. Pashley NRT: An inexpensive effective cryoprobe (for pediatric care). *Ann Otorhinolaryngol* 1982; 91:204.
4. Pashley NRT, Kranse CJ: Cleft lip, cleft palate and other fusion disorders. *Otolaryngol Clin North Am* 1981; 14:125–143.

CHAPTER 29

Rhinoplasty

Approach of

Howard W. Smith, M.D., D.M.D.

In operative nasal surgery, there are basically three areas of concern from a technical aspect: the tip, the dorsum, and the septum. It is interesting to note that among various excellent operators, each will express an area where he or she experiences the most difficulty. Almost none of the outstanding rhinoplasty surgeons has a set technique for each case. They do, in general, have a basic approach, which has to be varied to meet each situation.

The purpose of this chapter is to tell what works well for me, not only in my practice but in my teaching as well. An operation that is repeated often with varied modifications seems simple to the operator, and the more skilled the operator is, the simpler the operation seems for the student. Should the student be learning from a surgeon with minimal experience, the operation will look much less simple.

The goal in rhinoplasty is to satisfy the esthetic demands of the patient and at the same time carry out a safe physiologic procedure. As in most instances in medicine, the patient makes most of the decisions. First, he or she determines that nasal surgery is desired. This may come at any time in life. It may be a long-desired procedure put off until financial circumstances made it possible, or the effect of aging may have created a desire for appearance improvement. The individual seeks a professional opinion, submits to an examination, receives advice, and then decides whether or not to have the surgery performed. The most challenging part in rhinoplasty, in my experience, is to carefully analyze the patient in terms of what that person is like, how the person selected me to do the surgery, and what the patient expects from the operation.

Many years ago, before rhinoplasty became a major part of my practice, a very lovely woman came to the office seeking surgery. She had a nose that I would have been proud to achieve as a postoperative result. She had a perfectly straight nose, a

straight septum, an appropriate tip, and a pleasant dorsum. I sent her away, stating that she looked perfectly acceptable to me and that surgery was not indicated. I was too young to explore all the reasons why she came or to appreciate a degree of surgical perfection that I did not possess at that stage in my professional career. Many years later I reviewed the photographs taken at that first inverview. With a greater degree of confidence in my work after many years of experience, I had an appreciation of the finer aspects of the operation. I could see defects that were not obvious to me at the time. Her tip was a bit dependent, there was a general downward slope of the dorsum toward the tip, and there was a widening of the nose in the lower portion of the nasal bones with lack of definition on oblique views. In retrospect, the patient was more sophisticated than I. However, I was pleased with my decision because my skill at that time would not have achieved the fine degree of improvement she desired.

Thus the patient will often have a perception of what type of nose he or she would like, this perception being achieved by looking at surgical results obtained by friends. Not all of these friends had gone to the same surgeon, so questions were asked of these friends. From a group, a particular surgeon is selected. Other approaches include calling a referral service, medical centers, county and state medical organizations, or even consulting the *Yellow Pages*. Occasionally a young adult is brought in by a parent stating that it is time for "Sally" to have her nose surgery, without regard to Sally's wishes or desires. The patient who has an operation solely to satisfy a parent may never like the result regardless of the degree of perfection.

It is important to recognize the background of each patient with respect to their endeavors to reach you as a surgeon. It is also important to recognize that the need for an operation may be transient. Having the procedure, in some instances, will fill

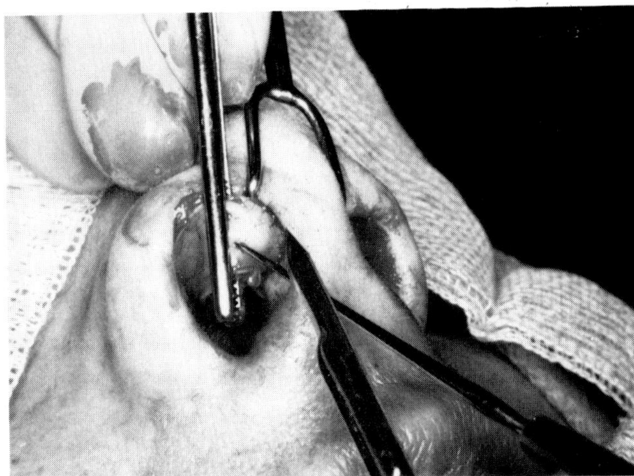

FIG 29–1.
Everted right lower lateral cartilage in preparation for complete division at the dome.

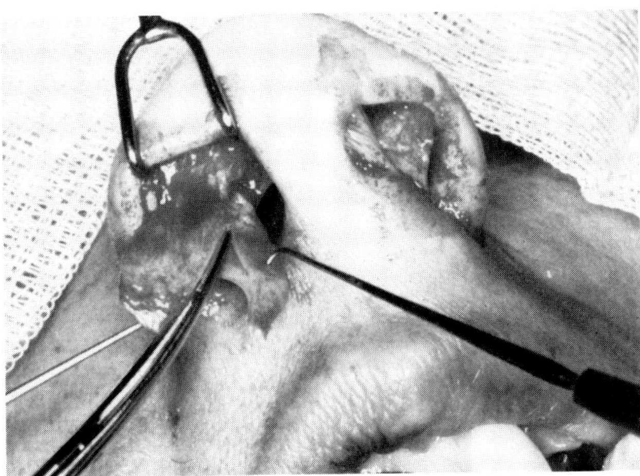

FIG 29–2.
Right lower lateral cartilage showing minimal removal of cephalic border.

most of the patient's requirement without strict regard to results. The person who has saved and saved and is now ready for the big occasion will be very fussy with the end result and will come in prepared with photographs of several current top models for discussion. It is very difficult to turn down patients, especially if a person wants surgery. You are obviously in the profession to do it, and the patient presents an interesting operative challenge. The patients with obvious psychologic problems are readily recognized, and appropriate consultation should be obtained. If the nose problem is beyond one's surgical capabilities, the case is one that cannot be improved or could even be made worse, or the patient is one who will never be satisfied, the case should be avoided.

I have been a student of rhinoplasty for more than 30 years and still seem to be learning. To be asked to write as an expert on rhinoplasty makes me wonder if I am qualified. Several years ago I was demonstrating a photographic technique to a well-known rhinoplasty surgeon with more than 30 years of experience. He asked how I performed tip surgery, saying that he was still dissatisfied with many of his results. So, it seems that all "experts" are continuing to learn.

SPECIFIC CHALLENGES

Reduction of the Overall Large Nose

Reducing the overall large nose can be a real challenge in some cases. The need is present in a patient with a nose that is, by itself, proportionately adequate but is just too large for the face. The danger is to end up with a nose that is smaller but wider, with round nostrils. It is difficult to write about all the various procedures, but in general I perform intercartilaginous incisions, complete transfixion incisions, and marginal incisions to facilitate delivery of the lower lateral cartilages. I divide the cartilage 2 to 3 mm lateral to the dome (Fig 29–1) including the vestibular skin, and reduce the cephalic border of each lateral crus minimally (Fig 29–2). I peel back about 4 mm of vestibular skin from the medial end of each lateral crus (Fig 29–3). Occasionally it is necessary to reduce the length of the lateral crura at the point of resection to help lower the tip (Fig 29–4). The medial crura are delivered, the intercrural connective tissue is removed, and the anterior borders are sutured (Fig 29–5). The medial crura are reduced to allow for reduction in height. Each medial crus can be crosscut to allow for bending (thus lowering the tip) but without cutting the attached vestibular skin (Fig 29–6). These reshaped medial crura can be palpated through the skin over the dorsum to check the progress of reduction. Often with an oversized nose, the skin over the tip may be thick and contain an excess of subcutaneous tissue. Exposure of the tissue is provided by pressing the tip externally on one side so that it presents in the opposite nostril.

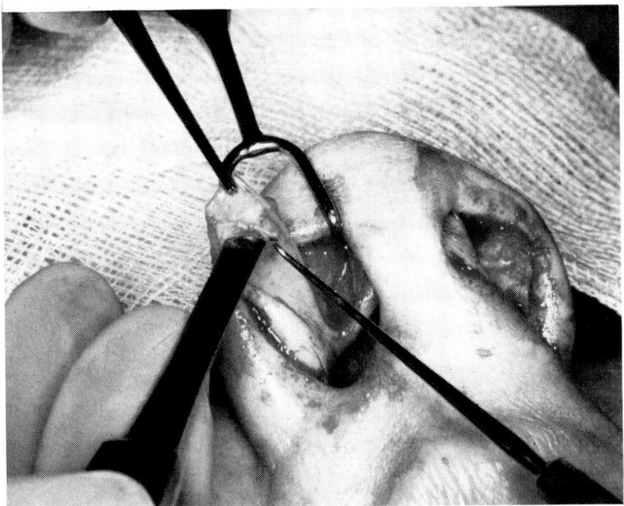

FIG 29–3.
Right lower lateral crus showing elevation of vestibular skin from the tip.

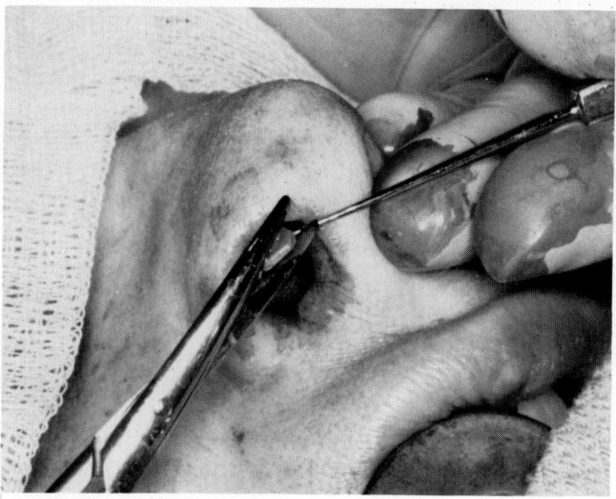

FIG 29–4.
Right lower lateral crus showing removal of a small segment to reduce the tip projection.

The exposed subcutaneous tissue can be trimmed with a small scissors. This procedure will also help narrow the tip and reduce projection. It will also tend to make the nostrils rounder. At this point, ala wedges can be removed to correct the nostril roundness (Fig 29–7), which also tends to further lower the tip. The remainder of the nose can then be proportionately reduced as in any rhinoplasty procedure of choice.

Delivery of the Lower Lateral Cartilages

The dome area may be difficult to deliver, the main cause of which is inadequate exposure. Three important areas must be incised. The intercartilaginous incision and the complete transfixion incisions are performed but are usually not the problem. The medial end of the marginal incision must be extended down the columella 4 to 5 mm below the dome area for exposure (Fig 29–8). The lateral aspect of the marginal incision must actually hug the cartilage and extend almost to the end of the cartilage. A third area of concern is the ligament of Pitanguay, which is a cord of connective tissue passing from the intercrural area back to the skin. This cord must be cut to allow both medial crura to be dissected and delivered into one nostril.

Fat Nasal Tips

Many fat nasal tips can be corrected. The excess may be heavy skin, but more frequently it is thick subcutaneous tissue. If the lower lateral cartilages are delivered, good access to the dorsum is achieved by pressing the dome skin on one side so the undersurface presents in the opposite nostril. Dr. Julius Newman developed and refined this technique without dividing the lower lateral cartilages.[1] It is, however, necessary to lower the cartilaginous dorsum to get freedom for this maneuver.

Wide Noses

Wide noses can be narrowed if there is sufficient sup-

porting tissue (bone and cartilage) over which to drape the skin. Wide undermining of the skin helps with redraping. Lateral osteotomies will help if there is sufficient height to the nose. Upper lateral cartilages must be divided from the septum to break the spring and allow the dorsal edge of each upper lateral cartilage to move medially and dorsally when the nasal bones are infractured. If the intercanthal area is narrow, the osteotomy can terminate where the wide portion of the nose ends, thereby creating narrowness only where needed.

Fragile Noses

Older patients have brittle bones. Chisel osteotomies will shatter the bone like glass if the operator is not careful to tap the chisel gently with the mallet. This brittle type of bone is in

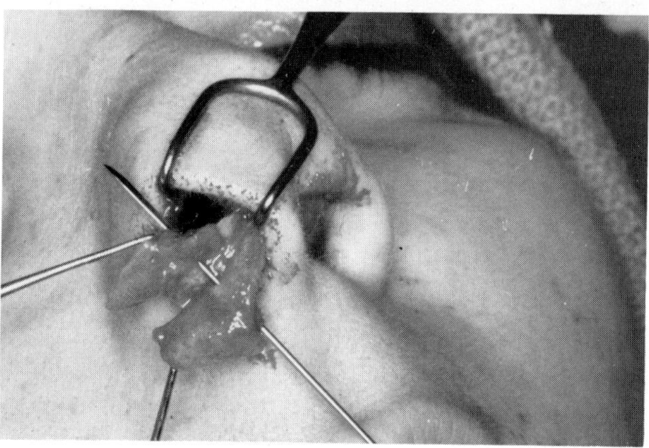

FIG 29–5.
Both medial crura of lower lateral cartilages showing suture of caudal border.

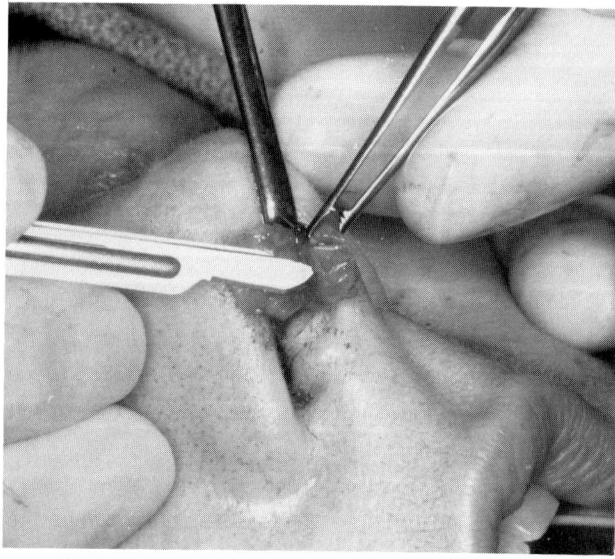

FIG 29–6.
Both medial crura showing crosscutting to soften the cartilage to avoid projection through the skin overlying the tip.

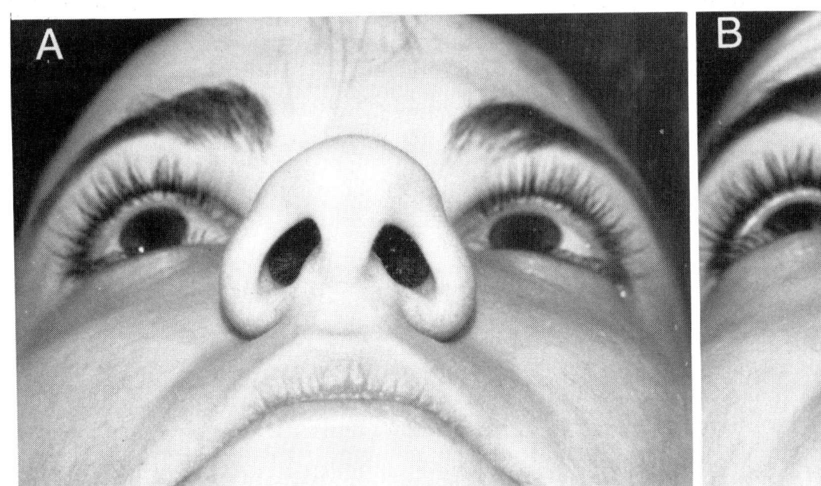

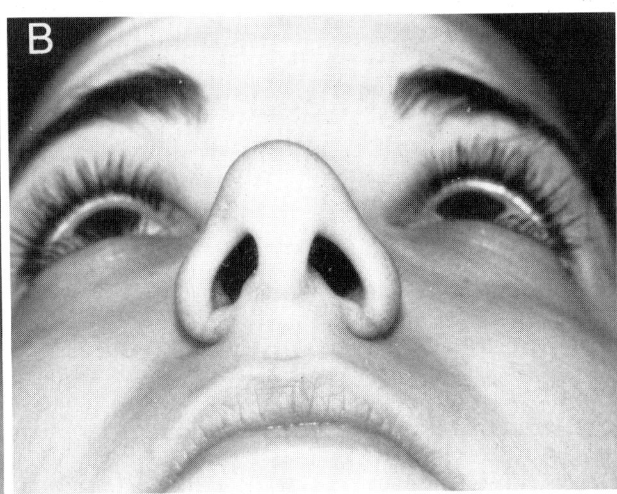

FIG 29–7.
A, nasal tip before removal of alar wedges. **B**, nasal tip in **A** after removal of alar wedges.

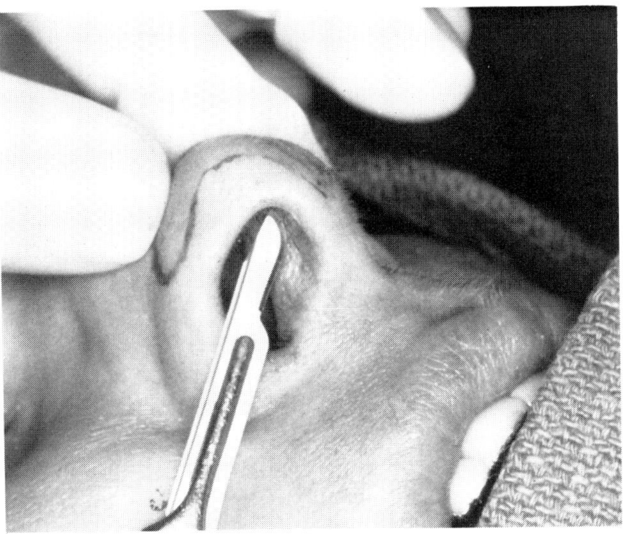

FIG 29–8.
Right nasal vestibule showing position of knife for making medial portion of marginal incision.

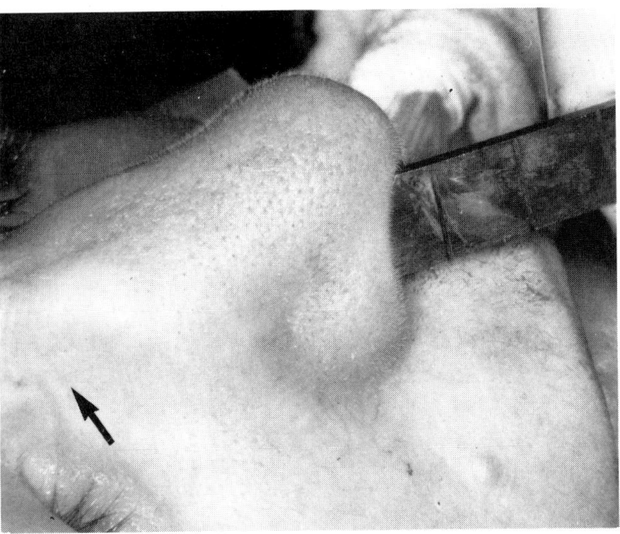

FIG 29–9.
Right side of nose showing position of the tip of a 12 mm chisel (*arrow*) used to elevate the right nasal bone laterally for mobilization.

sharp contrast to the bone of the young patient who may require total mobilization of the bones rather than simple infracture. Greenstick fractures, which tend to occur in the young patient, often spring back to leave the patient with an open roof. This can be avoided by performing both outfracture and infracture to adequately mobilize the bones (Fig 29–9).

Asymmetric Lower Lateral Cartilages

The lower lateral cartilage contribution to asymmetry of the tip is quite easy to recognize. In many instances the form of the cartilage can be observed. In most instances one can readily palpate the cartilage asymmetry. This condition is most often seen in postoperative cases. I believe the main reason for asymmetry is the use of the transcartilage approach to reduce the cephalic border. This is essentially a blind procedure where the dome cannot be observed, and the amount of tissue left behind cannot be accurately determined. Buckling occurs if too much is removed, thus allowing one side to produce a knuckle or sag. The unequal tips can be corrected by delivering the lower lateral cartilages by way of the intercartilaginous and marginal incisions and dividing the cartilages unequally to create equal-sized medial crura.

Over the years I have experienced fewer cases of tip asymmetry using a dome division technique. This technique is easy to teach, can be mastered easily, and does not lend itself to as many errors in judgment as other techniques.

Rim Creep

Alar creep is a postoperative condition whereby the alar rim retracts up the side of the nose, leaving too much columella exposed on lateral view. It can be prevented by not removing too much of the cephalic border of the lower lateral cartilages. When a great deal of rotation of the tip is required and the tip shifts upward, some alar creep cannot be avoided. The skeletal structure gap created by excess cartilage removal allows the vestibular skin to shrink. The scar tissue from healing causes a cephalic contraction of the ala margin. This condition can also be caused by excess removal of the caudal edge or tip of the upper lateral cartilage. This excess of cartilage removal also leaves a void, causing the ala rim to retract upward as vestibular skin contracts during healing.

Pinched Nose Appearance

The pinched nose may exist preoperatively, but most often it is a postoperative complication. Its cause, in my opinion, is too much removal of the caudal end of the upper lateral cartilage. This cartilage skeletal framework deficit, along with the mucosal loss, creates a void internally. Thus, healing occurs with contracture in all directions, causing essentially a depression along with ala creep. I avoid removing the caudal end of the upper lateral cartilage, even in noses that I want to reduce in overall length. I am willing to remove the curl or scroll often seen on the cartilage, but unless the scroll is contributing to excess width, I leave it to strengthen the edge of the lower lateral cartilage to keep the valve open.

Regrowth of Cartilaginous Dorsum

Cartilage does not readily lend itself to reduction by filing or rasping. An exception may be using a very sharp carbide rasp. The cartilage is deformed or flattened like cutting grass with a dull lawn mower, where the grass simply bends over and is not cut. When healing takes place, the cartilage seems to straighten up and resume its preoperative appearance, hence, the "regrowth" of the cartilaginous dorsum. To avoid this complication of undesirable effect, I try to remove cartilage excess in the dorsum area with either a Caplan scissors or a sharp no. 15 Bard Parker blade. I avoid the blades made by American Safety Razor, because they lack a belly, which aids in trimming the cartilage.

Wide Cartilaginous Dorsum

The preoperative wide cartilaginous dorsum can be a challenge. If reduction is required, the removal of the dorsum may leave a wide gap, closure of which cannot be achieved by simply bringing the two medial edges of the upper lateral cartilages together. This wide cartilaginous dorsum may be composed of a thick, T-shaped junction of the upper lateral cartilages with the septum.

To avoid the postoperative problem of a wide cartilaginous dorsum, I separate the upper lateral cartilages from the septum before attempting to reduce the height of the cartilaginous dorsum. The cut edges of the upper lateral cartilages will often rise up so that their true height may be appraised. Lowering of the septal portion of the cartilaginous dorsum may present a problem when scissors such as the Foman, Cottle, Caplan, or Becker are used. The edge to be cut is pyramidal, with the widest part at the dorsum. Scissors tend to slide down this pyramid and remove an excess of cartilage. To avoid doing this, I trim the sides of the septum at the dorsum with a sharp no. 15 Bard Parker blade. This thins the cartilage to create a flatness on the lateral surfaces for the scissors to contact.

Dermal Hump

When the upper lateral cartilages are divided and the cartilaginous dorsum is lowered with scissors, often the mucosa covering the septum is redundant. This tissue may rise above the level of the cartilaginous dorsum when the cast is applied to the nose. After the cast is removed, this tissue remains above the level determined at surgery for a proper tip-dorsum relationship. It may even be worse when mucosal tunnels are made and the dorsum of the septum and the medial edge of the upper lateral cartilages are trimmed to lower the dorsum. It can produce a sizeable mucosal mass postoperatively that resembles early formation of a polly beak. I believe that the mucosa should be trimmed along with the cartilage to produce a more accurate result.

Wide Bony Dorsum

After medial and lateral osteotomies and infracture are performed, the nasal bones often resist coming together to create a narrow bony dorsum. I perform two maneuvers to get the nasal bones to lie close to the bony septum. The first is to slightly angle the medial osteotomy laterally to leave intact a wider medial portion that contains the bony septum. This makes it easier to complete the superior fracture of the medial and lateral osteotomies for nasal bone mobilization. The other maneuver is to use a flat diamond rasp (Peet) to reduce the width of the bony septum at the medial osteotomy site. It may be necessary to outfracture the nasal bones first to provide room for the rasp. The irregular bone surface created by the osteotomy smooths down nicely with the rasp and also makes it possible to further narrow the dorsum by filing both sides of the septum.

Septal Hematoma

Septal hematomas are usually avoided in the routine septal operation because the mucoperiosteum is attached superiorly and inferiorly, and elevation around a spur often perforates the paper-thin mucoperichondrium, thus affording drainage. In the open rhinoplasty technique where the twisted caudal end of the quadrilateral cartilage is exposed on both sides, there is no superior attachment, and it is unlikely that there will be a perforation in this area. The septal space created anteriorly can easily accumulate a large hematoma even if packing is used. This hematoma has the potential of creating a septal abscess with dire effects on the remaining nasal cartilages.

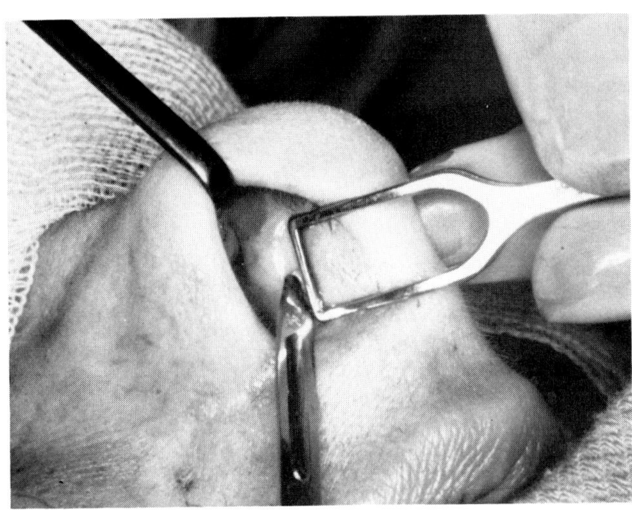

FIG 29–10.
Right vestibule showing use of columella clamp and knife to make right hemitransfixion incision.

To avoid creating space for a hematoma, I suture the septal mucoperichondrial layers together using mattress sutures, which pass through the remaining septal cartilage.

Nasal Incisions for Septal Surgery

Incisions employed to perform septal surgery are often made in an inappropriate location, making the elevation of the mucoperichondrial flaps difficult for lack of a clear view of the operative site. The teachings of Cottle et al. were to provide one with an excellent concept of tunnels.[2] In practice this concept is reduced to one tunnel, since it is easier to see into one large tunnel than it is to see with the tunnel constricted by decussating fibers passing from one side to the other through the junction between the vomer and quadrilateral cartilages. Edgar Holmes, in his teachings and writings in the mid-1950s at the Massachusetts Eye and Ear Infirmary, used a very good approach.[3] An incision is made in the mucoperiosteum on one side at the caudal end of the quadrilateral cartilage. A columella clamp is placed on this to stretch the tissue, so it is easy to expose the pericondrium of the septum (Fig 29–10). A small pocket is made by elevating posteriorly to allow minimal bleeding to accumulate without obscuring vision. Continued elevation is performed inferiorly along the caudal end of the septum to the vomer lateral to the nasal spine and out 4 to 5 mm onto the anterior surface of the pyriform aperture of the floor of the nose. A small sharp elevator (Cottle preferred) is used to expose the free edge of the pyriform aperture and elevate periosteum back toward the septum along the posterior surface of the pyriform ridge. This approach makes it possible to reach the vomer and avoid crossing a small recess lined with mucoperiosteum, thus creating a perforation. With the entire area elevated along the caudal end of the septum and side of the vomer, the entire mucoperichondrial-mucoperiosteal flap can be elevated posteriorly to and beyond the perpendicular plate of ethmoid bone, cutting the decussating fibers as elevation progresses posteri-

orly, thus providing excellent vision. Elevation is not carried up to the cartilaginous dorsum but stops about 1.5 cm below the cartilaginous dorsum. Quadrilateral cartilage and perpendicular plate of ethmoid bone are removed as needed. Mucosa is not elevated on the opposite side of the septum anteriorly or dorsally, so that the caudal 1 cm and dorsal 1.5 cm of quadrilateral cartilage has mucoperichondrium attached on one side. If it is necessary to bring the caudal end of the septum back into the midline, a portion of this section can be cut out inferiorly to allow the caudal end of the septum to be placed back behind the spine. A small triangle of cartilage with the apex pointed toward the tip of the septum at the dorsum will facilitate swinging the cartilage in line behind the columella. In other words, the caudal end of the quadrilateral cartilage is weakened so that it can be influenced by the straight columella. The remaining quadrilateral cartilage along the dorsum, if curved, may be vertically incised almost to the dorsum to allow it to swing back toward the midline. The incisions just described and excisions leave behind sections of the quadrilateral cartilage that have mucoperichondrium intact on one side.

General Versus Local Anesthesia

During training and early days of practice teaching, local anesthesia was employed for all of my rhinoplasty cases. It consisted of bilateral infratrochlear, external nasal, and infraorbital blocks using 1% lidocaine (Xylocaine) with epinephrine 1:100,000. The same local anesthetic was used to infiltrate the intercartilaginous, marginal, and transfixion incision areas. The base of the columella was also injected along with the pyriform aperture at the end of the inferior turbinate.

Cocaine powder moistened with epinephrine 1:1,000 was applied to the nasal mucosa at the end of the middle turbinate (sphenopalatine ganglion area) and at the internal surface along the site of the medial osteotomies.

In time, great improvements were made in the delivery of general anesthesia and the employment of agents safe to use with epinephrine. My choice of anesthesia today is all of the previously mentioned local and topical anesthesia employed under general anesthesia, with an oral endotracheal delivery system. I found that the bleeding is less using the combined local and general anesthesia technique.

Avoidance of Nasal Mucosal Perichondrial Perforations

One way to get a nasal perforation is to have poor visibility due to poor lighting. With advancing age, good lighting becomes a must for all operators. One of the best lights I have found is the new Lawson line provided by Aztec Corporation. It is a high-intensity cool-fiber optic headlight system with a see-through mirror. Another feature is the opportunity to place lenses in the see-through mirror hole, which will further improve vision.

One area for frequent mucoperiosteal perforations is along the quadrilateral cartilage-vomer junction, where the cartilage is deflected from the septum to overlie and extend below the upper edge of the vomer. I found that incising the cartilage along the upper edge of the vomer and then dissecting underneath the strip of cartilage that is parallel with the vomer allows the cartilage to ride up. This strip of cartilage is easily peeled from the overlying mucoperichondrium. By going under the cartilage instead of around it, I can readily avoid a perforation. One other precaution is in the removal of spurs with sharp pieces of bone. On removal, the sharp pieces of bone can easily incise the elevated mucoperichondrium and enlarge a small perforation.

Polly Beak Secondary to Nasal Bone Infracture

In many rhinpolasty procedures, the tip surgery is performed first, and the cartilaginous and bony dorsum are lowered to establish the proper profile. After lateral and medial osteotomies are performed and the nasal bones are infractured, it is necessary to reexamine the dorsal edges of the upper lateral cartilages. In some patients the infracture rotates the nasal bones, causing the dorsal edge of the upper lateral cartilage to assume a higher position. Failure to recognize and lower this new addition to the height of the cartilaginous dorsum can give rise to a polly beak deformity.

SUMMARY

The previously listed challenges represent some of the many problems that arise in performing cosmetic facial plastic surgery. Recognition of a problem often prevents a subsequent complication. Some problems may not be solved in one operation, and the possible need for secondary surgery should be introduced to the patient preoperatively.

REFERENCES

1. Ward PH, Berman WE (eds): Retrograde eversion tip rhinoplasty, in Plastic and Reconstructive Surgery of the Head and Neck. St Louis CV Mosby Co, 1984, vol I, pp 103–107.
2. Cottle MH, et al: The maxilla-premaxilla approach to extensive nasal septum surgery. *Arch Otolaryngol* 1968; 68:301–313.
3. Holmes E: Rhinoplasty in Montgomery WW (ed): *Surgery of the Upper Respiratory System*. Philadelphia, Lea & Febiger, 1971, vol I, pp 357–399.

Rhinoplasty

Approach of

M. Eugene Tardy, Jr., M.D.

NASAL DORSUM

Profile Alignment

Aligning the nasal dorsum into a pleasing and natural profile line commonly requires accurate assessment and proper reduction, augmentation, or reorientation of the three anatomic components contributing to dorsum anatomy: the alar cartilages, the cartilaginous septum, and the bony pyramid (Fig 29–11). Each component will need to be surgically modified to result in a gentle unbroken line from the nasofrontal angle to the tip-defining point. If tip projection or cephalic rotation of the nasal base (tip) is planned during the surgical event, it is preferable to create this modification first, since any permanent alteration in tip projection will impart significantly on the type and degree of profile realignment carried out.

The relative thickness of the overlying nasal soft tissues (epithelium, subcutaneous fat, and musculoaponeurotic system) influences decisions about appropriate profile alignment. Thick sebaceous skin with its associated abundant subcutaneous tissue generally camouflages any ultimate dorsal irregularities quite well but requires many months to several years to thin and redrape adequately. Exquisitely thin skin with sparse subcutaneous tissue cushions and hides even the slightest profile irregularity poorly, often thinning quickly in the postoperative

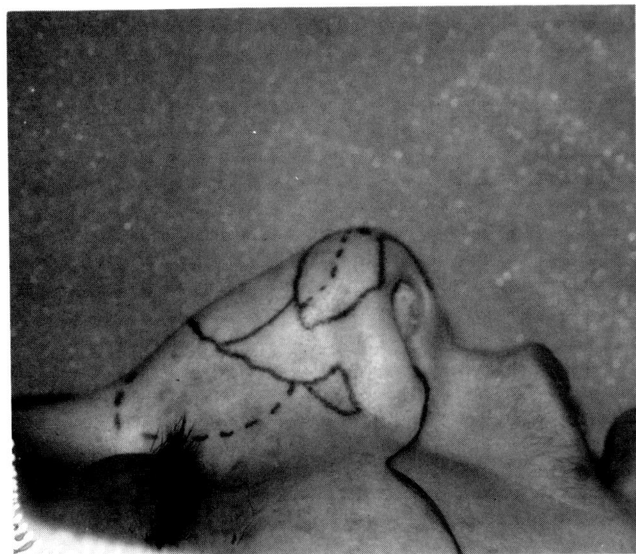

FIG 29–11.
Nasal dorsum on profile view is comprised of three anatomic components: the bony dorsum, the cartilaginous dorsum, and the lower lateral cartilage configuration. Each component needs to be surgically modified to result in an appropriate, pleasing profile line.

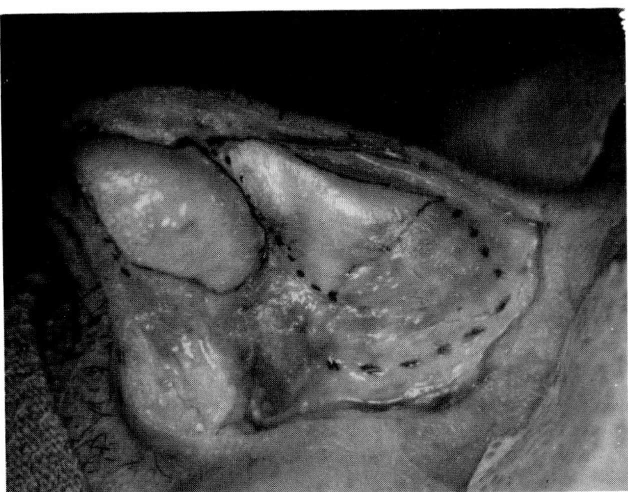

FIG 29–12.
Overlying epithelium and subcutaneous tissue of the nasal profile varies at different levels over the nasal dorsum, being thinnest at the osseocartilaginous junction and thickest in the immediate supratip area. Straight-line skeletal profile reduction will therefore ordinarily not result in an ideal profile; rather, the varying thickness of skin and subcutaneous tissue must be taken into consideration when reducing the cartilaginous and bony profile appropriately.

period to reveal vexing visible or palpable imperfections. An ideal skin-subcutaneous tissue epithelial covering exists between these two extremes, providing excellent cushioning while healing with pleasing definition.

Since the overlying epithelium–fat–superficial musculoaponeurotic system (SMAS) complex is of variable thickness at various levels of the nasal dorsum (thinnest at the rhinion,

thickest in the immediate supratip area), it follows that differential increments of bone and cartilage will need to be removed to accommodate the individual patient's anatomy (Fig 29–12).

Profile alignment is initiated by appropriate tip surgery. Stable tip refinement, rotation, and especially tip projection are prerequisites for accurate profile alignment. During the course of tip surgery, the soft tissues over the cartilaginous dorsum are elevated up to the osseocartilaginous junction with sharp knife dissection, carefully elevating sharply intimate to the perichondrium of the cartilaginous dorsum in the all-important sub-SMAS plane, a vital nasal dissection plane relatively devoid of vascular structures and nerves. Less postoperative scarring ensues when this valuable dissection plane is sought and exploited.

Elevation of the periosteum from the bony dorsum is carried out with the sharp Joseph periosteal elevator, elevating first over the left nasal bone and then over the right, ultimately bringing the two distinct dissection pockets into continuity with the Metzenbaum scissors. Elevation ensues laterally only sufficient to gain access to and ultimately remove the nasal bony hump. Wide undermining is reserved for older, nonelastic skin and some revision rhinoplasties.

In these proper supraperichondrial subperiosteal dissection planes, bleeding is essentially nonexistent, affording accurate visualization and surgical alignment of the bony and cartilaginous dorsum.

If the nasofrontal angle is in need of modification (deepening), a 2 mm osteotome is tapped transcutaneously in the midline into the bone at the site of the desired angle break (Fig 29–13). By progressively angulating the microsteotome laterally right and left, the root of the nasal bone is scored and weakened, creating a bony dehiscence at which the cephalic extent of bony hump removal will now be defined. This maneuver is atraumatic, is precise, and leaves no visible scar. The tiny incision

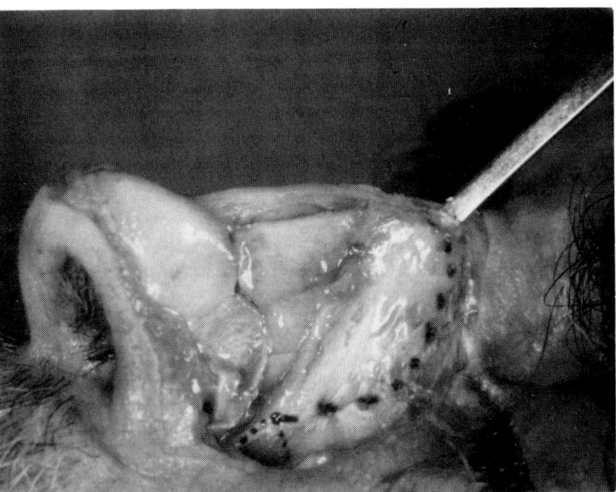

FIG 29–13.
An ideal and accurate method of positioning the new nasofrontal angle (when deepening of this angle is required) is transcutaneous passage of a 2 mm osteotome to score the cephalic margins of the nasal bone. This allows bony hump removal at precisely the position where the new nasofrontal angle is to be.

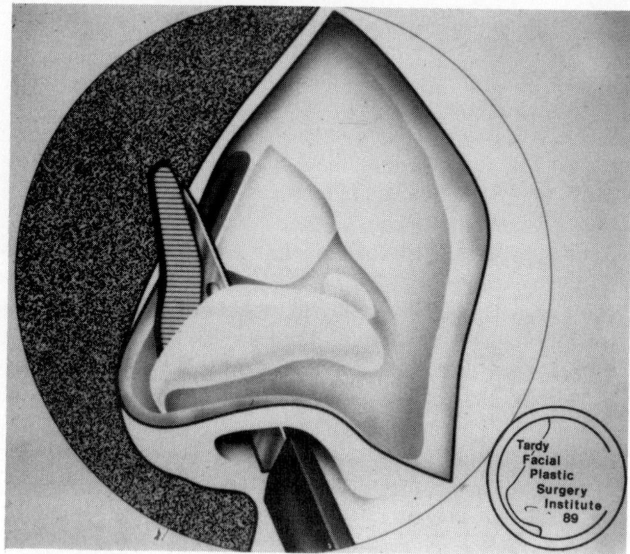

FIG 29–14.
Incremental reduction of the supratip cartilaginous dorsum is a safe and ideal method for creating a pleasing tip-supratip relationship.

(less than 2 mm after skin retraction) is closed with a single Steri-strip tape or suture of 6-0 mild chromic catgut.

Hump removal (proper alignment) next ensues using one of two approaches: incremental or en bloc.

Once the exposed dorsum is visualized with the aid of the thin Converse retractor and a strong fiberoptic headlight, the osseocartilaginous junction is palpated with the knife blade.

If the incremental approach is chosen, slivers of the cartilaginous dorsum are removed with the no. 15 knife down to and around the anterior septal angle until the desired tip-supratip relationship is created (Fig 29–14). In women, a gentle rise of 2 to 3 mm from the dorsum to the tip-defining point is generally ideal, whereas in men a straighter line or gentle convexity is preferred. Establishing this relationship incrementally demands that the surgeon have confidence in the long-term stability of the newly created tip projection and that the intraoperative prediction is not spuriously enhanced by the effects of local anesthetic and tissue edema. The incremental method additionally exposes the exact amount of bony hump to be removed to complete ideal profile alignment, thus providing a high margin of error and extreme safety. Depending on the extent of hump removal required, portions of the dorsal edges of the upper lateral cartilages abutting the septal dorsum will also be removed with each increment. Unless it contributes to a twist of the cartilaginous pyramid, no virtue exists in cutting the upper lateral cartilages away from the septum by dividing their common microperichondrial bridge, an unnecessary maneuver potentially damaging to the nasal valve.

If the en bloc method of hump removal is chosen (usually in larger humps), the knife is plunged horizontally through the osseocartilaginous junction and drawn caudally through the cartilaginous dorsum to a calculated point caudal to the anterior septal angle, thus providing a space into which a razor-sharp Rubin osteotome is seated. Removal of the bony extent of the hump (ordinarily less than the cartilaginous contribution) en-

sues by driving the osteotome cephalically to the intended site of the ultimate nasofrontal angle (Fig 29–15). The entire hump is removed en bloc and inspected for irregularities, which often provide clues to asymmetries or previous fractures.

After either method of profile alignment, gentle palpation of the dorsal skin with the forefinger moistened with hydrogen peroxide provides clues about any invisible excrescence or irregularity. Cartilage excesses are smoothed with the no. 15 blade, and the bony dorsum is refined with the aid of a sharp tungsten carbide rasp. A final inspection of the tip-supratip relationship for ideal profile alignment completes this phase of the rhinoplasty procedure (Fig 29–16).

Micro-osteotomes

Osteotomies during rhinoplasty have traditionally been accomplished with large (10 to 14 mm) guarded osteotomes, effective but highly traumatic instruments. In the continual search for atraumatic techniques generating minimal or no bleeding and ecchymosis, I strongly prefer sturdy 2 to 3 mm micro-osteotomes for both medial-oblique and curved lower lateral osteotomies. Equally effective as their larger counterparts, micro-osteotomes impart a delicacy and atraumatic nature to the most traumatic event in rhinoplasty, creating little, if any, injury to the soft tissues surrounding the nasal bones and maxillary ascending processes. The periosteum is largely preserved, thus maintaining an important supportive sling of strong tissue across the bony fracture lines. Improved postoperative bony stability results.

Medial-Oblique Osteotomies

To establish the exact site of backfracture of the lateral bony sidewalls, the surgeon employs medial-oblique osteoto-

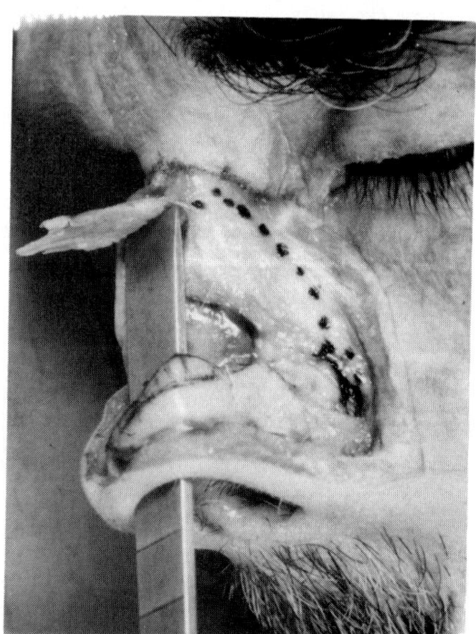

FIG 29–15.
Thin, sharp Rubin osteotome allows precision in reduction of a bony hump. Final refinement is accomplished with a sharp tungsten-carbide rasp.

bony margins, monitored throughout the rasping process by frequent palpation by gloved finger moistened with peroxide.

Low Lateral Osteotomies

The intent of lateral osteotomies is to surgically narrow the nose rendered flat and broad as a consequence of hump removal without overcompromise of the cross-sectional internal airway. Low curved lateral osteotomies answer this need admirably by maintaining the dimensions of the lower airway along the floor of the nose while aesthetically narrowing the nasal bridge to restore balance, height, and refinement to the dorsum (Figs 29–17 and 29–18).

With a small nasal speculum, the sharp edge of the ascending process of the maxilla is embraced at or just above the attachment of the inferior concha. The 2 or 3 mm osteotome is lightly driven through the soft tissue overlying the bone, temporarily crushing the incision site and eliminating bleeding associated with the traditional knife incision at this highly vascular site. As the surgeon directs the inclination of the micro-osteotome in a gently curving manner, the instrument is driven gently upward until the backfracture, predetermined by the previous medial-oblique osteotomy, occurs. A distinct difference in sound and bony resistance develops when the fracture occurs. Minor finger pressure completes the lateral osteotome

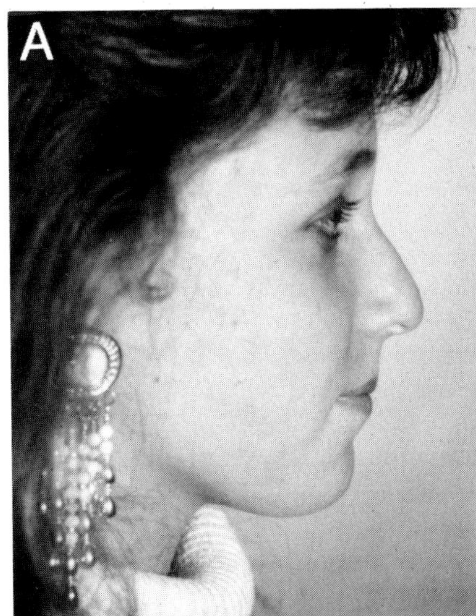

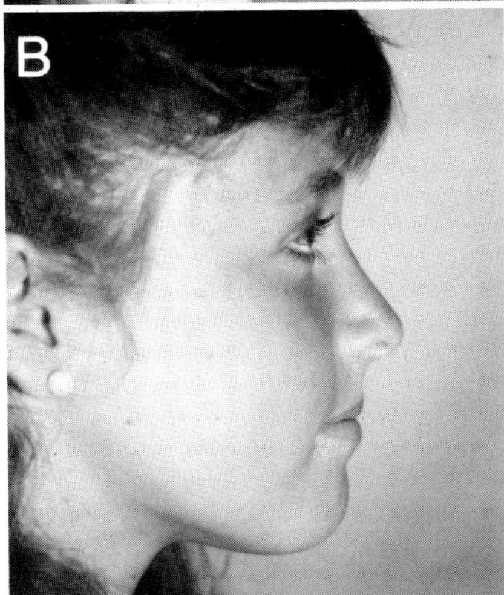

FIG 29–16.
A, preoperative appearance of inappropriate profile. **B,** appropriate and natural profile alignment 1 year after surgery.

mies prior to bony infracture (Fig 29–17). A 3 mm osteotome is seated at the cephalic extent of the hump removal (or at the caudal end of the nasal bones if no hump removal has been necessary) parallel to the septum. At an angle of 15 to 20 degrees, the osteotome is gently driven cephalically and laterally until the desired site of the intended bony backfracture is reached.

Creating this surgical dehiscence in bone thus aids in controlling the eventual narrowing influence created by lateral osteotomies, minimizes or negates the trauma occasioned by forceful manual pressure during traditional infracture maneuvers, and ensures that unwanted eccentric fractures are avoided in more distal parts of the nasal bones. In addition, the so-called rocker formation is completely avoided by surgically establishing the exact lines of osteotomy.

Smoothing of the cut margins of the bony dorsum finalizes profile alignment. Sharp tungsten-carbide down-cutting rasps, angled obliquely, provide a smoothing refinement to the cut

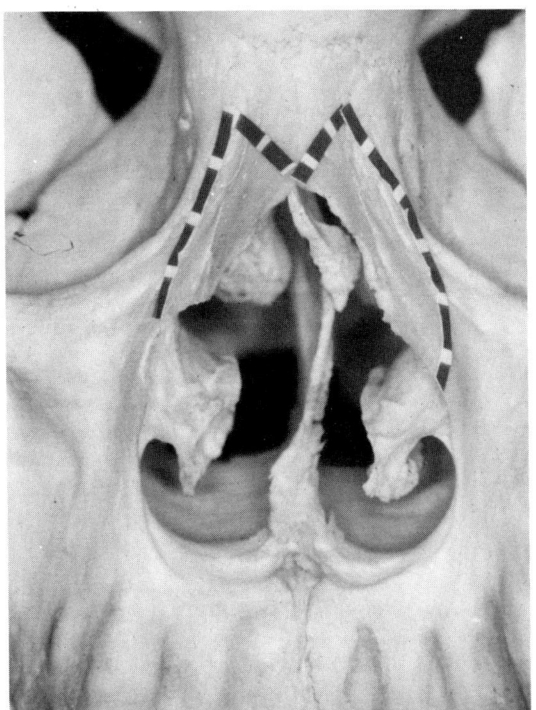

FIG 29–17.
Dotted line indicates intended siting of medial oblique and low curve lateral osteotomies on the bony skeleton. Note that the osteotomies begin relatively high on the ascending process of the maxilla, curve more deeply into the ascending process, then advance more medially to encounter the previously created medial oblique osteotomies, which course approximately 15 to 20 degrees away from the midline.

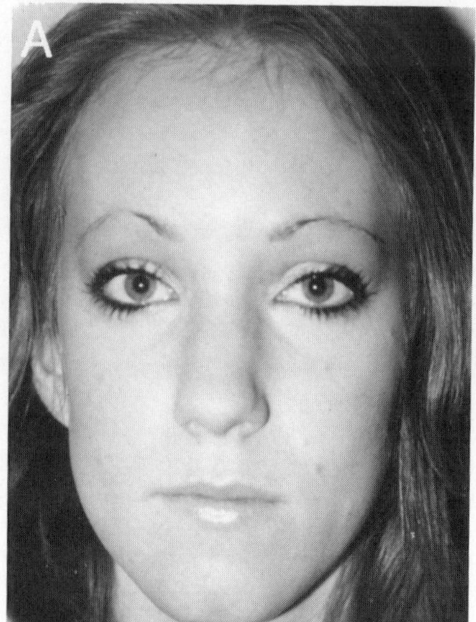

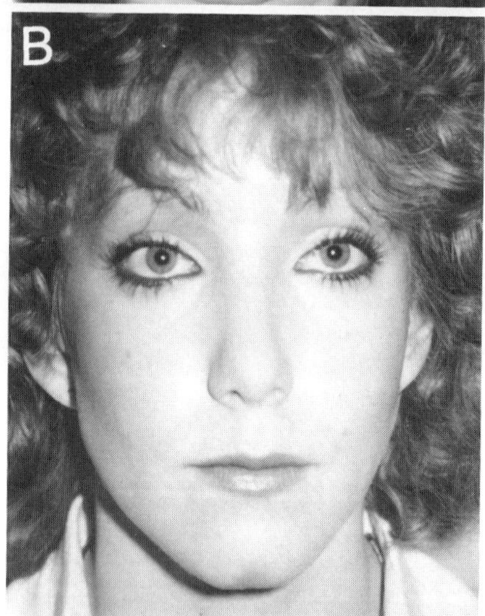

FIG 29–18.
A, preoperative appearance before significant osteotome narrowing of the nose for ideal refinement. **B,** postoperative appearance of nose narrowed by medial oblique and low curve lateral osteotomies, 5 years after repair.

in a controlled manner. Maintaining the periosteum intact on either side of the fracture line provides a substantial stabilizing influence on the fractured bony sidewalls, essentially eliminating overnarrowing and bony instability. Moreover, little trauma occurs to the overlying and underlying soft tissue mass, limiting injury and essentially eliminating bleeding as a consequence of the osteotomies.

Constant finger pressure over the osteotomy sites by the surgical assistant is maintained while final suturing occurs. This valuable maneuver further aids in the avoidance of postoperative swelling and ecchymosis.

In severely deviated noses in which the bony pyramid consists of one concave and one convex lateral sidewall, double osteotomies provide a mechanism to completely mobilize and

properly align the deviated bony pyramid. When indicated, the osteotomy positioned higher on the lateral bony sidewall is best accomplished first (while the bones are still stable) before the major lateral osteotomy is carried out.

Augmentation Techniques

If augmentation of the nasal dorsum is indicated, my preference is exclusively for implanting autogenous cartilage derived from the nasal septum or external auricle. Thick septal cartilage serves well for single-layer or multiple-layer grafts but, in saddle noses in particular, is not always available in sufficient quantity to serve adequately. The cavum-cymba concha complex of the external ear possesses an abundant storehouse of spare parts for augmentation and sculpturing of the nasal profile (Fig 29–19). Commonly cartilage is employed for layered augmentation of the bony or cartilaginous dorsum, whereas sculptured segments of curved cartilage grafts are highly useful for elevation of the deep nasofrontal angle, the nasal tip (either as onlay or infratip lobule grafts), the columella, and the columellar-labial angle (Fig 29–20).

Less frequently, residual segments of the alar cartilages, temporalis fascia, dermis, or mature scar tissue may be useful in improving alignment and contour. Alloplastic nasal implants are assiduously avoided in nasal reconstruction.

If a laminated graft of two or more layers is required, the sculptured pieces are secured to one another by 5-0 mild chromic catgut sutures or tissue glues. In the majority of noses in need of augmentation, precise soft tissue pockets are developed in the immediate dorsal supraperichondrial and subperiosteal planes to exactly accommodate the required implant of appropriate size and shape. If, during the course of operation, it has

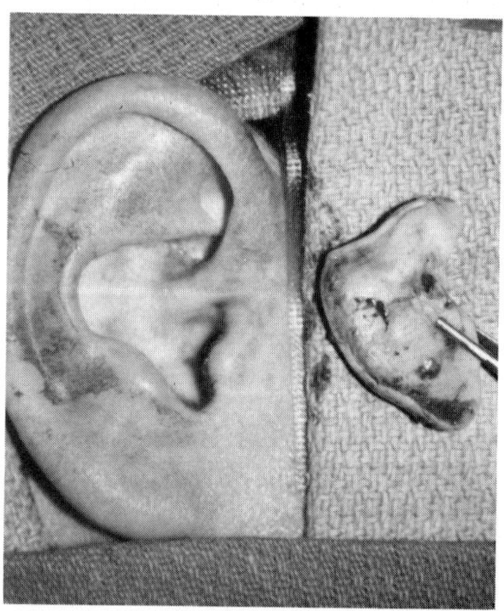

FIG 29–19.
Cavum–cymba-concha complex of the auricle yields superb tissue for nasal augmentation and defect effacement. The incision is most commonly sited medial to the antihelical prominence. When the overlying skin is replaced and sutured with fine suture material, healing is ideal and little scar is apparent months later. No change in the shape of the auricle occurs so long as the antihelical fold is maintained intact.

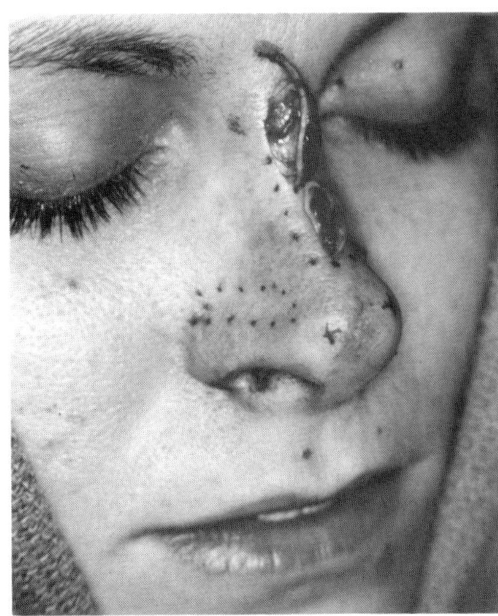

FIG 29–20.
Revision rhinoplasty is accomplished with multiple segments of auricle cartilage implants. Autogenous cartilage persists and maintains its shape, strength, and integrity.

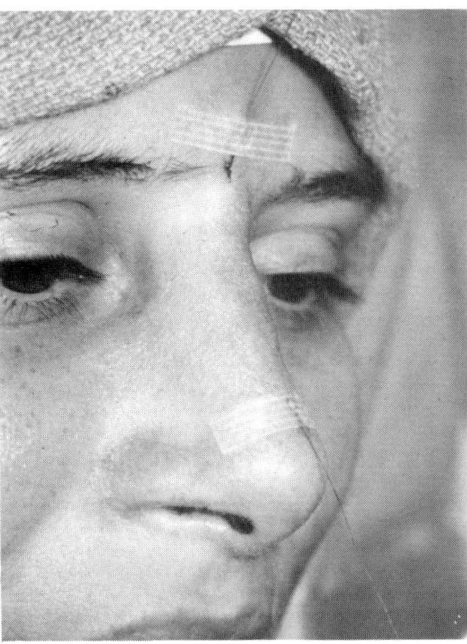

FIG 29–21.
Pull-out sutures of 5-0 mild chromic catgut suture are demonstrated in a patient who has undergone removal of a large alloplastic implant, creating a larger than ideal subcutaneous pocket. The sutures are used to maintain the ideal position of the auricular cartilage implant for 4 to 5 days, then trimmed at their epithelial exit site and allowed to retract into the skin.

been necessary to develop more substantial undermining of the overlying soft tissues, the cartilage implant is secured cephalically and caudally by transcutaneous pull-out sutures penetrating the skin and secured by temporary Steri-Strips (Fig 29–21). At 5 to 7 days, the sutures are cut flush to the skin and allowed to retract back into the soft tissues. Sufficient graft stability exists at this time to eliminate internal suture stabilization.

All lateral edges of cartilage grafts must be meticulously beveled by shave-excision and sanding (the Bovie unit scratch pad makes a convenient sanding tool) to eliminate visible or palpable edges following ultimate skin shrinkage (Fig 29–22).

NASAL TIP

Selection of Approach

Because of the wide diversity of anatomy found in the nasal tip, no single set of incisions, approaches, or techniques is routinely applicable. In each patient, an analysis consisting of inspection and palpation is required to calculate the operative scheme best suited to the anatomy encountered. Included among the critical aspects to be determined are (1) the degree and magnitude of the tip support mechanisms (Table 29–1), (2) skin

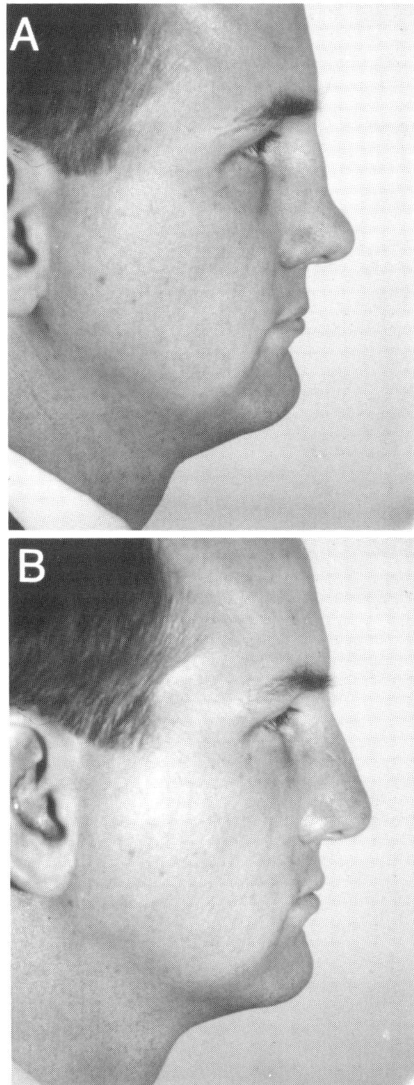

FIG 29–22.
A, preoperative saddle nose deformity. **B,** reconstructed nose after auricular cartilage implant.

TABLE 29–1.
Tip Support Mechanisms

Major
1. Size, shape, and resilience of medial and lateral crura
2. Medial crural footplate attachment to caudal border of quadrangular cartilage
3. Attachment of upper lateral cartilages (caudal border) to alar cartilages (cephalic border)

Minor*
1. Ligamentous sling spanning paired domes of alar cartilages
2. Cartilaginous septal dorsum
3. Sesamoid complex extending support of lateral crura to pyriform aperture
4. Attachment of alar cartilages to overlying skin and musculature
5. Nasal spine
6. Membranous septum

*Because of extreme anatomic variability, a "minor" tip support may assume the importance of a more major support.

thickness, (3) need for additional tip projection, (4) need for tip rotation, and (5) alar cartilage asymmetry. With this information determined, a decision regarding the best and most appropriate incisions, approach, and sculpturing technique is determined, based entirely on a *graduated systematic anatomic approach* (Fig 29–23). A clear preference exists for preserving the natural anatomy of the nasal tip, fundamentally reorienting the tip structures whenever the anatomy will allow rather than resecting. In the majority of patients, a substantial portion of residual complete strip of alar cartilage is preserved bilaterally, interrupted strips being reserved for those instances when marked rotation or significant retroprojection is required.

When the anatomy will allow (symmetric cartilages requiring modest reduction), a *transcartilaginous approach* is always preferred because of its conservative, atraumatic nature and predictable healing potential (Fig 29–24).

If a broad, trapezoid, boxy tip is encountered, or if significant asymmetry is encountered, a *delivery approach* is preferred, allowing further analysis and correction of the deformity under direct binocular vision and enabling bimanual repair. Narrowing refinement of the tip cartilages is effectively achieved with transdomal sutures of 4-0 clear nylon to permanently alter the shape and orientation of the cartilages without resorting to the unpredictables inherent in healing when interrupted strips are chosen (Fig 29–25).

The *external* or *open approach* to nasal surgery is an exclusive approach used for cause in a very limited number of specific situations:

1. Severe nasal twist
2. Marked tip asymmetry
3. Nasal tip overprojection
4. Cleft lip–nose complex
5. Septal perforations (large)
6. Foreshortened nose
7. Complex nasal augmentation
8. Teaching and demonstration

It may be of extreme value in unusual tip deformities or when wide exposure of the nasal anatomy is required to adequately correct major deformities. However, a price is paid for employing the open approach: wider dissection of normal structures with potentially unfavorable healing, more postoperative edema and swelling, diminished ability to fine-tune profile subtleties, a longer operation, and an external scar.

When significant cephalic rotation is indicated, as in the

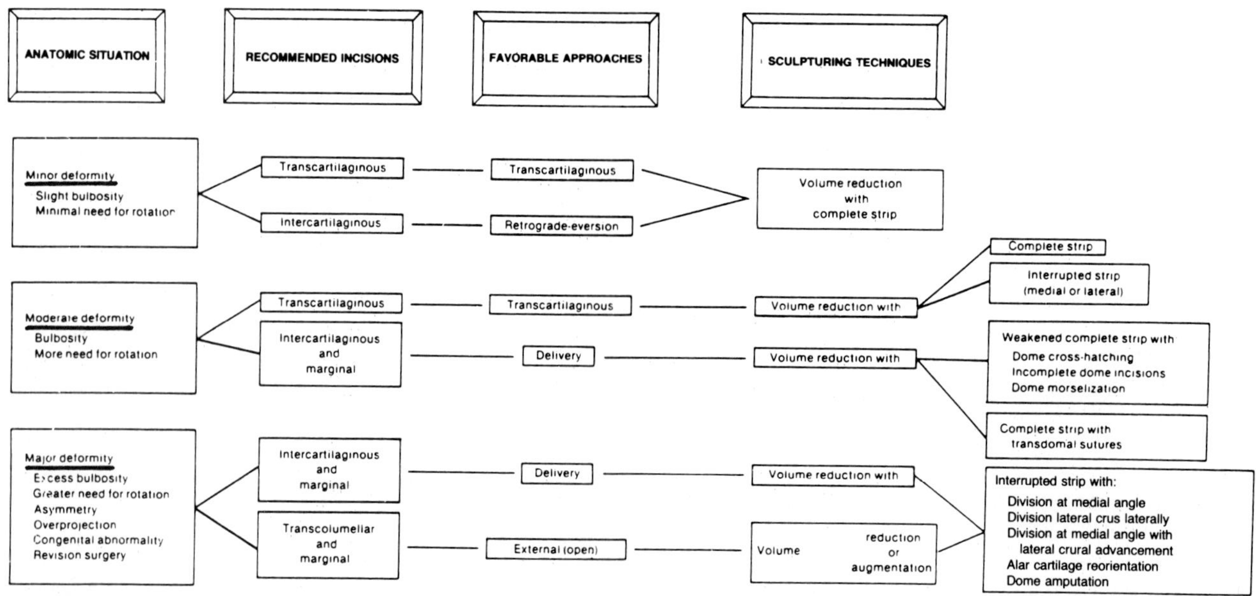

FIG 29–23.
Operative algorithm useful in selecting incisions, approaches, and techniques of nasal tip surgery. In every case the patient's anatomy dictates the selection. As the deformity worsens or becomes more abnormal, a graduated approach is taken to correct it.

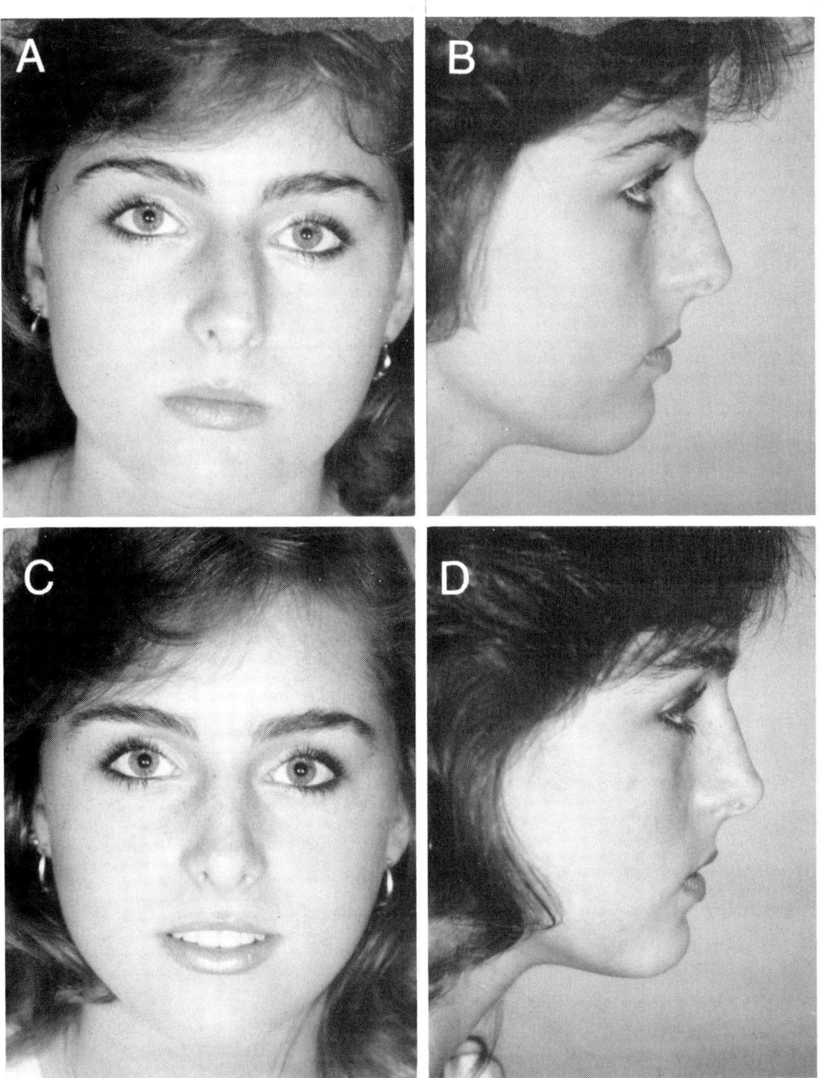

FIG 29–24.
A, preoperative appearance of patient with deviated nose in need of modest refinement of the nasal tip. **B,** preoperative lateral view. **C,** appearance 2 years after nasal straightening and tip refinement with a transcartilaginous approach, maintaining a generous intact com-plete strip of lower lateral cartilage. **D,** postoperative profile. No ce-phalic rotation has occurred, excellent tip projection is maintained, and the tip-supratip relationship is ideal.

so-called plunging tip, controlled calculated rotation of the nasal tip is carried out using a form of interrupted strip. After delivery and conservative volume reduction of the alar cartilages, a tri-angle of lateral crus (base upward) is excised from the far lateral portion of the lateral crus. Suture closure of the cartilaginous void thus created restores the integrity of the alar cartilage and results in a predictable degree of stable cephalic rotation (Fig 29–26). Invariably significant upward rotation will demand one or more of the adjunctive techniques valuable in rotational concepts, including caudal septal shortening, excision of re-dundant vestibular skin and mucous membrane, excision of the caudal margins of the upper lateral cartilages (if too long), and possible shave-excision of the caudal margin of overly convex medial crura.

The addition of permanent cartilage plumping grafts to open the columellar-labial angle may be valuable in providing the illusion of rotation without actually shortening the central dimensions of the nose, preserving a longer, more elegant struc-ture (Fig 29–27). If necessary, cartilaginous struts inserted through a lateral paracolumellar stab incision assist in filling out the columellar-labial angle as well as providing additional tip sup-port.

COMPLICATIONS

In general, untoward results in rhinoplasty may be dimin-ished by careful, accurate analysis and conservative, meticulous surgery. Preserving what is aesthetically pleasant in the nose while modifying that which is unpleasant is a useful philosophy of nasal surgery. Complications are invariably more likely when aggressive, nonconservative surgical maneuvers are unwisely employed without regard for tip support mechanisms, long-term healing changes, and well-known rhinoplasty surgical principles.

Saddle Deformity

The saddle deformity refers to any depression, from minor to profound, that spoils the natural unbroken line of the nasal dorsum. Overreduction of the cartilaginous dorsum relative to the nasal tip projection as well as loss of sufficient support of the dorsum consequent to septoplasty represent iatrogenic causes for saddle noses. In practice, external nasal trauma constitutes the most common etiology of saddle nose deformity. As chem-

ical substance abuse becomes more prevalent in society, increasing numbers of patients whose septal perforations lead inexorably to dorsal support collapse are encountered.

Autogenous cartilaginous grafts serve well for permanent, safe correction of nasal dorsum skeletal deficiencies. Since septal cartilage is generally not available for implantation, the external auricle is more commonly used as the source for a wide variety of supportive and sculpturing grafts for repair. As described previously, single- or multiple-layer grafts may be required to adequately efface the skeletal deficiencies encountered.

The gentle curves of the cavum-cymba concha complex may be surgically exploited to reconstruct a natural-appearing dorsum and may be relied on for permanent correction (Fig 29–28). Moreover, cartilage grafts stand up well to subsequent nasal trauma, an ever-present possibility in patients who are

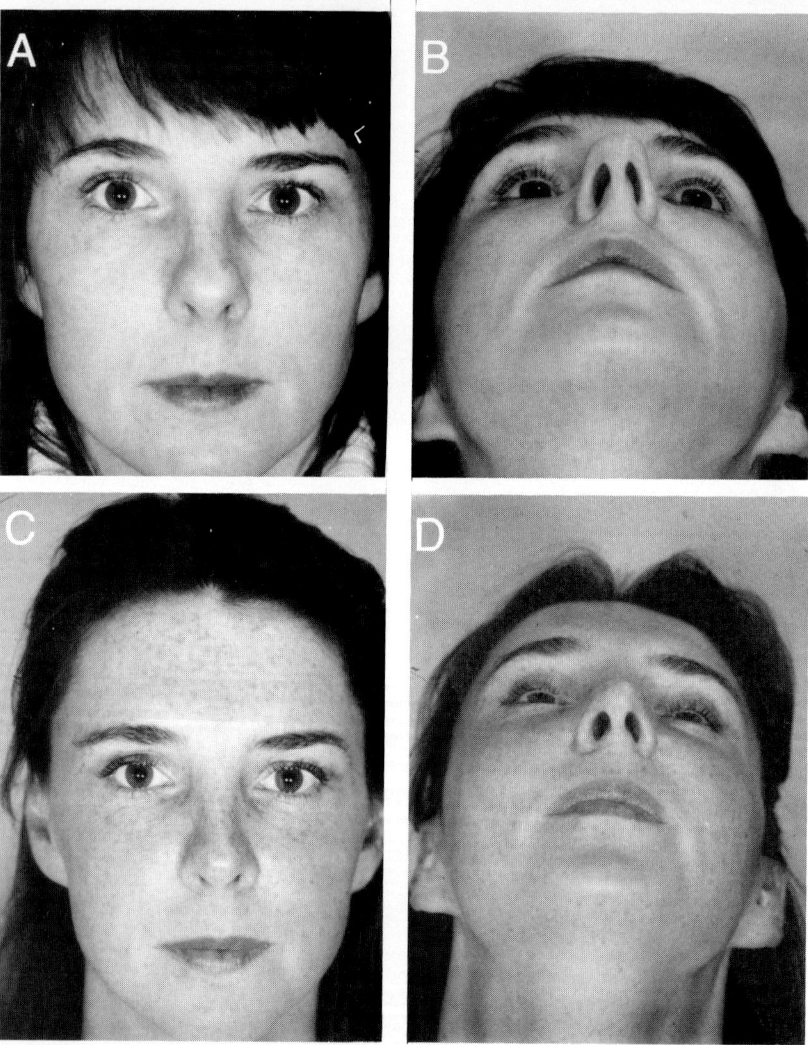

FIG 29–25.
A, preoperative appearance of patient with bulky lower lateral cartilage creating an overprojected nose. **B,** base view demonstrating trapezoidal, asymmetric nature of tip with overprojection and tall, slitlike nostrils. **C,** 18 months after repair using the delivery approach for volume reduction of the lower lateral cartilage, maintaining a complete strip of lower lateral cartilage. The cartilage has been refined and narrowed by a single 4-0 clear nylon transdomal suture. **D,** postoperative repair demonstrates retropositioning of the tip, correction of the overprojection, and triangular refinement of the nasal base.

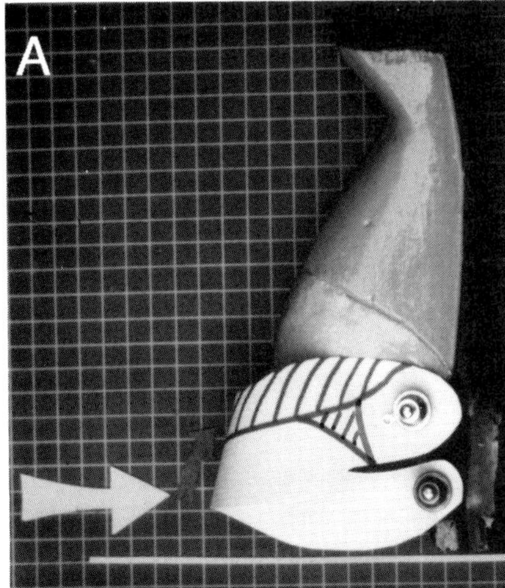

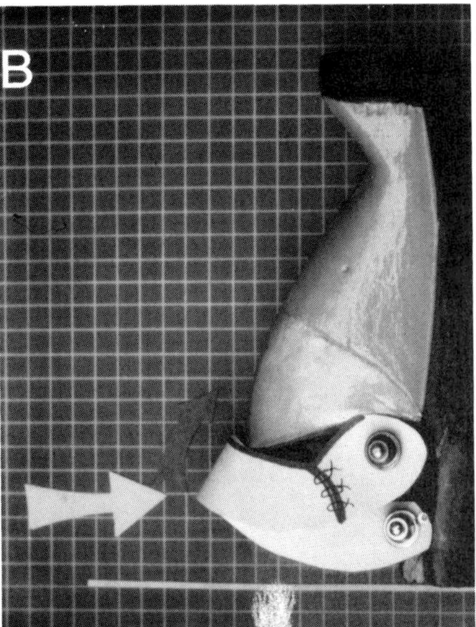

FIG 29–26.
A, rhinoplasty model of one form of safe and predictable nasal tip rotation after volume reduction of the cephalic margin of the alar cartilage, a triangular wedge of cartilages excised laterally in the lateral crus, allowing cephalic rotation. **B,** predictable cephalic rotation of the alar cartilage after wedge resection of the lateral crus in its lateral, most extent portion, repairing the defect and restoring the integrity of the lower lateral cartilage with fine sutures.

active and athletic (such is not the case with alloplastic implants, which have no place in our surgical philosophy).

Ear cartilage grafts may be harvested through posterior or anterolateral approaches. When substantial cartilage is required, an incision sited just medial to the antihelical fold provides excellent access for harvesting of the entire cavum and cymba concha and heals inconspicuously. As long as the antihelical fold is not violated (since it represents the skeletal buttress of the external ear), no change in the shape or orientation of the external ear develops. Cartilage grafts of up to 3.5 cm are commonly available from the external ear after the age of 6 years, when the ear has already achieved 80% of its final adult growth. Incision closure accomplished with 5-0 mild chromic catgut

suture obviates the need for eventual suture removal, and a sandwich bolster dressing of Telfa held by a single transauricular suture of 4-0 white Tevdek for 3 to 5 days effectively splints the healing ear, eliminating any potential dead space between the skin flaps.

Polly Beak Deformity

Reversal of the appropriate tip-supratip profile relationship (where the tip leads the supratip profile line by 1–3 mm) results in various degrees of the classic polly beak deformity. Two forms of this deformity exist: the dreaded soft tissue polly beak and the largely correctable cartilaginous variety.

The latter complication almost invariably results from a combination of postoperative tip ptosis (loss of tip support and projection) and inadequate reduction of the cartilaginous dorsum during primary rhinoplasty. Sacrifice of the tip support mechanisms without cause remains the principal preventable

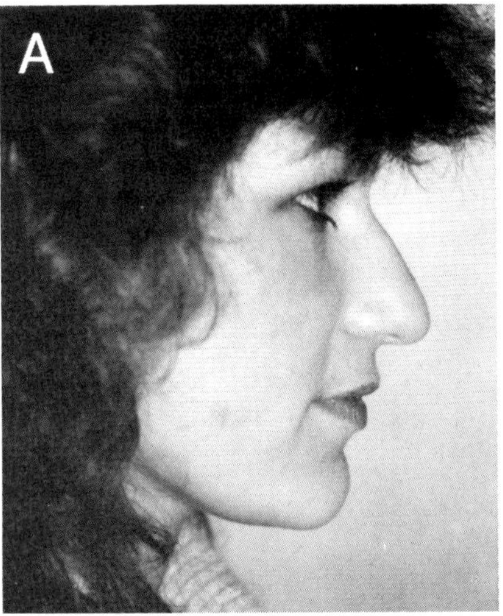

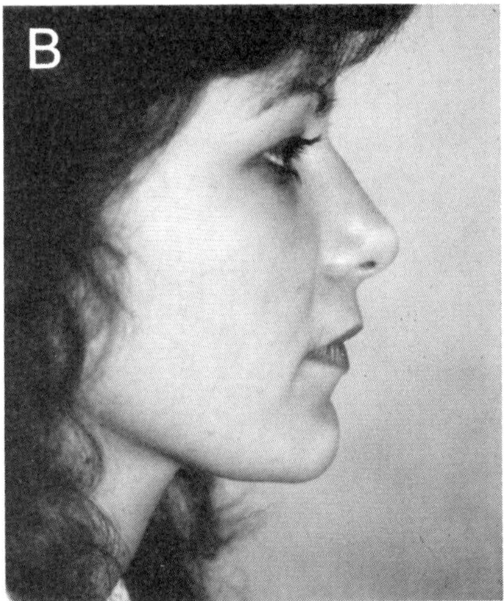

FIG 29–27.
A, preoperative appearance of elongated, plunging nose with acute nasolabial angle. **B,** 2 years after nasal tip rotation with the technique demonstrated in Figure 29–26, improved by augmentation of the acute nasolabial angle with permanent cartilage "plumping" grafts.

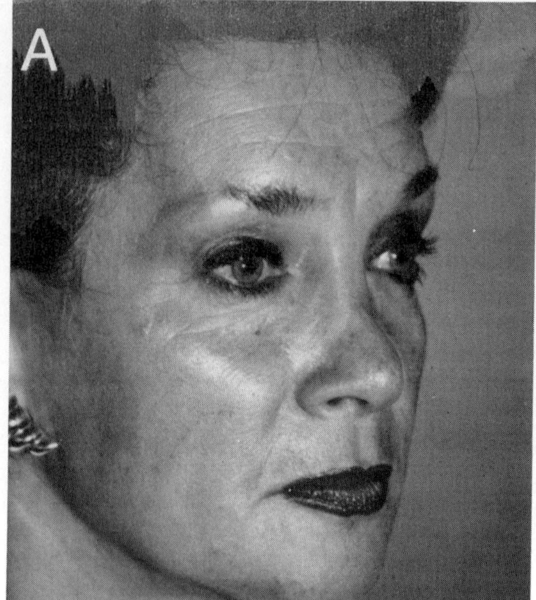

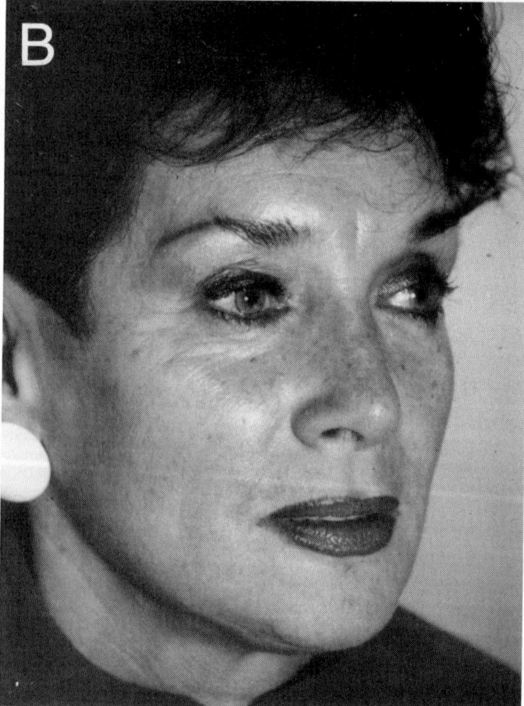

FIG 29–28.
A, saddlenose deformity after extrusion of alloplastic implant placed over the nasal dorsum in a patient before revison rhinoplasty. **B,** 2 years after dorsal augmentation and reconstruction with auricular cartilage grafts.

cause of tip ptosis. Appropriate correction of this complication is generally not difficult and involves a combined reduction of the cartilaginous dorsum with supportive tip projection to an ideal level (Fig 29–29). Through an intercartilaginous incision carried modestly around the anterior septal angle (which often is found inappropriately high), the cartilaginous dorsum is in-

spected and reduced with sharp knife excision until the profile level is judged appropriate. Any excess scar or upper lateral cartilage prominence is removed.

Projection of the ptotic nasal tip may then be carried out with one or more of a variety of tip projection techniques, including onlay tip grafts, infratip lobule grafts, cartilage columellar struts and suture refinement, and projection of the alar cartilage. domes.

Soft tissue polly beak deformities are much more difficult to adequately correct, since they commonly are encountered in patients with thick, sebaceous skin, poor skeletal support to the dorsum, and a tendency to form abundant scar tissue. Overreduction of the alar cartilages and bony-cartilaginous skeleton of the nose predisposes to this problem. Correction is often limited, involving the principles described earlier in conjunction with an overall augmentation of the whole nose to adequately support the overlying thick skin.

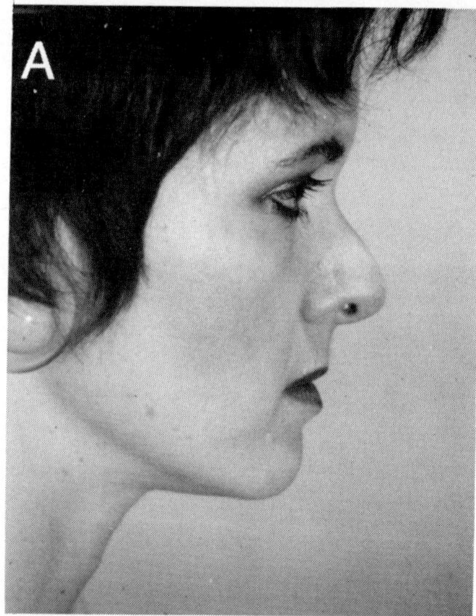

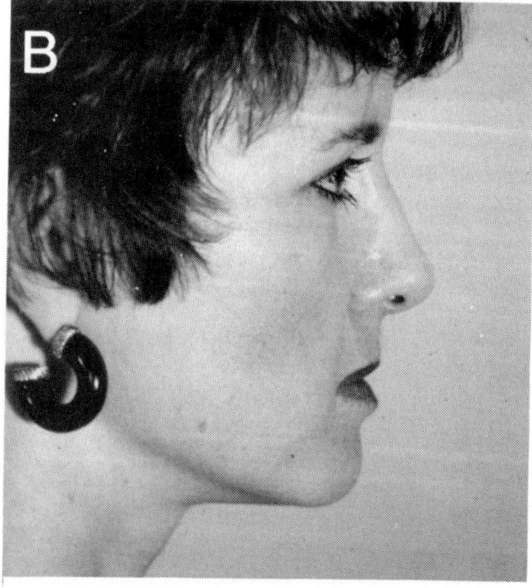

FIG 29–29.
A, classic supratip polly beak deformity complicated by overreduction of the bony dorsum and loss of nasal tip support. **B,** 1 year after reconstruction of the nose and nasal dorsum with augmentation of the bony profile defect, reduction of the cartilaginous polly beak deformity, and cartilaginous support of the nasal tip projection.

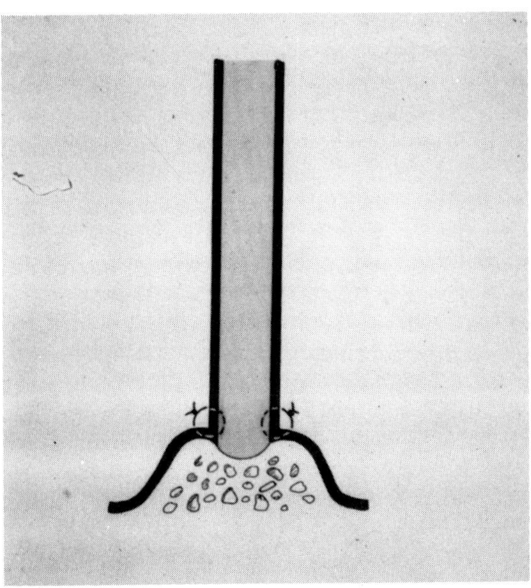

FIG 29–30.
After realignment and reconstruction of the nasal septum, permanent suture fixation of the caudal septum to the periosteum of the nasal spine is effective in providing an "internal splint" to permanently stabilize the position of the quadrangular cartilage in the midline.

Retracted Columella

Following rhinoplasty, retraction of the columella is an uncommon condition, occurring more frequently in the classic saddle nose deformity developing after significant nasal trauma or septal hematoma with infection. Correction most commonly requires substantial augmentation and effacement with autogenous cartilage. If the caudal quadrangular cartilage is displaced or buckled into the nasal cavities, caudal septoplasty with replacement of the distal quadrangular cartilage into the columella restores normal columellar anatomy. Suture-fixation of the caudal septum to the periosteum of the nasal spine with a permanent 4-0 clear nylon suture secures the long-term stabilization of the repositioned cartilage (Fig 29–30).

If augmentation of the columella is required, autogenous cartilage from the auricle is harvested and laminated or rolled into a strong, substantial implant designed to satisfactorily restore an adequate columellar profile and appearance. Invariably slight overcorrection is necessary to counter the influence of soft tissue edema (from local anesthetic and surgical tissue trauma) on the ultimate repair. A substantial soft tissue pocket in the columella between the medial crura is dissected in retrograde fashion through a left modified Killian incision created at the junction of the vestibular skin of the columella and the septal mucous membrane. The caudal septum is freed and isolated. Suture fixation of the implant to the caudal septum and the intercrural pocket stabilizes the graft and provides immediate columellar effacement. If the columellar-labial angle is overly acute, additional small free cartilage grafts placed in the inferior recesses of the intercrural pocket provide an additional profile refinement.

Bossae

Bossae of the nasal tip, single or bilateral, are defined as unsightly cartilage prominences or sharp edges visible through thin tip skin. They may become visible shortly following surgery but much more commonly make their appearance gradually many months following tip rhinoplasty (Fig 29–31). Bossae occur less commonly in patients with thick skin, which tends to camouflage irregularities or asymmetries of the underlying sculptured cartilage.

A frequent cause for bossae that manifest themselves in the early postoperative period is the injudicious use of interrupted strip techniques in thin-skinned patients with strong alar cartilages. The interrupted alar cartilage strip may be influenced asymmetrically by the perverse effects of scar healing and contracture, twisting and buckling the flail cartilage segments variably. Conversely, bossae are encountered in patients in whom complete strip techniques have been employed inexpertly, and excessive volume reduction of the alar cartilages results in an insubstantial width of the residual complete strip. Patients at risk for this complication generally manifest three conditions that predispose them to the gradual development of bossae: (1) extremely thin skin, (2) large thick alar cartilages, and (3) a wide intercrural distance between the tip defining points. If residual complete strips of less than approximately 5 mm are created in such patients, inexorable scar contracture over time may gradually pull the overweakened residual lateral crus medialward, creating unsightly (and often asymmetric) bossae, or knuckles of cartilage, clearly visible through thin skin.

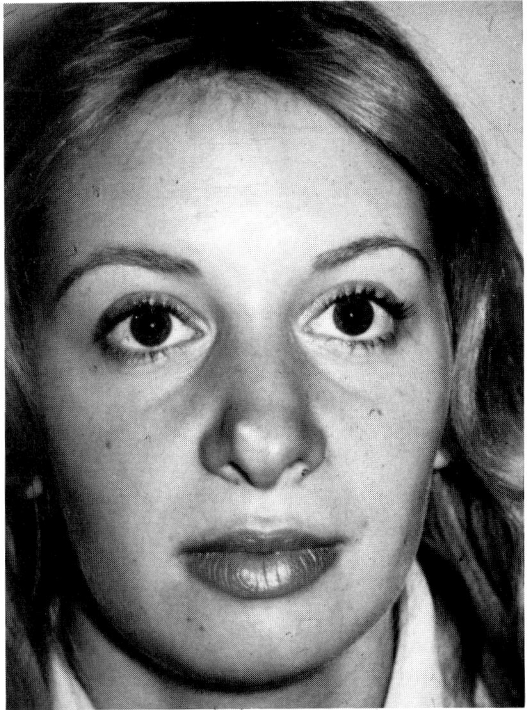

FIG 29–31.
Bossa formation in a patient before revision rhinoplasty. Exploration revealed complete strip preservation of the left lower lateral cartilage but interruption of the right lower lateral cartilage residual strip.

Bossae correction (or camouflage) requires exploration through bilateral marginal incisions. Once the magnitude and anatomy of the deformity are evident, shave excision of the sharp edge may be all that is required to create a smooth cartilaginous edge (too much shave excision reduction may result in an unwanted lowering of the tip defining points and spoiling of an otherwise elegant profile). In tip deformities of greater magnitude, reconstruction of the tip ensues with small, curved segments of onlay auricular cartilage, fashioned to recreate the natural contours of the dome. Unnaturally thin skin with sparse subcutaneous tissue may be favorably thickened and cushioned with one or two layers of temporalis fascia sutured between the cartilage and the overlying dermis.

Rhinophyma

The management of this progressive unsightly nasal condition involves both surgical and medical treatment. In patients with highly sebaceous nasal skin with early development of an apparent tendency toward full-blown rhinophyma, topical tretinoin (Retin-A) treatment diminishes or retards the progression of this skin disease in a substantial number of patients. Because of its intense drying effects on sebaceous gland activity, this product is useful in the postoperative management of individuals requiring surgical excision.

Full-blown rhinophyma with nasal distortion is managed by shave-excision of the rhinophymatous tissue with the Shaw (heated) scalpel. After local anesthesia is completed with 1% lidocaine and epinephrine 1:100,000, a sculpturing shave-excision procedure is gradually and incrementally carried out, resecting all visible hypertrophied tissue down to the depths of the deep, overlarge sebaceous glands. The Shaw scalpel possesses significant advantages in this procedure in that bleeding is immediately controlled throughout, and considerably improved visualization of the deeper tissues is afforded. Improved accuracy of the surgical shave-excision thus occurs. In the postoperative period, the avoidance of eschar and scab formation facilitates earlier healing and a return to normal activities. The operated nose is covered with a thin layer of neomycin sulfate (NeoDecadron) ophthalmic ointment kept in place with three layers of Adaptic gauze. The dressing is soaked away in 48 to 72 hours with peroxide, and daily ointment applications are continued until epithelialization ensues.

CHAPTER 30

Mentoplasty

Approach of

Howard W. Smith, M.D.

RECOGNITION

Cosmetic consideration of the chin for the majority of patients is primarily a matter of too much or too little protrusion. There are, however, mandibular deformities either acquired or congenital whereby the chin is not in the midline with an associated malocclusion, most often a crossbite. Malocclusion occurs in patients with either a protrusive chin or a retrusive chin, well documented in Angle's orthodontic classifications.[1] In the protrusive chin, the lower lip and chin relationships are relatively normal. In the retrusive chin with malocclusion, the chin–lower lip relationship is not normal.

For the purposes of this discussion, mentoplasty will be considered in those patients having normal occlusion. Rarely does the patient complain that his or her chin is too short or too pointed. The majority of patients present for revision of the nose and are unaware that the chin makes a significant contribution to facial disharmony.

I question new patients carefully about what they do not like about their face, being careful at the initial stage of the interview not to express my opinion. I examine the nose carefully, recording all defects as seen from the side, front, base, and oblique positions. I take lateral x-ray films of the face. This is essentially a true lateral sinus x-ray view that is unconed, making it possible to see the whole face. The x-ray exposure time is reduced to the amount required for lateral exposure of the nose. The x-ray, which is processed in about 90 seconds, provides an analysis of the nasal bones, the nasal spine, the tip of the mandible, and the lips as well as the chin. A tracing of this film provides a good profile of the face. Markers can be placed on the patient to identify the Frankfort horizontal line at the time of taking the x-ray film. These markings will serve as a guide to lay out standard facial analysis lines. The Frankfort

horizontal line is drawn on the tracing, and a perpendicular line is dropped from it, passing through the apex of the nasal labial angle. From this simple tracing, facial compartments and, most important, the lip-chin profile area as it relates to the nose can be drawn. It is at this time that I discuss the possibility of augmenting the chin. The essential landmarks in the chin-lip complex are the subnasale line, the lip line, the sublabial crease, and the prominence of the chin. The ideal situation is explained to the patient and the effect of an implant traced on the paper for comparison (Fig 30–1).

It is at this planning stage that problems can be recognized and unwanted results avoided. These unwanted results in an otherwise successful operation relate to the following.

Sublabial Crease.—Most patients who could benefit from a chin implant have a shallow sublabial crease. The placement of a medium-sized implant will create a new and pleasing sublabial crease. If the crease is already deep and the lip is full, the addition of an implant to the chin will cause an unacceptable chin-lip relationship readily appreciated on both the front and lateral facial views.

Pointed Chin.—Patients with a thin face and a narrow jaw often have a receding chin that is pointed. The addition of an implant will accentuate this pointed chin, even if the implant extends far laterally. The profile view is improved, but the front facial view is not.

Chin Dimples.—Many patients have an attractive dimple in the chin. The addition of a smooth, curved implant will eradicate the dimple, and only after it is gone will the patient wish it were back. This problem has been addressed by Dr. Benito Rish, and his implant provides for a dimple relationship.[2]

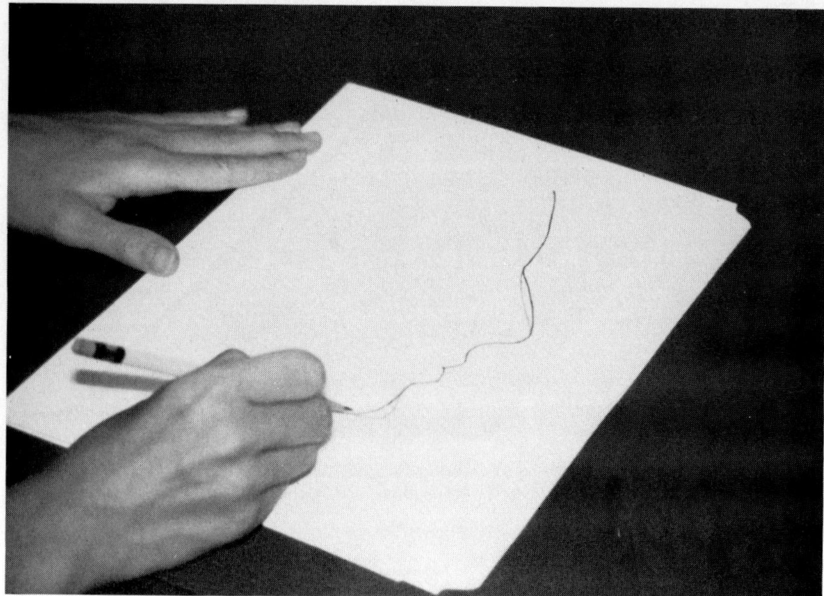

FIG 30–1.
X-ray profile tracing showing pencil sketch of reduction of the nasal dorsum and augmentation of the chin.

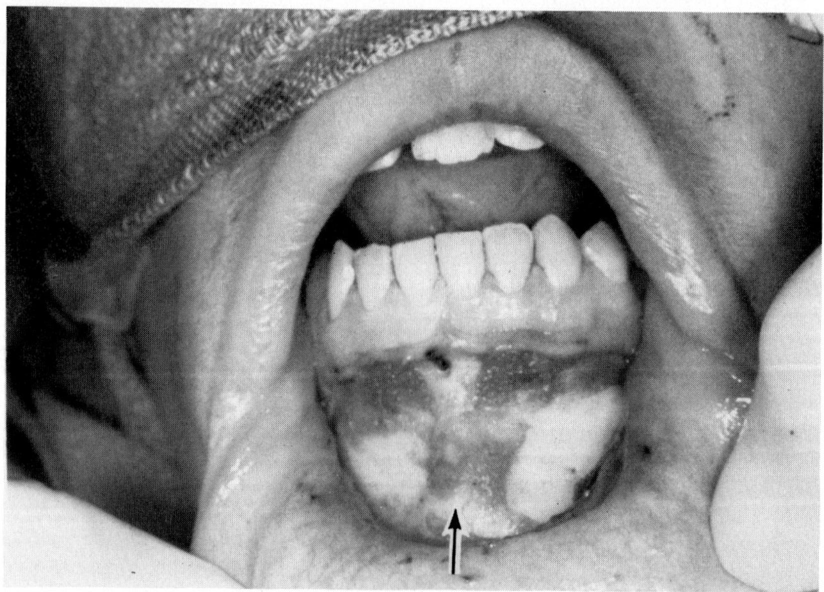

FIG 30–2.
Anterior surface of the mandible showing the ridge *(arrow)* often present in the midline.

The smooth silicone rubber (Silastic) implants can be fashioned to resemble a Rish implant and thereby avoid removing the dimple.

Prominent Bony Mental Symphysis.—This bony variance in the midline of the mandible may not be recognized until surgical exposure of the bone is completed (Fig 30–2). The problem may be palpated and recognized if the overlying soft tissue of the chin is thin or soft. This may influence the type of

implant employed. The solid acrylic type of implant that is inserted through a small submental incision may not seat properly. The implant, which is inserted beneath the mentalis muscle either subperiosteally or over the periosteum, will hug the bone on the insert side but cannot return with the same closeness to the mandible on the opposite side after being brought back and centered. Thus, one side will be close to the mandible, and the other will jut out into the soft tissues between the symphysis and the mental foramen. If the pocket is made large enough to avoid this, the implant will teeter on this bony prominence and eventually seat itself on one side or the other or in a diagonal position.

Implant Selection.—Too often a larger implant than can be easily implanted is selected. Although the size increase may seem relatively small, the size of the pocket has to be made considerably larger. The curvature of the mandible, even without a pointed symphysis, has to compare favorably with the implant or it will not seat evenly. Too large an implant will exaggerate the chin and upset the sublabial crease relationship to the lip.

Edentulous Patients.—Augmentation of the chin in edentulous patients should be attempted with great care or totally avoided. The position of the denture margin in the labial sulcus should be checked. The amount of alveolar resorption may cause the denture to lie low and leave insufficient room for an implant. Future resorption of the alveolar ridge may significantly lower the denture rim into the labial sulcus and cause erosion and exposure of the implant. The insertion of an implant in people wearing dentures, even if there appears to be adequate space for it to rest below the denture, will tend to dump the lower lip into the mouth and create a peculiar relationship of the lower lip to the upper lip, especially when the patient smiles.

AUGMENTATION MENTOPLASTY

The operative procedure for augmentation mentoplasty may be performed either intraorally or through a submental crease incision. In either case, it is essential to avoid the mental nerve by drawing lines on the skin to define the position of the mental foramen (Fig 30–3). The mental foramen can also be felt in many patients by palpating in the labial sulcus between the first and second premolars. A perpendicular line dropped from the pupils will cross the mandible at about the position of the mental foramen. The selected implant is placed on the skin and traced with a skin marking pen to also determine the size of the pocket necessary to receive the implant, and its relationship to the mental nerve can readily be appreciated (Fig 30–4).

When the intraoral approach is used, a midline incision is made in the lip, avoiding the need for a horizontal incision in the labial sulcus. The incision is made through the mucosa and thin subcutaneous tissue. The muscle fibers are separated with a small scissors, being careful to stay away from the external skin in the sublabial crease area. The pocket may be made either above or below the periosteum. Lateral pockets are made below the mentalis on each side with special elevators. This allows the paired mentalis muscles to retain the implant at the proper level. It is essential to make the entry route and pockets sufficiently large to accommodate the implant. It is better to have a smaller implant than one that is too large, which during insertion may cause tearing of the vertical incision so that the tears create a horizontal incision in the labial sulcus. This tear weakens the retentive value of the mentalis muscle, which may allow extrusion of the implant. I find that Silastic implants are easier to use intraorally than the firmer acrylic implants.

I prefer the submental approach for inserting implants. This route makes it easy to insert either the hard implant of the Rish acrylic type or the soft Silastic implants. In general, I like the shape of the Rish implant, and for the patient with a relatively wide jaw and a flat mental area, the Rish implant is easy to insert and centers nicely, giving the jaw a fullness rather than a pointed roundness. It can be pushed in to an excess on one side and then allowed to come back to the other side after shoehorning

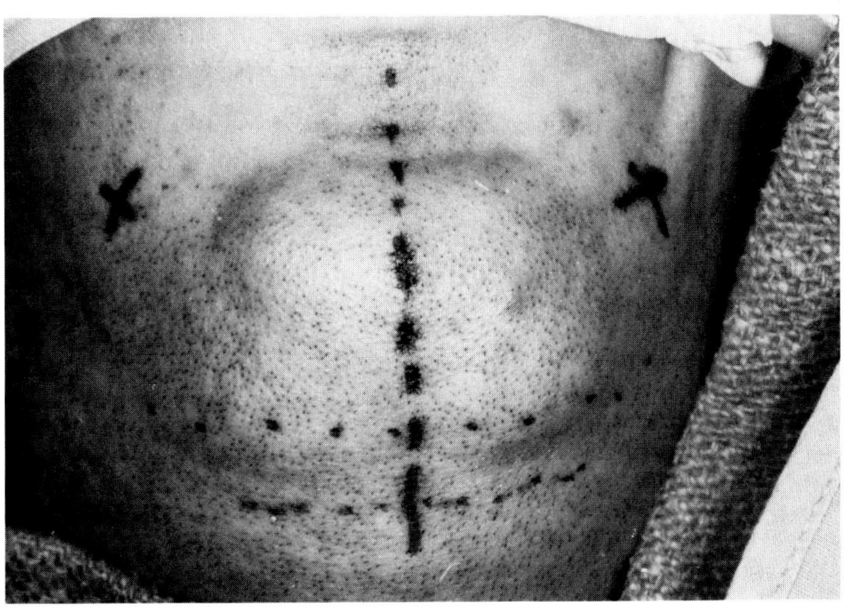

FIG 30–3.
Chin showing position of both mental foramina (marked by Xs).

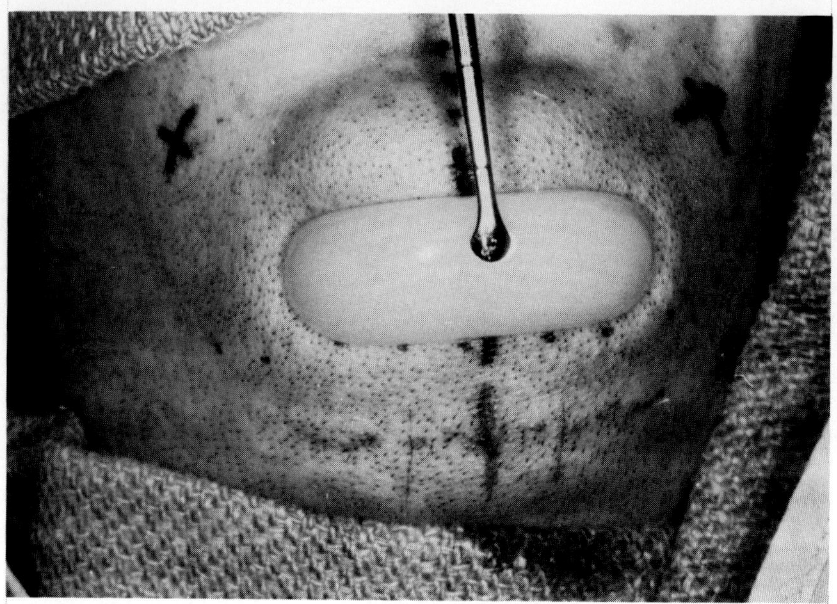

FIG 30–4.
Chin with overlying Silastic implant being traced onto the skin to determine dissection pocket location and size.

in the other tip. (I use a McKenty elevator for this, which works quite nicely.) This implant is easily centered. Care must be taken to trim the tips of the implant if it is too long and to be sure that the tip of the mandible is relatively flat. If not, the implant, on return to the midline, will engage the soft tissue and end up low against the jaw on the insert side and high (away from the jaw) on the return side. Patients are quick to perceive this undesired effect. The Silastic implant, in comparison, can be cut on its back side by removing a V-shaped section to weaken the stiffness and allow the soft tissue of the chin to compress the implant against the mandible. The Silastic implant can also be modified in the same fashion as the Rish implant to preserve or create a dimpled effect and to provide the patient with substance to the whole chin area rather than just the symphysis. The Silastic implant can be led in with sutures of 2-0 chromic catgut to get it centered accurately. The implant can have punch holes in it, which aid in the retention. In either instance, the skin incision and the soft tissue incisions are staggered. Immediately after insertion, the area can be compressed by using $\frac{1}{2}$-in Steri-Strips. Too large a pocket allows for hematoma formation and possible abscess formation. All patients are given antibiotics, and all are investigated thoroughly for bleeding tendencies. It is my impression that infection and extrusion are associated primarily with hematoma formation and excess edema. Mental nerve injury should not occur from careful elevation and insertion of a prosthesis.

Adequate positioning of the implant is a must. Even though the implant may be centered, it is hard to tell if one side is higher than the other. Malpositioning is embarrassing and the chief cause for removal, which requires a whole new operation. Often, taking out the implant requires waiting several months and then repeating the procedure. Trying to insert a new implant into the same pocket modified only on its relationship to

the mandible will allow the soft tissue curvature already made by the previous implant to assert its influence on the new implant and create the same defect.

AUGMENTATION MENTOPLASTY WITH A SLIDING GENIOPLASTY

This operation is ideal for those patients who do not desire a foreign body implant and are agreeable to a more extensive operative procedure. Essentially the same results can be obtained. The procedure is performed intraorally. The incision is horizontal, staying away from the labial sulcus by placing the incision on the lip side about 4 mm anterior to the depth of the labial sulcus. This incision thus leaves a cuff of tissue anterior to the sulcus so that sutures used for closure do not cross the depth of the sulcus and leave webs that allow food to collect. The incision starts in the region of the first premolar on one side and extends along the lip to the opposite side. The elevation is made subperiosteally to the level of the intended cut in the mandible. The mental nerve is carefully identified on both sides. Vertical grooves are made with a small drill on the mandible in the center and on each side about 1 cm from the midline so that the fragments will remain oriented when separated. A horizontal incision is made in the bone, being careful to stay well below the apices of the incisor and canine teeth. This bone incision is about 0.75 to 1 cm high anteriorly and tapers as it goes backward to end laterally at the border of mandible below the mental foramen. Thus, a wedge of bone (horseshoe shaped) is freed from the undersurface of the body of the mandible, leaving intact the muscular attachments along the inferior border (Fig 30–5). This segment of bone is freed up and advanced so that the posterior cortex of the inferior fragment can be wired to the anterior cortex of the body of the mandible. The previously drilled markings on the anterior surface of the mandible with a small drill serve as a guide to line up the drill holes in both fragments. A 24-gauge stainless steel wire is used for the immobilization (Fig 30–6). The most important part of this procedure other than to avoid the mental nerve is to have a suitable saw. Both the Hall and Stryker companies manufacture thin blades that come in straight and right-angle variations and

make the bone cuts an easy procedure. It may be necessary to tailor the ends of the inferior fragments in cases where the jaw tapers sharply toward the symphysis so that the advanced horseshoe-shaped piece does not protrude laterally and cause either a palpable or visual protruberance.

Augmentation mentoplasty can be varied by advancing the distal or freed segment and at the same time inserting a piece of iliac bone in the horizontal saw cut to reduce the tendency

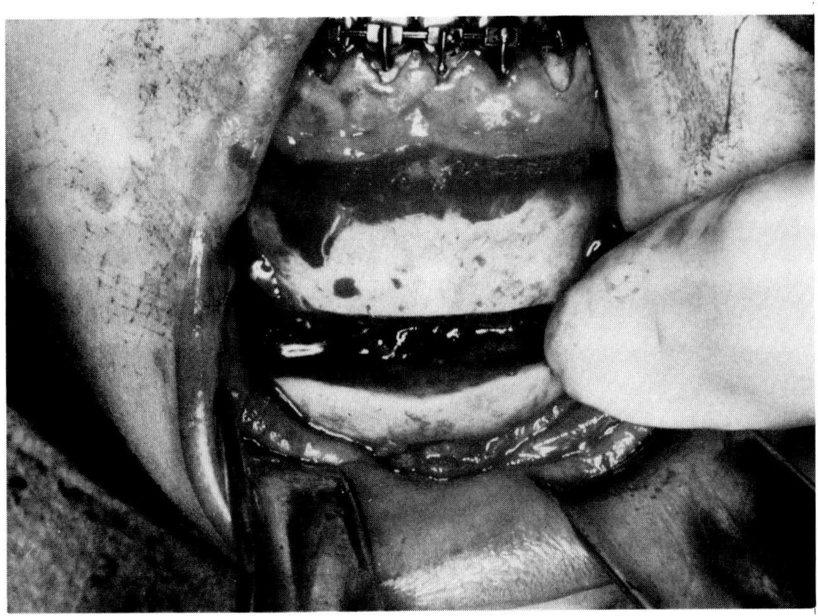

FIG 30–5.
Mandible showing horizontal bone cut in preparation for advancement.

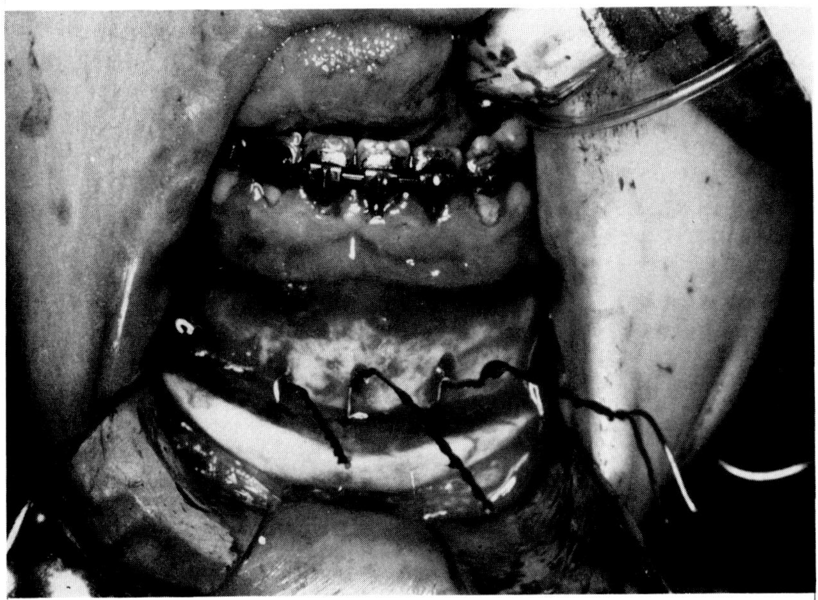

FIG 30–6.
Mandible in Figure 30–5 showing segment wired in an advanced position.

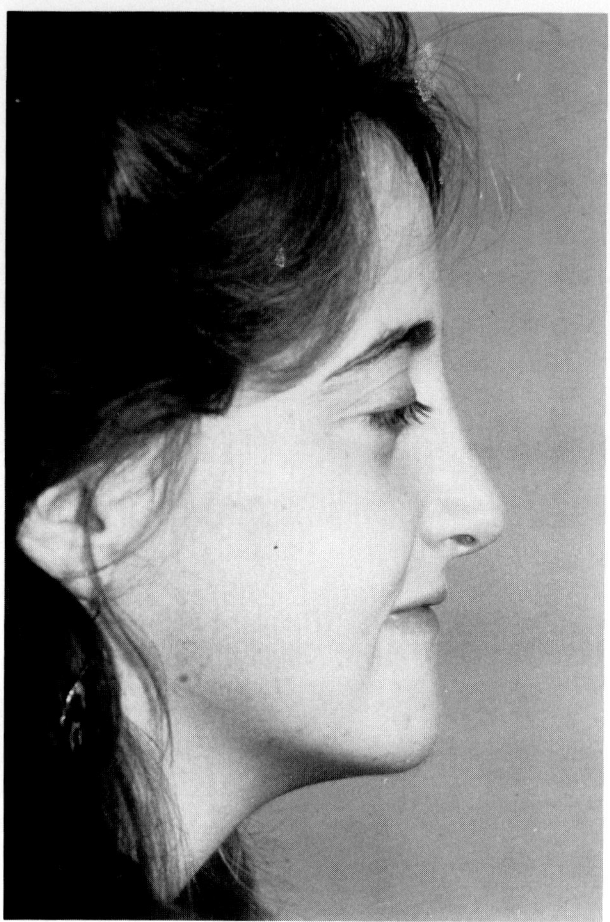

FIG 30–7.
Lateral view of patient showing a loss of sublabial sulcus following posterior sliding genioplasty.

to deepen the sublabial crease. Fixation of the bone graft is done in the same manner as that employed in the forward positioning of the inferior segment.

REDUCTION MENTOPLASTY

There are several ways to perform reduction of the excessively protruding chin in the presence of normal occlusion. These methods fall into two general categories: (1) to reduce bone and (2) to reduce soft tissue. When considering reduction of the chin, one cannot ignore the effect such reduction will have on lip competence, the sublabial crease, and the submental crease.

Simple reduction of the prominent bone at the symphysis of the mandible can be achieved easily by use of surgical burs or using an oscillating or sagittal saw. A less simple reduction is to perform a sliding osteotomy whereby a wedge of bone, created by a horizontal saw cut, is positioned in the reverse manner compared with a forward-sliding osteotomy. One variation is to make two horizontal cuts and remove the inner segment, thus reducing the vertical height of the chin in the

area below the sublabial crease. In any event, the effect may look satisfactory on the operating table, but over time several changes occur that cause alarm for the patient and lead to a nonacceptable result:

1. Flattening or complete loss of the sublabial crease. Reducing the bony prominence of the mandible allows the soft tissue of the chin to reposition itself in a posterior inferior direction, causing distortion of the sublabial crease (Fig 30–7).

2. Flattening of the lower third of the face. After a prominent chin is reduced, the lateral tissues of the face in the lower third take on a degree of prominence that makes the lower third of the face seem wider and flatter (Fig 30–8).

3. Cervical fullness. It occurs particularly with the posteriorly sliding osteotomy. The bony substance plus the attached musculature are compressed into the submandibular area laterally, creating an unattractive fullness (Fig 30–9).

4. Soft tissue ptosis. With resection of the mandible anteriorly, the ungloving of the mandible detaches the muscles. They do not reattach firmly to the reduced volume of bone. The volume of soft tissue that is unreduced sags inferiorly and overlaps the submental crease. In time this sagging resembles a soft tissue goatee (Fig 30–10).

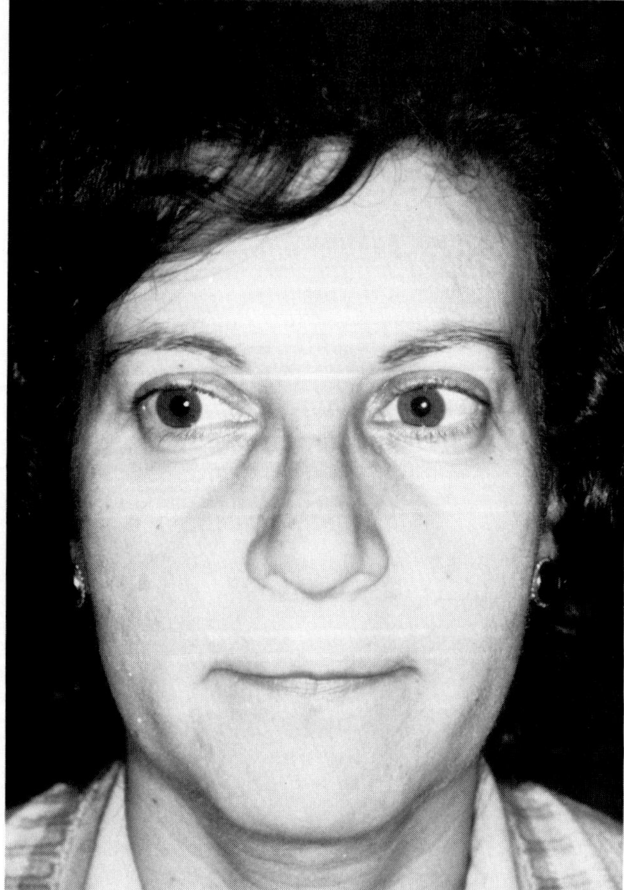

FIG 30–8.
Anteroposterior view of patient showing flatness of the chin area following reduction mentoplasty.

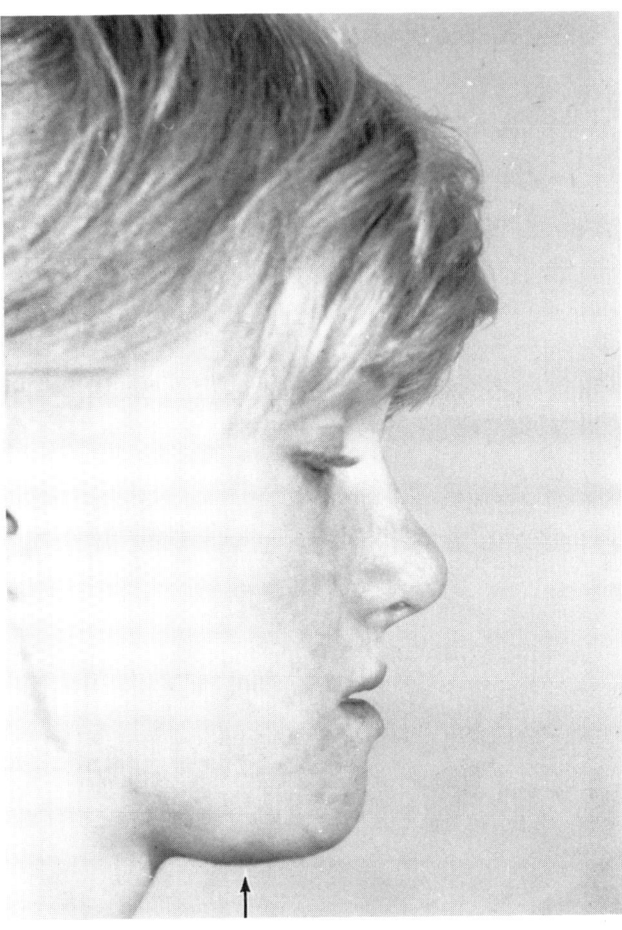

FIG 30–9.
Lateral view of patient showing submandibular fullness following posterior sliding genioplasty.

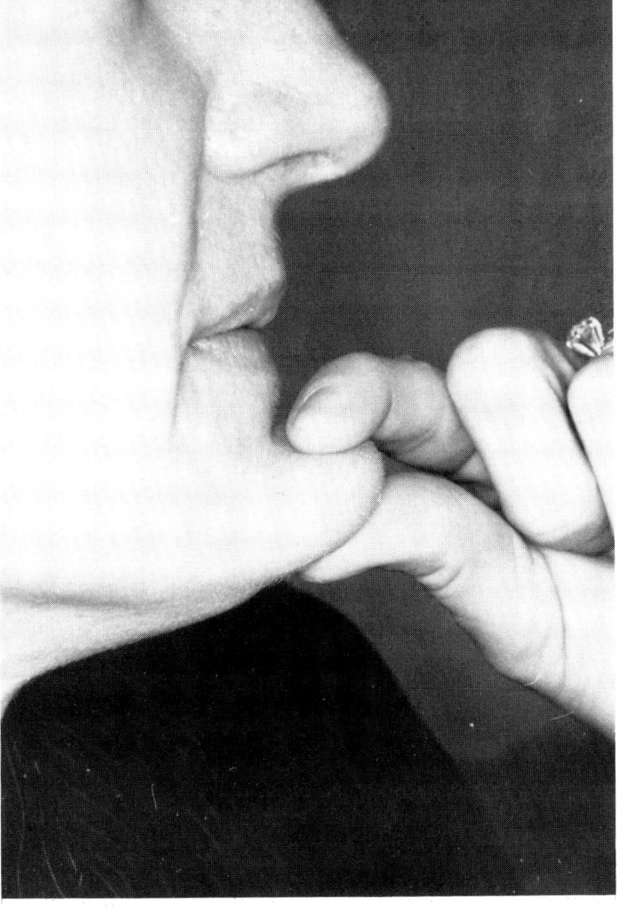

FIG 30–10.
Lateral view of patient showing chin ptosis following reduction mentoplasty.

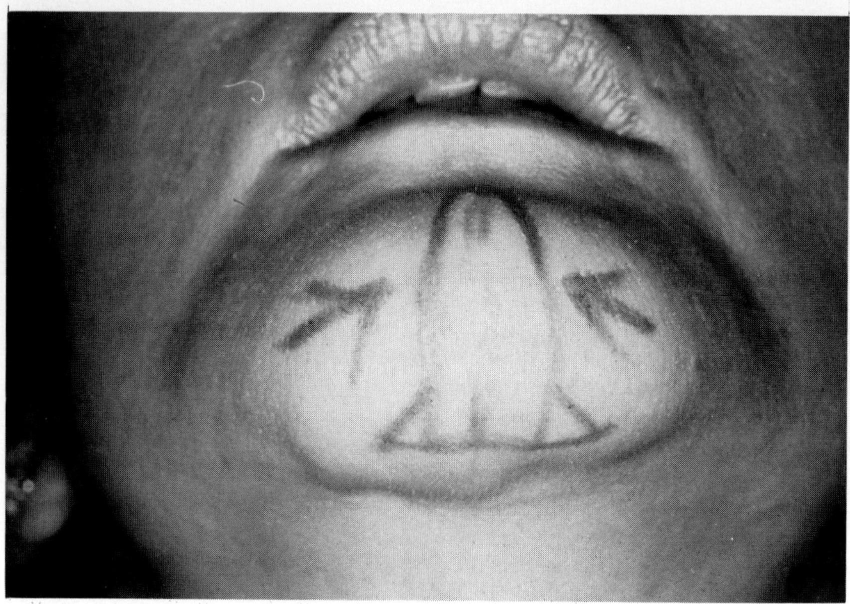

FIG 30–11.
Dorsum showing markings for excision of skin, subcutaneous tissue, and muscle to reduce chin ptosis.

The need for reduction mentoplasty involving soft tissue can be predicted in some young people by looking at the prominence of the chin and early formation of a deep submental crease. With time these tissues sag, and if a face-lift is performed at some later date, the defect will be exaggerated. The condition can be predicted quite accurately in patients having a reduction mentoplasty. A follow-up evaluation 5 to 10 years after the surgery will confirm the need for surgical correction of chin ptosis.

The technique for correction of chin ptosis depends on analysis of the tissues involved. The skin in the confined area below the sublabial crease extending to the inferior border of the mandible and extending laterally to the commissures of the mouth is thick and nonshrinkable. This tissue sags and overlaps the submandibular or submental crease. It can be actually grasped in the hand and moved about readily like an appendage. The fatty subcutaneous tissue is thick and nonmoveable. The muscles in the area are nonfunctioning for the most part, except for the orbicularis oris, which is slightly above this tissue. The removal of submental fat with or without a facelift will only make the soft tissue ptosis appear worse. In the procedure for surgical correction of chin ptosis, it is essential to remove a portion of all three layers. A triangular section of tissue with the apex at the sublabial crease based inferiorly on the submental crease can be removed, thus reducing the soft tissue ptosis without disturbing lip competence or disturbing the sublabial crease (Fig 30–11). In most instances, the patient is willing to swap a soft tissue goatee for a minimal vertical scar in the midline of the chin.

At the present time I am not in favor of performing a reduction mentoplasty by reducing the mentum or repositioning the bone at the inferior border of the mandible.

REFERENCES

1. Mathog RH: *Maxillofacial Trauma.* Baltimore, Williams & Wilkins, 1984, pp 116–117.
2. Rish B: Profile—plasty report on plastic chin implants. *Laryngoscope* 1964; 74:144.

Mentoplasty

Approach of

M. Eugene Tardy, Jr., M.D.

TECHNIQUE

For more than 23 years, only soft silicone bag chin implants have been employed in my practice for chin augmentation. Manufactured by Heyer-Schulte and McGhan, these soft malleable prostheses simulate the soft tissues of the chin area and are almost impossible to palpate after several months of healing of the overlying tissues (Fig 30–12). A 12 to 14 mm incision created in the submental area is preferred for access to the anterior mandible; no implant has ever been lost from infection or rejection using this approach, whereas the literature documents a small percentage of infections developing in patients in whom the intraoral route has been chosen. Antibiotic coverage during the perioperative period is indicated whenever foreign bodies are introduced into the facial skeleton.

All patients wash their face with hexachlorophene (pHisoHex) the evening before and the morning of surgery, thus arriving in the operating room surgically clean; the chin and neck are painted (but not scrubbed) with povidone-iodine (Betadine) solution. In the sitting position, several landmarks are marked: the exact midline of the chin, the lateral extent of the intended implant augmentation bilaterally, and the site of the submental incision. It has been observed over the years that curvilinear incisions placed just posterior to the submental crease heal less conspicuously than those sited in the crease itself.

The patient's color photographs are projected greater than life size on the wall of the operating room, ensuring an ideal visual reference during the augmentation procedure. Local anesthetic consisting of 2 to 3 mL of 1% lidocaine (Xylocaine) with epinephrine 1:100,000 provides satisfactory anesthesia without distortion of the chin tissues. If the chin augmentation accompanies rhinoplasty, the chin is operated first to maintain sterility and to allow the local anesthetic placed in the nose sufficient time to exert maximum vasoconstriction.

The submental incision, no more than 12 to 14 mm long, is carried through the skin and fat but stops short of the muscular layer. Excess fat, common in younger patients, is trimmed away from the incision (and frequently from the submental area as well) to better define the cervical-mental area (Fig 30–13). The incision is tracted upward (toward the anterior chin) with a wide double-pronged hook to expose the muscle overlying the pogonion. With the Bovie cautery, the site of the intended incision through the muscle is cauterized to minimize bleeding. The incision to gain access to the chin is thus placed away from the skin incision, staggering the eventual wound closure, a useful surgical principle whenever implants are placed. The incision is next carried through muscle and periosteum, elevating the latter layer from the anterior mandible sufficiently laterally to create a precise subperiosteal pocket for the intended implant.

Little bleeding occurs with this approach, thus limiting postoperative swelling and facilitating direct-vision surgery. The proper size gel Chin Dacron-backed implant is then selected and soaked in gentamycin (Garamycin) solution prior to insertion. Overaugmentation is a significant complication and must be avoided. With the aid of the thin, malleable Siegel retractor, the implant, because of its soft, flexible nature, is easily shoehorned into the prepared pocket through the small incision.

The chin and submental area undergo careful inspection and palpation with the peroxide-moistened finger to ensure symmetry and correct position of the implant using the projected photographs as an ideal reference. Closure of the staggered incisions is effected using muscular and subcutaneous sutures of 5-0 Dexon; the skin is approximated with a running intradermal suture of 6-0 Prolene. A light pressure dressing of Conform gauze wrapped around the chin and the skull provides support and light pressure for 24 hours, ensuring partial jaw immobilization and minimizing edema.

COMPLICATIONS

Asymmetry is perhaps the most common complication of chin augmentation, although not of a sufficient degree to warrant reoperation. Preoperative asymmetry of the mandible is a very common occurrence, and patients must be religiously made aware of this variation from normal. As stated, no implants have ever required removal because of infection or rejection. Broad-spectrum antibiotic coverage is maintained for 3 days postoperatively and then discontinued. Early postoperative hematoma formation is important to avoid since it predisposes to infection or potential shifting of the implant. Following the strict dissec-

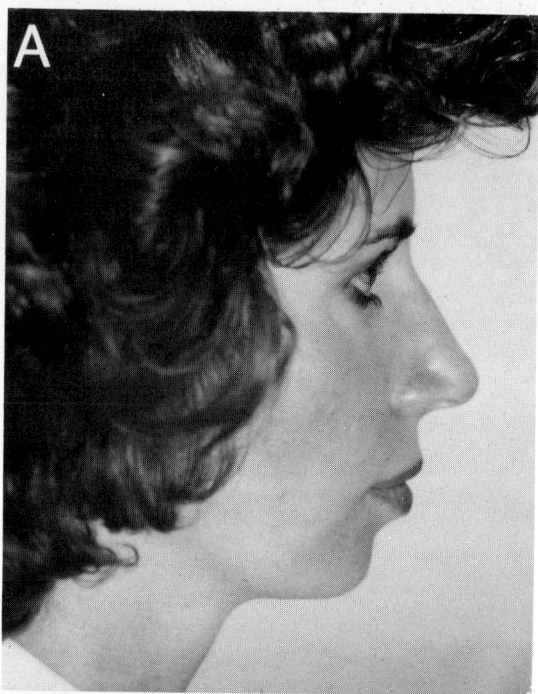

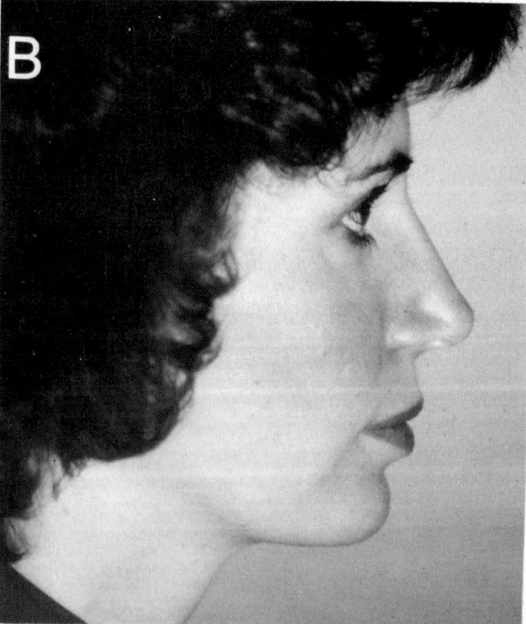

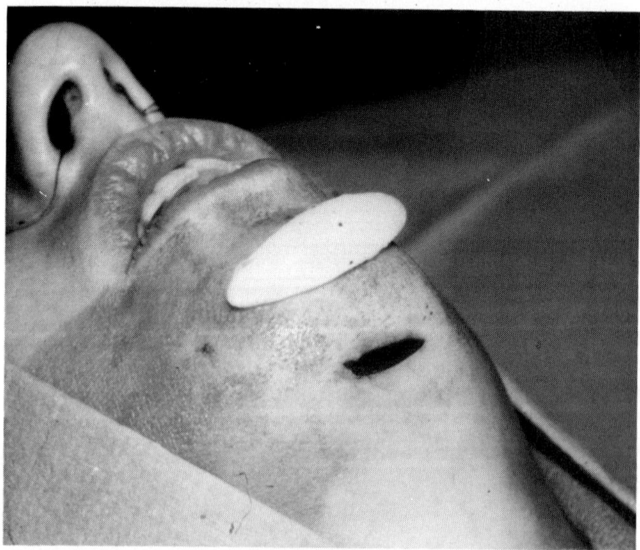

FIG 30–12.
Gel chin implant positioned over retrognathic chin in preparation for insertion through a small submental incision.

FIG 30–13.
A, preoperative appearance of patient with significant retrognathia. **B,** 2 years after correction of retrognathia with gel chin implant. Excess submental fat has been removed to improve the cervicomental angle.

tion principles previously recounted effectively limits this possibility. No instance of mental nerve injury has been encountered, probably because of the strength and resilience of this large sensory nerve. Palpating and marking the site of the mental foramen at the outset of the operation guards against potential injury.

Augmentation mentoplasty combined with submentoplasty (excision or liposuction of excessive submental fat) are operations that complement each other well and may be performed through the same small incision. It is vital, however, to guard against overexcision of submental fat to avoid an onerous midline cervical depression. Sufficient fat should remain on the dissected skin flap to not only protect the subdermal plexus but to maintain a smooth cervicomental profile line as well (see Fig 30–13).

CHAPTER 31

Rhytidectomy and Blepharoplasty

Approach of

J. Regan Thomas, M.D.

and

M. Sean Freeman, M.D.

RHYTIDECTOMY

Rhytidectomy, or facelift, is not a single procedure but, rather, a combination of procedures using a variety of techniques that are individualized for each patient based on age, tissue, and anatomic requirements into a single surgical plan. As with all cosmetic surgery, patient selection and initial patient evaluation are key components of successful surgical results. An accurate evaluation of the patient's individual physical requirements as well as emotional stability and capacity for realistic expectations must be assessed prior to surgery.

An ideal face-lift patient might be categorized as the patient who is thin, with strong bone structure, fair skinned, and in an age group that has retained some elasticity and resiliency of the skin and subcutaneous tissues. The opposite end of the patient spectrum would be an obese individual with poor facial bony definition, dark, thick, oily skin, perhaps with thin hair, and with less than realistic surgical expectations. Most patients fall somewhere within these two ranges, and a decision as to how to approach them, again, must be individualized.

The goals of face-lift surgery should include the following: tightening of redundancy and fullness in the submental and cervical regions; tightening and elevating nasolabial lines, smoothing and improving the contour of the mandibular line, particularly in the jowl area; and accomplishing an overall elevation and resupport of sagging facial and cheek tissues. Again, depending on the individual patient, additional procedures may be required. These frequently include blepharoplasty, which

will be discussed later in this chapter, and forehead lift, or brow lift. Many patients also benefit from adjunctive techniques, including facial peel or dermabrasion, particularly in the perioral areas. In some patients, bony augmentation such as cheek implants are used. These are generally secondary procedures done after a given period of healing following a blepharoplasty. Chin implants and certain patients with poor mandibular cervical angles or ptotic chins will benefit from a chin implant at the time of face-lift.

Surgical Procedure

Preparation

As with all cosmetic procedures, rhytidectomy is typically reserved for the patient in stable health. A complete history and physical examination are obtained and routine laboratory tests, including complete blood cell count, urinalysis, and SMA-12 profile are obtained prior to surgery. The patients also receive an electrocardiogram and chest radiograph if they are more than 40 years old. All patients have been asked to refrain from taking aspirin-containing products or vitamin E (other than what might be contained in a multiple vitamin) for 2 to 3 weeks prior to surgery. No prophylactic antibiotics are required, and the patient is asked to take nothing by mouth from the evening prior to surgery.

The operation is typically done as an outpatient procedure. In the outpatient preoperative waiting area, the patients have their hair prepared. Hair is parted along anticipated surgical incisions and then braided or taped to keep it from being in the way during surgery. No hair is shaved.

Incision sites are outlined with a surgical marking pen with the patient in the upright position. Specific areas of redundancy or those spots that will require submental and cervical liposuction are outlined at this time. Many of these areas are not easily observed once the patient is in the reclining position, and it is important to identify these areas prior to the surgical procedure (incision sites for blepharoplasty or other procedures are marked at this time as well). Often a premedication is given by the anesthesiologist during this period to begin the process of analgesia-anesthesia.

Anesthesia

Although occasional patients are given general anesthesia, the routine rhytidectomy patient is given a combination of local infiltration and continuously monitored intravenous analgesia. Specific agents are selected by the anesthesiologist based on the patient's age, weight, and state of health, but, in general, a twilight sleep anesthetic regimen is used intravenously. The patients are at a deeper level of sedation briefly during the times when the local anesthetic is injected and are then titrated at their comfort level with a lighter level of sedation during the remainder of the procedure. All patients are monitored, including blood pressure. A cardiac monitor and a pulse oximeter are generally utilized.

Local infiltration then proceeds in a stepwise fashion, infiltrating one area of the procedure. After surgery is accomplished in that region, the next area is infiltrated to minimize the amount of local anesthetic given at any one time. This technique also maximizes the longevity of the local agent. One percent lidocaine (Xylocaine) with epinephrine 1:100,000 is infiltrated along incision areas and 0.5% lidocaine with epinephrine 1:200,000 is infiltrated in those areas to be undermined. The incisions are initially infiltrated, and then the undermined areas are infiltrated in a fanlike fashion from this now anesthetized skin. The level of infiltration should be in the immediate subcutaneous plane just below the dermis. Following injection, 10 to 15 minutes is allowed to pass prior to initiating the procedure to allow for the appropriate epinephrine effect to begin.

Submental Lipectomy and Liposuction

Most patients benefit from submental liposuction. Those patients with a large amount of fat receive aggressive liposuction in this area. Those with lesser amounts of submental adipose undergo liposuction that is used primarily to free up the submental tissues for better draping and support. The key advantage to liposuction in the submental area is that fat can be removed through a relatively small incision. Liposuction also allows the surgeon to do a superior job of making a smooth contoured transition from the areas treated to the more peripheral areas as well as to avoid removing too much fat in the midline leaving an unsightly hollow area postoperatively. Some patients will require resection or plication of the platysma to correct the

platysmal bands, and in these situations following submental liposuction, the incision is enlarged enough to allow the medial margins of the platysma to be visualized and treated.

Liposuction is accomplished through serially enlarging liposuction cannulas beginning with 2 mm cannulas. Paths and tunnels are created in a fanlike direction in the submental area. The lateral range for liposuction is the anterior edge of the sternocleidomastoid muscle. The attachments to the skin make it more difficult to go beyond this area. The inferior limit to liposuction is usually the first cervical rhytid. Careful attention is made when one is liposuctioning in the jowl area not to create a notch over the mandible and to allow for a smooth mandibular line. Following creation of the 2 mm tunnels, a 4 mm cannula is passed to enlarge these tunnels, again done without active suction being used. Finally, a 6 mm cannula is used. Its passage is now facilitated by having created tunnels through the serially enlarged cannula use. Active suctioning is now pursued. Suction should be at approximately 1 atm of negative pressure, and fat is removed with a to-and-fro action of the cannula. Pressure and manipulation of the subcutaneous tissue by the opposite hand not holding the cannula are used to aid fatty tissue into the cannula opening. It is important to keep the cannula opening away from the dermis to avoid later ridging in the postoperative state. Once the submental area is completed, the patient is observed for symmetry or any areas of persistent fullness or asymmetry. These areas are suctioned again to obtain the optimum result. The wound is generally closed with one layer using interrupted 6.0 Prolene sutures. There is rarely any bleeding following liposuction using this technique. Once liposuction has been completed, attention is turned to the rhytidectomy incisions and creation of the face-lift flaps.

Rhytidectomy Incisions

There are many alternatives described for face-lift incisions, and the technique for any individual patient must be planned based on the patient's anatomy, including the hairline. Other considerations include the requirements of the face-lift procedure and such additional factors as whether they have had prior surgery. In general, however, the incision is placed so that it incorporates three areas: temporal, periauricular, and postauricular. The temporal component of the incision is made in a curvilinear fashion starting at approximately the point behind the temporal hairline superior to the attachment of the external auricle and is a curvilinear line going a variable distance superiorly. The periauricular incision connects with this line at the superior attachment of the auricle and follows the natural periauricular junction of the ear with a marked indentation at the area of the incisura above the tragus. It then continues in front of the tragus in the natural crease, tightly hugging the attachment of the lobule and extending behind the ear just above the sulcus on the conchal portion of skin. In men, especially those with heavily bearded skin, the preauricular part of the incision is made in a straight line fashion slightly anterior to the ear to avoid pulling bearded skin back against the tragus in an unnatural way.

The postauricular incision is carried superiorly to a level

just above the height that would correspond to the level of the external auditory canal. The line of incision then crosses to the hair-bearing postauricular area to a slightly superior plane to this point. The junction of the incisions at the postauricular area is joined with a small V-shaped dart that falls into the sulcus and is used to avoid a tight bridle-like scar. The postauricular incision goes into the hairline and extends posteriorly again in curvilinear fashion running inferiorly and entirely within hair-bearing tissue.

Flap Development

We have found it useful to think of development of the face-lift flap in three component stages: (1) incision development, (2) undermining, and (3) hemostasis. This is sometimes referred to, particularly in training environments, as "three regions–three times around." "The first time around" is aimed specifically at developing and initiating the incision beginning in the temporal area, moving to the periauricular area, and ending in the postauricular area. In the hair-bearing areas of the temporal and occipital regions, careful attention is made to bevel the incision to avoid hair follicle damage. As noted earlier, in the region of the ear above the tragus, the incisural area is exaggerated to break up the scar line and better camouflage the scar. At this time, only major bleeders are cauterized, and the progress of the incision is not stopped.

The "second time around" the flap is elevated. Here the flap is undermined and elevated to the extent predetermined on the individual patient. Again, the attention is directed specifically at undermining and elevating the flap, and only significant bleeders are cauterized and dealt with at this time to facilitate a stepwise progression in development of the flap. When the flap has been elevated in all three regions, the "third time around" is aimed at specific hemostasis using the bipolar cautery. The wound is rendered completely dry and without any evidence of active bleeding. Typically, no drains are required because of this careful attention to detail.

The amount of undermining of the flap varies and is individualized with the patient, but most often the temporal area is elevated to a point just beyond the hairline. It does not extend in the area between the hairline and the brow above the zygomatic arch to avoid possible injury to the facial nerve branch. It has been our experience that appropriate tightening and redraping of the tissues in this area can be accomplished well with this degree of undermining while at the same time providing for a safer procedure. Undermining in the facial cheek areas is typically moderate in its extent. A variety of techniques by various surgeons range from minimal undermining to extensive undermining going all the way to the nasolabial groove and lateral lip commissure. We prefer a more limited procedure, especially when combined with superficial musculoaponeurotic system (SMAS) plication. Undermining typically extends 4 to 5 cm in this region from the incision site. There are several advantages to this type of flap development, including avoiding the distal branches of the facial nerve as they become more superficial peripherally. Also, the more limited amount of undermining leaves less potential space for hematoma development. Undermining is accomplished through scissors dissection using a face-lift scissors with semisharp outer edges and a slightly blunted tip in a spreading action. Direct vision is then used to connect the individual undermined areas.

Superficial Musculoaponeurotic System Support

Resupport of the SMAS layer is a key ingredient to developing both initial good results from the face-lift and longer lasting results. Use of the SMAS layer for resupporting facial tissues also allows minimal tension on the skin edges in the visible areas of the preauricular incision site. If the patient has significant adipose tissue in the facial regions, open liposuction is used over the SMAS layer. In this technique the facial flap is retracted, and using the liposuction cannula with its fenestration against the SMAS surface, the operator removes fatty tissue superficial to the SMAS layer with a to-and-fro suctioning of the 6 mm liposuction cannula. This typically results in an easily observed glistening SMAS layer, which is then either grasped and plicated using interrupted 3-0 PDS sutures or is undermined and excised with the free edges and closed with the same suture in patients with more significant laxity. The PDS suture allows for significant strength to maintain this level until full healing has occurred, and then the suture is resorbed. To date, this has not created suture spitting problems. The SMAS level extends inferiorly to become confluent with the platysmal layers, and they are handled as part of the SMAS complex and retracted posterior superiorly. Much more tension can be placed on the SMAS layer than could be used on the skin layer, and thus a superior pull and redistribution of tissue can be accomplished without fear of unsightly scars. It should be noted that in most patients this retraction and repositioning of the SMAS and platysmal edges will sufficiently correct submental platysmal banding and deformity. That, combined with the previously accomplished submental liposuction, allows the submental and cervical mandibular areas to be corrected without significant incisions in the submental areas.

Tailoring of the Skin Flap

As noted earlier, the support of the SMAS level reduces the amount of tension in the preauricular areas of the skin flap. Skin can now be redraped in a posteriosuperior direction again. Once the skin is in position with moderate tension in the hair-bearing area, two key sutures can be placed. The first is at the junction of the temporal and preauricular incision at the superior attachment of the helix. The second key suture is placed at the junction of the postauricular incision with the sulcus of the postauricular area. Once these sutures have been placed, the skin flaps can be tailored and the excess excised. Closure in the hair-bearing areas is done in a single layer using stainless steel skin staples. The preauricular region is tailored so that the wound edges fit exactly, and there is no need for tension on them. A running intracuticular 5-0 Prolene suture is used for this region. A running 5-0 Prolene suture is used in the postauricular sulcus, and again, skin staples are used in the postauricular hair-bearing regions. Careful attention is made as the hair-bearing posterior incision is tailored to realign the hairline and avoid a step-off deformity.

Dressings

The rubber bands or tape are removed from the hair. Any dried blood or soap is rinsed, and the hair is combed out. Polymyxin B sulfate (Polysporin) ointment is applied to the suture lines, and a layered dressing is applied. This consists of fluffed gauze squares over the area of the incisions and facial flaps, as well as in the submental area. This layer is followed with a Kling gauze wrap and then a Coban secondary wrap. The dressing is applied so that it covers from the occiput under the chin and covers all facial and postauricular areas in turbin-like fashion. Note that although submental liposuction, particularly as an individual procedure, is sometimes described as requiring taping afterward, no taping is done here. In fact, taping may be contraindicated when combined with a facelift in that the submental taping would be actually pulling against the elevated facial flaps and would be counterproductive.

Postoperative Activity

Patients are provided with an oral pain medication, usually acetaminophen with codeine (Tylenol no. 3) and, after observation in the outpatient recovery area, are allowed to return home. They are asked to sleep with their head elevated at about 45 degrees and for the next 2 weeks to avoid strenuous exercise of heavy lifting. The patients return to the office the following morning, and the dressing is changed. The flaps are inspected for hematoma or other postoperative sequelae, and the dressing is reapplied. The patients again return the following morning, at which time the dressing is removed. If the flaps and incisions appear to be doing well, the dressing is left off, and the patient begins to wear an elastic support under the chin for the next 2 weeks. The patients may then wash their hair and are asked to clean their incisions and reapply their antibiotic ointment twice daily. The periauricular sutures are removed at 7 days, and the staples are removed at 2 weeks. During this interim, patients may apply makeup and return to normal activities within that 2-week period.

Complications

The most frequent postoperative sequelae statistically is hematoma.[1] Most hematomas are minor, but it is important to inspect the area and be prepared to treat a hematoma if more significant ones should arise. Careful hemostasis during the time of the procedure is of major importance in prevention, and occasionally a drain is used postoperatively in the patient who has persistent oozing or in whom hemostasis has been difficult to achieve. Baker et al. in a review of rhytidectomy summarized 12 other articles that stated the individual surgeon's incidence of large hematoma following rhytidectomy.[2] Individuals reported percentages of hematoma ranging from 0.8% to 5%.[2–5] It appears that hematomas may be more likely with more extensive flap undermining, and we believe that by using shorter flaps, the incidence of hematoma may be kept to a minimum. Webster published his experience with 221 consecutive rhytidectomies and had a hematoma rate of 0.9%.[6]

Small inactive hematomas can, at times, be treated by aspiration or sometimes expressed through the incision line after removing several sutures. More major active hematoma formation requires surgical intervention to avoid loss of skin flap viability.

Skin flap necrosis is another reported complication of facelift but should be an unusual occurrence. Most surgeons agree that this is a greater risk in those patients who are active smokers. Apparently, smoking deteriorates the vascular supply to the skin flap, at least at the capillary level, putting these patients at greater risk. Less tension on the skin flap is provided by using an SMAS layer. Peterson reported a published study that showed that when an extensively undermined side of a facelift was compared with one with less undermining, the extensively undermined side had 80% of the reported complications. There were no discernible differences in the aesthetic results obtained by either procedure.[7] Should flap necrosis occur, the area should be treated with conservatism, keeping the area moist and allowing it to heal by granulation and secondary intention. Fortunately, most of the time these appear in the postauricular areas, where they may not be as noticeable. Once final healing has been obtained, secondary scar revision can be pursued if required.

Unsightly Scars

Hypertrophic scarring and wide unsightly scars are a function of both tension on the suture line and an individual response to healing. In general, as in other wounds, the more tension placed on the skin in terms of wound closure, the more likely this will be a problem. For clearly hypertrophic, or keloidlike scars, intralesional steroids can be used. We prefer 10 mg of triamcinolone acetonide (Kenalog)/mL. For widened scars, surgical resection and then multilayered closure without tension following adequate wound maturation is the treatment of choice. A more conservative face-lift procedure with greater reliance on the SMAS support, as described by Webster and others, again, seems to help in avoiding these complications.[8–10]

Facial Nerve Injury

A serious complication of rhytidectomy is injury to the facial nerve. The literature reports incidence of injury to the nerve ranging from 0.5% to 2.6%[11,12] The most frequently injured branch of the facial nerve is the temporal, followed by the marginal.

Injury to the facial nerve is avoided in our technique by several actions. First, the proper plane of elevation is maintained throughout the procedure. Actual avoidance of danger regions during flap elevation helps ensure that the facial nerve is not harmed. If one does not undermine into the area of the temporal branch between the hairline and the lateral brow above the zygomatic arch, it would be unusual to encounter the nerve. Similarly, if only moderate facial flap elevation is used, the more distal branches of the nerve as they become more superficial are likewise avoided. Second, bipolar cautery is used throughout the procedure so that the current is localized and not allowed to radiate where it could do other damage, as would be the case with monopolar cautery.

Preoperative evaluation and careful photographic documentation of facial asymmetries and weaknesses are valuable tools that aid in the prevention of preexisting nerve problems.[13]

These conditions should be documented and pointed out to the patient as they occur. A history of facial weakness or Bell's palsy should, likewise, be noted in the chart in case the patient should have a recurrence of these problems in the postoperative period.

Other Nerve Injuries

Injury to the sensory nerves is typically of less consequence than injury to the facial nerve. Many patients will have a transient numbness in the area of the cheek or lower half of the ear during the early postoperative course, which usually disappears in 2 to 6 weeks. This may be particularly annoying for men because shaving in this area becomes difficult. Significant areas of numbness can be avoided by not injuring the great auricular nerve. During surgery care should be taken when one is dissecting over the sternocleidomastoid muscle inferior to the ear where this nerve is most superficial. Injury to the great auricular nerve can result in a permanent loss of sensation in the lower half of the ear and surrounding area. If dissection has extended into a deeper than usual surgical plane, other nerve injuries, such as injury to the 11th cranial nerve, are possible.

Earlobe Distortion

Too much tension on the earlobe area may widen the scar at this point or pull the ear in an inferior direction, producing a "satyr ear" or "pixie ear." This is an obvious sign of face-lift surgery and one that is difficult to camouflage. It is best avoided by draping the skin at the time of surgery so that it is well tucked up beneath the ear in a hammock-like fashion. There should not be tension on the earlobe during closure. If it occurs postoperatively, reexcision in this area with a tuck-up, or advancement, of skin will usually correct the problem. In patients with minimal earlobe development prior to surgery, creation of an earlobe is possible to avoid this problem in that anatomic situation.

Alopecia

If the flap is undermined in hair-bearing areas in too superficial a plane, damage to the hair follicles may result in permanent hair loss. Likewise, permanent alopecia may occur from vascular compromise from undue tension in the hair-bearing portion of the flaps. Cautery may be another cause of hair loss secondary to hair follicle damage. Utilization of bipolar cautery throughout the procedure will help minimize this. Fortunately, most hair loss is temporary and will return over 3 to 9 months.

In areas of hair loss, particularly around incision sites, small hair transplant autographs may be helpful. Likewise, a transposition of small, local hair-bearing flaps or simply advancement of the hair line, may correct the problem. Topical hair-stimulating medications such as minoxidil (Rogaine) have been suggested, but adequate experience as to their usefulness is not now available. In situations where the actual hair follicles have been damaged rather than are in simple telogen effluvium, these patients would not be expected to benefit from topical treatment.

In patients who have undergone prior face-lift procedures, the superoposterior advancement of the hairline may give the appearance of hair loss because of unnatural location of hair-bearing skin. In these cases, a modification of the face-lift incision should be considered to avoid further relocation of the hair-bearing skin, particularly in the preauricular, or sideburn, tufts.

BLEPHAROPLASTY

Preoperative Evaluation

Patient selection is important, particularly in cosmetic blepharoplasty patients. Certainly, only those physical complaints that can be reliably corrected by blepharoplasty should be selected, and those that do not respond well to surgery should be avoided. Equally important is a well-motivated patient with reasonable and realistic expectations for this elective cosmetic procedure. Although most of the clinical conditions that are collectively called "baggy lids" by the patient can be corrected, several problems cannot be surgically helped. Typically, dermatochalasis and aging skin changes along with protuberant fat pads and obicularis muscle hypertrophy can be corrected through outpatient surgery.[14]

The patient should be evaluated and counseled as to the degree of involvement from brow ptosis. The upper lid anatomy can be significantly affected by the level of the brow. Failure to correct brow ptosis in the clinically significant patient will result in a less satisfactory blepharoplasty result. Occasionally, simple correction of the brow will allow one to avoid upper lid blepharoplasty.

Brow lift can be pursued with a coronal approach, a mid-forehead lift, or a direct browpexy. The coronal brow lift that necessitates an incision posterior to the hairline (or at times at the hairline) shares the risk of most complications associated with rhytidectomy. These include hematoma, unsightly scarring, hair loss, and nerve damage.[15] The mid-brow lift, or browpexy (direct eyebrow lift), has additional problems, including visible scars.[16] With the direct brow approach, there tends to be a less natural elevation of the eyebrows, which, postoperatively, can be quite displeasing to the patient.[17] All of these procedures can result in numbness of the anterior scalp, which results from division of the supratrochlear nerve branches. Fortunately, sensation generally returns over a number of months, but numbness may sometimes be permanent. Frequently, itching is experienced as healing takes place.

A number of conditions will not be improved by surgery. These include a range of both local and systemic disorders that result in lid edema. Those edematous states are related to either metabolic disorders or allergic problems and, of course, will continue even after surgery. Hyperpigmentation and darker skin color in the periorbital area will not be corrected by blepharoplasty.

History of allergies related to medications and specifically the local anesthetics should be identified. Those patients who are taking aspirin or any medications with anticoagulant properties should cease intake of the medications for at least 2 weeks prior to surgery. It is a good idea to have the eyes checked prior to surgery, including documentation of visual acuity, level of moisturization of the eyes, and any preexisting ophthalmic problem. Those patients with a weak lower lid tarsus should realize that some type of lid-tightening or lid-shortening procedure must be added in addition to blepharoplasty to avoid postoperative problems. In addition, any suggestion of ptosis of the upper lids should be evaluated, and an additional procedure beyond blepharoplasty would be required to correct those patients.

Surgical Technique

Blepharoplasty of the Upper Lid

In the upright position, the upper lid should be marked and the surgical plan outlined since the reclining patient will change the appearance of the anatomy. The upper lid crease, which typically corresponds to the superior edge of the tarsal plate, is outlined with a fine line marker, and the line of the excision is extended laterally with an upward rotation of the line as it extends farther toward the lateral orbital rim. An attempt is made to avoid extending the excision beyond the lateral orbital rim into the thicker periorbital skin. Fat pads of the upper lid are located and marked over the area of prominence. Both sides should be marked independently, in that asymmetry and variation from one eye to the other is not unusual. Incisions that extend medially beyond the concavity of the junction of the nose to the lid should be avoided, or a risk of a webbed scar will be encountered. If a browlift is to be included, these incisional markings should be done in the upright position preoperatively as well.

With the patient's eyes closed, the redundant skin is grasped with the blades of smooth forceps, and the amount of excess skin is estimated and similarly marked.[18] Local anesthetic, which is typically 1% lidocaine (Xylocaine) with epinephrine 1:100,000, is infiltrated using a 27-gauge or smaller needle. An attempt is made to avoid distortion of the upper lid by not overinjecting. The skin incisions are made following the planned operative marks, and the skin to be resected is grasped and retracted medially while countertraction is maintained in the subcutaneous plane. Hemostasis is obtained with bipolar cautery or disposable ophthalmic heat cautery. The same procedure is done on the opposite lid.

In those patients with particularly heavy skin and a poorly defined upper lid crease, resection of a small strip of orbicularis muscle will be helpful. Attention is given to avoid superficial levator aponeurosis, and resection of boicularis muscle only as performed. Resection of this small strip of muscle will help the skin adhere to this layer and further demarcate a lid crease. No deep sutures are used for closure in this area. If the patient has clinically observable fat pads, a superficial stab excision through the muscle layer with spreading will allow the septum to be opened, the fat clamped and resected, and the base cauterized. No individual closure of the muscle layer is required following this maneuver.

The wound is closed with a running intracuticular 6-0 Prolene suture. The medial and lateral ends of the suture are left long so that they can be tacked to the skin with a small surgical tape.

Blepharoplasty of the Lower Lid

The lower lid blepharoplasty may be performed by elevating separate flaps (the skin flap followed by muscle excision) or combining it with what is typically known as the skin-muscle flap technique. Most frequently the skin-muscle flap technique is used. It separates the skin and orbicularis musculature from the septum orbitali and the orbital contents.

The lower lid is marked at the same time as the upper lid with the patient in a preoperative upright position. A planned line of incision several millimeters below the lashes is identified and extended laterally and superiorly to blend with the natural skin creases. Just as in the upper lid, an attempt should be made to avoid significant lateral extension beyond the orbital rim into thicker skin. Protruding fat pads are marked for later ease in identification.

After local anesthetic is infiltrated, the skin is incised along the line parallel with the lower lid lash line as marked preoperatively. The skin-muscle flap is developed using small curved blunt scissors. The plane of dissection is beneath the level of the orbicularis muscle but superficial to the septum orbitali and is continued from lateral to medial to a point corresponding with the medial puncta. Inferiorly, the dissection is extended down to approximately the level of the orbital rim. Hemostasis is obtained using bipolar cautery. A small bulb irrigator is often helpful to keep the field clear while hemostasis is being obtained.

At this point the septum orbitali and its underlying fat pads are in direct view. If the amount of fat protrusion is minimal, a direct cauterization of the septum orbitali may effectively tighten the septum and replace the fat back into normal position.[19] This is accomplished with a sweeping motion of the cautery over the most protruding area, in effect, creating cauterized stripes until a flat septal appearance is accomplished. In those patients who do not benefit from the cautery technique (e.g., those with excessive amounts of fat), fat pads may be approached openly and excised. The septum is opened directly above the fat compartment, and without traction the fat is allowed to extrude into the wound. The base is clamped with a small hemostat. The excess fat is cut away and its base cauterized with electrocautery. It is important that the fat be grasped with forceps beneath the hemostat before the hemostat is released. The fatty stump is inspected for bleeding, and if any is present, it is cauterized before the stump is allowed to retract back into the orbital contents. This is completed for all three compartments, medial, central, and lateral, as required.

The skin-muscle flap is now redraped and a smooth configuration of the lid is attained. It is important to avoid over-resection of the skin muscle flap in the vertical direction. The flap is redraped in a laterosuperior fashion. Often in a young patient who has had primarily a fat pad problem, minimal skin may need to be resected. Conservativism is always favored in the lower lid. Avoid an overaggressive resection with too much vertical shortening. This could result in ectropion and should be in the mind of the surgeon at this point in the procedure.

Following a resection and redraping of the skin, the muscle level is grasped and a 5-0 Vicryl suture used to suture the muscular layer in a suspensory fashion to the orbital periosteum at the level of the lateral canthus.[20] Following resection of excess skin and muscle and placement of the suspensory suture, the wound is closed in one layer. An ophthalmic antibiotic ointment is placed on the suture lines of the upper and lower lids, and small ice pads are placed over the eyes for the next 4 to 12 hours postoperatively. No other dressings are used.

Postoperative Care

The sutures are removed at 4 to 7 days, and the eyes are kept moisturized with antibiotic ointment until that time.

Shortening of the Horizontal Lid

When horizontal lid laxity exists in the blepharoplasty patient, a horizontal lid shortening maneuver must be contemplated. Preoperative identification of these patients generally is through an abnormal lower lid snap test. In this group of patients, a full-thickness lid-shortening procedure avoids scleral show and ectropion postoperatively.

The procedure is accomplished following elevation of the skin or skin-muscle flap. A pentagonal block may be resected lateral to the limbus. This procedure is essentially a modified Kuhnt-Szymanowski procedure. To determine the width of the resection (which is usually 3 to 4 mm), the lateral-most half of the pentagon is made first, allowing the medial segment to overlap and identifying the amount of redundancy. The medial portion is then resected and the wound closed.

The wound is approximated with 6-0 silk sutures at the area of the pentagonal resection. Sutures should not go through the conjunctiva. Additional augmentation can be gained by placing a single 6-0 Vicryl suture through the tarsal plate. The silk marginal sutures are left long enough to be brought out over the skin flap and anchored inferiorly with a Steri-Strip. The skin flap or the skin-muscle flap is then handled as described earlier and closed in routine fashion. The marginal sutures, however, are left in place for a full 7 days.

Complications

As in all surgeries, complications can occur in blepharoplasty even with appropriate precautions and in the best of hands. Fortunately, serious complications are uncommon and, when they do occur, can generally be managed successfully. A discussion of several areas that would be included as complications follows.

Vision Loss

Perhaps the worst complication of blepharoplasty is vision loss or complete blindness. Fortunately, this is extremely rare. The mechanism has not been totally identified but is presumed to be from retrobulbar hemorrhage leading to intraorbital and intraocular pressure, compromising the circulation to the optic disk and central retinal artery.[21–23]

Ectropion

Ectropion is a more common complication and a distressing problem following blepharoplasty of the lower lid.[24] Ectropion may be related to excessive removal of skin in the vertical direction. A frequent, and perhaps less frequently recognized, problem, however, is the failure to treat laxity of the eyelids. The snap test preoperatively is a useful guide to determine if lids that do not spring back to coapted position against the globe when pulled out should be shortened or tightened as part of the procedure. Minor degrees of ectropion generally improve with time, and the use of taping and massage, in addition to forceful squinting exercises, will frequently clear the problem without further surgery.

Dry Eye

Most patients will have a temporary dryness of the eyes, which generally will not be a problem. However, prolonged dryness of the eye or an eye that was preoperatively dry and now exacerbated following surgery can result in corneal irritation. Lubricants and artificial tears along with patching are helpful techniques in preventing subsequent ophthalmic problems until normal moisturization has returned.

Lagophthalmos

Lagophthalmos is less frequent than problems with the lower lid and tends to be related to excessive skin excision of the upper lid. When permanent, it is best corrected by placement of a thin full-thickness skin graft on the area. Other causes of lagophthalmos may be related to damage to the orbital septum or may involve the orbital septum with suturing.

Ptosis

It is important to check for ptosis during the preoperative eye evaluation. Postoperative ptosis may be temporary and due to edema, hematoma, or reversible injury to the levator aponeurosis, as from cautery. Many patients will have had a preoperative ptosis and not recognize it and only begin to notice it postoperatively if it is not corrected. In this situation, it is not a complication of cosmetic surgery but a condition that will not be improved without additional procedures. Postoperative ptosis should be treated conservatively and ophthalmic correction of levator repair considered if it does not appear to be responding.

Unsightly Scars

The thin skin of the lid usually heals with acceptable scars. However, just as in other anatomic sites, hypertrophic or contracted scars may occur. Fortunately, most of these resolve with conservative treatment, but small scar revisions may, at times, be required.

REFERENCES

1. Thomas JR: Complications of aesthetic surgery, in Johns ME (ed): *Complications in Otolaryngology–Head and Neck Surgery.* St Louis, CV Mosby Co, 1986.
2. Baker DC, Aston SJ, Guy CL, et al: The male rhytidectomy. *Plast Reconst Surg* 1977; 60:514–522.
3. McGregor MW, Greenberg RL: Rhytidectomy, in Goldwin RN (ed): *The Unfavorable Result in Plastic Surgery:*

Avoidance and Treatment. Boston, Little, Brown & Co, 1972, pp 335–344.

4. Conway H: The surgical facelift—rhytidectomy. *Plast Reconst Surg* 1970; 45:124–130.

5. Pitanguy I, Ramos H, Garcia L: Filosofia Technica e Complicacoes das Ritidectomiaa Atrávas de Abservacas e Analise de 2600 Casos Pessoalis Consecutivos. *Rev Bras Cir* 1972; 62:277.

6. Webster GV: The ischemic facelift. *Plast Reconst Surg* 1972; 50:560–562.

7. Peterson R: The role of the platysma muscle in cervical lifting, in Goulion D (ed): *Symposium of Surgery of the Aging Face.* St Louis, CV Mosby Co, 1978.

8. Webster RC, Davidson TM, White MF, et al: Conservative facelift surgery. *Arch Otolaryngol* 1976; 102:657–662.

9. Webster RC, Smith RC, Smith KF: Extent of undermining of skin flaps. *Head Neck Surg* 1983; Jul/Aug: 525–534.

10. Webster RC, Smith RC, Smith KF: Facelift, part 3: Plication of the superficial musculoaponeurotic system. *Head Neck Surg* 1983; Nov/Dec: 696–701.

11. Baker TJ, Gordeon HL, Mosienko P: Rhytidectomy—a statistical analysis. *Plast Reconst Surg* 1977; 59:24–30.

12. Baker TJ, Gordeon HL: Complications of rhytidectomy. *Plast Reconst Surg* 1967; 40:31.

13. Thomas JR, Tardy ME, Prezkop H: Uniform photographic documentation in facial plastic surgery. *Otolaryngol Clin North Am* 1980; 13:367.

14. Cook TA: Baggy eyelids, in Gates G (ed): *Current Therapy in Otolaryngology–Head and Neck Surgery 1986–1987.* St Louis, CV Mosby Co, 1987.

15. Johnson CM, Willett JM: The coronal foreheadlift: Present status. *Adv Ophthalmol Plast Reconstr Surg* 1983; 2:1971.

16. Johnson CM, Waldman SR: Mid foreheadlift. *Arch Otolaryngol* 1983; 109:155.

17. Brennan HG: Management of the ptotic brow. *Otolaryngol Clin North Am* 1980; 13:272.

18. Thomas JR, David WE: Pinch technique blepharoplasty for the upper eyelid. *Ear Nose Throat J* 1977; 65:40–42.

19. Cook TA, Dereberry J, Harrah R: Reconsideration of fat pad management in lower lid blepharoplasty surgery. *Arch Otolaryngol* 1984; 110:521–524.

20. Webster RC, Davidson TM, Reardon EJ, et al: Suspending sutures in blepharoplasty. *Arch Otolaryngol* 1979; 105:601–604.

21. Jafek BW, Kreiger AE, Morledge DM: Blindness following blepharoplasty. *Arch Otolaryngol* 1973; 98:366.

22. DeMere M, Wood T, Austin W: Eye complications with blepharoplasty or other eyelid surgery. *Plast Reconstr Surg* 1974; 53:634.

23. Kelly P, May D: Central retinal artery occlusion following cosmetic blepharoplasty. *Br J Ophthalmol* 1980; 64:918–923.

24. Hamako C, Baylis HI: Lower eyelid retraction following blepharoplasty. *Am J Ophthalmol* 1980; 89:517–521.

Rhytidectomy and Blepharoplasty

Approach of

J. Richard Casuccio, M.D.

The cosmetic surgeon must be perceptive and observant. Because much of cosmetic surgery training consists of long hours of watching accomplished specialists, with few opportunities for hands-on experience, students must be technically accomplished before beginning such training. They must be able to translate visual images into coordinated hand motions. Unlike sculptors, who can test their ideas and techniques in plaster, cosmetic surgeons must transcribe their mental images directly into an aesthetic operative result. Thus an honest appraisal of one's surgical talents is the first act of humility for the cosmetic surgeon. Establishing their limitations and knowing their capability to correct a patient's particular physical concern is a responsibility they owe both themselves and their patients. They should be perceptive about a patient's true desires and willing to refuse surgery to a patient with unrealistic expectations. They should see problems before they occur, and be able to rectify them should they occur. Being sympathetic, articulate, and occasionally quick-witted can be helpful in achieving a graceful solution to a difficult situation.

I am not advocating that surgeons go out and make mistakes

for the sake of experience. Rather, a cosmetic surgeon should have a broad surgical background with many good experiences and some bad from which to learn and grow. I expect that a formidable number of those experiences will be guided and supervised by a tutor, whose valuable knowledge can become the future tools of the surgical student. Cosmetic operations are reasonably standardized, and some are technically easy; but the difference between the novice and the expert is less likely to be a matter of talent and more a reflection of the surgeon's powers of observation, the ability to recognize a potential problem and avoid it, and the ability to learn from one's own mistakes and the mistakes of others. I hope to illustrate this philosophy with a summary of my approach to the cosmetic patient and the methods I use to minimize the potential for complications in face-lift and blepharoplasty operations. Inasmuch as the perfect face-lift and blepharoplasty have yet to be defined, each surgeon must establish which techniques are best for him or her and the patients. Many texts are available through which students of cosmetic surgery can learn of the variety of surgical procedures for the face. I will not reiterate what is already written, nor recommend any single technique. Instead, my goal will be demonstration of a thought process that is dedicated to achieving a noticeable improvement for each patient, with minimal risk of surgical complications.

PATIENT SELECTION

My approach to cosmetic surgery starts by knowing the cosmetic patient as an individual, and it begins at the moment of introduction. I try to learn about his or her concerns and motivations, priorities, and problems. I like to know both the medical and personal backgrounds and how the patient expects his or her life-style to change after aesthetic surgery. I need two interviews to become comfortable with a patient, and hopefully during that time the patient will become comfortable with me. In the first interview I let the patient do most of the talking. I take a medical history, perform an examination, explain the options briefly, and allow the patient to take over the conversation. At the end of the session I invite the patient to talk to my staff about any financial questions they may have. Brochures are provided, and the patient is invited to return when a decision has been made as to the surgery desired.

I invite opinions of the patients from my staff, and am frequently impressed at their insight. Patients are at times more open and perhaps more truthful with office personnel, whom they feel they do not have to impress.

In the second interview I do much of the talking, explaining the surgery and, most important, what should and should not be expected from a cosmetic operation. My staff has accused me on occasion of trying to talk the patient out of having surgery, but in truth this has rarely happened. More to the point, by using this two-interview process I have been able to expose inconsistencies between a patient's requests and desires that make cosmetic goals impractical. I am thus warned to avoid surgery on that person. On other occasions I have brought patients to realize that cosmetic surgery or myself as a surgeon is not what they truly want, and they return to their life more learned about themselves or more knowledgeable about the type of surgeon they would like to have.

Good patient selection is not ideal patient selection, and cosmetic surgeons must be competent to address a multitude of situations, providing each patient with the reasonable expectation of improvement. The key word here is improvement; no one should expect miracles.

EXAMINATION

My examination begins the moment the patient and I are introduced. I observe the way the patient walks and sits, the way he or she speaks, gazes, blinks, squints, frowns, and smiles. I examine their posture and try to read their body language. Once the patient identifies the reason for the visit, all of the visual information I have accumulated serves as an assay for the depth of feeling that the patient has for the problem. Also important is how quickly the patient can come to the point when defining what exactly he or she does not like about their physical self. In short, I must know the patient's mind, and I must know it accurately so that I can direct my attentions to the patient's needs. I am not interested in correcting features that are of little concern to the patient.

From this point, the examination is continued in front of a mirror. I use either a wall mirror or a simple hand-held mirror. I believe that the mirror examination is essential because it allows the surgeon to see the patient as the patient sees himself or herself. Though human beings are blessed with binocular vision, they cannot look at themselves in three dimensions. Whether by reflection, photography, or television, we see ourselves as flat objects. It is from this perspective that we must study our patients to gain insight to their anatomic concerns and to discuss solutions from a common frame of reference.

To further evaluate the patient's face, I frequently take photographs. This not only provides a two-dimensional record that can be studied later but isolates the face from the surrounding distractions. I can see the face as a whole in isolation and can mentally analyze each of the features that contribute to or detract from facial aesthetics. Occasionally I will look at the patient through the camera viewfinder with only one eye open. I am amazed at how often I notice some subtle anatomic nuance that would otherwise be missed. Conversely, if I have done all of these things and still cannot see a problem, the patient is most likely fixated on his or her face and is not a good candidate for cosmetic surgery.

When the examination is completed and after the findings are studied and digested, I define the realistic surgical possibilities for the patient. I can then choose the technique that will give me the best chance of accomplishing the goal. Unfortunately, the techniques that one might employ to achieve benefit and minimize complications when doing a face-lift or blepharoplasty are varied and nonspecific. Ideally, science should guide the hands of surgeons, telling them which operations are beneficial and which techniques are safe. Ideally, this would be done through a series of well-controlled studies with arduous scrutiny of the results before any conclusions are made. But cosmetic surgery, unlike other surgical disciplines, does not conform neatly to the precepts of the scientific method. Controls are difficult to establish, and the results are difficult to analyze objectively. As a result, much of the literature has been dedicated to empirical observation and personal impression, and this is the best that can be offered for the foreseeable future and perhaps forever.

My single recommendation for dealing with this dilemma is that the cosmetic surgeon draw on his or her own education and surgical experiences. By the time a surgeon enters cosmetic practice, he or she has considerable understanding and a broad repertoire of cosmetic, reconstructive, and functional procedures for the face and eyelids. By keeping a wide-angled perspective and refusing to become narrowed by nip-and-tuck surgery, one can develop the technical refinement needed to be an accomplished cosmetic surgeon. This critical assimilation of previous observations and personal experiences allows the surgeon to develop a style that is both competent and predictable. The following is my approach to the face-lift operation, which has evolved over 8 years and continues to evolve as my experience grows.

RHYTIDECTOMY

Face-lift incisions are reasonably standardized,[1,2] but there are as many minor variations as there are surgeons performing the operation. I am not aware of any rules, but certainly it is desirable to place the incisions where they are concealed best yet allow a healthy facial flap to be elevated easily. My approach is to begin the incision in the hairline about 4 cm above the high point of the ear. It then continues anteriorly in the preauricular crease, around the lobule, leaving a 2 mm cuff of facial skin, and behind the ear just posterior to the postauricular sulcus to the level of the tragus. Finally, a gradual 90-degree turn is made posteriorly, and a 4 to 5 cm cut across the hairline concludes the incision. I am comfortable with this incision, but I must be cognizant of two potential problems. The first concern stems from my preference to conceal my incisions in the hairline; therefore I do not want to elevate the flaps so thinly that I injure the hair follicles and cause noticeable alopecia. The second potential problem is failure to align the hairline properly after flap advancement.

I elevate a flap that is not too thin by restricting the elevation to very definable planes. I do not use SMAS dissection, but I do use the SMAS as a landmark for appropriate plane for flap elevation. The SMAS represents that fascia that overlies both the muscles of facial expression and the facial nerve; thus dissection above this fascia protects these structures. The SMAS also continues as the galea aponeurotica superiorly and is contiguous with the platysma muscle inferiorly. With experience, this relatively bloodless sheet of fascia is recognized easily. I make a superior incision down to the level of the galea, which is well below the hair follicles. From here the temple can be elevated safely. I dissect no farther than the hairline, because further dissection does not improve the result, and may lead to facial nerve injury, since the nerve resides in this plane; however, as the dissection approaches the root of the zygoma, further caution is warranted. Although the temporal branch of the facial

nerve becomes superficial (penetrates the fascia) as it crosses the zygoma, it is still subfascial at the zygomatic root. Careful dissection will free the fascia from the skin, but an extra margin of safety can be achieved by bluntly defining and separating this plane by placing a piece of gauze on the fingertips and sweeping the fascia away from the skin.[3] Below the zygoma, I use the classic scissors dissection technique of spreading and cutting.

The dissection behind the ear follows the same principles, but there are a couple of nuances that I would like to share. The SMAS does not extend behind the ear, or at least current anatomic research has not defined such a continuation. To avoid developing a flap that is too thin and causing hair loss behind the ear, I incise down to the fascia that overlies the mastoid periosteum. The dissection divides this superficial fascia, which is then elevated with the facial flap to protect the vascularity of the facial skin. Again, elevation in this plane is commonly bloodless, and the hair follicles are well protected by the thickness of the flap. As the dissection approaches the tendinous portion of the sternocleidomastoid muscle, the tough fibrous attachments that connect the overlying skin to the underlying periosteum must be sharply divided. When the posterior border of the sternocleidomastoid muscle is recognized, the dissection is stopped. Continuing in this plane would undermine the platysma muscle. The facial (preauricular) dissection is now continued inferiorly over the platysma, where it will eventually open into the posterior dissection along the border of the platysma. The two planes are connected by transsecting the superficial cervical fascia in a safe and relatively bloodless area. This approach of flap elevation depends on definite landmarks (sternocleidomastoid muscle, platysma, zygoma) and definable planes (galea aponeurotica, mastoid fascia, SMAS). The goal, as ever, is a good result via a safe and comfortable technique.

The *pixie ear* is perhaps the telltale sign of face-lift surgery. To avoid the pixie ear I keep a 2 mm cuff of facial skin attached to the lobule.[3] When the facial flap is advanced, I bury the ear under the flap and keep it there until the flaps are secured to adjacent and nondissected skin above and behind the ear. Thus tension is diverted away from the lower half of the ear. Once satisfied with the lift of the facial flaps, I trim away the excess skin. If I err, it is on the side of conservatism, excising too little rather than too much. The skin edges surrounding the earlobe should fall together in perfect approximation. Sutures are placed to maintain epidermal alignment and not to provide support.

If a pixie deformity occurs, the easiest way to resolve the problem is to separate the lobule from the face and close the facial incision in a V-Y fashion. The anterior limb of the V is undermined where the posterior limb is not. In this way the closure is made slightly behind the earlobe, where a natural shadow would fall. The lobule can then be tailored as needed and closed on itself. The resulting scars will be visible but less noticeable than the pixie deformity, and can be camouflaged with earrings or makeup. The timing of such revision depends on the surgeon's honest estimation of what went wrong. If the pixie ear was the result of a technical error, such as an excessive excision of skin, it may be addressed as soon as it is noted, perhaps at the time of the original surgery. If the cause is less clear, a period of observation allows the deforming forces to come to equilibrium, which then allows a more predictable reconstruction.

As a senior medical student rotating on the plastic surgery service, I can remember the department chairman speaking of the face-lift as the antigravity operation. If an operation is to be designed to oppose gravity, the techniques used should reflect this goal. In face-lift surgery, the facial flaps can be advanced posteriorly or rotated superiorly. Either direction will improve the facial definition by removing the excess tissue and tightening the remaining skin; but since humans walk upright and since few spend much of their day recumbent, a superiorly rotated flap is a more logical choice to counteract the downward forces that contribute to sagging jowls and farrowed skin. Such rotation gives better definition to the jawline and the upper part of the neck. The continuity of the hairline is maintained, and this is of particular benefit for those of us who bury the incisions within the hairline above and behind the ear. It also minimizes the postauricular redundancy of skin (dog ear) that can be a nuisance to remove. I think it gives a more natural look.

The elevation and tailoring of the SMAS is an intriguing idea based on some excellent anatomic studies.[4] It has been touted to improve the lift of facial tissues, particularly in the perioral area, and has been credited with increasing the duration of such results. I no longer use it. The effect of an SMAS lift is obvious on the operating table, but I have yet to see a definable benefit in the early postoperative period. I concede that this may be a reflection of my technique and training, but I trust my powers of observation, and for me to add an extra dissection to a procedure that carries a small but definite risk to the facial nerve, I must see a difference. In terms of facial improvement, results with or without SMAS lift appear similar to me during the first 6 months to 1 year after surgery, and I have concluded that the extra effort and time are not worth the risk. I concede that the SMAS may increase durability of a face-lift, but I have found no compelling data in that regard.

The single best improvement to my face-lift technique has been the addition of suction lipectomy. Previously I struggled with the removal of fat from the neck, which was made difficult by poor visibility and bleeding that was often difficult to control. Lumpiness of the neck due to retained clumps of fat was a continual source of frustration. I now minimize problems by adding liposuction techniques to the face-lift. The use of both a 1.8 mm three-port cannula and a 2.4 mm two-port cannula allows blunt elevation of the skin of the neck through a small stab incision just beneath the chin. Suction then can be applied to remove fat uniformly, avoiding bleeding and skin irregularities. The fatty double chin can be noticeably reduced, and in many cases (those without platysmal bands) this may be all that is needed to refine the neck. The same technique can be adapted to the cheeks, jowls, and perioral area to minimize the need for scissors dissection when the facial nerve is known to be superficial. After completing the standard flap elevation, which dissects and elevates a flap from the incisions to an imaginary line drawn from the zygomaticotemporal suture line to the antegonial notch, the suction cannula is passed beneath the skin and above the SMAS under direct vision.[5] Pretunneling is done so as to parallel the seventh nerve, and depending on the fullness of the cheeks, suction may or may not be used. If the cheeks are chubby, a more aggressive lipectomy may be needed, and it can be done by reorienting the cannula some 45 to 60

degrees to the previous tunnel tracts and continuing with the suction. Though some authors[5, 6] have suggested doing this through stab incisions made in the nasolabial fold, I most often do it through the facial incisions by reorienting the cannula to parallel the nasolabial fold. Further lipectomy of the neck, if needed, also can be done through this lateral facial approach where the upper part of the neck can be suctioned horizontally, thus satisfying the cross-suctioning principle. If a more extended flap elevation is needed for contouring purposes, it is now done easily by pushing away the subcutaneous attachments to the skin with an open scissors. For me, blunt cannula dissection and liposuction have shortened the time of surgery and made my results more consistent, with less bleeding and risk of facial nerve palsy. These techniques also allow me to elevate a facial flap while maintaining a maximum number of vascular and neural attachments. Again, if we recognize the paucity of data, when a limited dissection of facial tissues can be done, albeit with a suction cannula, it would seem logical that the opportunities for complications also would be limited.[7]

BLEPHAROPLASTY

Perhaps my two most vivid memories from medical school are admonitions from a couple of internists for whom I have great respect. The first was the advice that physicians should pursue a medical mystery as Sherlock Holmes would pursue a criminal investigation. After reading *The Annotated Sherlock Holmes,*[8] I realized that Holmes is less a detective and more a physician. His techniques are organized, his reasoning deductive, and his observations complete. He is knowledgeable beyond his area of specialization. More to the point, the characters of Holmes and Watson are the latent egos of Doyle, who was a practicing physician. He used his understanding of late 19th century medicine, particularly the discipline of physical diagnosis, to develop a fictional physician who solved social riddles rather than medical ones.

The second admonition is basic and easy to remember, but I am afraid it is often forgotten. It was quoted by a learned but frustrated professor who was visibly irritated by his case review of a patient who had received improper treatment. With irritation deep in his voice, he beseeched his students to remember that regardless of their choice of specialty, they should never forget that they are first and foremost physicians.

A patient desiring cosmetic blepharoplasty deserves our expertise, which should extend beyond the technical to include a lucid evaluation of the patient's needs, desires, and limitations. Lest we be replaced by some less-educated technician, as has already happened in some countries, we should maintain our ability and right to carefully examine our patients. We should be able to look beyond the obvious to find the obscure that could undermine surgery that is otherwise perfect.

Blepharoplasty is a highly reliable and beneficial cosmetic operation. Yet patient selection, reasonable goals, and the proper choice of technique are the keys to successful eyelid surgery. Perhaps every patient who has an interest in this procedure desires the wrinkle-free, smooth, and pristine skin of their early teenage years, eyelids without puffiness, and eyes that are not sunken. Realistically, that is not possible for the 50-year-old who is slightly overweight, who has had a lifetime of sun exposure, whose eyelids are chronically puffy, and whose skin is cobblestoned and furrowed. This appearance does not make the individual less a candidate, but the goals for this patient must be defined so that there is an equitable compromise between what is desired and what can be achieved.

The first step toward improved eyelid appearance starts with an understanding of how the eyelids age. The particular tissue changes that have occurred over time will determine the type of correction that will best benefit the patient. Next the surgeon must identify those peculiar signs that can predispose to a less than optimum result. Finally, a mental review of the various techniques available is needed to determine the operation that best satisfies the patient's needs.

The evaluation begins with a definition of the problem. For example, if the patient complains that he or she always looks tired because the eyelids are puffy and sag, the surgeon must determine whether this puffiness is due to herniated orbital fat, chronic eyelid edema, thickened and redundant skin, or a combination of some or all of these. This is done by a careful analysis that is both visual and tactile.

Once a feel for the problem is established, the surgeon must look for all the signs that set traps for the casual and occasional plastic surgeon. This instinct for the pitfalls comes with training and experience and can prevent a straightforward operation from becoming a disaster. For the blepharoplasty operation, it starts with an acute knowledge of orbital and periorbital anatomy and continues with understanding of the pathophysiology of that region. The surgeon should know the physical examination of this area with precision and should be cognizant of the variety of treatments, medical as well as surgical, that are applicable to the periorbital tissues. In short, look for problems carefully.

The examination includes the obvious checks of pupillary responses and extraocular eye movements. Measurements of the interpupillary and intercanthal distances are taken. Upper eyelid excursion is measured, and the locations of the palpebral margins are noted in relationship to the iris. A Schirmer test is done, and a fluorescein test is performed if there is a history or signs of eye irritation. The eyelids and the globes are studied for any lesions, asymmetry, or abnormality of position. Visual fields can be checked quickly by standing eye to eye with the patient. From arm's length, a bright point of light is moved from a variety of directions toward the space between the patient and the examiner; both should see the light at about the same time. Visual acuity can be checked by either a reading test or a standard eye chart. Even the fundi are examined, if for no other purpose than to quantify any concurrent medical problems. Though such an examination is time consuming, I recommend that the surgeon complete the examination himself or herself rather than ignoring it or deferring it to the patient's ophthalmologist. Eyelid abnormalities are often subtle in the older population and may not be of great concern to either the patient or eye specialist; however, eyelid surgery in such a patient could amplify the problem, making it more noticeable and bothersome. A multitude of potential problems can be ruled out by careful examination of the patient. Dry eye, minor conjunctival

and corneal abrasions, eye allergies, ptosis, lid lag, ectropion, entropion, enophthalmos, and proptosis are some conditions that can turn a cosmetic blepharoplasty into a nightmare. Should anything be found abnormal, the appropriate consultation or treatment is recommended, and cosmetic surgery is deferred until the problem is rectified.

If all is fine except for signs of aging, the evaluation progresses to quantifying the aesthetic problem and choosing those techniques that will best suit the patient's needs. Gentle probing and poking and pulling of the eyelids help to tell the surgeon the limits of surgery. Slight pressure applied to the upper eyelid may demonstrate the herniation of fat into the lower lid. Similarly, pressure to the lower lid or lateral canthus may magnify the herniation in the upper lid. Remember, the protrusion of fat into the eyelids is recognized during the examination and is not caused by the examination. The manipulations should amplify the hernia already present and not create one, since there is no reason to remove eyelid fat for prophylaxis. Chronic eyelid edema, usually noted in the lower lids, is distinguished by slow reinflation of the skin after it is squeezed for a moment. When the eyelid is as decongested as possible, it can be studied for underlying fat herniation. The eyelids should be examined while the patient gazes upward with the mouth wide open. This, better than any other test, will give the surgeon the best idea of how much skin, if any, can be safely removed from the lower eyelid. Based on these manipulations, assisted by the mirror examination and photographs, a map can be drawn highlighting the critical eyelid features. Thus a blueprint of the operation is made. The type of incision and approach to be used, the location and amount of fat to be removed, and the excess skin and muscle to be excised are all illustrated. When the surgeon walks into the operating theater the goals are well outlined. The changes in the patient's face that occur after the patient assumes a recumbent position or after the induction of general anesthesia can often be misleading; however, if the surgeon is equipped with the map, he or she will not lose direction.

Many times I have heard blepharoplastic surgeons comment that they always remove equal amounts of fat from both orbits or that they remove only fat that spontaneously herniates from the orbit after the septum is opened, swearing that they never chase fat. In addition, I have noticed a tendency among eyelid surgeons to use the same flap for lower eyelid blepharoplasty regardless of the amount or type of tissue to be removed. I am sure this surgery by rote works in a number of cases, but it is neither scientific nor artistic. The purpose of plastic surgery is to satisfy the individual needs of the patient, whether they be physical or mental, with surgery that is unique to them. That is why there are few standard operations in reconstructive surgery. This principle should be utilized in cosmetic surgery as well. My recommendation to any surgeon venturing into this field is that he or she be well-versed in all the techniques, cosmetic as well as reconstructive, and know how and when to use them. When the problem is baggy eyes caused solely by fat herniation, why chance an ectropion by excising skin? The simple removal of fat through a transconjunctival approach will suffice.[9] As an alternative, fat can be removed through a subciliary incision after a skin-muscle flap is elevated. There is no need to extend the incision beyond the lateral canthus if there is no need to excise skin. When a small amount of redundant skin is apparent, an excision of the composite of excess of skin and muscle is preferred. A skin-muscle flap is elevated through the subciliary approach. The lateral limb of the incision is kept short so that the motor nerve to the orbicularis oculi is not injured.[10] After upward and lateral advancement of the flap, a narrow strip of skin and muscle, usually not more than 5 mm, is excised.

Although infrequent, there are occasions when the lower lid skin is highly redundant and the predicted skin excess will be substantially greater than 5 mm. I suggest that the best, and perhaps only, solution to this situation is blepharoplasty using the skin flap technique. I am least fond of this approach, because it requires that the muscle belly of the orbicularis be divided to expose the orbital fat. Bleeding, which must be meticulously controlled in eyelid surgery, is a common and annoying feature of the skin flap technique. On occasion the injured muscle forms a scar that adheres to the skin flap, creating a small dimple or linear depression in the central lower eyelid. If fine, absorbable sutures are used to close these muscular fenestrations, they may leave small but visible bumps in the skin. Both of these problems are certainly minor considerations, which can be easily corrected later with surgical touch-up, and should not deter a surgeon from using the technique if it will best serve the patient.

The upper lid blepharoplasty is a straightforward operation well illustrated in a number of texts.[10] My thoughts concerning this procedure are about planning. The majority of plastic surgeons examine patients for blepharoplasty while they are sitting in a chair, but when it comes to making the critical markings for surgery the patients are most likely lying down. There is no question that the facial highlights change as body position changes. The upper eyelid redundancies that are so obvious during the office examination are difficult to see when the patient is on the operating table. At times I find myself guessing at the proper position of the upper incision. That incision is obvious when the markings are made preoperatively with the patient sitting or standing.[11]

I prefer to do a blepharoplasty with the patient awake so that I can enlist the patient's help throughout the procedure. This is truest when I am prepared to excise skin and muscle from the lower eyelids. At that moment I have the patient open the mouth widely and look upward. What was an excessive amount of skin a moment earlier may now be only a few millimeters. A few millimeters with an ounce of conservatism is all that should be excised. If the patient is under general anesthesia or heavily sedated, as may be the case if a face-lift is being done at the same operation, I support the patient's mouth open with a 40 mm bite block. For both the upper and lower lids, I exercise more caution and excise slightly less tissue than I would if the patient were awake. Minor corrections can be made easily 6 months later in the office, with local anesthesia.

Few complications are more disconcerting than the appearance of an ectropion following lower lid blepharoplasty. It may occur after any procedure that makes an incision in the lower lid, regardless if skin has been excised or not. The cause is often not clear, but I have generally found it to be most likely due to one of four reasons: (1) underlying senile ectropion, (2) excision of too much lower lid skin, (3) inadvertent elevation

of both eyelid and cheek skin as a single flap, and (4) accidental dehiscence of the incision after the sutures are removed.

If an ectropion is noted, the eye must be checked for adequate lubrication and protection, and the appropriate therapy prescribed if a corneal abrasion or conjunctival irritation is noted. In most cases a few drops of artificial tears every 2 to 4 hours and nightly taping of the eyelids closed will suffice. In others, antibiotic ointment and an ophthalmologic consultation may be needed. In rare occasions, particularly if the ectropion is noticed during the first or second day after surgery and the cause is from a small subcutaneous hematoma or a dehiscence of the suture line, the retracted skin can be reelevated and redraped with as little manipulation as possible. If this is not the case or if it is not feasible, I recommend a period of observation so long as the eye has adequate protection. In an atmosphere clouded by anxiety, the physician must act sympathetically to allay fears and to instill a sense of confidence to the patient that the situation is under control and the ectropion, though a complication, can be remedied.

Ectropion is an example of a difficult complication, not because it requires sophisticated surgery to correct it, albeit it can, but because it may require no treatment at all. With minor lower lid ectropion there is lower lid conjunctival show and scleral show below the iris but functional competence of the lid and full protection of the globe. My usual approach to this problem is to do nothing surgically for 3 to 6 months. Instead, I recommend light massaging of the involved eyelid and nightly taping of the lids closed with a bandage. Of the ectropions I have seen as a result of either cosmetic or traumatic surgery, nearly all have resolved spontaneously without need for further surgery, and surprisingly, even some more major ectropions have improved to the degree where if any surgery is needed, it is relatively minor. If a major ectropion requires skin grafting, the donor skin best suited for this purpose is from the upper eyelid so long as excess skin is available. Postauricular skin is a lesser choice. When an ectropion occurs because of the elevation or excision of too much skin or the failure to recognize an underlying condition that predisposes to ectropion, the surgeon should first recognize the mistake and learn from it, and then proceed with the appropriate correction. The greatest challenge is the careful nurturing of the physician-patient relationship, which is built on mutual confidence and respect, a trust that will allow the patient to wait through many weeks of frustration to achieve the expected good result.

I would like to explore two final ideas that parallel my theme of good results by careful planning, excellent technique, and thorough understanding of the problem and its solutions. I will borrow from Dr. Ralph Millard as written in his text *The Principalization of Plastic Surgery*.[12] In one of the early chapters he explained his preference for doing a face-lift before blepharoplasty, and lower lids before upper lids. I use the same approach, but my reasoning is basic. I proceed from the most grueling part of the operation to the least so. Among my peers, a variety of approaches are used, most based on personal quirks, as were mine. Millard, however, is much more pragmatic. The face-lift, though not an operation for eyelid abnormalities, will nonetheless alter the position of the lateral eyelid skin. If blepharoplasty is done first, the original orientation of the lateral excision is altered, perhaps to a less than optimum location. When the face-lift is done first, the eyelid incisions remain where they were made. Millard fashions pressure dressing to the face immediately after completing the lift and before starting the eyelid surgery. This simple maneuver may limit the potential for facial hematoma while the blepharoplasty is being done.

The lower eyelids are more prone to postoperative problems than the upper eyelids. As mentioned earlier, a faux pas of lower lid surgery is the inadvertent or miscalculated excision of too much skin. If the lid closed primarily, or if tissue is advanced from the cheek to compensate for the loss, ectropion is likely after surgery. The usual treatment for this problem is the application of a full-thickness skin graft, preferably from the upper eyelid. An upper lid blepharoplasty will harvest a graft that can be tailored for application to the lower lid. Thus the complication can be avoided. If the upper eyelid skin is harvested first, an inadequate amount of skin may have been taken when, with foreknowledge, extra skin could have been harvested safely. As illustrated by Millard,[12] good surgeons know how to plan well, economizing their efforts and time to achieve an aesthetic goal.

REFERENCES

1. Smith JW: Cosmetic surgery of the aging face, in Grabb WC, Smith JW (eds): *Plastic Surgery,* ed 3. Boston, Little, Brown & Co, 1979.

2. Barton FE Jr: Rhytidectomy. *Select Read Plast Surg* 1985; 3:1–20.

3. Berggren R: Personal communication, 1985.

4. Jost G, Levet Y: Parotid fascia and face lifting: A critical evaluation of the SMAS concept. *Plast Reconstr Surg* 1984; 74:42.

5. Hetter GP, Herhahn FT: Adjunctive or isolated lipolysis of the face and neck, in *Lipoplasty, the Theory and Practice of Blunt Suction Lipectomy.* Boston, Little Brown & Co, 1984.

6. Mladik RA: Lipolysis combined with facial rhytidectomy, in *Lipoplasty, the Theory and Practice of Blunt Suction Lipectomy.* Boston, Little, Brown & Co, 1984.

7. Webster RC, Kazda G, Hamdam US, et al: Cigarette smoking and face lift: Conservative versus wide undermining. *Plast Reconstr Surg* 1986; 77:596.

8. Baring-Gould WS: *The Annotated Sherlock Holmes.* New York, Clarkson N. Potter, 1967.

9. Rees TD: *Aesthetic Plastic Surgery.* Philadelphia, WB Saunders Co, 1980.

10. Tessier P, Rougier J, et al: Esthetic surgery of the eyelids, in *Plastic Surgery of the Orbit and Eyelids.* Chicago, Year Book Medical Publishers, 1981.

11. Beekhuis GJ: Blepharoplasty. *Otolaryngol Clin North Am* 1980; 13:225–236.

12. Millard DR Jr: *The Principalization of Plastic Surgery.* Boston, Little Brown & Co, 1986.

CHAPTER 32

Otoplasty

Approach of

Richard T. Farrior, M.D.

and

Edward H. Farrior, M.D.

There are a number of satisfactory techniques for correcting the protruding ear. Surgeons should not be married to a single technique, nor should they be critical of techniques used by others without valid reasons or without having given a different technique a fair trial. In large part, otoplasty surgeons are treating themselves as they seek near perfection and, more realistically, a corrected natural-looking ear. For the significantly prominent ear, most patients will be satisfied if this prominence is corrected without the patient giving a great deal of attention to the contour, postauricular sulcus, or slight irregularities.

On the other hand, surgeons should seek the best possible result and have more than one technique in their armamentarium. As stated before, both the profession and the public are becoming better informed regarding the procedure, therefore becoming quite naturally more critical of the final results.

All simple suture techniques, setback procedures, or methods requiring cartilage incisions should not be universally accepted or rejected. The simple suture technique is quite satisfactory for the less resilient auricular cartilage; where some contour of the antihelix already exists, there is an adequate helical rim, and the deeply cupped concha is not a problem. Should there be a deep conchal cup, the suture technique alone is less than ideal in that to correct the concha, the antihelix must be made too wide. If the helix and associated scaphoid fossa are poorly developed, there is too much flatness posterior to the newly created antihelix or in the area of the helix. A good combination, especially in many young children, is the combined simple suture technique and conchal setback procedures.

Setback procedures, in truth, may be considered camouflage techniques in that the contour or lack of contour of neither the antihelix nor conchal cavity is corrected.

The next step would then be to reduce the concha by the excision of concha, thereby requiring incisions through the cartilage. Cartilage incisions are not sinful, nor are they to be condemned simply because in some hands they are improperly placed. Cartilage incisions and techniques for weakening the cartilage must be precisely made and created to follow the natural contour of the auricle. When properly executed, incisions effectively break the cartilage spring and assist in precise contouring and reducing the cupped deep concha. We have advocated for many years an *advancing,* or *progressing, operation* that uses the technique best suited for the particular ear based on analysis of the pathological anatomy and the resilience or stiffness of the individual cartilage.

The technique chosen would progress from the simple suturing technique through extended incisions. From the suture technique, one would advance with the addition of conchal setback or reduction and weakening of the spring before incisions are elected. If there is satisfactory contour of the antihelix, conchal reduction only may be done using a modified mattress suture. With the extension of incisions, weakening techniques, and additional sutures, a more severe deformity without contour and even with thick and resilient cartilage can be corrected.

Techniques for weakening the cartilage spring may include removal of longitudinal cartilage wedges, parallel beveled cuts in the cartilage extending the length of the antihelix, or thinning by shaving and dermabrasion of the cartilage. None of these techniques goes through the cartilage and therefore does not violate the perichondrium on the anterior surface. All are created in our hands on the posterior surface of the cartilage.

In regard to incisions and excisions of skin, we prefer to

work over the area of the antihelix on the posterior surface and not to disturb the auriculomastoid sulcus. We prefer to avoid extensive dissections and resections of tissue over the mastoid, as in some conchal setback procedures.

The technique we first advocated remains useful and reliable and has withstood the test of time.[1] The technique used takes into consideration essentially all variables and pitfalls and will provide uniformly good results. If one were required to use a single technique, the surgeon, the patient, and the patient's family would be satisfied with the results. It requires thorough knowledge of the anatomy of the external ear and precise placement of the incisions and sutures. Although it is more complicated than is necessary for some ears by requiring knowledge of the anatomy and attention to detail, the young surgeon, if prepared and knowing what goals to strive for, can make modifications according to the complexity of the abnormality.

We will reemphasize that a progressing technique from the simple suture technique to an extended technique, especially where necessary for the resistant aspect of the ear, is our approach. Uniform for each otoplasty is the elliptical dumbbell incision, the marking of the new antihelix with Keith needles, and the outline of the antihelix from the posterior surface by light scoring with the knife. One then progresses from the simple horizontal suture technique around this outline.

Only three of the several references from the senior author's writings are included.[1–3] This is done intentionally to further direct the reader for more detail rather than for the historic aspect of things. The original article made a comparison to many of the techniques done at that time.[1] The references within that first article are both historic and still of technical value. This publication was based on the early experience and coordinated with critical clinical analysis and cadaver dissections. As developed in the other two articles, modifications and extension of the technique were developed. Among these, the most significant is the use of sutures that include the anterior and posterior borders of the newly created antihelix. This more effectively rolls the antihelix compared with the previous technique, which simply joined the scaphoid fossa and concha with the new antihelix overriding. On occasion with stiff cartilage this made the new antihelix too flat. The references in the other two articles fairly well update the current thinking that surrounds the original technique and emphasizes a progressing technique to "make the punishment fit the crime."[2, 3] More scientifically expressed, the procedure selected is correlated with the variables of the pathologic anatomy.

TECHNIQUE

The surgical techniques used are presented without an attempt to review the entire subject. The major point to be made, once again, is that our technique is truly a composite of operations advancing from simple suturing with conchal and fossa triangularis setback sutures to extended complete and partial incisions, conchal reduction, weakening or breaking of the spring, trimming of the caudal helicis, and extension of incisions into the inferior crus and on around the dome of the ear under the helix. The complexity of the procedure performed depends on the deformity encountered, the stiffness of the cartilage, and the ability of the surgeon. Anesthesia and skin incisions are carried out in the same fashion in each modification of the technique.

Anesthesia

After adequate preoperative sedation is obtained or general anesthesia induced, the pinna is infiltrated with 2% lidocaine and epinephrine 1:100,000. In the patient under local anesthesia, it is certainly more important to reduce the actual and perceived number of needle sticks. Our initial injection is made in the midportion of the postauricular sulcus (Fig 32–1,A). The needle is then passed both inferiorly and superiorly in the postauricular sulcus, blocking the greater auricular nerve inferiorly and raising a wheal at the auricular temple sulcus superiorly. The needle is then passed anteriorly, ballooning the skin of the lateral cartilaginous canal. From the same puncture the needle is passed over the posterior surface of the auricle. Next, the needle is placed in the wheal superiorly and passed in the preauricular soft tissue to the level of the tragus with blocking of the anterior auricular nerve (Fig 32–1,B). The last puncture is made to mark the superior extent of the skin incision at the junction of the midportion of the new superior crus of the antihelix at the helix. Infiltration of the remaining portion of the posterior surface of the pinna is performed from here (Fig 32–1,C). After adequate time has been allowed for anesthesia and vasoconstriction, the incision is performed.

Skin Incision

The skin incision is made on the posterior surface of the auricle and does not cross, reach, or involve the postauricular sulcus, preserving the natural auricular mastoid crease. The incision assumes the configuration of an elliptical dumbbell (Fig 32–2), with the midportion of the medial and lateral incisions running parallel and slightly closer together than the superior and inferior extents. This prevents the pinched-back appearance at the midportion of the helix. The skin is then grasped at the superior point with a skin hook or forceps and excised in a plane between the perichondrium and the subcutaneous tissue. If there is concern about the amount of skin to be excised, the lateral incision is made, and a skin flap is elevated. The skin is redraped at the completion of the procedure with excision of redundant skin at that time. We do advocate a subcutaneous closure with 5-0 Vicryl prior to placement of the running subcuticular 5-0 nylon.

Identification of Anatomic Landmarks

Since the most common and significant abnormality necessitating otoplasty is the absence or reduction of the antihelix or the antihelical fold, therefore scaphoid fossa, the surgery is aimed at the creation of an antihelix. If one keeps this in mind, it beomes quite obvious that the incisions or modifications of the posterior cartilage need to create a natural antihelix and

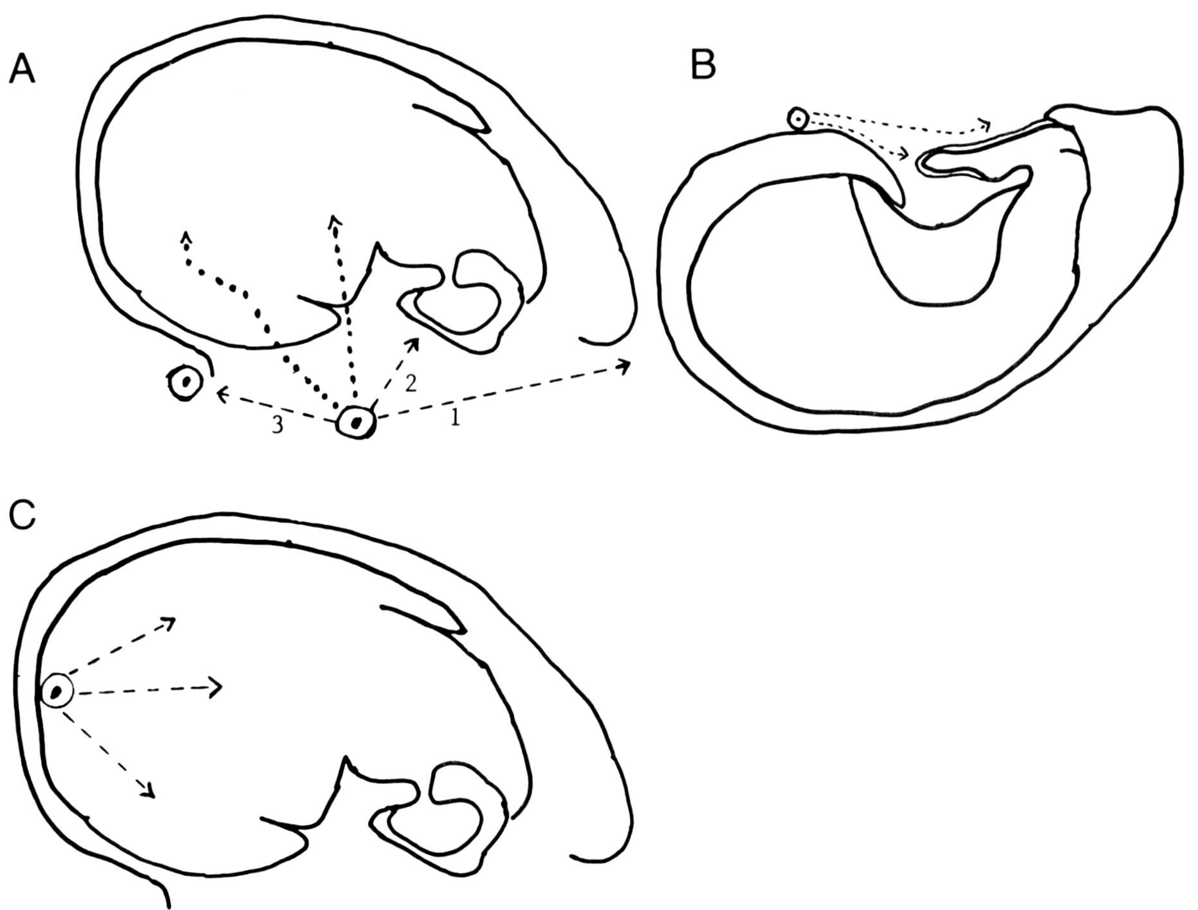

FIG 32–1.
A, postauricular injection in nerve block: *(1)* infiltration and block of the greater auricular nerve, and *(2)* infiltration to the lateral portion of the cartilaginous canal, and *(3)* infiltration and wheal at the auricular temporal sulcus. Dotted lines represent infiltration of the posterior surface of the auricle. **B**, needle is placed in the wheal superiorly and passed in the preauricular soft tissue to the level of the tragus with blocking of the anterior auricular nerve. **C**, completion of infiltration of the posterior surface of the auricle with needle stick to mark the superior extent of the skin excision at the junction of the midportion of the new superior crus of the antihelix at the helix.

superior crus. Straight cutting needles are placed through specific locations on the anterior pinna to identify them posteriorly.

In placing these needles, one marks the reconstructed anterior border of the antihelix and superior crus. Needles are placed as such: (1) at the desired new anterior border of the superior crus adjacent to the helical rim, (2) at the junction of the superior and inferior crus in the triangular fossa, (3) at the junction of the inferior crus and antihelix proper on the conchal rim (Figs 32–3 and 32–4), and (4) at the inferior antihelix in the margin of the conchal rim (see Figs 32–3 and 32–4). A fifth needle is sometimes placed along the posterior border of the antihelix at the level of the inferior crus to determine the exact width of the antihelix at this point. No marking solution is used. From this point, the posterior surface of the cartilage is scratched just distal to the needles to mark the new anterior border of the antihelix and superior crus (Fig 32–5). The partial incision on the anterior border of the superior crus is not carried across the inferior crus. From this point on the operation is modified to the specific needs of the individual. Frequently, a scratch will

also be placed on the posterior surface of the scaphoid fossa to mark this lateral landmark (see Fig 32–5).

Technique

The Farrior technique results from a graduated approach to the structure, support, and deformity encountered, resulting in a composite of procedures. The complexity of the procedure varies depending on the thickness and resilience of the cartilage, depth and cupping of the concha, existing convexity of the antihelix, existing concavity of the scaphoid fossa, degree of development of the helical rim, and the pillar effect of the inferior crus. We will attempt to describe the procedure in a logical, graduated fashion, starting at the point of completion of anesthesia, skin incisions, marking of anatomic landmarks, and scratching of the posterior cartilage at the anticipated anterior border of the antihelix and superior crus (see Fig 32–5). These are done the same in all procedures.

The simplest form of otoplasty we use is the suture tech-

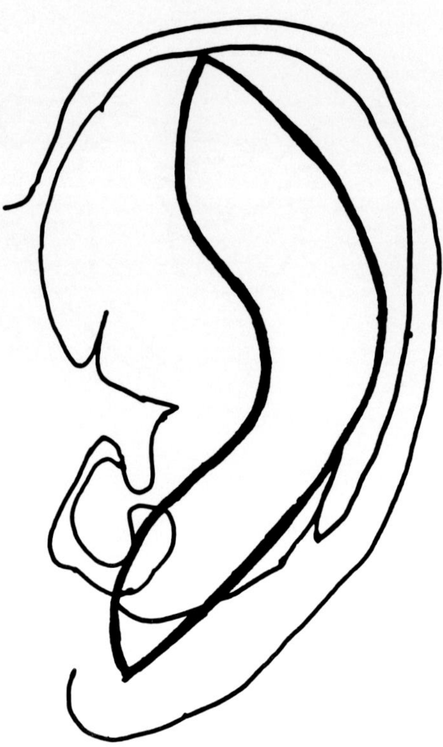

FIG 32–2.
Skin incision and excision in the shape of an elliptical dumbbell.

nique as popularized by Mustardé.[4] For this a 4-0 Mersilene suture on an Ancor 1844 no. 5 needle is used. A horizontal mattress suture is placed paralleling the antihelix from the scaphoid fossa to the conchal rim in a radial fashion (Fig 32–6). An additional suture may be passed from the posterior to anterior border of the superior crus. These sutures should not penetrate the perichondrium on the anterior surface of the pinna. Simple suturing technique is frequently accompanied by conchomastoid suturing. It is important to place these sutures in the concha cavum, concha cymba, and triangular fossa (Fig 32–7). Care must be taken to place the mastoid portion of the suture posteriorly to avoid narrowing the external auditory meatus.

The next step in our progression is dependent on the resilience of the cartilage and is performed prior to placement of sutures. Cartilage weakening techniques include wire brush dermabrasion, longitudinal beveled incision, longitudinal wedge excisions, cartilage shave, fish scale incisions, and scoring of the anterior surface. We prefer longitudinal beveled incisions and would discourage any surgery on the anterior surface of the cartilage. Two to three longitudinal beveled incisions are made the full length of the antihelix extending into the superior crus. Additional beveled incisions are made in the superior crus but do not cross the inferior crus (Fig 32–8). These cuts should not extend through the entire thickness of the cartilage. The bevel is angled from proximal to distal on the posterior surface. The horizontal mattress sutures are then applied (Fig 32–9).

Next in the progression is reduction of the deep or cupped concha. Conchal reduction is preferred to conchomastoid suturing because of preservation of a normal external auditory

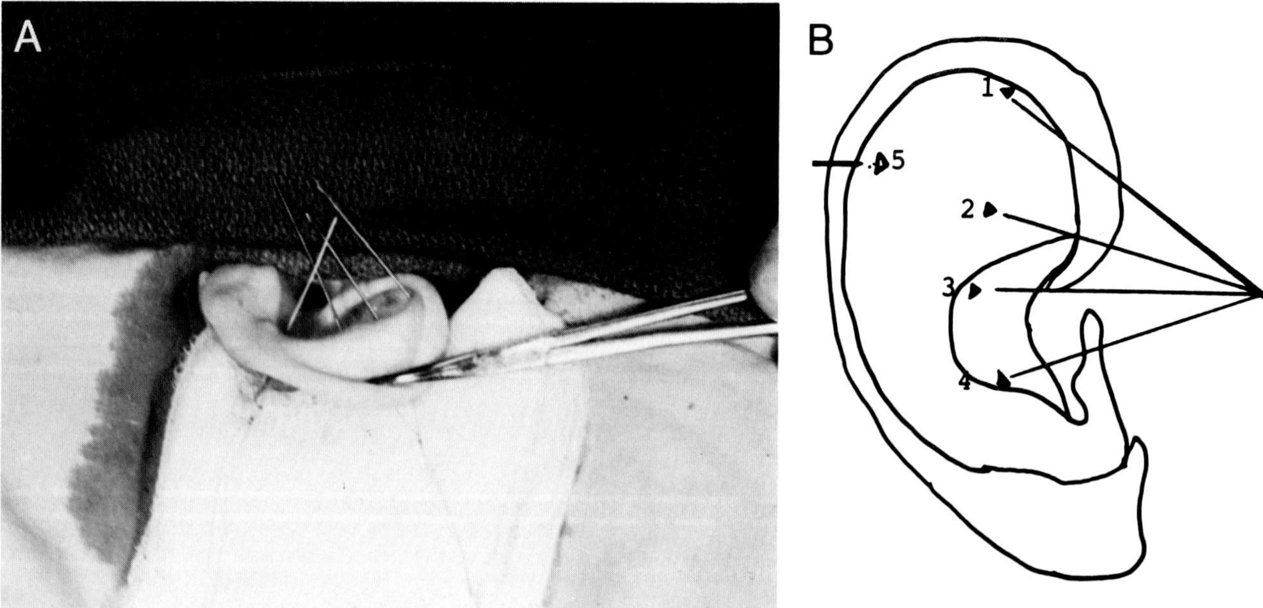

FIG 32–3.
A, placement of the Keith needles to the anterior surface of the helix marking. **B,** the desired new anterior border of the superior crus adjacent to the helical rim *(1)*, the junction of the superior and inferior crus in the triangular fossa *(2)*, the junction at the inferior crus and antihelix proper on the conchal rim *(3)*, and the inferior antihelix in the margin of the conchal rim *(4)*. The needle is sometimes placed at the posterior border of the antihelix at the level of the inferior crus *(5)*.

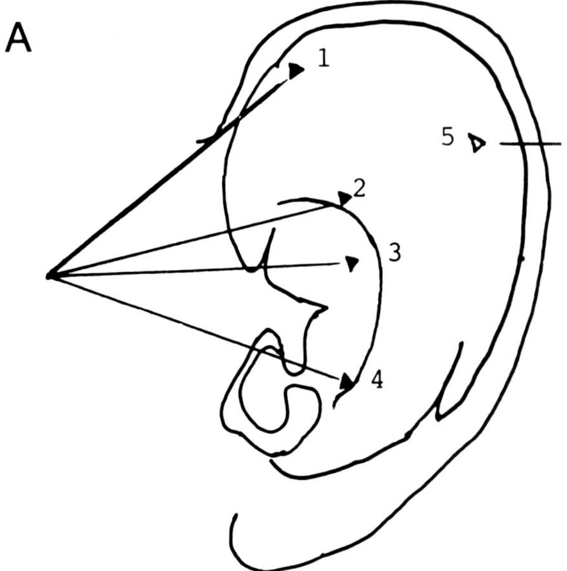

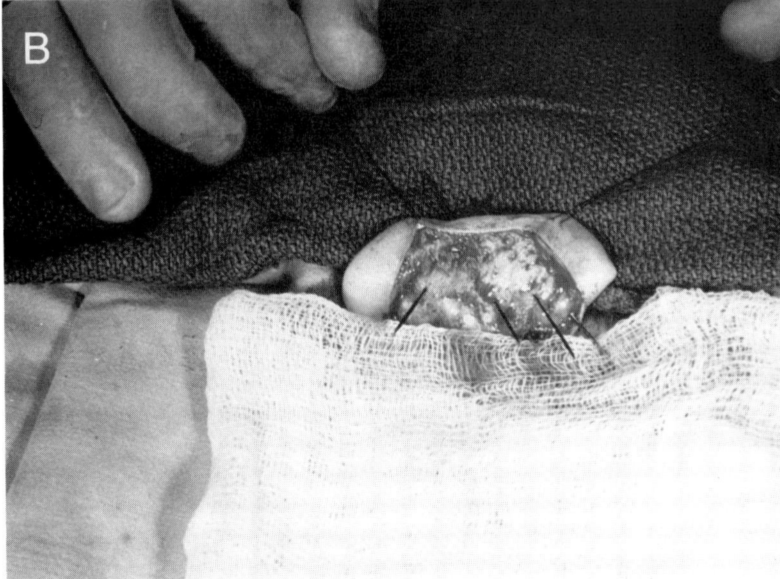

FIG 32–4.
Posterior views of the placement of the Keith needles.

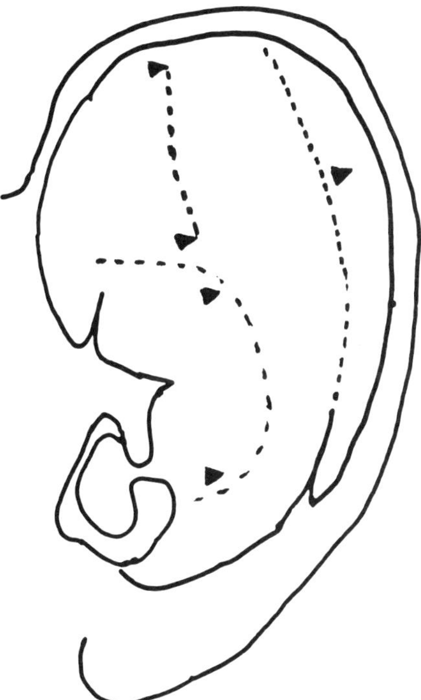

FIG 32–5.
Scratching of the posterior surface of the cartilage just distal to the needles to mark the new anterior border of the antihelix and superior crus. The partial incision on the anterior border of the superior crus is not carried across to the inferior crus. A mark is also placed on the posterior surface of the scaphoid fossa to identify this lateral landmark.

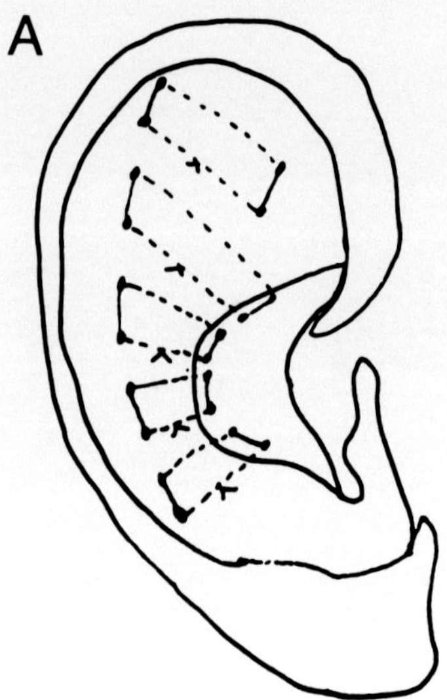

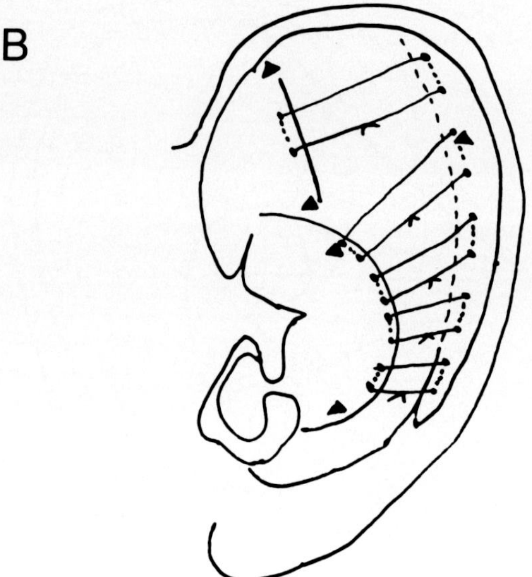

FIG 32–6.
A, anterior surface of the auricle with horizontal mattress sutures placed in a radial fashion from the scaphoid fossa to the rim of the concha, the most superior suture being optional. **B,** posterior surface of the auricle with radially placed horizontal mattress sutures.

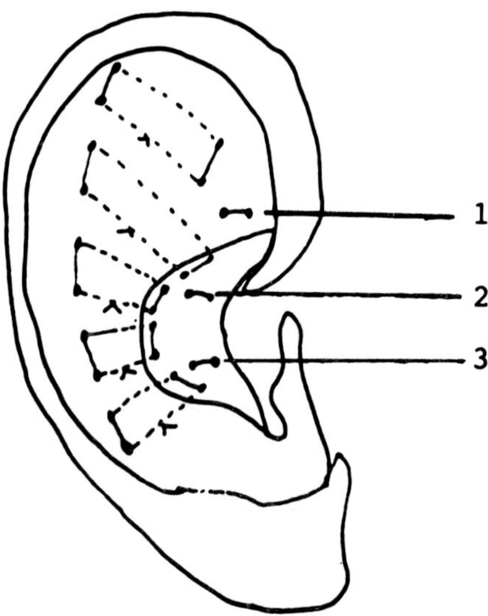

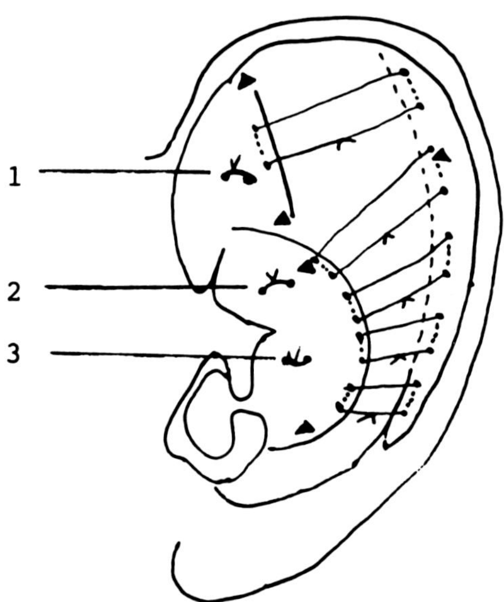

FIG 32–7.
Anterior and posterior surface of the auricle with placement of the conchomastoid setback sutures: *(1)* the triangular fossa, (2) the concha cymba, and *(3)* the concha cavum.

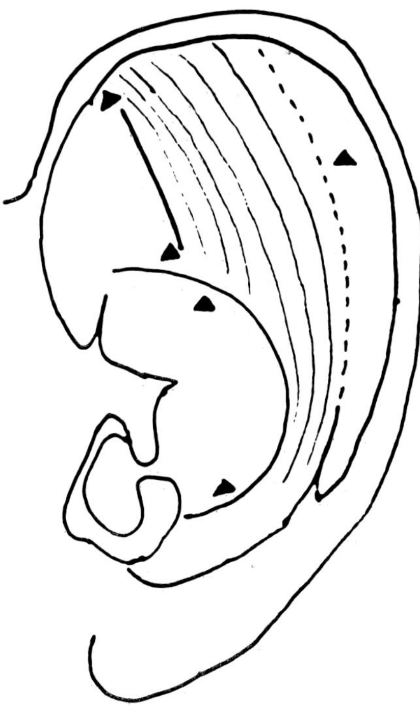

FIG 32–8.
Posterior surface of the auricle with longitudinal beveled incisions in the antihelix and superior crus.

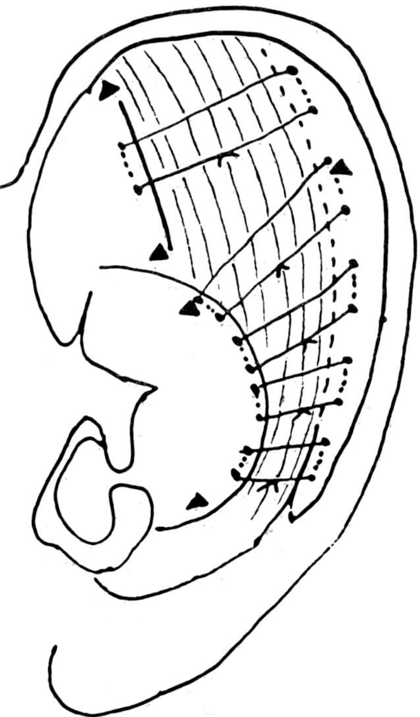

FIG 32–9.
Horizontal mattress sutures on the posterior surface of the auricle after scoring the antihelix and superior crus with beveled longitudinal incisions.

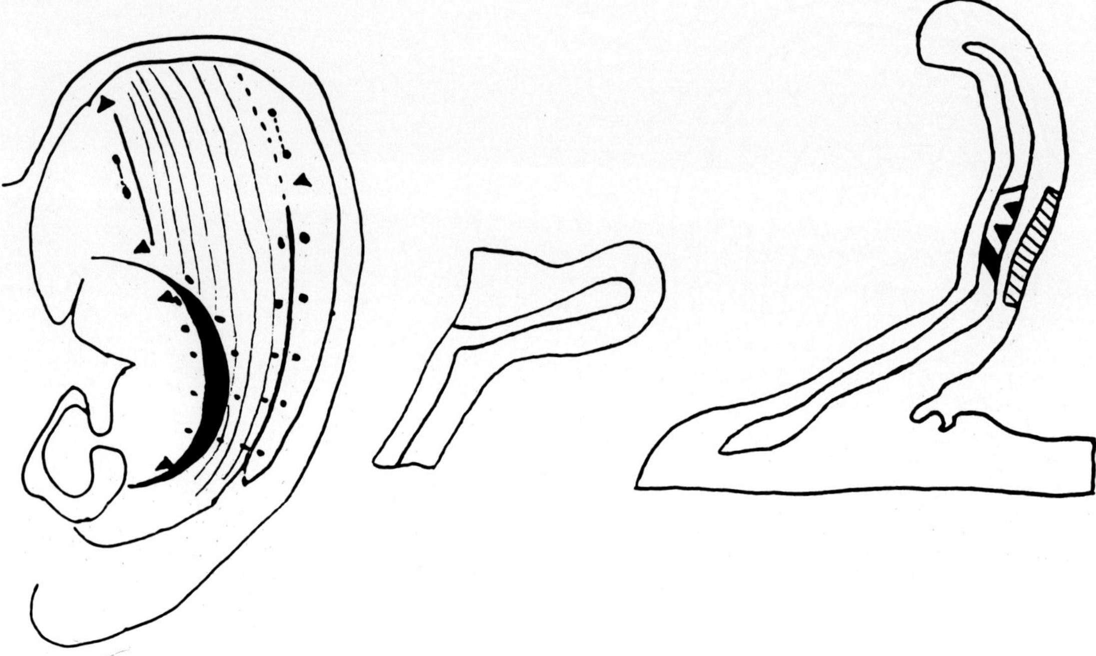

FIG 32–10.
A, incision on the crescent of the cartilage at the junction of the concha and anterior border of the antihelix. **B,** the incision is made in the cartilage, beveling from proximal to distal to enhance smooth contouring of the overlying cartilage of the new antihelix.

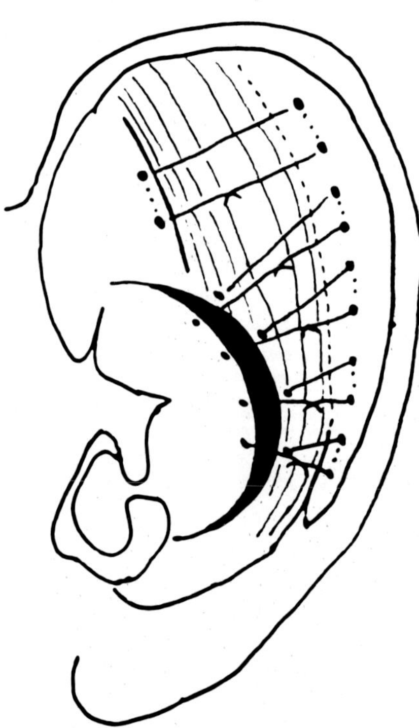

FIG 32–11.
Modified horizontal and vertical mattress sutures placed in a radial fashion.

canal meatus and the more permanent result. Conchal cartilage is excised around the conchal rim, with the lateral incision corresponding to the anterior border of the antihelix and beveling from proximal to distal (Fig 32–10). The suture is then modified to combine a horizontal and vertical mattress suture. The horizontal segment is in the cartilage of the scaphoid fossa and parallel to it, with the vertical segment picking up the anterior antihelix and the reduced conchal cartilage (Fig 32–11). A horizontal mattress suture is frequently used at the superior crus, as previously described.

Those patients lacking an antihelix, and therefore a scaphoid fossa, would qualify for the next additional step. This would be a through-and-through incision along the scaphoid fossa, extending superiorly to the level of the junction of the crura (Fig 32–12). This incision can be carried further superiorly if necessary and is beveled from distal to proximal to allow blending of the new antihelix with the underlying cartilage (Fig 32–13). When a through-and-through incision is made at the scaphoid fossa and conchal rim, a vertical mattress suture is used (see Fig 32–12). This is applied by grasping the anterior border of the cartilage within the scaphoid fossa, the posterior border of the new antihelix, the anterior border of the new antihelix, and the conchal rim.

The previous description is the Farrior otoplasty as initially presented, including (1) reduction of the conchal rim; (2) incision through the cartilage in the scaphoid fossa to the level of the junction of the crura; (3) weakening of the spring with parallel beveled incisions, or as initially described, resection of beveled wedged strips of cartilage, following the new antihelix and superior crus, not crossing the inferior crus; and (4) vertical

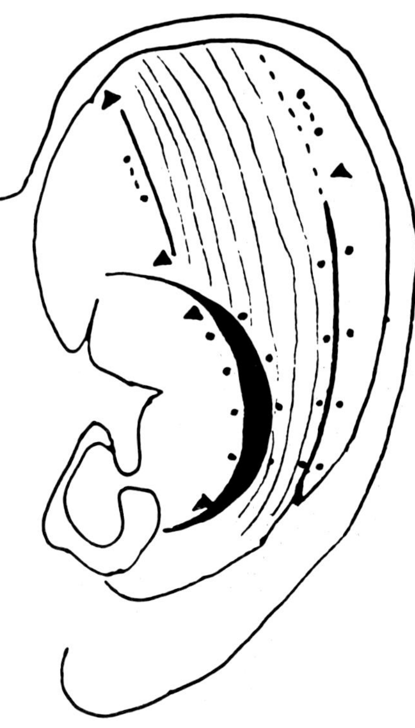

FIG 32–12.
Incision along the scaphoid fossa, extending superior to the level of the junction of the crura. Vertical mattress suture grasping the anterior border of the cartilage within the scaphoid fossa, the posterior border of the new antihelix, the anterior border of the new antihelix, and the conchal rim is used when a through-and-through incision is made within the scaphoid fossa.

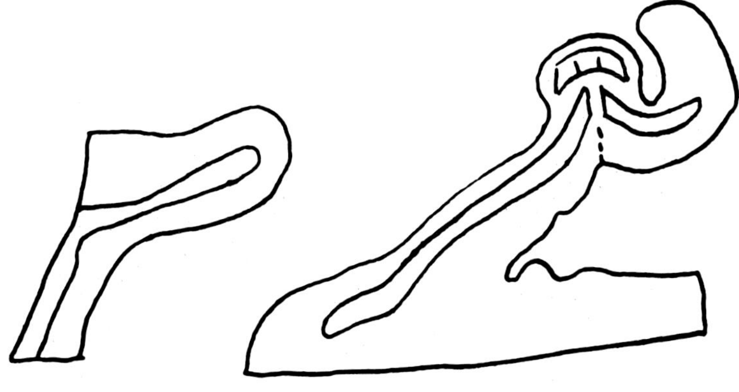

FIG 32–13.
Beveling of the anterior and posterior border of the antihelical rim to allow blending and camouflage on the anterior surface of the auricle.

mattress sutures. No incisions are made through the cartilage of the superior crus, and no sutures are placed across the superior crus in the original technique.

Modifications or additions to this technique may be required. In the ear where the superior portion above the junction of the crus is resistant to contouring, it may be necessary to extend the scaphoid fossa incision above the level of the junction of the crura. If there is a marked pillar effect from the inferior crus, one may want to extend the scaphoid fossa incision around the dome of the ear under the overhang of the helix (Fig 32–14).

If the inferior portion of the ear is prominent, it may require trimming or resection of the cauda helicis. Resection of the cauda helicis is seldom done. It is helpful to have a remnant of the cauda helicis to place the inferior mattress suture through. If the lobule itself is enlarged, the incision on the posterior pinna can be extended to resect a portion of the lobule.

Dressing and Postoperative Care

After the postauricular incision is closed, the dressing is applied. The incision is dressed with antibiotic ointment and fine mesh gauze. Cotton strips and small balls are then moistened in mineral oil and molded to the contour of the triangular fossa, the scaphoid fossa, the concha, and the postauricular

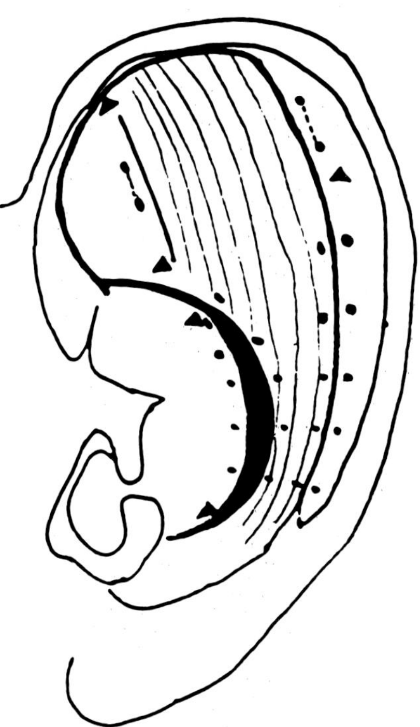

FIG 32–14.
For the particularly stubborn ear, it is sometimes necessary to extend the scaphoid fossa incisions superior to the junction of the crura. It may also be necessary to extend the conchal rim incision into the inferior crus to the level of the junction with the helix. It may even be necessary to connect these two incisions around the dome of the ear beneath the overhang of the helix.

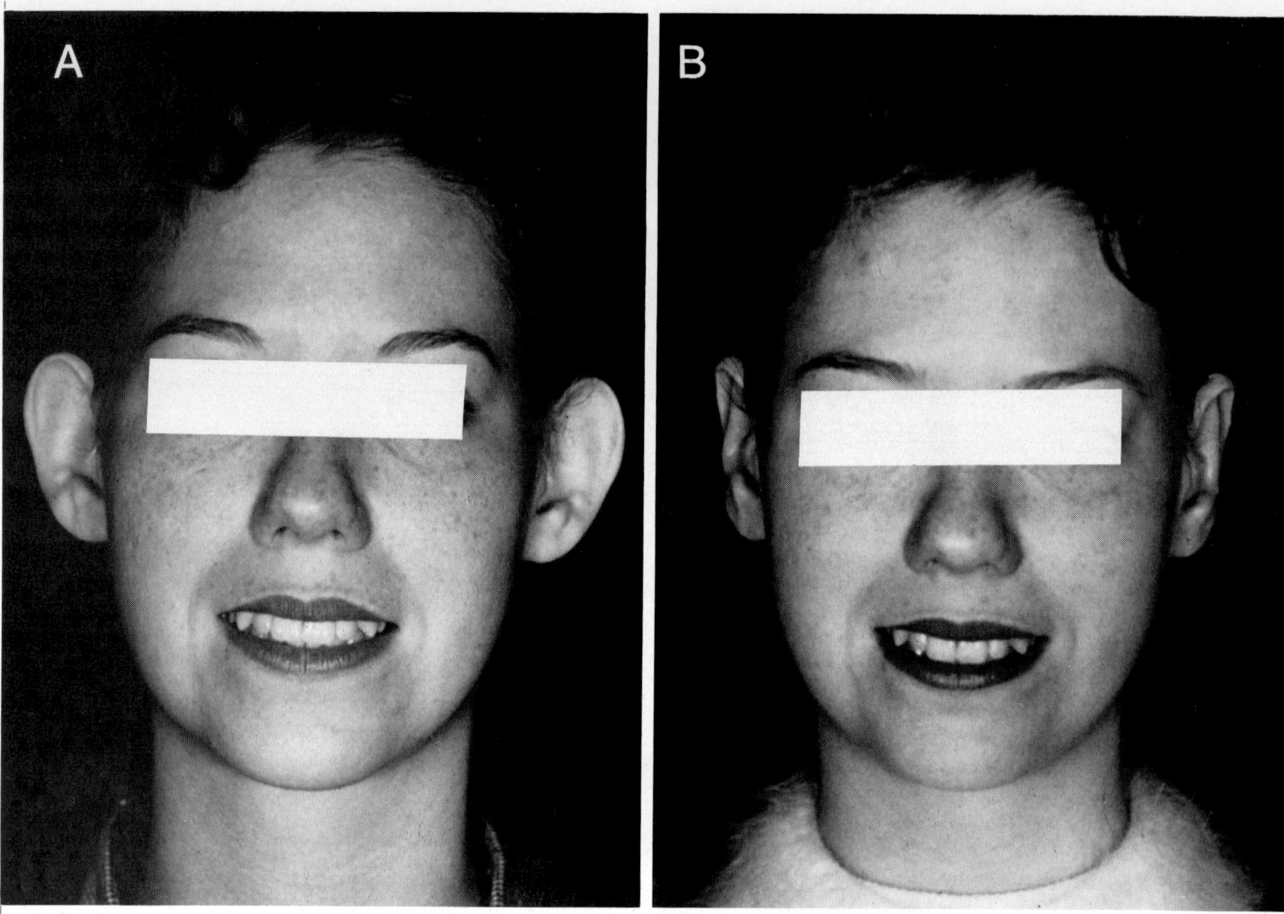

FIG 32–15.
Preoperative (**A**) and postoperative (**B**) frontal and preoperative (**C**) and postoperative (**D**) oblique views of a patient who underwent the standard Farrior otoplasty with reduction of the conchal rim, incision through the cartilage and the scaphoid fossa to the level of the junction of the crura, weakening of the spring with excision of wedged strips of cartilage and vertical mattress suturing.

sulcus. A fluff is placed over each ear and a secure wrap-around dressing applied. The dressing is changed on the fourth postoperative day. The contour cotton is left in place if clean. The entire dressing is removed at 1 week, and at that time the patient is encouraged to sleep with a stocking cap or headband to avoid inadvertent trauma to the ear. The subcuticular nylon suture remains in place for 10 to 14 days.

Many criticisms of the Farrior otoplasty have been based on its complexity. We would argue that the technique is not complex but complete (Fig 32–15). There are numerous simpler and faster ways to correct the lop ear deformity, but none of these addresses the contributing factors to auricular protrusion as completely or anatomically. The Farrior otoplasty is based on recreating the normal anatomy of the anterior ear while assuring a strong lasting result. Anyone willing to familiarize themselves with the topographic anatomy of the ear will be able to perform this technique without difficulty. It is important to remember that there is no one technique used but, rather, a sequence of additional steps graduated according to the deformity.

SUMMARY

This chapter has been designed to give the reader a practical and applicable understanding of the various techniques for otoplasty, selecting those techniques applicable for the majority of ears.

The advancing or progressing technique cannot be overemphasized as one attempts to select the best procedure for a particular ear. Although it was beyond the present subject, it should be mentioned that many of the techniques incorporated can also be incorporated in correcting the cupped or constricted ear and with reductions in the actual size of the ear, as in true macrotia.

As we have critically evaluated the multiple new techniques that have been presented through the last 30 years, we have in no way seen any reason to abandon the original technique as it has been modified. If anything, time has reemphasized the value of the technique, including as a teaching vehicle. The original technique requires that the surgeon learn the external anatomy and learn to be precise in executing the method. If

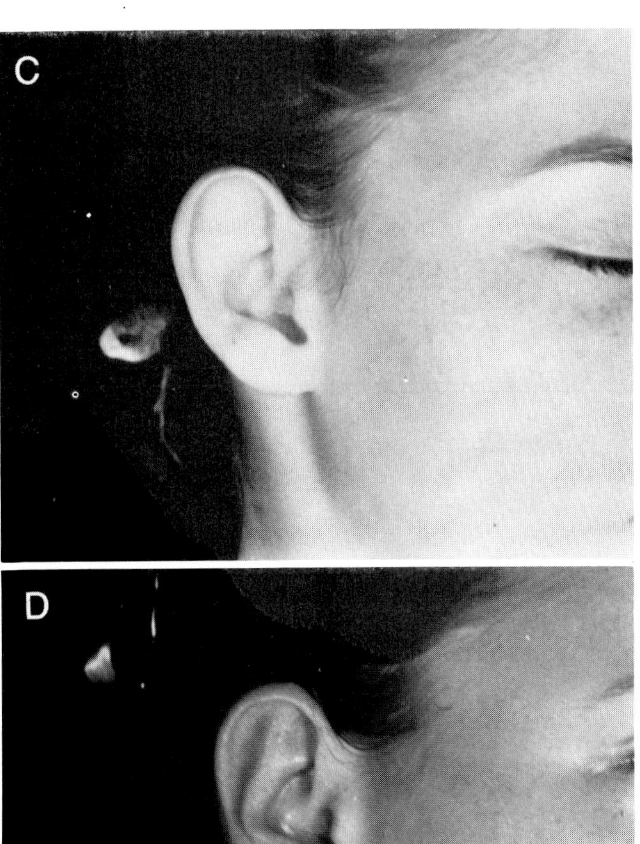

the technique were used for all ears generally, the patient and the surgeon would be pleased. I would recommend the procedure for the young surgeon until experience allows him or her to modify with either a simpler or more advanced technique.

Although incisions through the cartilage may be avoided where possible, precise incisions are not to be condemned. The original technique combines many of the features that (1) use the suturing techniques, (2) weaken the spring, (3) incise the cartilage to break the spring, and (4) reduce the deeply cupped concha.

It is our hope that readers will find both principles and techniques that they can apply to their own surgical armamentarium and take to their own patients.

REFERENCES

1. Farrior RT: A method of otoplasty. *Arch Otolaryngol* 1959; 69: 400–408.
2. Farrior RT: Otoplasty: Surgery for protruding ears, in English GM (ed): *Otolaryngology,* rev ed. Philadelphia, Harper & Row, Publishers, 1984.
3. Farrior RT: Modified cartilage incisions in otoplasty. *Facial Plast Surg* 2:109–118.
4. Mustardé JG: The correction of prominent ears using simple mattress sutures. *Br J Plast Surg* 1963; 16:170.

SUGGESTED READINGS

1. Luckett WH: A new operation for prominent ears. *Surg Gynecol Obstet* 1910; 10:635.
2. Converse JM, et al: Technique for surgical correction of lop ears. *Plast Reconstr Surg* 1955; 15:411.
3. Furnas DW: Correction of prominent ears by conchamastoid sutures. *Plast Reconstr Surg* 1968; 42:189.
4. Feuerstein S: A technique of otoplasty. Paper presented at the First International Symposium, New York, 1970.
5. Rothfeld ID: Suture technique of otoplasty. *Arch Otolaryngol* 1969; 89:883.
6. Wright WK: Otoplasty goals and principles. *Arch Otolaryngol* 1970; 92:568.

Otoplasty

Approach of

Sidney S. Feuerstein, M.D.

The technique of otoplasty to be presented in this chapter, in reality, represents a combination of the salient features of many techniques described over the past 60 years.[1-9] The prime objective has been to place the protruding auricle into a proper and permanent position with a normal relationship to the skull, especially the re-creation of the normal auricular anatomy when viewed from its lateral aspect.

COMPLICATIONS

Prior to presentation of the specific technique, it may be useful to present a variety of complications observed in the past that guided us in developing a technique that hopefully prevents these undesirable complications. Reprotrusion of the ear, in my experience, has been a common occurrence following the utilization of the "suture only" technique as described by Mustardé (Fig 32–16).[9] "Sharp lines" of the cut concha were commonplace in techniques of Barsky[2] and Kitlowski[3] (Fig 32–17). Necrosis of the conchal and antihelical cartilage has occurred when the postoperative dressings were placed too tightly (Fig 32–18). Granulomas of the postauricular skin over a permanent suture have been noted, especially when the buried sutures are placed in close proximity to the skin incisions (Fig 32–19). Morselization of the antihelix through a postauricular incision has been used to break the spring. Note the pebbled effect of the lateral surface from perichondrial regeneration following morselization (Fig 32–20). Another common postoperative complication has been the creation of the "telephone ear" when viewed from the front. This complication is most commonly secondary to excessive removal of postauricular skin and conchal cartilage (Fig 32–21).

One final complication, which fortunately is not commonplace, is the formation of the postauricular keloid (Fig 32–22). These occur more commonly in darker-skinned patients. It is recommended that catgut sutures not be used for skin closure, and excessive wound tension should be avoided.

TECHNIQUE

Several considerations relating to the general philosophy of management of the protruding ear should be discussed. Usually the protruding ear is congenital in origin and concerns the absence of adequate unfolding of the antihelix in the third month of gestation. As a result, one usually notes that the projection of the inferior crus from the skull exceeds the normal 35 degrees, and, in addition, the conchal-scaphal angle may exceed the normal 90 degrees. Thus, we have found that a cartilage cutting technique is most essential to recreate the normal relationship of the inferior crus to the skull and, second, the normal 90-degree relationship of the conchal margin with the scapha of the antihelix.

The possibility of creating a telephone ear is minimized by first creating a mastoid pedicle skin flap. Skin is not removed at this initial phase of the surgical procedure (Fig 32–23). The cartilage incision between the concha and antihelix is then outlined, and the antihelix is completely separated from the concha, which allows for adequate posterior location of the auricle and ultimate fixation in its desired position. Conchal setback sutures are now inserted to fix the conchal cartilage to the firm mastoid periosteum (Fig 32–24). Following this fixation of the concha to the mastoid, vertical mattress sutures are inserted at three levels of the antihelix and fixed to the cut edge of the concha as noted in Figure 32–25.

On completion of the otoplastic procedure, the frontal appearance of the auricle should be evaluated to determine if any abnormal protrusion of the antitragus or lobule exists. Prominence of the antitragus could readily be reduced by wedge excision of some of its cartilage. The lobule may also be tailored by direct excision of skin.

Hemostasis during the procedure should be meticulously observed. Bipolar cautery prevents excessive use of chromic catgut ties. Insertion of a small Penrose drain is recommended, because, in my experience, there is always a collection of blood in the postoperative dressing for 24 hours. Local anesthesia has

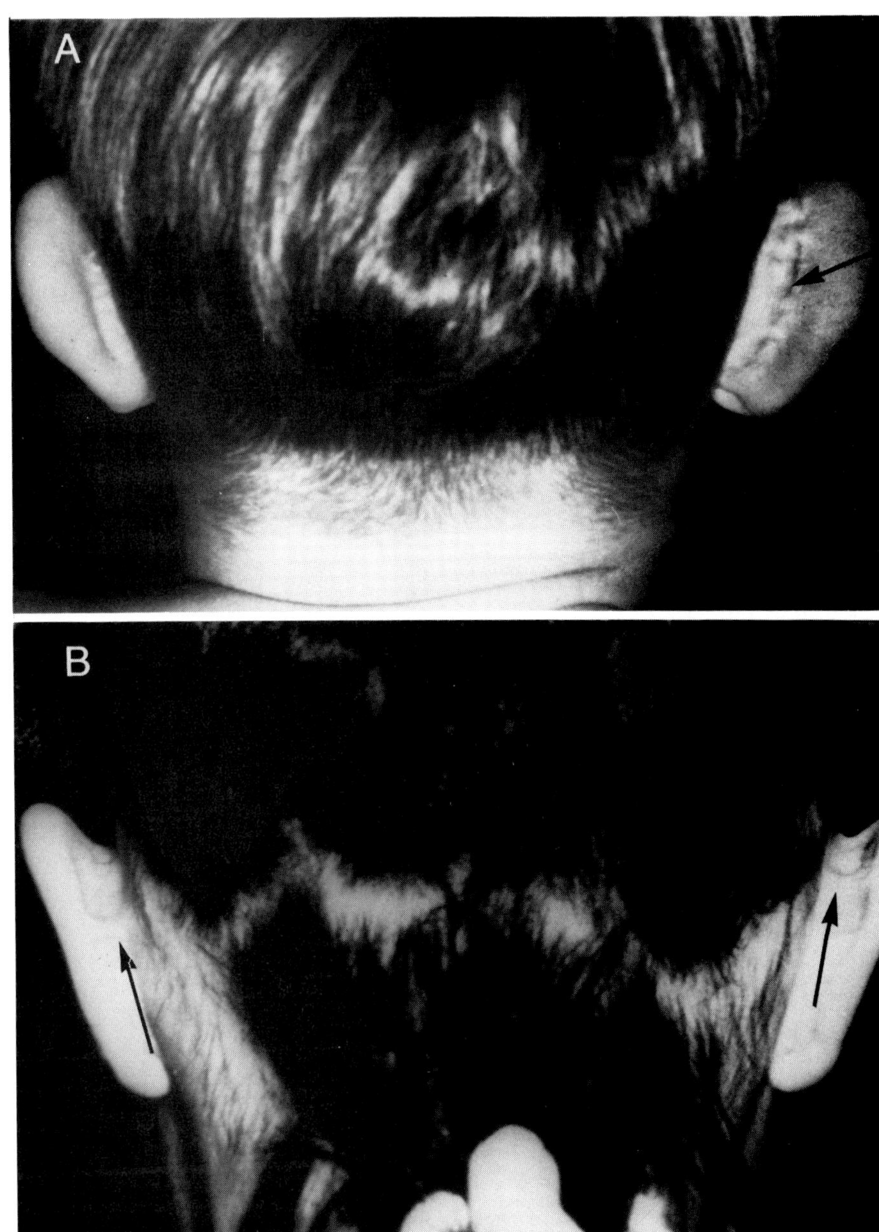

FIG 32–16.
A, posterior view following suture only technique. Note outline of sutures under incision *(arrow)*, which appear to be stretching 6 months following surgery. **B**, another patient following suture only technique with a suture granuloma behind left ear *(arrow)*. (From Feuerstein SS: *Facial Plast Surg* 1986; 2:142–150. Used by permission.)

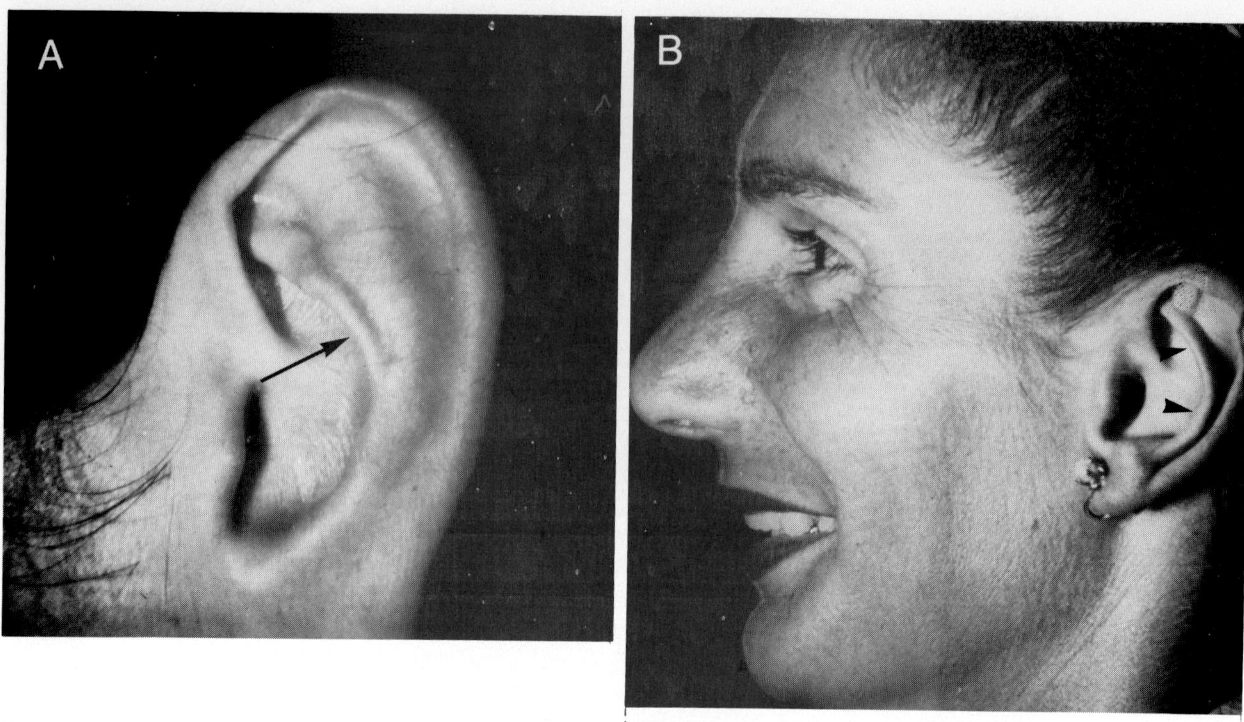

FIG 32–17.
A, postoperative lateral view with telltale sharp line of incised concha *(arrow).* **B,** another postoperative patient following cartilage cutting and tubing technique *(arrows).* (From Feuerstein SS: *Facial Plast Surg* 1986; 2:142–150. Used by permission.)

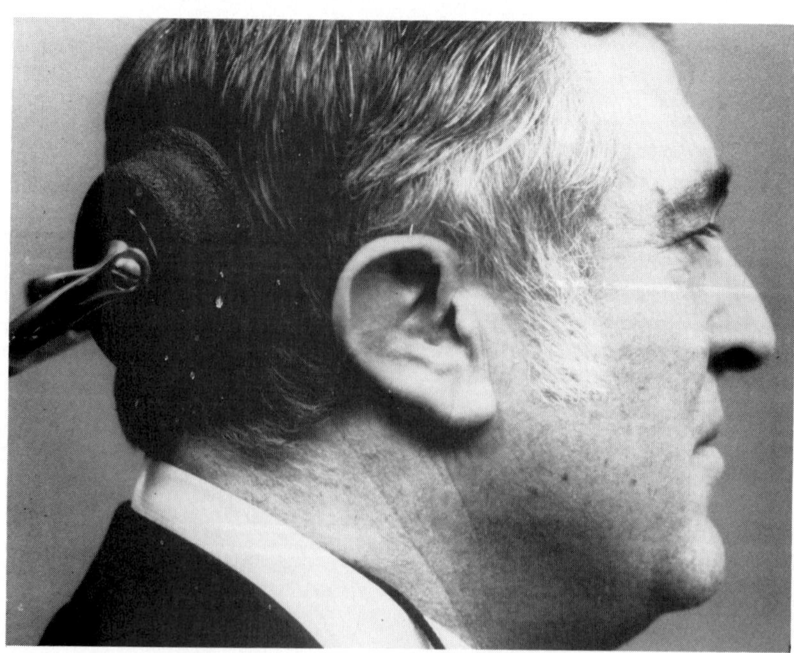

FIG 32–18.
Postoperative patient 50 years following otoplasty. Note conchal and antihelical deformity secondary to necrosis associated with tight dressing. (From Feuerstein SS: *Facial Plast Surg* 1986; 2:142–150. Used by permission.)

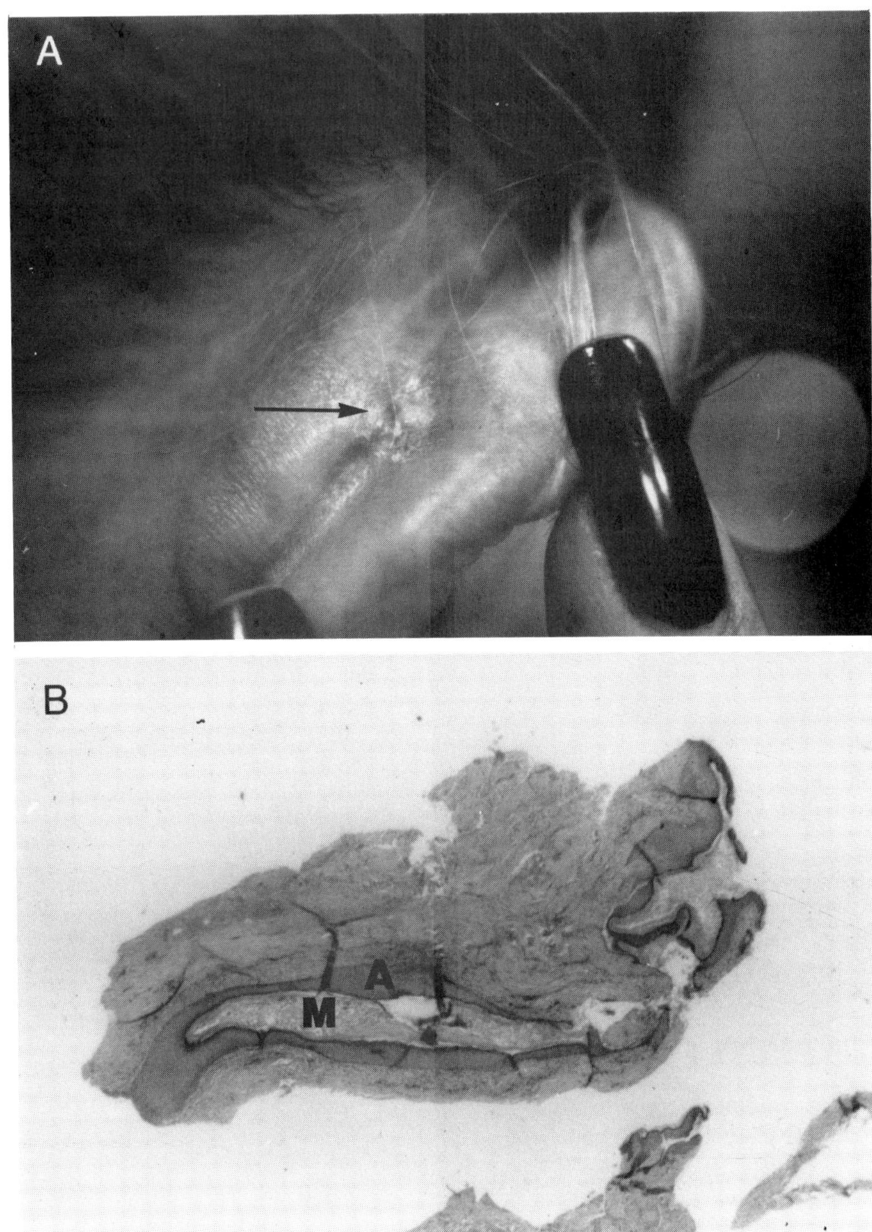

FIG 32–19.
A, postauricular suture granuloma in patient in Figure 32–16, B. **B**, Laboratory section of tissue demonstrating wall *(A)* of suture tunnel with cholesterol crystal *(M)* in lumen and surrounded by granulation tissue. (From Feuerstein SS: *Facial Plast Surg* 1986; 2:142–150. Used by permission.)

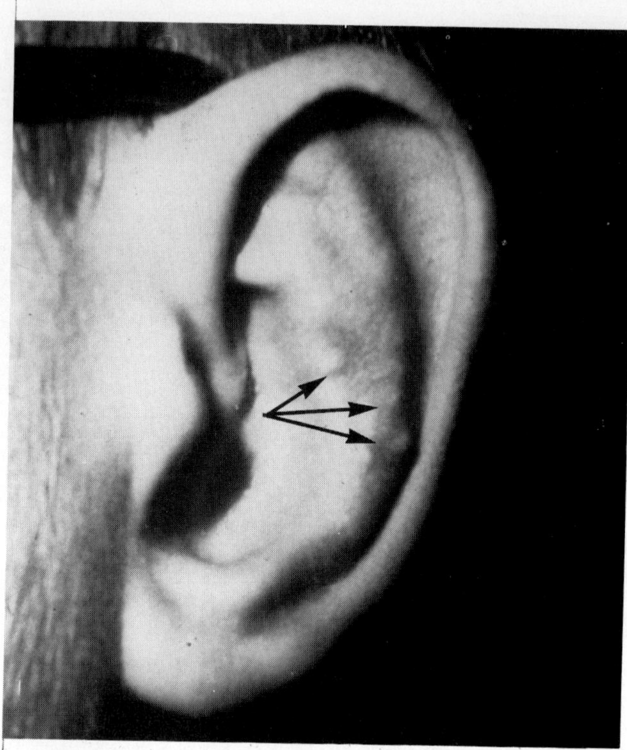

FIG 32–20.
Pebbled effect of antihelix *(arrows)* following morselization. (From
Feuerstein SS: *Facial Plast Surg* 1986; 2:142–150. Used by per-
mission.)

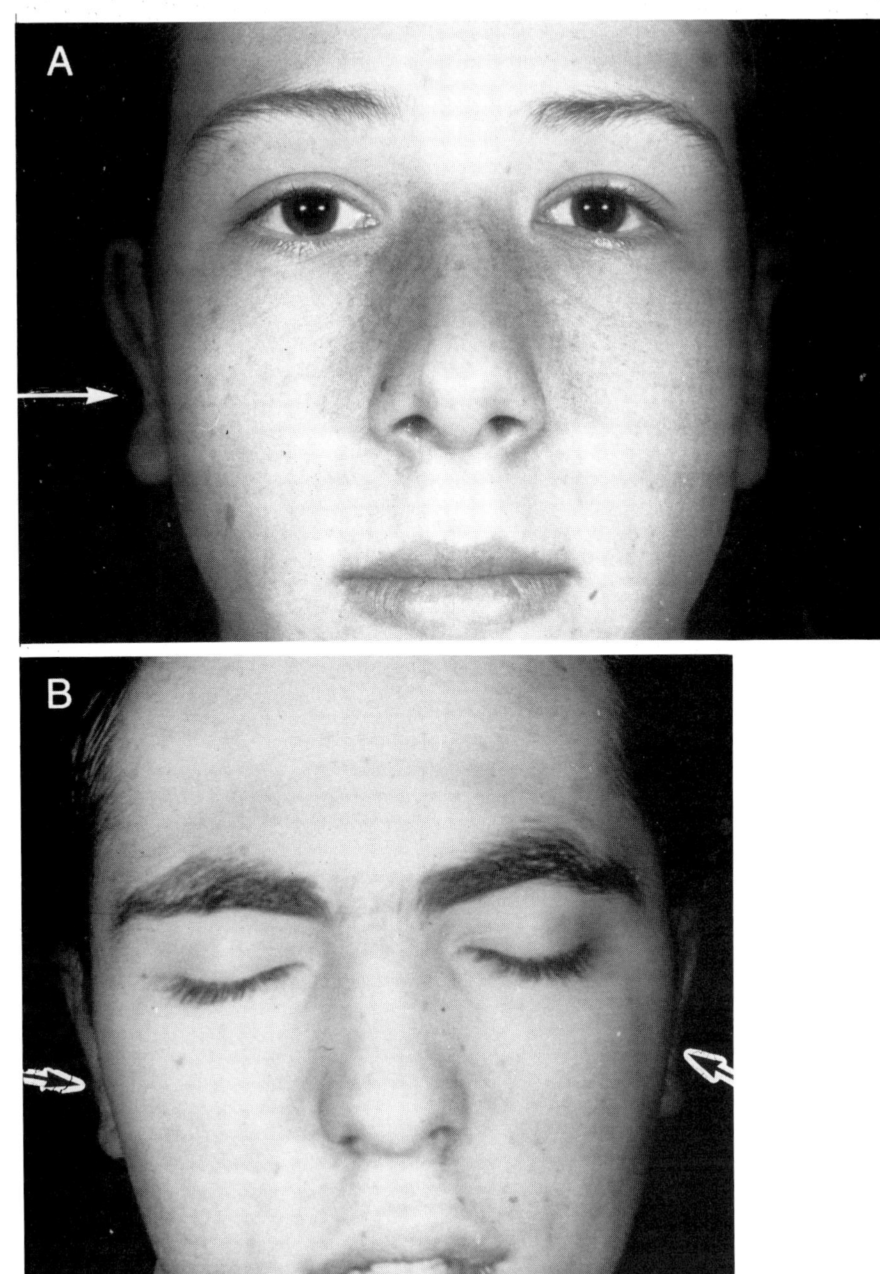

FIG 32–21.
A, postoperative frontal view demonstrating telephone ear on right side. **B,** moderate telephone ears *(arrows)* following excessive removal of conchal cartilage and postauricular skin. (From Feuerstein SS: *Otolaryngol Clin North Am* 1974; 7:136. Used by permission.)

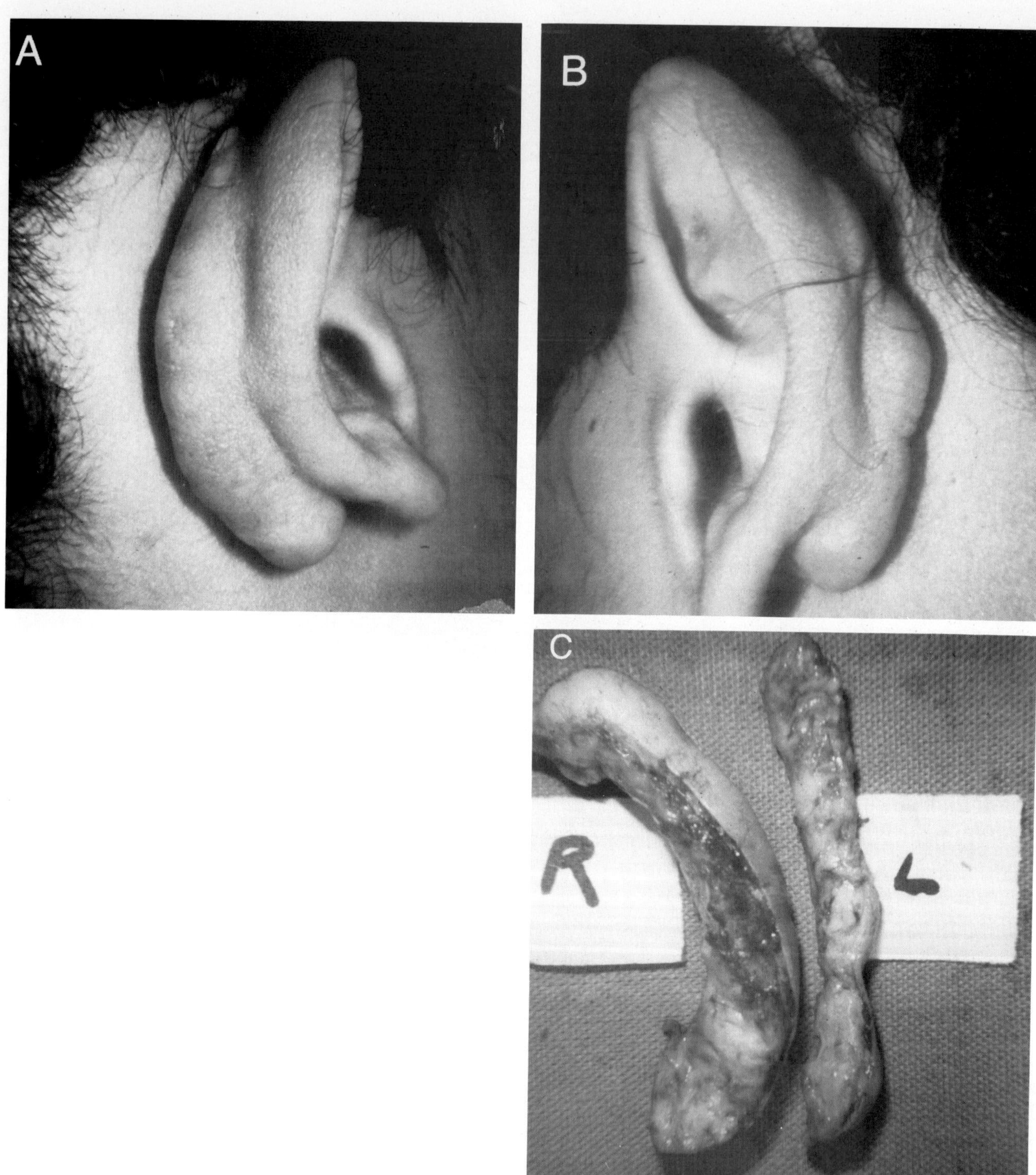

FIG 32–22.
A, postoperative keloid right ear 1 year following surgery. **B**, Same on left ear. **C**, Excised keloids. Patient received superficial radiation therapy. (From Feuerstein SS: *Facial Plast Surg* 1986; 2:142–150. Used by permission.)

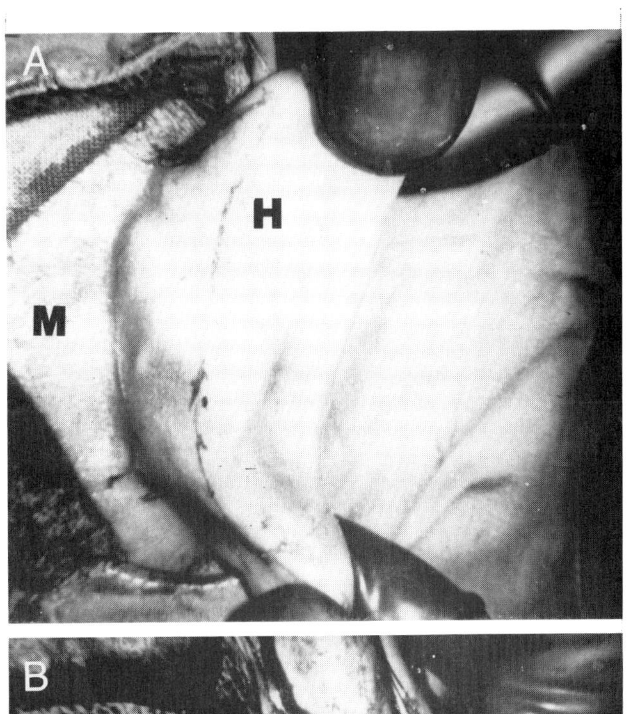

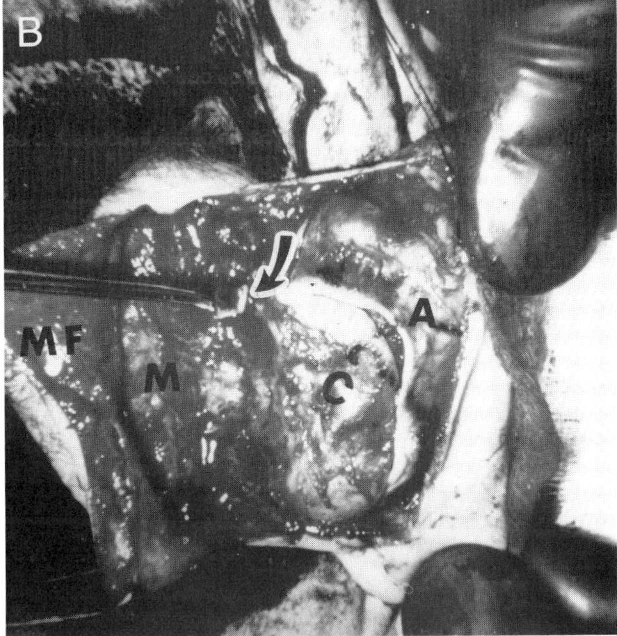

FIG 32–23.
A, mastoid pedicle flap is outlined. Note mastoid area *(M)* and antihelix-helix region *(H)*. **B,** mastoid flap *(MF)* is dissected, exposing mastoid bone cortex (M). Conchal cartilage *(C)* is separated from antihelix *(A)* by conchal incision. Note removal of cartilage segment at junction of inferior crus with helical crus *(arrow)*.

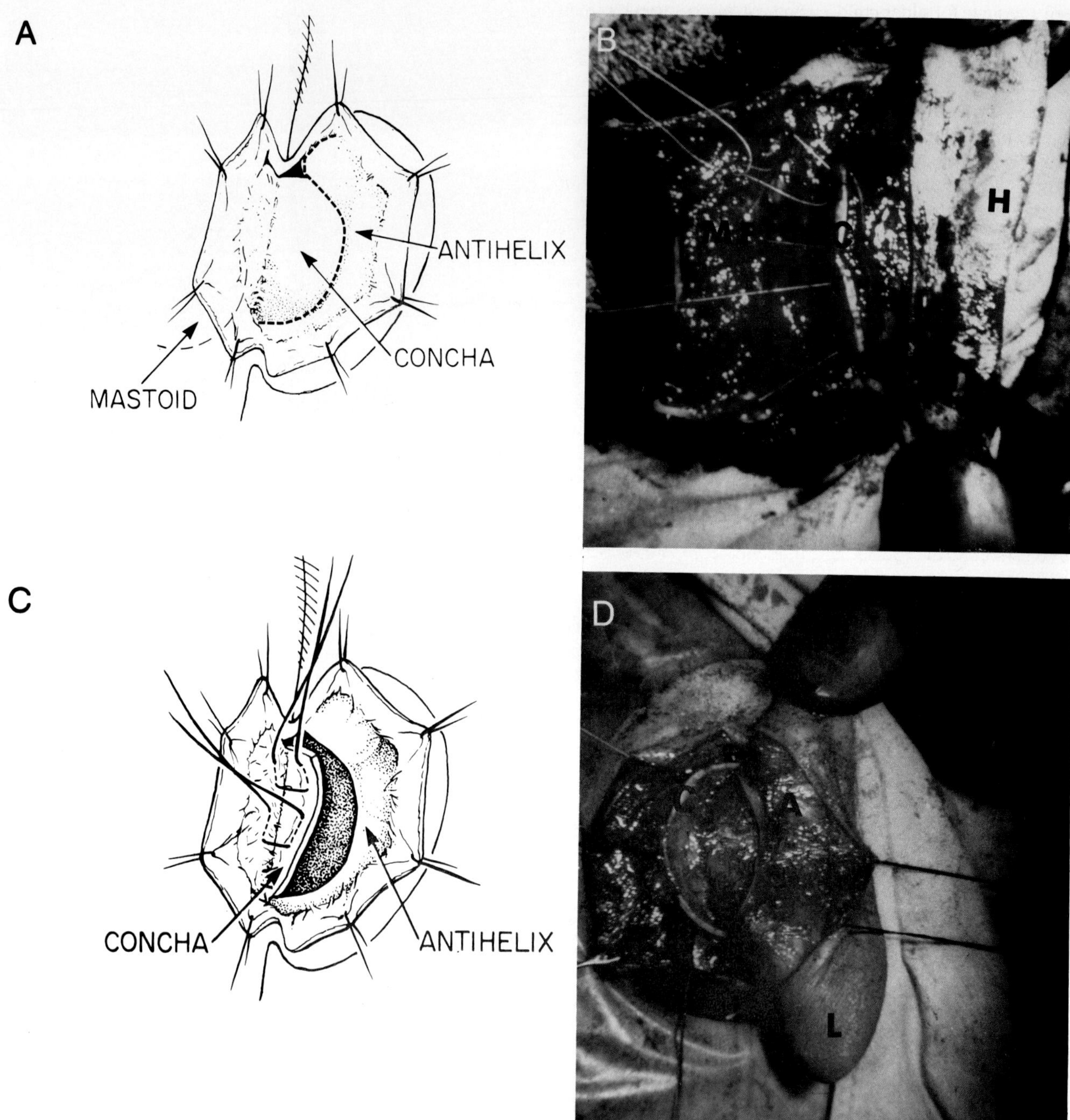

FIG 32–24.
A, complete separation of antihelix from concha. Note removal of cartilage segment at junction of inferior crus with crus of helix *(solid triangle).* **B,** conchal setback sutures are inserted in conchal cartilage *(C)* and fixed to mastoid periosteum. Note mastoid pedicle flap *(MF)* and helix *(H).* **C,** insertion of conchal setback sutures. **D,** conchal cartilage *(C)* in fixed position to mastoid. Note antihelix *(A)* and lobule *(L).* (From Feuerstein SS: *Facial Plast Surg* 1986; 2:142–150. Used by permission.)

been adequate for older children and adults. Children less than 7 or 8 years of age would most likely require general anesthesia. Postoperatively, the drain is removed in 24 hours, and it is recommended that a complete dressing be applied. If the patient complains of pain, it is best to remove the dressing and inspect the ear for any abnormal reaction.

A protective dressing over the ear is recommended for about 1 week, following which a headband can be used for approximately 1 week during sleeping hours.

Figure 32–26 shows an 8-year-old patient preoperatively and 1 year postoperatively and then at 18 years' follow-up. The maintenance of the normal appearance of the ears over this 18-year period is demonstrated.

CONCLUSION

The described technique of otoplasty in this chapter is a combination of the desirable features of many techniques previously described. The key that should be stressed is the basic premise that the embryologic defect must be corrected; the abnormal relationship of the inferior crus with the skull is to be adjusted; and the conchal and antihelical compartments must be placed into normal relationship.[10–13]

Only small amounts of cartilage are sacrificed, and all incisions are concealed so that another dictum in plastic surgery is carefully observed, namely, the repair of one defect should not create another. Complete mobilization of the conchal and antihelical auricular compartments is stressed, allowing only minimal tension on the sutures, whose primary function is to maintain the repositioned cartilage in its permanent position until sufficient fibrous tissue has formed.

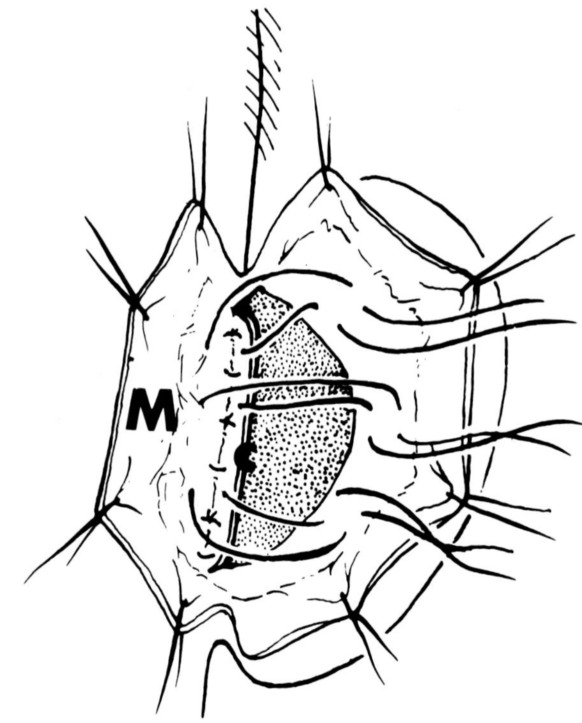

FIG 32–25.
Conchal cartilage fixed to mastoid periosteum. Vertical mastoid sutures fix antihelix over the cut conchal edge. Note mastoid pedicle flap *(M)* and cut edge of concha *(C)*. (From Feuerstein SS: *Otolaryngol Clin North Am* 1974; 7:141. Used by permission.)

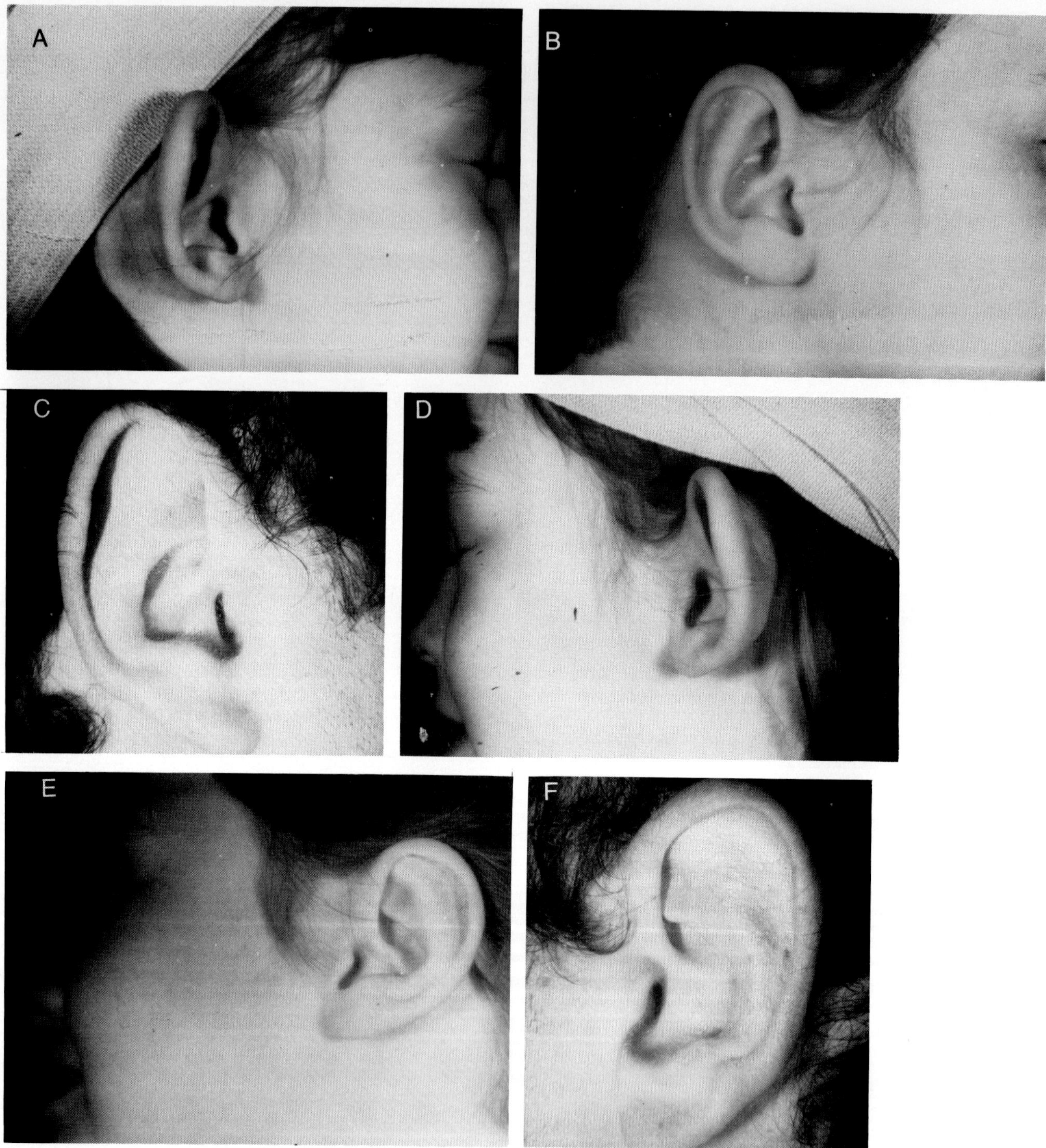

FIG 32–26.
A, preoperative 8-year-old girl demonstrating abnormal inferior crus projection in right ear. **B,** same patient 8 months following otoplasty. **C,** same patient 18 years following surgery. **D,** same patient showing preoperative view of left ear. **E,** same patient 8 months following otoplasty. **F,** same patient 18 years following surgery.

REFERENCES

1. Luckett WH: A new operation for prominent ears based on the anatomy of the deformity. *Surg Gynecol Obstet* 1910; 10:635–637.
2. Barsky AJ: *Plastic Surgery.* Philadelphia, WB Saunders Co, 1938, p 178.
3. Kitlowski EA, Davis JS: Abnormal prominence of the ears: A method of readjustment. *Surgery* 1937; 2:835–848.
4. Furnas D: Correction of prominent ears by concha-mastoid sutures. *Plast Reconst Surg* 1968; 42:189–193.
5. Feuerstein SS: Management of the inferior crus in otoplasty. *Eye Ear Nose Throat Monthly* 1958; 37:385–389.
6. Young F: Correction of the abnormally prominent ears. *Surg Gynecol Obstet* 1944; 78:541–550.
7. Becker OJ: Surgical correction of the abnormally protruding ear. *Arch Otolaryngol* 1949; 50:541–560.
8. Farrior RT: A method of otoplasty; normal contour of the antihelix and scaphoid fossa. *Arch Otolaryngol* 1959; 69:400.
9. Mustardé JG: The correction of prominent ear using simple mattress sutures. *Br J Plast Surg* 1963; 16:170.
10. Feuerstein SS: Combined technique of otoplasty. *Laryngoscope* 1969; 79:1118–1131.
11. Feuerstein SS: Importance of differential diagnosis in otoplasty. *Eye Ear Nose Throat Monthly* 1960; 39:732–734.
12. Feuerstein SS: Revision techniques in otoplasty. *Otolaryngol Clin North Am* 1974; 7:133–144.
13. Feuerstein SS: Complications and revisions in otoplasty. *Facial Plast Surg* 1985; 2:142–150.

CHAPTER 33

Cervicofacial Liposuction

Approach of

Douglas D. Dedo, M.D.

CLOSED LIPOSUCTION OF THE FACE

Preoperative Evaluation

Several areas of the face have been treated with liposuction to reduce the subcutaneous layer of fat that gravitates with age. These localized collections of fat may occur anywhere but usually concentrate in the malar bags, cheek-lip folds, buccal space, and jowls. Since each one of these has a distinct etiology and anatomy, each requires specific management and treatment.

Malar Bags

In reality, these are not true collections of fat but pseudobags because of their development. They form from an inferior ptosis of the subcutaneous fatty layer that cascades into the cheek-lip fold. A trough, or depression, runs from the medial canthus to the angle of the mandible. The malar bag forms the superior border of this depression and should not be reduced since malar augmentation is one of the solutions to facial rejuvenation. The preferred treatment of the malar pseudobag is not to remove it but to camouflage it with sublabial cheek implants to eliminate the depression along its inferior border. Injectable fillers (fat, collagen) in this diagonal trough also work but, unfortunately, are not as permanent as the Alloplastic material.

Cheek-Lip Folds

This anatomic unit (erroneously called nasolabial folds) has been subjected to liposuction with regular-sized cannulas[1] (3/16 in or 5 mm) to minicannulas (14-gauge needle, 3 mm), with disastrous results. More complications have occurred with liposuction in this area than any other place. Instead of the desired result of reducing the fullness of the cheek-lip fold and depth of the groove, single or multiple troughs that run in and parallel to the original fold have been created.

These depressions form because the cushion of fat has been sufficiently reduced to permit adherence of the dermis to the underlying mobile facial musculature. Prevention of this complication is, first, not to treat these folds with liposuction. However, if they develop, the two treatment alternatives are excision (which must be done bilaterally) of the pseudogroove and cheek-lip fold or filling of the iatrogenic rhytid. Unfortunately, present-day fillers (fat, collagen) offer only a temporary solution because they are absorbed over time. The gravitational pull of the skin and fat over the tethered orbicular fascia that runs from the nose to the chin with subsequent formation of full cheek-lip fold is not amenable to liposuction.

Buccal Fat

Individuals with a full, round face who lack definition of the malar areas are candidates for transoral buccal fat extraction. This fat fills the buccal space that is formed by the masseter muscle laterally and the buccinator muscle medially. As described by Newman et al., a stab incision is made opposite the first molar in the buccogingival sulcus.[2] The open-ended blunt suction cannula is placed in the incision and directed posteriorly and parallel to the inferior rim of the maxilla to enter the buccal space. The suction is turned on and the cannula gently withdrawn, pulling the buccal fat into the incision. It then is gently teased out with forceps and suction cannula. Care is taken not to destroy the septae or blood vessels. An alternative method is to clamp the stalk of the fat pad and cauterize the base after excision to prevent hematoma formation. Selection of individuals for buccal fat removal should be limited to those with full, round cheeks and poorly developed malar prominences. Preoperative assessment can be achieved by having the patient purse the lips and gently suck inward. The resultant concavity demonstrates the area of buccal fat removal.

Jowls

The fascia of the facial musculature is densely adherent to the mandible posterior to the notch of the facial artery and anterior to a line drawn inferiorly from the oral commissure. The gap between these fascial attachments identifies the jowl that forms from ptosis of the subcutaneous layer of fat. It can be judiciously reduced with liposuction. The safest technique is to direct the facial 3/16 in. cannula to the center of the jowl fat with the vacuum off. It can be approached inferiorly from the submental incision, laterally from the subauricular incision, or after elevation of the face-lift flaps. It is important to stabilize, pinch, and retract the jowl fat laterally as the cannula is gently inserted into the center. After the vacuum is turned on, three or four strokes are made as the stabilizing hand squeezes the fat into the cannula. It is important not to try to remove all the jowl fat or to reduce the fullness by tunneling over it beneath the skin. Both of these approaches will produce irregular contouring along the mandible. By removal of a central core of fat, the jowl area will shrink in fullness, contract, and leave a satisfactory jawline. As the size of the jowl increases (directly proportionate to age), the skin reaches a limit beyond which it will not contract adequately. In these patients, concomitant face-lift and superficial musculoaponeurotic system (SMAS) tightening are required to produce a youthful jawline.

OPEN LIPOSUCTION OF THE FACE

Once the temporal, preauricular, cervical, and occipital flaps of the face-lift have been elevated, the subcutaneous layer of fat, intimately attached to the SMAS, becomes readily accessible. Small isolated collections and thick layers of subcutaneous fat (particularly noticed in round-faced individuals) are thinned under high vacuum by simply rubbing the cannula briskly over the fat as if scrubbing it. As the SMAS layer is skeletonized, it can be undermined, excised, and advanced or simply plicated on itself. Open liposuction extends superiorly to the zygomatic arch and anteriorly over the parotid gland along a vertical line that will be plicated posteriorly to the preauricular area. Extension of fat removal beyond this imaginary line into the cheek-lip fold risks creating subcutaneous dimples and irregular contouring. Inferiorly the sculpting of fat runs into the neck. Along the mandible, the cushion of fat is thinned and not totally eliminated to prevent a step deformity. Below the border of the mandible the platysma is cleaned sufficiently to expose the platysma muscle fibers. This fat removal accentuates and redefines the jawline posteriorly, a hallmark of a youthful neck.

If the open technique is used with face-lifting, the thickness or roll of a plicated SMAS is reduced. Furthermore, the raw surface area created when the fat is removed may fibrose and heal more firmly when it is sutured on itself than when two layers of fat are sutured together.

CLOSED LIPOSUCTION OF THE NECK

Introduction and subsequent refinement of closed cervical liposuction have revolutionized cosmetic surgery of the neck and cervicomental contour. The operative challenge in closed liposuction of the neck is the identification of the ideal candidate. It is one who is young with good skin turgor and elasticity with a submental collection of fat who could tolerate a chin implant. Patients with wrinkled inelastic skin will not achieve satisfactory contraction of the skin after liposuction. As a result, the obtuse cervicomental contour has been converted to a neck covered with hanging loose skin. The chin implant will accomplish two things: (1) it helps take up any slack in the skin, and (2) it enhances the neckline by giving the illusion that the neck is longer. As the age of the patient approaches 40 years or more, they are advised that a face-lift may be required to sufficiently tighten the cervical skin.

Another challenge in cervical liposuction is identification of the pathologic platysma muscle. Frequently the patient will want closed liposuction for an obtuse cervicomental contour. As the edema subsides after liposuction, the anterior platysma bands become visible due to the muscle being skeletonized from fat removal. Treatment of this postoperative sequela is best accomplished with a full face-lift and submental tuck.[3] Prevention is achieved by identifying preoperatively the contribution of the platysma to the submental fullness. Voluntary grimacing and contraction of the platysma will help identify the muscle and the fat. When visible or palpable cords are present, the platysma muscle must be manipulated in some way to produce a satisfactory postoperative result.[4]

Lax, thick skin and ptotic musculature may masquerade as fat in the neck. Following liposuction, there is no postoperative improvement or change. These patients are usually men with short necks, thick skin, and heavy hair follicles. Well-developed platysma and accessory muscles (e.g., in wind musicians) contribute to the fullness. Subsequent face-lifts even with SMAS-platysma tightening do not completely correct the problem. Prevention and subsequent counseling are by preoperative identification, which is extremely difficult.

Ptotic submandibular glands will produce fullness in the submandibular triangle. Following cervical liposuction, two round bulges are seen. Palpation of the cobblestone gland surface confirms the diagnosis. Usually these glands are obvious preoperatively on inspection and palpation of the neck. Showing them to the patient and telling them of postoperative enhancement will avoid unnecessary explanations after surgery. When they are identified and pose a problem (either preoperatively or postoperatively), several alternatives exist, none of which gives a perfect result. Suspension of the gland with a 2-0 braided suture from the anterior border posteriorly to the mastoid fascia exposes the marginal mandibular nerve to potential injury without adequate results. Tightening the platysma with a submental tuck and posterior advancement over the sternocleidomastoid fascia should theoretically eliminate the bulging. Unfortunately, one of the reasons the glands have become ptotic is the absence of a significant platysma muscle to hold them up, and when it is manipulated, the fibers are themselves atrophic and weak.

Surgical Technique

The surgical technique of closed liposuction is begun with the patient in the sitting position. Symmetric tunnels are drawn on the neck and face where the fat is to be removed. The lateral boundary in the neck is the anterior border of the sternocleidomastoid muscle. Inferiorly, the cricoid cartilage is usually the anatomic landmark, but should there be a collection of fat in the suprasternal notch, it is also marked for subsequent treatment. The mandible is the superior border unless the jowl is to be reduced. In the latter instance, the jowl fat is circumscribed on its periphery with a marker and seen to end posteriorly at the mandibular notch for the facial artery. The local is infiltrated in the area to be treated. Incisions are placed in the subauricular and first submental crease. Should liposuction be combined with a face-lift and submental work, the incision is placed posterior to the first submental crease to facilitate exposure. The cannula is placed into the incision, vacuumed off, and pushed to the end of the tunnel as the other hand, in this case usually the left hand for right-handed individuals, pinches and pulls the skin laterally. The cannula is placed on top of the platysma muscle and not deep to it. Once the vacuum is turned on, short strokes of the cannula are made so that it traverses only the distance between the fingers of the left hand as they squeeze the fat into the cannula. It is best to think of the cannula as a battering ram that breaks up the fat being stabilized with the other hand. Once the fat is removed at the end of the tunnel, the left hand is advanced up the neck to stabilize the next segment and so on until the tunnel has been treated back to the incision. The second tunnel is now approached by again inserting the cannula (with the vacuum off) on top of the platysma as the opposite hand stabilizes and retracts the skin laterally. The tunnels fan out from the submental incision. The second and third array of tunnels radiate out from beneath each lobule to create a cross-hatching effect over the neck. The opening of the cannula is always away from the skin to prevent dermal injury, and the tunnels themselves are never connected with a sweeping motion across the neck.

The jowl fat may be approached from the submental incision. To prevent injury to the marginal mandibular branch of the facial nerve, the cannula is again placed in the incision with the vacuum off. As the cannula tip advances over the mandible, it is directed away from the underlying bone and superficially into the skin to protect the nerve. Again, the jowl is pulled outward and stabilized as the cannula is shoved into the center of the fat. The vacuum is turned on, and short strokes of the cannula between the fingers are made to create a central reduction in the volume of fat that allows for contraction of the jowl onto itself.

Once the entire cervical area has been treated, the skin and subcutaneous layers are palpated, pinched, and rolled between the fingers to feel for areas of irregularity or incomplete fat removal. Should such an area be felt, the cannula is reinserted and the fullness reduced.

Since there are no vital neurovascular structures in this insulating layer of fat, there should be no significant bleeding or nerve injury. There have been no published reports of permanent nerve injury. Significant hematoma formation has not been reported.[5] However, should the cannula be placed deep to the platysma muscle, theoretical damage to the thin-walled internal jugular vein is possible. By constantly feeling the tip of the cannula between the fingertips, it is possible to immediately note an increased thickness of the folded skin due to the platysma muscle beneath it. After closed liposuction of the neck, a bulky pressure dressing is placed on the neck. It is changed the next day after surgery and left in place another 3 to 4 days. An orthopedic stockinet is rolled into a chin strap and worn for another 7 days after removal of the dressing. Should liposuction be done as an adjunctive procedure to face-lift, the routine regimen for face-lift dressings is followed.

Following resolution of the edema and skin contracture, small irregularities may be seen or palpated. The operator should wait a minimum of 6 months before treating any depression or mounds in the face and neck. Persistent fullness due to a collection of fat may be injected with 10 mg of triamcinolone/mL through a 30-gauge needle. An alternative is aspiration of the fat collection with a 16-gauge needle on a 10 mL syringe under local anesthesia. Depressions are more difficult to treat and will require collagen or autogenous fat injections, which are only temporary.

A phenomenon observed in early patients to improve and prolong the results of liposuction is to encourage even a small weight loss during the first or second year following surgery. Those patients who lose weight seem to metabolize and mobilize the traumatized fat more readily than those who maintain or gain weight, resulting in a thinner neck and improved cosmetic result.

ANCILLARY PROCEDURES OF LIPOSUCTION SURGERY

Debulking Flaps

Following reconstructive surgery and adequate maturation of the flap, the recipient area may be too bulky or thick. Subcutaneous fat and edema account for this excessive bulk and are frequently seen with myocutaneous flap reconstruction of the head and neck. Under local or general anesthesia, the cannula is inserted through a short incision to fan out over the flap and defat it. The skin usually contracts adequately. However, if it becomes too redundant following the debulking procedure, simple direct excision and closure will correct the problem. Liposuction should not be done at the time of primary reconstruction for fear of damaging the perforating vasculature that supplies the overlying skin.

Lipoma

Lipomas are particularly amenable to excision with liposuction. The circumference of the lipoma is marked. After infiltration of local anesthesia, a 1 to 1.5 cm incision is made at the most inconspicuous edge of the lipoma. Scissors spread the incision to facilitate introduction of the cannula. The fat of the lipoma has a different consistency from the surrounding layer and is readily squeezed into the aspirating cannula as it repeatedly batters the tumor. Following fat reduction of the lipoma, one can feel the capsule move around under the skin. It should be palpated and moved up to the incision. The capsule is grasped with a hemostat through the incision and peeled out from under the skin. Concomitant insertion and aspiration with the cannula into the capsule while it is being pulled out will further debulk it to facilitate its removal. Once the capsule has been removed, the area is repeatedly squeezed and palpated for any residual pieces of capsule. If found, they are moved up to the incision for subsequent removal as before. The incision is closed and a bulky pressure dressing applied for 4 days.

Autograft Fat Transfer

The natural aging process leaves furrows and depressions as the facial skeleton is absorbed, with concomitant skin and subcutaneous atrophy. These changes, combined with traumatic and postoperative deformities, need to be filled to improve form and function. For years fat grafting has been tried with little permanent success. Since the development of liposuction, there was renewed interest in using fat as a reconstructive tool. However, results have been disappointing so far as long-term survival is concerned. The technique involved harvesting the fat with a sharp 14- or 16-gauge needle attached to a syringe. Fournier makes a point to avoid injecting the donor or recipient area with local anesthesia.[6] Instead, ice packs and nerve blocks are used for anesthesia. Once the fat is harvested, it is rinsed with normal saline in the syringe and the latter expelled from the syringe prior to fat injection. The recipient area is marked and the fat injected as the needle is withdrawn, trying to overcorrect the deficiency by 30%. Approximately 2 to 4 mL of fat are injected in any one area. Besides the problems with absorption, one case of blindness has been reported following injection of the glabellar area.[7] Although initial experience seems to reproduce prior fat grafting results, many approaches and investigations are being conducted to try to find a way to prolong and improve the effects of autograft fat transfer.

CONCLUSION

Liposuction is an effective and safe technique to remove subcutaneous fat. It is safer and faster than using direct excision and, when combined with other surgical procedures, will enhance the postoperative result.

REFERENCES

1. Illouz WG: *Liposuction: The Franco-American Experience.* Beverly Hills, Calif, Medical Aesthetics, 1985, Chapter 13.
2. Newman J, Nguien A, Anderson R: Liposuction of the buccal fat pad. *Am J Cosmetic Surg* 1986; 3:1–4.
3. Dedo D: Liposuction and the platysma muscle. *Arch Otol* 1986; 112:306–308.
4. Dedo D: Management of the platysma muscle after open and closed liposuction of the neck in face-lift surgery. *Facial Plast Surg* 1986; 4:45–56.
5. Newman J, Dolsky RL: Evaluation of 5,458 cases of liposuction surgery. *Am J Cosmetic Surg* special issue no 1, 1986, pp 37–41.
6. Fournier PF: *Body Sculpturing Through Syringe Liposuction and Autologous Fat Re-injection.* Samuel Rolf, Int'l., United States of America, 1987, p 78.
7. Teimourian B: Correspondence, in *Plastic Reconstructive Surgery,* August 1988, p 361.

Cervicofacial Liposuction

Approach of

Julius Newman, M.D.,

and

Mani Nambiar, M.D.

The contour and shape of the face are influenced by the amount and distribution of adipose tissue in these regions. Conventional lipectomy has been included in cervicofacial aesthetic procedures since the work of Passot in 1919,[1] but unsightly scars make conventional lipectomy unappealing. Suction lipectomy for body sculpturing was made popular by Illouz in the early 1980s.[2] Newman and colleagues subsequently applied the technique to the cervical and facial areas, and have since improved and refined suction lipectomy of the face and neck and coined the term liposuction in 1982.[3–6] At the present time, liposuction has been used at the melolabial mound, the malar sad pad, the buccal fat pad, the jowl, the submental area, and other areas of the neck. It is also used in conjunction with and to facilitate other cervicofacial cosmetic procedures such as mentoplasty, malarplasty, and rhytidectomy.

CERVICOFACIAL LIPOSUCTION

Anatomy of the Adipose Tissue of the Face and Neck

To perform liposuction with confidence and precision, one must understand the distribution of adipose tissue and its relation with surrounding important structures. In the face, adipose tissue relevant to liposuction is found in the subcutaneous layer, the buccal space, the malar sad pad, the melolabial mound, and the glabellar fold.

The subcutaneous fat is described and located on both sides of the SMAS, which is in continuity with the frontal and temporal muscles superiorly and with the platysma caudally. The anatomic concept of SMAS is vague and recently challenged by Jost et al., who consider it an "anatomic impossibility."[7] Subcutaneous adipose tissue is superficial to the parotid fascia, the masseter muscle, and the muscles of facial expression. Important structures such as the branches of the facial nerve, facial vessels, and the parotid duct are covered by parotid fascia and muscle. The melolabial mound, the glabellar fold, and the malar

sad pad represent excessive accumulations of subcutaneous adipose tissue in the respective areas.

The buccal fat pad is located in the buccal space, which is formed by the buccinator muscle medially, the masseter muscle laterally, and the mandibular ramus inferiorly. The parotid duct is an important structure in the buccal space, which penetrates the buccinator muscle and enters the mouth opposite the maxillary second molar. Branches of the buccal nerve, a branch of the trigeminal nerve, are also found in the buccal space, supplying sensation to the buccal mucosa. The facial artery and vein, after crossing the superior portion of the masseter muscle, anastomose with the anterior facial vessels along the anterior border of this muscle superficial to the buccal fat pad.

In the neck, adipose tissue is located on both sides of the platysma, which is invested by two layers of the superficial cervical fascia (Fig 33–1). The platysma is a long, oblique, flat muscle whose fibers run vertically on both sides of the neck, extending from its origin at the pectoralis major and deltoid muscles in the infraclavicular area to its insertion into the aponeurosis of the facial muscles (Fig 33–2). In about 60% of the population, the fibers of the platysma interdigitate in the midline at the submental region from the chin to the hyoid bone. Below this region, the anterior borders of the platysma separate and extend posteriorly in an oblique fashion. The lateral borders of the platysma blend into the fascia of the sternocleidomastoid muscles. The platysma is innervated by cervical branches of the facial nerve. A number of anastomoses exist between the cervical branches and the mandibular branches of the facial nerve, supplying the muscles of facial expression. The mandibular branch of the facial nerve lies deep to the platysma at the level of the mandibular ramus in 80% of the population. In the other 20%, this branch is located 1 to 1.5 cm below the mandibular margin (Fig 33–3).

The external jugular vein descends from the mandibular angle toward the clavicle, becoming covered by the platysma as it encounters the lateral border of this muscle (Fig 33–4).

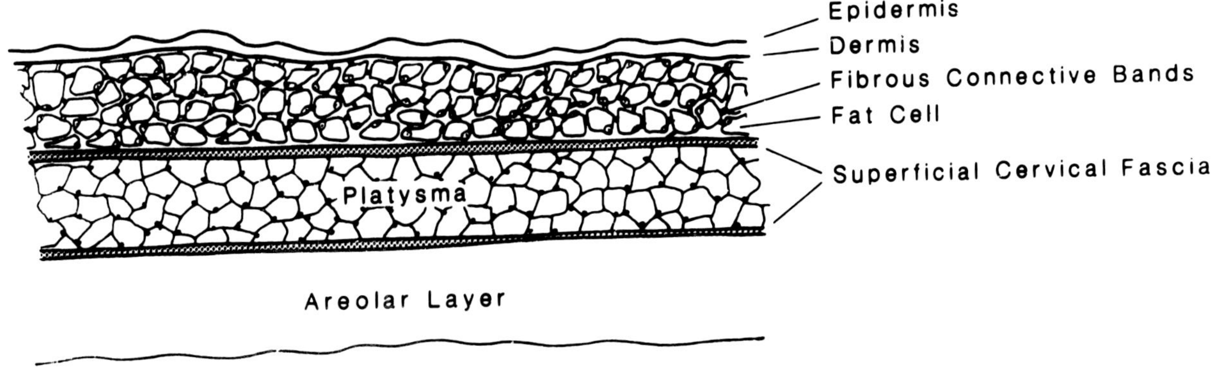

FIG 33–1.
Fascial layers of the neck.

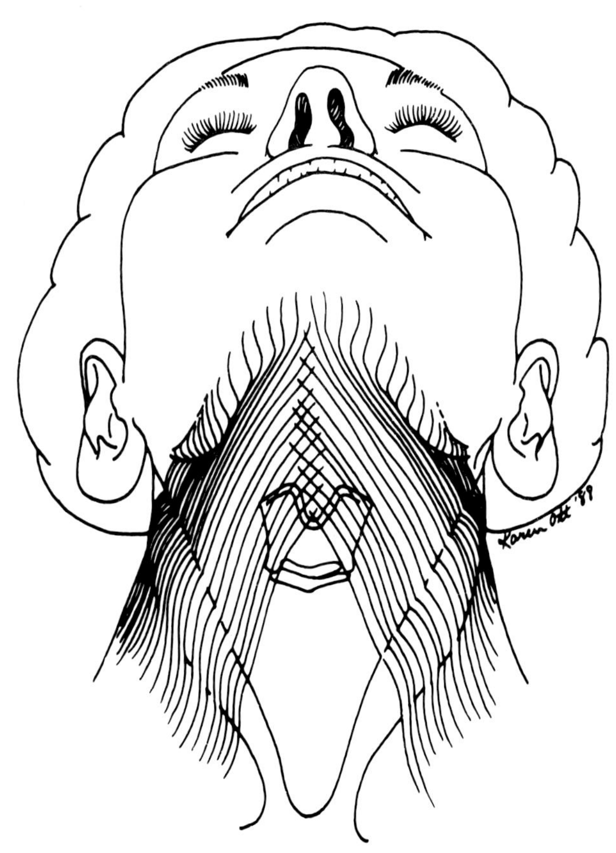

FIG 33–2.
Anatomy of the platysma muscle.

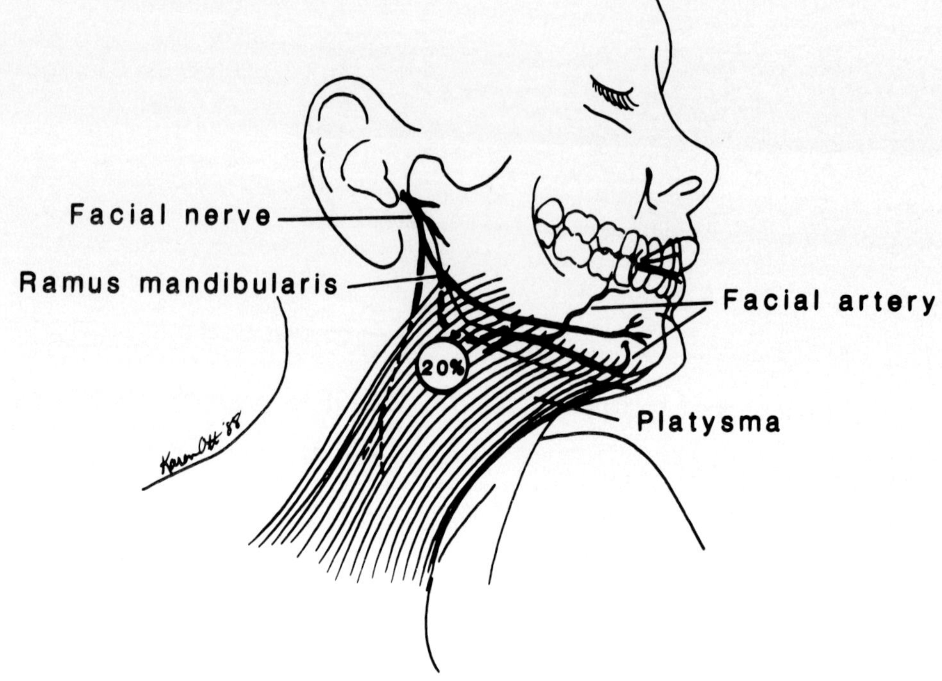

FIG 33–3.
Relationship of the mandible to the mandibular branch of the facial
nerve.

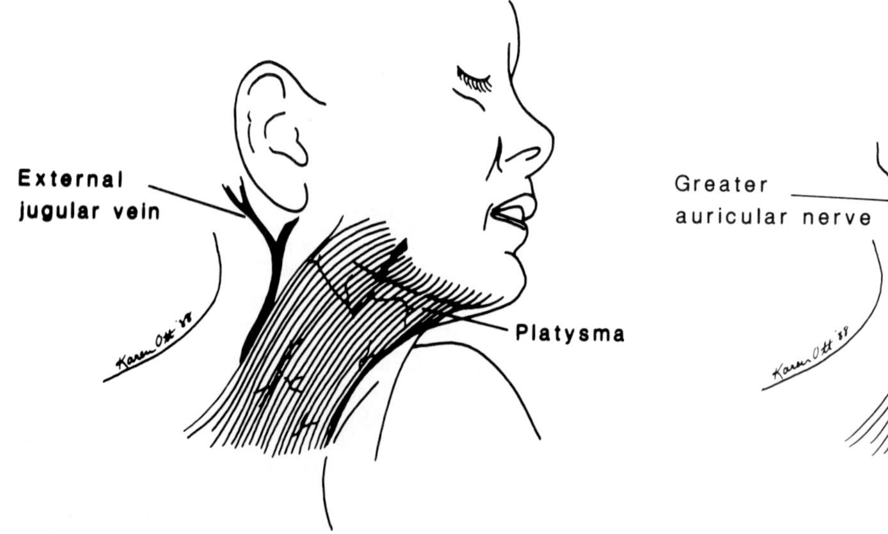

FIG 33–4.
Relationship of the external jugular vein to platysma.

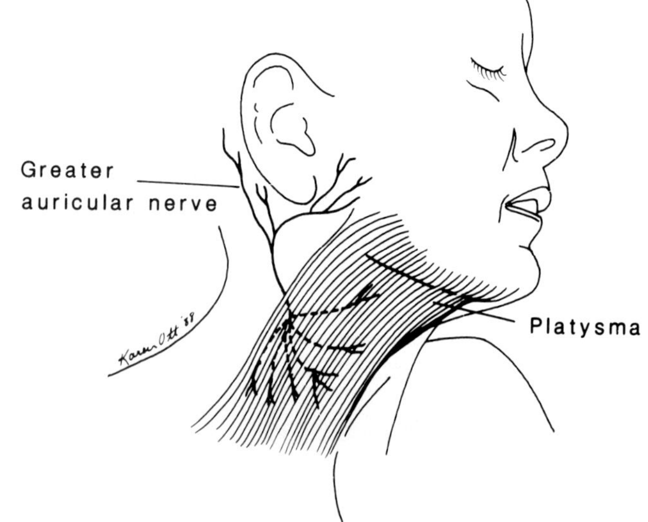

FIG 33–5.
Relationship of the greater auricular nerve in the neck.

The greater auricular nerve is similarly covered by the platysma
(Fig 33–5). Both the external jugular vein and the greater auricular nerve are under the superficial fascia where not covered
by the platysma. All other major vessels are well beneath the
platysmal layer.

In the subdermal adipose tissue, there is a fibrous septal
network connecting the dermis to the platysmal superficial fascia (see Fig 33–1). Liposuction is generally performed on this
layer of fat.

There is another adipose deposit in the neck relevant to

Instruments and Equipment

The cannulas used for cervicofacial liposuction have been modified to make adherence to the principles already outlined easier. The Newman quick connect spatula internal Luer-Lock liposuction cannula system comprises four cannulas 15 cm long and 4, 5, 6, and 8 mm in diameter (Fig 33–6). They are designed with a universal Luer-Lock handle for quick connection. These handles can also be attached to a syringe for easy irrigation and cleaning (Fig 33–7). The tip of the cannula is blunt and flattened in a spatula shape to prevent dermal injury and to stay easily within the subcutaneous layer. The blunt tip also prevents injury to nerves, arteries, and veins by pushing them to the side as the cannula is passed through the tissues. The suction port of the cannula is located 180 degrees away from the skin to avoid injury to the dermal undersurface.

Included in the Newman cannula series is a guided buccal

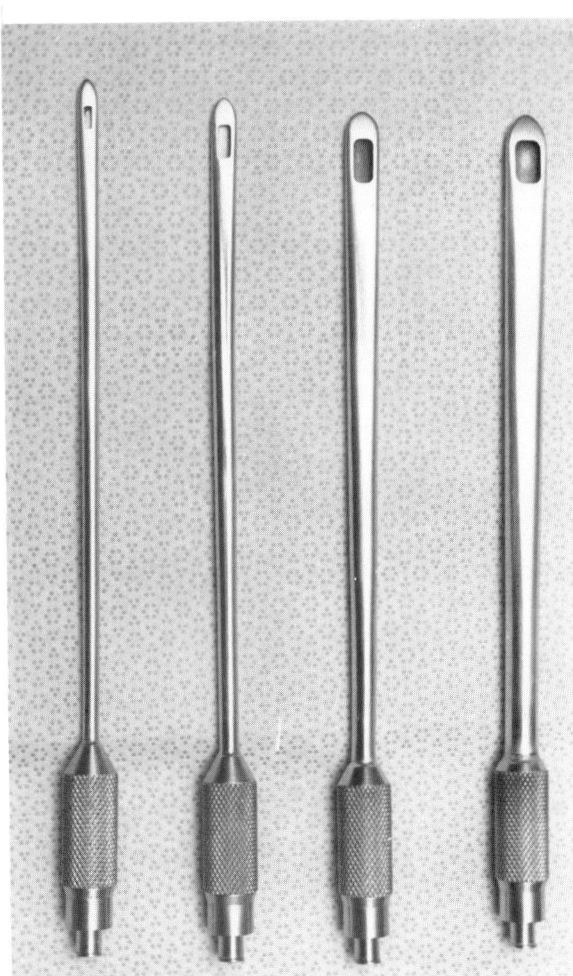

FIG 33–6.
Newman quick connect Leur-Lock spatula cannula system.

liposuction located in the submental region deep to the platysma. It is this adipose tissue that causes the double chin appearance when excessive accumulation occurs.

Concepts

Unlike body liposuction where tunnels are created in the fatty tissue to cause compression and flattening of certain areas, facial liposuction involves removal of all excess fatty tissue. At times this creates a skin flap that needs to be redraped over facial core structures. Facial and cervical skin has a rich blood supply and lymphatic drainage. The skin in these areas can be widely undermined and defatted without fear of skin necrosis.

Several important principles must be kept in mind to achieve satisfactory results: (1) to prevent injury to the dermal layer; (2) to preserve a small amount of subdermal fat, which is necessary to maintain cutaneous lymphatic drainage, skin sensation, tonicity and trophicity; and (3) to prevent injury to deep structures by being sure to stay within the subcutaneous layer and avoid penetration of the cervical fascia and platysma muscle.

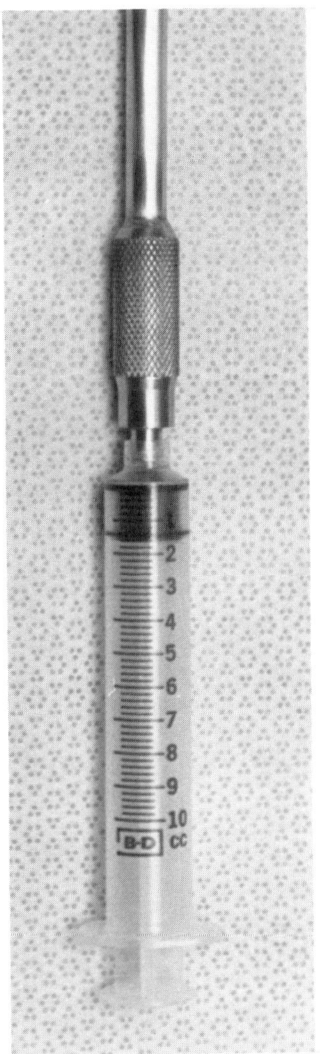

FIG 33–7.
Attachment of a cannula to a syringe for irrigation.

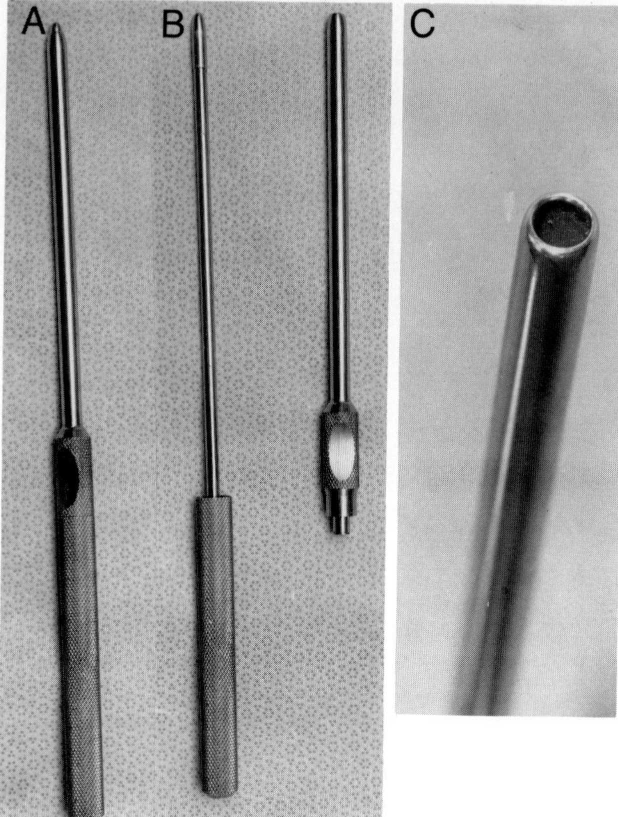

FIG 33–8.
A, guided buccal-jowl extractor; **B**, separated buccal-jowl extractor; **C**, open tip of the buccal-jowl extractor.

and jowl extractor (Fig 33–8). This is a blunt, open-ended 6 mm suction cannula with a round-tipped stylet. It allows atraumatic entry into the buccal space.

Two specially designed spatula needles (Fig 33–9) measuring 8 and 15 cm are used for infiltration of local anesthesia. Their shape makes it easier to stay within the proper tissue plane than with conventional needles.

The suction machine is a 0.5 hp, double-diaphragm unit (Fig 33–10) that generates 1 atm of negative pressure, which it reaches within 5 to 6 seconds.

The tubing connecting the cannula to the suction machine is the routine suction tubing found in most operating rooms.

Preoperative Evaluation

The choice of patients for cervicofacial liposuction is very selective. The face and neck are evaluated for abnormal accumulations of subcutaneous fat. Facial skin tone, elasticity, and redundancy are also evaluated. Age, although not a contraindication for cervicofacial liposuction, is an important factor involving skin tone and elasticity.

The midface is examined to determine the presence of an enlarged melolabial mound and deep smile lines. The size of the sad pad is determined. The cheek contour is examined in conjunction with the malar prominence superiorly and buccal

fat pad inferiorly. Full cheeks, combined with a normal to flat malar eminence giving a chipmunk appearance, can be improved with buccal suction possibly combined with malar implants.

The lower part of the face and the neck are evaluated for jowl prominence, submental fat accumulation, skin tone, and degree of skin sagging of the neck.

Generally, in younger patients with good skin tone and isolated fat accumulation, submental liposuction can be performed alone with good results. In older patients, platysma bands, so-called turkey neck, and sagging neck and jowls appear and worsen with age. Submental liposuction alone will not be of benefit. Depending on the redundancy and elasticity of the skin, total neck suction and flap redraping (the closed neck lift) or a liposuction assisted rhytidectomy must be performed.

The preoperative evaluation also focuses on the chin and cheekbones in relation to the patient's facial profile. A fat neck

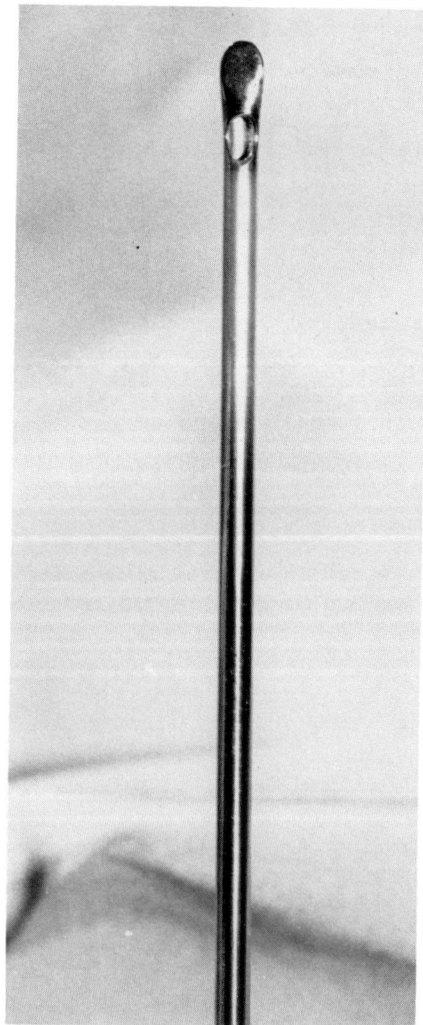

FIG 33–9.
The Flattened tip of the spatula needle.

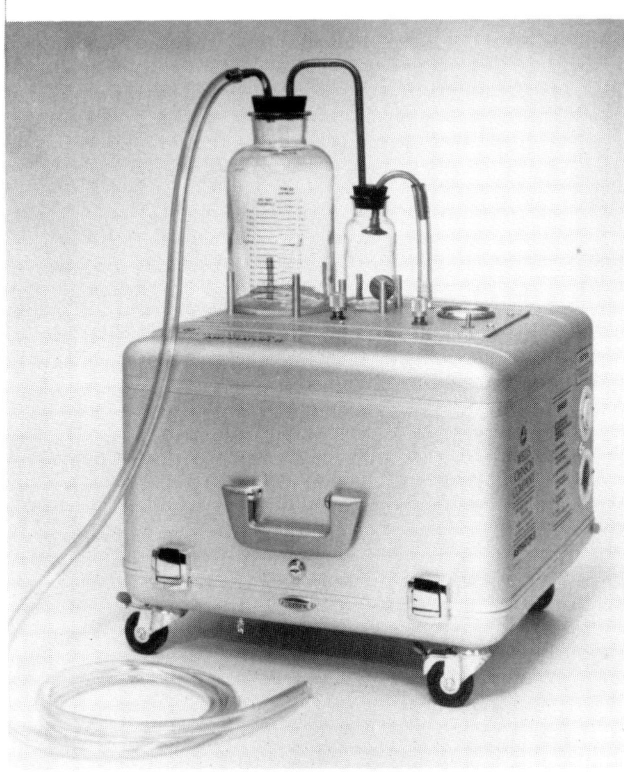

FIG 33–10.
The 0.5 hp suction machine.

and recessive chin give an unpleasant look to the face. In many instances, the neck almost comes to the edge of the recessive chin line. As an adjunct to liposuction of the neck, insertion of a hard acrylic chin implant gives better definition to the neck-chin angle.

Preoperative Preparation

The head and neck areas are washed with a disinfectant soap, and a first-generation cephalosporin is given intravenously prior to the procedure. While the patient is in the sitting position, the areas of abnormal fat accumulation and the incisions are marked with an indelible pen. General or local standby anesthesia may be used, depending on the surgeon's preference, the extent of the surgery, and the equipment and staffing of the facilities.

Areas marked for incision are infiltrated with a solution of 2% lidocaine (Xylocaine) with epinephrine 1:100,000. The areas to undergo liposuction are infiltrated with a diluted mixture of anesthetic. Mixing 50 mL of 1% lidocaine with 1:100,000 epinephrine in 450 mL of normal saline gives a final mixture of 0.1% lidocaine with epinephrine 1:1,000,000. The technique of infiltration will be described in the discussion of each technique.

Techniques

Submental Fat Pad

Indications.—

1. Restoration of the neck-chin angle
2. Young age group (not absolute)
3. Good skin tone and elasticity
4. Isolated submental fat accumulation

Preoperative Preparation.—The extent of the fat bulge and submental incision are marked with the patient in the sitting position. Infiltration is with 2% lidocaine with epinephrine 1:100,000 into the fat pad and extending only 2 or 3 cm into the surrounding area.

Surgical Technique.—A 0.5 cm incision is made in the submental crease. A subcutaneous tunnel is started with a small blunt scissors. The 4 mm spatula-tipped cannula is inserted into the tunnel, and the cannula is connected to machine suction. With the right hand as the pusher and the left hand as the guider, the cannula is pushed back and forth radially throughout the submental fat pad. A 5 mm spatula-tipped cannula is inserted, and the process is repeated. During the suctioning process, the thickness of the subcutaneous tissue is palpated by gently pinching the skin between two fingers to determine the thickness of the treated area. Subplatysmal fat can sometimes be extracted in the midline using the 6 mm cannula, creating further definition of the chin and submental region. The skin is closed with Steri-strips.

The dressing consists of three layers of Webril covered by three layers of French tape. These are held in place by an elastic face-chin-neck support garment (Fig 33–11). This dressing is worn for 5 days, after which it is replaced by two tennis headbands, which the patient is instructed to bring to the office (Fig 33–12).

Closed Neck Lift

Indications.—

1. Restoration of the neck-chin angle
2. Older age group (not absolute)
3. Some sagging of anterior neck skin
4. Submental fat accumulation
5. Not enough sagging skin to justify full face-lift

Purpose.—The closed neck lift combines submental liposuction with wide undermining of the skin of the anterior neck. The undermining creates a totally free skin flap in which the spatula cannula can sweep across the anterior neck skin without inhibition by subcutaneous attachments. The skin of the neck is then redraped and held in place with dressings so that scarring causes the skin to adhere to the underlying fascia in a more desirable, tighter fashion.

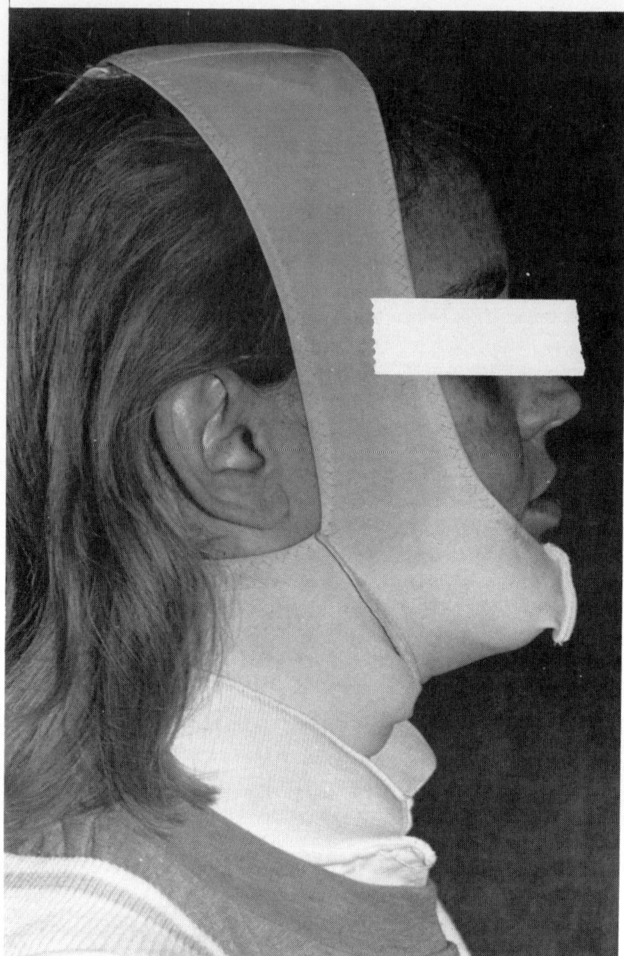

FIG 33–11.
Facial-chin-neck support garment.

Preoperative Preparation.—The extent of the area to be undermined as well as the incision are marked preoperatively with the patient in the sitting position. A small skin wheal is made with 2% lidocaine with epinephrine 1:100,000 in the submental crease for the incision. A 0.5 cm incision is made and a tunnel created with a small blunt scissors (Fig 33–13). Diluted anesthetic solution of 0.1% lidocaine with epinephrine 1:1,000,000 is then infiltrated using the specialized spatula needles. The entire anterior neck to the sternocleidomastoid muscles laterally and the suprasternal notch inferiorly is infiltrated with this solution.

Surgical Technique.—The 5 mm spatula-tipped cannula is inserted into the incision, and submental liposuction is carried out similar to the technique of the submental fat pad. However, if the neck is thin with little fat, the machine suction is turned off. The 6 mm cannula is then inserted, and the entire anterior neck skin is undermined without suction (Fig 33–14,A) so that there are no tunnels or septae connecting the skin to the underlying fascia. If there is a lot of fat in the neck, the suction

can be maintained during this part. The cannula should be able to sweep across the neck subcutaneously (Fig 33–14,B).

Through the same incision, the 8 mm cannula is inserted in the subplatysmal plane in the midline by using the left hand to push the tip of the cannula cephalad (Fig 33–15). This is to suction any fat that may have retracted under the platysma with the patient in the supine position. The cannula is maintained in the midline so as not to damage any structures found laterally such as the submandibular branch of the facial nerve.

The incision is closed with Steri-Strips, and the same dressing used in the submental fat pad suction is used. Again, the patient wears this dressing for 5 days, and it is replaced with two tennis headbands in the office.

Buccal Fat Pad and Jowl Extraction

Indications.—

1. Fat, bulky cheeks in patients of all ages
2. In conjunction with malarplasty in patients with flat malar areas and bulky lower half of cheeks to accentuate a higher cheekbone look

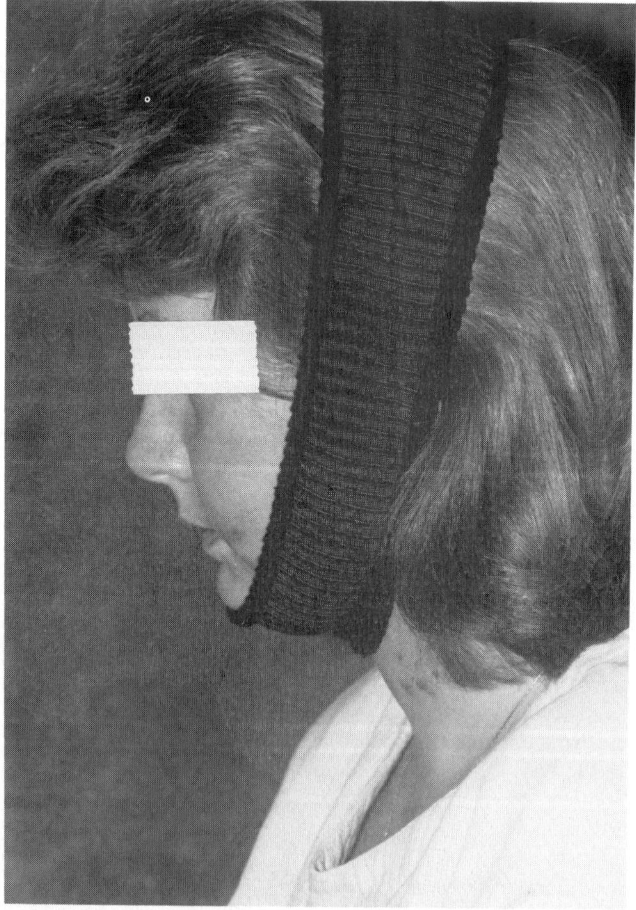

FIG 33–12.
Tennis headbands in proper position for prolonged neck support.

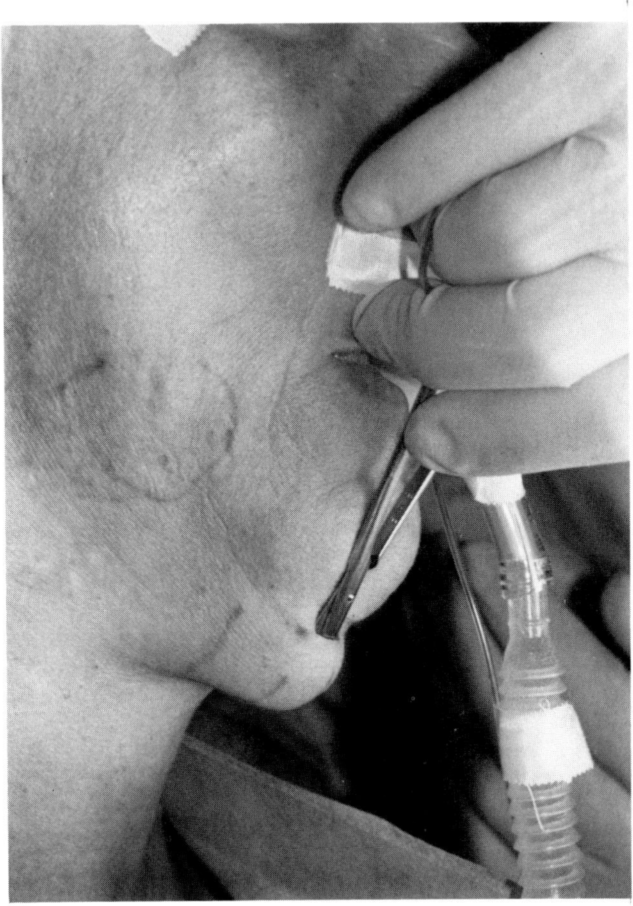

FIG 33–13.
All tunnels are begun with blunt scissors.

3. In older patients, sagging of the buccal fat pad into a more inferior position, creating the jowl (Fig 33–16), which is removable only by this approach

Preoperative Preparation.—A small mark over the cheek prominence may be all that is necessary since the buccal fat pad is a deep structure. Infiltration anesthesia with 2% lidocaine with epinephrine 1:100,000 is performed on the buccogingival sulcus between the second molar and the parotid duct orifice. The easiest way to find this area is to count back six teeth starting with the first incisor on each side.

Surgical Technique.—A 5 mm incision is made in the buccogingival surface at the point infiltrated with lidocaine (Fig 33–17). The specially designed buccal-jowl extractor is inserted into the buccal space (Fig 33–18). Entry into the space can be felt as the extractor pops in. The stylet is removed, and the extractor is attached to machine suction. The buccal-jowl fat pad is then pulled out of the space where an assistant gently teases out the pad with two smooth DeBakey forceps (Fig 33–19). The pad is broken up with the forceps and suctioned out. Bleeding is minimal, and the incision is not closed.

When buccal fat pad suction is combined with malarplasty, a Caldwell-Luc incision is made for the malarplasty. The buccal fat pad is extracted through the lateral aspect of the incision as described, and the malarplasty is performed in routine fashion.

Sad Pad

General Principles.—During the aging process, a combination of fat accumulation and sagging skin is seen on the gravitational line of the malar region. This area cannot be corrected with conventional face-lift or blepharoplasty procedures.

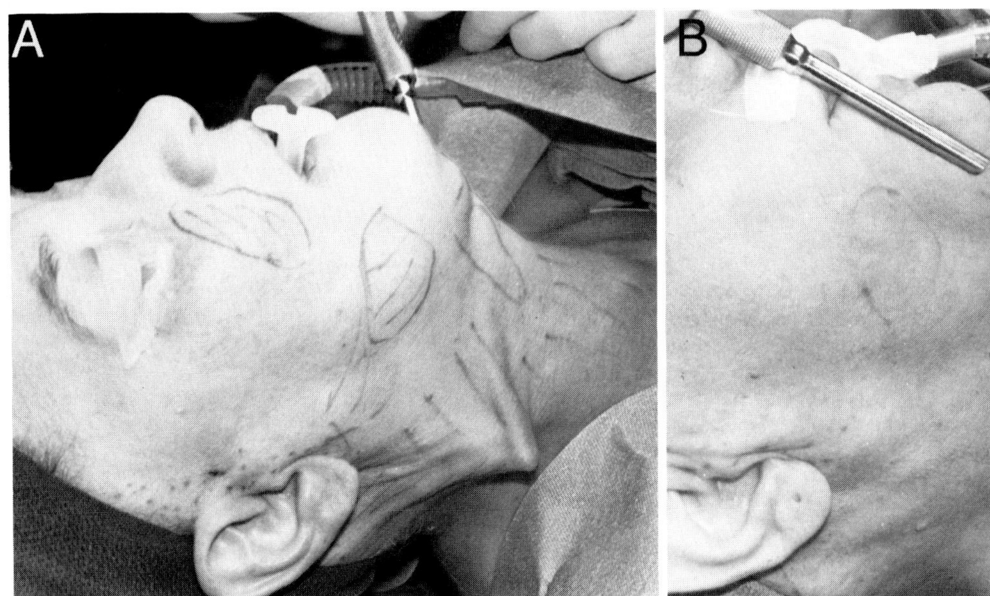

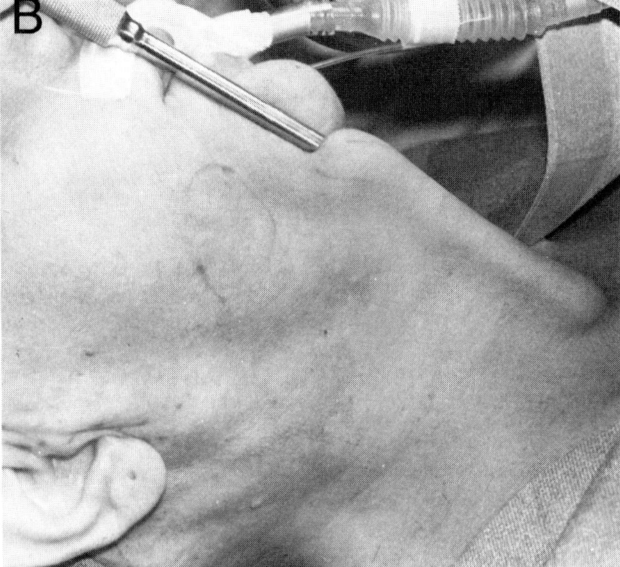

FIG 33–14.
A, undermining of the neck to the sternocleidomastoid laterally using the spatula cannula. **B,** undermining to the suprasternal notch.

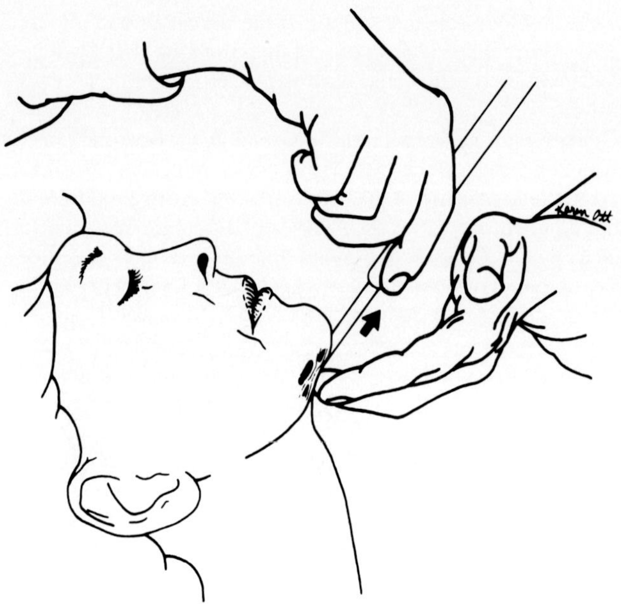

FIG 33–15.
Guiding the 8 mm cannula into the subplatysmal space in the midline.

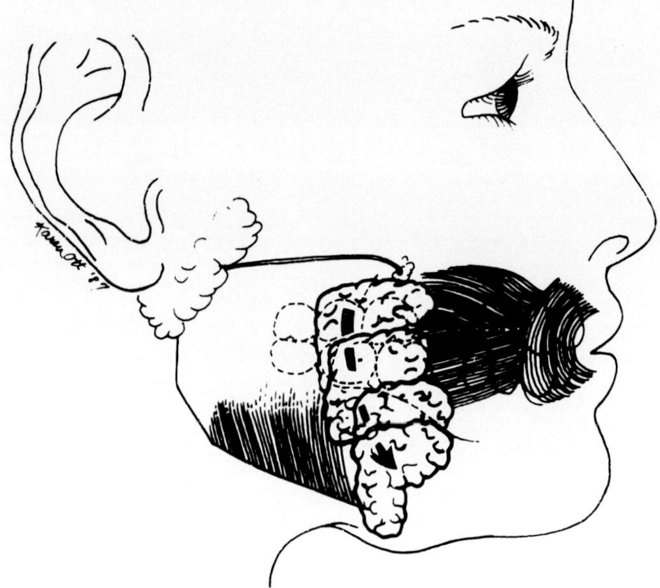

FIG 33–16.
The buccal fat pad descends with age to form the jowl.

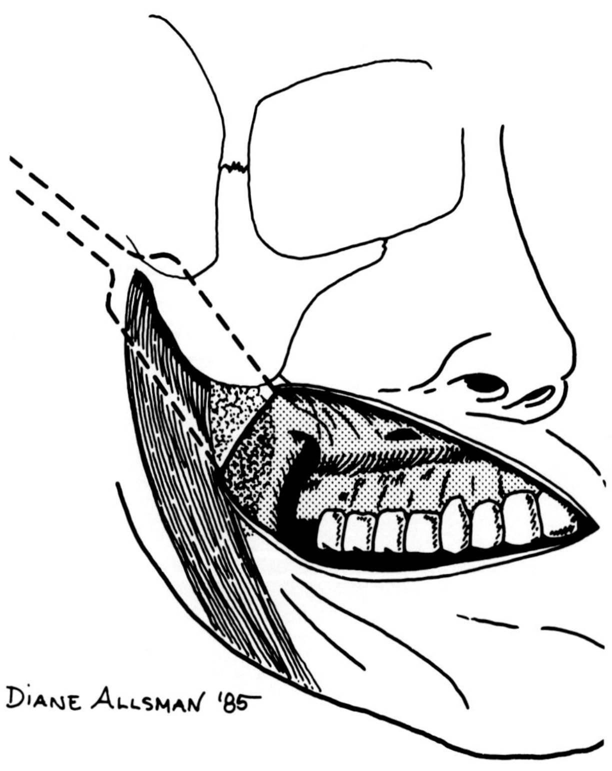

FIG 33–17.
Placement of the incision for buccal-jowl extraction.

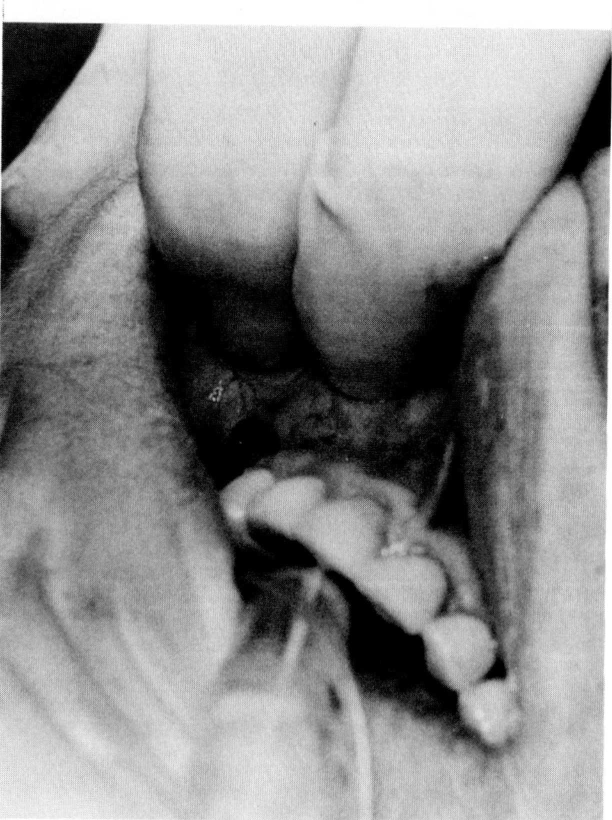

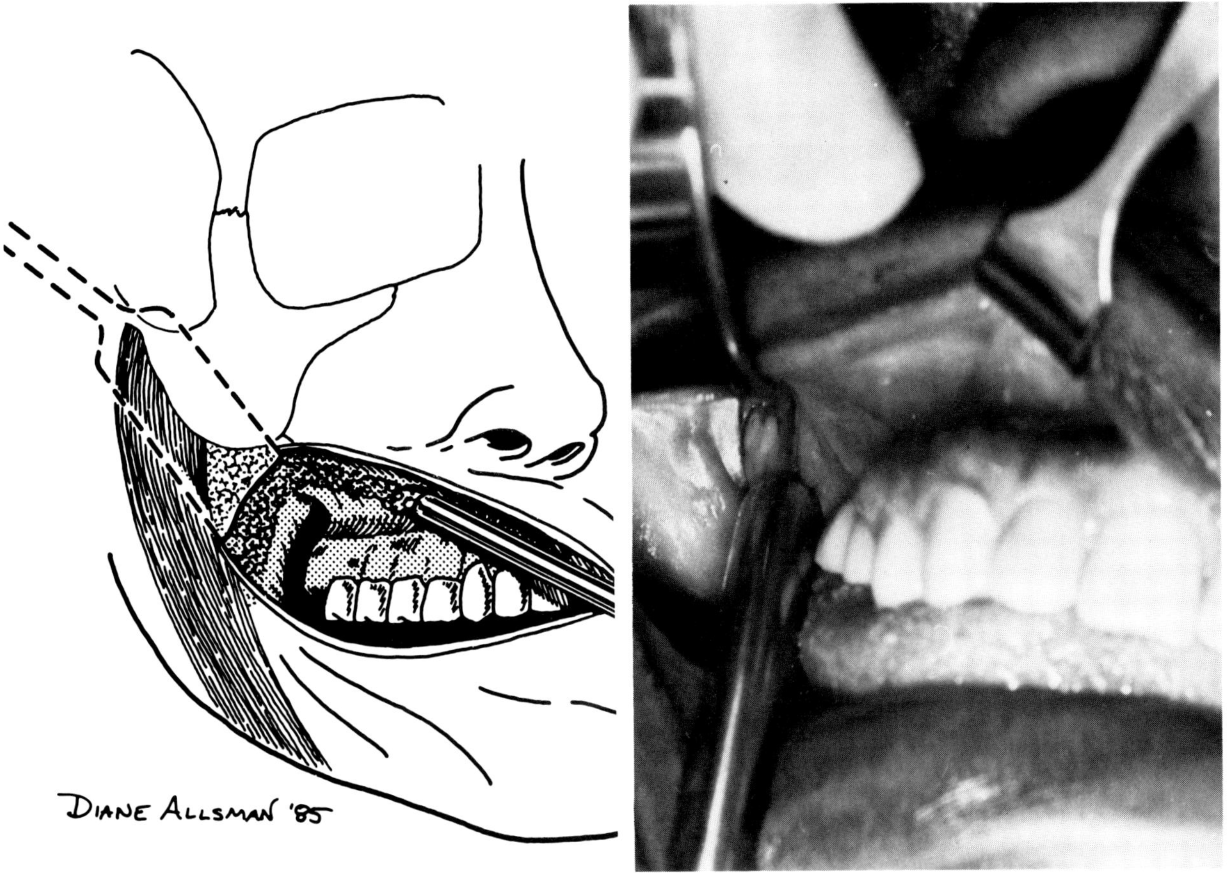

FIG 33–18.
Insertion of the extractor into the buccal space.

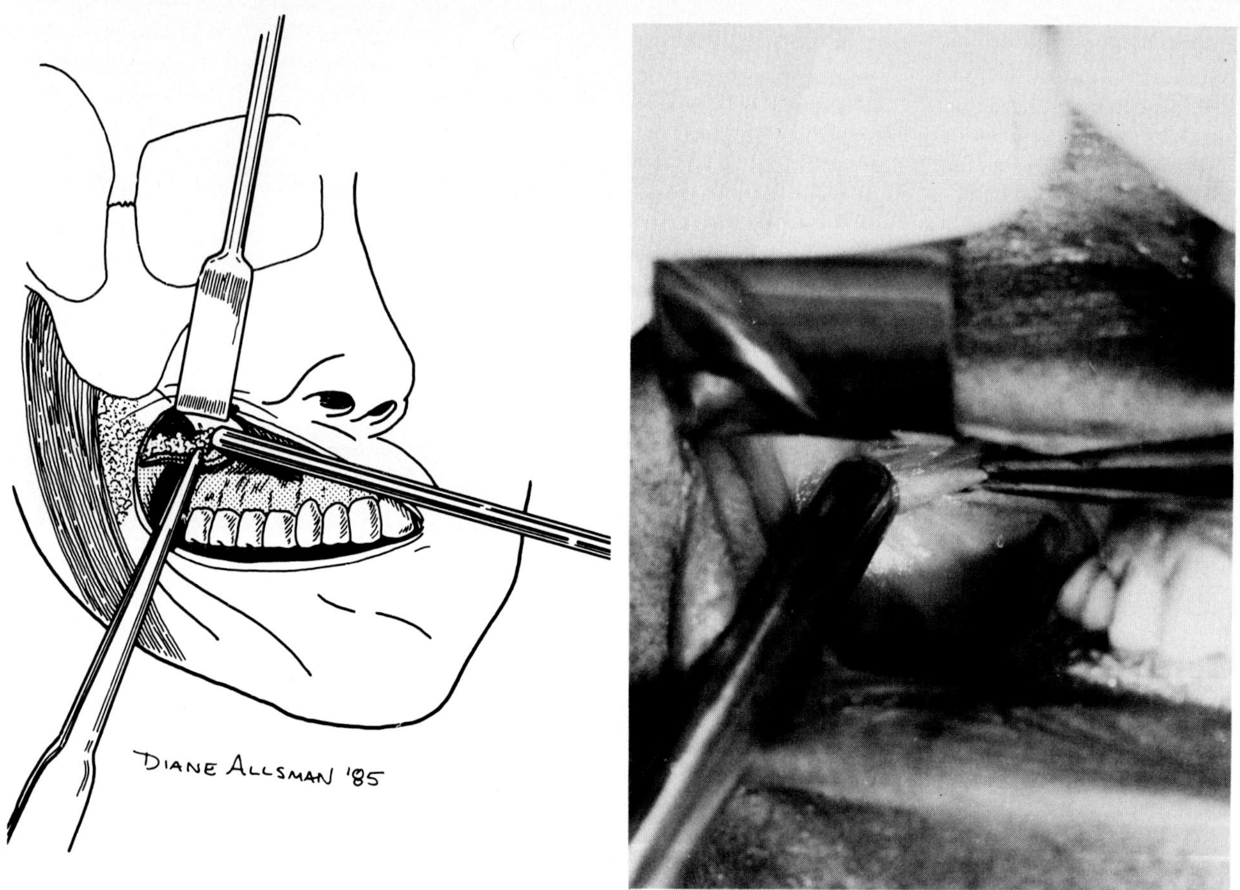

FIG 33–19.
Removing the fat pad with DeBakey forceps.

scarring of the subcutaneous tissues and flattening of these mounds. Prominent cheek rolls are seen in all age groups. This procedure is effective in diffusing prominent smile lines.

Preoperative Preparation.—The prominent melolabial mound is marked beyond the crease line. The areas of infiltration anesthesia include the intranasal vestibule and the subcutaneous tissue of the melolabial mound and surrounding tissue for 2 to 3 cm.

Surgical Technique.—A stab incision is made in the nasal vestibule similar to a lateral osteotomy incision. A subcutaneous tunnel is created with a scissors, and then a 4 mm cannula is inserted (Fig 33–22) to create radial tunnels into the cheek. The tunnels should extend beyond the crease line of the melolabial mound. It is important to keep the opening of the extractor turned down away from the dermis to prevent dermal injury and scarring. The 5 mm cannula may be inserted next to remove any larger fat globules missed by the 4 mm cannula.

The stab wound is left open, and no dressing is applied. A melolabial compression device is applied to maintain pressure postoperatively (Fig 33–23).

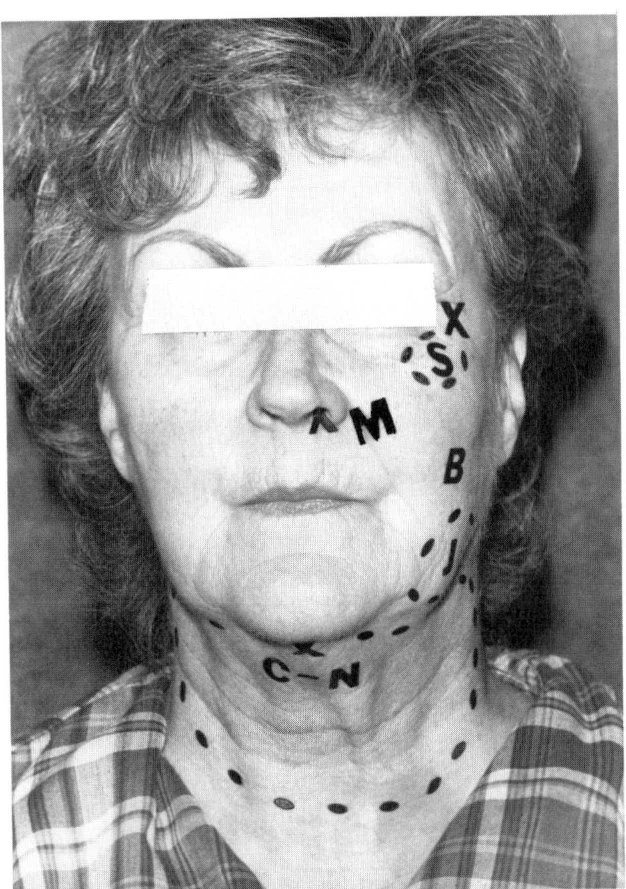

FIG 33–20.
Facial markings for areas designated for liposuction: (*S*) sad pad, (*M*) melolabial mound, (*B*) Buccal fat pad, and (*J*) jowl.

Liposuction of these regions actually is meant to scarify the subcutaneous tissue in this region to cause flattening of the skin.

Preoperative Preparation.—The sad pads are marked with the patient in the sitting position (Fig 33–20). Infiltration anesthesia is made with 2% lidocaine with epinephrine 1:100,000. The incision line at the orbital rim near the lateral canthus of the eye and the subcutaneous tissue of the sad pad are infiltrated.

Surgical Technique.—A stab wound is made in the area described earlier in the direction of the crow's-feet lines. A small subcutaneous tunnel is made with a blunt scissors. A 4 mm cannula is inserted and gently advanced throughout the malar region (Fig 33–21). The cannula tip is palpated throughout the procedure to avoid deep penetration, which could injure the infraorbital nerve, and anastomosing ramifications of the zygomatic and buccal branches of the facial nerve. The stab wound is closed with Steri-Strips.

Melolabial Mound Extraction

General Principles.—Liposuction of the melolabial mound extracts minimal fat but breaks up the subcutaneous attachments of the skin and induces depression of the cheek roll by causing

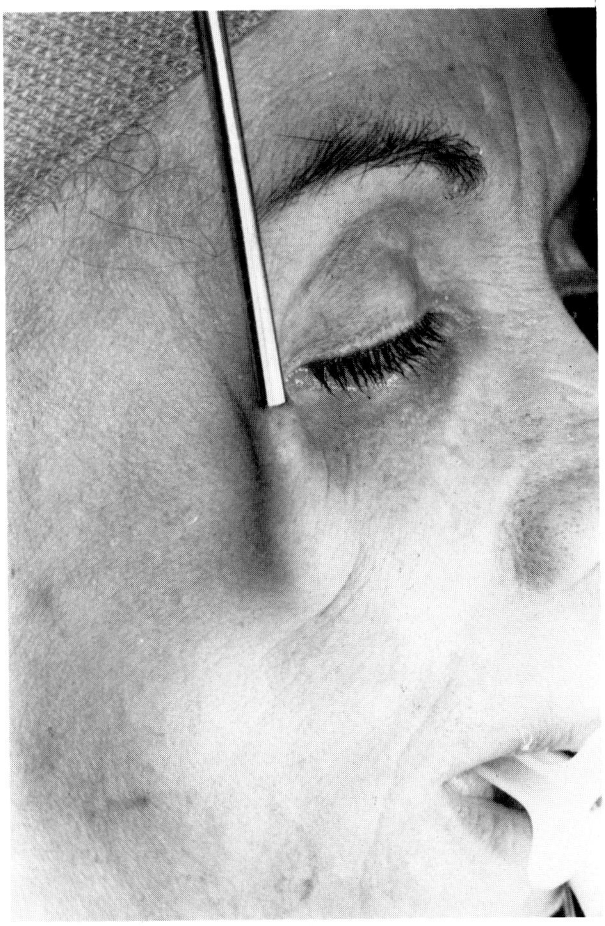

FIG 33–21.
Sad pad suctioning.

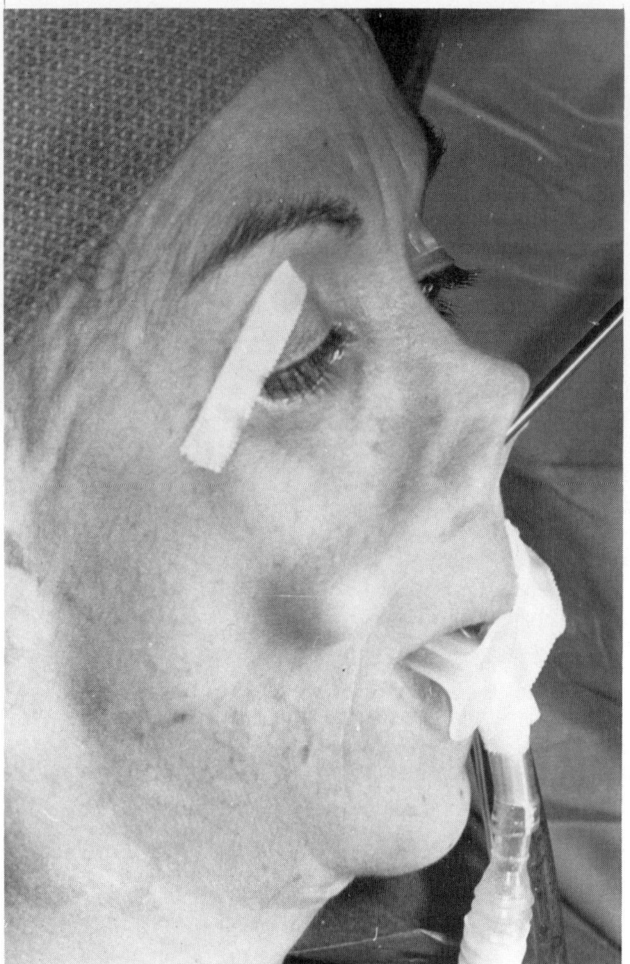

FIG 33–22.
Melolabial mound suctioning.

Cervicofacial Liposuction in Conjunction With other Cosmetic Procedures

Rhytidectomy

When a face-lift procedure must be performed, liposuction can be used to assist in creating skin flaps and removing fat that would be very difficult to remove using conventional techniques. The liposuction-assisted rhytidectomy is a quicker method with less risk of injury to major structures.

Preoperative Preparation.—The patient is marked in the sitting position. The planned incision as well as areas of loose hanging skin and fat are marked. Five incisions are planned and injected with 2% lidocaine with epinephrine 1:100,000. An incision is made in the submental crease, in the infralobule crease of the ear, in the pretragal region, the posterior cervical area, and the posterior conchal region. Using the spatula needles, diluted 0.1% lidocaine with epinephrine 1:1,000,000 is infiltrated throughout the neck, face, and posterior cervical regions.

Technique.—*Closed Liposuction.*—From the submental incision, a 6 mm spatula cannula is passed with suction, freeing the anterior neck skin laterally to the sternocleidomastoid muscles as in the closed neck lift. Next, through the infralobule incision the fat accumulation at the mandibular ramus and lateral neck are suctioned. It is important to keep the tip of the suction cannula pointing and tenting the skin so as not to damage underlying structures. In this region the submandibular branch of the facial nerve can be damaged by deep suction. Through the pretragal incision, the 4 mm cannula is used to suction fat from the cheeks and temporal areas. At this point the suction machine is turned off. The 4 mm cannula is inserted into the posterior mastoid incision, and with a sawing motion, the skin is separated from the mastoid and sternocleidomastoid muscle fascia (Fig 33–24). Finally, the 4 mm cannula is passed, without suction, through the posterior conchal incision to free the attachments of the infralobule region (Fig 33–25).

After raising the skin flap, the operator can visualize the tunnels created by the liposuction cannulas (Fig 33–26). These

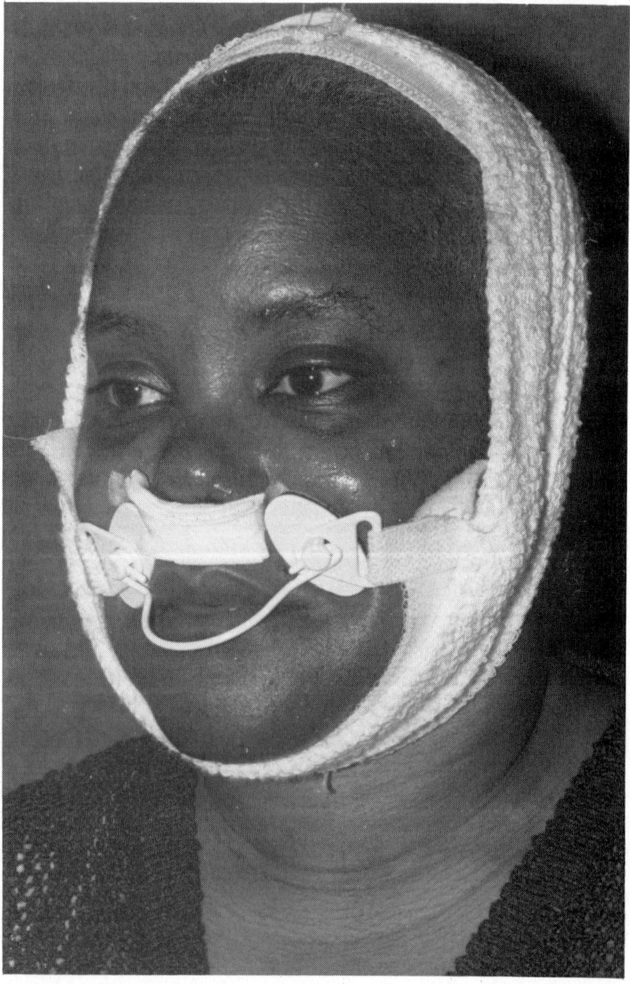

FIG 33–23.
Melolabial mound compression device.

Preoperative Preparation.—The submental crease and area of the neck to be suctioned are marked with the patient in the sitting position. Infiltration of the incision is performed with 2% lidocaine with epinephrine 1:100,000. A 2 to 3 cm incision is made in the crease. The neck is infiltrated with diluted lidocaine with epinephrine solution using the spatula needles.

Surgical Technique.—Submental or full neck suction is performed as described earlier. After suctioning, a hard acrylic chin implant is inserted through the same incision in the routine manner. The wound is then closed with two or three buried subcutaneous absorbable sutures, and the skin is closed with a continuous subcuticular suture of 5-0 nylon.

Dressings are similar to those used with the closed neck lift; however, two rolled 2 × 2 in. gauze sponges are taped between the implant and the lower lip.

Malarplasty

Liposuction of the buccal fat pad in conjunction with malarplasty can impart a better appearance by thinning the lower aspect of the face and giving more prominence to the malar regions. This reverses the hound dog look, giving the patient a more energetic appearance. The technique is described in the section on buccal fat pad suction.

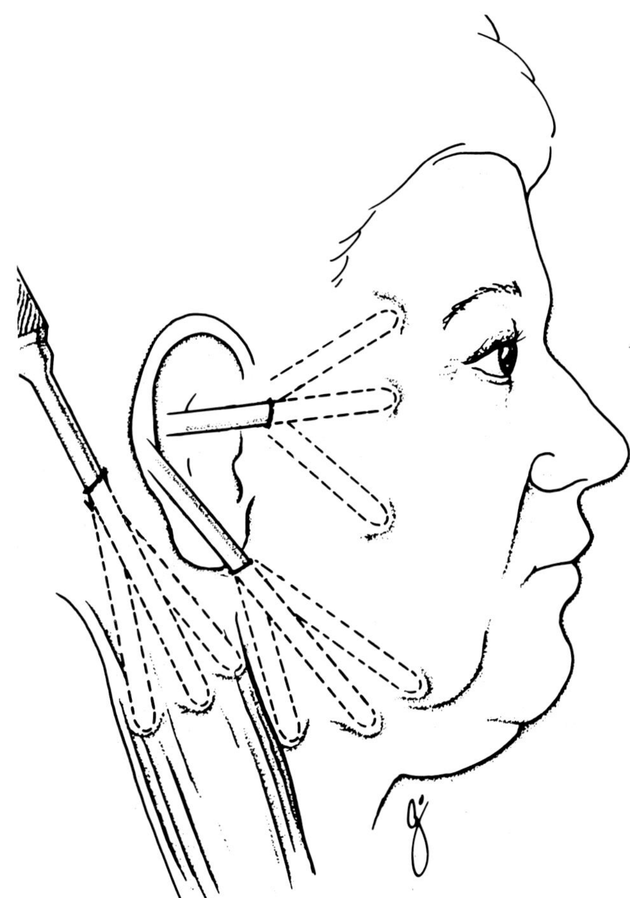

FIG 33–24.
Schematic view of the three incisions around the ear used during the suction-assisted face-lift.

tunnels can then easily be connected with scissors, creating a large skin flap in much less time than it would take during a conventional face-lift procedure.

Open Liposuction.—Once the entire skin flap is raised, any residual fat can be removed from the sternomastoid fascia with an 8 or 10 mm spatula cannula. The spatula cannulas are especially good for this procedure since the opening of the cannula is located on only one surface of the cannula, and full suction can be created to remove fat. DeBakey forceps are used by the assistant to break up any lobules of fat that are adherent to the fascia. Occasionally one has to turn the cannula over and suction excess hanging fat from the undersurface of the skin flap. One must be sure not to get too vigorous so as not to completely defat the dermis.

Mentoplasty

Liposuction of the neck when combined with mentoplasty can give better definition to the neck-chin angle. Sometimes slightly drooping skin of the submental region can be tightened with insertion of a chin implant as well as submental liposuction.

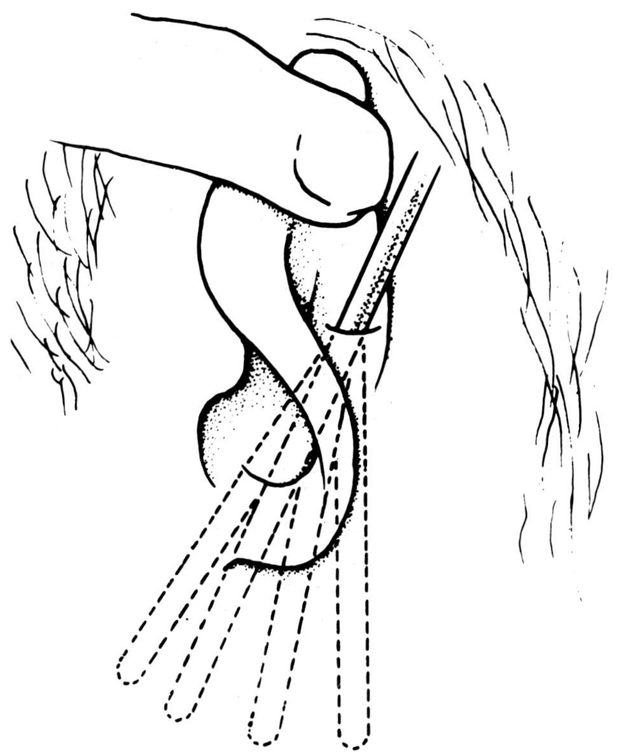

FIG 33–25.
Schematic view of the posterior conchal incision.

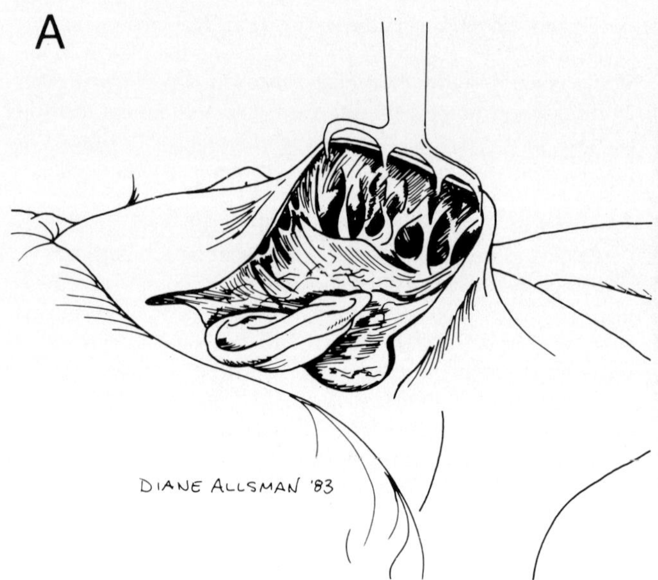

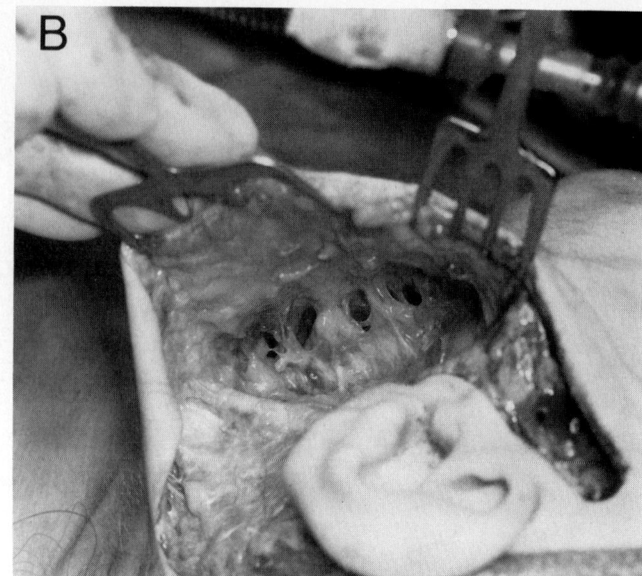

FIG 33–26.
A, visualization of the subcutaneous tunnels created during liposuction shown schematically. **B**, visualization of the subcutaneous tunnels intraoperatively.

Complications

Skin Complications

Skin dimpling and wrinkling from dermal injury, vertical wrinkling from taping, and skin reactions to tape are the most frequent complications of cervicofacial liposuction.

Early experience of facial liposuction with round-tipped cannulas showed that dermal injury can be sustained from too vigorous suctioning. It causes scarring and excessive adherence of the skin to the underlying tissue, resulting in linear skin dimpling and wrinkling. Since the introduction of the flat spatula–shaped cannulas in which the opening is on only one side of the cannula and is kept downward toward the fascia and away from the skin, the problem of dermal injury has been virtually eliminated.

Vertical wrinkling of submandibular and submental skin is caused by applying tape directly to the skin to remold these areas after liposuction. This problem has been reduced to a minimum by applying a layered dressing of Webril and French tape. This dressing is replaced in 5 days with two tennis headbands placed in the coronal plane under the chin to support the skin of the neck for 2 weeks postoperatively.

The most common complication used to be skin reaction to molding tape manifested by itching, blister formation, and excoriation of the skin. Early removal of the tape and replacement with elastic headbands have reduced the incidence of this complication.

Hematoma and Seroma Formation.—Major bleeding is rarely encountered because of the use of the blunt-tipped spatula cannulas. These cannulas tend to push aside the fibrous septae that contain blood vessels. Penetration of the cannula into the platysma muscle can cause bleeding; therefore, it is important for the operator to keep the tip of the cannula point-

ing toward the skin and to stay within the subcutaneous layer.

Seroma formation is extremely unusual postoperatively since compression of the suctioned region is maintained for 2 weeks.

Nerve Injury.—Injury to the mandibular branch of the facial nerve can occur during vigorous suctioning during the closed neck-lift or face-lift procedure (Fig 33–27). However, this is a transient problem, and motor function always returns to normal.

Infection.—Because of the rich blood supply in the face, infection has not been a problem in cervicofacial liposuction. In addition, all patients are given prophylactic antibiotics in the form of a first-generation cephalosporin intravenously preoperatively. They are continued on antibiotic therapy for 5 days postoperatively. One infection occurred in a patient with buccal fat pad suctioning, and it resolved easily with a short course of antibiotics.

Conclusion

Cervicofacial liposuction is an effective surgical method for aesthetic sculpturing of the face and neck. It can be performed on both men and women with practically no age limitation. The operative procedure lasts 10 to 20 minutes and requires only a small stab wound, which can be well hidden in preexisting skin folds, behind the ear, or within the nose or mouth. When it is performed in conjunction with other cosmetic procedures such as the rhytidectomy, most of the dissection work is performed by the cannulas, and the operative time is markedly shortened. Minimal trauma and stress allow for the patient's early return to routine activities.

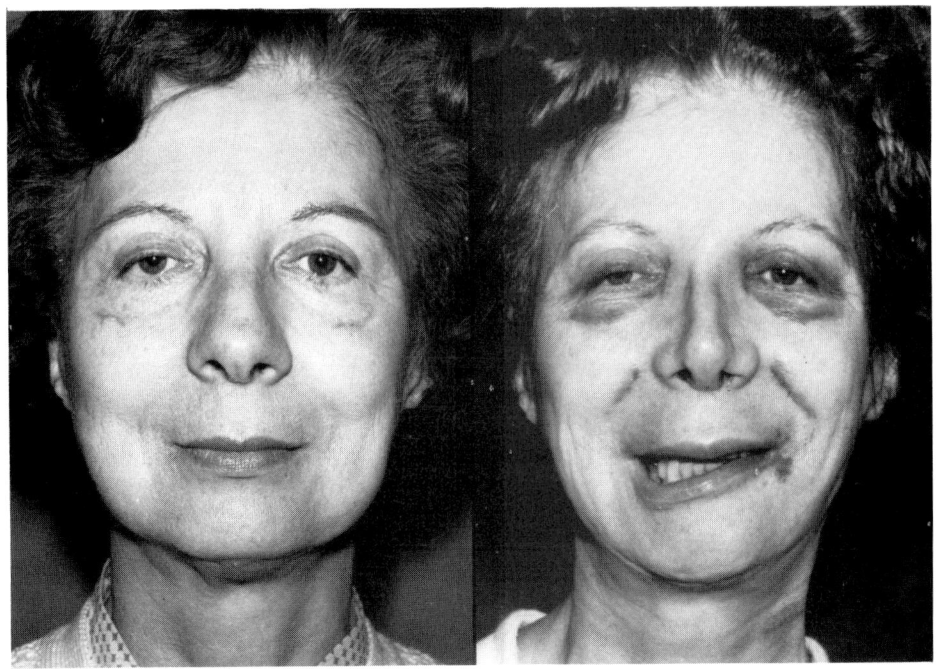

FIG 33–27.
Temporary left facial palsy related to trauma to the submandibular branch of the facial nerve.

Patient acceptance of cervicofacial liposuction has been excellent since there is minimal morbidity and quicker return to normality than with excisional lipectomy methods. Proper use of cannulas, an understanding of the facial cutaneous-adipose complex, and careful patient selection and operative planning are general guidelines for pleasing cosmetic results.

Figures 33–28 through 33–35 show preoperative and postoperative photographs associated with the various cervicofacial liposuction procedures.

LIPOTRANSPLANT SURGERY

In 1893 the first free fat transplant was performed by Neuber,[8] in which he transplanted free fat from the upper extremity to a depressed area in the face. In 1911, a German researcher named Brunings placed small pieces of fat in a syringe and injected them to correct postrhinoplasty deformities.[9] Many experiments have been performed to evaluate and successfully demonstrate the ability of fat to be transplanted. In 1977, Illouz[2] introduced a simplified and safe method of fat removal known as liposuction, and since then there has been an abundance of fat available for transplantation.

Today fat is used as a subcutaneous implant to fill in defects of the face and body. Atrophy of facial fat and underdevelopment of facial bony prominences as well as depressed scars can be filled with a patient's own fat.

Evaluation

Patients are evaluated for facial lipotransplantation in the

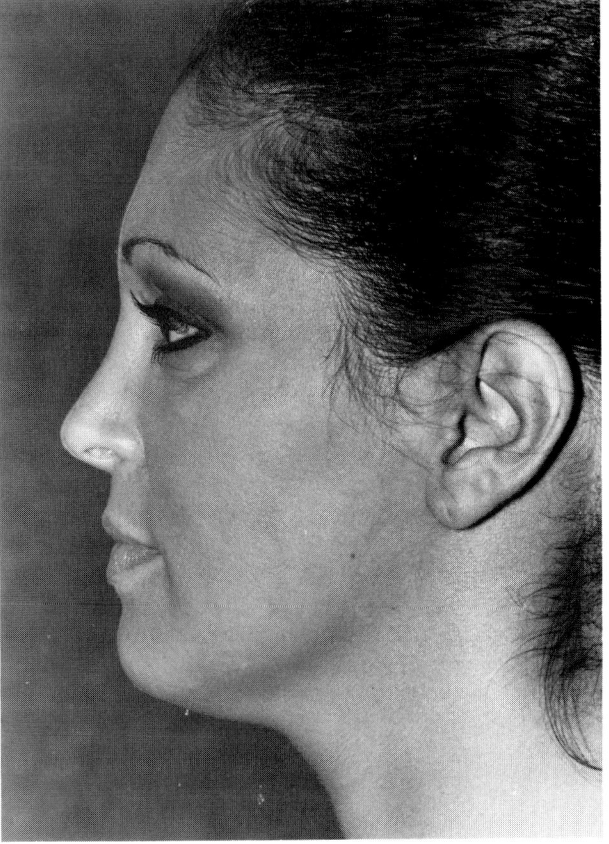

FIG 33–28.
Preoperative view before submental liposuction.

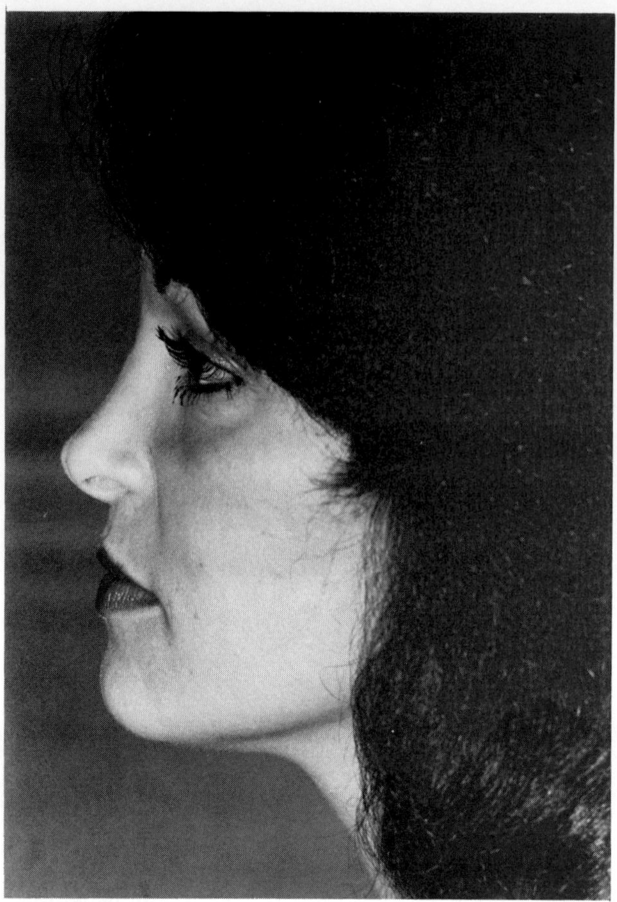

FIG 33–29.
Postoperative view after submental liposuction.

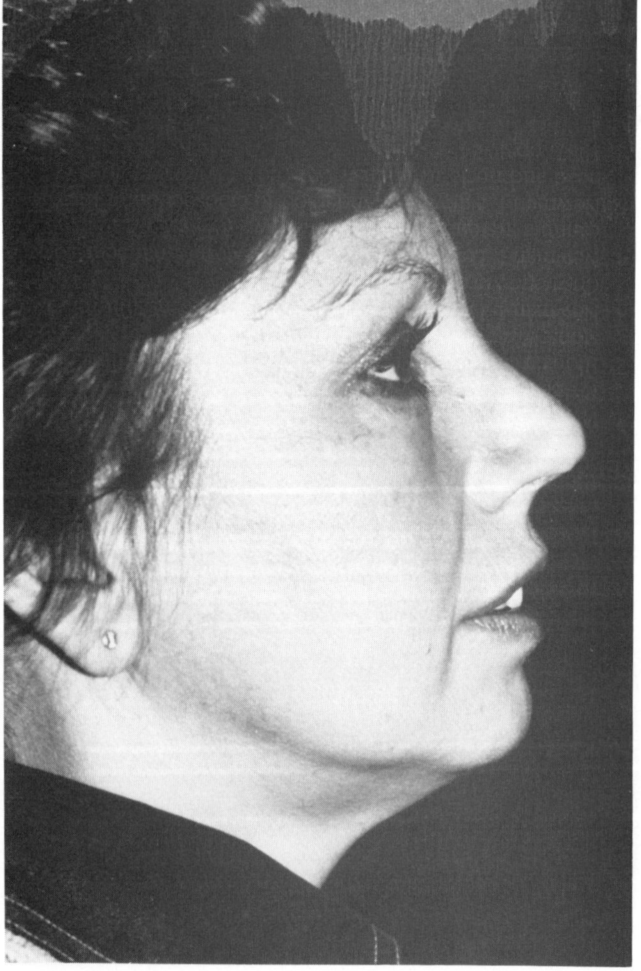

FIG 33–30.
Preoperative view of a patient needing chin implant and closed neck lift.

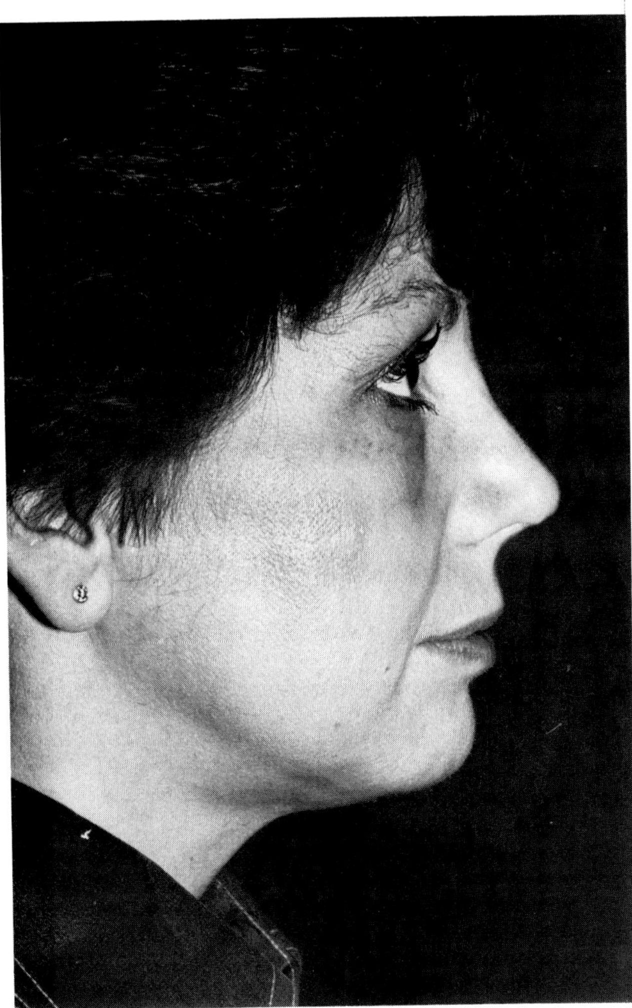

FIG 33–31.
Postoperative view after chin augmentation and closed neck lift.

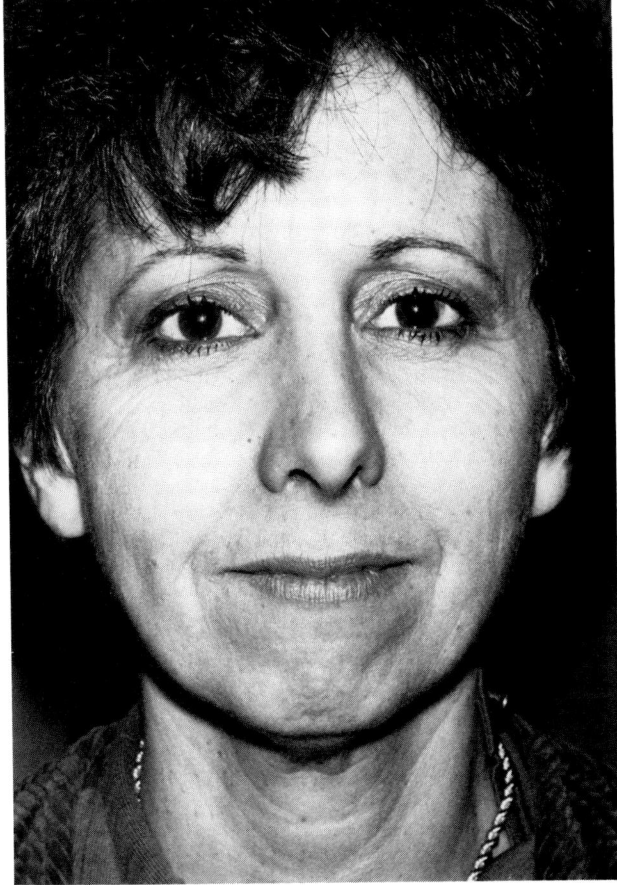

FIG 33–32.
Preoperative anterior view prior to closed neck lift and chin implant.

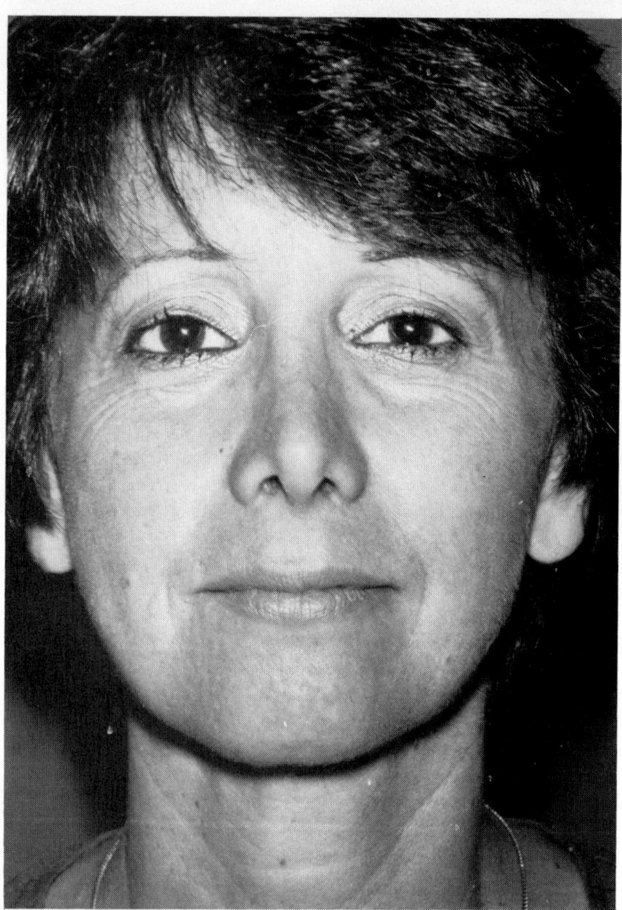

FIG 33–33.
Postoperative anterior view shows improvement of hanging neck skin.

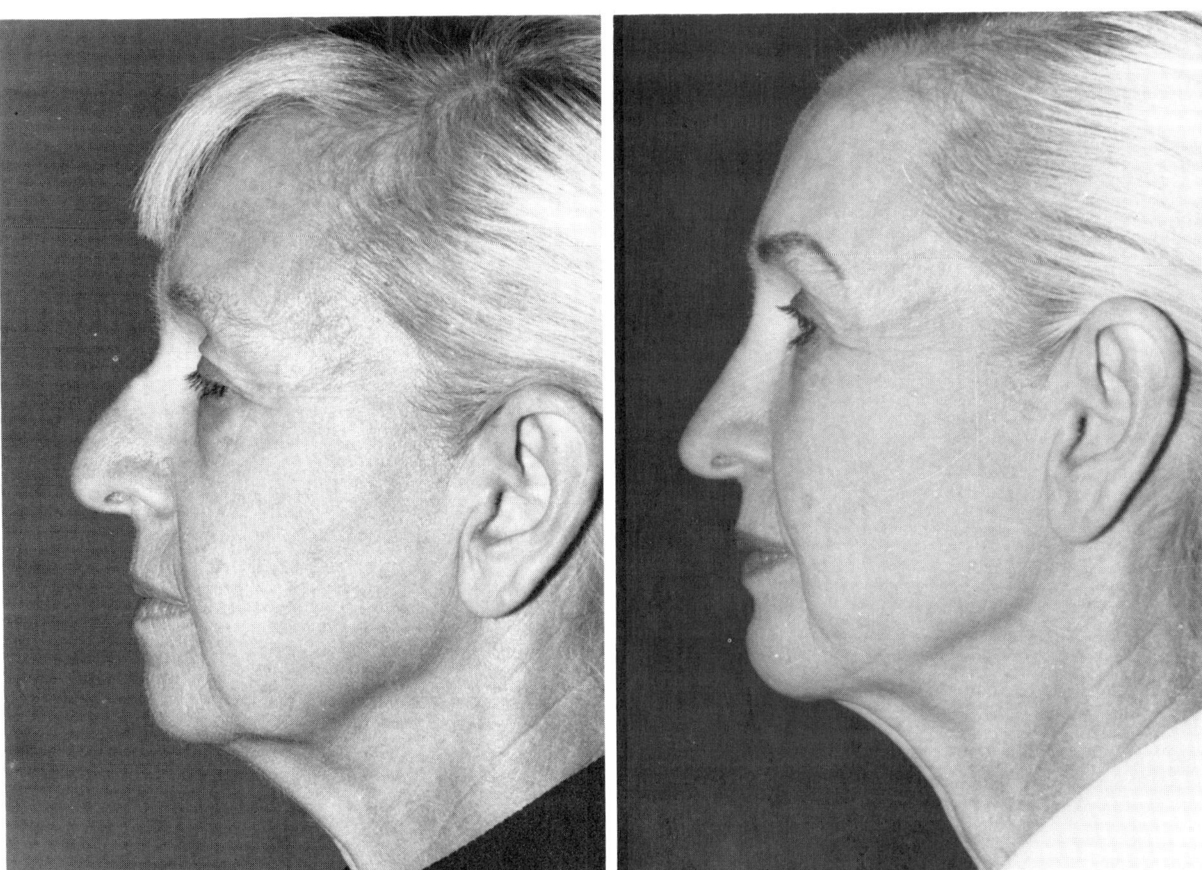

FIG 33–34.
Preoperative and postoperative views in a patient who underwent jowl liposuction and chin augmentation.

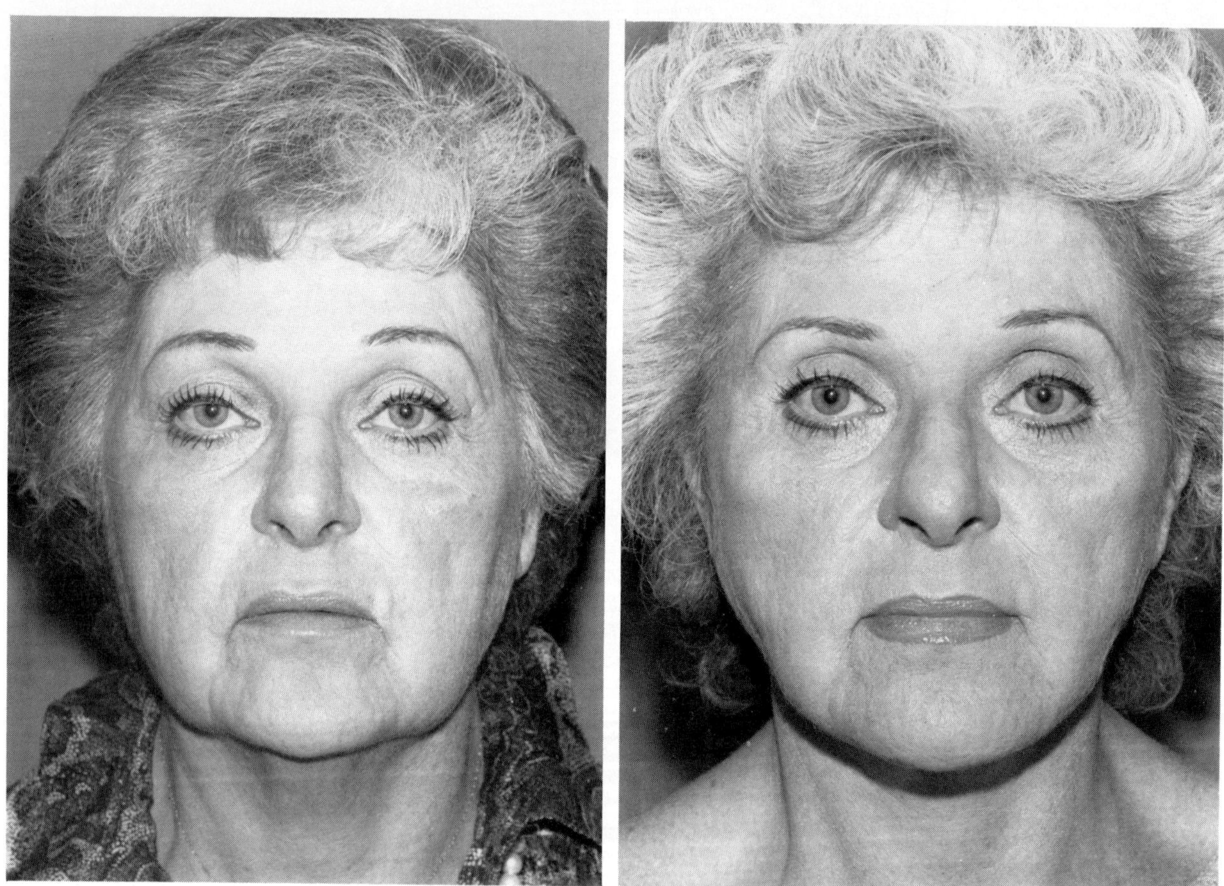

FIG 33–35.
Preoperative and postoperative views after liposuction-assisted facelift and jowl extraction.

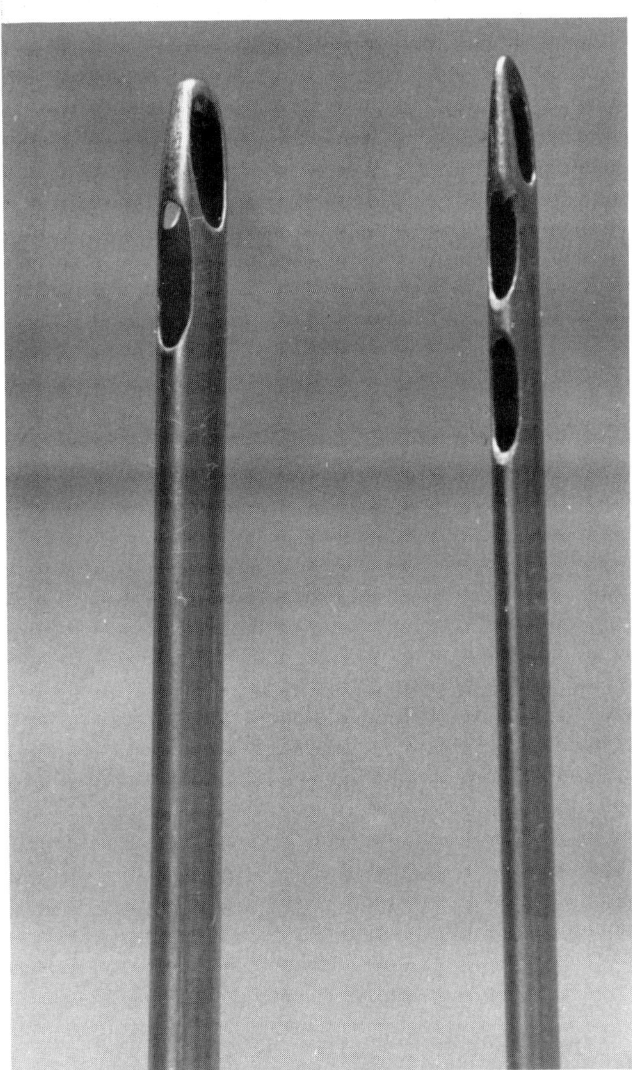

FIG 33–36.
Zaki trivalve semisharp 4 mm suction cannula used for fat harvesting.

same manner as those for facial liposuction. The patient is examined in the sitting or standing position. The glabella is evaluated for deep furrows that may be filled in with fat. The malar regions are evaluated for fullness. This area is especially responsive to fat implantation and is often combined with buccal extraction to reverse the sagging hound dog look. Smile lines can be softened with injection of fat as well as the ptotic chin.

Of course, the abdomen and thighs must be evaluated for the presence of adequate quantities of fat for transplantation. A surprising number of patients will request fat injection to the face and have very little donor adipose tissue.

Instruments and Technique

The first step in fat transplantation is harvesting. The donor sites are prepared and draped as for liposuction. Antibiotics are given intravenously preoperatively and continued for 5 days postoperatively. Diluted local anesthesia of 0.1% lidocaine with epinephrine 1:1,000,000 is infiltrated into the donor areas. A 4 mm trivalve semisharp cannula is used for fat harvesting (Fig 33–36). Wall suction instead of machine suction is used to minimize trauma and damage to the fat cells. Connected in-line between the cannula and the wall suction is a collecting system. This is a simple Leukens trap that can be easily changed when full (Fig 33–37). After the fat has been collected, it is treated for implantation. The fat is washed in a mixture of 1,000 mL of lactated Ringer's solution with 100 units of regular insulin (Fig 33–38). This removes blood, serum, destroyed fat cells, and free lipids removed during suctioning. The insulin stabilizes the fat cell membrane. Removing these substances produces clean fat, which causes less tissue reaction when injected.

The cleaned fat is then placed in the barrel of the New-Jet Lipo-Injector. This is an instrument designed specifically for fat injection, which is composed of a stainless steel hand-activated ratcheting handle with interchangeable needles and specimen barrels (Fig 33–39). The injector barrel has a capacity of approximately 8 mL. The plunger is gear driven for smooth control of fat injection. The barrel has a special Leur-Lock adapter that

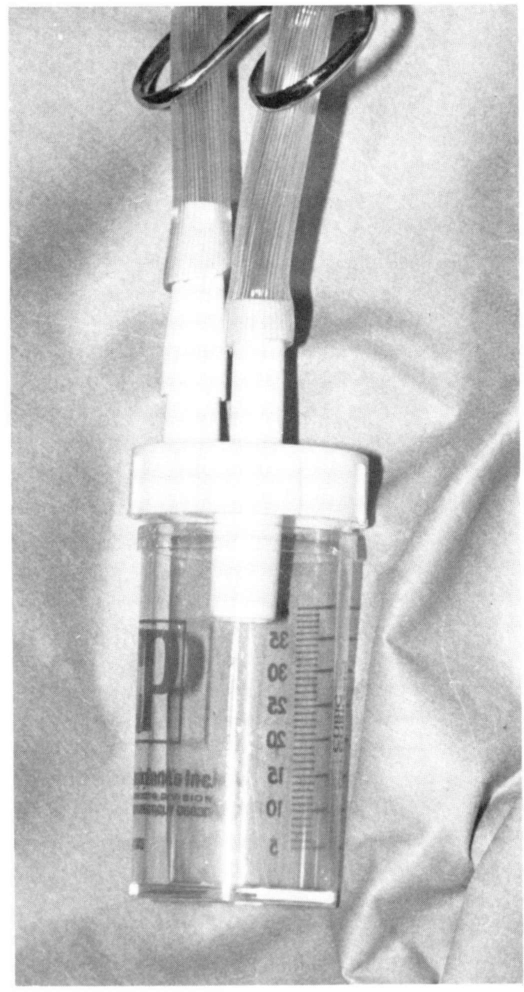

FIG 33–37.
Leukens trap used for fat collection.

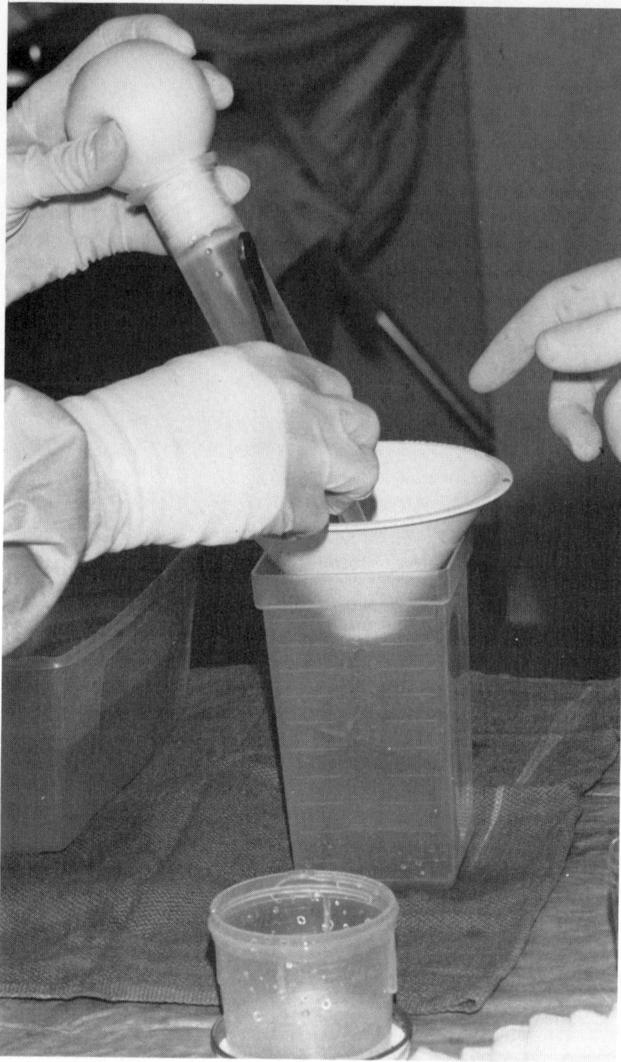

FIG 33–38.
Fat is washed with 1,000 mL of lactated Ringer's solution with 100 U of regular insulin.

secures the needle during the high pressures required for fat injection. This is especially important when one is injecting around the face and eyes.

A 16- or 18-gauge stainless steel bullet needle is used for injecting fat. These needles are specially designed blunt needles with a side opening located approximately 0.5 cm from the tip of the needle. The needles are blunt so that important structures such as nerves, arteries, and veins are not injured or accidentally cannulated. There is no opening at the tip of the needles so that coring of tissue does not occur during insertion of the needle. The opening is located well away from the tip of the needle so that in case a vein is accidentally cannulated, the fat will not be injected intravenously.

Specific sites of injection include the melolabial groove, the inframalar groove and malar region, the ptotic chin, the glabellar furrows, and forehead frown lines. Depressed scars and traumatic or surgical defects may also be sites for fat in-

jection. No local anesthetic is injected into the recipient sites so as not to distort the area.

Fat implantation of the melolabial groove is approached through the mouth at the midline of the upper lip near the frenulum or directly through the skin near the area (Fig 33–40). The needle is inserted in the subdermal plane throughout the extent of the defect. Fat is injected as the needle is withdrawn. The area is overfilled only slightly since there will be some reabsorption of the injected fat. However, if the area is overfilled too much and a lot of the fat takes, the patient will be left with a poor result. Once the desired amount of fat has been injected, the operator molds the fat into the desired contour with his or her fingers.

In the region of the inframalar groove and malar region, the needle enters the skin over the arch of the zygoma. The needle is advanced medially in the subdermal plane, and fat is injected as the needle is withdrawn (Fig 33–41). Once the desired amount of fat is injected, it is molded into the desired shape. The area is overfilled as previously described.

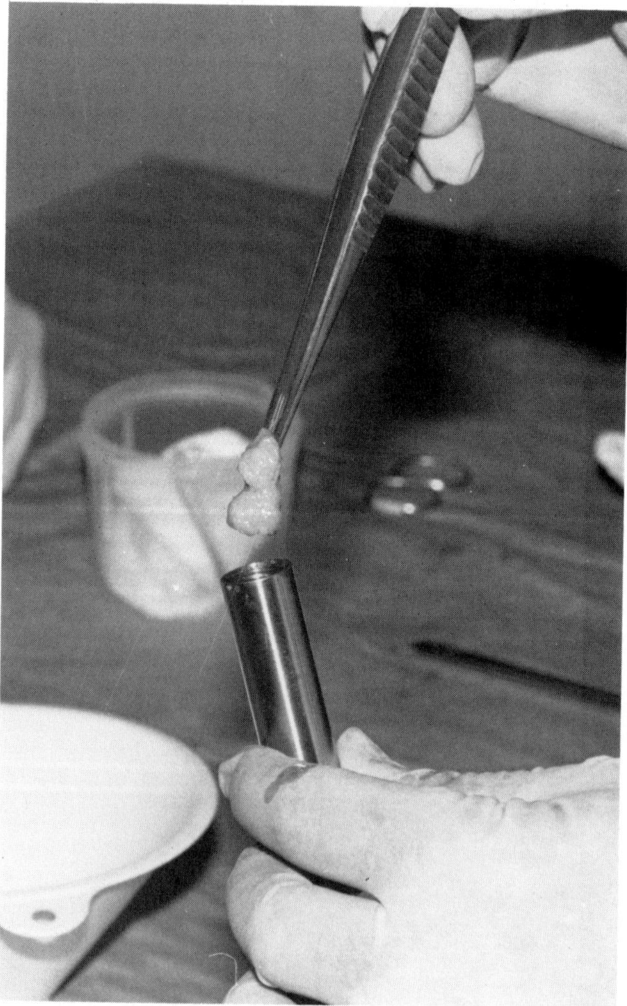

FIG 33–39.
The washed fat is placed in the New-Jet Lipoinjector barrel.

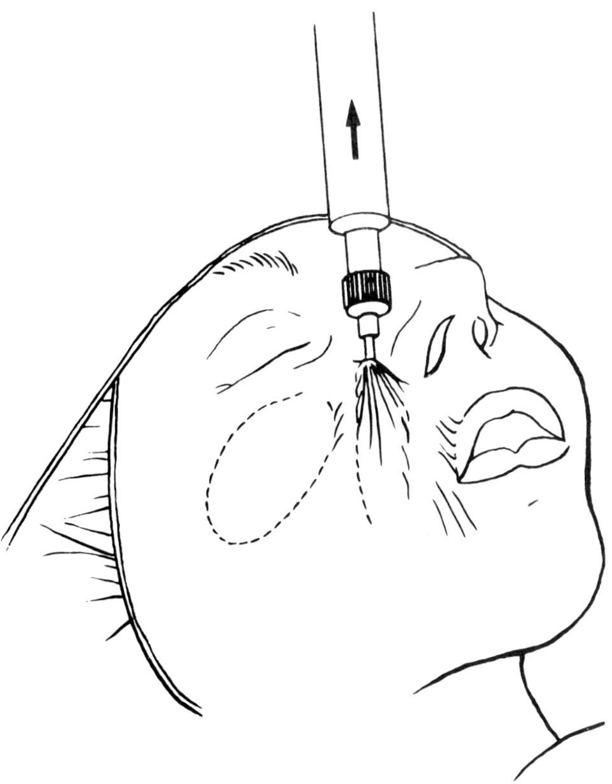

FIG 33–40.
Injection of fat into the melolabial mound as the injector is withdrawn.

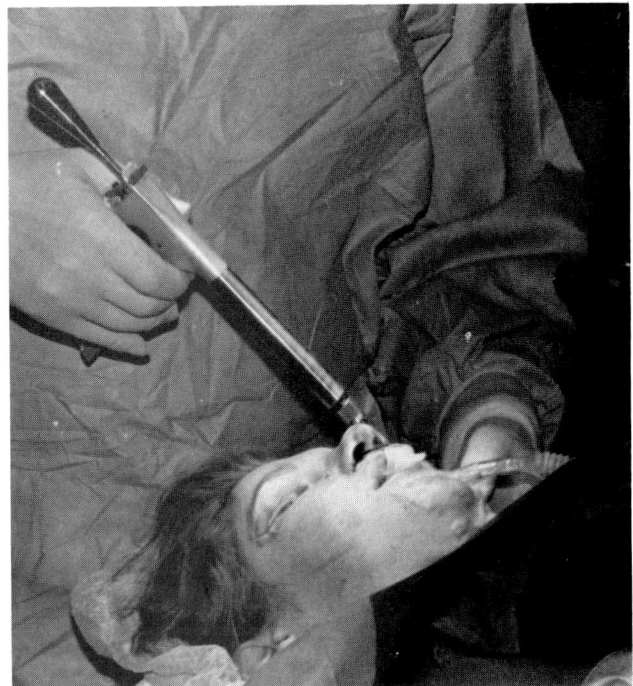

FIG 33–41.
Injection of fat into the malar region.

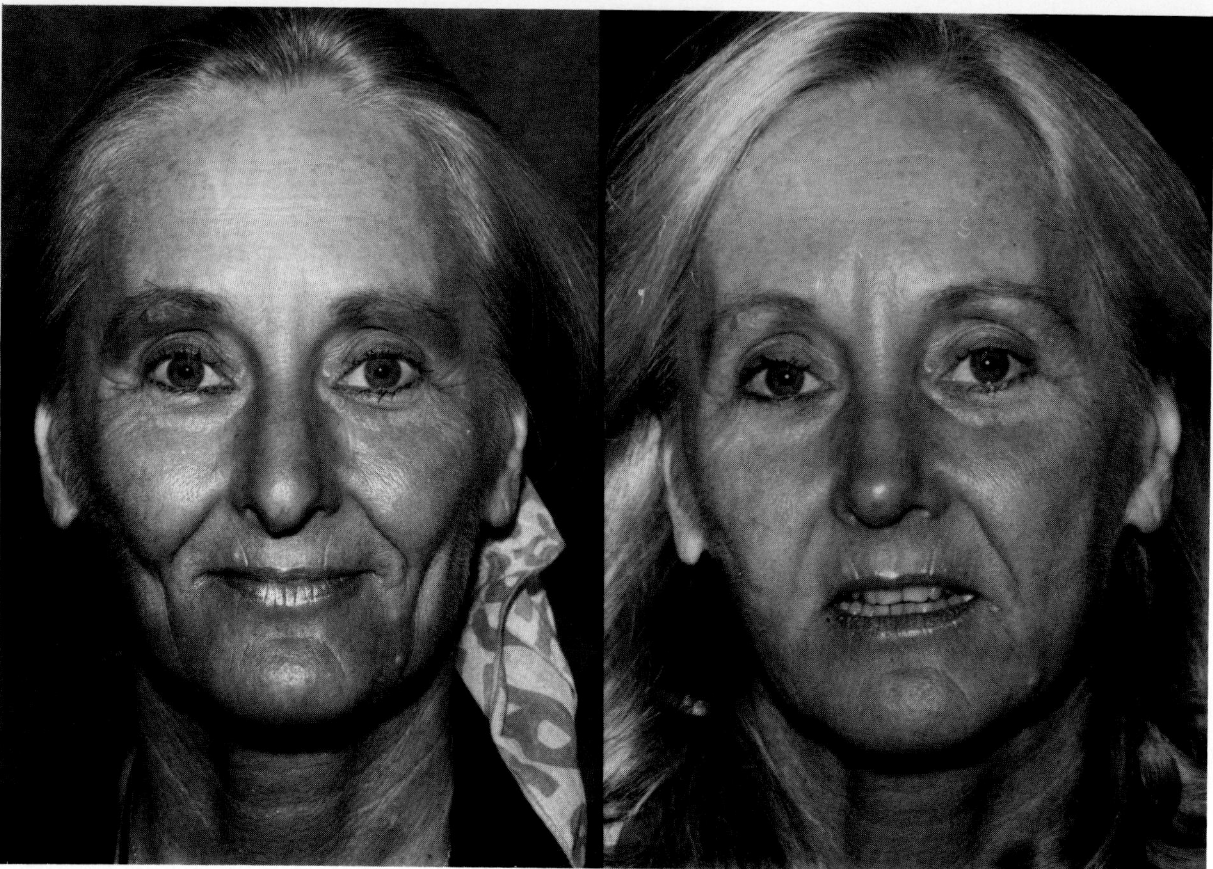

FIG 33–42.
Preoperative and postoperative views after lipotransplants to deep cheek grooves.

In older patients, the chin may lose its forward projection and sag inferiorly, producing the ptotic chin. This can be corrected by injecting fat into the areas of the submental crease and chin sides.

Defects and scars can be greatly improved with fat transplantation. A small serrated knife blade or myringotomy blade is inserted in the subcutaneous plane to free adherent scar tissue and elevate the depressed area. It also creates a space for the fat graft. Fat is then injected into this area in a similar fashion as already described.

Glabellar furrows and forehead lines must be undermined in a similar fashion to depressed scars, otherwise the lines will be accentuated. The needle is inserted at the root of the nose inferior to the glabella for injection of these regions.

Postoperative Care

No dressings are required or desired so that the injected sites are not deformed by the bandages. The needle insertion sites do not need to be sutured. Antibiotics are continued for 5 days postoperatively. Only mild pain medication is required. The areas are examined on a regular basis for up to 1 year.

Results

Gratifying results have been obtained by using this method of fat transplantation (Fig 33–42). In our series of 350 patients, we have noted that 60% to 70% of the grafted material has survived for more than 1 year. One episode of cellulitis occurred when buccal fat was extracted through the oral cavity and then injected into the inframalar groove. This resolved easily with oral antibiotics. Resorption rates of 30% to 60% have been reported. Complete resorption of the fat implant within 6 weeks has been noted in only 30% of the population. Long-term stability of the fat implant is currently under investigation; however, if the implant survives for 6 months postoperatively, the chances of long-term survival are good.

Conclusion

Fat transplantation is a satisfactory method for correcting multiple soft tissue deformities. At present time, no antigenic response with repeated fat transplant has been reported. The complication rate is negligible. Presently, continuous research is being conducted to reevaluate and improve fat transplantation.

REFERENCES

1. Passot R: La chirurgie esthetique des rides du vihsage. *Presse Med* 1919; 27:258.
2. Illouz YG: Fat cell "graft": A new technique to fill depressions. *Plast Reconstr Surg* 1986; 78:122.
3. Newman J: Liposuction surgery: Past, present, future. *Am J Cosmetic Surg* 1984; 1:19.
4. Newman J, Levin J: The quick connect internal Leur-Lock cannula system. *Am J Cosmetic Surg* 1988; 5:17.
5. Newman J, Nguyen A, Anderson R: Liposuction of the head and neck, in English GM (ed): *Otolaryngology.* 1987, pp 1–24.
6. Newman J, Levin J: Facial lipo-transplant surgery. *Am J Cosmetic Surg* 1987; 4:131.
7. Jost G, Levet Y: Parotid fascia and face lifting: A critical evaluation of the SMAS concept. *Plast Reconstr Surg* 1984; 74:42.
8. Neuber F: Fat grafting. *Chir Kongr Verb Disch Ges Chir* 1910; 39:188.
9. Brunings. Cited by Broeckaert and Steinhaus.
10. Chajchir A: Liposuction fat grafts in face wrinkles and hemifacial atrophy. *Aesthetic Plast Surg* 1986; 10:115.

CHAPTER 34

Periorbital Reconstruction

Approach of

Terry L. Fry, M.D.

The periorbital area is possibly the most challenging area for reconstruction in the head and neck. This area is a focal point for facial expression and emotion, pinpointing it for even unintentional scrutiny. A primary focus on functional rehabilitation often yields the simultaneous gain of cosmetic rehabilitation. Functional reconstruction requires symmetry of the orbits, imperative for clear stereoscopic vision in all fields of gaze, as well as functional symmetry of the ocular adnexae. The upper and lower lids not only protect the globe but also propel tears laterally to medially, providing continual lubrication and cleansing while also providing a pumping mechanism to evacuate these tears and debris down the lacrimal system.

A brief review of the medial canthal region is appropriate prior to discussing repair of this area. The medial canthal tendon is not the simple ligamentous attachment of the upper and lower lid tarsi to the anterior and posterior lacrimal crests as is often depicted. In fact, the superficial lateral portion of this ligament attaches to the upper and lower lid, pretarsal and preseptal muscles, as well as the orbicularis muscles.[1] The more deeply situated lateral component of the medial canthus is composed of the upper and lower heads of Horner's muscle, which originates from the area of the posterior lacrimal crest and has muscle attachments to its accompanying canaliculi and the medial end of the tarsus (Fig 34–1). The lacrimal sac, which is surrounded by periosteum, is situated between these superficial and lateral portions of the medial palpebral ligament. The sac's lateral periosteal covering serves as partial origin of the upper and lower deep heads of the preseptal muscle. These deep heads of the preseptal muscle exert lateral traction on the lacrimal sac, creating a negative pressure within it. Meanwhile, lateral to medial closure of the lid milks the pool of tears along the palpebral margin into the area of the lacrimal puncta. Capillary action, with its direction of flow controlled by the negative lacrimal sac pressure, carries tears through the upper and lower

canaliculi. Tear movement is further augmented by the action of the superficial and deep heads of the pretarsal muscles, which close the ampullae and shorten the canaliculi.[1] The only simple ligamentous portion of the medial canthus is the most anterior medial portion, which attaches to the ascending process of the maxillary bone anterior to the anterior lacrimal crest. It is unusual that traumatic or surgical defects interrupt only this most anterior ligamentous structure, and it is intriguing that simple suture repositioning of this complex medial canthal area gives acceptable results in the majority of patients. Nevertheless, knowledge of this anatomy and its function will allow the surgeon to inform patients of the potential for morbidity following trauma or surgical excision of the medial aspect of the eyelids or the lacrimal sac area, as well as allow for specific goals in reconstruction.

The goals in the reconstruction of central eyelid defects are globe protection, maintenance of a film of cleansing tears, and cosmesis. Any defect involving as much as one half of the total lid can be repaired with an Esser flap, analogous to the Abbe-Estlander technique of the lip.[2] A full-thickness, marginally pedicled lid flap measuring one half the horizontal length of the original defect but the full vertical width is rotated 180 degrees from the central portion of the uninvolved adjacent eyelid (Fig 34–2). Care should be taken to maintain 5 mm of marginal pedicle because the blood supply is approximately 3 mm from the lid margin. The graft is secured with a three-layer closure, with care to avoid strangulation of its vascular pedicle. The donor site is closed primarily. This technique requires a second stage for release of the vascular pedicle at 18 to 21 days but is much more reliable than a free graft and fulfills all functional and cosmetic requirements if it is carefully performed. The lid defect is shared equally by upper and lower lids, maintaining symmetry, but necessarily shortening the palpebral fissure compared with the unaffected opposite eye. If this is a

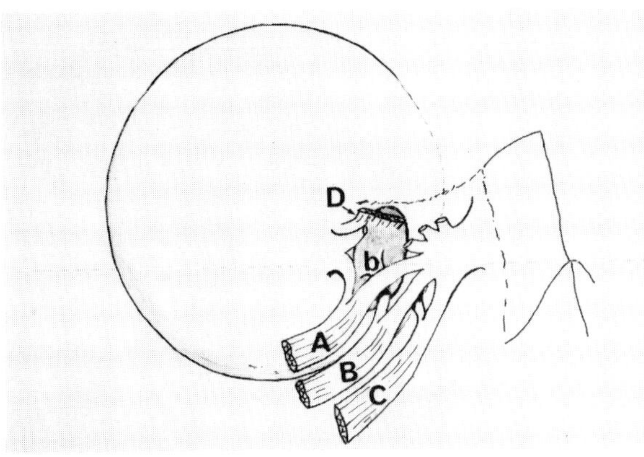

FIG 34–1.
Medial canthal tendon's superficial lateral portion attaches to the pretarsal (*A*), preseptal (*B*), and orbicularis (*C*) muscles. Horner's muscle (*D*) originates from the area of the posterior lacrimal crest and its accompanying canaliculi of the lacrimal sac (shown in gray). The preseptal muscle has attachment (*b*) to the periosteum surrounding the lacrimal sac to create a negative pressure within the sac during lid closure. (For simplicity, the upper lid musculature and both canaliculi have been omitted.)

serious cosmetic blemish, the lids of the opposite eye may be proportionally shortened with simple pentameter wedge excisions. Full-thickness central lid losses measuring one fourth the length of the lid or less may be closed primarily in this same fashion (Fig 34–3).

Loss of central portions of the eyelid with an intact lid margin is best reconstructed with similar tissues. Full-thickness skin loss should be replaced with lid skin from an uninvolved lid in the older patient or from postauricular skin in a child. This graft should be bolstered and the lid immobilized with a tarsorrhaphy or dressing for 7 to 10 days. Loss of eyelid skin and tarsus, leaving intact conjunctiva, is best replaced with a composite graft of posterior conchal skin with its adherent conchal bowl cartilage.

Free conchal cartilage grafts for the lower lid are preferable to borrowing tarsal cartilage from the upper lid because this avoids possible detachment of the upper lid levator muscle,

which may result in ptosis, and avoids upper lid distortion, which may result from excessive loss of upper lid tarsus.

Lower lid defects can often be most simply closed by a sliding facial flap, perhaps requiring lateral canthal release if the lid margin is involved in larger defects (Fig 34–4).

This latter technique provides vascularized skin for reconstruction after complete lower lid loss. This facial flap ideally is lined with either buccal or labial mucosa or full-thickness maxillary sinus mucous membrane with its periosteum for less contracture.[3] Auricular conchal cartilage can be used to replace the tarsus if the lid lacks resilience.

These concepts also apply in reconstruction of the entire upper lid. A switch flap of the entire lower lid may replace the upper lid, whereas the lower donor site is repaired with facial advancement flap and free graft of mucous membrane.

Should more than one half of the length of upper lid be missing, one must identify the proximal edge of the levator muscle and attach it to the grafted tarsus for proper lid function. Smaller lid losses usually preserve enough undisturbed levator to avoid ptosis.

ECTROPION REPAIR

The method for correction of ectropion is based on identifying the source of ectropion. Cicatricial ectropion may complicate periorbital trauma wherein insufficient lid skin produces lid eversion. These deformities require complete scar release, followed by a skin graft approximately 50% larger than the resulting defect. A bolster and temporary tarsorrhaphy improve results by avoiding bunching of the graft with lid motion.

A similar repair is used for ectropion resulting from excessive skin removal during blepharoplasty. Because eyelid skin is best replaced with eyelid skin, some surgeons save excised upper lid skin in a refrigerated antibiotic solution for 14 days following blepharoplasty for the rare situations of untoward results.

Paralytic ectropion is most appropriately handled as a severe senile or involutional ectropion wherein both loss of orbicularis muscle tone and tarsal lengthening have produced lid

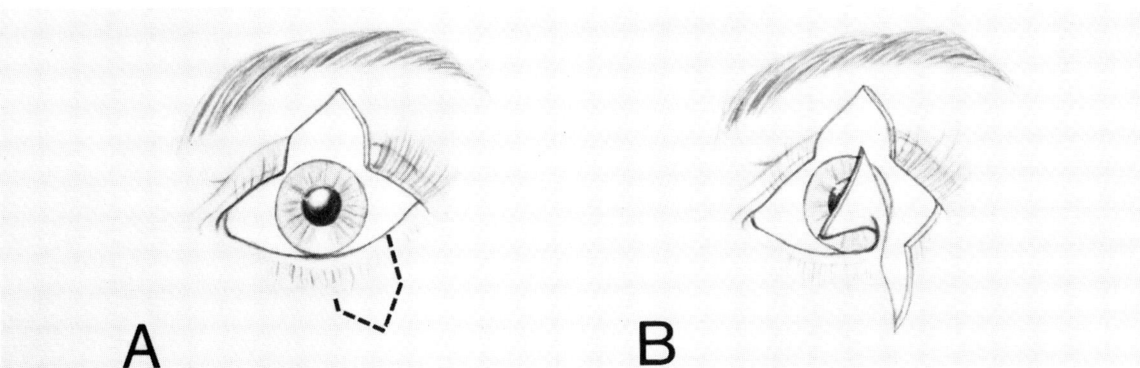

FIG 34–2.
A, full-thickness flap is designed to measure approximately one half of the opposing lid defect but its full vertical height. **B**, maintenance of a 5 mm marginal pedicle is crucial to flap survival.

FIG 34–3.
Pentameter wedge excision allows primary closure of smaller lid defects without notching.

eversion. Calculated repair of both components is best handled by a technique described originally by Kulent[4] and Szymanowski.[5] This procedure requires a preoperative assessment of lid excess. This is best determined after topical anesthesia of the conjunctival sac, which allows two forceps to grasp the lid, folding the excess sufficiently to bring the conjunctiva snugly against the globe (Fig 34–5,A). Measurement of this folded excess allows the design of a triangle (whose base equals the excess) in the skin lateral to the lateral canthus. The base of the triangle is directed temporocephalically from the lateral canthus. The medial side of the triangle is approximately one and one half times the length of the base and perpendicular to it in an inferior direction. The lateral ends of these two lines are connected, completing the triangle.

At this point, the lid may be injected for anesthesia and hemostasis. The skin triangle is removed prior to dividing the lateral two thirds of the lid along the gray line (Fig 34–5,B). (This is initiated with a scalpel and completed by blunt scissors dissection between the tarsus and overlying skin-muscle. Extremes of lid eversion require that the lid split be carried more medially, closer to the punctum.) The skin muscle layer should be freed sufficiently to allow easy advancement laterally to fill the triangular defect. Forceps folding of the tarsoconjunctival flap now allows for accurate, but conservative, triangular resection of this tissue (Fig 34–5,C). The base of the triangle is along the lid margin, and the apex is directed inferiorly. Closure of the tarsoconjunctiva is best done with woven, nonabsorbable 4-0 or 5-0 suture with all knots against the external surface of the tarsus and extreme care taken to achieve good approximation without notching. The skin-muscle layer is now drawn superolaterally to close the triangular skin defect following excision of the excess marginal cilia (Fig 34–5,D). A 5-0 stitch of nonabsorbable suture is used to firmly attach the new ciliary margin of the lower lid to the lateral canthal angle, and the triangular skin defect is closed with interrupted fine 6-0 sutures. Dissolution of absorbable suture requires local tissue inflammatory reaction and should be avoided in the thin skin of the eyelid to minimize erythema and swelling.

Some patients additionally require a lateral canthopexy if the lateral canthal attachment is lax. Care should be taken to place the positioning suture medially within the orbital periosteum deep to the ideal lateral canthus to snug the lid up onto the globe.

Early, minimal ectropion of the punctum may be easily corrected by a horizontal elliptical excision of the conjunctiva. This superficial excision is carefully performed just below the ampulla, avoiding injury to the drainage system.

REPAIR OF THE EPICANTHAL FOLD

Epicanthal folds may be congenital or posttraumatic. A simple Z-plasty or multiple Z-plasties with the central limb along the fold is the simplest technique for repair (Fig 34–6). If the canthus is also displaced inferiorly, a single Z-plasty is preferred, and the more superior angle is enlarged to allow for overcorrection. This latter situation requires detachment of the medial portion of the canthus, followed by permanent suture reattachment in a more cephalic position (Fig 34–7).

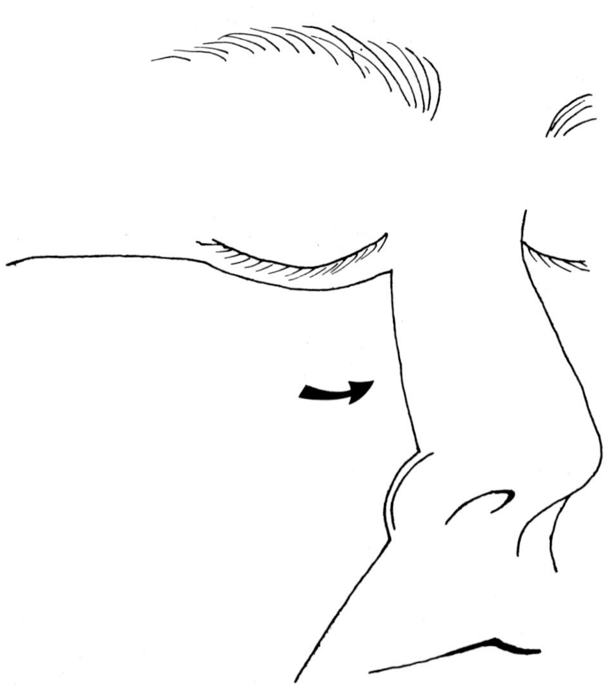

FIG 34–4.
Sliding facial flap can be used to resurface massive lower lid as well as lateral nasal defects.

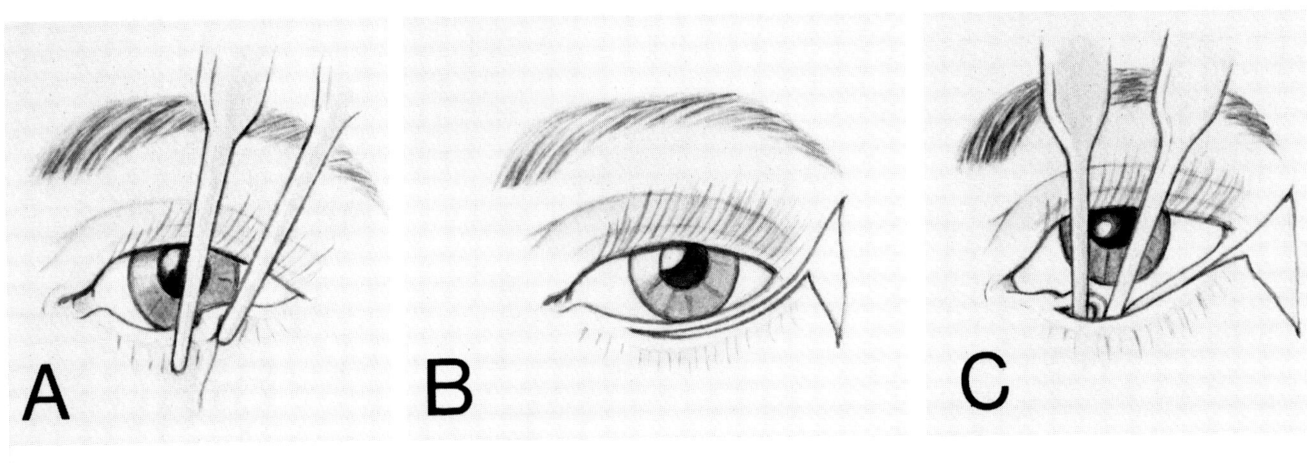

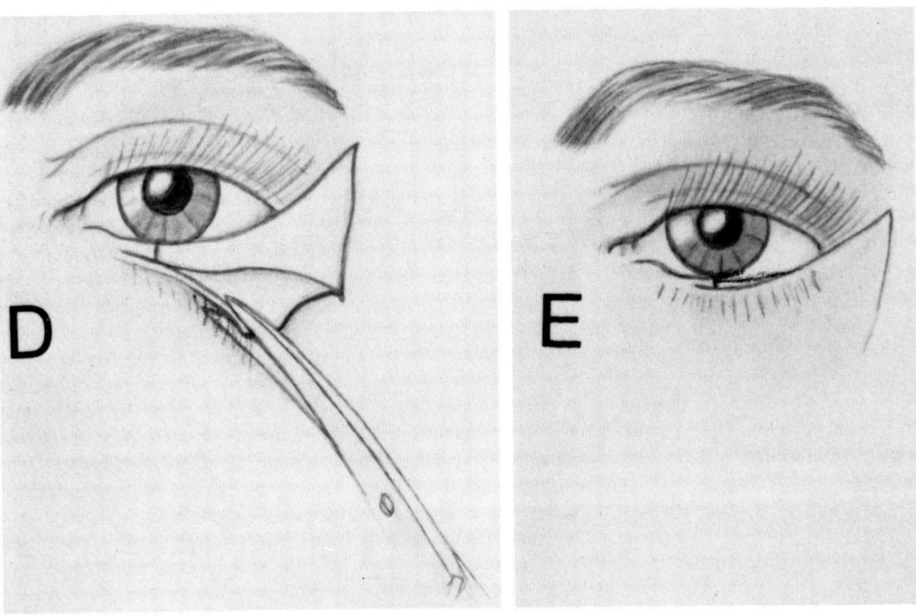

FIG 34–5.
Repair of paralytic ectropion. **A,** grasping the lid with two forceps allows estimate of the length of lid excess. **B,** an appropriately designed lateral skin triangle is excised prior to separation of the lateral lid along the gray line. **C,** grasping the tarsoconjunctival flap with two forceps allows for accurate excision of the lid excess as a triangle. **D,** excess marginal cilia are trimmed prior to closure of the skin triangle with lateral advancement of the skin-muscle layer of the lid. **E,** corrected paralytic ectropion.

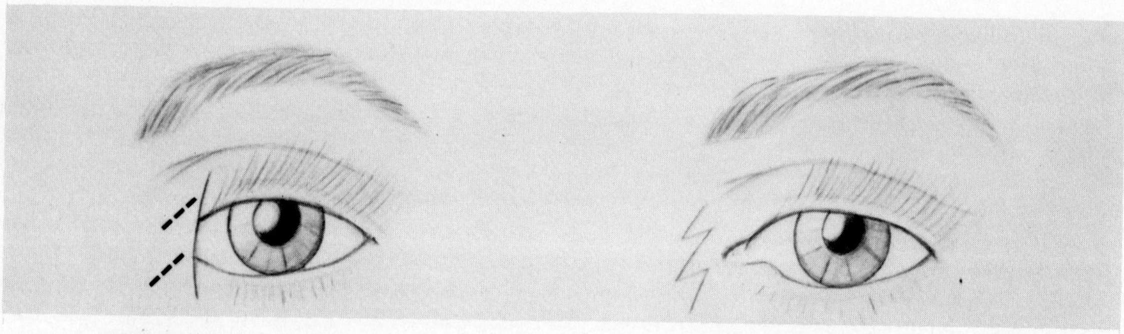

FIG 34–6.
Z-plasty repair of an epicanthal fold.

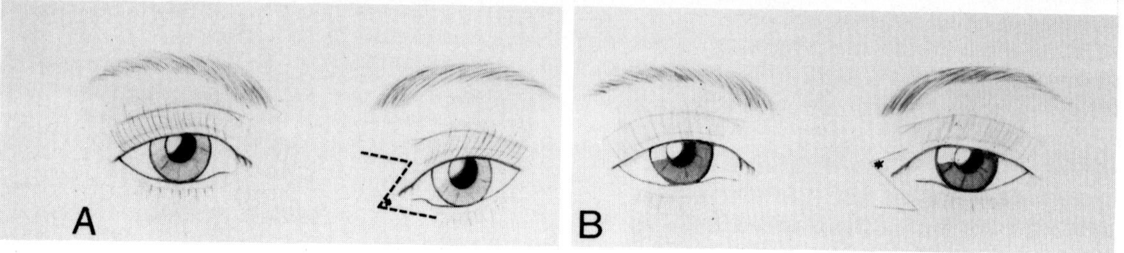

FIG 34–7.
A, inferiorly displaced medial canthus is best repaired by a Z-plasty repair with the medial canthus incorporated in the lower triangular flap *(asterisk).* **B,** permanent suture secures the superiorly repositioned medial canthal flap to the orbital periosteum.

EXOPHTHALMOS

Ophthalmic Graves' disease is the most common etiology of exophthalmos. The increased intraorbital tension is primarily secondary to progressive extraocular muscle enlargement due to lymphocytic infiltration and edema, which may progress independent of control of thyroid dysfunction. The increasing muscle mass impedes venous and lymphatic return, further aggravating orbital congestion, leading to progression of proptosis and chemosis, as well as the already limited extraocular motion. Progressive fibrosis of the levator and Müller's muscle further aggravates the widened palpebral fissure and promotes keratitis and eventual panophthalmitis with progressive loss of vision.[6] Similar clinical appearance may be seen with orbital pseudotumor, lymphoma, metastatic disease, infectious involvement of the orbit, cavernous sinus thrombosis, or vascular malformations in the orbit or cavernous sinus areas. These etiologies may be easily identified by history or physical examination. They are readily differentiated by coronal computed tomography (CT) with contrast.[6] The coronal CT not only documents the extraocular muscle enlargement in Graves' ophthalmopathy but also gives sinus detail and hopefully documents lack of chronic sinus disease.

The evolution of surgical decompression is nicely summarized in numerous texts.[7–9] However, the procedure that best fulfills the criteria for salvage of visual acuity, decrease in intraorbital pressure, corneal protection, cosmesis, and avoidance of postoperative complications such as orbital pulsation is that described by Walsh and Ogura.[10] A standard Caldwell-Luc procedure allows entry into the ethmoid air cells approximately 1 cm anterior to the junction of the posterior and medial walls of the maxillary sinus. As with any ethmoidectomy procedure, the surgeon should be well trained in the sinus anatomy to avoid injury to the ethmoidal arteries, the optic nerve, and the cribriform plate. Ethmoid exenteration is followed by careful removal of the lamina papyracea, avoiding disruption of the orbital periosteum. Removal of the orbital floor is easily accomplished after careful bony thinning with a mastoid bur. The path of the infraorbital nerve is readily identified. Copious irrigation and preservation of the nerve's bony canal avoid postoperative paresthesia in the midface and upper lip. The bony orbital floor both medial and lateral to the nerve can be bluntly removed after proper thinning. Linear cuts in the orbital periosteum to allow orbital fat prolapse are a prerequisite to adequate decompression. These posterior to anterior cuts are initially performed high in the area of the ethmoids with an otologic sickle knife. The sequential progression of these cuts from superomedially to inferolaterally along the orbital periosteum allows for visibility during the procedure. Prolapsing fat will progressively interfere with visualization, and therefore periosteal cuts should be carefully performed in sequential fashion. An exophthalmometer will aid in obtaining symmetry in bilateral decompression as these cuts are made. Milder degrees of exophthalmos may require only ethmoidal decompression, whereas unilateral disease may require an intact orbital periosteum lateral to the infraorbital nerve to avoid diplopia. Horizontal incisions in the periorbita may be necessary in the more extreme degrees of proptosis. This technique, allowing for spontaneous prolapse, avoids injury to the extraocular muscles and optic nerve. The procedure is completed with creation of a standard nasal antral window.

Marked improvement is seen in the immediate postoperative period and often continues for up to 4 months. Patients are generally cautioned to see their otolaryngologist for any subsequent sinusitis for early institution of medical therapy.

PTOSIS

Optimal surgery for ptosis requires preoperative assessment of etiology and degree of ptosis. Simple traumatic detachment of the levator is easily remedied with good results. The upper lid is infiltrated with 1% lidocaine and epinephrine 1:100,000. An incision is made through skin and orbicularis just below and paralleling the superior margin of the tarsus. This is facilitated by grasping the lid with an Ehrhardt clamp. The skin-muscle flap is elevated inferiorly, stopping well short of injury to the marginal cilia. The superior skin-muscle flap is elevated sufficiently to expose the thickening of the septum orbitale as it fuses with the underlying levator. (This thickened band usually lies just above the tarsal border and extends horizontally and slightly downward in a nasal direction.) This orbital fascia is bluntly undermined and then separated from the levator. As the fascia retracts, orbital fat may prolapse and require amputation to avoid subsequent irregular thickening of the lid. Identification of the detached levator may be facilitated in the awake patient by the muscle's motion as the patient attempts to elevate the eyelid. Several double-armed sutures of 5-0 nonabsorbable, white woven suture are placed in mattress fashion 2 to 3 mm from the detached edge of the levator and through the upper tarsal border (see Fig 34–9,B). The tension on these sutures is adjusted such that the two upper lids occupy the same position over the upper limbus as the patient looks forward. The lid skin is then closed with care to include a bite of levator along the superior tarsal border (Fig 34–8). This maneuver assures appropriate position of the supratarsal fold.

Repair of unilateral ptosis secondary to partial atrophy of the levator is less rewarding. Normal levator action requires symmetric opening and closing of both eyes, equal distance between the lids in all fields of gaze, symmetric movement of both lids with upward and downward movement of the globe, and absence of lid lag. These goals are more easily met with the lesser degrees of ptosis and good levator function. Therefore, preoperative counseling should follow measurement of the number of millimeters of ptosis as well as the amount of upper lid excursion from patient downward to upward gaze. In general, the more lid excursion, the more conservative the levator resection. For example, with 10 mm or more of lid excursion (implying good levator function), the amount of levator resection often approximates the number of millimeters of ptosis. However, with lesser amounts of lid excursion, one must overcorrect the ptosis in anticipation of less than optimal levator function. Absence of levator function in paralysis disqualifies the patient for levator resection procedures. Overall, operative results often inversely reflect the amount of anticipated levator resection, with lag ophthalmus being the most common sequela following levator resection for marked ptosis and poor levator function.

As with all surgically correctable lesions, there are a multitude of acceptable techniques. The anterior approach, as previously described for traumatic levator separations, is applicable for all degrees of ptosis (with levator mobility) and avoids conjunctival interruption with its potential for corneal damage or granulation.[11] Conjunctival approaches for excision of Müller's muscle are effective in only the mildest degrees of ptosis. No more than 2 mm of lift can be expected, and best results are seen in patients who preoperatively respond to 10% phenylephrine (Neo-Synephrine) hydrochloride placed in the conjunctival sac.

Following preoperative estimation of the amount of levator resection, the pretarsal incision, skin muscle dissection, and separation of the orbital fascia from the levator are accomplished as described in foregoing paragraphs. However, as a caution, one should place a 4-0 black silk suture around the superior rectus muscle (identified by lifting the lid up while pulling the globe down) to avoid injury to this muscle during extensive dissections. At this point, the lid should be everted and the conjunctiva injected with local anesthetic in such a fashion as to balloon it away from Müller's muscle directly anterior to it. If epinephrine is used, the additional 2 mm of lift created by Müller's muscle must be remembered in determining subsequent length of levator resection. Müller's muscle is then buttonholed along the lateral superior marginal edge

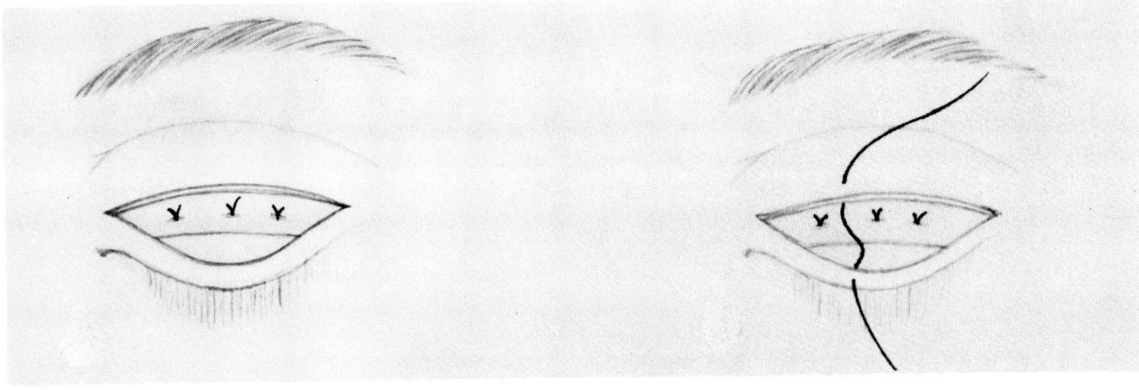

FIG 34–8.
Lid skin is closed with care to include a bit of levator along the superior tarsal border to assure correct position of the supratarsal fold.

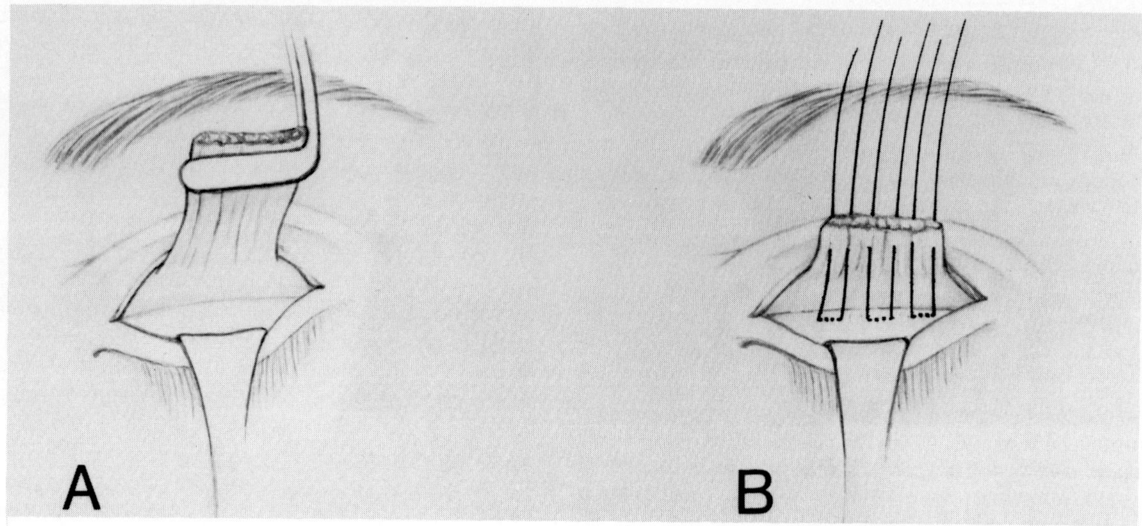

FIG 34–9.
A, levator and Müller's muscles are grasped in a ptosis clamp and carefully dissected from the underlying conjunctiva. **B,** trimmed edge of the levator is secured with permanent mattress sutures to the upper tarsal border.

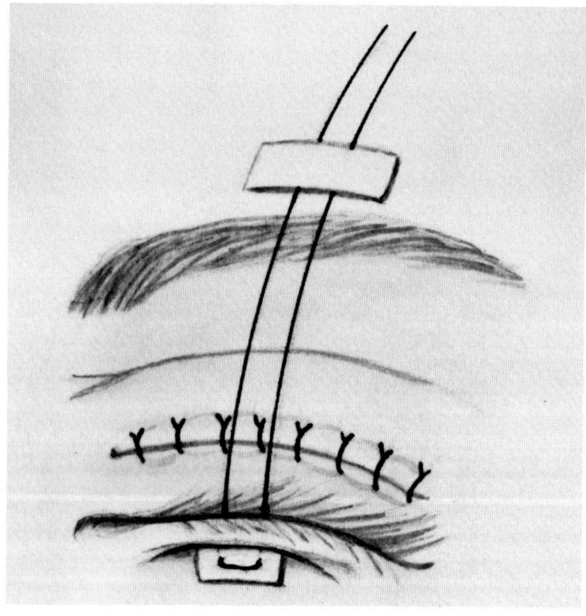

FIG 34–10.
Frost suture is placed through the lower lid and taped superiorly for protection of the cornea postoperatively.

of the tarsus and bluntly dissected away from and avoiding damage to the underlying conjunctiva. This blunt dissection is terminated at the medial end of the tarsus by again pushing through the levator muscle complex anteriorly. A ptosis clamp can be placed through this tunnel to grasp both levator and Müller's muscle just prior to dividing their insertions to the upper tarsal border. Lifting the ptosis clamp (Fig 34–9,A) allows careful dissection of Müller's muscle away from the conjunctiva. When more than 12 mm of levator resection is anticipated, extensive anterior and posterior dissection allows identification

of the medial and lateral horns of the levator. The lateral horn is best palpated after lifting the ptosis clamp medially. This is cut by using superolaterally directed blunt scissors along the orbital wall. Lifting the ptosis clamp laterally allows palpation and division of the medial horn and check ligament. Care must be taken to avoid injury to the superior rectus muscle (identifiable by the 4-0 black silk suture) during posterior dissection and division of the medial levator attachments. An immediate give to the levator is sensed if these attachments are properly divided. Any adhesive bands between the orbital rim and the levator should also be transected. Three double-armed 4-0 Vicryl sutures can now be spaced along and approximately 6 mm below the superior tarsal margin in horizontal mattress fashion.

The amount of levator resection is again estimated, with an assistant placing the globe in the position of forward gaze with the upper lid margin resting at the superior corneal limbus. Gentle draping of the levator allows estimate of the amount needing resection to position the cut edge along the superior tarsus. The previously placed tarsal sutures are appropriately spaced through the levator complex approximately 2 mm proximal to the estimated line of resection (Fig 34–9,B). The excess levator is excised. A single throw in each of the sutures allows for adjustment in the height of the lid with the globe in a forward-gaze position. The knots are now secured with additional throws. The superior lid skin may require modest trimming prior to closure as depicted in Figure 34–8,B to assure a good supratarsal fold.

A Frost suture is used to lift the lower lid for corneal protection in the postoperative period (Fig 34–10). It can often be removed after 3 days due to spontaneous corneal protection by the heavy, edematous upper lid. The operated eye should be patched at night for several weeks to avoid corneal trauma. Exposure keratitis is a rare postoperative problem if the patient preoperatively demonstrates a good Bell's phenomenon. Sur-

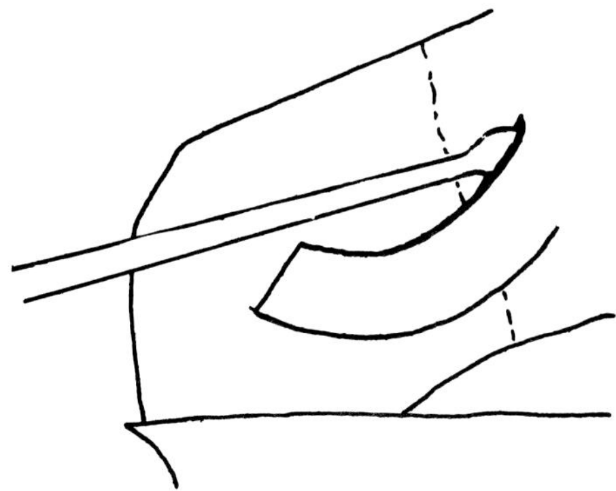

FIG 34–11.
Mucoperichondrial-periosteal flap is elevated from the nasal septum. The correct plane is easily identified if dissection is begun over the perpendicular plate after bullous infiltration of local anesthetic in this plane.

gical intervention for overcorrection or undercorrection should be postponed for 3 months, because early evaluations are often erroneous.

DACRYOCYSTORHINOSTOMY

Epiphora may result from loss of punctal contact with the globe even very early in ectropion, which typically begins medially. Epiphora is also a manifestation of palsy of the orbicularis muscle with loss of the lid motion necessary to efficiently milk the ribbon of tears across the palpebral fissure. Epiphora may result from traumatic or infectious obstruction of the proximal canaliculi, the lacrimal sac, or the nasolacrimal duct. Excessive tearing due to overproduction or stimulation of the lacrimal gland may present with a similar clinical picture. All of these entities can be readily identified with a thorough examination, which may require punctal probing and irrigation, dye studies, or even radiologic evaluation.[12]

Complete obstruction of the proximal canaliculi such as that following severe trauma or surgical resection of tumor is variously handled with glass tubes or sundry shunting procedures. My choice is a shunt consisting of a medially based inferior flap of conjunctiva anastomosed to a flap of nasal septal mucoperichondrium. The latter is easily developed after a careful subperichondrial injection of lidocaine with epinephrine 1:100,000 along the ipsilateral nasal septum. The mucosa of the lateral nasal wall, including the area superior to the middle turbinate and the inferior sulcus of conjunctiva, is also infiltrated with the vasoconstrictive anesthetic. A crescent-shaped mucoperichondrial flap with its base posterior and midway up the septum and a width of 1 cm is outlined sharply and elevated with a Cottle elevator (Fig 34–11). The correct plane of dissection is best accomplished by beginning posteriorly where the base of the flap overlies the perpendicular plate of the ethmoid. Similarly, the proper plane of anesthetic injection is also simplified by beginning in this area where one readily feels the needle contact bone just prior to injection. The distal free corners of the flap are then tagged with 5-0 Vicryl for later ease in placement (Fig 34–12). A medially based conjunctival strip

measuring approximately 15 mm long and 1 cm wide is elevated with sharp scissors following initial scalpel incision for outline. Blunt dissection medially beneath this flap identifies the lamina papyracea. Chisel cuts through this bone, with care to be below the level of the medial canthus, allow use of Haejaks or back-biting bone rongeurs to enlarge the opening and advance it inferomedially through the anterior ethmoid air cells and into the nasal cavity. Ideal entrance into the nasal cavity is just anterior to the middle turbinate or as a second choice above the level of the middle meatus and through the substance of the middle turbinate. The tunnel between orbit and nasal cavity should be no smaller than 1 cm in diameter. Passage of a wire loop from orbit to nasal cavity allows for easy retrieval of the Vicryl sutures into the orbit. The two flaps are then sutured end to end under direct vision (Fig 34–13). The conjunctival portion and more distal end of the septal flap can even be tubed with the mucosa placed luminally. A short silicone rubber (Silastic) tube may be gently placed within the new conduit to optimize the lumen during healing, but is not necessary. The new conduit is then gently withdrawn toward the nasal cavity. Antibiotic ointment–coated absorbable gelatin sponge (Gelfoam) is gently

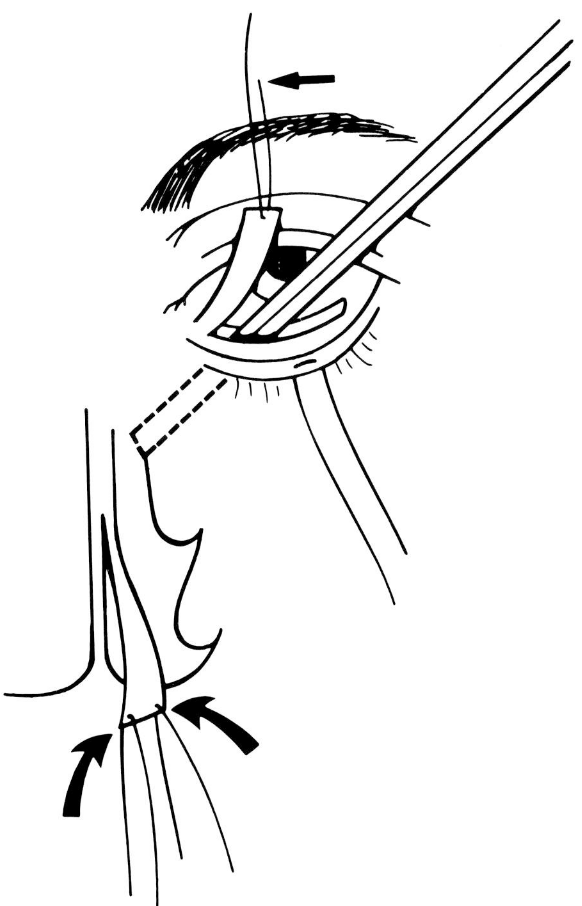

FIG 34–12.
Sutures are placed in the free corners of the septal flap *(large arrows)*. A medially based conjunctival strip is elevated *(small arrow)*, allowing chisel cuts through the lamina papyracea.

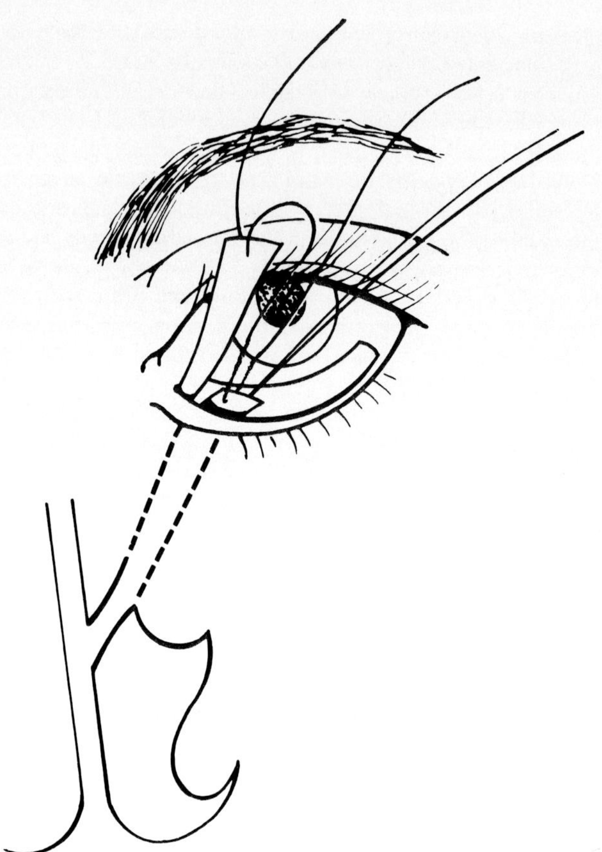

FIG 34–13.
Septal and conjunctival flaps are sutured end to end under direct vision.

placed in the nasal cavity, and the patient is given antibiotic ophthalmic solution to use during the first postoperative week. Placement of the nasal end of the transethmoid tunnel in the more posterior (second choice) position decreases the incidence of crusting in the more patent nose. Use of a septal mucoperichondrial flap is advocated because of the greater ease in visualization and the greater available length, which is appreciated at the time of anastomosis and "tubing."

In the more ideal situation, the lacrimal drainage system is often patent through the level of the lacrimal sac. This situation, where no prior trauma or surgical ablation has distorted the area, is more often seen and handled by an ophthalmologist with a dacryocystorhinostomy procedure, of which there are many. Surgical expertise in the nasal cavity often adds a measure of success and ease to this operation. Visibility is facilitated by injections of anesthetic with epinephrine 1:100,000 or 1:200,000 in the lateral nasal cavity and the medial canthal areas whether the patient is to be awake or asleep for the procedure. A curvilinear incision through skin and periosteum is made between the medial canthus and the bridge of the nose. Bipolar cautery is advantageous in obtaining a dry surgical field before proceeding. The lateral periosteum can be easily elevated to the level of the anterior lacrimal crest with a small periosteal elevator. Traction sutures are placed through the periosteum. The

entire anterior lacrimal crest should be exposed before an attempt is made to elevate the more tightly adherent periosteum along this landmark. Inadvertent injury to the lacrimal sac during this maneuver can lead to frustration later on. Fortunately, the sac itself is easily elevated from the lacrimal fossa. The bone of the lacrimal fossa is gently fractured with a small chisel to allow removal of the entire bony fossa with small back-biting bone rongeurs. Extra care taken here to avoid laceration of the underlying mucosa is rewarded by a dry surgical field. A brief pause to inject more of the vasoconstrictive anesthetic between the bone and underlying mucous membrane is also helpful. The lacrimal sac is then opened by placing the point of the blade of delicate tissue scissors in the lumen of the opening to the nasolacrimal duct at the inferior aspect of the sac. The sac can be opened by fashioning an anteriorly based rectangular flap.

Attention is now turned to the intranasal aspect of this procedure. A mucoperiosteal flap with its base near the anterior tip of the middle turbinate is developed over the area corresponding to the nasolacrimal fossa where previous bone removal allows identification by palpation or transillumination. Placement of a 4-0 Vicryl suture in the free end of the lateral nasal flap facilitates its delivery into the orbital aspect of the wound, where it is sutured to the posterior edge of the opening into the lacrimal sac. The anteriorly based lacrimal sac flap is similarly sutured to the free edge of the lateral nasal mucosa. This flap technique of staggering the suture lines avoids the synechiae of opposed suture lines within the lumen of the new drainage route. A thin strip of Silastic sheeting or soft tubing can be placed from the sac to the nasal cavity by securing it to the anterolateral aspect of the sac with a 5-0 plain chromic suture. This stent also helps the surgeon avoid catching the deeper wall of the new mucosal channel while suturing the anterior flap to the nasal mucosa. This stent can best be maintained in position if a 5-0 nylon suture secures its nasal extension.

The patient is given antibiotic ophthalmic drops to use three times daily during the first postoperative week and longer if any sign of purulent conjunctivitis exists. The Silastic stent is easily removed 7 to 10 days later when its superior chromic attachment has dissolved.

An endoscopic approach for dacryorhinostomy in an effort to avoid a skin incision has also been advocated.[13] I am concerned that creation of a mucosal conduit under direct vision improves results and therefore offsets the minor criticism of a cosmetic skin incision. This technique, however, should be considered initially in keloid formers.

REFERENCES

1. Zide BM, Jelks GW: *Surgical Anatomy of the Orbit.* New York, Raven Press, 1985, pp 41–46.
2. Fox SA: *Ophthalmic Plastic Surgery.* New York, Grune-Stratton, 1976, pp 345–350.
3. Fry TL, Woods CI: Readily available full-thickness mucous membrane graft. *Arch Otolaryngol Head Neck Surg* 1987; 113:770.

4. Kulent H: *Beitrage zur Operationen Augenheilkunder.* Jena, G. Fischer, 1883, pp 45–55.
5. Szymanowski J: *Handbuch der Operationen Chivurgie.* Berlin, Braunschweig, 1870, p 243.
6. Ogura JH, Thawley SE: Orbital decompression of exophthalmos. *Otolaryngol Clin North Am* 1980; 13:29.
7. Rowe LD, Dedo HH: Ophthalmic surgery in malignant exophthalmos. *Otolaryngol Clin North Am* 1981; 14:449.
8. Lucente FE, Biller HF: *Surgery of the Paranasal Sinuses.* Philadelphia, WB Saunders Co, 1985, p 241.
9. Converse JM, Krupp S: *Reconstructive Plastic Surgery.* Philadelphia, WB Saunders Co, 1977, pp 970–971.
10. Walsh TE, Ogura JH: Transantral orbital decompression for malignant exophthalmos. *Laryngoscope* 1957; 67:544–568.
11. Fox SA: *Surgery of Ptosis.* New York, Grune & Stratton, 1968, pp 32–118.
12. Moazed KT, Cooper WC: *Surgery of the Paranasal Sinuses.* Philadelphia, WB Saunders Co, 1985, pp 228–229.
13. Rice DH: Endoscopic intranasal dacryocystorhinostomy—a cadaver study. *Am J Rhinol* 1988; 2:127–128.

Periorbital Reconstruction

Approach of

Ira D. Papel, M.D.

RECONSTRUCTION OF EYELID DEFECTS

General Considerations

When an eyelid or part of an eyelid is lost to tumor resection or trauma, both aesthetic and functional considerations must be addressed in reconstruction designs. The eyelids, together with the eyebrows, contribute greatly to facial expression and convey emotions such as fear, joy, and fatigue. They also protect the cornea from drying and help with tear drainage. The upper eyelid is the major protector of the cornea, and its absence can lead to drying, ulcerations, and eventual blindness. During sleep the globe rotates up (Bell's phenomenon), primarily covered by the upper lid. A defect in the lower lid will cause epiphora and conjunctival irritation. For these important indications, reconstruction of eyelid defects is essential to protect the integrity of the globe and preserve vision.

In recent years, the specialty of Mohs' chemosurgery for epidermal tumor resection has proved to be safe and effective for facial lesions.[1] Recurrence rates, especially for locally recurrent lesions, are considerably lower than with traditional wide excision. I routinely collaborate with a Mohs surgeon on most facial malignancies located in vital areas such as the periorbital region. Reconstructive considerations are then developed based on the actual tumor-free defect, not on the desired defect as anticipated before resection. Restoration of the protective function of the lids is the first priority, followed by aesthetic considerations.

Central Defects

Central eyelid lesions up to 25% in young people can be repaired with primary closure. In older patients with more laxity in their lids, defects up to 40% can be repaired, especially if a cantholysis procedure is included. When defects are repaired with this method, certain principles need to be observed to obtain an optimal result. A major advantage of direct closure is that the normal lash line is preserved. In preparing the defect for closure, one must use parallel incisions perpendicular to the lid margin instead of a pie-shaped defect. These parallel incisions should encompass the entire vertical height of the tarsus. When combined with a careful layered approximation, this technique will reduce the chances of a vertically contracted scar, which presents as notching of the lid margin or buckling of the remaining tarsal plate (Fig 34–14). If a lateral cantholysis is necessary to reduce tension on the wound, a horizontal incision is made over the lateral orbital rim, and the appropriate segment of the lateral canthal tendon is dissected until the wound closes easily. The tarsal plate is then approximated with

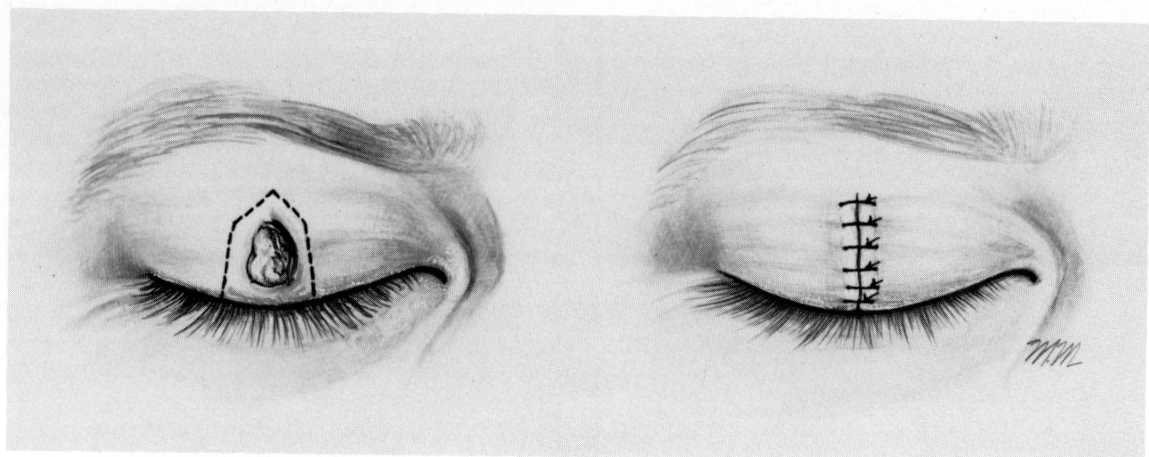

FIG 34–14.
Full-thickness pentagonal excision for primary closure of an eyelid defect.

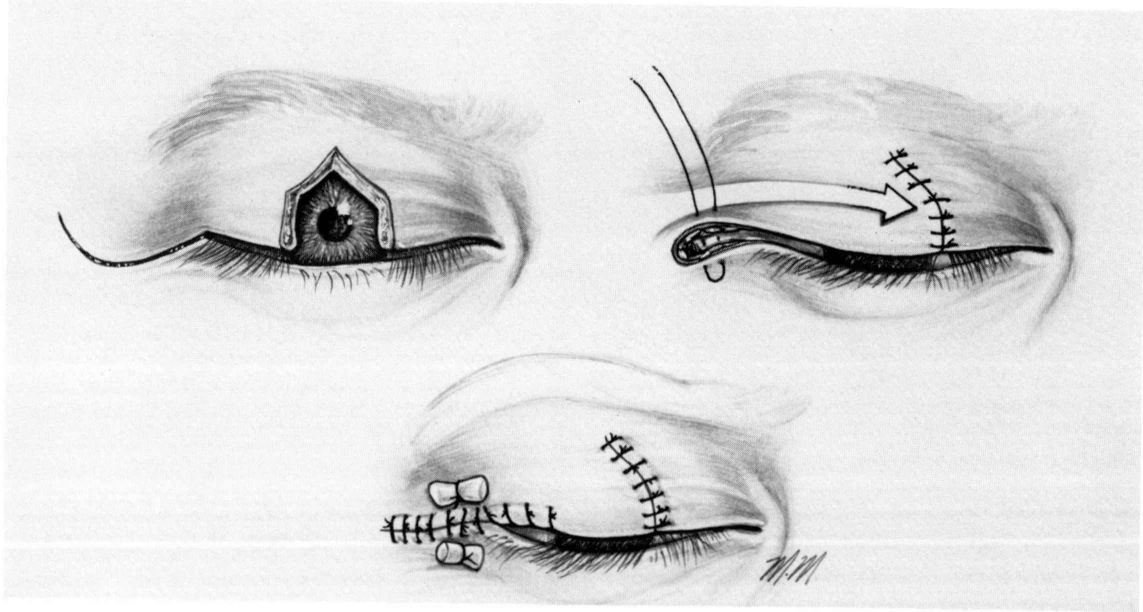

FIG 34–15.
Tenzel flap for central eyelid defects of 40% to 60% of eyelid length.

7-0 silk sutures with the knot buried anterior to the plate. The skin-muscle layer is then approximated with 6-0 Novafil interrupted sutures. The lash line is everted by use of a vertical mattress suture. For central defects comprising 40% to 60% of the eyelid, a Tenzel semicircular advancement flap provides reliable and consistent results.[2] This is a skin-muscle flap that advances tissue from the loose area around the lateral orbital rim. For this reconstruction to be successful, there should be at least a remnant of tarsal plate in the lateral defect. It can be used for either upper or lower eyelid defects with equal ease. In the design of the initial flap incisions, the only difference is the rotation of the incision either superior or inferior from the lateral canthus. To illustrate an upper lid defect, one draws a line from the lateral canthus arching downward into a crow's-foot line. The line then sweeps upward toward the lateral brow

but not more lateral than the brow. The skin-muscle flap is elevated, and a lateral canthotomy of the upper tendon is carried out. The flap is rotated into position, and the lid margins are approximated. A mattress suture is placed at the lateral lid margin into the periosteum of the lateral canthal tendon to help provide support and contour to the new lid. The lateral wound is closed, and any dog-ears are excised in the temporal region (Fig 34–15). A variation of this technique is to use a Z-plasty in the temporal area to further camouflage the incision and provide length if necessary.

Composite grafting can be used to reconstruct fairly large eyelid defects. Up to 8 mm can be harvested from a contralateral lid and can be expected to survive well under a skin-muscle flap.[3] When it is combined with a lateral canthotomy on the recipient side, defects up to 50% of an eyelid length may be

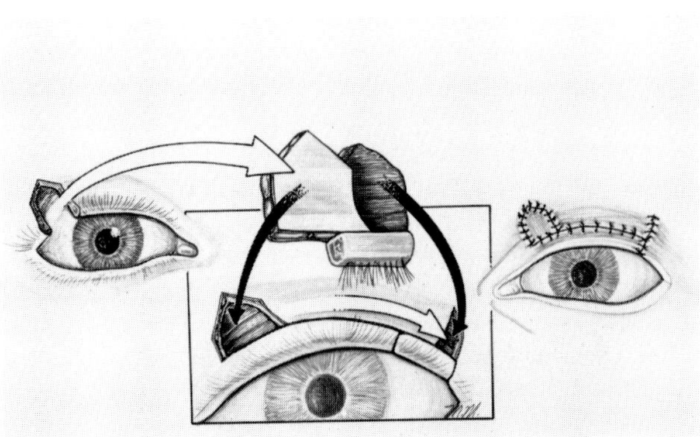

FIG 34–16.
Method of composite grafting from the contralateral eyelid.

corrected. The advantage of this technique is that very similar tissue can be transplanted to provide a very natural appearance. Due to the difference between eyelash lengths (longer on upper lids) grafts between upper and lower lids are not recommended. The main disadvantage of composite grafts is that an otherwise normal lid must be disturbed. This is also a problem with any lid-sharing technique.

The surgical technique of composite grafting includes harvesting a pentagon-shaped graft from the donor lid, usually lateral to the limbus. The donor site is closed primarily as any other lid defect. The anterior skin is then removed to bear the orbicularis muscle beneath. The graft is sewn into the recipient tarsal defect with fine sutures, and a skin flap is elevated on the recipient lid and placed over the composite graft's exposed muscle. The skin from the composite graft is then placed into the defect left by the covering flap (Fig 34–16).

A time-tested method of central eyelid reconstruction is the tarsoconjunctival flap as utilized in the Hughes procedure.[4] This reconstruction uses a tarsoconjunctival flap reflected from the superior tarsus into the lower eyelid defect to provide a posterior lamella. The usual anterior coverage has traditionally been provided with a full-thickness skin graft over the pedicled flap. Doxanas has recently proposed mobilizing a bipedicled orbicularis muscle flap into the defect and placing the full-thickness skin graft anterior to the muscle to provide a more vascular recipient site and also better thickness and mobility in the reconstructed eyelid.[5] This reconstruction works better for lower lid defects due to the more generous size of the superior tarsus. The donor skin can be harvested from either the upper lid or postauricular area.

Lid-sharing procedures are of great value for large defects of the upper lid. When they are combined with rotation flaps as described by Mustardé, near-total or total upper lid defects can be replaced by rotating normal lower lid tissue into the defect.[6] The cheek flap and a chondromucosal graft from the nasal septum will replace the support and covering of the lower lid. In general, the upper lid is not sacrificed to supply the lower due to the important protective function of the upper lid.

Marginal Eyelid Defects

Medial canthal lesions quite often involve portions of both

lids. The lacrimal drainage apparatus and the supporting structure of the medial canthal tendon must also be considered. When tumor resection is performed in this area, aggressive margins are suggested due to the rich lymphatic drainage and the closeness of adjacent structures such as cribriform plate and ethmoid sinuses, where recurrence could be lethal. Full-thickness resection, including periosteum and possibly nasal bone, may be indicated. Reconstruction may rely on regional skin flaps or tarsoconjunctival swing flaps with full-thickness skin graft coverage. If the medial canthal tendon is sacrificed, support can be obtained by raising a periosteal flap as a replacement or by fixing the nasal bones with wire. Reconstruction of the lacrimal apparatus is usually delayed until tumor control is assured and the need for increased lacrimal drainage is determined. In the majority of cases epiphora is not a major problem. In medial canthal reconstruction, the most difficult task is to create a medial palpebral angle that is of normal shape and contour. A rounding of the angle is commonly seen as final healing occurs.

The median forehead flap provides a large amount of tissue of good thickness and color match for the medial canthus. The flap can be split at the distal end to provide skin for both upper and lower eyelids. Variations of this flap include the glabellar flap and the island flap techniques. When the donor flap is designed, it should be slightly wider and longer than the measured defect to be reconstructed. The need for medial canthopexy should be determined at this time so that this can be accomplished before the flap is turned into final position. If canthopexy is required to prevent a telecanthus, either transnasal wire fixation or a periosteal flap reconstruction should be performed. Repair of the conjunctival defect to provide lining to the reconstructed eyelid area can usually be accomplished by advancement and direct suture of the conjunctival edges. If insufficient conjunctiva is available, free grafts of nasal mucosa may be necessary on the inner side of the forehead flap. The flap is then rotated into position, trimmed, and sutured using a layered closure (Fig 34–17). A dog-ear may form over the bridge of the nose. This deformity can be excised if the blood supply to the flap is not endangered, but a secondary procedure to tailor this area may be necessary. For large defects where much of either eyelid must be removed, the forehead flap may be supplemented by cheek flaps and other reconstructive techniques. For small defects, an island forehead flap may be used to reconstruct the medial canthal area.

An alternative technique of medial canthal reconstruction is a sliding tarsoconjunctival flap surfaced by either a full-thickness skin graft or a rotation skin flap. It provides a natural posterior lamella to the eyelid and can be covered with the most suitable source of skin available at the time of reconstruction. This procedure involves fashioning a superior tarsoconjunctival flap with an incision 3 to 4 mm from the lid margin extending from the limbus to the free edge of the defect medially. The flap is then rotated and sutured to the periosteum or bone near the medial canthus. The same considerations of medial canthopexy hold here as earlier. Anterior coverage is fashioned from either a full-thickness skin graft, median forehead rotation flap, or glabellar flap. The flap is divided and tailored 2 weeks later (Fig 34–18).

Lateral canthal defects are much rarer than medial canthal

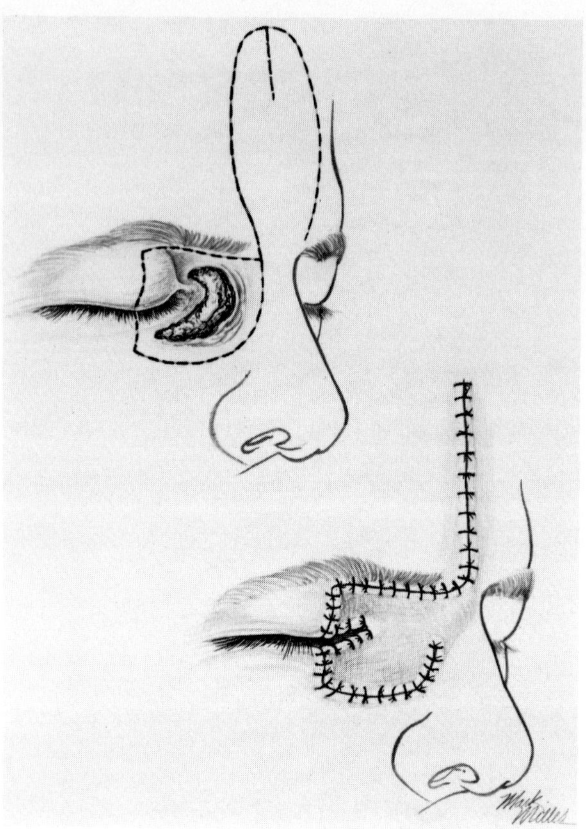

or central eyelid tumors. Unlike the medial canthus, however, there is not an abundance of regional skin that can be mobilized for reconstruction. Full-thickness skin grafts can be used for partial-thickness defects, but when the orbital rim is exposed, a local flap will be necessary. If the lesion is confined to the lower lid, cheek rotation flaps can be used for reconstruction. When both lids are involved, the reconstruction will need to use a lateral forehead flap or a tarsoconjunctival flap with skin coverage. Regardless of the method selected, the lateral canthal tendon area should be reestablished with regard to both vertical and horizontal position. If the lateral canthus is not firmly established, the palpebral fissure will have a rounded appearance, and the eye will have a slanted unnatural appearance. The lateral canthus can be reestablished with a periosteal mattress suture or wire fixation to the orbital rim.

The lateral forehead flap[7] for canthal reconstruction can be split to provide two-lid coverage. After mobilization of the flap, the conjunctiva can usually be closed primarily, but a nasal mucosal flap may be required in some cases. The skin flap is then tailored and sutured into position. A periosteal suture is usually required at the lateral canthus. Due to the relative immobility of the lateral brow area and the possibility of eyebrow distortion, primary closure of the donor site is rarely indicated. Skin graft coverage is usually required (Fig 34–19). The tarsoconjunctival flap with full-thickness skin graft can provide excellent coverage with slightly less bulk than the lateral forehead flap. The technique is similar to the medial canthal method already described (Fig 34–20).

FIG 34–17.
Median forehead flap for reconstruction of medial canthal defects including both eyelids.

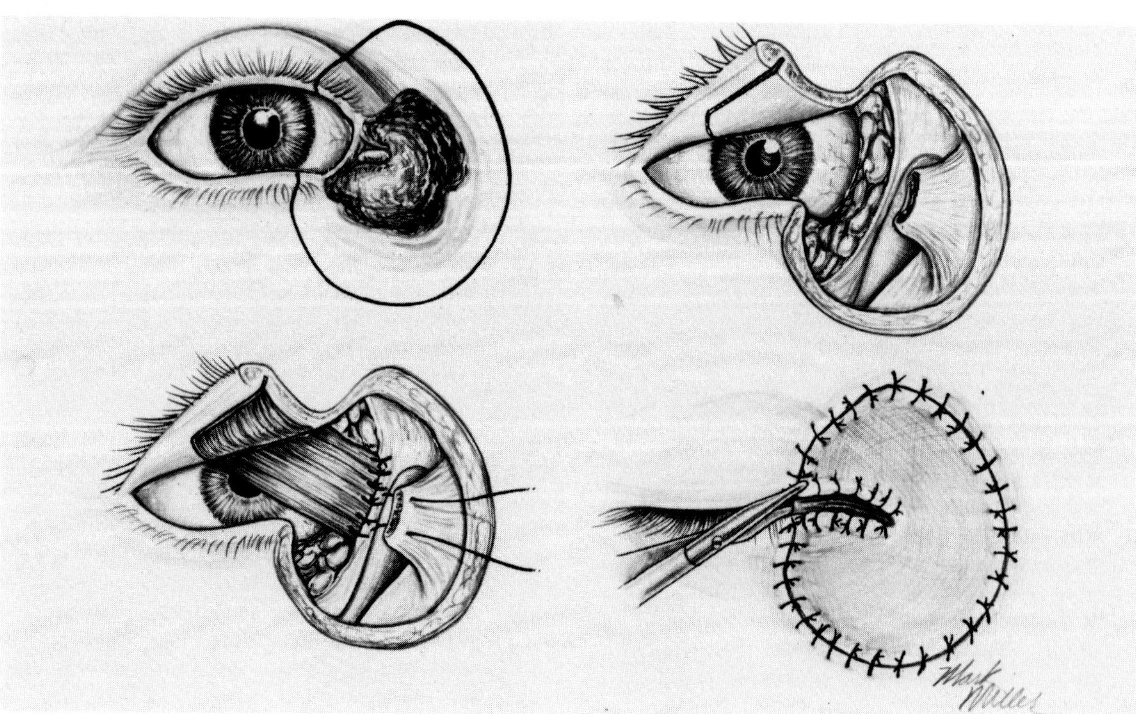

FIG 34–18.
Tarsoconjunctival flap and full-thickness skin graft for medial canthal reconstruction.

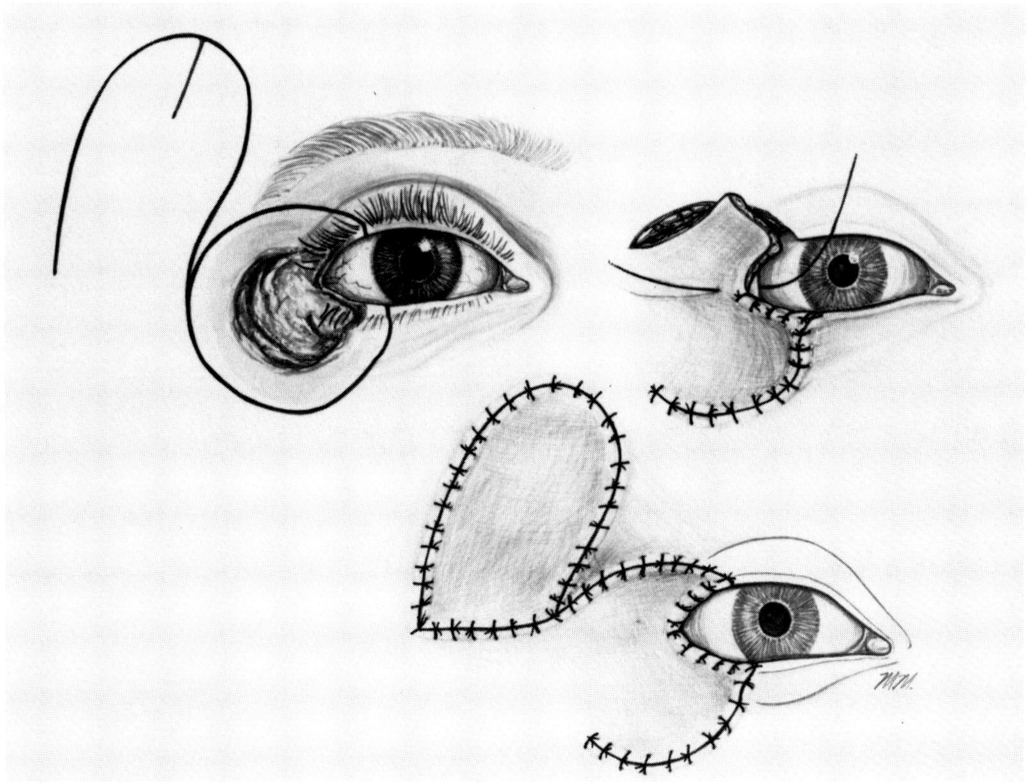

FIG 34–19.
Lateral forehead flap for canthal reconstruction. The donor site is repaired with a skin graft.

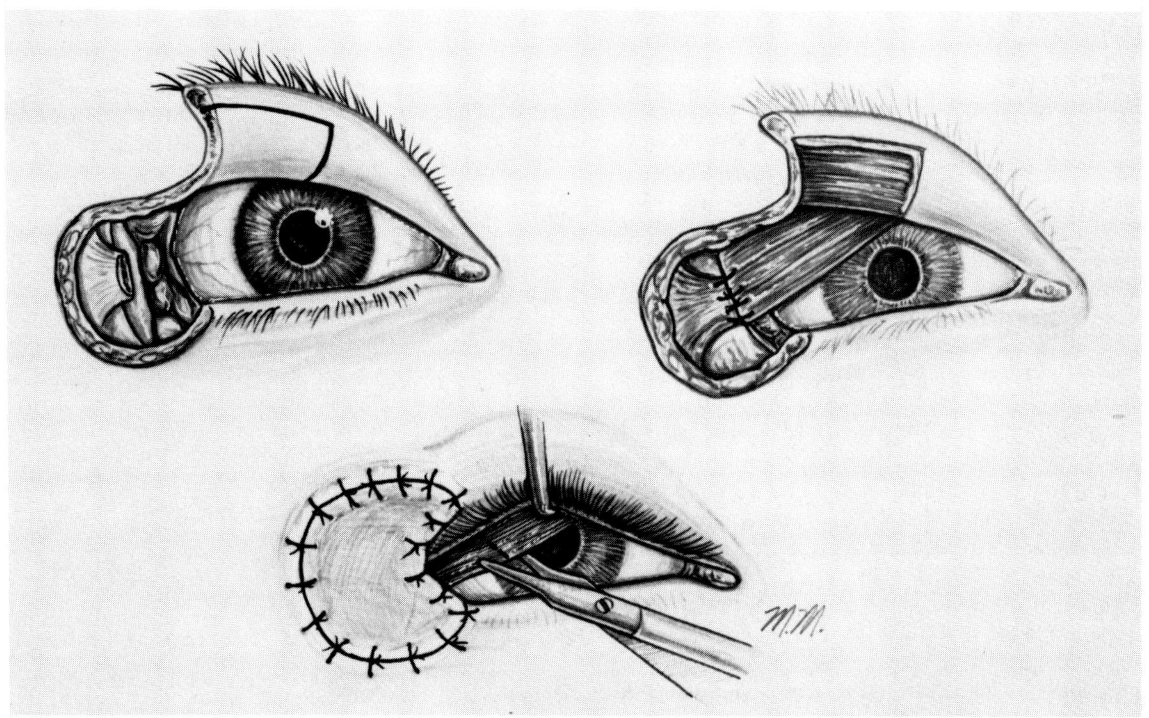

FIG 34–20.
Lateral canthal reconstruction using a tarsoconjunctival flap. The flap is divided after 2 weeks to recreate the palpebral fissure.

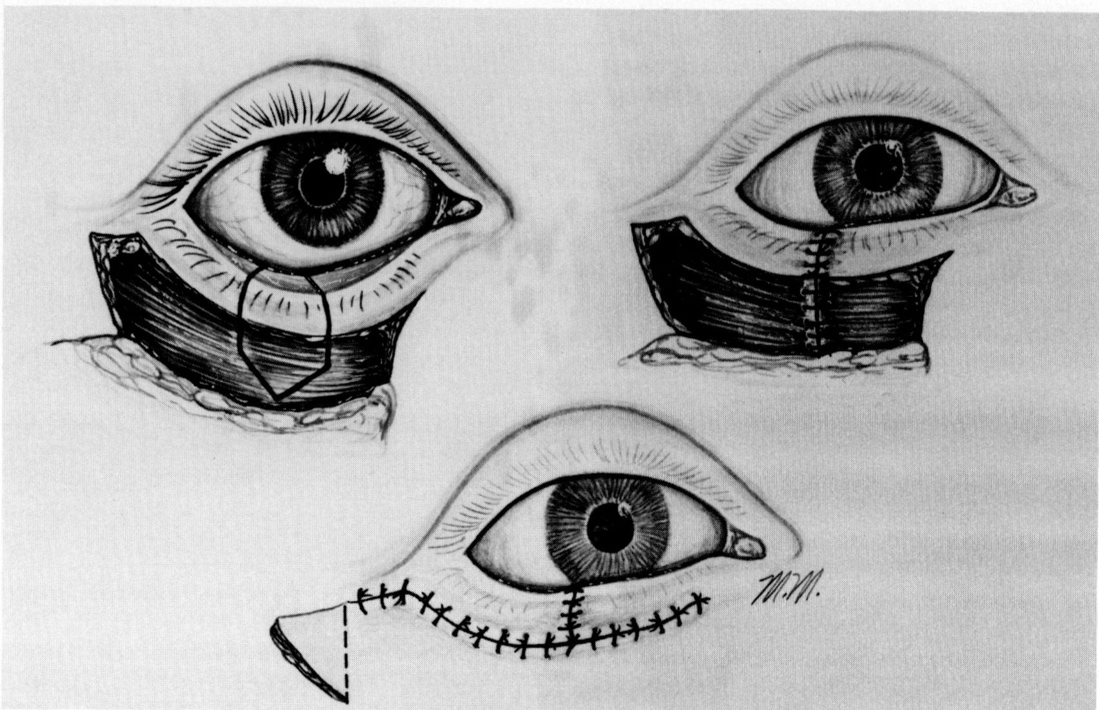

FIG 34–21.
Shortening the lower lid using a pentagonal wedge resection under a sliding skin flap.

Ectropion

Ectropion of varied etiologies must be recognized by surgeons performing facial plastic and reconstructive procedures. This pertains to both preoperative and postoperative evaluation. Careful examination and observation before eyelid surgery is performed can prevent complications and often add to the desired surgical result.

Involutional lower lid ectropion is attributed to laxity of the lower lid tissues. The effects of gravity and decreased strength of the orbicularis may lead to an increased length of the lid and malposition. The canthal tendons must also be evaluated for laxity and position before effective surgical therapy can be planned. When the lid is evaluated for laxity, the pinch test is helpful.[8] If the lid can be easily pulled 6 mm from the globe, laxity is present. The snap text also helps to evaluate the tone of the lower lid. In this test the lower eyelid is pulled away from the globe, and the elasticity of its return to the globe surface is observed.[9] A swift return indicates normal function, whereas a slow return may indicate a potential for ectropion. Scleral show beneath the limbus and rounding of the lateral palpebral fissure are also signs of involutional changes.

Surgical repair of involutional ectropion concentrates on shortening of the lower eyelid and canthal tendon tightening. The most common method of lid shortening has been the wedge resection.[10] In this procedure a lower lid skin flap is raised from an incision 2 mm below the lash line. A pentagonal wedge is then resected lateral to the limbus by first making the lateral incision and then pulling the lid temporally to measure the correct length to be resected. This length is usually about 8 mm. The wedge is resected, and the tarsus is reconstructed with careful approximating sutures. The skin flap is redraped and the excess trimmed as during blepharoplasty (Fig 34–21). This procedure is indicated if there is no evidence of lateral canthal tendon laxity.

When the lateral canthal tendon is noted to be lax, with or without lengthening of the lower lid, a procedure to tighten or reposition the tendon must be designed. The lateral strip technique allows for accurate tightening and positioning of this area.[11] This procedure is initiated by making a lateral canthotomy incision and performing an inferior cantholysis to release the lower lid. The lid is draped laterally, and the anterior lamella is raised as a medially based flap as far as the lid shortening will require. The area of conjunctiva that will be buried is then scraped off with a sharp knife. The tarsus is attached to the lateral orbital rim slightly superotemporal to the old attachment area. The lateral tarsus is attached to the periosteum with a 4-0 Mersilene or equivalent permanent suture. The orbicularis and skin are trimmed and closed in separate layers to eliminate any dog-ear formations (Fig 34–22).

Cicatricial ectropion is caused by any deficit of anterior lamella of the lower lid. This situation may occur after burns, trauma, or as a result of overresection during cosmetic blepharoplasty. A simple test for adequate vertical height of the lower lid is to grasp the lid margin and pull superiorly. If the margin cannot reach more than 2 mm above the inferior limbus, insufficiency of the anterior lamella exists and surgical correction is indicated. For isolated scars secondary to trauma, lengthening and camouflage may be gained by the use of a properly designed Z-plasty. Burns and blepharoplasty complications will usually require the use of full-thickness skin grafts. If upper lid skin is available, it provides a graft of excellent thickness and color match. The second choice is skin harvested from the retroauricular area. The graft is excised after infiltration of local anesthetic, and all subcutaneous tissue must be trimmed from the undersurface before being placed into the lid defect. An incision is then made 2 mm below the lash line, and all scar tissue is dissected free from the wound edges to allow full relaxation of the lid and release of the orbital septum. The defect is measured, and a graft one and one half times the size of the defect is designed and placed into the wound. The graft is fixed into position using 6-0 mild chromic interrupted sutures. A bolster dressing is placed over the graft using the uncut ends of every fourth chromic suture. Telfa or petrolatum (Vaseline) gauze provides a good nonstick dressing. A Frost suture may be placed to further immobilize the lid and graft during the first few postoperative days (Fig 34–23). The bolster is removed after 4 days, and local wound care is started. For surgeons performing lower lid blepharoplasty, it may be wise to save all skin resected in normal saline for several days after the procedure. Upper lid skin should also be saved if four lid procedures are carried out. In the early postoperative period, impending ectropion can often be recognized and corrective measures taken using the saved skin from the original procedure. Careful preoperative diagnosis of involutional ectropion and lateral canthal tendon weakness may help the surgeon avoid postoperative compli-

cations. Lid shortening and lateral tarsal strip procedures can be combined with cosmetic blepharoplasty to improve function and appearance for the patient.

Congenital ectropion is a rare form of cicatricial ectropion in which there is deficient skin in all four eyelids. This deformity usually requires retroauricular skin grafts to all four lids, often in two sessions.

Ptosis

Blepharoptosis of the upper eyelids is defined as a drooping of the lid to a point where it covers 1 to 2 mm of the superior limbus. The measurement of ptosis in unilateral disease can be ascertained by measuring the vertical height of the palpebral fissure on the involved side and comparing this to the normal eye. In ptotic superior lid, the supratarsal fold is usually higher than in the normal eye or is absent. Measurements should be taken in forward, upward, and closed positions so that the amount of levator function can be assessed. Ptosis can be graded into three categories: 1 to 2 mm is mild, 3 mm is moderate, and 4 mm is severe. Levator function is described as excellent if excursion is 13 to 15 mm, is fair at 5 to 7 mm, and is poor at 2 to 4 mm. Both of these measurements are important for proper preoperative evaluation.

To properly assess a ptotic lid, one must consider the relative anatomy. The superior orbital septum is a fascial layer that

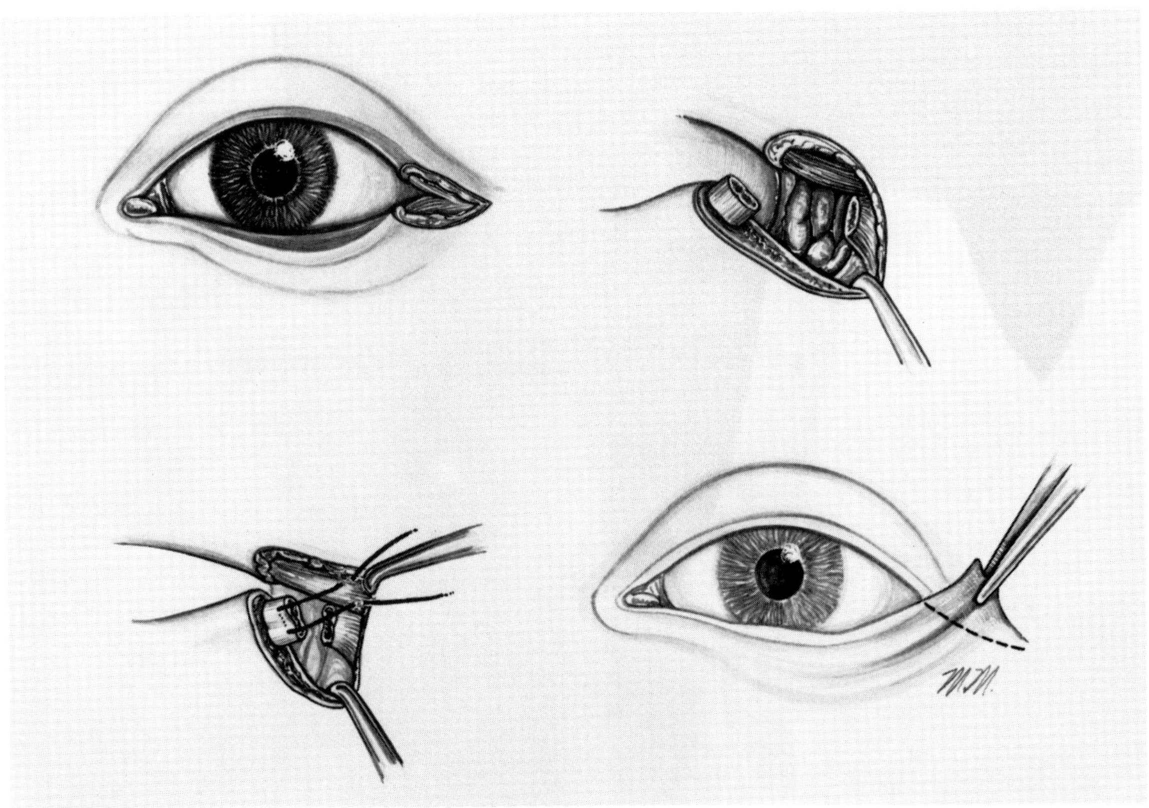

FIG 34–22.
Lateral strip technique for shortening and repositioning of the lateral canthus.

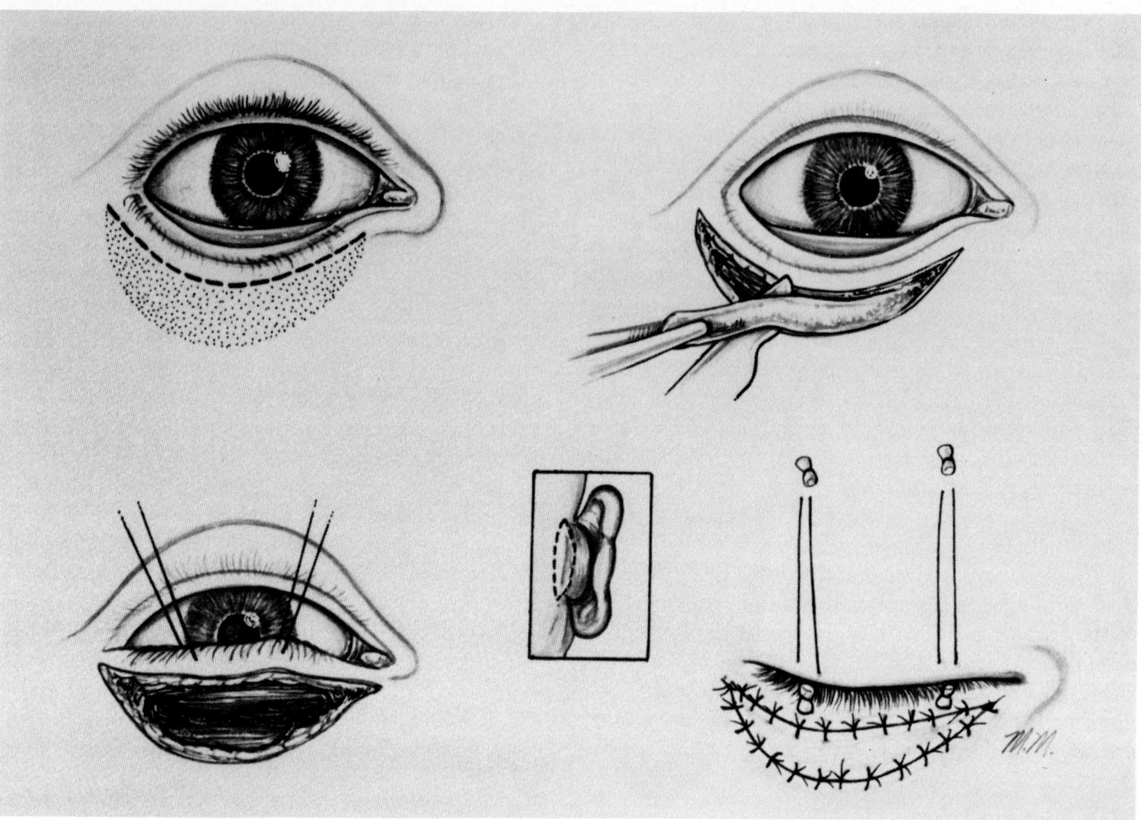

FIG 34–23.
Full-thickness skin graft for repair of lower lid ectropion.

extends from the superior orbital rim and joins the levator aponeurosis just before its insertion into the tarsal plate. Just deep to the orbital septum lies the preaponeurotic fat that covers the levator aponeurosis. This fatty tissue is commonly removed during blepharoplasty, and a surgeon unaware of the intimate relationship to the levator apparatus may cause injury and resultant ptosis. The levator apparatus itself is comprised of the 40 mm levator muscle of the upper eyelid and its attached 15 mm aponeurosis. The apparatus is covered in part by Whitnall's ligament, which stretches from the superior oblique pulley to the lacrimal gland capsule. Müller's muscle is an involuntary smooth muscle, which is innervated by the sympathetic system and helps to maintain tone of the upper lid. This muscle provides 1 to 2 mm of lid elevation and, thus, the ptosis observed with Horner's syndrome. The levator is supplied by the third cranial nerve and aids in voluntary raising of the upper lid. All of these structures must be considered in the evaluation and treatment of blepharoptosis.

Otolaryngologist–head and neck surgeons usually encounter blepharoptosis as a complication of maxillofacial trauma or blepharoplasty. Dermatochalasia may also cause a degree of ptosis in patients who are about to undergo elective procedures, and this should be recognized preoperatively. In the majority of acquired ptosis cases, the pathology will ultimately be detachment of the levator aponeurosis from the tarsal plate.[12] In acquired ptosis, the defect is usually not due to levator weakness but to mechanical disruption. In severe cases of dermatochalasia, the constant extra weight on the junction between the levator aponeurosis and the tarsal plate can cause stretching or breaking of the delicate connecting fibers. Traumatic detachments in this area can be caused by orbital fractures with hematoma, radical frontoethmoidectomy procedures, tumor ablation, or elective cosmetic and functional eyelid surgery. The surgical correction of acquired ptosis usually involves reattachment of the levator to the tarsal plate. Congenital ptosis, which involves weakness of the levator muscle, usually requires levator resection or advancement. Occasionally a blepharoplasty patient has a temporary or permanent ptosis postoperatively even when the levator apparatus has been meticulously preserved. There is evidence that a myotoxic effect from local anesthesia may explain these cases.[13]

The surgical approach to acquired ptosis is usually through a blepharoplasty-type incision with local anesthesia. The correct amount of skin resection is measured by comparison to the normal side. After the skin excision, a narrow strip of orbicularis is resected across the wound to expose the orbital septum. The septum is then divided where appropriate, and the preaponeurotic fat is either resected or retracted to expose the levator aponeurosis beneath. This layered approach to the levator system provides a safe and controlled exposure even in patients with prior trauma or surgery in the area. The tarsal aponeurotic junction area can then be inspected by retracting the pretarsal orbicular muscle from the superior tarsal plate. If a detachment is recognized, the repair can be made at this point by suturing the levator aponeurosis to the tarsal edge using interrupted 6-0 chromic catgut. The repair can be checked by comparing the lid height to the normal side. In patients with other levator dysfunction such as Horner's syndrome, muscle denervation, or congenital ptosis an advancement of the levator muscle onto the tarsal plate may be necessary (Fig 34–24).[14] The advantages of this type of levator repair over other methods include the preservation of Müller's muscle, no resection of potentially active levator muscle, and the possibility of reversal if overcorrection is noted postoperatively.[15] In nontraumatic primary cases of acquired ptosis and in congenital ptosis, resection of the levator muscle may be indicated.

Epicanthal Fold Repair

Epicanthal folds are extra folds of skin that may lie over the medial canthus area. These may occur as congenital abnormalities such as Down's syndrome or other craniofacial abnormalities. In many areas of the world, especially in Asia, the absence of an epicanthal fold would be considered abnormal. The occurrence in the Asian population is 2% to 3%. Epicanthal folds may also occur after traumatic injuries to the orbital region or after cosmetic blepharoplasty where the upper incisions extend too far nasally. The surgical management of these folds follows the same principles. Also to be considered is the condition of the medial canthus. If the canthal tendon has been displaced, this will need to be corrected to restore a normal shape to the palpebral fissure.

The double Z-plasty as popularized by Mustardé[16] has become the most common method of eliminating epicanthal folds when the medial canthus is in good position. This method has the effect of transferring the excess amount of skin in the horizontal direction to the vertical while maintaining the position of the medial canthus. If work on the medial canthus is necessary, it can be performed through the same incisions. This procedure is performed by marking a horizontal incision through the epicanthal fold over the medial canthus. Incisions are then planned along the lid margins for approximately 8 mm, and the area is widely undermined. The Z-plasties are designed with incisions passing superior and inferotemporally from the horizontal incision at 60-degree angles. Final incisions are made passing nasally at 45 degrees to the previous incisions. The flaps are widely undermined and are transposed. The skin closure is performed with 6-0 Novafil or Prolene sutures (Fig 34–25). Sutures are usually removed after 5 to 7 days.

Other techniques for epicanthal fold elimination have been described. The method of Roveda,[17] which employs a Y-V flap technique, has been used in recent years. The disadvantage of

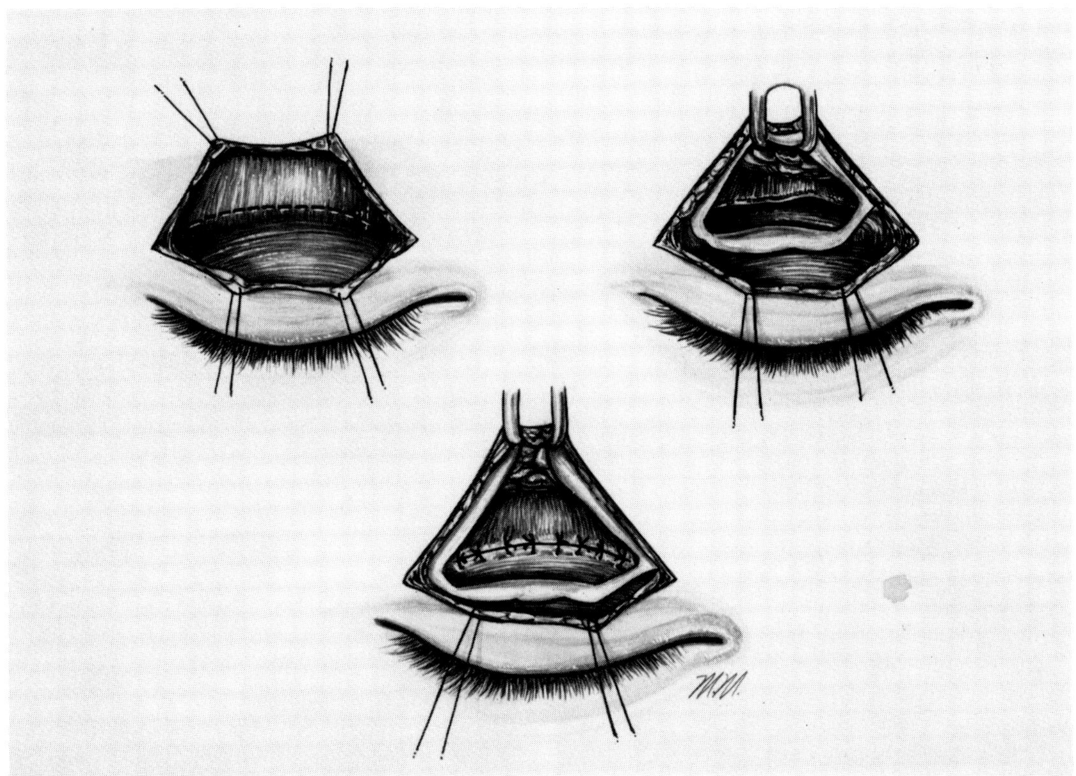

FIG 34–24.
Exposure of the levator system and tarsal plate for repair in ptosis cases.

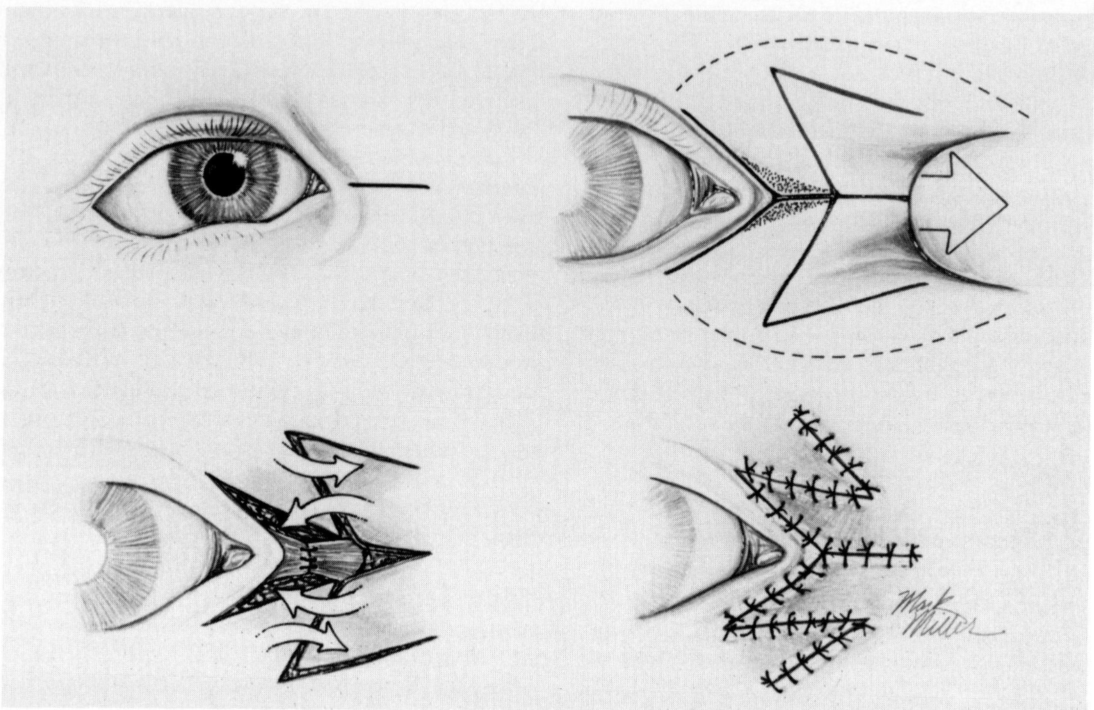

FIG 34–25.
Double Z-plasty for repair of epicanthal folds.

this method is the tendency to form a bridle scar due to the concave incision located nasally. All of the Y-V techniques have this drawback but are simpler to perform than the double Z-plasty.

REFERENCES

1. Mohs FE: Micrographic surgery for the microscopically controlled excision of eyelid cancers. *Arch Ophthalmol* 1986; 104:901–909.
2. Tenzel RR, Stewart WB: Eyelid reconstruction by semicircular flap technique. *Trans Am Soc Ophthalmol Otolaryngol* 1978; 50:1165.
3. Putterman AM: Viable composite grafting in eyelid reconstruction. *Am J Ophthalmol* 1978; 85:237.
4. Hughes WL: A new method for rebuilding a lower lid. *Arch Ophthalmol* 1937; 17:1008–1017.
5. Doxanas M: Orbicularis muscle mobilization in eyelid reconstruction. *Arch Ophthalmol* 1986; 104:910–914.
6. Mustardé JC: Reconstruction of the upper lid, in Brent B (ed): *The Artistry of Reconstructive Surgery*. St Louis, CV Mosby Co, 1987, pp 167–173.
7. Jackson IT: Local flaps, in *Head and Neck Reconstruction*. St Louis, CV Mosby Co, 1985.
8. Hill JC: Analysis of senile changes in the palpebral fissure. *Trans Ophthalmol Soc UK* 1975; 95:49.
9. Schaefer AJ: Lateral canthal tendon tuck. *Ophthalmology* 1979; 86:1879.
10. Smith B, Bosniak S, Sachs M: The management of involutional lower lid ectropion, in Smith B, Bosniak M (eds): *Advances in Ophthalmic Plastic and Reconstructive Surgery*. New York, Pergamon Press, 1983, vol 2.
11. Anderson RL, Gordy DD: The tarsal strip procedure. *Arch Ophthalmol* 1979; 97:2192.
12. Pearl RM: Acquired ptosis: A reexamination of etiology and treatment. *Plast Reconstr Surg* 1985; 76:56.
13. Rainin EA, Carlson BM: Postoperative diplopia and ptosis. *Arch Ophthalmol* 1985; 103:1337.
14. Carraway JH, Vincent MP: Levator advancement technique for eyelid ptosis. *Plast Reconstr Surg* 1986; 77:394.
15. Beard C: Editorial discussion. *Plast Reconstr Surg* 1986; 77:403.
16. Mustardé JC: *Repair and Reconstruction in the Orbital Region,* ed 2. New York, Churchill Livingstone, 1980.
17. Roveda JM: Epicanthus et Blepharophimosis, Notre, Technique de Correction. *Ann Oculist* 1967; 200:551.

CHAPTER 35

Facial Flaps

Approach of

William W. Shockley, M.D.

Few surgical challenges are as intriguing and stimulating as the design, creation, and implementation of facial flaps. Each surgeon has his or her own preferred techniques for facial reconstruction. The methods of reconstruction available and favored by the surgeon will vary with the surgeon's expertise, experience, and familiarity with the options available. This chapter will outline my perspective with its inherent bias. I hope to demonstrate some of the reconstructive options available through a "how and why I do it" approach. Naturally, there are different methods available than those discussed here, and the reader is encouraged to become acquainted with these alternatives.

Perhaps the single most important question when one is contemplating reconstruction after ablative surgery is not how to reconstruct but whether to reconstruct. The following discussion will highlight the philosophy of ablation and reconstruction, because the principles of one cannot be fully explored without consideration of the other.

The impetus of this chapter is not to examine the full spectrum of facial flaps but to limit the discussion to the operative challenges that exist. This chapter will concentrate on three issues: (1) the management of skin neoplasms, (2) the preferred techniques in nasal reconstruction, and (3) the options in management of midfacial defects. In this context, although the discussion will center around facial flaps, the role of skin grafts, composite grafts, regional flaps, free flaps, and prosthetics will also be addressed.

TREATMENT TECHNIQUES FOR SKIN CANCER

Basal Cell Carcinoma

It is well known that markedly different forms of basal cell carcinoma (BCC) exist. The vast majority are benign in their behavior and can be cured in 95% of cases with the first therapeutic modality. However, some lesions are stubbornly aggressive and may ultimately lead to death. The surgeon must be mindful of the risk factors involved with BCC when determining appropriate ablative techniques.

I use surgical excision for all lesions. The advantages include histologic confirmation of tumor eradication as well as healing per primum. The four methods generally employed are:

1. Excision in the office setting
2. Surgical excision with frozen section control
3. Surgical excision with permanent section control
4. Mohs' surgery

The initial assessment of the lesion should take into account several important risk factors. These include its clinical presentation, size, histology, location, and other prognostic factors such as whether it is recurrent or radiation induced. The features associated with a worse prognosis are:

1. Size greater than 2 cm
2. Aggressive histology
3. Location in fusion plane
4. Recurrence
5. Radiation-induced lesion

Generally one can assimilate this information to determine whether the lesion falls into a low-, intermediate-, or high-risk category.

Once this decision has been made, the appropriate setting and method of treatment can be chosen. For example, in dealing with a 1-cm nodular basal cell of the forehead, one would find excision and primary closure in the office setting to be appropriate, expedient, and cost effective. The specimen is oriented and marked for the pathologist. If a positive margin is recognized, the surgeon may reexcise the area involved or simply observe the area, based on his or her judgment.

Lesions that are larger than 2 cm, have ill-defined borders, or are located in high risk regions and those with aggressive histology (i.e., morpheaform, basosquamous) should be treated with due respect. They will have a greater tendency to recur, and the initial treatment setting offers the best chance for curing the cancer. The high-risk locations include the nose, medial canthal areas, and periauricular regions. Once again, surgical judgment will dictate the preferred method of treatment. Lesions of intermediate risk may be excised with frozen section control and reconstructed after histologic confirmation.

Lesions considered to be high risk should be treated with Mohs' surgery if at all possible. This would include tumors of morpheaform histology, those adjacent to vital structures, recurrent tumors (particularly in a field of previous irradiation), and those invading embryologic fusion planes.

In many communities, Mohs' surgery is not available. In this situation, surgical excision with permanent section control may be appropriate. This technique is useful for high-risk lesions, for those lesions in which frozen sections would be too time consuming, or in tumors where bone is resected and histologic confirmation is difficult to determine. With this method, the tumor is resected with 1 to 2 cm margins, and the specimen is oriented for the pathologist and appropriately marked. The wound is packed with a nonadherent gauze and a dressing applied. A few days later, once permanent sections are available, attention can be directed to specific areas identified as having positive or close margins.

I seldom employ radiotherapy as the primary modality of treatment. It has been useful in palliation of some patients with advanced lesions and has been used as an adjunctive measure in patients with positive margins following major resections. The carbon dioxide laser is beneficial in palliation of extensive exophytic or ulcerative lesions requiring frequent dressing changes. The CO_2 laser can often debulk the tumor and form an eschar that will enhance patient hygiene and diminish the amount of nursing care needed.

Squamous Cell Carcinoma

It is my philosophy that squamous cell carcinoma (SCC) of the skin should always be treated with surgical excision. Although early lesions may behave in a fairly indolent manner, there is always the potential for lesions of this histology to demonstrate virulent characteristics. Although they are uncommon, I have seen lesions less than 1 cm metastasize to regional lymph nodes and subcutaneous lymphatics. Since it is difficult to predict this type of behavior, it seems prudent to histologically confirm complete tumor removal.

Once again, therapeutic decisions will be based on lesion size, configuration, degree of infiltration, and structures involved. For small lesions (<1 cm) with minimal invasion, excision in the office should be satisfactory. The precautions and techniques are the same as those outlined previously. For larger lesions, those with ill-defined borders, those adjacent to cos-

metically important structures, and those requiring more than primary closure, resection is undertaken in the operating room with frozen section control. The role of Mohs' surgery in high-risk lesions has been addressed and is reemphasized here.

Generally, prophylactic lymph node dissection is not worthwhile, given the low incidence of metastasis. In some circumstances, postoperative radiotherapy is indicated for highly aggressive lesions requiring major resections involving the nose, maxilla, and orbit. The surgeon's experience will help determine which patients will benefit from adjunctive therapy. Other indications for postoperative radiation therapy are:

1. Positive margins if (a) further surgery is not feasible and (b) "maximal" surgery has been done
2. Perineural or perivascular invasion (in selected cases, based on clinical judgment)
3. High risk of recurrence despite normal margins

In these cases, the nodal groups at risk should be included in the fields to diminish the incidence of regional recurrence.

Keratoacanthoma

This neoplasm is recognized by its rapid growth phase and characteristic morphologic features. Keratoacanthoma (KA) tends to occur in the elderly, and typically the pattern of tumor behavior exhibits three phases: growth, plateau, and involution.[1] During the initial phase, the tumor demonstrates rapid enlargement for 6 to 8 weeks. Keratoacanthomas present as dome-shaped nodules with a central keratin crater. Typically, lesions are 1 to 2.5 cm in diameter, and the nose is the most common site to be affected in the head and neck. Although a classic KA should involute with time, there are potential problems associated with the wait and see approach.

The disadvantages of waiting for involution include:

1. Despite generous biopsies, the pathologist is often unable to distinguish with assurity squamous cell carcinoma from KA.
2. The growth phase may not be complete, and the tumor may grow to a larger size during the period of observation.
3. The time for involution is greatly variable.
4. The resultant scarring and distortion resulting from involution is likewise unpredictable.
5. There remains some controversy as to whether these neoplasms can "transform" into a squamous cell carcinoma.

For these reasons, the recommended treatment for KAs is surgical excision. They are usually well demarcated, and 2 to 5 mm margins are acceptable when KA is confirmed with frozen section control. Resections often result in fairly large cutaneous defects and routinely require some form of reconstruction.

Malignant Melanoma

The treatment of choice for malignant melanoma is surgical

excision. There are, however, controversies concerning the issues of preferred margins of resection, the role of elective lymph node dissection (ELND), and the role of adjunctive therapy. Due to multiple cooperative efforts and the use of sophisticated biostatistical techniques, great advances have been made in identifying those features that most profoundly affect the ultimate outcome.

The prognostic factors that significantly impact survival are:

1. Tumor thickness
2. Ulceration
3. Pathologically positive nodes
4. Location
5. Growth pattern

It is generally accepted that in stage I melanoma (i.e., a localized lesion without evidence of regional or distant metastasis), the single most important feature is tumor thickness. Thus, most therapeutic decisions are based on the identification of the risk factors just listed, with tumor thickness being the predominant prognosticator. Using this malignancy profile, one can characterize lesions as low risk (thin lesions), moderate risk (intermediate thickness lesions), and high risk (thick lesions).

My decisions regarding management are based on the level of risk posed by a given neoplasm. The initial step is to establish the diagnosis by performing an excisional biopsy with 2 mm margins. If the lesion cannot be simply excised, a generous incisional biopsy can be undertaken with the tissue taken from the most suspicious region of the lesion (e.g., the darkest, the most ulcerative, or the most nodular). Results of the biopsy confirm the clinical diagnosis and provide information about the growth pattern (lentigo maligna melanoma, superficial spreading, or nodular), the thickness, Clark's level, and other histologic features. Based on this information, the level of risk can be assessed, and this will provide the surgeon a rationale on which to construct a game plan.

The appropriate margin of resection for malignant melanoma has been recently addressed.[2–4] Most surgeons are well aware that local recurrence is not the major problem in melanoma. In a review of nearly 3,600 patients, the local recurrence rate was only 3.2%.[2] Margins of resection are based primarily on tumor thickness (Table 35–1). For thin lesions (<0.75 mm) the recommended margin is 1.0 to 1.5 cm; this results in a 2 to 3 cm defect. It may be safe to be even more conservative with thin lesions because the recurrence rate for this subset of melanomas is 0.01%.[2] For lesions of intermediate thickness, the margin of excision is 1.5 to 2.0 cm, yielding defects of 3.0 to 4.0 cm in diameter. High-risk lesions (>3.5 cm) are excised with 2.0 to 3.0 cm margins but are narrowed somewhat to maintain the integrity of nearby structures of cosmetic and functional importance. There is no proof that margins of resection beyond 2 cm increase local control or survival rates.

The role of ELND in the treatment of stage I melanoma is currently a hotly debated subject. The arguments for and against elective nodal dissection are beyond the scope of this chapter. If there is a role for elective lymphadenectomy, it appears that

TABLE 35–1.
Recommended Margins of Resection*

Tumor Thickness, mm	Classification	Margin of Resection, cm
<0 .76	Thin	1.0–1.5
0.76–3.50	Intermediate	1.5–2.0
>3.50	Thick	2.0–3.0

*These are purely estimates and should be individualized for a given location and associated risk factors.

the group of patients most likely to benefit are those with lesions 1.50 to 4.0 mm thick.[5,6] This group has a relatively high risk of regional metastasis without an inordinately high risk of distant metastasis. If elective lymph node dissection is contemplated, the following criteria should be satisfied:

1. Good surgical risk
2. Predictable lymphatic drainage
3. Non-midline location
4. Consider surgery for (a) lesions 0.76 to 1.50 mm with high-risk features and (b) lesions 1.50 to 4.0 mm

The surgeon should be very familiar with the literature on ELND before making this decision, because the data on the survival benefits of ELND for head and neck melanoma are inconclusive.

NASAL RECONSTRUCTION

It should be emphasized prior to any discussion concerning nasal reconstruction that a conscious determination must be made that the patient is disease free and will likely remain so. The first question in nasal reconstruction is not how to reconstruct but when to reconstruct. Some defects are best left open for a period of observation to prevent delayed diagnosis of recurrence.

The nose is well known as the site in the head and neck that is most prone to recurrent cutaneous carcinoma. There are several reasons for this. First, since the nose is of paramount cosmetic importance, resections tend to be more conservative than in other regions of the head and neck. Second, there is no subcutaneous tissue to form a buffer to deep invasion. Once tumor penetrates the dermis, the perichondrium and periosteum is involved. These layers tend to serve as barriers to tumor spread temporarily, and the tumor infiltrates along these planes in a centrifugal manner. Later in the neoplastic process, the underlying cartilage and bone may be invaded as well. Third, embryologic fusion planes in and around the nose serve as pathways for surreptitious spread of carcinoma. This concept has been fully described by Panje and Ceilley.[7]

Alar Defects

These defects are quite intriguing; they are often small enough that the surgeon is a bit reticent to use a flap for reconstruction. Yet the survival of composite grafts is not pre-

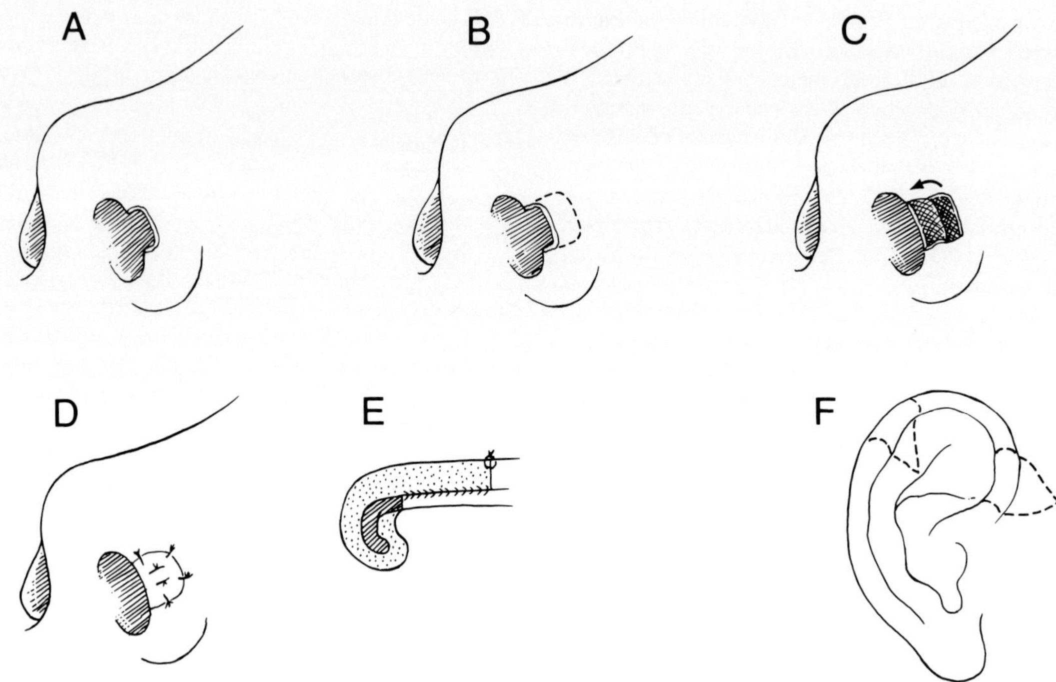

FIG 35–1.
Composite graft for alar rim reconstruction. **A,** defect of alar rim. **B,** turn-in flap site. **C,** flap turned down and in place. (Surface area for graft contact crosshatched.) **D,** composite graft in place. **E,** cross section showing graft in contact with dermis of turn-in flap and its donor site. **F,** donor sites for composite grafts.

dictable. For alar rim defects like the one shown in Figure 35–1, I favor the use of composite grafts employing a modified technique as outlined in the caption. The modifications are modeled after those described by Baker.[8] At the time of resection, the defect is left open, and the skin is sutured to the mucosa. After at least 4 weeks of healing, reconstruction can be contemplated. Turn-in flaps are created based on the mucocutaneous junction of the defect. These will provide the inner lining as well as a blood supply to the deep surface of the graft.

A composite graft is obtained from the ear. It is always better to take a graft slightly larger than needed so it can be trimmed to fit. The graft is cut to the appropriate size and shape of the new defect. (Remember the cutaneous defect is now somewhat larger due to the use of the turn-in flaps.) The undersurface of the skin of the graft and cartilage are removed such that there is cartilage only in the actual rim of the new ala. The donor site favored by Baker[8] incorporates preauricular skin with the chondrocutaneous graft. This allows about 75% of the graft to be in contact with viable tissue. When the modified technique is used, the composite graft can attain a blood supply not only at its periphery but also from its deep surface. The graft is sutured in place with 6-0 nylon. A minimum of sutures are used, and care is taken not to compromise the tissue by tying them too tightly. One or two mattress sutures of 5-0 chromic are placed through and through to coapt graft to flap and obliterate any dead space. Postoperatively iced saline-moistened dressing pads are applied by the patient to the area of repair for 48 hours. Meticulous wound care is mandatory. Although the success rate is not 100%, it is far superior to the standard

approach. Defects larger than 1.5 cm are usually reconstructed in another manner, although Baker has reported a greater than 90% success rate in grafts up to 3.5 cm.

If the alar defect approximates the alar groove (i.e., abuts the cheek), an alternative method may be appropriate. This approach is adapted from Stucker.[9] In these cases, a nasolabial flap folded on itself to create an inner and outer lining can be designed (Fig 35–2). At the "fold" the skin is deepithelialized. The two edges of the flap are sutured together to form the new alar rim. The nasolabial flap must be based inferiorly and should be long enough that the thinner skin along the nose and cheek can be incorporated. Often another flap (e.g., a glabellar or cheek flap) will be necessary to close the secondary defect.

More extensive defects of the ala are reconstructed with a midline forehead flap with the tip folded on itself, the fold serving as the new rim. This requires at least two stages, and commonly the reconstructed area requires refinement, debulking, or both.

More lateral alar defects that are not through and through can easily be reconstructed with a nasolabial flap. Superiorly based flaps are favored to take advantage of the thicker skin adjacent to the nasolabial fold, because some defects in this area are relatively deep. Occasionally, advancing a simple cheek flap into the defect can preserve the anatomic units of the nose, nasomaxillary junction, and cheek.

Tip Defects

Cutaneous defects of the nasal tip present a reconstructive

challenge. Small rotational flaps are seldom applicable in this region because the adjacent "nondistensible" nasal skin prevents gaining the customary advantage of primary closure of the donor site. Another disadvantage of using adjacent flaps is that the secondary scarring is unacceptable. Nasolabial flaps are too bulky and require a second stage.

For these reasons, I prefer a composite graft for nasal tip resurfacing. An ideal graft for this location is the perichondrial cutaneous graft (PCCG). The consistency, color, thickness, and enhanced viability make it a superlative option for isolated tip defects. This composite graft has been popularized by Stucker and co-workers, and its advantages have been realized in both the laboratory and clinical settings.[10, 11] The anterior conchal skin has become the favored donor site because of the adherence of the perichondrium to the skin. This secondary defect is resurfaced with a postauricular island flap.

Technique

1. Since the most common deficits result from ablative cancer surgery, they tend to be circular in nature. Ideally the tip should be reconstructed as a cosmetic unit of the nose. These defects should be recontoured in such a fashion that symmetry

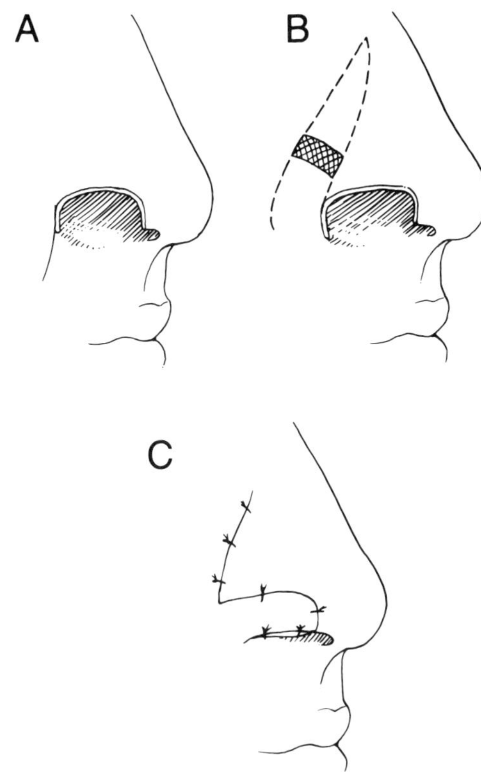

FIG 35–2.
Deepithelialized flap for alar rim reconstruction. **A**, alar rim defect. **B**, nasolabial flap with crosshatching at deepithelialized segment. **C**, flap in place, folded on itself with edges sutured.

is created, even if this necessitates removal of normal skin (Fig 35–3). The long-term advantage of a natural appearance of the tip will outweigh any disadvantage of further tissue loss.

2. The resultant defect should be recreated with a template, and it should be applied to the conchal region. The contemplated graft is then marked out, and the area is infiltrated with 1% lidocaine with epinephrine 1:100,000 (Fig 35–4,A).

3. An incision is made around the periphery of the graft. This incision can be easily hidden behind the antihelial fold and tragus. The depth of the incision is down to cartilage (through perichondrium).

4. A Cottle elevator used to identify the subperichondrial plane at the inferior aspect of the concha (Fig 35–4,B). The dissection is completed out to the limits of the incision, and the graft is harvested.

5. The conchal skin defect is marked out posteriorly using the sulcus as a reference for the midpoint of the island flap. The center of the flap should lie over the postauricular muscle, which can be seen as a band crossing the sulcus at its midpoint when the auricle is pulled forward (Fig 35–4,C). The central portion of the conchal cartilage is removed and discarded. The postauricular island flap is then marked out as an ellipse that includes the defect within its boundaries (Fig 35–4,D).

6. After incising through skin and subcutaneous tissue, the operator undermines the flap circumferentially toward to center for about 1 cm. This leaves the island flap pedicled on the postauricular muscle and its accompanying blood supply. The flap is then rotated anteriorly through the cartilagenous defect and sutured into place (Fig 35–4,E). The postauricular fusiform defect is closed in a vertical direction, resulting in a slightly more shallow sulcus (Fig 35–4,F). The transposed skin provides an excellent cosmetic result. A cotton roll is fashioned and placed anteriorly into the conchal bowl, and another is placed posteriorly in the sulcus. Coaptation is accomplished with two or three large nylon mattress sutures. A mastoid dressing is an alternative to this method but is more time consuming, less effective, and more cumbersome.

7. The PCCG is sutured into place with 6-0 chromic or nylon sutures. A bolster is not used, but two or three sutures are placed through the graft in a quilting technique.

8. Postoperatively, the patient is instructed to apply iced saline-soaked gauze pads to the area for 48 hours. This may help in the take of the graft, but more important, it provides a mechanism to minimize the crusting that occurs.

The results of this technique have been gratifying, and with proper technique, graft take has a predictably high rate of success (Fig 35–5). If the limits of the PCCG are extended beyond the concha, grafts up to 3 cm in size can be harvested.

An alternative technique for closure of tip defects is use of the sliding dorsal nasal flap (SDNF). This method is useful when secondary scarring is not a major consideration. Generally, it is reserved for older patients in whom scars are much less noticeable due to the loss of elasticity of the skin. This technique moves skin from the nasal dorsum into the lower third of the nose and takes advantage of the natural redundancy of the skin in the intercanthal and glabellar regions (Fig 35–6).

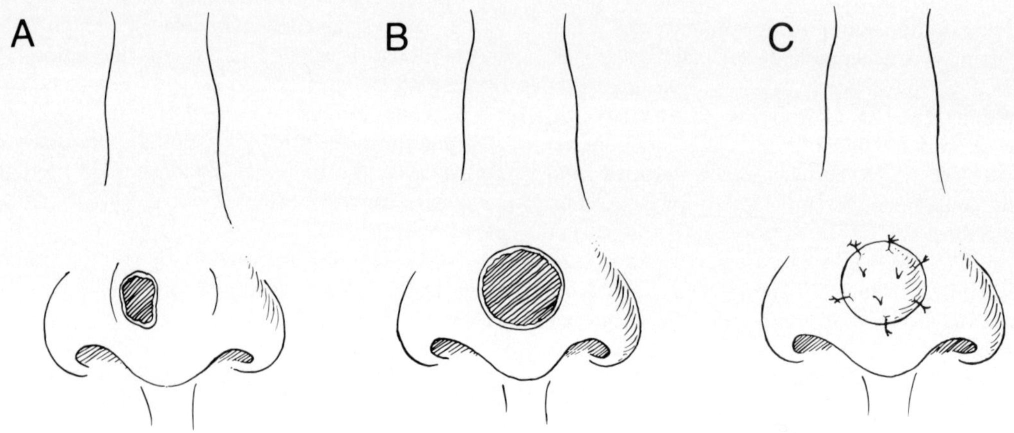

FIG 35–3.
Perichondrial cutaneous graft reconstruction of nasal tip defect. **A**, resultant defect after cancer resection. **B**, creation of symmetric defect. **C**, PCCG sutured in place. Central mattress sutures obviate bolster.

The proposed incision begins at the lower border of the tip defect and proceeds laterally to the nose-cheek junction. It then follows this line into the medial canthal region and becomes incorporated into a glabellar flap with the inverted V centrally located between the brows. Dissection is in a subcutaneous plane in areas where fat exists and in a supraperichondrial supraperiosteal plane over the nasal skeleton. The flap is then rotated down into the defect. A counterincision is sometimes necessary to minimize the dog ear that results. The defect is closed, resulting in an inconspicuous vertical scar. The scar along the nasomaxillary groove is usually imperceptable.

Through-and-Through Defects

Nasal defects that involve the internal (mucosal) and external (cutaneous) surfaces of the nose represent a challenge for the reconstructive surgeon. There is a theoretical advantage of replacing the inner lining with mucosa, but there appears to be little clinical advantage. Although there are certain methods described to transpose mucosa, such as septal flaps, I prefer not to violate the septum. No problems have been encountered with the use of skin to line through-and-through defects, presumably because the remainder of the nasal cavity provides abundant tissue for proper humidification and lubrication.

The midline forehead flap (MLFF) is the workhorse flap in reconstruction of through-and-through defects (Fig 35–7). This flap has an axial blood supply and provides a muscle layer that is readily graftable. The flap is extremely reliable and results in a minimal secondary deformity.

The MLFF is equally versatile for providing either the inner or outer replacement lining. The primary options include (1) MLFF as cutaneous lining, graft for inner lining; (2) MLFF as inner lining, graft for cutaneous defect; and (3) turn-in flap for inner lining, MLFF as outer. The flap will sustain a split-thickness skin graft, a dermal graft, a full-thickness graft, or a PCCG. All of these options have been used effectively in different clinical situations.

The technique is familiar to most surgeons and has been previously described in greater detail.[12] The flap is marked out using two parallel vertical lines that converge at the hairline. (Caution must be used, because any hair that is transposed will likely survive.) To ensure adequate length, the surgeon mimicks the rotation of the proposed flap by using a gauze template of equal length stabilized at the base. The incisions are made through the skin, subcutaneous tissue, frontal muscle, and galea. The flap is elevated in a supraperiosteal plane. Care is taken to avoid trauma to the supratrochlear vessels that provide the blood supply to this axial flap. The flap is then somersaulted 180 degrees for use an an inner lining or laterally rotated 180 degrees for external coverage. If insufficient length or excessive tension results, backward rotation provides the maximal length by avoiding the kink that results from the standard rotational maneuver.

The forehead deficit is closed primarily. As long as the flap width does not exceed 3 cm, this is usually not a significant task. If use of a wider flap is anticipated, preoperative tissue expansion is an option, as is grafting with planned serial excision. To enhance closure, vertical incisions on the undersurface of the frontalis muscle and galea may enhance skin distensibility enough to permit primary closure. The vertical dimension of

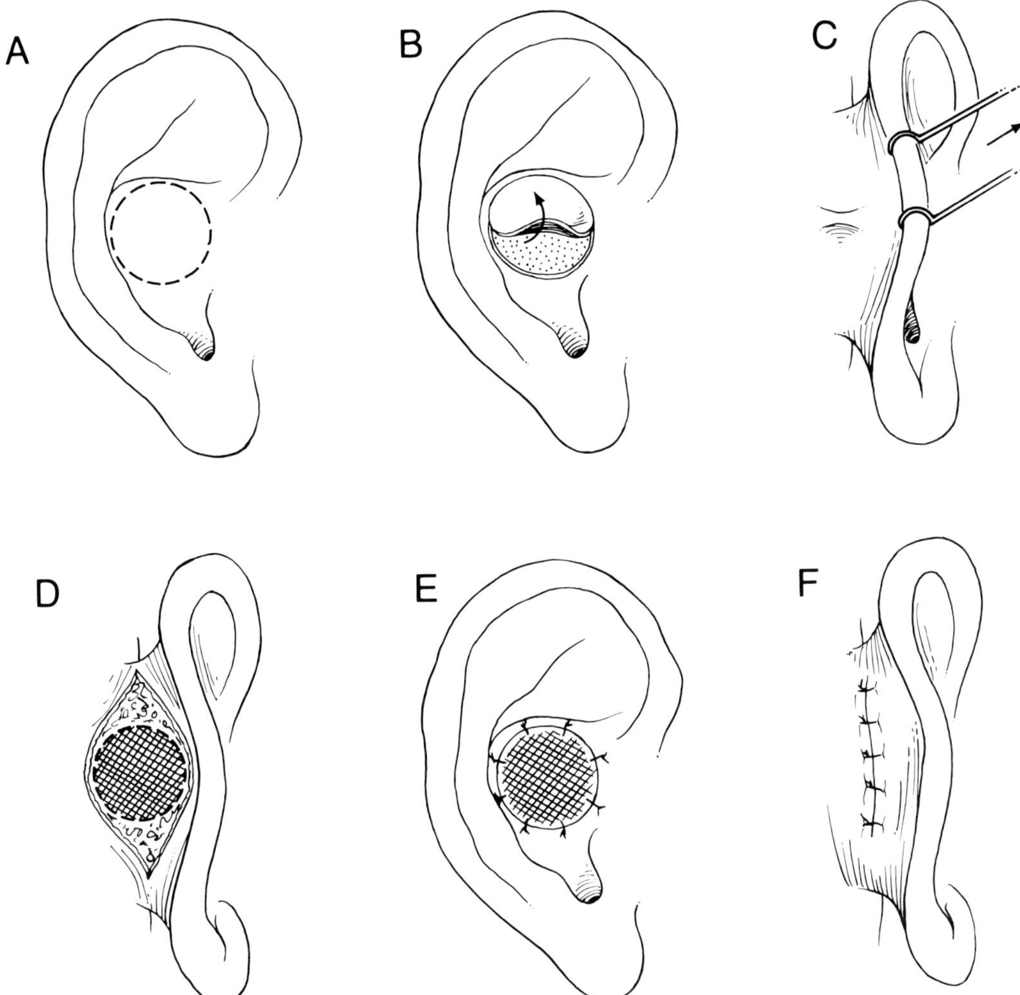

FIG 35–4.
Perichondrial cutaneous graft-harvesting and secondary reconstruction. **A**, donor site for PCCG. **B**, subperichondrial plane established. **C**, postauricular muscle band. **D**, postauricular island flap to fill-in defect. **E**, island flap rotated into place. **F**, postauricular flap site closed.

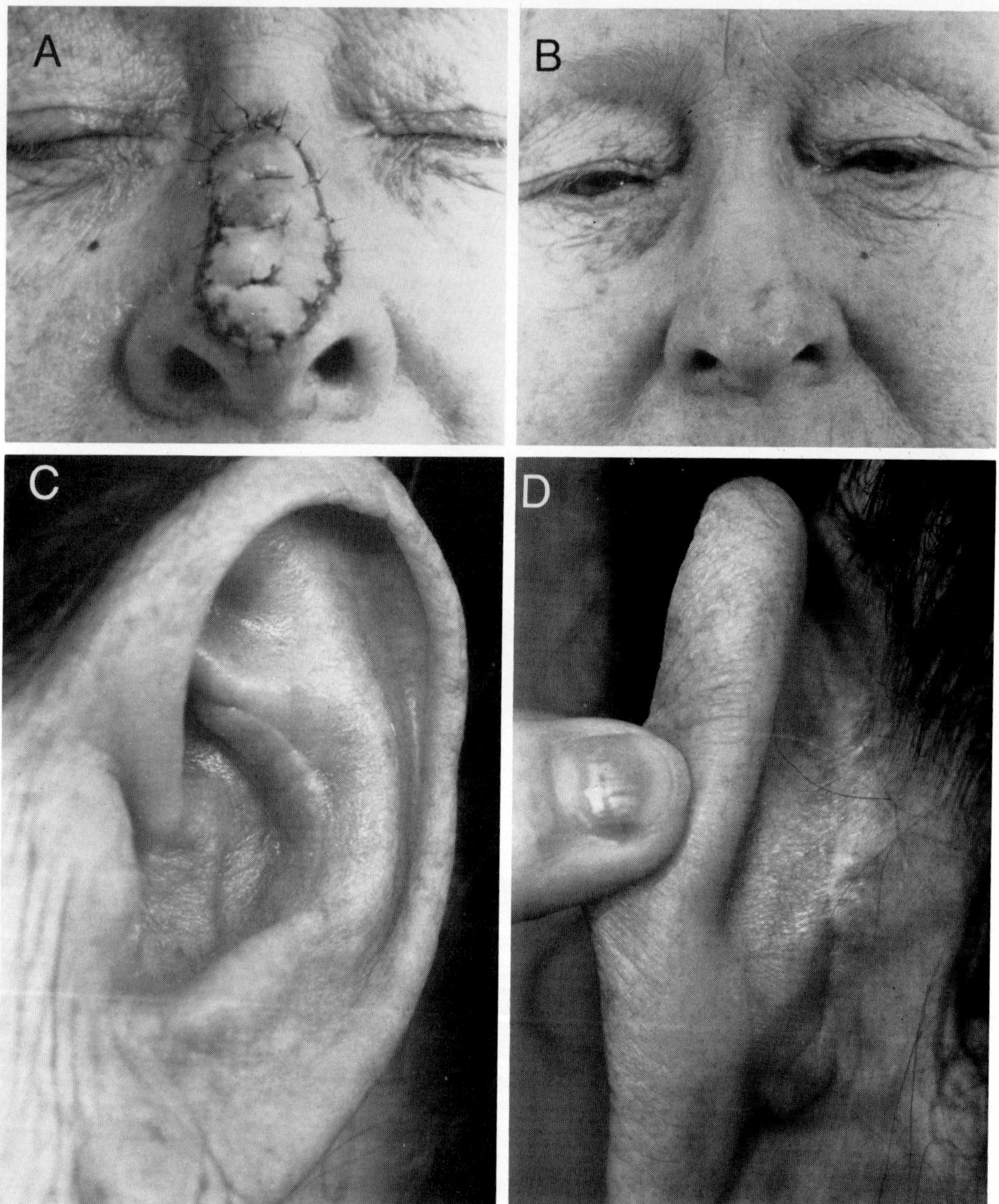

FIG 35–5.
A, perichondrial cutaneous graft. Graft in place following resection of basal cell carcinoma. **B,** result 2 months following surgery. **C** and **D,** postoperative appearance of ear.

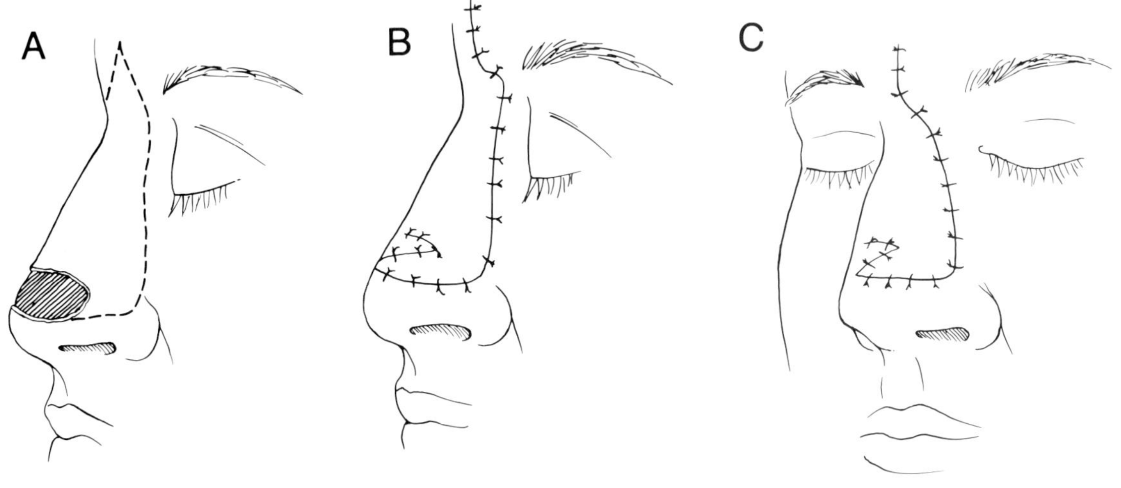

FIG 35–6.
Sliding dorsal nasal flap. **A**, nasal tip defect. SDNF marked out. **B**, SDNF rotated into position. **C**, counterincision to reduce dog ear.

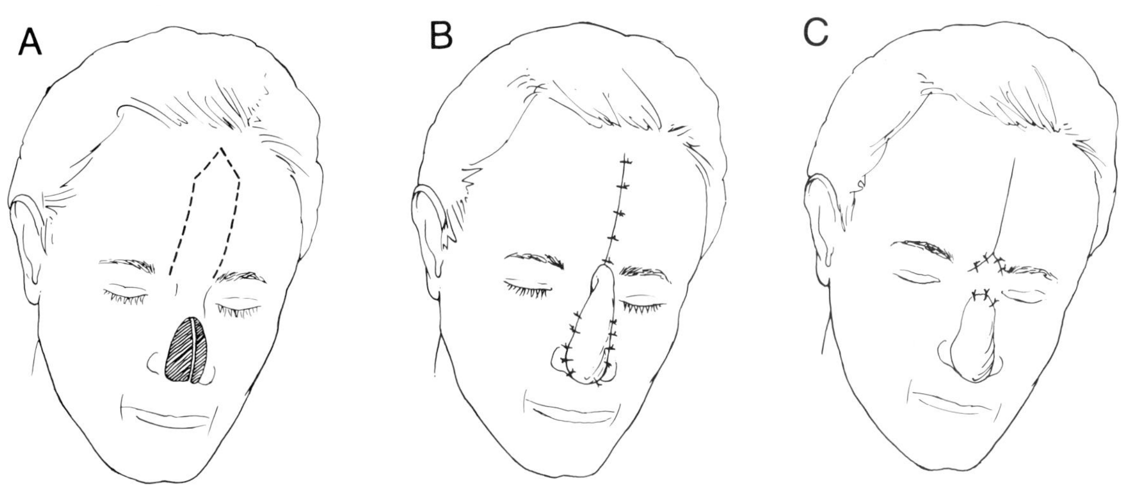

FIG 35–7.
Midline forehead flap reconstruction. **A**, defect in lower half of nose. MLFF marked out. **B**, MLFF lined with dermal graft provides external coverage. (Note kink at base of flap.) **C**, flap divided and defect closed. Skin returned to forehead no higher than eyebrow level.

the flap may be limited in patients with a short forehead and low hairline. In these cases, the flap can be designed in a more oblique direction to gain additional length.

When the MLFF is used for external coverage, preference is given to dermis as the lining graft. In this case the graft is "pie-crusted" and sutured to the undersurface of the flap. The cutaneous portion of the flap is sutured to two thirds of the circumference of the defect. Three weeks later the pedicle is divided, and the remainder is tailored to the defect. The flap is returned only to the level of the brows. Any skin above this line

is discarded because replacement leads to a less acceptable cosmetic result (Fig 35–7,C).

When a PCCG provides a superior color match, the MLFF is turned to line the inside of the nose. In this instance, the PCCG is sutured to the flap as well as to the edges of the defect.

Nasolabial island flaps are appropriate for inner lining in certain laterally placed defects. Turn-in flaps can also be used, but I prefer not to use these at the time of resection so that the base of this random flap will have a better blood supply. When turn-in flaps are used, a cheek advancement flap is planned so that its apposition with the MLFF will recreate the natural nose-cheek junction.

There are inherent limitations with the MLFF. Not only is a second stage required, but the horizontal and vertical dimensions are limited. Lymphedema of the reconstructed area is common and usually takes several months to resolve. Local injection of steroids may be helpful in the treatment of the problem, and debulking may be necessary.

Total Nasal Reconstruction

Only the experienced reconstructive surgeon should embark on a course of total nasal reconstruction. There are numerous judgments to be made, and miscalculations may result in further harm to a patient who has already been devastated by a socially debilitating facial deformity.

The first question to be answered is *whether* to reconstruct. A defect of this magnitude logically results from a tumor that has a significant risk of recurrence. My personal philosophy is to wait 1 to 2 years before reconstruction, depending on the level of risk. If a suitable period of observation has elapsed, or in the event of a traumatic defect, options in management can be discussed with the patient.

A suitable prosthesis is the best option for some patients. A good prosthetic appliance is often cosmetically superior to tissue reconstruction. Some patients may be unwilling or unable to undergo the multiple procedures often required to attain an acceptable result. Other patients have an unrealistic view of what their "new nose" will look like. In these situations, prosthetic rehabilitation is preferable to total nasal reconstruction.

If reconstruction is the selected option, the surgeon must evaluate the defect and determine the most appropriate series of surgical maneuvers that will be necessary. The sequence of these efforts will also be of vital importance. Once this assessment is complete, the expected course of events and their timing should be discussed with the patient. A realistic appraisal of the expected final result should also be emphasized.

The typical defect requiring total nasal reconstruction (TNR) is a through-and-through defect from the caudal margin of the nasal bones to the cutaneous portion of the upper lip. The defect spans at least the pyriform aperture and may extend beyond it.

The key to success in reconstituting this deformity is establishing an architectural framework that will support the soft tissues and provide the needed vertical dimension to the nose. If the nasal bones and cartilagenous septum are intact, the anticipated result will be good, possibly excellent. If there is a significant septal deficiency, both the patient and the surgeon should be prepared for suboptimal (often disappointing) results.

Establishing skeletal support for nasal reconstruction is no easy task. Millard has described the use of a septal advancement flap that provides dorsal support and caudal projection.[13, 14] Burget has outlined a rather intricate construction of a foundation consisting of struts, battens, buttresses, and braces.[15] Our experience would indicate that no method is universally reliable in recreating the missing structural framework. Some authors advocate soft tissue reconstruction first, followed by insertion

of cartilage and bone grafts at a later stage. This technique is foreordained to fail. In those few patients who initially have an acceptable result, this skeletal foundation inevitably weakens as the grafts resorb, bend, and warp under the pressures of time, contraction, and gravity.

When a suitable infrastructure is present, best results are obtained using forehead flaps and their modifications. The seagull-shaped forehead flap as described by Millard is useful in providing a new nasal dorsum as well as providing tissue for the ala and columella (Fig 35–8).[13, 14] The internal lining can be established by grafting the flap, turn-in flaps, endonasal mucosal, or chondromucosal flaps. The latter two techniques have been described in more detail elsewhere.[15, 16]

The Converse scalping flap has been used for many years in TNR, and many surgeons who regularly use this flap are able to obtain acceptable results.[17] However, my preference is the Millard seagull-shaped forehead flap. The advantages of the latter are that it can be done more easily under local anesthesia, the interim deformity is more readily accepted by the patient, and the defect can be closed primarily. The Converse flap is bulky, is difficult to care for, is associated with more blood loss, and necessitates a skin graft over the forehead defect. The cosmetic result at the donor site is less acceptable than the T scar associated with the Millard flap.

An alternative method is to use the midline forehead flap fashioned to cover the deficiency of the lower two thirds of the nose. Instead of using turn-in flaps, the MLFF itself is used as the internal lining. The flap is flipped back 180 degrees and sutured to the circumference of the nasal defect (Fig 35–9). A vertical midline incision is made in the flap, which is used as a groove for the septum. Sutures through the dorsal septum and this incision allow coaptation of the septum and flap. The outer surface of the flap (frontalis muscle) is grafted with a full-thickness skin graft. A few stab incisions are made in the graft prior to application.

The graft is then stretched slightly over the convexity of the flap as it drapes over the septum. This tension helps to prevent a hematoma and obviates the need for a bolster. Iced saline compresses cool the graft and provide a mechanism to prevent crusting and absorb the minimal oozing of blood and serous fluid that inevitably occurs.

Although experience with this latter technique in TNR is limited, it has worked well in those cases in which it has been used. An additional advantage of this technique is the added length gained by rotating the flap backwards instead of laterally. Cosmetic results are very acceptable as long as symmetry is maintained. The color match is surprisingly good, and the pink hue may be accounted for by the redness of the underlying muscle.

Prior to undertaking TNR, one should correct any deformities outside of the nasal defect. Those secondary defects that extend into the cheek or upper lip should be reconstituted up to the normal anatomic boundaries of the nose. This may entail cheek advancement flaps laterally or a nasolabial flap for reconstructing a partial upper lip deformity.

Once the defect is narrowed to the confines of the nasal floor and pyriform aperture, the agenda for nasal reconstruction

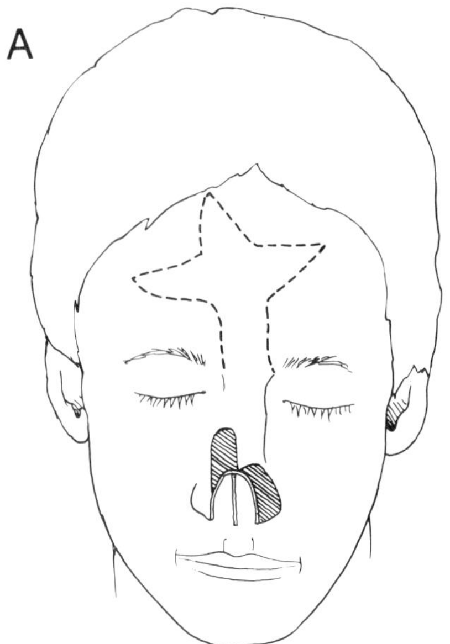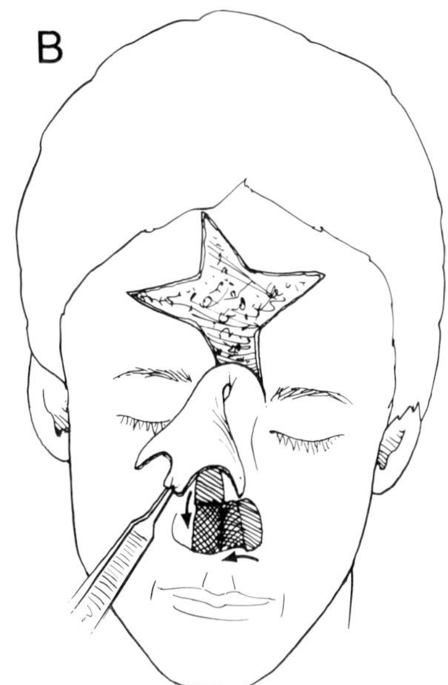

FIG 35–8.
Millard seagull-shaped forehead flap. **A**, defect in lower half of nose. Proposed turn-in flaps hatched. Seagull-shaped flap outlined. **B**, turn-in flaps for nasal lining crosshatched. Forehead flap elevated and rotated.

can be formulated. If deficiencies in the skeletal framework exist, they are addressed by the methods previously mentioned. Once a stable infrastructure is present, decisions are made regarding the establishment of the endonasal lining. In general, the most expedient and reliable methods are the most desirable. For the cutaneous defect, careful planning is mandatory to envision and create a flap of suitable length, width, and orientation. The design must also account for the deficits involving the ala and columella. Proper execution of this process demands meticulous tissue management and postoperative care. Total nasal reconstruction can be gratifying to patient and surgeon, although a surgical misadventure is disastrous. Multiple revision surgeries are often necessary to attain optimal results.

MIDFACE RECONSTRUCTION

The patient with a massive midface defect presents a nearly overwhelming task for the reconstructive surgeon. This deformity most commonly results from either a single ablative procedure or multiple resections that have been undertaken over a period of years. Occasionally, a seemingly curable lesion repeatedly recurs and, as the surgeon chases the tumor, the face is gradually eroded by a cycle of malignancy and resection. Most head and neck surgeons have encountered the patient with this disease process and are familiar with this frustrating sequence of events. A smaller group of patients who demonstrate significant midfacial defects are the victims of self-inflicted gunshot wounds.

Midface defects encompass a wide range of deformities. As a result, the preoperative assessment begins by simply taking inventory: What structures are present, and which ones are missing? It is assumed that every patient in this category has extensive, if not total, loss of the nose. Coexisting soft tissue deficits may include the eye, adnexae, medial canthus, lips, cheeks, and glabella. Structural losses may include the premaxilla, palate, maxilla, septum, nasal bones, and orbital rims. With the endless combination of defects that can be encountered, it is impossible to provide a cookbook approach to reestablishing the bony-cartilaginous framework and cutaneous coverage. Each case must be carefully and thoughtfully evaluated with a tally of assets and debits.

Before reconstruction is planned, it is prudent to determine the appropriate timing. In cancer patients, the urge to immediately reconstruct must be tempered. I favor delayed reconstruction so that a surveillance for recurrent neoplasm will be optimal. If prosthetic rehabilitation is available, it can be used until definitive reconstruction is undertaken. As alluded to, a maxillofacial prosthesis may be a reasonable alternative to further surgery in many patients.

In managing defects of the midface, two unifying principles should be foremost in the surgeon's mind: to reestablish function and to recreate the normal facial units. In other words, plans should include surgical maneuvers that will eliminate ectropion, reestablish lacrimal drainage, provide for oral competance, resolve palatal deficiency, and restore nasal breathing. Prioritization is a necessary process, and perfection is never attained, but rehabilitation of the patient is the desired endpoint.

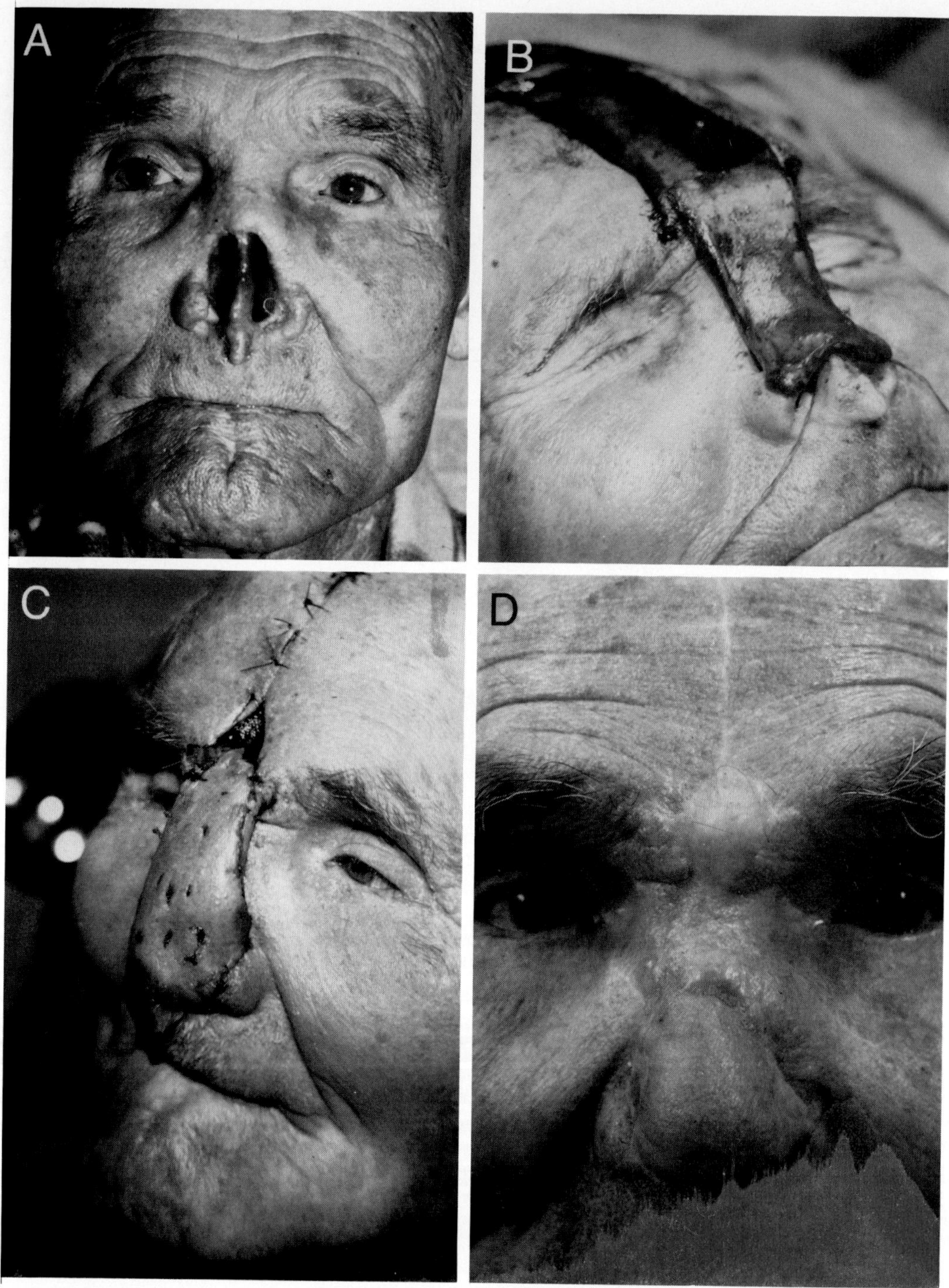

FIG 35–9.
Back-flip flap. **A**, nasal defect prior to reconstruction. **B**, midline forehead flap rotated backwards 180 degrees; prior to application of full-thickness skin graft. **C**, result at 6 weeks. **D**, final result. (Further augmentation obtained by rotating pedicle down onto nasal dorsum.)

Coupled with this attempt at functional restoration is the endeavor to resurface the areas of deficiency by rebuilding in anatomic units. The ideal is to recreate the nose, lips, and cheeks as well as their junctional landmarks.

In general, my preferred reconstruction for significant upper lip defects is the Karapandzic flap. It provides immediate restoration of the oral sphincter and provides continuity to the vermillion and sufficient length to the upper lip. Medial canthal and adnexal problems are managed with full-thickness skin grafts. If epiphora is a problem, the lacrimal drainage system is reconstituted over silicone rubber (Silastic) tubes cannulated through the upper and lower puncta, lacrimal sac, and duct. Cheek flaps should be advanced medially to the pyriform aperture or its former vicinity. Patience in reconstruction by using serial advancement of skin in multiple-staged procedures can often provide necessary coverage for the most extensive defects. Palatal and premaxillary defects can best be closed by using a palatal prosthetic appliance. It can provide sufficient projection to the upper lip as well as to obturate the hole in the palate.

As outlined earlier, total nasal reconstruction should be undertaken as an entity by itself. Preference is given to the midline forehead flap. Regional and free flaps have been used to cover massive midface defects. However, despite multiple surgical procedures to refine, debulk, and contour this amorphous mass of tissue, the end result is usually disappointing to patient and surgeon. The problems with establishing a sound foundation for the nose have been discussed. For bony defects of the orbital rim, delayed insertion of iliac crest bone grafts is a reasonable option. By affixing these to adjacent bones with miniplates, one can enhance a secure bony union.

SUMMARY

There are numerous alternative techniques not discussed, but I have outlined those I favor. The keys to success lie in thoughtful preoperative assessment, cautious planning, meticulous surgical technique and postoperative wound management, a concept of the necessary stages and sequence of events, and a realistic idea of the results that can be attained.

REFERENCES

1. Swanson NA, Grekin RC: Recognition and treatment of skin lesions, in Cummings CW, Fredrickson JM, Harper LA, et al (eds): *Otolaryngology—Head and Neck Surgery.* St Louis, CV Mosby Co, 1986, pp 241–260.
2. Urist MM, Balch CM, Soong S-J, et al: The influence of surgical margins and prognostic factors predicting the risk of local recurrence in 3445 patients with primary cutaneous melanoma. *Cancer* 1985; 55:1398–1402.
3. Milton GW, Shaw HM, McCarthy WH: Resection margins for melanoma [editorial comment]. *Aust NZ J Surg* 1985; 55:225–228.
4. Day CL, Mihm MC, Sober AJ, et al: Narrower margins for clinical stage I malignant melanoma. *N Engl J Med* 1982; 306:479–481.
5. Urist MM, Balch CM, Soong S-J, et al: Head and neck melanoma in 534 clinical stage I patients: A prognostic factors analysis and results of surgical treatment. *Ann Surg* 1984; 200:769–775.
6. Day CL, Lew RA: Malignant melanoma prognostic factors 7: Elective lymph node dissection. *J Dermatol Surg Oncol* 1985; 11:233–239.
7. Panje WR, Ceilley RI: The influence of embryology of the mid-face on the spread of epithelial malignancies. *Laryngoscope* 1979; 89:1914–1920.
8. Baker DC: Massive chondrocutaneous grafts for nasal reconstruction. Paper presented at the International Conference on Head and Neck Cancer, Baltimore, July 24, 1984.
9. Stucker FJ: Personal communication, 1982.
10. Stucker FJ, Portuese WA, Shockley WW: The perichondrial cutaneous graft: A ten year clinical experience (submitted for publication).
11. Portuese WA, Stucker FJ, Shockley WW, et al: The perichondrial cutaneous graft: A study of the revascularization process. *Arch Otolaryngol Head Neck Surg* 1989; 115:705–709.
12. Shockley WW, Stucker FJ, Bryarly RC: Local forehad flaps in facial reconstruction, in *Plastic and Reconstructive Surgery of the Head and Neck: Proceedings of the Fourth International Symposium.* St Louis, CV Mosby Co, 1984, pp 896–905.
13. Millard DR: Reconstructive rhinoplasty of the lower half of the nose. *Plast Reconstr Surg* 1974; 53:133–139.
14. Millard DR: Reconstructive rhinoplasty for the lower two thirds of the nose. *Plast Reconstr Surg* 1976; 57:722–728.
15. Burget GC: Surgical restoration of the nose, in *Current Therapy in Plastic and Reconstructive Surgery.* St Louis, CV Mosby Co, 1988, pp 400–412.
16. Weisman RA: Septal chondromucosal flap with preservation of septal integrity. *Laryngoscope* 1989; 99:267–271.
17. Converse JM, McCarthy JG: The scalping forehead flap revisited. *Clin Plast Surg* 1981; 8:413–434.

Facial Flaps

Approach of

H. Clif Patterson, M.D.

For the majority of cases, adjacent flaps are used to close significant excisional facial defects. Although the occasional large excision might require a skin graft, a regional flap (scalp sickle, scalping, median forehead), or a distant flap (deltopectoral or myocutaneous), this chapter will address commonly used, simple, and reliable adjacent flaps. Such flaps are necessary only when the wound is located in an area where the lack of tissue laxity precludes undermining and direct closure along the favorable skin tension lines. Most flaps exploit the facial regions in which there is lax and available tissue to transfer coverage to an adjacent region without compromise of key anatomic landmarks with donor site closure. Frequently used donor sites are the lower part of the cheek and the jowl, the glabella, the cheek-lip groove, and the upper part of the cheek beyond the lateral canthus area. The objective one must keep in mind is to provide skin that is similar in color, texture, and hair-bearing potential to that previously excised.

NOMENCLATURE

Nomenclature of local flaps is determined by their mode of transfer. Advancement, rotation and transition flaps, or combinations of these, are the most commonly used.[1]

Advancement flaps are perhaps the least employed of the three because they are fashioned by tissue undermining and advancement in a straight line along the same line as the defect. This maneuver usually creates two linear scars and protrusions on either side of the base of the flap due to the length discrepancy between the flap and the flap plus defect dimension (Fig 35–10), both of which can be unfavorable in the final result. Smaller advancement flaps can be useful for reconstruction of missing eyebrow tissue, adhering to the tenet of replacing hair-bearing (brow) tissue with like tissue. Larger flaps, again oriented horizontally along favorable skin tension lines, might be exemplified by two half forehead flaps advanced medially to close a midline forehead defect. This same principle of two advancement flaps on opposite sides of a defect is applied to upper or lower lip defects to accomplish straight line closure of the remaining lip tissue (see Figs 35–21 and 35–22). Here,

the nasal base-lip and cheek-lip boundary is used to hide one limb of the advancement incision.

Rotation flaps, most useful for closure of triangular defects, are created by the transfer of tissue through an arc into the recipient site (Fig 35–11). Such flaps are, by necessity, large and require extensive undermining. The principle of halving or Burow's triangle excisions are useful for closure of the unequal lengths created. Resurfacing of large cheek defects is accomplished by these large flaps (see Figs 35–26 to 35–28). Closure of medial cheek and nose-cheek junction defects can be accomplished by an inferiorly or superiorly based flap with incision lines along the landmark junctions of the lower eyelid–lateral canthus areas and cheek-lip groove–lateral oral com-

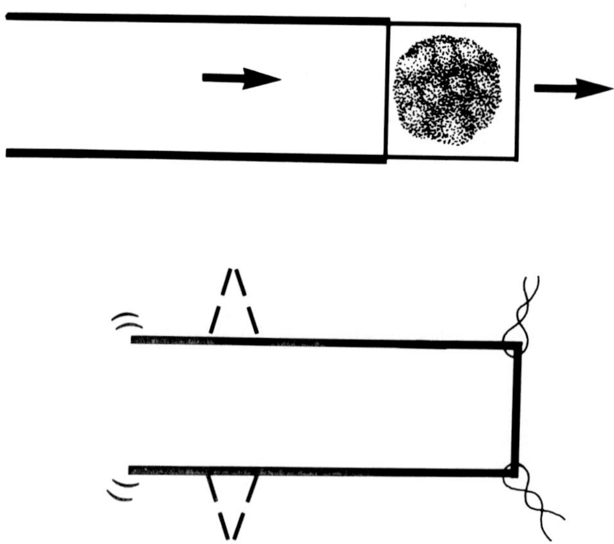

FIG 35–10.
Rectangular advancement flap. Note protrusions formed on outside of the base of the flap due to discrepancy of tissue lengths after closure. Burow's triangle excision is often necessary to equalize these lengths.

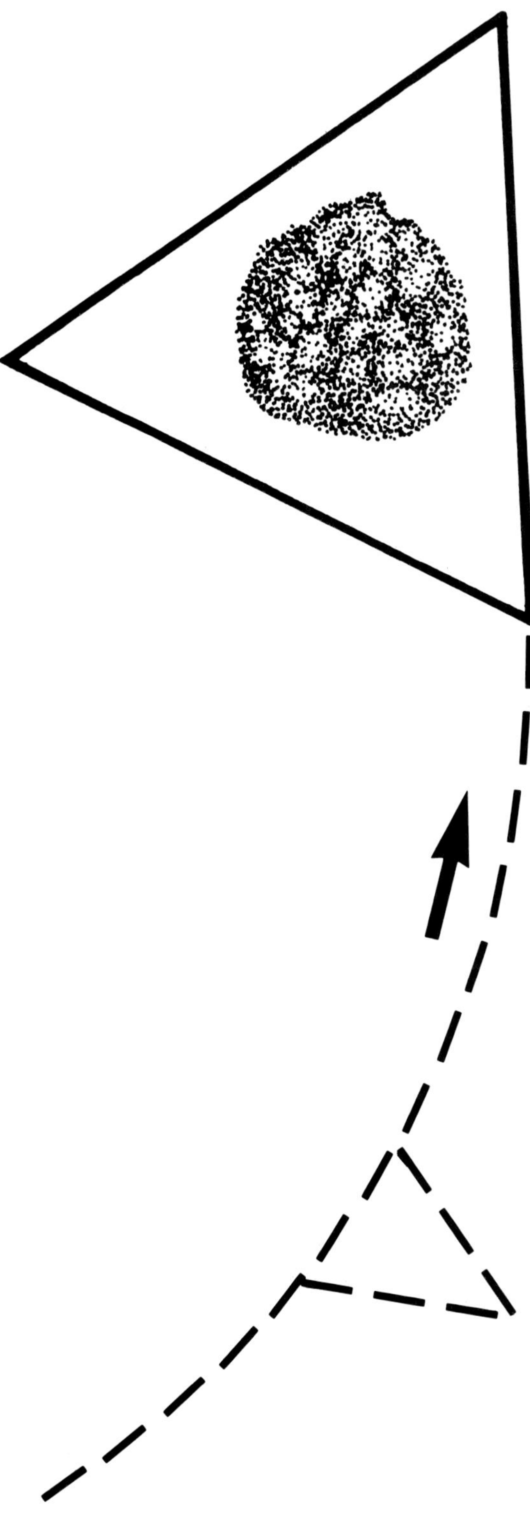

FIG 35–11.
Rotation flaps require extensive undermining and are usually large. Many clinical problems require a combination of a rotation and advancement flap. Note Burow's triangle excision to equalize unequal wound edge lengths.

missure–neck crease areas, respectively.[2] Actually, the face-lift employs two cheek-neck rotation flaps to redrape the excess cheek-neck skin.

Transposition flaps provide the surgeon an opportunity for creativity. Defined as flaps that are transposed over an adjoining piece of tissue, they are the most versatile and commonly used flaps for small- to medium-sized defect reconstruction. I find them particularly applicable for nasal, cheek, temple, and chin defects.[1–3] Advantages are the variety of geometric designs available, the ability to disperse wound tension along several directions, a breaking up of the lines of closure, and minimal dog ear formation. The classic transposition flap is outlined in Figure 35–12. The rhomboid, 30-degree transposition or some variation of these geometric designs is my workhorse solution to the most commonly encountered facial defects after benign or malignant lesion excision (Fig 35–13). Other transposition flaps, such as the median forehead, nasolabial, and bilobed are employed for larger reconstructions. They will be discussed as they apply to selected problems.

Specific anatomic portions of the face have varied requirements for reconstruction, such as hair-bearing (moustache area)

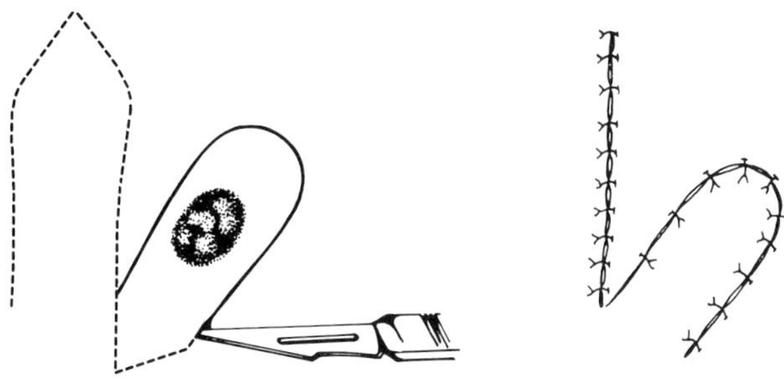

FIG 35–12.
Classic transposition flap. Skin and subcutaneous tissue transposed over an intervening bridge of skin to close a defect. The donor site is closed directly.

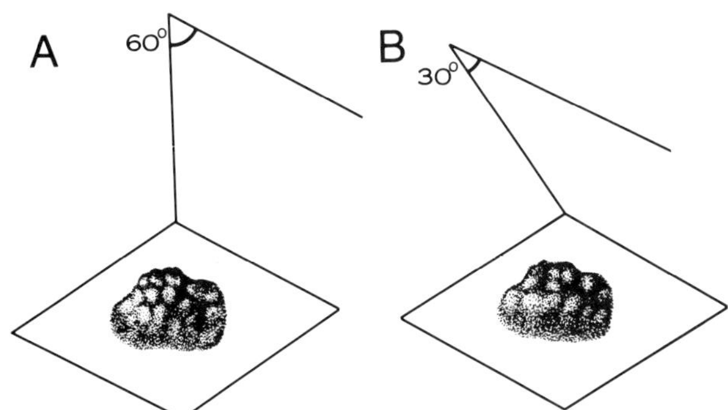

FIG 35–13.
The rhomboid (**A**) or 30-degree transposition flap (**B**) can be oriented in several different ways to take advantage of shared tensions, favorable skin lines, or anatomic boundaries.

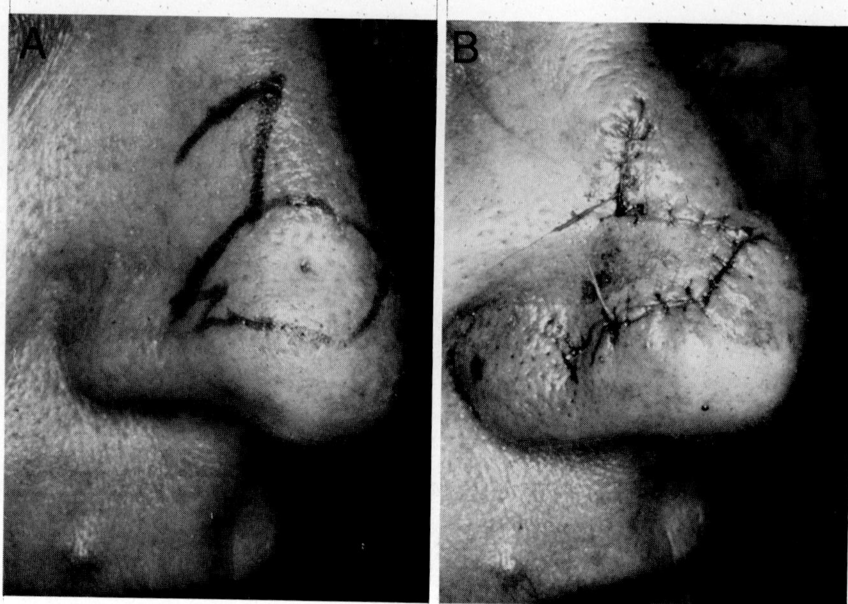

FIG 35–14.
Modified rhomboid (30-degree transposition) flap with M-plasty (**A**). Nasal tip elevation will gradually return to a more normal orientation due to the constant force exerted by the cartilaginous nasal skeleton (**B**). (Courtesy of R.C. Webster, M.D.)

or non-hair-bearing (medial cheek), heavy sebaceous gland population (lower part of nose), or thin eyelid skin. One way to discuss facial flaps is to focus on these anatomic regions and describe reliable reconstructive patterns for each.

NOSE

Nasal tip defects are nicely resurfaced with nasal skin of similar texture, color, and cutaneous gland populations by modified rhomboid, bilobed, or banner flaps. For example, the transposition flap in Figure 35–14 uses dorsal lateral skin. Medial cheek laxity is taken advantage of since the majority of the closure tension is at the donor site. The nearby lower eyelid and cheek-lip groove are unchanged.

Bilobed nasal flaps exploit the laxity of the dorsal nasal and glabellar tissues, as well as the resistance of the nasal skeleton to permanent distortion. Tardy et al. quote Zimary's practical description of a bilobed flap as "consisting of two lobes separated by more or less of an angle and based upon a common pedicle" (Fig 35–15).[4] The two similarly sized lobes rotate approximately 90 degrees and so share wound closure tension along two axes at approximately right angles to each other. A smaller bilobed nasal flap is illustrated in Figure 35–16.

The glabellar region provides a generous amount of non-hair-bearing, thinner skin for reconstruction of superior and lateral nasal, medial canthal, and medial eyelid defects. Fortunately, this is especially so in older individuals, because they usually are the ones requiring neoplasm excisions. Simple advancement with Burow's triangle excisions, V-Y advancement, or a transposition flap are possibilities, depending on the need. The donor site closure is forgivingly concealed in the favorable

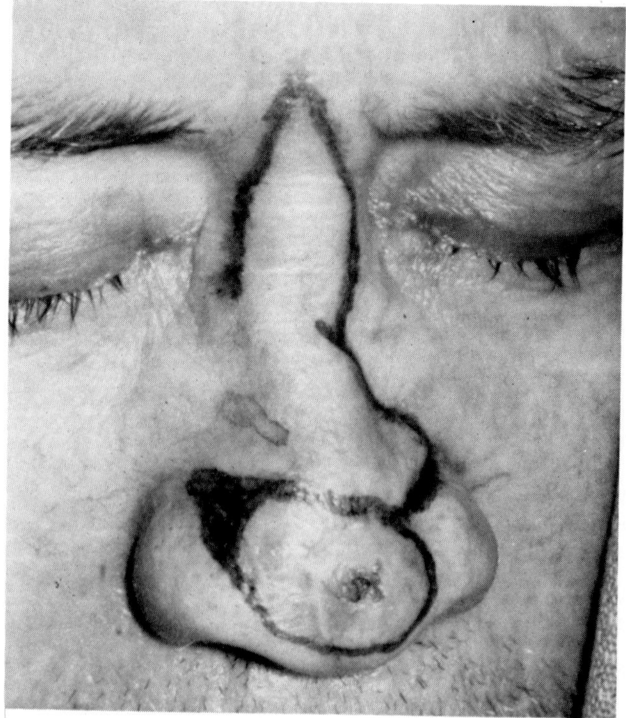

FIG 35–15.
Nasal glabellar bilobed flap for resurfacing a nasal tip defect after excision of a BCC.

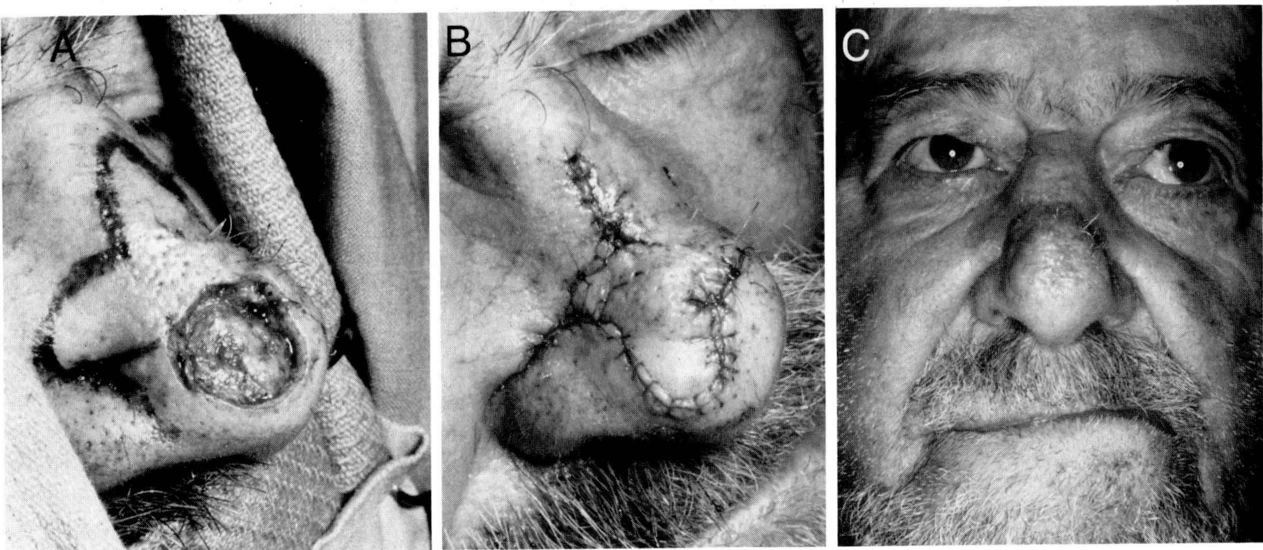

FIG 35–16.
A, nasal bilobed flap for closure of a defect after BCC excision. **B**, closure; **C**, 6 months postoperatively.

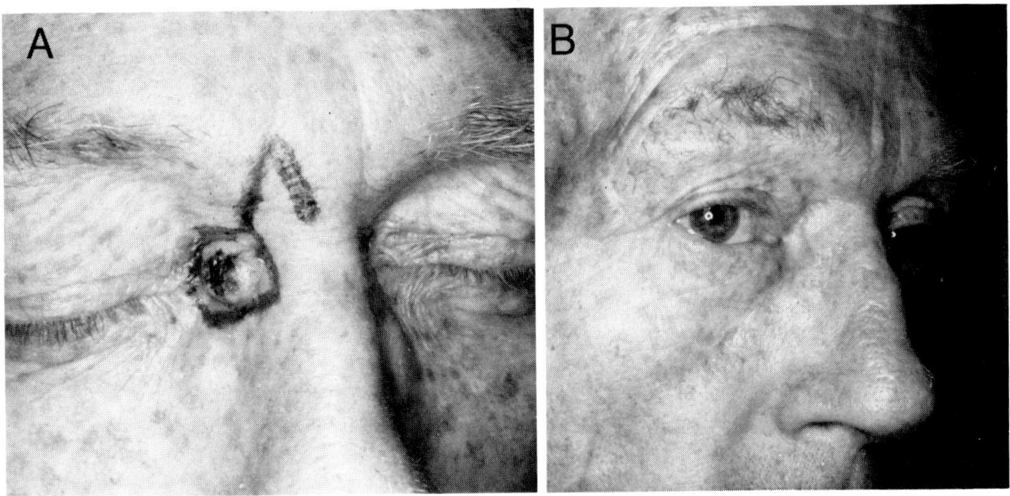

FIG 35–17.
A, modified Romberg flap outlined for reconstruction after excision of a KA. Donor site closure assumes the majority of closure tension and orients the resultant scar within a glabellar frown line. **B**, results 7 months postoperatively. (From Patterson HC: *Otolaryngol Head Neck Surg* 1983; 91:263–270. Used by permission.)

skin creases between and above the brows. I prefer the modified Romberg (Fig 35–17) or bilobed flaps (Fig 35–18) in this region. If the eyebrows meet in the midline, this flap would not be appropriate since hair-bearing skin would be transferred to a non-hair-bearing recipient area.

Lateral and central nasal defects, as well as nasal alae and tip reconstruction, provide an opportunity for the popular, superiorly based *nasolabial flap.*[5] Well-vascularized, non-hair-bearing medial cheek skin and subcutaneous tissue are transposed after tumor margins have been cleared. Undermining and donor site closure are accomplished so that the resultant scar will lie along the previous nasolabial or cheek-lip groove. Problems with nasolabial flaps include obliteration of that cheek-lip groove, protrusions of the inferior limit of the donor site, and "trap door" contracture of the transposed flap. For these reasons, I prefer alternative solutions, such as local nasal flaps (glabellar or nasal transpositions and banner flaps) or rotation-advancement of a large medial cheek flap for central and lateral nasal lesions. Alar reconstruction, if not done with a distant flap or free composite graft, does, however, often require a naso-

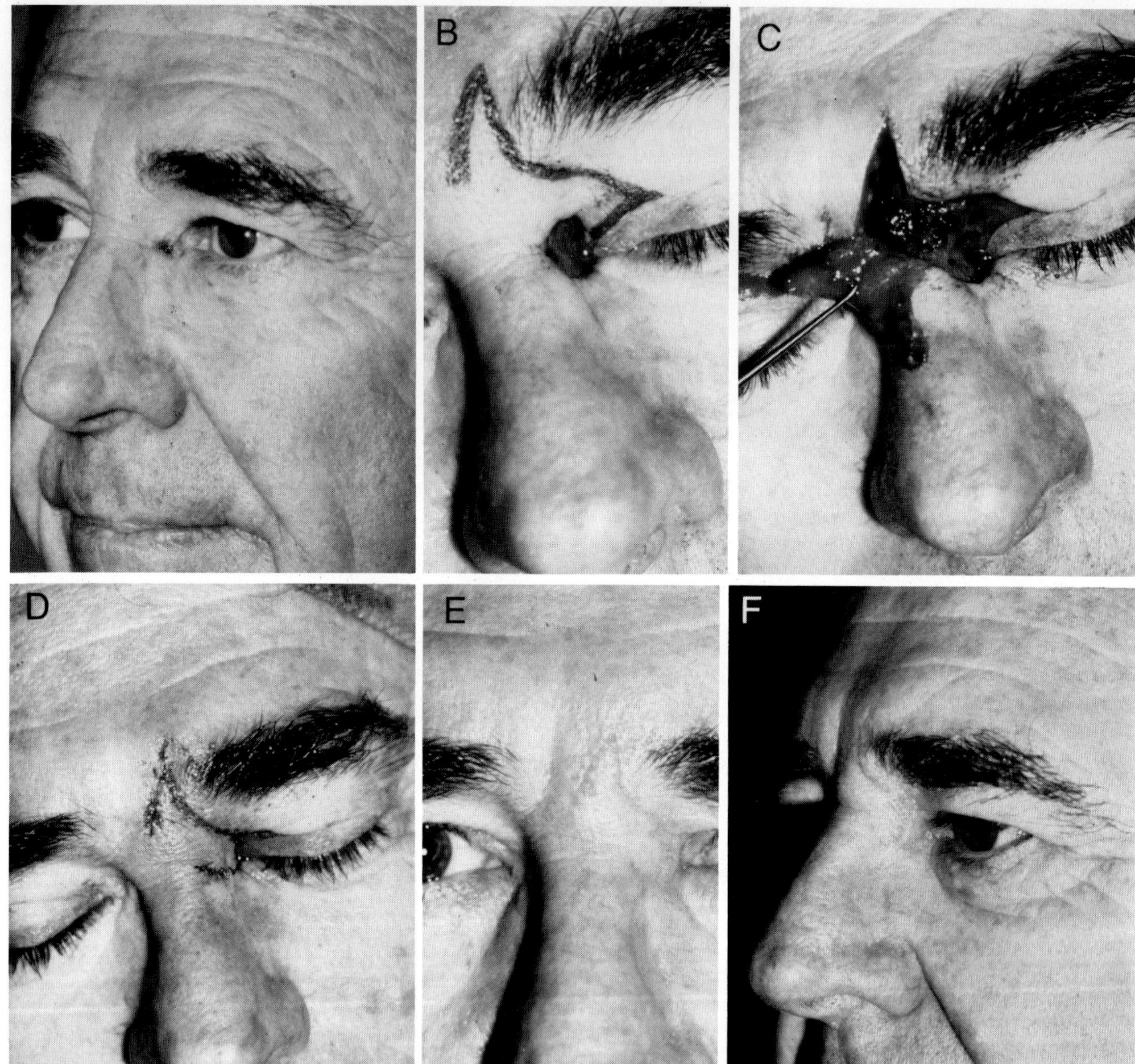

FIG 35–18.
Bilobed glabellar flap provides thin upper eyelid skin for the medial canthus and thicker skin for advancement onto the nasal dorsum. The glabellar portion is actually a V-Y advancement to decrease tension on the defect closure. **A**, BCC, medial canthal–lateral nasal area; **B**, outline of upper eyelid–glabellar bilobed flap; **C**, elevation; **D**, transposition; **E** and **F**, results 2 months postoperatively.

labial flap that might require possible subsequent revisions. Figure 35–19 nicely illustrates the planning and execution of a superiorly based nasolabial flap. Note that the dog ear, or standing cones (see Figs 35–19,D and F), are excised away from the base of the flap so as not to compromise its vascular supply.

Inferiorly based nasolabial flaps are good choices for columellar, nasal base, and upper lip defects in which the lip vermillion is not excised.[5] The flap illustrated in Figure 35–20 closes such an upper lip–base of nose defect without distorting the oral commissure. Another flap that might have been useful

in this case would have been a rotation flap of lateral upper lip skin and muscle, with the donor incision following the cheeklip groove (Karapandzic's principle).[6] It provides a more dynamic and functional result with moustache-bearing skin rather than a relatively static, non-hair-bearing flap.

The earlier principle of using like tissue to replace like tissue is evident in Figure 35–21. This large squamous cell carcinoma required removal of upper lip musculature, most of the columella, and a significant volume of the nose-lip juncture and right ala. The skin bridge between the vermillion and the

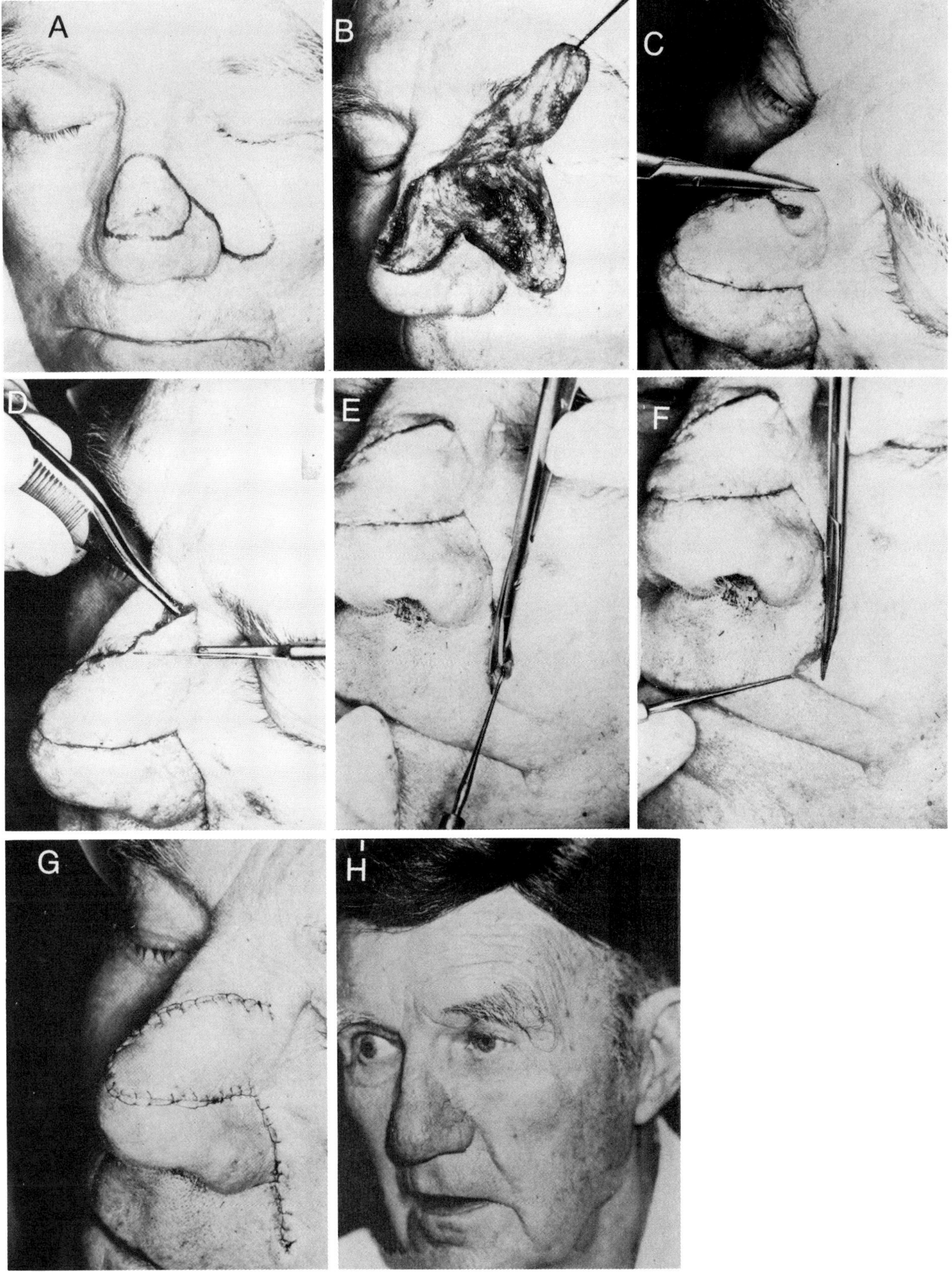

FIG 35–19.
A, proposed excision for recurrent BCC outlined, superiorly based nasolabial flap marked. **B**, flap raised, cheek undermined in subcutaneous plane. **C**, standing cutaneous cone at rotation point of flap incised away from base of flap. **D**, excision of redundant tissue. **E**, small standing cutaneous cone at distal end of donor site incised. **F**, redundant tissue excised. **G**, final closure. **H**, results 6 months postoperatively. (From Becker FF: *Nasolabial flaps,* in *Facial Reconstruction With Local and Regional Flaps.* New York, Thieme Medical Publishers, 1985, pp 12, 13.

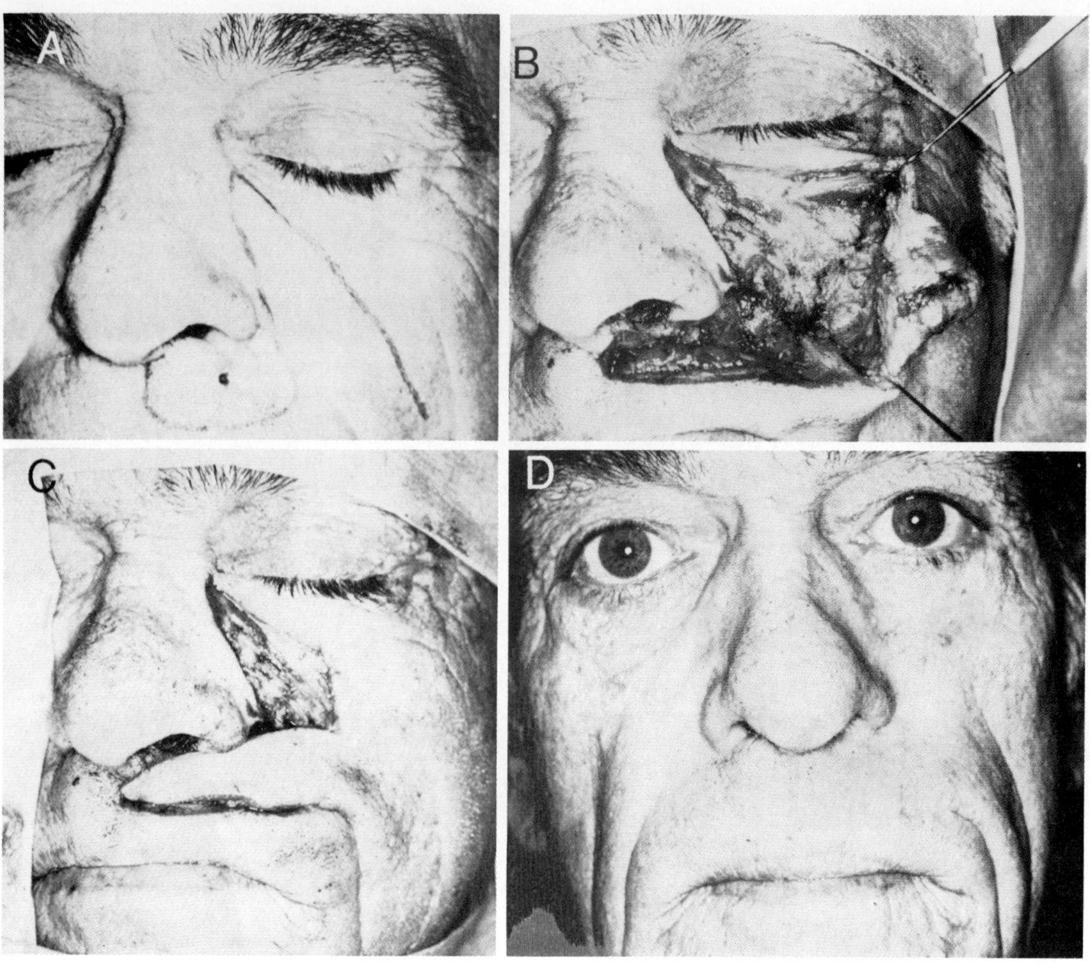

FIG 35–20.
A, proposed excision of tumor outlined, inferiorly based nasolabial flap marked. **B**, tumor excised, flap and lateral cheek undermined. **C**, flap rotated into place, donor site close primarily. **D**, results, 6 months postoperatively. (From Becker FF: *Nasolabial Flaps, in Facial Reconstruction with Local and Regional Flaps.* New York, Thieme Medical Publishers, 1985, p 17. Used by permission.)

defect was excised and the upper lip closed with bilateral advancement flaps. The incisions were concealed along the boundaries of the vermillion border and the nasal base–cheek lip groove areas. In this case, the columella was resurfaced with a full-thickness postauricular skin graft.

Combinations of the aforementioned flaps are often necessary for reconstruction after more extensive resections, as exemplified in Figure 35–22, a patient with a recurrent BCC after prior treatment with external beam radiation therapy. It is highly recommended that recurrent, sclerosing (morpheaform), or large cutaneous carcinomas with indistinct margins be removed by specialists versed in microscopically controlled (Mohs') excision techniques.[7] Such a premise is especially true for malignancies located in the columella-alar base, temple, postauricular sulcus, medial canthus, and external auditory meatus areas. Mohs' excision excels in margin control and tissue preservation, both extremely important requirements prior to reconstruction of defects with flaps. This Mohs' excision defect demonstrates the loss of a significant amount of the columella,

nasal tip, and alar tissue (see Figs 35–22,B–D). A banner flap, borrowing healthy glabellar and nasal dorsum skin, was advanced inferiorly for closure of the nasal tip defect. Bilateral upper lip advancement flaps were used to close the upper philtrum defect. Septal mucosa was advanced to cover exposed septal cartilage (see Fig 35–22,E). Once again, well-vascularized adjacent tissue similar in texture, color match, and function is borrowed to cover the defect.

On occasion, the magnitude of nasal excision is such that more tissue volume, cartilage composite flaps, or flaps able to support a skin graft on their deep surface are required. These *regional flaps* transpose more distant tissue into the recipient site, examples of which are the MLFF and tempororetroauricular flap.

The *midline forehead flap* (Fig 35–23) is a richly vascularized musculocutaneous flap that has been used for subtotal nasal and medial cheek resurfacing since nasal amputation prompted reconstructive attempts in India many centuries before Christ. Nourished by supratrochlear arteries from the in-

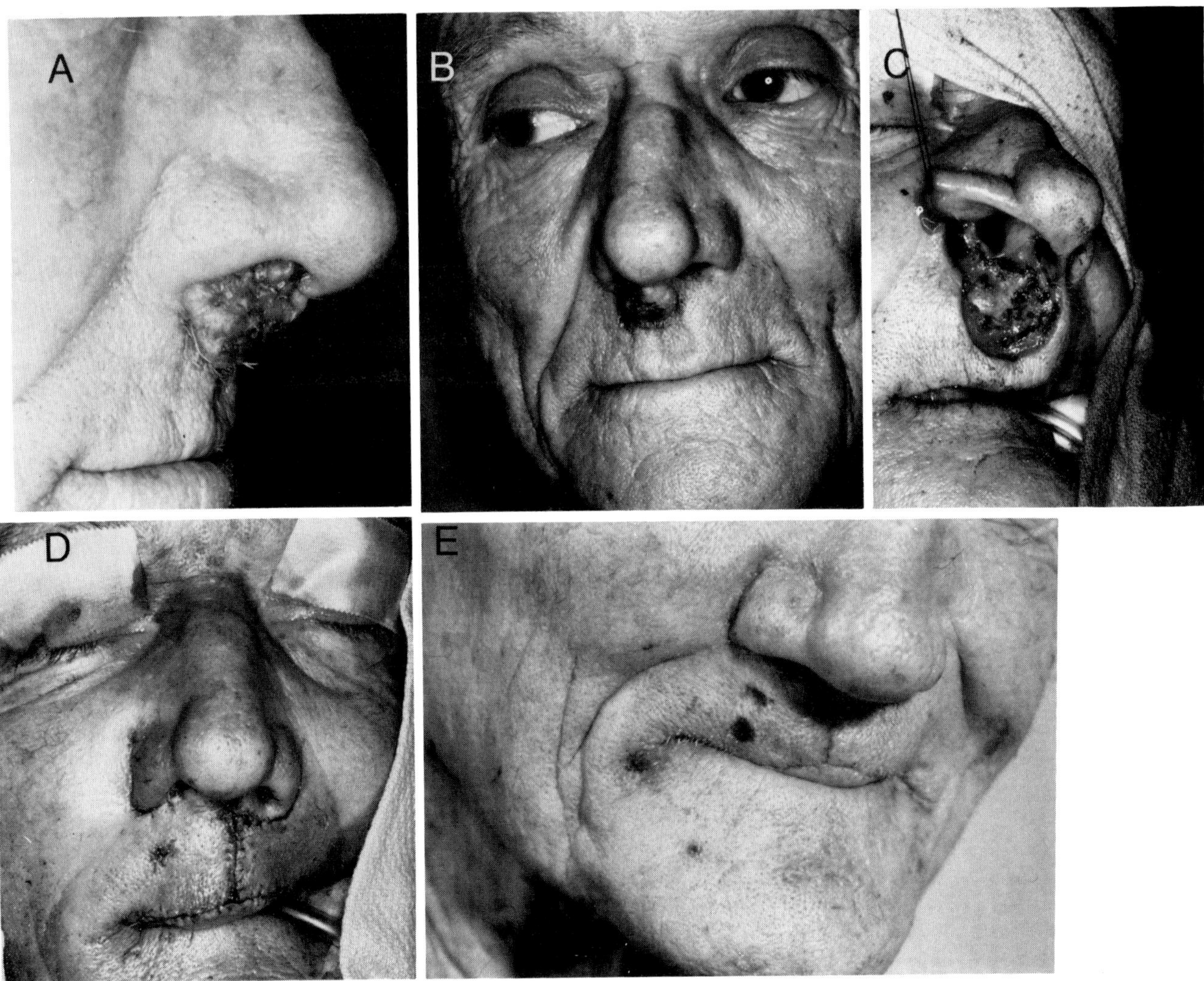

FIG 35–21.
A–C, excision of SCC of the columella, nasal base, and upper lip. **D,** bilateral orbicularis oris myocutanous advancement flaps close the lip and nostril sill defect. **E,** results 2 weeks postoperatively.

ternal carotid system and angular arteries from the external carotid artery, this flap is perhaps without comparison for dependability. A width of 2.5 to 3.5 cm and length dependent on the distance between the intercanthal area and widow's peak of the scalp is available. The plane of dissection lies beneath the subgaleal tissue but superficial to the frontal bone periosteum, with care taken in the lateral areas of the root of the nose to avoid trauma to the nutrient vessels. Greater length can be gained by division of one of the vascular pedicles. Donor site closure is accomplished by subgaleal undermining and advancement of both lateral forehead edges together into the midline. Pedicle division is appropriate 2 to 3 weeks after transposition. The entire nasal dorsum, large medial canthal–lateral nasal defects or lower nasal defects can be resurfaced. The distal pedicle of these flaps may be skin grafted for intranasal relining in situations where through-and-through defects are present.

One such case is illustrated in Figure 35–23. This gentleman had received radiation therapy to his nose and right medial canthal area 15 years previously for an unknown neoplasm. His presenting problems were a nasolacrimal duct–cutaneous fistula (see Fig 35–23,A), a nasal cutaneous fistula (see Fig 35–23,B), and radiation damaged and deformed nasal and medial canthal area tissue. A split-thickness skin graft was sutured to the distal MLFF and the flap delayed for 10 days due to the questionable radiation damage to its base. A dacryocystorhinostomy (see Fig 35–23,E) was performed coincidentally with flap transposition into the excised damaged tissue site. The skin-grafted portion served as an inner lining for the nose. A portion of the unused pedicle was replaced into the glabellar region. His 1-year postoperative result (see Figs 35–23,F and G) includes an additional debulking procedure to the transposed tissue. In retrospect, the flap delay was probably not necessary and did seem to cause a loss of elasticity (and possibly more lymphedema) of the distal flap, and therefore would not be recommended.

The *tempororetroauricular flap,* though more difficult and time consuming for both the surgeon and the patient, has the advantage of avoiding visible donor site scars on the face.[8] Skin or a compound flap of skin and cartilage is transposed from the postauricular and mastoid area on a pedicle containing the posterior branch of the superficial temporal artery and its anastamoses with the retroauricular artery. The most appealing application of this flap is nasal alar reconstruction, but it also can be used for nasal, cheek, or eyelid defects. The thin skin

and cartilage from the auricle are ideal for alar defects, as is demonstrated in Figure 35–24. This patient had also had a radiation failure for a recurrent basal cell carcinoma of the right ala and subsequently had the area excised. Because of its recurrent history, he was advised not to have it reconstructed, and so lived with the defect for several years. A turn-down flap was created from the nasal skin superior to the defect to provide an inner lining, and a compound retroauricular skin and auricular cartilage flap was transposed to the recipient site. Three weeks later, a tourniquet test confirmed revascularization of the distal flap, and the bridge of scalp tissue was returned to its normal location. The raw areas had been dressed with non-

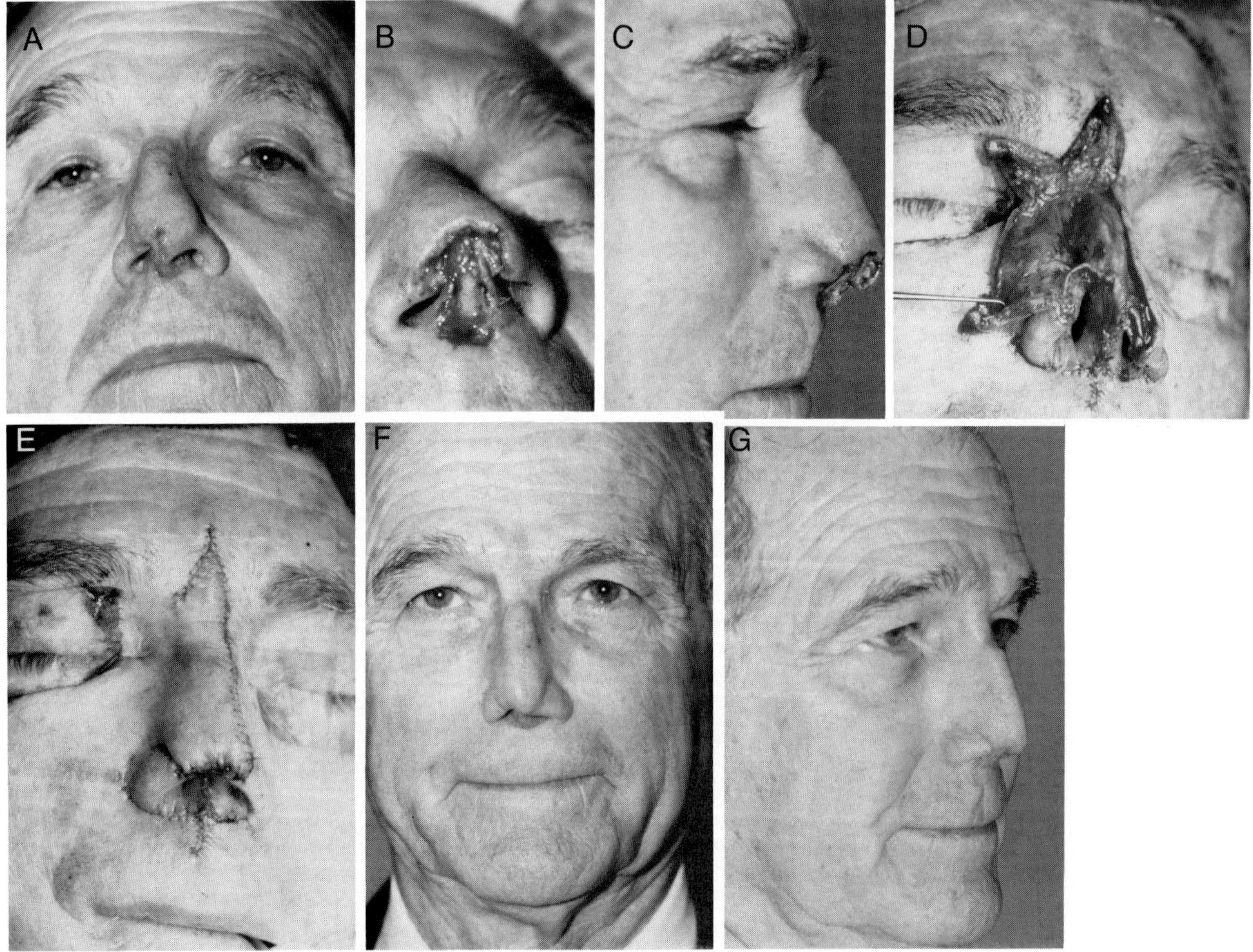

FIG 35–22.
A, recurrent BCC after radiation therapy 2 years previously. **B–D,** after Mohs' controlled excision. **E,** banner flap is elevated; upper lip–nasal base and columella are closed by advancement techniques, and Banner flap is advanced into defect. **F** and **G,** results 6 months postoperatively.

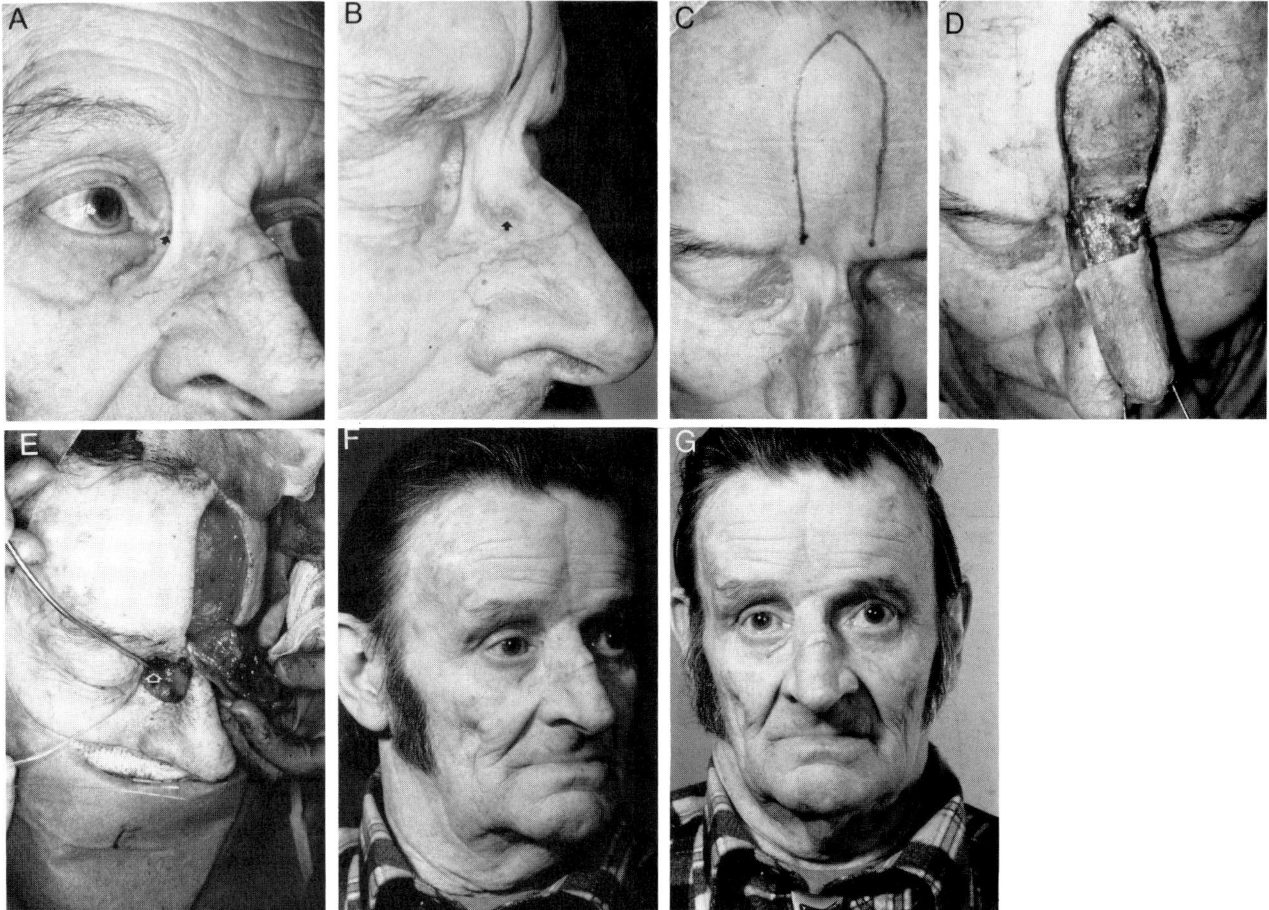

FIG 35–23.
A, radiation damaged nasal–medial canthal area with associated lacrimal duct–cutaneous fistula *(arrow)* and, **B**, nasal cutaneous fistula *(arrow)*. **C**, MLFF outlined; **D**, split-thickness graft sutured to the distal pedicle and the flap delayed for 10 days. **E**, dacryocystorhinostomy *(arrow)* performed, and flap transposed. Patient had one debulking procedure performed prior to his 1-year postoperative photographs, **F** and **G**.

adherent gauze during the interim. Obvious drawbacks of this flap are the hesitancy of the patient to appear in public between stages, the operating time involved with both stages, and simply the need for a two-stage repair. However, it does offer an alternative to the riskier free compound grafts, the donor site scars inherent in an adjacent, local flap reconstruction, and the loss of the cheek-lip groove if a nasolabial flap is chosen.

Although regional (scalping forehead) and distant (trapezius, latissimus dorsi) myocutaneous flaps have been used for total nasal reconstruction, I prefer prosthetic management in these cases. With the possible exceptions of a massive benign neoplasm or a traumatic nose loss, the perinasal area is possibly at risk for a local recurrence and in all probability has been irradiated. Multistaged reconstruction is thus risky, is cost ineffective, and never looks as good as a well-done prosthesis. As exemplified in Figure 35–25, a prosthesis might be a superior solution for all concerned.

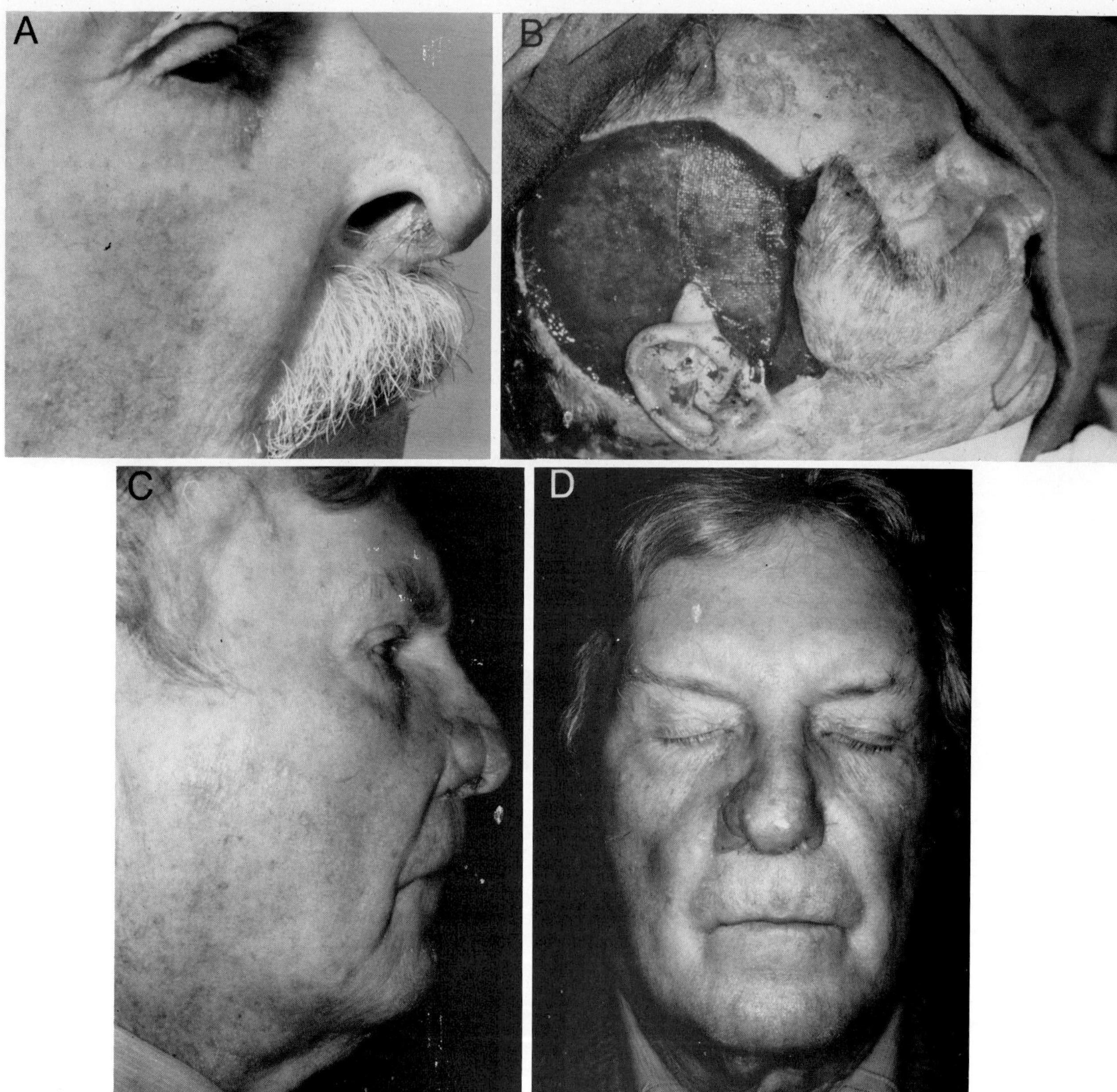

FIG 35–24.
A, alar defect of several years' duration after excision of a radiation failure recurrent BCC. **B**, transposed compound (auricular akin–cartilage) tempororetroauricular (Washio) flap is used to resurface a turn-down flap from the superior aspect of the alar defect. **C** and **D**, results 1 month postoperatively.

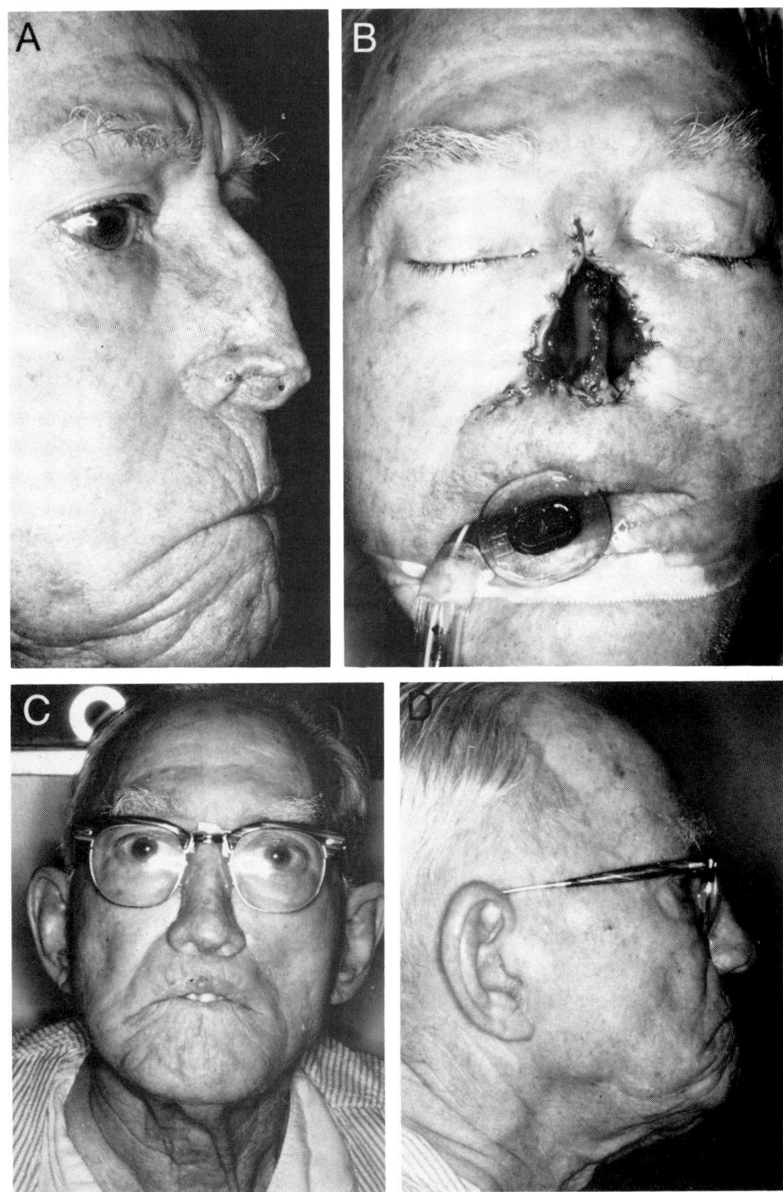

FIG 35–25.
A, recurrent nasal BCC and SCC in a previously operated on and irradiated nose. **B**, total rhinectomy, **C** and **D**, immediate rehabilitation with a nasal prosthesis.

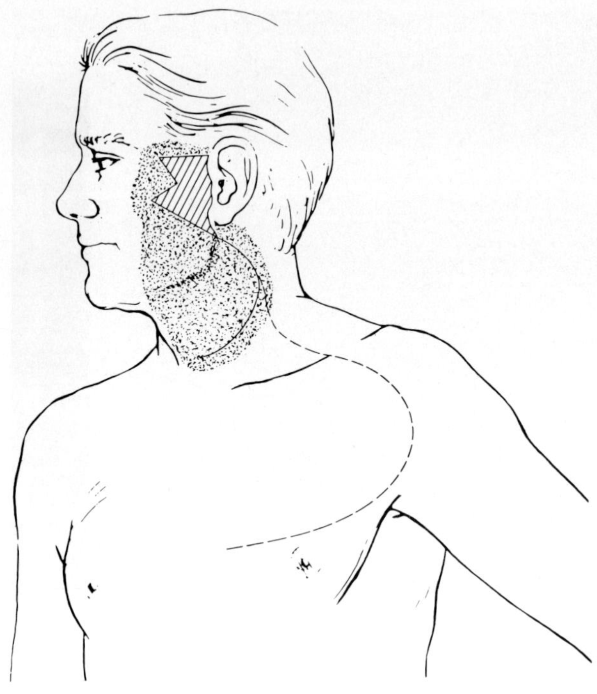

FIG 35–26.
Cheek-neck rotation flap is outlined by a solid line. Dotted line outlines possible cervicopectoral flap if needed. Defect to be closed is cross-hatched; area of undermining is stippled. Note basic triangular defect with anterior M-plasty. (From Patterson HC: *Otolaryngol Head Neck Surg* 1983; 91:263–270. Used by permission.)

CHEEK

The cheek contains loose skin that is amenable to several different flap designs, particularly rhomboid or 30-degree transposition flaps oriented appropriately along the favorable skin tension lines. Breaking up the scar is particularly important in this area of gently convex contour, where anatomic boundaries are not in close proximity to camouflage the scars.

Larger defects of the temporozygomatic-cheek area can be nicely reconstructed with a *cheek-neck rotation flap* (Fig 35–26), where the arc of rotation scars are hidden along the cheek, auricle, and neck crease boundaries.[9] A triangular excisional defect is created and closed with a large rotation flap using the principle of halving for closure of the inequal wound edge lengths. In addition, elevation of such a flap affords access to deeper structures, such as the parotid or node-bearing tissue, which often needs to be addressed when one is dealing with periparotid malignancies. The platysma is included in the lower portion of this flap. Figure 35–27 illustrates this flap in an elderly patient with two cutaneous SCCs of the posterior cheek region associated with positive periparotid lymphadenopathy. Superficial parotidectomy and upper cervical node dissection were possible with this approach.

A patient with an extensive morpheaform BCC of the auricle and preaurical area who underwent Mohs' microscopic controlled excision and reconstruction with a large rotation flap is shown in Figure 35–28.

EYELID, EAR, AND CHIN

Eyelid, ear, and chin defects are no different than other areas in that they require similar tissue to that excised for appropriate chromatic and texture match, but they do present the problem of important landmark distortion if local flaps are not planned appropriately. For eyelid defects, one must always orient the closure tension horizontally so that lagophthalmos or ectropion are avoided. For this reason, two opposing advancement flaps are often used. The laxity of upper eyelid tissue provides a rich resource of skin for transposition flaps in either canthal area, as shown in Figures 35–18 and 35–29. In Figure 35–29, the vector of maximum donor site closure tension is oriented lateral to the lateral canthus to avoid lid distortion.

A generous amount of non-hair-bearing and relatively lax skin located behind the ear provides an excellent tissue match for the auricular skin. Figure 35–30 demonstrates a bilobed flap for closure of a moderate-sized defect. One could argue that a skin graft might be just as effective, but a separate donor site, more operative time, and problems with contracture are potential drawbacks.

In Figure 35–31, a large basal cell carcinoma of the chin is excised and the defect reconstructed with a modified rhomboid flap. Several variations in design are possible. The one chosen takes advantage of the junction between the lip and the chin to conceal the donor site closure scar. Overall, the broken scar is less noticeable than a straight or curvilinear one.

Although local flaps provide significant advantages over skin grafts for most reconstructions, grafts remain a reasonable and occasionally superior option in selected cases. I believe the cosmetic result of small full-thickness grafts placed in small nasal tip defects is better than direct approximation of the wound edges or a local flap (Figs 35–32 and 35–33). The retroauricular skin is often remarkably similar to the thinner nasal tip skin in those patients with relatively nonoily skin and is a favorite graft donor site. Serendipity proves frequently to be a poignant teacher, as demonstrated in the unplanned final result (Fig 35–34). This lesion was referred as an SCC but historically and clinically appeared consistent with a keratoacanthoma (KA).[10] The decision was made to excise it with close margins and graft the resultant defect, and then to reconstruct at a later date if indicated by a 1-year disease-free interval. Supraclavicular full-thickness skin was used for the graft. The final diagnosis was KA, and the patient was satisfied with the result; therefore, no further surgery was necessary.

Auricular defects in which the helical rim has been preserved are also easily and appropriately resurfaced by full-thickness skin grafts, preferrably from the upper eyelid or retroauricular sulcus. Removal of a significant amount of cartilage beneath the graft is advised so that the free graft is rapidly nourished (Fig 35–35).

Finally, pathologic considerations will, on occasion, dictate

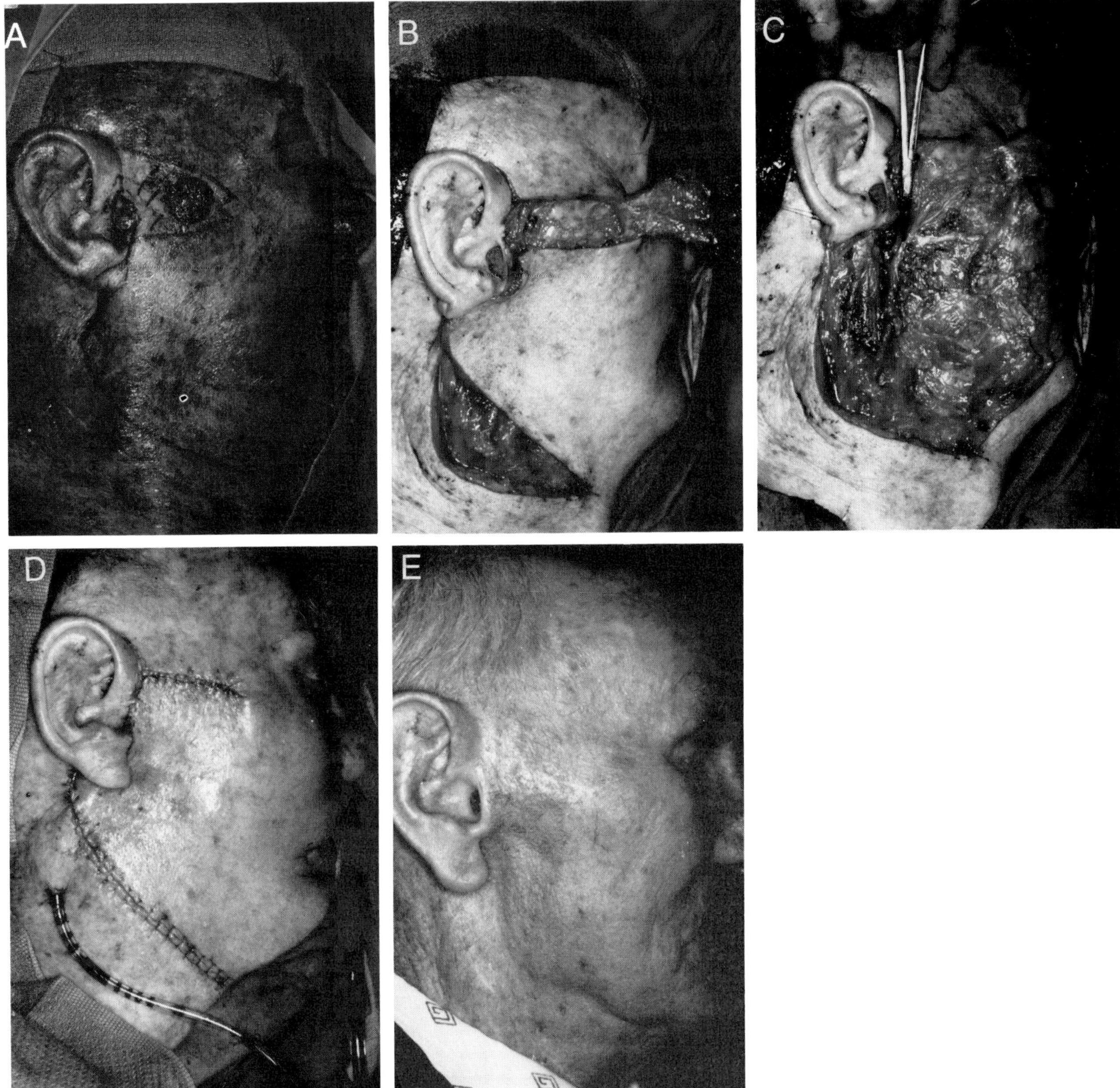

FIG 35–27.
Squamous cell carcinomas of the preauricular area with parotid metastasis. **A**, cheek-neck rotation flap for exposure and immediate reconstruction is outlined. **B**, superficial parotidectomy and exploration of upper part of neck. **C**, clamp identifies seventh nerve. **D**, closure and, **E**, results 6 months postoperatively. (From Patterson HC: *Otolaryngol Head Neck Surg* 1983; 91:9. Used by permission.)

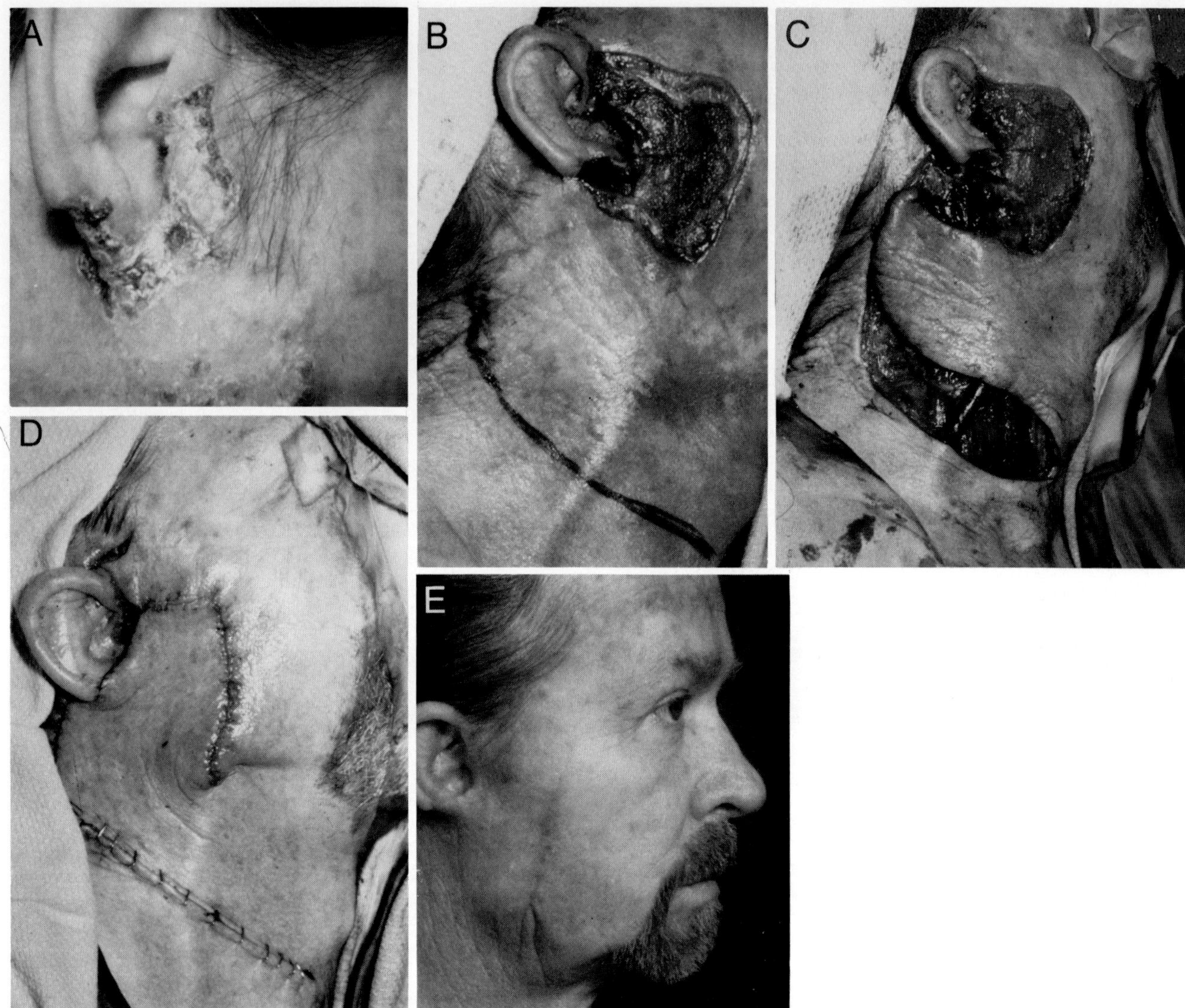

FIG 35–28.
Morpheaform BCC (**A**) excised by Mohs' microscopic controlled excision (**B**). Rotation flap elevated (**C**) and transposed in addition to a V-Y closure superiorly (**D**). Results 4 months postoperatively (**E**).

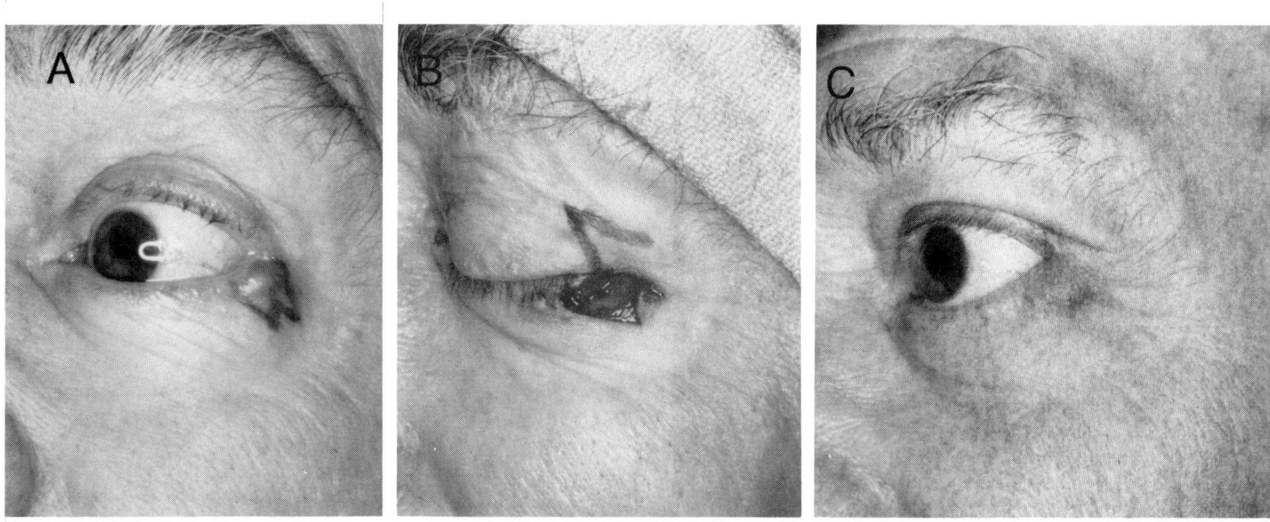

FIG 35–29.
A and **B**, benign adenoma of lower eye lid with proposed excision and 30-degree transposition flap outlined. **C**, results 2 weeks postoperatively.

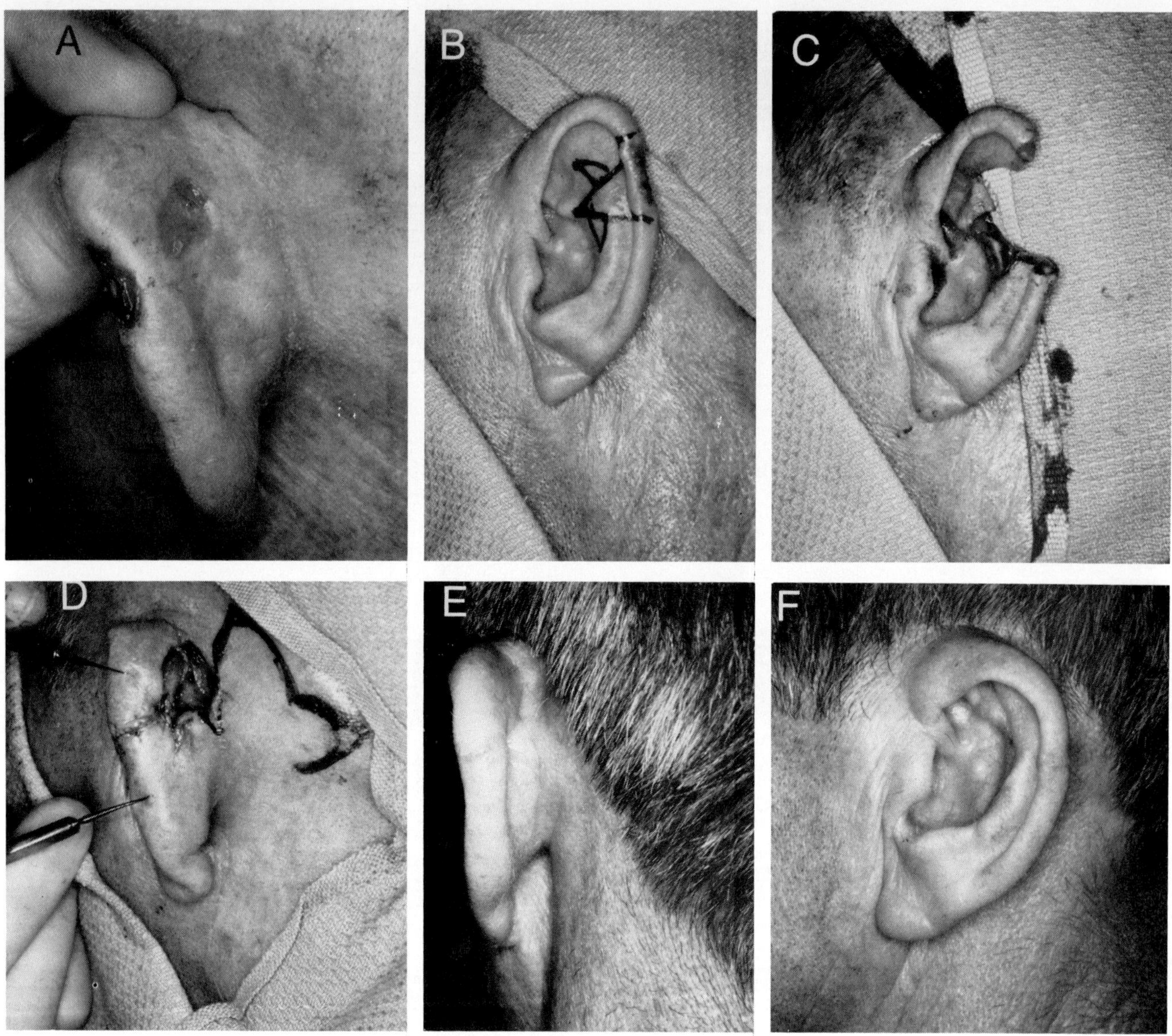

FIG 35–30.
A, BCC of the auricle with **B**, proposed wedge excision. **C**, defects closed primarily. **D**, defect closed with a bilobed flap from the hairless retroauricular area. **E** and **F**, results 2 months postoperatively.

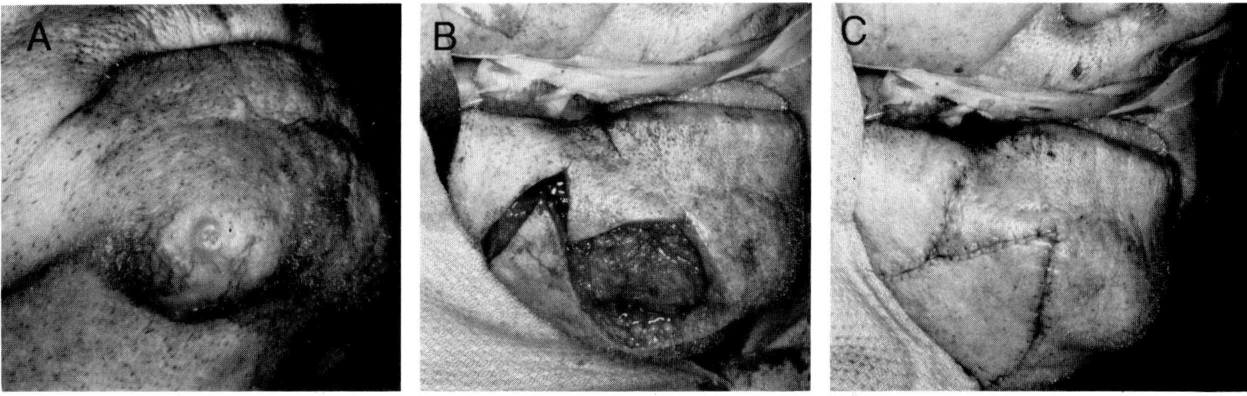

FIG 35–31.
A, BCC of the chin is excised and reconstructed with a modified Romberg flap. **B** and **C**, note scan placement along anatomic boundary lines and breaking up of the resultant suture lines by sharing closure tensions in several different directions.

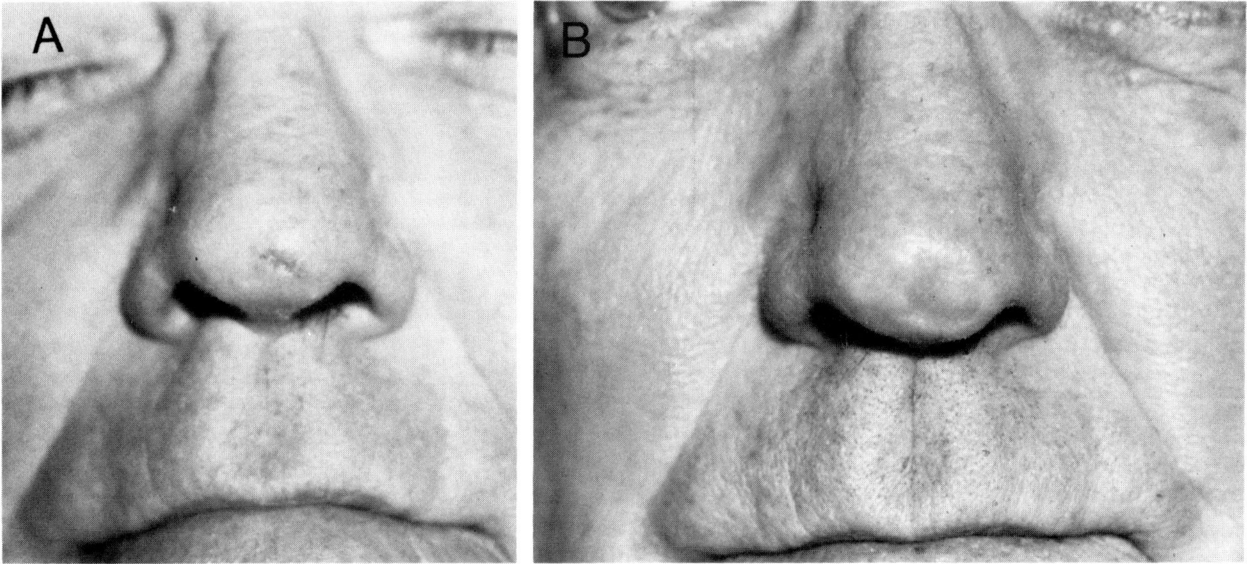

FIG 35–32.
A, excision of this BCC and, **B,** full-thickness grafting with retroauricular skin provide a very acceptable result.

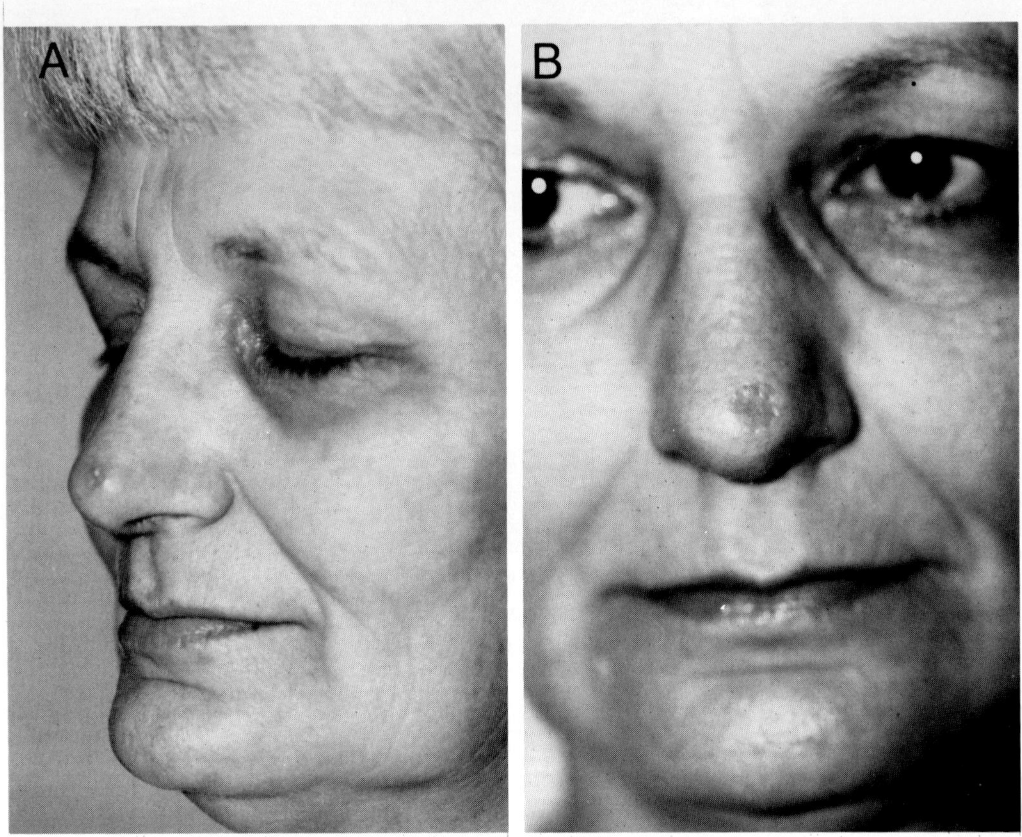

FIG 35–33.
A BCC (**A**) excised and reconstructed with a full-thickness skin graft. (**B**).

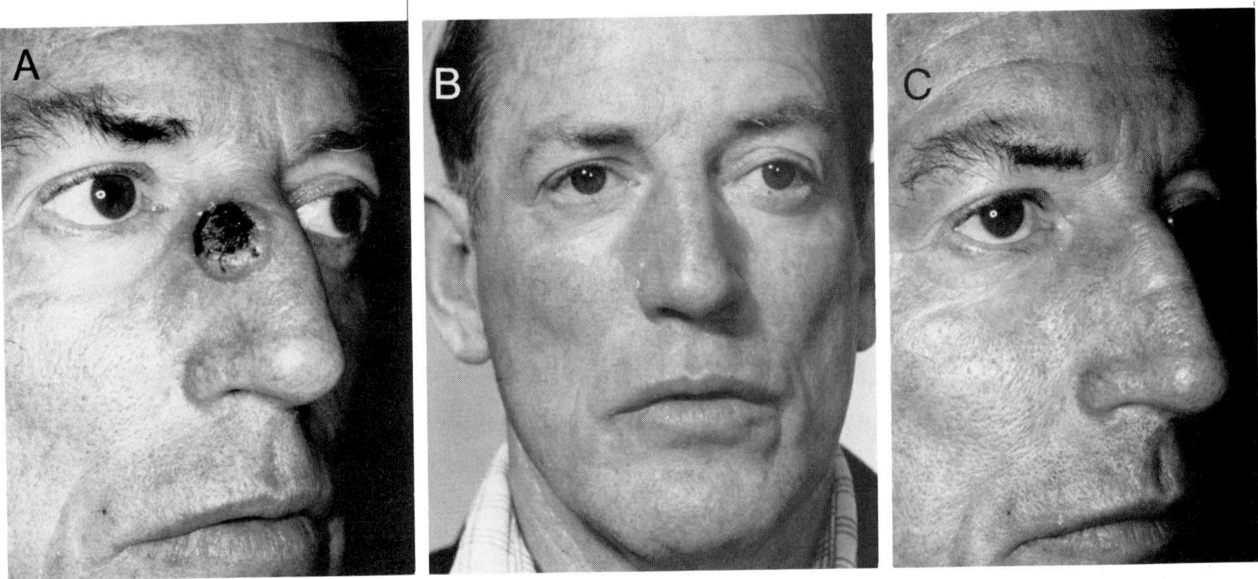

FIG 35–34.
A, KA excised with close margins and the defect resurfaced with a supraclavicular full-thickness skin graft. **B** and **C**, results 1 year postoperatively. (From Patterson HC: *Otolaryngol Head Neck Surg* 1983; 91:263–270. Used by permission.)

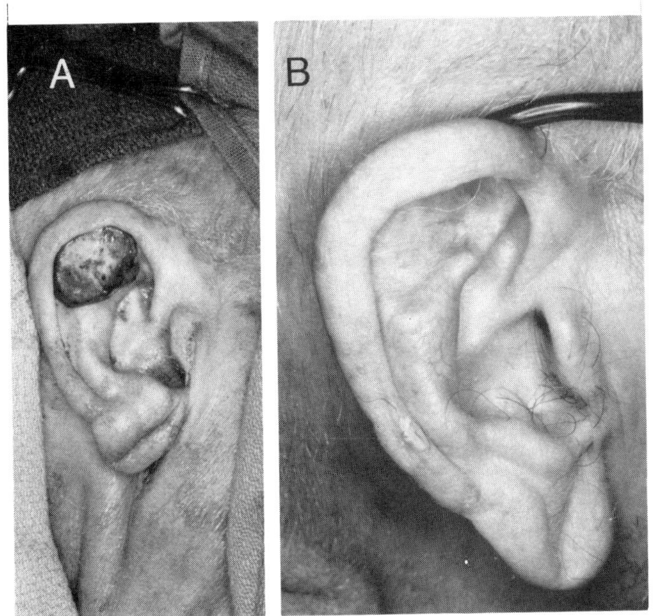

FIG 35–35.
Full-thickness grafts from the upper eyelid or retroauricular area resurface partial auricular defects where the helix is spared quite nicely.

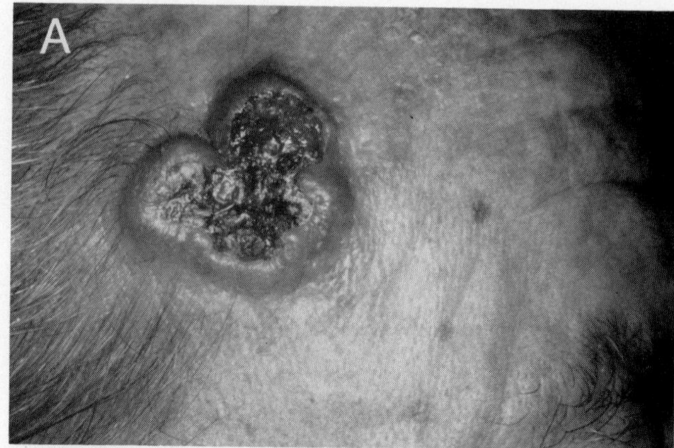
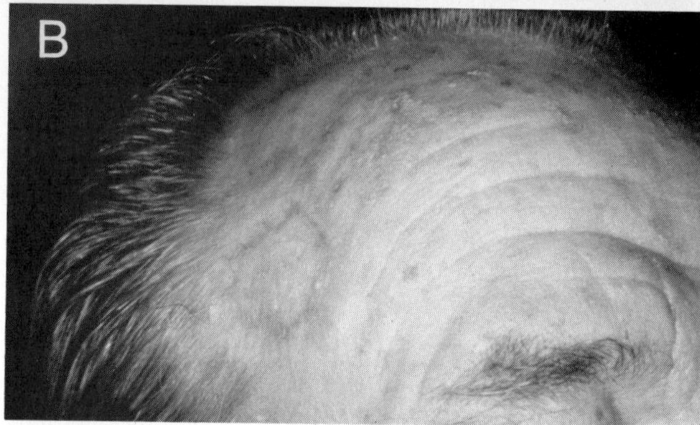

FIG 35–36.
A, poorly differentiated SCC of the temple. **B,** after excision and split-thickness skin grafting. Note wound edge contracture.

that split-thickness grafts are indicated in spite of the poor color and texture match, decreased sensation, and possible need for a later flap reconstruction inherent in grafting. Melanoma[11] or aggressive SCCs, especially if large, serve as examples (Fig 35–36). The patient surgeon will eventually be provided the opportunity to create a local or distant flap to reconstruct such defects after an appropriate disease-free interval has passed.

REFERENCES

1. Davidson TM, Webster RC, Gordon BR: *The Principles and Dynamics of Local Skin Flaps. A Self-Instructional Package.* Rochester, Minn, American Academy of Otolaryngology–Head and Neck Surgery, 1977.
2. McGregor I: Local skin flaps in facial reconstruction. *Otolaryngol Clin North Am* 1982; 15:77–98.
3. Becker FF: Rhomboid flap in facial reconstruction. *Arch Otolaryngol* 1979; 105:569–573.
4. Tardy ME, Thomas JR, Paschow MS: Adjacent skin flaps for facial reconstruction. *Ear Nose Throat J* 1981; 60:37.
5. Becker FF: Nasolabial flaps, in *Facial Reconstruction With Local and Regional Flaps.* New York, Thieme Medical Publishers, 1985, pp 9–19.
6. Karapandzic M: Reconstruction of lip defects by local arterial flaps. *Nr J Plast Surg* 1974; 27:93.
7. Thomas Jr, Goslen B: Effective use of the team approach in facial malignancy. *Facial Plast Surg* 1987; 5:1–92.
8. Maillard GF, Montandon D: The Washio tempororetroauricular flap; its use in 20 patients. *Plast Reconstr Surg* 1982; 70:550–559.
9. Patterson HC, Anonsen C, Weymuller EA, et al: The cheek-neck rotation flap for closure of temporozygomatic-cheek wounds. *Arch Otolaryngol* 1984; 110:388–393.
10. Patterson HC: Facial keratoacanthoma. *Otolaryngol Head Neck Surg* 1983; 91:263–270.
11. Medina JE, Byers RM, Batsakis JG: *Malignant Melanoma of the Head and Neck.* Rochester, Minn, American Academy of Otolaryngology–Head and Neck Surgery Continuing Education Program, 1984, pp 23–26.

CHAPTER 36

Facial Reanimation

Approach of

Harvey M. Tucker, M.D.

The human face is its owner's window on the world. Through it one receives information and impressions of and from one's surroundings. Like most windows, the face works in both directions, returning its wearer's thoughts and feelings in the form of facial expressions. As a result, any unwanted change in facial appearance has impact not only in the real sense that it interferes with accurate communication but, more important, in the individual's perception of how negatively his or her altered appearance will affect those with whom the individual comes into contact. As a result, facial palsy or paralysis is of importance to the physician not only because it may be a sign of major pathology but because of the often devastating effect it may have on the patient's psychologic well-being.

Facial paralysis may result from trauma to the facial nerve anywhere in its course intracranially, through the temporal bone, or in its extracranial course or from any of several disease states that involve it separately or because of its proximity to other structures. Once it is determined that paralysis cannot be expected to resolve spontaneously and that the underlying disease state is either controlled or is not likely to cause further difficulty, attention can be given to rehabilitation of the palsy itself.

SPECIFIC SYNDROMES

Bell's Palsy

Bell's palsy is the single most common diagnosis associated with facial paralysis (60%).[1] It is presumed to be a viral neuropathy,[2,3] perhaps due to herpes simplex virus. By definition, Bell's palsy is a spontaneous, unilateral paralysis in which all other identifiable causes have been excluded. Topographic testing can sometimes localize the lesion to various sites along the peripheral course of the nerve, but the most common localization is to the region of the geniculate ganglion. This primary site of involvement probably is secondary to the presence of the nerve cell bodies of the special visceral afferent taste fibers in the ganglion, via which nerves the causative virus is thought to gain access. Thus, the palsy results from pressure of swollen sensory nerve cell bodies on the motor fibers within the rigid confines of the fallopian canal.

The usual course of Bell's palsy is complete, spontaneous recovery without treatment in at least 70% of patients, beginning within 3 months of onset.[4] All patients realize some degree of recovery; if not, the diagnosis is probably incorrect, and some other cause for the palsy must be sought. Because of such a high spontaneous rate of recovery, the efficacy of any form of treatment, whether surgical or medical, is very difficult to assess.

Medical treatment of Bell's palsy now revolves about (1) management of the eye to avoid corneal drying or abrasions and (2) steroids used to decrease swelling and inflammation of the nerve, thus seeking to minimize long-term damage and to speed up recovery of function.[5–7] Definitive evidence to prove that steroids make any real difference in the outcome of this disease is not yet available but there is general agreement that steroids reduce discomfort and generally do no harm. Adjunctive measures such as electrical stimulation of the facial nerve and muscles, physical therapy, and vasodilators have been of even more questionable value.

Surgical management of Bell's palsy is also controversial. Most current thinking is that if surgical decompression is to be of any value, it must include the geniculate ganglion (if not the entire nerve),[8] except in those infrequent cases where topognostic testing clearly indicates a more distal lesion. Adequate decompression is best accomplished via the middle cranial fossa and combined mastoidectomy approach, although many patients can be managed by the postauricular approach[9] when tearing is intact and the mastoid is well pneumatized.

Timing of surgical intervention also appears to be critical.

Recommendations varying from immediate "emergency" decompression[10] to intervention only for complete nerve degeneration[11] as indicated by electrical studies have appeared in the literature. Timing of surgery based on careful diagnostic assessment and comparison of electrical testing such as minimal and maximal excitability over a 2- to 3-day period after onset of complete paralysis seems to make sense, however, in the absence of firm findings to support the other approaches.[12]

Ramsay-Hunt Syndrome

Herpes zoster oticus results in unilateral facial palsy characterized by pain, which often precedes onset of paralysis, and the presence of erythema, blebs, or both in the distribution of the sensory components of the facial nerve. Multiple cranial nerve involvement is more common than in Bell's palsy. Evaluation and management are essentially the same as for Bell's palsy. Steroids are helpful in relieving severe pain, but strong analgesics are often necessary as well.

Melkersson-Rosenthal Syndrome

Alternating and recurring facial palsies, recurrent edema of the face, lips, and eyelids, cheilitis, and fissured tongue are the hallmarks of this symptom complex of unknown origin. Hereditary factors are often implicated. Since paralysis usually recovers fairly well, at least in the first few episodes of palsy, a conservative approach seems justified. In those few cases wherein electrical testing suggests that degeneration is imminent, decompression may be indicated.

PARALYZED EYELID

Regardless of eventual return of function, loss of tonus or blink reflex can result in serious injury to the eye. It is imperative, therefore, that close attention is paid to protection of the eye from the beginning of any paralysis that involves it.

Surgical intervention should be considered if the paralysis is expected to last more than 6 months or when there is a poor Bell's phenomenon, anesthesia of the cornea, and dryness of the eye (called the BAD syndrome). Widely used techniques include (1) palpebral springs, (2) upper lid gold weights, (3) canthoplasty or lid shortening procedures, and (4) muscle-fascia sling reanimation.

Palpebral Spring and Gold Weights

The use of palpebral springs and gold weights has been championed in the literature by Levine et al.[13] Although my personal experience with this technique is limited, it appears to be a valid approach and may be even more helpful to gain further improvement when it is used in conjunction with other procedures, such as temporal muscle slings.

Wedge Resection

Lower lid shortening is readily accomplished by a simple V-shaped wedge resection of the lower lid, followed by direct approximation. This is especially useful in elderly patients who may exhibit some degree of drooping of the lower lid even before the onset of paralysis.

Medial Canthoplasty

Medial canthoplasty can be even more effective.[14] In this technique, probes are placed in each lacrimal punctum to protect them. Skin is removed just lateral to the inner canthus on both lids to reveal the canthal tendon. The tendons are joined with nonabsorbable sutures, which may be removed in about 10 days. The procedure can be reversed with a scissors in the office.

Temporal Muscle–Fascia Sling

The procedure that has been most reliable for static and dynamic eyelid rehabilitation in my hands has been the temporal muscle–fascia sling. This approach provides simultaneous tightening of the lower lid, improved dynamic eye closure, and, in time, neurotization of the orbicular muscle with further dynamic improvement.

Technique

An incision is made within the hairline, vertically from the level of the zygomatic arch to the insertion of the temporal muscle. Scalp flaps are developed at the level of the surface of the temporalis fascia to expose most of the muscle. When the procedure does not include reanimation of the rest of the face (see later discussion), a single, full-thickness, inferiorly based flap of temporal muscle and fascia approximately 2 cm wide is developed. In this manner, the blood supply and the innervation from fifth nerve motor fibers (both of which come from below) are preserved. Fascia is elevated from the external surface of the flap from below upward, preserving the attachment of the fascia to the distal end of the muscle flap. It is often advisable to strengthen this attachment with one or two nonabsorbable sutures.

A tunnel is developed by blunt dissection from beneath the anterior scalp flap to the orbital rim, and a crow's foot incision is made into it at a point just superior to the outer canthus of the eye. With a fine curved hemostat, a tunnel is created deep to the skin of the lower eyelid from the crow's foot incision laterally to the inner canthus of the eye medially. A small stab wound is made at this point, and a doubled 2-0 silk suture is grasped by the hemostat and withdrawn through the lower eyelid tunnel. The loop of suture is divided so that, in effect, two silk sutures now reside in the eyelid tunnel to provide a backup in case the first suture breaks. The previously prepared muscle-fascia pedicle is delivered under the anterior scalp flap to the outer crow's foot incision. Two nonabsorbable sutures are used to affix the distal end of the muscular portion of the flap to the underlying orbicular muscle at a point slightly above the outer canthus of the eye.

One of the silk sutures is threaded into a needle and is then affixed to the end of the fascia strip. Traction on the suture leads the fascia strip through the lower eyelid tunnel until it can be grasped through the stab wound at the inner canthus. One or two white Dexon sutures are used to affix the fascia to the periosteum of the adjacent nasal process of the maxilla or to the canthal tendon. The excess fascia is removed, the remaining silk guide suture is removed, and all incisions are closed. A drain is placed in the scalp incision.

This technique may be modified by splitting the fascial strip longitudinally and leading the second strip through a similar tunnel made in the upper eyelid. This means of rehabilitation of the eye provides immediate static support to the lower lid. Within 1 or 2 weeks, tightening of the temporal muscle contracts the muscle pedicle, effectively drawing the outer point of fixation of the fascial sling laterally, thus raising the lower lid. Finally, after several months there is further restoration of tonus and eye closure because of neurotization of the orbicular muscle with fifth nerve motor fibers that invade it from the temporal muscle strip.

PARALYZED ORAL COMMISSURE

Many techniques exist to rehabilitate the paralyzed oral commissure, largely because none of them is totally satisfactory. If an ideal method existed, it would: (1) achieve perfect return of voluntary and mimetic function, (2) require only one stage, (3) provide separate motion of the mouth and eye, (4) recover function in a short time, and (5) do so without serious deficit to other head and neck functions.

In approximate order of preference, the methods available to restore oral commissure movement are:

1. End-to-end anastomosis of ipsilateral facial nerve
2. Interpositional grafting of facial nerve
3. Cranial nerve VII-VII crossover
4. Crossover from other cranial nerves (e.g., cranial nerve XII)
5. Nerve-muscle pedicle from cervical nerves
6. Dynamic slings (e.g., temporal, masseter)
7. Static slings
8. Minor tailoring techniques

Generally, the best results are achieved when the facial nerve itself (no. 1 and 2) can be used as a source for reinnervation, since whatever activity results will be appropriate and spontaneously mimetic. Synkinesis, mass action, and loss of nerve fiber population at anastomotic sites are all problems commonly seen with this means of rehabilitation. It is imperative that there be no tension between anastomosed ends of the nerve. Therefore, even though quality of return of function is generally inversely proportional to the number of anastomoses necessary, it is better to use an interpositional graft than to attempt an end-to-end anastomosis of a severed facial nerve under tension. It is also important to use the smallest number of sutures necessary and, of the finest material possible, to achieve good approximation of the segments. Good results with facial nerve grafting within the temporal bone, where no sutures are generally used since there is no motion to distract the approximated nerve ends, support the view that the smallest possible number of sutures is best.

Cranial Nerve VII-VII Crossover

Cranial nerve VII-VII crossover seems like a desirable method for rehabilitation, but it is not usually suitable by itself for total rehabilitation, except possibly in very small children. In adults, the length of nerve graft and the time necessary for regeneration of nerve from one side to the other usually results in very little return of function. I find this approach most useful as a second-stage, adjunctive procedure to gain improved motion and spontaneous mimetic activity when superimposed on some other means of basic reanimation, such as nerve-muscle pedicle or temporal muscle–fascia sling (see later discussion).

Technique

A graft of approximately 10 cm is obtained from the greater auricular nerve (although any suitable source will do). Bilateral incisions are made in the nasoalar creases and extended for a short distance into the nasolabial creases as well. With sharp and blunt dissection, the fibers of the levator muscle of the corner of the mouth are identified and elevated. Branches of the buccal division of the facial nerve will be encountered in the fat pad immediately deep to this muscle. Once identified grossly, they can be confirmed (at least on the normal side) using an electrical nerve tester. On the paralyzed side, even after prolonged loss of function, it is usually possible not only to find the nerve branches anatomically but to observe muscular activity in response to electrical stimulation, provided that the nerve tester is set at 5 to 7 mamp.

Under an operating microscope, the branches of the facial nerve on the normal side are traced proximally as far as possible. The nerve graft is led through a tunnel created bluntly between the cheek incisions just beneath the nasal spine. The buccal division is transected on the normal side, and an end-to-end anastomosis of the proximal portion of this branch to the nerve graft is accomplished using a minimum number (two or three) of 10-0 nylon sutures. The facial nerve branches previously identified on the paralyzed side are likewise traced proximally and divided. The end of the nerve graft is anastomosed to the distal portion of this nerve branch, again using 10-0 nylon sutures. The wounds are closed meticulously after first placing small drains.

The slight weakness created on the normal side by severing peripheral branches of the buccal division of the facial nerve actually improves symmetry initially. Moreover, within several months this weakness usually recovers. Return of function usually begins on the paralyzed side in 2 to 4 months, but as much as 1 year has been necessary in some ultimately successful cases. Some degree of useful return of function has been achieved in 80% of my cases, although the amount of motion can vary from barely detectable improvement to almost normal function. When superimposed on a previously successful baseline procedure, such as nerve-muscle pedicle reinnervation or temporal muscle–fascia sling, it can add significantly improved ability to elevate the corner of the mouth, as well as an automatic trigger that does not require that the patient think about smiling.

Cranial Nerve XII-VII Crossover

Cranial nerve XII-VII crossover is probably the most widely used basic procedure for total facial rehabilitation when the facial nerve itself is not available. Its disadvantages include (1) mass action that does not separate eye closure from oral commissure function, (2) at least temporary slurring of speech due to unilateral tongue paralysis, and (3) a relatively long time lapse before return of function. Adjunctive reinnervation procedures such as VII-VII crossover cannot be used with this technique, since it occupies the neural tubules with XIIth nerve fibers, thus making them unavailable for other means of reinnervation. Recent modifications in technique using only part of the XIIth nerve have minimized tongue weakness and have limited the number of cases in which return of function is more of a grimace than a controlled smile.

Technique

A parotidectomy type of incision is usually employed. The distal portion of the facial nerve is identified. The posterior belly of the digastric muscle is retracted superiorly to expose the XIIth nerve at the point where it passes medial to the muscle. It is mobilized proximally and distally so that an ample length of nerve can be exposed. The nerve is partially transected as far peripherally as possible. The superior half of the nerve is mobilized posteriorly to create a pedicle long enough to reach the distal segment of the facial nerve when transposed superiorly. The posterior belly of the digastric and the stylohyoid muscles may be transected, if necessary, to gain sufficient length of nerve. An end-to-end anastomosis without tension is carried out under the operating microscope using two or three sutures of 10-0 nylon. If the peripheral facial nerve transection is beyond the main trunk where major branches have diverged from each other, the XIIth nerve pedicle may be separated longitudinally into two or three branches for individual anastomosis, as necessary. Supporting sutures of any suitable material may be used to anchor the epineurium of the XIIth nerve segment to underlying fascia to relieve tension and the effects of gravity or motion on the suture line. The incision is closed over a suction catheter drain.

Return of function may begin as soon as 3 to 4 months after surgery, but 6 months to 1 year is more common. Most patients achieve significant improvement in tonus and at least some motion, although it is often mass action of the entire face. Unwanted movement during talking or eating is also sometimes a problem.

Nerve-Muscle Pedicle

Nerve-muscle pedicle technique derived from branches of the ansa hypoglossi nerve to strap muscles in the neck can be used to selectively reanimate muscles about the mouth. This approach arrests denervation atrophy or fibrosis, restores tonus, and can provide useful return of motor function, without synkinesis of the eye. Moreover, return of function is generally apparent in 2 to 4 months, with further improvement possible for as much as 6 months thereafter. Since this approach does not involve the facial nerve itself, it can be undertaken even in cases where spontaneous recovery is still possible. It also permits secondary improvement by nerve VII-VII crossover technique. Denervation of the strap muscles does not impart any clinically significant deficit.

Although this approach has been very useful as a baseline procedure on which further improvement can be superimposed with secondary procedures, it has not often provided sufficient voluntary movement to attain full rehabilitation by itself. Nevertheless, it remains one of the two procedures of choice for initial facial rehabilitation in my hands (the other being temporal muscle–fascial sling (see later discussion).

Technique

A skin crease incision is made midway between the lower border of the thyroid cartilage and the clavicle on the side of paralysis. The sternocleidomastoid muscle is retracted to expose the jugular vein, on whose surface the ansa hypoglossi can be identified. The anterior belly of the digastric muscle is divided, and the nerve traced inferiorly, identifying and mobilizing the branches to the sternothyroid and sternohyoid muscles as they are encountered in sequence. Two or three nerve-muscle pedicles can be developed by excising blocks of muscle approximately 3 mm on a side, including the nerve branch at the point where it enters the muscle. These are developed back to the main trunk of the descendens hypoglossi, which, in turn, is elevated from the jugular vein to the point where it arises from the hypoglossal nerve itself. If necessary to provide adequate length, the descendens cervicalis (posterior) limb of the loop of the ansa hypoglossi may be sectioned, since it contains relatively few of the fibers destined for the strap muscles. A second incision is made parallel to the mandibular margin about one finger-breadth below it and overlying the anterior portion of the submaxillary fossa. Superior and inferior flaps are developed, the upper one permitting access to the orbicular, depressor, levator, and risorius muscles about the corner of the mouth. The previously prepared nerve-muscle pedicles are delivered into the upper incision, and the pedicles are individually sutured to the surface of the exposed muscles of facial expression using one or two sutures of 5-0 nylon. Depending on the number of pedicles available and their relative lengths, the levator-risorius, orbicularis, and depressor muscles of the corner of the mouth are reinnervated in order of importance. Since they are essentially nonfasciated, simple onlay of the nerve-muscle pedicle to the underlying facial muscle is adequate. Both incisions are drained and closed carefully.

Return of tonus, visible motor function, or both may be seen as soon as 2 months after surgery, but 4 months is more often the case. Once movement is detected, further strengthening can be achieved by dynamic tensing exercises (grimacing) for 10 or 15 minutes several times daily over several months.

Dynamic Slings

Dynamic slings have become more popular recently, largely through the reported experiences of Rubin[15] and May.[16] Although the masseter muscle has been used with some success, its direction of pull is not really appropriate. Therefore, the temporal muscle is usually agreed on as the best source for this type of dynamic reanimation.

Technique

The temporal incision is made as described earlier for reanimation of the eye. When the entire temporal muscle has been exposed, it is elevated from its attachments to the skull from above downward, leaving its blood supply and fifth nerve innervation intact at the level of the zygomatic arch. The muscle can be incised full thickness to create three separate flaps if both the mouth and eye are to be reanimated simultaneously. Development and anchoring of the fascial extensions of the muscle strips is as previously described. After reanimation of the eye, tunnels are created subcutaneously with large Kelly hemostats from just below the zygomatic arch to reach (1) the upper lip at a point just lateral to the apex of the vermilion-cutaneous margin at the cupid's bow and (2) the outer corner of the mouth. Incisions are made in the mucocutaneous junction at each of these points, and doubled 2-0 silk guide sutures are withdrawn through each of them. The loops are divided so that a backup suture is left in each wound. One of the guide sutures is attached to the distal end of the fascial strips, which are then led through their respective tunnels. Vigorous retraction of the mouth upward to create a pronounced grimace showing the maxillary teeth and gingiva is necessary so that the muscle fascia strips can be anchored to the underlying lip tissue with white Dexon sutures under sufficient tension. The scalp incision is drained, the guide sutures are withdrawn, and the remaining facial incisions are closed. Tape strips can be applied to further support the grimace that has been created.

Over the 3 to 5 days following surgery, the grotesque snarl will gradually descend, hopefully to a position symmetric with the intact side. It is virtually impossible to overcorrect with this technique, and one is much more likely to end up with insufficient elevation of the corner of the mouth at rest. Within 1 to 2 weeks, successfully reanimated patients will be able to elevate the corner of the mouth when they tense the temporal muscle. Initially this is often achieved by clenching the teeth, but in time most of them learn to accomplish it without actually tightening the other jaw muscles.

I have recently had several very gratifying results by beginning with temporal muscle–fascia sling reanimation, followed in 6 months to 1 year by VII-VII crossover. This latter procedure not only strengthens movement about the mouth without synkinesis of the eye but also seems to provide a spontaneous trigger to initiate appropriate movement of the mouth in response to emotional stimuli.

Tailoring Procedures

Several minor tailoring procedures are available to gain additional improvement after major reanimation has been obtained by one or more of the previous approaches. In my practice, the most useful of these has been Z-plasty repositioning of the corner of the mouth.

Technique

Under local or general anesthesia, incision is made along the mucocutaneous margin of both the upper and lower lip, meeting at the outer corner. These incisions are full thickness, save only for the mucosa, which can be left intact. A third incision is made from the nasolabial crease at the point to which the oral commissure is to be repositioned, diagonally anteroinferiorly to meet the medial end of the upper lip mucocutaneous incision. The flap containing the outer corner of the mouth is transposed with the upper lip skin flap thus described and sutured in layers. The underlying mucosa slides along to assume an appropriate new position inside the mouth.

REHABILITATION PYRAMID

Since no single rehabilitation procedure is likely to provide fully satisfactory results, the surgeon should have an orderly game plan or sequential menu of techniques that may achieve superior restoration of facial function in the aggregate. This process can be likened to an Aztec step pyramid, the base of which is a procedure described to arrest degeneration, provide muscle tonus, and whatever degree of voluntary motion can be achieved. The next step in the pyramid may then be designed to further improve both motion and automatic control, and the third and possibly subsequent steps may be tailoring procedures aimed for fine-tuning or regional further improvement. The process of mounting higher steps on the pyramid (assuming no intervening health or personal issues) stops when either the patient says, "I am satisfied," or when the physician says, "I don't think we can achieve anything further."

REFERENCES

1. May M: *The Facial Nerve.* New York, Thieme Medical Publishers, 1986, chapter 9.
2. Tomita H: Viral etiology of Bell's palsy, in Fisch U (ed): *Facial Nerve Surgery.* Birmingham, Ala, Aesculapius, 1977.
3. Djupesland G, et al: Viral infection as a cause of acute peripheral facial palsy. *Arch Otolaryngol* 1976; 102:403–406.
4. Pietersen E: The natural history of Bell's palsy. *Am J Otol* 1982; 4:107–111.
5. Brown JS: Bell's palsy: A five-year review of 174 consecutive cases: An attempted double-blind study. *Laryngoscope* 1982; 92:1369–1373.
6. Stankiewicz JA: Steroids and idiopathic facial paralysis. *Otolaryngol Head Neck Surg* 1983; 91:672–677.
7. May M: The use of steroids in Bell's palsy: A prospective controlled study. *Laryngoscope* 1976; 86:1111–1112.
8. Fisch U: Surgery for Bell's palsy. *Arch Otolaryngol* 1981; 107:1–11.
9. May J: Total facial nerve exploration: Transmastoid, extralabyrinthine and subtemporal indications and results. *Laryngoscope* 1979; 89:906–916.
10. Bumm P, et al: Residual palsy and synkinesia after facial nerve decompression surgery, in Graham MD, House WF (eds): *Disorders of the Facial Nerve.* New York, Raven Press, 1982, pp 257–263.

11. Pulec JL: Early decompression of the facial nerve in Bell's palsy. *Ann Otol Rhinol Laryngol* 1981; 90:570–577.
12. Hughes GB: *Textbook of Clinical Otology.* New York, Thieme Medical Publishers, 1985, p 250.
13. Levine RE, et al: Ocular complications of seventh nerve paralysis and management with the palpebral spring. *Am J Ophthalmol* 1972; 73:219.
14. Levine RE: Management of the eye after acoustic tumor surgery, in House WF, Luetje CM (eds): *Acoustic tumors.* Baltimore, University Park Press, 1979, vol 2, pp 105–149.
15. Rubin LR: Temporalis and masseter muscle transfer, in May M (ed): *The Facial Nerve.* New York, Thieme Medical Publishers, 1986, chapter 37.
16. May M: Surgical rehabilitation of facial palsy: Total approach, in May M (ed): *The Facial Nerve.* New York, Thieme Medical Publishers, 1986, chapter 39.

Facial Reanimation

Approach of

Newton J. Coker, M.D.

NERVE DECOMPRESSION IN ACUTE PARALYSIS

Idiopathic Facial Paralysis

Bell's palsy is a self-limited disorder with a typical clinical presentation. Patients develop a rapidly progressive facial weakness that worsens within the first 3 weeks. Expected findings include facial weakness involving all divisions of the facial nerve, a numbness sensation in the face, and occasionally retroauricular pain, hyperacusis, and epiphora.

Peitersen followed the natural course of idiopathic facial paralysis in 1,011 patients and found that compared with the age of the population at large, patients from ages 20 to 69 years showed a marked increase in the incidence of the disorder.[1] Men and women were affected equally, except in the fourth and fifth decades of life, when there appeared to be a male predominance. In his study, almost one third of patients experienced an incomplete paralysis or paresis. The remaining individuals, however, developed a complete paralysis. By the third week following the onset of facial dysfunction, 85% of all patients demonstrated spontaneous remission. Nevertheless, 15% of patients progressed to total nerve degeneration and showed a late return of function, not until the third or fourth month following the onset. Those patients with late remission developed the sequelae of faulty nerve regeneration, namely, weakness, synkinesis, contracture, or tics. Seventy-one percent of all patients regained normal function of the facial musculature. Sixteen percent developed moderate or severe sequelae and were more likely to be those patients demonstrating complete degeneration by electrical testing.

All patients with Bell's palsy demonstrate some recovery of facial movement. Another etiology must be sought in those patients with no return of function. The most common true cause of a facial paralysis misdiagnosed as "Bell's palsy" is tumor. This should be suspected in all cases of slowly evolving facial weakness or cases of complete paralysis with no recovery.

Evaluation

Because the etiology remains unproved, a diagnosis of Bell's palsy requires the exclusion of all known causes of facial paralysis. An otologic, head, and neck examination with cranial nerve assessment and inspection of the entire pharynx and larynx should be performed on all patients. Findings other than lower motor neuron paralysis of the facial nerve and conjunctival inflammation due to exposure are rare.

Indicated studies include pure tone and speech audiometry with acoustic reflex testing and for those individuals with a complete paralysis a radiographic evaluation of the temporal bone, preferably high-resolution and contrast computed tomography (CT) of the temporal bone and posterior fossa. Schirmer's test documents the amount of tearing on the involved side so that aggressive eye care can be initiated before corneal exposure symptoms develop.

A number of electrophysiologic tests have been proposed

to follow the degenerative phase: the minimal (nerve) excitability test, the maximal stimulation test, and electroneurography. All are useful only in the acute phase of the paralysis (i.e., the first 3 weeks). In many ways, serial electroneurography as shown by Esslen[2] and Fisch[3] confirms what Peitersen[1] reported in the natural course of Bell's palsy, namely, that the disorder runs its course within 2 to 3 weeks of onset. By the end of 3 weeks, the nerve either has begun recovery with deblocking of neuropraxic motoaxons (and regeneration of injured motoaxons) or has completely degenerated. With complete facial nerve degeneration, no muscle movement is visible by minimal excitability or maximal stimulation testing, and the compound action potential is absent on electroneurography. Electromyography will show fibrillations and no voluntary motor unit potentials.

The minimal excitability test, maximal stimulation test, and electroneurography are unnecessary for an incomplete paralysis or paresis. The patient with complete paralysis within 3 weeks of onset is screened with the minimal excitability test. Stimulation with square-wave pulses over the main trunk of the facial nerve establishes the minimal amounts of current necessary to evoke just perceptible muscle contractions. A threshold difference of 3.0 to 3.5 mamp or greater between comparable stimulation sites over the facial nerve traditionally has been considered an indicator of poor prognosis for return of facial function. Once the thresholds approximate 3.0 mamp, electroneurography is preferred. Repeated suprathreshold stimuli over the main trunk lead to synchronous firing of all intact motoaxons. The peak-to-peak amplitude of the compound muscle action potentials recorded from facial musculature of comparable sites on the healthy and affected sides of the face are used to quantify the amount of neural degeneration. Prognosis for functional recovery is good as long as degeneration does not exceed 90% as measured by electroneurography. When the degree of degeneration is 95% to 98%, satisfactory recovery can be expected in approximately one half of the cases. If degeneration exceeds 98%, the prognosis for normal return of facial function is uncertain.

Although many theories have been proposed, the causative agent or precipitating event is still unestablished. Only a few temporal bones have been studied histopathologically during the acute phase of the disease. Fowler demonstrated edema, disruption of axons, and intraneural hemorrhage,[4] and Proctor et al. found marked edema of the nerve in the internal auditory canal with constriction of the nerve at the point where it leaves the internal auditory canal and enters the bony fallopian canal.[5] The common event appears to be inflammatory with edema of the meatal, labyrinthine, and geniculate segments of the nerve, entrapment of the nerve at the meatal foramen, vascular compromise with intraneural hemorrhage, disruption of the axons, and degeneration and demyelinization distal to the internal auditory canal. This point of entrapment has been demonstrated electrically by intraoperative electromyography.[6] Sunderland has classified neural injuries according to the pathophysiologic events that affect the peripheral nerve and its connective tissue.[7] The first-degree (neuropraxic), second-degree (axonotesis), and third-degree (neurotmesis) injuries occur in Bell's palsy, and often a mixture of the three is present. The magnitude of the third-degree injury with its inherent loss of axons and endo-

neurial tubules ultimately determines the grade of sequelae in recovery.

Medical Management

Many agents have been advocated for the treatment of Bell's palsy; however, the efficacy of all medications remains controversial, because controlled clinical trials are lacking. The efficacy of all treatments needs to be compared with the outcome of natural remission. Nevertheless, steroids are a logical choice in view of the inflammatory events present, but studies conflict as to their value. If used, steroids should be instituted as early as possible after the onset of the paralysis and only in the acute phase of the disease (<3 weeks' duration). Steroids are not recommended in insulin-dependent diabetics or in patients with previous tuberculosis exposure. Their use in the pregnant patient is warranted in the second and third trimesters with proper obstetric consultation. Oral prednisone initiated at 1 mg/kg/day, followed by a 10-day tapered course, is commonly administered.

Careful attention must be paid to the protection of the eye, particularly in patients with complete paralysis and diminished lacrimation. Ophthalmic lubricants and methylcellulose drops used generously, along with eye patching during sleep, are usually sufficient to prevent exposure keratitis and corneal scarring. A temporary tarsorrhaphy may be necessary in the elderly patient with total degeneration.

Pitfalls.

1. Tendency to overdiagnose "Bell's palsy" without a complete evaluation to exclude other causes of facial paralysis.
2. Late use of steroids. The disorder runs its course within the first 3 weeks, so the use of steroids thereafter is probably not beneficial.
3. Lack of aggressive eye care early in the course of the paralysis to prevent exposure keratitis.
4. Failure to follow the patient until maximal recovery of 12 to 18 months.

Surgical Management

The rationale for surgery in Bell's palsy is based on the role of entrapment in the pathogenesis of the paralysis and not on the possible etiologic agent. Histopathologic studies, gross findings at surgery, and intraoperative electrical testing have demonstrated that the nerve is entrapped at the narrowest part of the fallopian canal, the meatal foramen. Edema can produce vascular compromise and disruption of axons, resulting in third-degree injury with faulty regeneration. Surgery attempts to relieve the point of entrapment to prevent the progression of injury from one level to another, namely, neuropraxia to axonotmesis to neurotmesis (third degree).[8]

The efficacy of surgery in reducing the sequelae of Bell's palsy continues to be questioned. General agreement has been reached that mastoid decompression alone has no role in the treatment of this disease.[9] If surgery is to be performed, it must be during the acute phase of the disease (within 21 days) when electroneurography demonstrates 90% or more degeneration.

A middle fossa approach is required to gain complete access to the entrapped nerve from the internal auditory canal to the geniculate ganglion.

One should remember that surgical decompression of the facial nerve for Bell's palsy is an elective procedure to enhance the quality of return of facial movement. To date, the surgery is investigational, and the patient should be so informed. Prerequisites for the surgery include a proper evaluation, a nerve exhibiting 90% or more degeneration by electroneurography within 3 weeks of the onset of paralysis, a patient less than 60 years of age, and informed consent. Contraindications to surgery include an infected field (e.g., chronic otitis), an only hearing ear, first trimester gestation, and high-anesthetic risk.

Surgical Technique

The patient is placed in a supine position with the head turned to the side such that the plane of the squamous portion of the temporal bone is parallel to that of the table. Seated at the top of the table, the surgeon looks at the top of the auricle in the inferior aspect of the field. A one-third to one-half scalp shave, followed by application of povidone-iodine (Betadine) and alcohol solutions prepares the field.

The incision is made in the incisura and carried through the fold of the superior attachment of the helix to the top of the ear. The incision is extended superiorly and slightly anteriorly in the scalp. The temporal muscle and the periosteum are incised and reflected. A 4 × 5 cm craniotomy flap is based on the root of the zygoma, which marks the level of the floor of the middle cranial fossa. The inferior edge of the craniotomy site should be lowered to the level of the middle fossa floor and widened at least 1 cm to each side to create greater access to the superior surface of the temporal bone.

The dura is carefully elevated and the arcuate eminence and the petrosal nerves identified. Aggressive exposure anteriorly usually leads to bleeding from the petrosal vessels or from the middle meningeal artery and its branches. Diamond burrs over the arcuate eminence delineate the blue line of the superior canal. The internal auditory canal can be located inferior to the meatal plane, a flattened surface of the temporal bone in an axis 60 degrees anterior to the axis through the superior canal. The location of the internal canal can also be recognized in an axis bisecting the angle formed by the petrosal nerves and the axis of the superior canal.

For the purposes of facial nerve decompression, the geniculate ganglion is exposed first by removing bone over the petrosal nerves and following these structures proximally. The ganglion is uncovered and the proximal tympanic segment of the facial nerve identified. The bone overlying the internal auditory canal is removed until the dura of the canal can be seen. The limits of the canal should be completely outlined prior to opening the dura. The most tedious step then involves removing bone overlying the labyrinthine segment of the facial nerve because the nerve can be quite angulated. Once this is accomplished, the dura of the internal canal is opened.

An edematous nerve with dammed axoplasm, injected vessels, and focal infarction at the meatal foramen are the classical findings. Erythema extends from the meatal foramen to the geniculate ganglion in most cases. The epineurium overlying the nerve in the labyrinthine and geniculate segments is incised to allow for the complete decompression of the entrapped nerve.

Once the decompression is complete, the internal auditory canal is closed with a muscle plug from the temporal muscle. The temporal lobe is allowed to resume normal anatomic position. The bone flap is secured in place by suturing closed the temporal muscle.

Pitfalls.

1. Failure to carefully identify anatomic landmarks.
2. Decompression of the tympanic and mastoid segments of the facial nerve. Transmastoid decompression is not indicated unless there is an absence of pathology in the labyrinthine and geniculate regions.
3. Late decompression. The purpose of decompression is to prevent complete degeneration and third-degree injury of the nerve; therefore, timely decompression based on electroneurography should be performed only within 3 weeks of the onset.

Herpes Zoster and Facial Paralysis

Ramsay and Hunt first described the association between this viral pathogen and facial paralysis.[10] Otalgia, facial paralysis, and a vesicular eruption over the sensory afferent distribution of the seventh cranial nerve to the external auditory canal and concha characterize Ramsay Hunt syndrome. Other presenting symptoms may include sensorineural hearing loss, tinnitus, and vertigo, which result from cochlear or eighth cranial nerve involvement. The syndrome rarely presents a diagnostic dilemma but can be mistaken for an external auditory canal tumor or infection, such as malignant otitis externa, when the vesicular eruption becomes secondarily infected and the diagnostic vesicles obscured. In questionable cases, elevated and convalescent antibody titers to herpes zoster help confirm the diagnosis. Variants to the syndrome do exist; other cranial nerves with sensory components may manifest the vesicular eruption coexistent with a facial weakness.

Even though herpes zoster is the second most common cause of acute facial paralysis, the natural history is poorly documented. Degeneration of the facial nerve with deterioration of facial function progresses rapidly within 3 weeks of onset, but unlike Bell's palsy, there is general agreement that a greater number of affected individuals progress to complete degeneration and ultimately demonstrate poorer return of facial function.

All infected individuals need a complete otologic, head, and neck examination with cranial nerve assessment. Recommended studies include pure tone and speech audiometry and brainstem evoked response testing in the presence of sensorineural hearing loss. Electronystagmometry or rotary testing should be considered for those patients experiencing dizziness.

Even though the etiology of the facial paralysis is established, the treatment of Ramsay Hunt syndrome remains controversial. Oral steroids have been a mainstay of management in the acute phase of the paralysis, usually in dosages prescribed for Bell's palsy. The efficacy of this empirical therapy remains unproved, and the dissemination of herpes zoster through the immunosuppressive effect of steroids, although a concern, has yet to be reported. Presently, intravenous acyclovir is an investigational agent. The development and use of antiviral agents ultimately will improve the prognosis for return of facial function in patients with Ramsay Hunt syndrome.

Interestingly, the site of facial nerve involvement seen at the time of surgery is similar to Bell's, namely, the geniculate and labyrinthine segments of the facial nerve. Proponents of decompression believe that entrapment, at least in part, plays a role in the progression of paralysis and recommend surgery for those patients who develop progressive degeneration (i.e., greater than 90% by electroneurography within 3 weeks of onset). The surgical management entails decompression of the meatal, labyrinthine, and geniculate segments of the facial nerve.

Melkersson-Rosenthal Syndrome

Yanagihara et al. have classified recurrent idiopathic facial paralysis into various types: unilateral recurrent, alternating bilateral, and recurrent bilateral[11]; and although it is less common in the Japanese population, the incidence in the Western population approximates 10%. Any recurrent paralysis should be suspect for Melkersson-Rosenthal syndrome, and the clinical diagnosis is established in those rare individuals who demonstrate two of four classic manifestations: (1) recurrent facial paralysis, (2) facial edema, (3) cheilitis, or (4) lingua plicata. Associated features include a familial predisposition, trigeminal neuralgia, and migraine headaches.

The presentation and course of the paralysis are similar to Bell's palsy except that in an individual with recurrent paralysis, the likelihood of a normal recovery of facial function becomes less probable with each recurrent episode, and, ultimately, the patient develops residual weakness and synkinesis.

The evaluation should include basic audiometry and, if the manifestations are not classical, a thin-section, high-resolution CT study of the temporal bone detailing the course of the fallopian canal to exclude any possibility of a facial nerve neuroma or other neoplasm mimicking idiopathic recurrent paralysis.

The cause of recurrent paralysis in the Melkersson-Rosenthal syndrome is unknown, but the presence of the disorder in families points to a genetic predisposition. The coexistence of migraine phenomena and facial swelling implicate vasomotor abnormalities in the genesis. Drug therapy for the paralysis is empirical. Oral steroids as prescribed for Bell's palsy are recommended. Middle cranial fossa decompression of the internal auditory canal, labyrinthine, and geniculate parts of the fallopian canal has been performed in recurrent cases of severe progressive paralysis, and findings at surgery are reportedly similar to Bell's palsy. Efficacy of any treatment for the paralysis remains unestablished. The absence of recurrent paralysis in those individuals who have undergone decompression will help establish the effectiveness of surgical decompression and add support to those who believe entrapment plays a pathogenic role both in this syndrome and Bell's palsy.

REANIMATION OF THE PARALYZED FACE

The primary goals of facial reanimation include:

1. Closure of the eyelids and protection of the cornea
2. Competence of the oral commissure
3. Tone and symmetry of the face
4. Voluntary movement
5. Limitation of synkinesis
6. Preservation of self-esteem

The techniques considered to accomplish these goals must take into account the etiology and duration of the paralysis, as well as the functional and emotional needs of the patient. The key to successful neural reanimation depends on the status of the mimetic musculature. Denervated muscle can survive more than 2 years without irreversible atrophy, and dynamic techniques should be performed whenever feasible. A slowly evolving paralysis secondary to neoplastic involvement of the facial nerve is an exception to this general rule; numerous neuromuscular units may be lost before the facial weakness becomes evident. In this situation, successful reanimation with neural reinnervation is less predictable. Electromyography and muscle biopsy should be considered in individuals with paralysis of greater than 2 years' duration. An absence of electrical activity, no fibrillations, no polyphasic motor unit potentials on electromyogram, and muscle atrophy on biopsy make successful reinnervation unlikely. Static methods of reanimation should be employed. The etiology of paralysis will play a definite role in the prognostication of return of facial function. Factors negatively influencing return of facial function following dynamic techniques include a neoplastic etiology of the paralysis, lesions of the nerve close to the facial motor nucleus, gunshot injuries of the temporal bone, irradiation, and poor medical condition of the patient.

If the continuity of the facial nerve has been lost or the nerve has sustained a severe traumatic injury (Sunderland's fourth degree or fifth degree), facial function will never be normal regardless of the method of reanimation. The reanimated face will exhibit limitations in voluntary movement and synkinesis if reinnervation techniques are performed. The subtlety of emotion or expression will be lost. Both the patient and the physician have to be aware of the limitations of these procedures in terms of restoring "normal" facial tone and function. Nevertheless, the outcome of these techniques can be entirely satisfactory in terms of accomplishing functional goals (i.e., competence of the eyelid and oral commissure), and voluntary movement in most cases can be very acceptable.

The techniques available to accomplish the goals of facial reanimation can be classified as dynamic or static. Dynamic procedures provide a new source of regenerating motoaxons to supply the denervated facial musculature or involve the use of a regional neuromuscular pedicle or neurovascular muscle free graft transferred and attached to a local blood and nerve supply in the face. Dynamic procedures include (in order of preference):

1. Direct end-to-end anastomosis with or without rerouting of the facial nerve
2. Interpositional grafts
3. Cranial nerve crossovers
4. Cross-face grafting

Static procedure include masseter and temporal muscle transfers, fascial slings, eyelid weights or springs, and various cosmetic procedures. Static procedures can restore tone and symmetry to the face but offer limited voluntary movement.

Neurorrhaphy Techniques

The best results for facial reanimation are achieved by direct end-to-end anastomosis of the facial nerve or interpositional grafting. The techniques for neurorrhaphy are similar for both. Whether or not a direct anastomosis can be done depends on the amount of tension at the anastomotic site. If the ends of the proximal and distal stumps can be approximated without tension, the direct anastomosis should be done. If tension is present, the option of rerouting may be considered. Rerouting of the facial nerve from the internal auditory canal to the distal mastoid segment is a practical consideration in transverse fractures of the temporal bone with sensorineural hearing loss and in translabyrinthine removal of cerebellopontine angle tumors when the continuity of the nerve has been lost. However, in most other situations, interpositional grafting should be performed. Rerouting entails removal of the nerve from the fallopian canal (and its blood supply), so the superiority of direct end-to-end anastomosis after rerouting over interpositional grafting remains to be demonstrated.

A perineurium-to-perineurium technique should be done when possible.[12] The epineurium on the ends of the nerves to be grafted should be removed approximately 5 mm to each side of the anastomotic site and then a slightly oblique cut with a very sharp blade made across the nerve stumps. The nerve ends are approximated and then joined with at least four to six fine monofilament sutures (9-0 or 10-0). An oblique cut is recommended to increase the surface area available for the regenerating neurofilaments crossing the anastomotic site.

When interpositional grafting is required, donor nerves can be harvested from the neck or lower extremity.[12] The greater auricular nerve courses over the sternocleidomastoid muscle in a direction bisecting a line between the mastoid tip and angle of the mandible. The sensory nerve travels from Erb's point toward the meatus of the external auditory canal. This nerve can provide 5 to 6 cm of donor material. The sural nerve can be identified behind the lateral malleolus adjacent to the lesser saphenous vein. If the nerve is followed proximally, more than 30 cm of graft can be obtained.

Return of function can try the patience of both the physician and patient. As a rule, clinical evidence of return of voluntary movement requires 12 to 18 months for grafts performed in the posterior fossa, 6 to 12 months for grafts in the temporal bone, and 3 to 6 months for grafts extracranially. Good tone and symmetry in repose are to be expected and usually precede voluntary contraction. Voluntary movement is quite satisfactory but occasionally may be weak in the forehead and lower lip.

Mass motion or synkinesis of the reinnervated facial musculature is to be expected because the growth of new axons across the anastomotic site and into the distal tubules is nondirected.

Pitfalls.

1. Closure under tension. An interpositional graft is preferred if tension between the nerve stumps is encountered. If it is closed under tension, the anastomosis will separate.
2. Epineurial closure. Perineurial closure is more difficult than epineurial. If necessary, epineurial closure can be used; however, the epineurium is the source of fibroblasts that can grow into the anastomotic site.
3. Nerve grafting in the cerebellopontine angle is very difficult because of the confines of the surgical field, the pulsation of the brain and cerebrospinal fluid, and a facial nerve that has no epineurium. The use of a collagen splint can prove helpful.

Cranial Nerve Crossover

The hypoglossal, accessory, and motor division or the trigeminal nerve have been used to provide sources of regenerating motoaxons. The hypoglossal-facial nerve crossover is the most common procedure for reanimation of the face when the proximal segment of the facial nerve is not available for grafting.[13] The crossover technique requires that the distal seventh cranial nerve be accessible and that the facial musculature be viable. The procedure is best for patients with paralysis of recent onset, although in many situations the crossover is a backup technique when neurorrhaphy techniques fail. The procedure must be performed before the distal facial nerve is fibrosed and the facial musculature has atrophied. Denervation atrophy is estimated to be complete 24 to 36 months following complete nerve degeneration. Electromyogram and muscle biopsies to confirm muscle presence should be performed in long-standing cases prior to surgery.

The cranial nerve XII-VII crossover is accomplished through a parotid incision with extension of the lower part of the incision anteriorly approximately 4 cm below the angle and body of the mandible. The facial nerve is identified entering the posterior parotid gland along the axis formed by the bisection of a line between the pointer of the tragal cartilage and the mastoid tip. The main trunk of the nerve is freed from the stylomastoid foramen to the pes anserinus. The hypoglossal nerve is identified in the neck medial to the tendon of the digastric muscle and freed from the surrounding tissue proximally from the occipital artery distally to its insertion into the tongue musculature. The nerve is cut at its most distal point and rerouted to the main trunk of the facial nerve, which has been transected at its most proximal point. The neurorrhaphy is then performed.

Movement usually appears 3 to 4 months after surgery. Good tone and symmetry can be anticipated. The eye is usually protected by a competent orbicular sphincter, and intentional movements of the face can be achieved by self-directed movements of the tongue. Varying degrees of mass movement will be evident. Unilateral denervation of the tongue rarely produces speech or mastication problems.

Pitfalls.

1. Tension at the anastomosis. Additional nerve length can be obtained by passing the hypoglossal under the digastric muscle.
2. Mass movement. Excessive mass movement in the midface may be reduced by clipping the buccal branches and directing the regenerating axons to the upper and lower halves of the face.

Cross-Face Grafting

The superior methods of reanimation include direct anastomosis or interpositional grafting of the facial nerve. Advocates of neuromuscular pedicles, reneurotization, and neurovascular muscle free grafts are few, and the experience is too limited to draw conclusions. Cross-face grafting, in theory, offers the best means of targeting functional areas (i.e., eye and mouth) for reinnervation by using less important branches of the contralateral nerve.

If large buccal and orbitozygomatic branches of the normal side are connected to the orbitozygomatic and mandibular branches of the denervated nerve via tunneled cable grafts (sural nerve), most of the goals of reanimation should be fulfilled: protection of the eye, oral competence, improved symmetry, emotional and voluntary movement, and limitation of synkinesis. However, the population of regenerating axons becomes too limited to provide forceful contraction. (Also, this is a criticism of neuromuscular pedicles and reneurotization.) The procedure may be considered for augmentation of symmetry in repose but not as a primary means of dynamic rehabilitation. The use of cross-face grafting with free flap muscle transfer is under investigation.

Static Reanimation of the Face

Masseter and temporal muscle transfers are used for patients with long-standing facial paralysis who have atrophy of the facial musculature or for those patients who lack a distal facial nerve for reinnervation. The results are inferior to the dynamic reanimation techniques, but muscle transfers can provide symmetry and contour to the face and fair sphincter action to the eye and mouth. I do not recommend temporal muscle transfer to the periorbital region, because results can be cosmetically unpleasing in terms of muscle bulk over the zygoma or fascial sling action around the eye. Masseter muscle transfer to correct the sagging oral commissure with cosmetic tarsorrhaphy or upper eyelid weights to provide eyelid closure is preferred management.

Masseter Muscle Transfer

An external approach to the masseter provides the best exposure. The parotid gland is reflected through a standard incision to gain access to the muscle medially. The muscle is detached from its insertion on the body of the mandible and rotated anteriorly toward the oral commissure. The neurovascular bundle entering the medial surface of the muscle passes between the condyle and coronoid process should be protected.

The deep fascial covering on the medial surface of the muscle and the periosteal attachments at the inferior border should be preserved. The subcutaneous dissection extends to the oral commissure. Separate external incisions are made in the nasolabial fold and in the lower lateral oral commissure and tunnels created to allow passage of the masseter muscle. The muscle is divided into two slips at the inferior border, and the ends are sutured to the upper and lower lateral orbicular region of the mouth.

An alternative to the use of the temporal muscle to reanimate the eye is masseter reanimation of the lower half of the face and the use of gold weight or spring implants as described by May.[14] Gold weights are recommended for patients with lid paresis, and springs are recommended for patients with total eyelid paralysis.

Pitfalls.—Pitfalls of the technique include a failure to overcorrect, because with time the face will sag. The end of the masseter muscle must be secured with several nonabsorbable sutures, preferably 4-0 monofilament, to prevent separation. Jaw movement should be restricted for 1 week postoperatively.

Gold Weight Implantation of the Upper Eyelid[14]

Following local anesthesia to the cornea and upper eyelid, a 1 cm incision is made in the tarsal-supratarsal fold. A pocket overlying the tarsus is created by tunneling through subcutaneous tissue and the orbicularis and levator muscles of the eye. A 1 by 5 by 10 mm 24-carat weight is secured in the pocket with 8-0 monofilament suture through three preexisting holes in the weight—two sutures to the septal tissue and one suture inferiorly to the tissue lateral to the tarsus. The wound is closed in two layers with absorbable suture.

Pitfalls.—Lid droop is one pitfall. Lid closure is overcorrected but tends to improve as the levator muscle strengthens.

Palpebral Spring[14]

A spring made of 0.3 mm round orthodontic wire looped once with two 4 cm arms is implanted through two incisions. One incision in the supratarsal fold is carried down to the tarsal plate. A second incision exposes the lateral orbital rim, and a spinal needle is used to pass the lower limb of the spring lateral to the tarsus. The fulcrum of the spring is secured to periosteum at the lateral canthus. The upper limb is sutured to the periosteum of the laterosuperior orbital rim. Finally, the lower limb is enveloped in 3 by 4 mm Dacron mesh and closed in a pocket over the tarsus.

Pitfalls.

1. Extrusion. Use of a larger-gauge or less malleable wire may lead to extrusion. The Dacron mesh is rec-

ommended to prevent extrusion of the lower limb of the spring.

2. Lid droop. If lid droop is not self-correcting, removal of the spring and use of an alternate technique should be considered.

The primary aim of eyelid reanimation is protection of the cornea. Factors predisposing the cornea to keratitis include complete paralysis, diminished lacrimation, poor patient compliance with medical management, lagophthalmos and ectropion, and hypesthesia (trigeminal). Lateral tarsorrhaphy is an effective means of protecting the cornea but, as a permanent measure, is cosmetically unacceptable to many patients. Alternative static measures include the use of the palpebral springs, gold weights, and canthoplasty to improve lid tone and function. When they are combined with secondary procedures such as blepharoplasty, rhytidectomy, or brow lifts, the cosmetic results are quite pleasing and superior to measures involving temporal muscle transfer.

REFERENCES

1. Peitersen E: The natural history of Bell's palsy. *Am J Otol* 1982; 4:107–111.
2. Esslen E: *The Acute Facial Palsies.* New York, Springer-Verlag, 1977.
3. Fisch U: Total facial nerve decompression and electro-neuronography, in Silverstein H, Norrell H (eds): *Neuro-logical Surgery of the Ear.* Birmingham, Ala, Aesculapius, 1977.
4. Fowler EP Jr: The pathologic findings in a case of facial paralysis. *Trans Am Acad Ophthalmol Otolaryngol* 1963; 67:187–197.
5. Proctor B, Corgill DA, Proud G: The pathology of Bell's palsy. *Trans Am Acad Ophthalmol Otolaryngol* 1976; 82:70–80.
6. Gantz BJ, Gmuer A, Fisch U: Intraoperative evoked electromyography in Bell's palsy. *Am J Otolaryngol* 1982; 3:273–278.
7. Sunderland S: *Nerve and Nerve Injuries,* ed 2. New York, Churchill Livingstone, 1978.
8. Fisch U: Surgery for Bell's palsy. *Arch Otolaryngol* 1981; 107:1–11.
9. May M, Klein SR, Taylor FH: Idiopathic (Bell's) facial palsy: Natural history defies steroid or surgical treatment. *Laryngoscope* 1985; 95:406–409.
10. Ramsay HJ, Hunt JR: Herpetic inflammations of the geniculate ganglion. A new syndrome and its aural complications. *Arch Otolaryngol* 1907; 36:371–381.
11. Yanagihara N, Mori H, Kozawa T, et al: Bell's palsy: Non-recurrent v recurrent and unilateral v bilateral. *Arch Otolaryngol Head Neck Surg* 1984; 110:374–377.
12. Fisch U: Facial nerve grafting. *Otolaryngol Clin North Am* 1974; 7:517–529.
13. Conley J: Hypoglossal crossover—122 cases. *Otolaryngol Head Neck Surg* 1977; 84:763–768.
14. May M: Gold weight and wire spring implants as alternatives to tarsorrhaphy. *Arch Otolaryngol Head Neck Surg* 1987; 113:656–660.

Infections of the Head and Neck

CHAPTER 37

Infections of the Oral Cavity

Approach of

Sally R. Shott, M.D.,

and

Robin T. Cotton, M.D.

Federal statistics show that 281,000 tonsillectomies, adenoidectomies, or both were performed in 1986, in contrast with the 629,000 similar procedures performed in 1976.[1] Obviously, in the past 10 years, the philosophy and approach to surgery on the tonsils and adenoids have changed substantially. Tonsillectomy has traditionally been one of the most frequent surgical procedures performed. As medical economics have become more of a reality, this procedure has been closely scrutinized, and specific indications for tonsillectomy and adenoidectomy have been established. Current indications for tonsillectomy or adenoidectomy include recurrent episodes of tonsillitis, more than four episodes per year. Chronic tonsillar hypertrophy in a patient with a physical examination consistent with cor pulmonale should be treated with tonsillectomy. Obstructive sleep apnea or severe upper airway obstruction that has not yet progressed to the more severe cor pulmonale or apnea syndromes should also be treated with tonsillectomy, adenoidectomy, or both. Because the pediatric population usually requires a general anesthesia for drainage for a peritonsillar abscess, we believe that tonsillectomy should be performed at the same time.

Hypertrophy of the tonsils and adenoids causing upper airway obstruction ultimately may influence dentofacial growth and configuration of the child. Surgery should be considered in children who are constant mouth breathers. Waiting for the child to outgrow their hypertrophied adenoids and nasal obstruction can have significant long-term effects on their facial appearance.

Any child under suspicion for a malignancy involving the tonsillar tissue should undergo a complete tonsillectomy as the minimum biopsy.

Relative indications for tonsillectomy include chronic pharyngitis, including those patients who have had chronic sore throats for more than 6 months with chronic cervical lymphadenitis who have been unresponsive to medical therapy. In addition, patients with halitosis believed to be secondary to persistent debris in the tonsillar crypts may benefit from tonsillectomy. Patients with poorly controlled diabetes or sickle cell anemia, exacerbated by recurrent tonsillitis, may benefit from tonsillectomy to stabilize their medical condition.

The issue of hypertrophied adenoids and their relationship to recurrent otitis media has been somewhat controversial. We believe that in a child who has a history of recurrent otitis media and evidence of nasal obstruction from a large adenoid pad, adenoidectomy is helpful in clearing purulent secretions from the entrance to the eustachian tubes.

OUTPATIENT VERSUS INPATIENT SURGERY

In the last 5 years, we have moved from performing all of our tonsillectomy and adenoidectomy surgery on an inpatient basis with preoperative admission and postoperative observation to performing the majority of the surgery on an outpatient basis. We do, however, have very specific indications for postoperative admission on the day of surgery after tonsillectomy and adenoidectomy are performed. Patients with any of the following preoperative factors are admitted postoperatively and observed overnight[2]:

1. Age less than 3 years

2. Transportation time from hospital more than 1 hour
3. History of obstructive sleep apnea
4. Coexisting medical problems
5. Social circumstances with inadequate postoperative adult observation

All other patients have their surgery performed on an outpatient basis.

If these criteria are followed, outpatient surgery for tonsillectomy and adenoidectomy is both a safe and cost-effective use of ambulatory surgery. In 1986, we performed a prospective study on 421 consecutive tonsillectomy or tonsillectomy plus adenoidectomy surgeries and found that those procedures performed on an outpatient basis were as safe as those performed with postoperative inpatient admission.[2] The critical period for immediate postoperative bleeding was approximately 4 hours after surgery, and, therefore, all patients remain in the surgical postoperative area for this length of time before being discharged.

In this study, we evaluated all patients who required readmission to the hospital following their surgery because of postoperative bleeding. Out of this group of 421 patients, 9 patients were readmitted following their surgery because of bleeding problems. Four of these patients had been admitted for 24 hours of observation following their surgery, and the remaining five had been performed on an outpatient basis. Although one of these patients presented with hemorrhage 36 hours after surgery, the remaining eight did not present until between 3 and 9 days postoperatively.

We also had 7 admitted patients in this group of 421 who required readmission because of dehydration and vomiting with poor oral intake. Of the seven patients, four had been admitted after their surgery for 24 hours observation and were not discharged until they were taking fluids well. The remaining three had gone home immediately after their surgery.

We found from this study that if one uses specific admission criteria, tonsillectomy and adenoidectomy can be performed quite safely as outpatient procedures. We stress, however, the importance of these very specific criteria for inpatient postoperative observation. It is important to evaluate a patient's need for postoperative admission not only from a medical standpoint but also from a social viewpoint. Poor access to follow-up health care as well as poor parental supervision or reliability are all valid reasons to keep a child in the hospital after surgery.

SURGICAL TECHNIQUE

All surgery is performed as same-day surgery unless there are extenuating medical circumstances. The patient is instructed not to eat or drink after midnight prior to surgery. The child is brought into the operating room, and general anesthetic with endotracheal intubation is instituted. A rolled towel is placed under the shoulders to achieve better extension of the neck. A Blair drape is used at the head and secured with a towel clip. A single sterile sheet drapes off the body. The table is turned approximately 45 degrees from anesthesia, and the surgeon sits at the patient's head. A Crowe-Davis mouth retractor is placed in the oral cavity. The retractor is attached to the Mayo stand for suspension. This retractor secures the endotracheal tube in position, and no taping of the tube is required. A Rae endotracheal tube provides the proper angle and is not kinked off by the Crowe-Davis mouth retractor. A red rubber catheter is passed through one nares and used to retract the soft palate. It is standard practice to palpate the hard palate to rule out an occult submucous cleft. A bifid uvula would also suggest this. In addition, examination of the pharynx and nasopharynx is performed for any significant pulsations suggesting an aberrant course of the carotid artery. The laryngeal mirror is used to visualize the adenoids. If the procedure includes an adenoidectomy as well as a tonsillectomy, the adenoidectomy is performed first. Adenoid curettes are placed under direct vision using the laryngeal mirror, and the adenoid tissue is removed. Emphasis is placed on removing the adenoid tissue blocking the posterior choanae. Although it is important to remove the laterally placed adenoid tissue that may be blocking the eustachian tube, one should not curette too far laterally, because this can cause scarring around the eustachian tube orifice. Several surgical sponges are placed in the nasopharynx to achieve hemostasis.

Attention is then directed to the tonsils. The majority of our tonsillectomies are performed using the electrocautery technique. A small piece of red rubber catheter is used to cover up most of the cautery blade except for the distal 1 cm. This protects the patient from any inadvertent burns. The tonsil is grasped with a straight Allis clamp and retracted medially. An incision is made through anterior pillar mucosa down to the capsule of the tonsil. The Allis clamp is then reapplied, incorporating the medial aspect of the anterior pillar and the lateral tonsillar capsule. Using the cautery as a dissector, staying right on the capsule, the operator removes the tonsil from the superior pole down to its inferior pole.

Electrocautery provides good hemostasis and allows the surgeon to stay right on the tonsillar capsule. Cautery into the tonsil does not cause significant bleeding as in the traditional dissection technique but, rather, causes the tonsil tissue to puff up like a piece of popcorn. This allows the surgeon to err on the side of going into the tonsil. The technique requires that the surgeon be very aware of the cautery instrument in his or her hand, because mild problems have incurred through careless cautery burns of the posterior tongue. If proper retraction is done with the Allis clamp and dissection is performed right on the capsule upon removing the tonsil, there is very minimal eschar present in the tonsillar fossa. Minimal cauterization in the resultant surgical wound means less postoperative pain.

It is important, however, for the surgeon to be familiar with all techniques of removing tonsils, because there are occasions when electrocautery removal of tonsils is not the best technique. This would include patients who have significant scarring and blunt dissection is required to best visualize the correct plane of the tonsillar capsule. In addition, if one encounters significant bleeding during the process of removing the tonsil requiring the tonsil to be removed before bleeding can be controlled, frequently electrocautery is not useful because it cannot conduct through fluid.

Hemostasis in the nasopharynx is then achieved using suction cauterization under direct vision with the laryngeal mirror. It is useful to release the traction of the Crowe-Davis mouth retractor for several minutes following the procedure to ensure that no vessels would bleed once the retraction was removed. A reexamination is performed on the tonsillar fossae and nasopharynx, and the Crowe-Davis mouth retractor and red rubber catheter are removed. The hypopharynx is suctioned of any loose blood. This minimizes the need for blind suctioning by the anesthesiologist before removal of the endotracheal tube.

General anesthetic is then discontinued. The endotracheal tube is removed and the patient transferred to the recovery room. If this surgery is to be performed on an outpatient basis, the child receives the equivalent of 24 hours of intravenous maintenance fluid in the next 4 to 5 hours that he or she remains in the hospital. This removes the responsibility on the parent's part of ensuring that adequate oral intake is taken during that first 24 hours. All patients are discharged with adequate supplies of pain medications as well as medication for nausea. Families are given a detailed guideline of adequate fluid intake in their instructions. No child is discharged unless he or she is starting to take some fluid. If there is evidence of severe nausea and vomiting, the patient is admitted and observed overnight.

All patients undergoing tonsillectomy are given a perioperative dose of parental ampicillin and then discharged home on 7 days of amoxicillin therapy. This is in line with the recent study at the Children's Hospital of Philadelphia that showed that such antibiotic coverage decreased the severity of pain, mouth odor, and poor oral intake after surgery.[3]

It is important with all tonsillectomy patients that parents are familiar with a plan of action should the patient bleed postoperatively. We instruct parents that if the child coughs or vomits blood any time after surgery, most commonly at the fifth to seventh postoperative day, they should return immediately to the emergency room where any hemorrhage can be controlled.

All patients who undergo outpatient surgery at our institution receive two postoperative telephone calls from our outpatient department nurses.

A few bits of information are helpful to parents and answer many of the common postoperative questions. Patients undergoing tonsillectomy will frequently have ear pain following surgery because of referred pain. Halitosis also is common. It is also useful to tell the parents to expect their children to have a whitish green covering of the tonsillar fossae for approximately 2 weeks after surgery. Parents frequently look into their children's mouths off and on for several weeks after surgery and are quite relieved when they find that this greenish coating is normal and not a sign of infection.

MANAGEMENT OF PERITONSILLAR ABSCESS

The treatment of acute peritonsillar abscess is a controversial topic. Controversies surround the roles of needle aspiration vs. incision and drainage vs. Quinsy tonsillectomy. We prefer to divide our treatment along the lines of pediatric patients and adult patients, because we treat these two populations differently.

In general, peritonsillar abscesses seem to follow a pattern of several days of throat pain, followed by some improvement, but then a resurgence of symptoms. The abscesses tend to occur unilaterally, and there does not appear to be any relationship to a history of chronic tonsillitis. The patient will usually present with complaints of pain on one side of the pharynx, frequently with an inability to handle their secretions. Trismus is often present because of inflammation around the pterygoid muscles. Ear pain is also frequently present because of referred pain. Examination of the patient reveals unilateral swelling of the soft palate and the anterior tonsillar pillar, with medial displacement of the tonsil. The uvula often crosses the midline toward the opposite side. Because of difficulties swallowing, the patient may be described as having a "hot potato" voice. Cervical lymphadenenopathy is usually more prominent on the side of the infection, and the patient may hold the neck toward that side.

It is theorized that abscesses develop from microabscesses within the tonsillar tissue, which then break out into the area of the superior pole with spread of the pus laterally and inferiorly along the capsule. With potential spread into the retropharyngeal and parapharyngeal spaces, recognition and immediate treatment of peritonsillar abscesses are imperative.

The treatment of a peritonsillar abscess in a child is inherently different from treatment of an adult because of the need of a general anesthetic to ensure safe and controlled treatment to the abscess. We believe that if the child requires a general anesthetic for drainage of a peritonsillar abscess, a tonsillectomy should be performed at the same time. This surgery is performed as a relative emergency. This means that all patients should have had nothing by mouth at least 6 hours prior to their surgery. We also prefer that the patient receive at least one dose of parental penicillin prior to performing the procedure.

Aspiration of the abscess is usually satisfactory in treatment of an adult. Because of the proximity of the carotid artery, we use an 18-gauge needle that has protective tape around it, exposing only the distal 1 cm. This protects the patient in case of inadvertent movement during the procedure. Spraying the proposed area of aspiration with benzocaine (Cetacaine) will provide some pain relief for this maneuver. The 18-gauge needle is then placed in the superior and lateral aspect of the tonsil. Too often failure comes from placing the needle too inferiorly and too far medially. If aspiration provides good evacuation of purulent material and immediate decrease in the medial bulge of the tonsil, this is all that is performed. The patient is then discharged home on penicillin therapy and reexamined within 24 to 48 hours. However, if minimal purulent fluid is obtained or significant medial deviation continues, incision and drainage are indicated. For this procedure, local infiltration with 1% lidocaine with epinephrine 1:1,000,000 is used for the patient's comfort but even more for hemostasis in this highly inflamed mucosal tissue. Once again, the needle used for infiltration of the local anesthetic is protected with a band of cloth tape except for a distal 1 cm to protect the patient from the needle inadvertently going too deep. A similarly protected no. 11 blade is used to incise the area of the superior lateral tonsillar pole. If an abscess cavity is present, it is usually easily entered. A hemostat is placed at the incision and spread into the abscess cavity. It is important that the patient be cooperative for this procedure. The suctioning of loose blood and the patient's own ability to protect their airway are imperative. The decision of outpatient antibiotic treatment vs. the inpatient therapy is, unfortunately, a matter of patient compliance. If the patient is believed to be reliable, he or she can be discharged home on oral antibiotics with follow-up within 24 to 48 hours in case of recurrence of the abscess. However, if there is any question of the patient's reliability, because of the potential spread of this abscess, the patient should be admitted and treated with IV antibiotics.

Indications for Quinsy tonsillectomy in an adult would include peritonsillar abscess in a patient with a history of recurrent tonsillitis. In addition, those patients with a recurrent abscess should be treated with a Quinsy tonsillectomy. Recurrent abscesses in this location have the potential for causing weakening or erosion of the carotid artery wall, which lies just 1 to 2 cm lateral from the tonsillar capsule. There is also an increased risk of jugular vein thrombosis in these recurrent cases.

FLOOR OF MOUTH INFECTIONS: MANAGEMENT OF LUDWIG'S ANGINA

In general, otolaryngologists as a group have had increasingly less experience in dealing with deep neck infections. Because of antibiotics, the patient is protected from infections that may have occurred in the preantibiotic era. However, these infections continue to be life threatening not only because of their potential for spread into the mediastinal structures but also because of their ability to cause rapid airway obstruction.

Ludwig's angina is an infection involving both the sublingual and submaxillary spaces. The sublingual space lies between the muscles of the floor of the mouth and the mylohyoid muscle. The submaxillary space is located in the area below the mylohyoid. The submandibular gland is present in between these two areas. The infection can easily involve both sides of the anterior neck by spreading across the anterior digastric muscle.

Most abscesses in this area are secondary to floor of mouth trauma or dental infections. Infections at the base of the tongue or involving Wharton's duct can also lead to this deep space abscess. Infections involving the mandibular premolars tend to involve the sublingual space, whereas the first and second molars will involve the submaxillary space.

Infections in the sublingual space alone are usually more localized, and though the tongue is pushed slightly upward and backward, there is rarely airway compromise. This localized abscess can be drained usually through the floor of the mouth directly, and recovery occurs most often without incident. However, if the infection spreads to involve the submaxillary space and then spreads to the opposite side, diffuse anterior neck swelling occurs, and Ludwig's angina is present.

This abscess has been described more often as a phlegmon rather than a true abscess, because the tissue is usually found to be rock hard and diffusely inflamed with no true localization

of pus. Incision into the anterior neck should include both submandibular spaces. The tissue is found frequently to be gangrenous, with a putrid smell. Serosanguinous, oozing fluid may be present as opposed to a localized pocket of purulent material.

In patients who develop Ludwig's angina, respiratory difficulties are paramount and should be addressed immediately. A tracheotomy performed under local anesthesia is usually indicated prior to neck drainage. High-dose parental antibiotics are also required.

The drainage procedure in Ludwig's angina consists of exposure of the submandibular and sublingual spaces. After the anterior neck is incised, the submandibular gland should be localized. Because of the woody edema of all involved tissue, precise tissue planes are difficult to delineate, and blunt dissection, with special attention to preserving the marginal mandibular and the hyperglossal nerves, is done. Attention must also be placed to determine if the infection has spread to contiguous neck spaces. This frequently will involve exposure of the carotid sheath and inferior dissection into the pretracheal space. If the infection has spread, it is imperative that these areas also be opened and drained.

After the anterior portion of the neck is drained, numerous drains should be placed. Wide exposure with wide drainage should be continued for several days. Frequently, irrigation of the wound is required to ensure adequate drainage. Removal of the drains should be very conservative. The woody edema may take weeks to months to resolve.

Ludwig's angina can be a life-threatening infection. In addition to the immediate risk of airway obstruction, there are possible complications of mediastinal extension as well as parapharyngeal extension. There have also been reported cases of osteomyelitis of the mandible secondary to this infection. An awareness of these potential problems should guide the physician to the proper evaluation and treatment.

REFERENCES

1. Regional variation in costs of tonsillectomy and adenoidectomy. *Stat Bull* Oct-Dec 1985.
2. Shott SR, Myer CM, Cotton RT: Efficacy of tonsillectomy and adenoidectomy as an outpatient procedure. *Int J Pediatr Otolaryngol* 1987; 13:157.
3. Telian SA, Handler SD, Fleisher GR, et al: The effect of antibiotic therapy on recovery after tonsillectomy in children. *Arch Otolaryngol Head Neck Surg* 1986; 112:610–615.

SUGGESTED READINGS

Paradise JL: Tonsillectomy and adenoidectomy, in Bluestone CD, Stool SE (eds): *Pediatric Otolaryngology.* Philadelphia, WB Saunders Co, vol 2, pp 992–1006.

Kornblut A, Kornblut AD: Tonsillectomy and adenoidectomy, in Paparella MM, Shumrick DA (eds): *Otolaryngology,* ed 2. Philadelphia, WB Saunders Co, 1980, vol 3, pp 2296–2299.

Infections of the Oral Cavity

Approach of

Margaret A. Kenna, M.D.

Acute infections of the oral cavity are common problems in otolaryngology. The management approaches to three of these entities, recurrent acute adenotonsillitis, acute peritonsillar abscess, and Ludwig's angina, have changed with the advent of antimicrobial therapy and orotracheal intubation. Surgery still plays a significant role in the therapy of these clinical conditions. However, better understanding of their natural history and etiology has led to more rational and stringent criteria for surgical intervention, with medical therapy being crucial in the overall treatment plan.

INFECTION OF THE TONSILS

Pharyngotonsillitis is a general term describing inflammation of Waldeyer's ring, which may extend to the cervical lymph nodes. Waldeyer's ring is composed of the faucial (palatine) tonsils, the adenoids, pharyngeal bands, and lingual tonsils.[1] Tonsillitis or adenotonsillitis are other terms for pharyngotonsillitis and indicate varying involvement of the portions of Waldeyer's ring among patients. The inflammation can be bacterial, viral, or fungal in nature, and the differing etiologies can be difficult to tell apart based solely on clinical signs and symptoms. Tonsil and adenoid surgery is considered for recurrent pharyngotonsillitis, secondary to recurrent or persistent bacterial infection, unresponsive to medical management. Tonsil and adenoid surgery for viral or fungal infection is very uncommon.

Bacterial adenotonsillitis occurs in all age groups but is uncommon under the age of 3 years or over the age of 50 years. In younger children, both the tonsils and adenoids are frequently involved, whereas in older children and adults, the tonsils are the main focus of infection, because the adenoids usually atrophy in later childhood. Signs and symptoms of acute infection include sore throat, dysphagia, odynophagia, fever, headache, otalgia, cervical lymphadenopathy, and malaise.[1] If the tonsils or adenoids become acutely enlarged with infection, airway symptoms may also occur, causing snoring, mouth breathing, and occasionally apnea. In most patients, some, but not all, of these symptoms may be present but often are constant

with each infection in a given patient. Missed school or work by the patient or parent, with frequent visits to medical personnel, can be significant contributors to the overall presentation of clinical illness and will add to the stress of recurrent sickness in a family.

Although most episodes of pharyngitis are viral, the episodes that are more severe tend to be bacterial.[2] Group A β-hemolytic *Streptococcus* (GABHS) is the most commonly isolated bacterial pathogen and appears to be more frequently isolated in children than in adults.[3] More recently, alpha and gamma streptococci, diphtheroids, *Staphylococcus aureus, Branhamella catarrhalis,* and *Hemophilus influenzae* have all been implicated as pathogens.[3] Brook et al. have also demonstrated the presence of anaerobes and β-lactamase-producing bacteria from core tonsillar cultures.[4] Documentation of bacterial infection in the pharyngotonsillar area at the time of presenting clinical illness not only helps in the immediate management decision but also establishes the natural history of sore throat illness in a given patient in an objective fashion. However, a positive throat culture should be associated with the clinical signs and symptoms of tonsillitis for it to be considered evidence of acute infection. Positive cultures in the absence of clinical illness most likely represent the carrier state and do not routinely need medical or surgical intervention.

Criteria for tonsil and adenoid removal vary greatly. In the 1984 report by Paradise et al. in the *New England Journal of Medicine,* criteria for tonsillectomy were very strict.[5] They demonstrated that children with seven documented episodes of pharyngotonsillitis in 1 year or five episodes in each of 2 years had less sore throats during the 2 years following surgery than a comparable nonsurgical control group. Many of the patients seen by pediatricians and otolaryngologists do not meet these strict criteria but still have considerable morbidity. The Pittsburgh group is now continuing the study evaluating children with less, but still significant, sore throat illness. Without documentation of illness, it can be very difficult to determine exactly how many episodes of sore throat a given patient has had. Paradise et al., as part of the previously mentioned prospective tonsillectomy and adenoidectomy study, followed 65 children with histories of recurrent throat infection for 1 year.[6] Only 11

"

children (17%) had subsequent episodes of sore throat with documented clinical signs and symptoms similar to their histories. On the basis of this study, it is reasonable to have documentation of sore throat illness prior to considering tonsillectomy.

In the office, it is difficult when one is faced with an unhappy parent or patient complaining of recurrent pharyngitis to not recommend surgery. However, tonsillectomy and adenoidectomy usually require general anesthesia, can have intraoperative and postoperative complications, require missed time from work or school, and may not always solve the original problem. Therefore, documentation of at least several of the sore throat episodes is needed to consider surgical intervention. Because the otolaryngologist is not the primary care provider, records from the referring physician or emergency room can often provide the needed documentation. The objective criteria utilized by Paradise et al. were oral temperature greater than 38.3°C, cervical adenopathy (enlarged [>2 cm] or tender lymph nodes), tonsillar or pharyngeal exudate, or positive culture for GABHS.[5] Other criteria to be considered would be elevated white blood cell count and throat culture positive for pathogens other than GABHS. Patients meeting the strict criteria of the Pittsburgh group will usually benefit from a tonsillectomy. If the patient has three to five episodes each year for 2 or more years, if they are well documented, and there is concurrent loss of work or school, they may also benefit significantly. Patients with only mild symptoms, even if recurrent, with a poorly documented history, or with possible other etiologies (e.g., allergy, smoking, viruses) are not good candidates for tonsillectomy, because the efficacy of tonsillectomy has not been proved in this group, and the risks may outweigh any benefit.

Preoperative evaluation should include, most important, a detailed history and physical examination. Complete blood cell count with platelet count, prothrombin time, and partial thromboplastin time, together with a thorough history, will rule out (or in) many significant bleeding problems. However, von Willebrand's disease is frequently not discovered by these studies, and a bleeding time is needed. A thorough history from both the patient and family will often raise the question of von Willebrand's disease, and further laboratory evaluation may then be obtained. All patients should be off aspirin and nonsteroidal anti-inflammatory therapy for 2 weeks prior to elective tonsil or adenoid removal.

Relative contraindications to tonsillectomy and adenoidectomy include documented blood dyscrasias, such as von Willebrand's or hemophilia; patients on anticoagulant therapy, including warfarin (Coumadin), heparin, aspirin, and possibly nonsteroidal anti-inflammatory agents; and patients with other systemic illnesses. In most patients with recurrent pharyngotonsillitis, tonsillectomy and adenoidectomy are relatively elective. However, there are exceptions, such as patients with prosthetic cardiac valves who have documented recurrent streptococcal infection. In this instance, concern about seeding the valve may be enough to perform the procedure, even if the patient is anticoagulated. Patients with insulin-dependent diabetes can also undergo these procedures safely but need close in-hospital monitoring of blood glucose levels. Patients with other systemic problems should be evaluated on a case-by-case

basis. Documentation of disease frequency and associated clinical signs and symptoms in these patients is extremely important, because these patients are at higher surgical risk in the perioperative and postoperative periods.

The technique of tonsillectomy has varied considerably historically[7] and continues to vary between practitioners. The two most commonly used procedures are Bovie tonsillectomy and dissection and snare removal. Bovie tonsillectomy works well for tonsils with a definite capsule and well-defined plane between the tonsil and surrounding muscular bed. It can be difficult, however, if the tonsils are small or scarred, the capsule is poorly defined, or the surgical plane is not evident. In these cases, blunt dissection is extremely useful and possibly safer in defining the plane between tonsil and fossa and becomes the technique of choice. Once the tonsil is pedicled at the inferior pole, Bovie, scissors, or snare is used to remove it. Hemostasis with all techniques should include packing the fossa with gauze sponges after tonsil removal. Most bleeding points can be cauterized using electrocautery suction devices. With the advent of electrocautery, sutures are used must less frequently and, in certain cases, may actually cause bleeding. Patients who have had Bovie tonsillectomy are sometimes believed to have slightly more pain and delayed bleeding than patients who have undergone dissection and snare removal, although this has not been documented in a prospective fashion. Using the Bovie technique, blood loss is minimal, usually 10 to 15 mL, compared with more than 100 mL in many cases of dissection and snare. When one is operating on small children or a patient who may have an increased risk of bleeding, use of the Bovie can be advantageous because of the minimal blood loss, with this benefit outweighing the possibly slightly increased risk of late bleeding. Bismuth subgallate, when applied to the tonsillar bed as a paste, appears to decrease the rate of postoperative bleeding, both early and late. Bismuth has recently been shown to activate Hageman factor (factor 12) and is currently being evaluated in a prospective clinical trial.[8] Both the cautery and dissection methods of tonsillectomy can be performed very expeditiously by an experienced surgeon. The disadvantages of the Bovie technique include unintended burns of the lips, tongue, and oral cavity, possibly increased postoperative pain, and possibly increased late hemorrhage. The advantages of dissection and snare include time-proved reliability and possibly decreased postoperative pain compared with the Bovie method. Disadvantages of dissection and snare include possibly increased intraoperative blood loss compared with the Bovie technique and possibly slightly higher early bleeding rate. Again, however, these two techniques have not been compared in a prospective, random fashion.

Adenoidectomy is often performed in conjunction with tonsillectomy for recurrent adenotonsillitis. Indications for adenoidectomy alone include recurrent or persistent adenoiditis, manifested by chronic nasal drainage. These patients, usually children, often have associated chronic ethmoid and maxillary sinusitis, which should be identified prior to surgery, because antral lavage may be performed at the same time as adenoidectomy. Other possible reasons for adenoidectomy include persistent middle ear effusion unresponsive to medical management,[9] nasal obstruction (suggested by snoring), mouth breathing, and sleep pauses. The symptoms of nasal obstruction may acutely worsen with each upper respiratory tract infection, when the adenoids (and tonsils) may become inflamed, enlarged, and obstructing. If the patient undergoing tonsillectomy also has nasal obstruction, persistent middle ear effusion, or recurrent sinusitis, adenoidectomy may be indicated and performed at the same time.

Prior to adenoid removal, the uvula and hard palate should be inspected and palpated. The presence of an obvious bony cleft palate, submucous cleft palate, or even a bifid uvula should make the surgeon very cautious, because persistent postoperative velopharyngeal incompetence may occur after adenoid removal. In patients with strong indications for adenoidectomy with some degree of clefting evident, only the adenoid tissue directly obstructing the choanae should be considered for removal. In this case, the patient and family should be informed preoperatively of the possibility of velopharyngeal incompetence after adenoid removal, and other treatment options should be considered. Even in patients without any degree of clefting, it is not uncommon for a patient to have transient voice change or nasal regurgitation of fluids after adenoidectomy secondary to a swollen and less mobile soft palate; however, this should resolve in 4 to 6 weeks.

Many methods of adenoid removal have been advocated. The soft palate should initially be elevated, preferably by red rubber catheters, and the nasopharynx inspected. Visualization with a mirror to establish size, possible infection, and degree of obstruction of the adenoid pad should be performed both before and after adenoid removal. Adenoid curettes and a St. Clair Thompson forceps, used separately or together, provide very effective adenoid removal, even in the posterior choanae. Hemostasis is provided by gauze packs and electrocautery suction.

There should be clear visualization of the posterior septum and both choanae after the adenoids are removed. Persistent bleeding from the adenoid bed may be caused by adenoid tags, and these should be removed under mirror guidance. If there is still bleeding after adequate adenoid removal, packing with gauze, microfibrillar collagen (Avitene), absorbable gelatin sponge (Gelfoam), bismuth, topical thrombin, or epinephrine-soaked sponges may be effective. Rarely, it may be necessary to leave a posterior pack in place for 24 to 48 hours.

At the end of tonsillectomy and adenoidectomy, before the patient awakens, it is essential to have a dry, nonbleeding operative field. Old blood should also be suctioned from the stomach prior to awaking from anesthesia. Both of these measures serve to prevent aspiration of blood in the immediate perioperative period, and good intraoperative hemostasis prevents continued and often overlooked oozing from the tonsil and adenoid beds. If there is persistent or diffuse bleeding from the tonsil or adenoid bed without an obvious cause, the patient should be evaluated for an occult coagulopathy or underlying bleeding disorder, and correction should be undertaken.

Postoperative care includes no vigorous activity and a diet of soft, cool, nonspicy foods. Antibiotics for several days postoperatively may lessen the risk of infection and hasten the patient's recovery.[10] Aspirin and nonsteroid anti-inflammatory medications should not be used for pain control because of increased risk of hemorrhage.

ACUTE PERITONSILLAR ABSCESS

Acute peritonsillar abscess is quite common, affecting primarily older children and adults, with reported age ranges of 3 to 79 years.[11,12] In the past, immediate tonsillectomy, or stab incision and drainage followed by interval tonsillectomy, have been the standard treatment choices. However, several recent studies indicate that incision and drainage, or needle aspiration, and systemic antimicrobial therapy are safe and effective treatment, although they have not been compared prospectively for recurrence rates and initial rate of reaccumulation of abscess.[11,13–15] These same studies base their management strategy on the fact that many patients with acute peritonsillar abscess have no significant prior history of tonsillitis and often go on to have no significant tonsillitis after resolution of their abscess.

In cooperative patients with peritonsillar abscess, stab incision and drainage or needle aspiration will provide adequate drainage of the abscess. Cultures should be obtained, and systemic antimicrobials, usually high-dose penicillin, should be given either orally as an outpatient or intravenously. Outpatient therapy is successful and safe if the patient is not dehydrated, has no associated complications, and will reliably return for follow-up. During the first few days of treatment, the patient should be evaluated for reaccumulation of pus, degree of trismus, ability to take liquids, recurrent fever, and onset of complications. If the patient is diabetic, immunocompromised, dehydrated, or unable to take adequate oral liquids, he or she should be treated as an inpatient with IV fluids and antimicrobials. Patients with decreased ability to care for themselves, such as young children, elderly patients, or patients with impaired mental status, should also be considered for admission.

If no pus is obtained at initial incision or aspiration, either (1) the patient has peritonsillar cellulitis and no abscess is present or (2) the abscess was missed. The patient should be admitted, rehydrated, and started on IV antimicrobial therapy. If there is localization of edema, erythema, and tenderness, incision or aspiration can be reattempted. If pus is obtained, the clinical course should be observed for 24 to 48 hours in the hospital while antimicrobial therapy is continued. If no pus is obtained, or if there is continued pain, fever, trismus, and drooling, tonsillectomy should be performed. Whether to perform the drainage procedure under local or general anesthesia depends on the patient. Uncooperative patients, especially young children, those with severe trismus, or those with airway compromise cannot undergo safe and successful drainage under local anesthesia. For these patients, general endotracheal anesthesia should be employed to ensure adequate drainage and airway protection from infected material and blood. If immediate tonsillectomy is performed, general anesthesia should be used for the same reasons.

The advantages of stab incision and drainage or needle aspiration are (1) either procedure can usually be performed under local anesthesia; (2) the complication rate is very low;

and (3) they can be performed in a timely fashion at the bedside or in the emergency room, thus eliminating the wait for operating room time. Cultures can be obtained with either procedure. Although the two procedures have not been compared side by side, the possible advantage of stab incision and drainage over aspiration is a wider area to allow adequate and continued drainage of the abscess cavity and prevent reaccumulation of pus. Needle aspiration may be slightly faster and possible with greater degrees of trismus than incision and drainage.

The indications for "hot," or quinsy tonsillectomy, have changed. The advent of effective and safe antimicrobials in the past 40 years permits successful medical therapy of most cases of peritonsillar cellulitis, and coupled with incision or aspiration, therapy of peritonsillar abscess. Immediate tonsillectomy is still the surgical treatment of choice in the presence of complications, including neck abscess, airway compromise, parapharyngeal or retropharyngeal space involvement, and venous thrombosis. Immediate tonsillectomy should also be considered for patients with peritonsillar cellulitis unresponsive to medical management and for patients with peritonsillar abscess who have not responded adequately to local drainage and systemic antimicrobials.

There is some controversy over whether unilateral or bilateral tonsillectomy should be performed for peritonsillar abscess.[12] Because there is a low incidence of bilateral abscess, bilateral tonsillectomy is recommended, especially if there is a past history of pharyngotonsillitis.

Interval tonsillectomy used to be standard after peritonsillar abscess.[16] However, several clinical studies have documented that 75% to 90% of patients with documented peritonsillar abscess will not go on to have another one.[14, 15] About 20% of patients with peritonsillar abscess will go on to have recurrent tonsillitis without abscess. The patients who develop recurrent peritonsillar abscess or tonsillitis often give a strong history of recurrent tonsil disease prior to the abscess. It is this group of patients who should be considered for interval tonsillectomy on the basis of recurrent pharyngotonsillitis as well as peritonsillar abscess or cellulitis. In this group of patients, hot tonsillectomy is worth considering, especially if the patient in uncooperative or has severe trismus, and general anesthesia is required for any surgical procedure.

LUDWIG'S ANGINA

In 1836, Wilhelm Frederick von Ludwig described a case of gangrenous induration of the tissues of the floor of the mouth and neck. Ludwig's angina (from the Latin angere, meaning "to strangle") is now defined as a rapidly spreading cellulitis of the sublingual and submaxillary spaces (which together comprise the submandibular space).[17] It is clinically indicated by brawny edema and induration of the suprahyoid area, tender swelling of the floor of the mouth, and edema, elevation, and posterior displacement of the tongue. Most of these infections are odontogenic in origin, with the second and third mandibular molars being most commonly involved. Severe periodontal disease has also been implicated, as well as trauma to the mandible and oral cavity, malignancy,[18] and foreign bodies.

In the preantibiotic era, death rates in patients with Ludwig's angina were high, with Ludwig reporting a 60% mortality rate.[17] Airway obstruction was usually the cause of death and continues to be the major complication.[19] Even before antimicrobial therapy, recognition of airway compromise, with intervention by tracheotomy, decreased the death rate in several series to less than 10%.

Using Grodinsky's criteria,[17] we can separate definite cases of Ludwig's angina from the other infections of the oral cavity and neck. In Ludwig's angina, there is cellulitis, not abscess, of the submandibular space, which:

1. Is usually bilateral and never involves only one space.
2. Produces gangrene with serosanguinous infiltration but very little pus.
3. Involves connective tissue, fascia, and muscles but not the salivary glands.
4. Is spread by direct extension, not lymphatics.

If a diagnosis of Ludwig's angina is established, the patients should be hospitalized and started on appropriate high-dose IV antimicrobials therapy. Many of these patients, because of inability to swallow and handle secretions, are markedly dehydrated on initial presentation and should be vigorously rehydrated. A source of infection, usually dental, should be sought, and extractions or local drainage should be performed if possible and appropriate.

The choice of antimicrobial therapy is based on direct culture, suspected bacteria, or both. Mixed cultures are very frequent. The most common aerobic organisms are *Streptococcus* and *Staphylococcus* species, and *Bacteroides* species are the most common anaerobe.[17, 18] Penicillin is still the most widely used and effective antimicrobial, although other agents may be needed based on initial clinical response and culture results.

The criteria for surgical intervention is nonresponse to medical management, including increased edema, odynophagia, dysphagia, and trismus, and persistent fever. Airway signs and symptoms are the most ominous and important. Stridor, cyanosis, increasing restlessness (from hypoxia), and marked lethargy (from increased carbon dioxide retention) are all signs of airway compromise and possible acute obstruction. If there is any evidence of impending airway decompensation, the patient should be observed in an intensive care environment and an artificial airway support considered. If airway problems are noted in the early stages, orotracheal intubation in the operating room, with anesthesia and otolaryngology personnel in attendance, is often possible.[20] Once this is accomplished, incision and drainage of the floor of mouth and any dental work can be accomplished without compromise of the airway. Early intervention for successful and safe intubation is needed. If the airway becomes acutely compromised because of massive glottal edema, trismus, brawny, enlarged floor of mouth, or cervical adenopathy, intubation by any route—oral, nasal, or guided by bronchoscopy—may be impossible, and urgent tracheotomy is required. This is life saving, but because the neck may be swollen and the patient agitated and hypoxic, tracheotomy in this setting is difficult and more dangerous. Once the airway is secure, systemic antimicrobials are continued, and slow recovery usually occurs. The endotracheal or tracheotomy tube should not be removed until the patient shows a definite clinical response with decreased soft tissue and glottal edema and decreased drainage from surgical sites.

Ludwig's angina in small children is very uncommon and may have an unusual etiology. In a report by Barkin et al., three out of four children were immunocompromised; *Pseudomonas aeruginosa* was isolated in two patients, *Candida albicans* was isolated in one, and *H. influenzae* was isolated in the fourth.[21] In the paper by Patterson et al., 2 out of 20 cases were children less than 3 years of age in whom no obvious underlying etiology could be found.[17] Finally, Shaw et al. recently reported a case of Ludwig's angina in a 5-year-old boy caused by *H. influenzae* type b and associated with uvulitis, epiglottitis, and retropharyngeal abscess. The management of Ludwig's angina in children should be the same as that in adults. However, uncommon etiologies should be aggressively sought in these patients for optimal management.

SUMMARY

The management of pharyngotonsillitis, peritonsillar abscess, and Ludwig's angina is presented. In most cases, surgical management should be accomplished in conjunction with appropriate and aggressive therapy.

REFERENCES

1. Zalzal GH, Cotton RT: Adenotonsillar disease, in Cummings CW, Fredrickson JM, Harker LA, et al (eds): *Otolaryngology—Head and Neck Surgery.* 1986, vol 7, pp 1189–1211.
2. Boat TF, Doershuk CF, Stern RC, et al: Acute pharyngitis, in Behrman RE, Vaughn VC (eds): *Nelson's Textbook of Pediatrics,* ed 13. Philadelphia, WB Saunders Co, 1987, pp 871–877.
3. Brook I, Foote PA: Comparison of the microbiology of recurrent tonsillitis between children and adults. *Laryngoscope* 1986; 96:1385–1388.
4. Brook I, Yocum P, Friedman EM: Aerobic and anaerobic bacteria in tonsils of children with recurrent tonsillitis. *Ann Otol Rhinol Laryngol* 1981; 90:261–263.
5. Paradise JL, Bluestone CD, Bachman RZ, et al: Efficacy of tonsillectomy for recurrent throat infections in severely affected children. *N Engl J Med* 1984; 310:674–683.
6. Paradise JL, Bluestone CD, Bachman RZ, et al: History of recurrent sore throat as an indication for tonsillectomy. *N Engl J Med* 1978; 298:409–413.
7. Kornblut A, Kornblut AD: Tonsillectomy and adenoidectomy, in Paparella MM, Shumrick DA (eds): *Otolaryngology* ed 2. Philadelphia, WB Saunders Co, 1980, vol 3, pp 2283–2301.
8. Maniglia AJ, Kushner H, Cozzi L: Adenotonsillectomy: A safe outpatient procedure. *Arch Otolaryngol Head Neck Surg* 1989; 115:92–94.
9. Gates GA, Avery CA, Prihoda TJ, et al: Effectiveness of adenoidectomy and tympanostomy tubes in the treatment of chronic otitis media with effusion. *N Engl J Med* 1987; 317:1444–1451.
10. Handler SD, Miller L, Richmond KH, et al: Post-tonsillectomy hemorrhage: Incidence, prevention and management. *Laryngoscope* 1986; 96:1243–1247.
11. Ophir D, Bawnik J, Poria Y, et al: Peritonsillar abscess. A prospective evaluation of outpatient management by needle aspiration. *Arch Otol Head Neck Surg* 1988; 114:661–663.
12. Christensen P-H, Schonsted-Madsen U: Unilateral immediate tonsillectomy as the treatment of peritonsillar abscess. *J Laryngol Otol* 1983; 97:1105–1009.
13. Herzon F: Permucosal needle drainage of peritonsillar abscess. *Arch Otolaryngol* 1984; 110:104–105.
14. Holt GR, Tinsley PP: Peritonsillar abscesses in children. *Laryngoscope* 1981; 91:1226–1230.
15. Herbild O, Bonding P: Peritonsillar abscess. Recurrence rate and treatment. *Arch Otolaryngol* 1981; 107:540–542.
16. Kornblut AD: Non-neoplastic diseases of the tonsils and adenoids, in Paparella MM, Shumrick DA (eds): *Otolaryngology,* ed 2. Philadelphia, WB Saunders Co, vol III, chapter 23.
17. Patterson HC, Kelly JH, Strome J: Ludwig's angina: An update. *Laryngoscope* 1982; 92:370–378.
18. Fischmann GE, Graham BS: Ludwig's angina resulting from the infection of an oral malignancy. *J Oral Maxillofac Surg* 1985; 43:795–796.
19. Moreland LW, Corey J, McKenzie R: Ludwig's angina. *Arch Intern Med* 1988; 148:461–466.
20. Allen D, Loughnan TE, Ord RA: A re-evaluation of the role of tracheostomy in Ludwig's angina. *J Oral Maxillofac Surg* 1985; 43:436–439.
21. Barkin RM, Bonis SL, Elghammer RM, et al: Ludwig's angina in children. *J Pediatr* 1975; 87:563–565.
22. Shaw KN, Marshall GS, Tom LWC, et al: Ludwig's angina caused by haemophilus influenzae type b. *Pediatr Infect Dis* 1988; 7:203–205.

CHAPTER 38

Cervical Space Infections

Approach of

J. David Osguthorpe, M.D.

ANATOMY

The deep cervical fascia consists of three layers: superficial, middle, and deep. The superficial layer originates from the spinous processes of the cervical vertebrae and extends around the neck as a continuous fibrous sheet, encircling two muscles (trapezius and sternocleidomastoid), two glands (submandibular and parotid), and two spaces (the posterior triangle and the suprasternal space of Burns), in other words, the "rule of twos." The middle layer encloses the viscera, including the laryngotracheal complex, esophagus, and thyroid gland. The deep layer envelopes the paraspinous muscles and vertebrae, attaching to the transverse process of the vertebrae laterally and splitting anteriorly into a prevertebral and an alar layer. Septae from all three layers of the deep cervical fascia contribute to the visceral-vascular space, commonly known as the carotid sheath, which encompasses the carotid artery, internal jugular vein, and adjacent lymph nodes, vagus nerve, and sympathetic trunk. There are a number of other potential spaces within the deep cervical fascia, many which intercommunicate and have boundaries determined by planes of the greatest resistance (Fig 38–1). There is not a universally accepted definition of these spaces, but this chapter will present the most common classifications.[1, 2]

The lateral pharyngeal space (pharyngomaxillary, parapharyngeal) has the shape of an inverted cone with its apex at the greater cornu of the hyoid and a base across the petrous portion of the temporal bone. It is bounded medially by the lateral pharyngeal wall (more posteriorly by the retropharyngeal space), laterally by the deep lobe of the parotid and the internal pterygoid muscle, and anteriorly communicates with the submandibular space. The lateral pharyngeal space is divided into two compartments by the styloid and stylopharyngeal aponeurosis. The anterior contains fat and lymph nodes, which drain the sublingual, submandibular, peritonsillar, and deep parotid regions, whereas the posterior, or vascular, compartment is traversed by the carotid sheath.

Spaces that involve the deep layer of the deep cervical facia are, from anterior to posterior, the retropharyngeal, the "danger" (visceral), and the prevertebral (Fig 38–2). The retropharyngeal space is situated between the posterior pharyngeal wall and the alar fascia, containing fat and lymph nodes that drain the posterior nose, paranasal sinuses, nasopharynx, soft palate, and eustachian tubes. It extends from the skull base to fuse (at approximately T1-2) with the middle layer of the deep cervical fascia surrounding the esophagus. Directly posterior to the retropharyngeal space and continuing inferiorly to the diaphragm is the danger space, filled with loose areolar tissue and usually infected only by direct extension from adjacent spaces. The prevertebral space contains little tissue and extends from the skull base to the coccyx between the prevertebral layer of the deep cervical fascia and the anterior longitudinal ligament of the spine.

CLINICAL PRESENTATION AND EVALUATION

An individual suspected of having a deep cervical space infection should be questioned regarding recent dental infections or manipulations, head and neck trauma, and infections of the upper respiratory tract, with particular emphasis on the nose, sinuses, adenoids, tonsils, ears, and salivary glands. Physical examination early in the course of infection may disclose little, because deep infections seldom cause brawny edema of the neck skin or externally palpable fluctuance until they are quite advanced. The mucosa overlying an affected space becomes boggy and inflamed, and there may be pain with neck rotation. In advanced disease, the patient's neck may be ex-

706

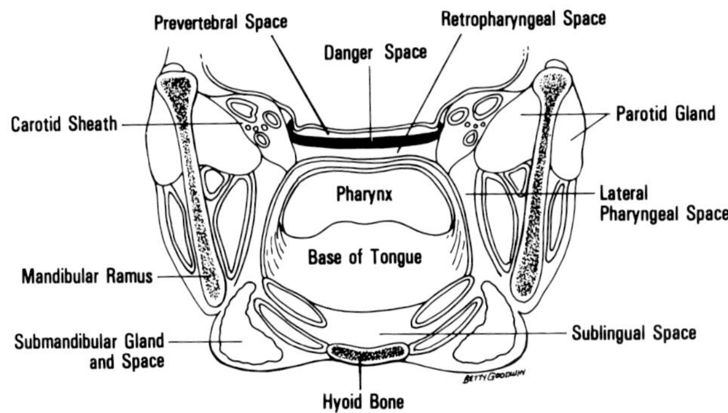

FIG 38–1.
Spaces formed by deep cervical fascia in a cephalad-angled section from hyoid bone through ramus of mandible.

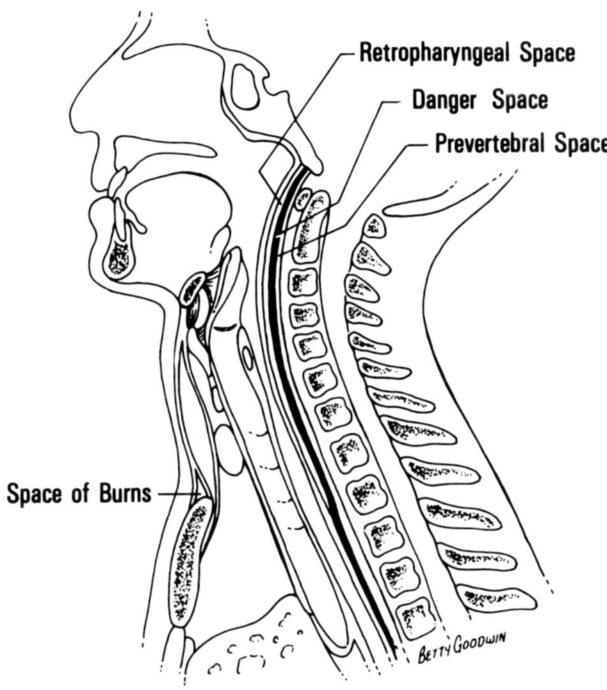

FIG 38–2.
Spaces formed by deep cervical fascia in a midline saggital section of the head, neck, and chest.

tended or tilted opposite the infection focus. Dysphagia and odynophagia occur earlier during the course of retroesophageal infections than those of the lateral pharyngeal space. Noisy breathing, a muffled voice, and difficulty with secretions evolve as the pharyngeal lumen narrows. Patients become dehydrated and have a steady, elevated temperature unless an internal jugular vein thrombosis develops, in which case the "picket fence" temperature spikes of septicemia become evident. Blood studies disclose a leukocytosis with a left shift and dehydration.

Enhanced computed axial tomography (CAT) provides excellent delineation of deep cervical infections, with the hypervascular areas of cellulitis and the internal jugular vein highlighted by the contrast material and any abscesses and air readily discernible as hypodense regions (Fig 38–3).[3,4] When CT is not readily available, the patient is uncooperative, or serial radiographic study is desired after an initial CT, a lateral plain roentgenogram of the neck will frequently delineate gross changes in the retropharyngeal, danger, and prevertebral spaces. There may be air or widening of the retropharyngeal soft tissue from cellulitis or abscess formation (Fig 38–4). The area overlying the second cervical vertebrae (C-2) on a lateral x-ray film averages 4 mm, and greater than 7 mm is abnormal in both children and adults. As a rule of thumb, the tissue should be about one third the width of the C-2 body in adults and equal to the width of the C-2 body in children. The distance between the C-6 vertebra and tracheal air column should not exceed 14 mm in children and 20 mm in adults, but interpretation of this region in infants is difficult.[5]

About one third of lateral pharyngeal infections originate from dental disease spreading posteriorly from the submandibular and sublingual spaces, with additional sources being tonsillitis or other oral, major salivary gland, and ear infections, such as petrous apicitis or Bezold's abscess, and trauma.[5–7] The anterior compartment is more commonly affected and manifests as trismus and medial displacement of the tonsil and adjacent oropharyngeal wall. A large peritonsillar abscess can be difficult to distinguish from a lateral pharyngeal space infection, with the former frequently leading to the latter if untreated. As a lateral pharyngeal infection advances, there is tenderness and brawny induration of the skin behind the angle of the jaw, and the posterior compartment containing the carotid sheath may be invaded. The posterior compartment is a much tighter space, and infection usually spreads by suppuration of lymph nodes along the jugular chain. As these nodes enlarge within the tight carotid sheath, dysfunction of cranial nerves IX through XII or Horner's syndrome may ensue. The internal jugular vein may thrombose as pressure increases inside the carotid sheath, with the carotid artery being most resistent to thrombosis or rupture (see Fig 38–4,A).

Of the three spaces formed of the deep layer of the deep cervical fascia, the retropharyngeal is most commonly subject to infection. Prior to atrophy of lymph nodes in this region at 4 to 5 years of age, paranasal and adenoid infections readily spread to this space. Early, the midline raphe may confine the disease, and the posterior pharyngeal mucosa bulges asymmetrically, but this weak barrier is quickly breached, and the mucosal inflammation becomes symmetric. Patients develop hypopharyngeal airway compromise and dysphagia much earlier than in lateral pharyngeal infections, and mediastinitis from a retropharyngeal process rupturing into the danger space is the most common avenue for neck infections to reach the chest. Prior to the development of effective medical therapy, the prevertebral space was often penetrated by tuberculosis of the spine, but currently most infections originate from trauma to the cervical spine or the surgical intervention for such. Contaminations of the prevertebral space may spread from the skull base to the coccyx, even presenting as a psoas abscess.

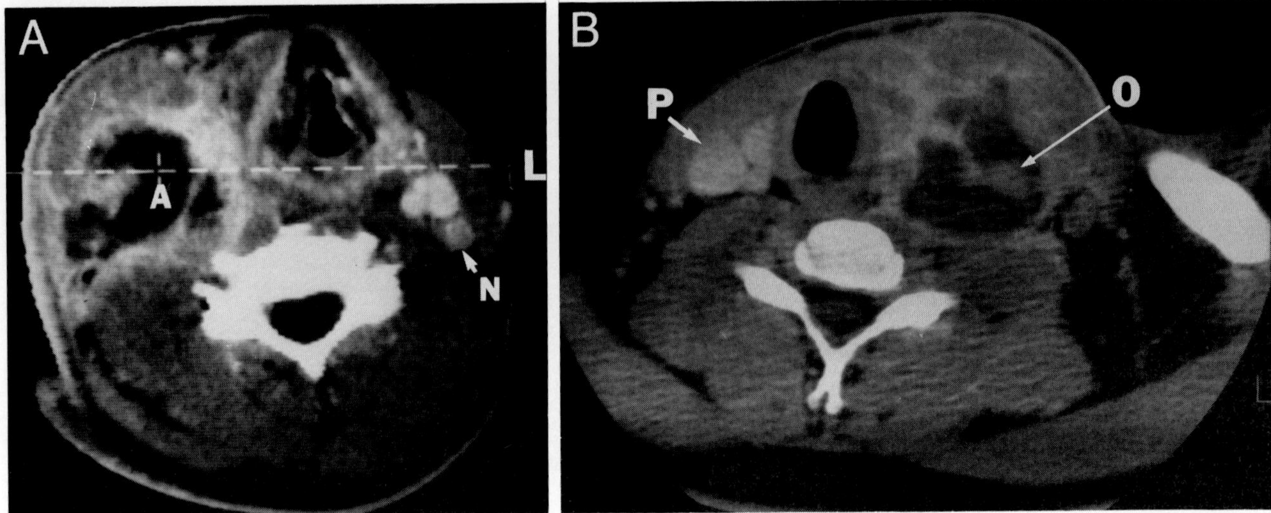

FIG 38–3.
A, enhanced CT scan of the neck at the level of the vocal cords demonstrates an abscess (suppuration of lymph node, *A*) that displaces the carotid sheath antermedially on the right, and an inflammatory node *(N)* just behind jugular vein on left. **B,** enhanced CT scan of neck demonstrating an occluded internal jugular vein (*O*) surrounded by an abscess on one side of the neck, and a patent, dilated vein (*P*) on the contralateral side.

Spread of infection between the deep cervical spaces develops along planes of least resistance, and the thin tissue separating these spaces readily ruptures as pus comes under pressure. Retrograde thrombophlebitis, sequential suppuration of lymph nodes along the cervical chain, embolization of thrombi, and bacteremia may also occur. Because all three layers of the deep cervical facia contribute to the carotid sheath, infections in any can involve this sheath, with a lateral pharyngeal origin being most frequent. Primary infection of the carotid sheath is unusual except in addicts using the internal jugular veins for narcotic injection.[8] A neck CT scan will frequently disclose small microabscesses or gas bubbles around particles along the injection tracts.

TREATMENT

The patient with a deep neck space infection should be hospitalized and provided intravenous (IV) hydration, mild-to-moderate analgesia (avoid excessive sedation), and antipyretics (only for temperatures more than 39°C because the fever proceeds other clinical responses of therapy). After blood cultures and needle stick aspiration of any abscess, the patient is given broad-spectrum antibiotics on an empiric basis, and such therapy can be appropriately tailored when culture results become available.[7, 9, 10] Approximately one third of all deep neck space infections are odontogenic in origin, and about one half of these are anaerobic, with most of the remainder being mixed aerobic-anaerobic flora. If the origin is cutaneous or nasal, the offending organism is likely *Staphylococcus aureus* or β-hemolytic *Streptococcus* in adults and *Hemophilus influenzae* in children. For community-acquired infections, IV penicillin (amoxicillin in

young children) is adequate for 80%, though the increasing incidence of bacterial resistance has prompted many to add metronidazole to obtain superior anaerobic coverage for odontogenic sources or to use cefoxitin in place of penicillin and metronidazole. For the penicillin-allergic patient, clindamycin

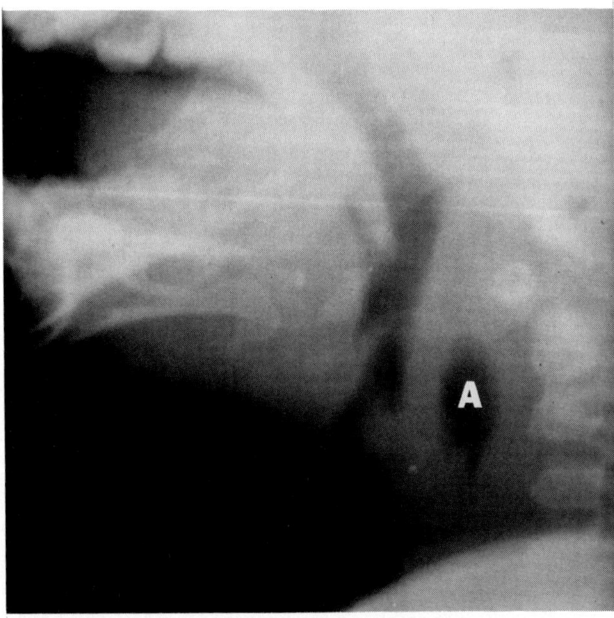

FIG 38–4.
Plain lateral neck roentgenogram in a 2-year-old child documents a retroesophageal air pocket (abscess *A*) and swelling of surrounding soft tissues (cellulitis).

is an excellent choice. A complete blood cell (CBC) count with differential establishes a useful baseline for following therapy, and serum electrolyte levels disclose any dehydration. At a minimum, soft tissue roentgenograms of the neck and chest are obtained, and CT is indicated in advanced disease.

Therapy is individualized depending on the patient's presentation and airway status. If the patient has an adequate oral airway with either cellulitis or a small abscess (<10–20 mL, which can be aspirated), observation for response to antibiotic therapy for 24 to 48 hours is sufficient. When there is a progression, failure to improve, gas formation in the soft tissues, or a large abscess, surgical intervention is indicated.[4–6, 10–14]

The surgical approach depends on the status of the patient's airway and the neck space or spaces permeated. The surgeon must be familiar with the planes of the cervical fascia and the anatomy of the involved spaces to minimize damage when approaching the abscess in an inflamed and distorted neck. The patient's oral airway is assessed, and those in active airway distress or with substantial trismus undergo tracheostomy. Those with less airway compromise are given intramuscular atropine to minimize secretions and undergo an awake intubation, with a bronchoscopy and tracheostomy setup in the operating room. With the patient in a semisitting position on the operating table, nasotracheal passage of a tube over a flexible endoscope can be quite useful for intubation of a marginal airway. If there is substantial anterior displacement of the posterior pharyngeal wall by an abscess, tracheostomy is prudent when general anesthesia is necessary, because rupture of the abscess during a traumatic intubation will cause aspiration.

For an uncomplicated abscess of the retropharyngeal, danger, or prevertebral spaces, a peroral approach under local anesthesia is appropriate in cooperative patients.[5, 6, 11, 15] Such a patient is placed in a Rose position and the operating table in Trendelenburg. The oral cavity is sprayed with a topical anesthetic, and a metal tongue depressor is used to visualize the pharynx. A 3 to 4 cm vertical incision over the most prominent bulge of the abscess affords entrance to all three spaces. A large tonsil suction must promptly evacuate the pus, and a long curved clamp can probe the cavity to break up loculations. For abscess cavities greater than about 20 cc (smaller in children), a $^1/_4$ to $^1/_2$ in. Penrose drain is positioned, with a pull-out suture, for 2 to 3 days to prevent early wound closure and pus reaccumulation.[15] A small nasogastric tube is placed, and the patient is given nothing by mouth for about 5 days. In uncooperative patients, either intubation or tracheostomy should be performed, with the cuff inflated before the incision to avoid pus aspiration.

For retropharyngeal, danger, or prevertebral abscesses that spread into the lateral pharyngeal space or inferiorly into the mediastinum, an external approach is mandatory. The classic approach was described by Dean in 1918, accessing the area through an incision along the anterior border of the sternocleidomastoid muscle.[5, 11] Today, one might place the upper portion of the incision over the body of the muscle and extend it inferiorly to the sternal notch and then across the midline to the contralateral side for bilateral neck drainage, if necessary (Fig 38–5).[3, 5, 11] In such a circumstance, the tracheostomy is

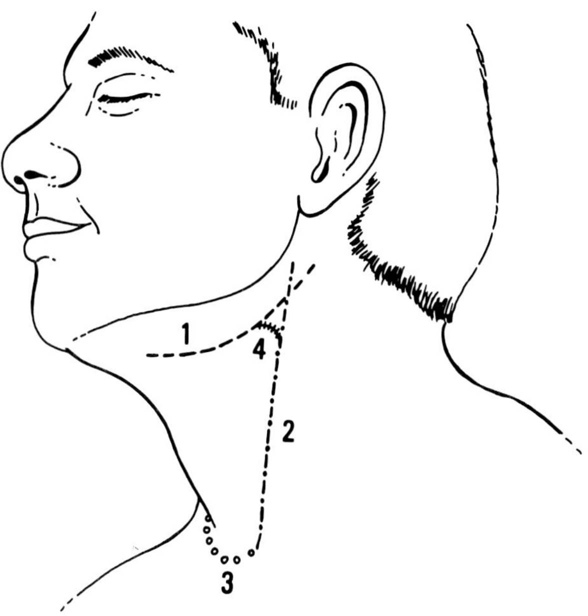

FIG 38–5.
Neck incisions for access to deep neck infections: (*1*) submandibular approach to lateral pharyngeal space, (*2*) along anterior border of sternocleidomastoid muscle to retropharyngeal/danger/prevertebral spaces, (*3*) extension across midline to drain both sides of neck (place tracheostomy at apex of apron flap), and (*4*) modification of incisions no. 1 and 2 for lateral pharyngeal abscess with extensive cervical spread (though incision no. 2 usually suffices).

placed at the apex of the "apron" flap. After the airway is secured, the planned incision lines are injected with 1% lidocaine (Xylocaine) with 1:100,000 epinephrine. The incision is carried through the skin and platysma, and the anterior border of the sternocleidomastoid muscle and the underlying carotid sheath are mobilized posteriorly. If the abscess is confined to the upper part of the neck, the hypoglossal and the superior laryngeal nerves are identified, and the larynx is retracted toward the contralateral side (Fig 38–6). The greater cornu of the hyoid is identified, and finger dissection is carried posteriorly, separating the superior pharyngeal constrictor from the alar fascia to access the retropharyngeal, danger, and prevertebral spaces, as needed. If the abscess has progressed inferiorly in the neck, the middle thyroid vein is ligated, the omohyoid muscle divided, and the trachea and thyroid gland retracted toward the contralateral side. Blunt (finger) dissection can proceed in the retropharyngeal space into the posterior mediastinum and in the pretracheal space to the tracheal bifurcation. The abscess is evacuated, cultures are taken, and the cavity is irrigated with an antibiotic solution (e.g., neomycin, bacitracin, polymyxin B sulfate). Any obviously necrotic tissue is debrided. For small abscesses, a Penrose drain is placed and the wound closed, but larger ones require continuous suction drainage (and intermittent antibiotic irrigation where appropriate) for 2 to 3 days postoperatively. When preoperative evaluation reveals soft tissue gas formation and inspection confirms myonecrosis, suction-irrigation is mandatory, and reexploration of the wound for further debridement is undertaken if the patient does not improve within 24 hours of the initial surgery.[10] In necrotizing anaerobic or mixed infections, hyperbaric oxygen therapy should be considered.

Infections of the lateral pharyngeal space are usually entered through a submandibular-type incision at the level of the hyoid, much as described by Mosher in 1929 (see Fig 38–5).[5, 7, 11] Due to inflammatory tissue edema, it is prudent to incise directly down to the hyoid, ligate the facial artery and vein, suture the superior stumps to the platysma of the upper skin flap, and then elevate a flap directly over the submandibular fascia and posterior belly of the digastric muscle to avoid inadvertent injury to the marginal mandibular nerve. Finger dissection is carried medially and superiorly from the lesser cornu of the hyoid along the stylohyoid muscle to access both compartments of the lateral pharyngeal space. The area between the internal pterygoid muscle, lateral pharyngeal wall, and styloid is readily opened by blunt dissection. If there is a large parapharyngeal abscess or the infection has originated from the submandibular or sublingual space, the submandibular gland is removed for better access to the involved spaces and improved drainage. As with posterior pharyngeal infections, the cavity is copiously irrigated with an antibiotic solution, and either a Penrose or suction-irrigation drain is placed. For infections involving both the lateral pharyngeal and retropharyngeal spaces, it is sometimes necessary to connect a submandibular incision with one along the sternocleidomastoid muscle to open up both the upper part of the neck and mediastinal inlet, though the latter incision alone usually suffices.[3]

COMPLICATIONS

Life-threatening complications of deep neck infections are most commonly related to airway compromise by an expanding abscess, aspiration from rupture into the pharynx, septicemia, shock, mediastinitis, internal jugular vein thrombosis, and carotid artery rupture. Such complications will occur with untreated or inadequately treated infections (i.e., inappropriate antibiotics or resistant organisms), failure to drain all loculations, and when there is progression of soft tissue necrosis by anaerobic or mixed organisms. The patient with a picket fence spiking temperature is evaluated for internal jugular vein thrombosis. Such thrombosis most frequently originates from the lateral pharyngeal space and may cause plethora of the ipsilateral face. Fundoscopic examination is generally unremarkable but results of the Tobey-Ayer test are positive. This test is performed by monitoring the cerebrospinal fluid (CSF) pressure via a lumbar tap while alternately placing manual pressure over the internal jugular vein suspected of thrombosis and the normal one on the contralateral side. When one vein is thrombosed, the CSF pressure will rise as the normal vein is compressed. The diagnosis is more easily made with an enhanced CT scan (i.e., internal jugular vein will not opacify), which can also delineate the upper and lower extent of the thrombosis. The patient with an internal jugular vein thrombosis should be surgically explored as soon as medically feasible. The vein is ligated below the thrombus prior to any other manipulation to avoid displacing the infected thrombus into the superior vena cava. If the upper extent of the thrombus is accessible in the neck, the vein can be ligated above this point and the clotted segment

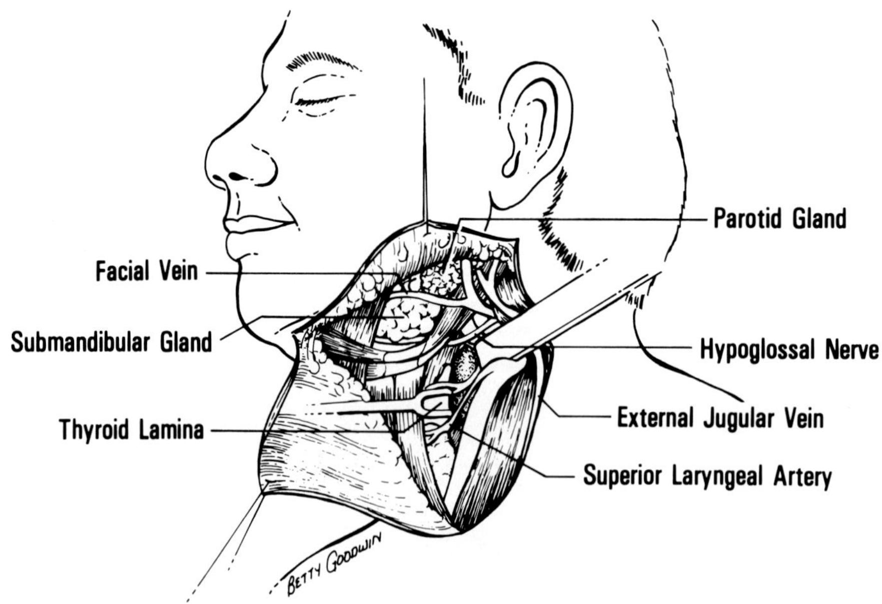

FIG 38–6.
Surgical exposure for a retropharyngeal abscess. Note posterior retraction of sternocleidomastoid muscle and carotid sheath to expose area between pharynx and vertebrae, with preservation of hypoglossal nerve and superior laryngeal neurovascular bundle. (Anterior retraction of thyroid cartilage with a double-pronged hook is helpful.)

removed. If the thrombus extends into the jugular bulb, a Fogarty catheter with a 3 cc balloon is threaded into or past the bulb via a small incision in the vein and inflated to block hemorrhage while the jugular vein is amputated at the mastoid tip and the bulb irrigated of infected clot. An antibiotic-soaked hemostatic pack, such as oxidized cellulose (Surgicel), is packed into the jugular bulb as the balloon is deflated and extracted. When stabilization of the pack seems necessary, the posterior belly of the digastric muscle is detached from the hyoid and sutured medially to the paraspinous fascia to form a sling under the jugular foramen. As an alternative, iodoform gauze may be packed into the foramen and slowly advanced beginning on the fifth to the seventh postoperative day.

Whenever the chest x-ray film demonstrates mediastinal spread of a neck infection, thoracic surgical consultation is obtained. Many can be successfully drained through the root of the neck by finger dissection in the pretracheal and retropharyngeal planes and then placement of suction-irrigation catheters into the involved mediastinal spaces[3]; however, tube thoracostomy may be necessary to drain widespread mediastinal purulence. Patients with such involvement frequently have dyspnea, substernal pain, and Hamman's sign (mediastinal crunch on auscultation). Caution should be exercised in interpreting a wide mediastinum from an anteroposterior chest roentgenogram, because it exaggerates the mediastinal width. When auscultatory findings and routine chest films suggest mediastinal involvement, the chest is scanned at the same time CAT of the neck is performed.

A major venous or arterial rupture from deep neck infection is infrequent, with the common and internal carotid arteries being most resistant. A vessel rupture may first manifest as a rapid expansion in neck swelling and concomitant airway compromise but more commonly presents as blood in the abscess cavity during surgical exploration. Pressure in the cavity in an inflamed, edematous neck will frequently limit the hematoma until the compartment is decompressed. The surgeon is alerted by blood in or around a deep neck abscess and, preferably, has already exposed the common carotid artery and the internal jugular vein below the abscess so these vessels can be controlled. If hemorrhage occurs, the cavity is packed with hemostatic gauze, and manual pressure is placed on the internal carotid artery low in the neck. Exposure of the internal jugular vein and carotid artery must be quickly obtained, with the placement of rubber vascular loops for atraumatic vessel control. Venous bleeding is controlled by ligation of the internal jugular vein above and below the abscess using the aforementioned technique with a Fogarty catheter if the jugular vein is difficult to control high in the neck. For an arterial bleed, the rubber loop around the common carotid artery is tightened and the external carotid artery ligated at the bifurcation. The common carotid loop should then be loosened to establish whether the hemorrhage has abated. The external carotid artery may also have to be ligated above the abscess, but ligation at the bifurcation should substantially diminish the rate of bleeding. If it does not occur, an internal carotid defect must be assumed, which, unfortunately, is the case in approximately 75% of major arterial hemorrhages associated with deep neck infections. If

the origin of the hemorrhage is in doubt, a 20-gauge angiocatheter may be threaded into the common carotid artery, and 10 mL of diatrizoate (Hypaque) may be forcefully injected as a lateral neck roentgenogram is obtained. An internal carotid artery rupture must be controlled by ligation above and below the defect. The contiguous abscess makes direct repair or a patch graft unlikely to succeed and puts the patient at great risk for a second hemorrhage (in a less controlled situation than the operating room). If the internal carotid artery is ligated, the patient is transfused to a normal hematocrit and kept well hydrated and oxygenated for at least the first 5 postoperative days.[16]

REFERENCES

1. Paonessa DF, Goldstein JC: Anatomy and physiology of head and neck infections, in Herzon FS (ed): *Otolaryngologic Clinics of North America.* Philadelphia, WB Saunders Co, 1976, vol 9, pp 561–580.
2. Lindner HH: The anatomy of the fasciae of the face and neck with particular reference to the spread and treatment of intraoral infections that have progressed into adjacent fascial spaces. *Ann Surg* 1986; 204:705–714.
3. Levine TM, Wurster CF, Krespi YP: Mediastinitis occurring as a complication of odontogenic infections. *Laryngoscope* 1986; 96:747–750.
4. Sacks JC, Gilmore WC: Closed percutaneous catheter drainage of a cervical abscess. *J Oral Macillofac Surg* 1985; 43:971–973.
5. Rabuzzi DD, Johnson JT: *Diagnosis and Management of Deep Neck Infections.* Washington, DC, American Academy of Otolaryngology–Head and Neck Surgery, 1978.
6. Dzyak WR, Zide MF: Diagnosis and treatment of lateral pharyngeal space infections. *J Oral Maxillofac Surg* 1984; 42:243–249.
7. Peterson LJ: Odontogenic infections, in Cummings CW, Fredrickson JM, Harker LA, et al (eds): *Otolaryngology— Head and Neck Surgery.* St Louis, CV Mosby Co, 1986, vol 2, pp 1213–1230.
8. Myers EM, Kirkland LS, Mickey R: The head and neck sequelae of cervical intravenous drug abuse. *Laryngoscope* 1988; 98:213–217.
9. Brook I: Microbiology of abscesses of the head and neck in children. *Ann Otol Rhinol Laryngol* 1987; 96:429–433.
10. Beck HJ, Salassa JR, McCaffney TV, et al: Life-threatening soft-tissue infections of the neck. *Laryngoscope* 1984; 94:354–362.
11. Levitt GW: Cervical fascia and deep neck infections, in Herzon FS: *Otolaryngologic Clinics of North America.* Philadelphia, WB Saunders Co, 1976, vol 9, pp 703–716.
12. Herzon FS: Needle aspiration of nonperitonsillar head and neck abscesses. *Arch Otolaryngol Head Neck Surg* 1988; 114:1312–1314.
13. Ophir D, Bawnik J, Poria Y, et al: Peritonsillar Abscess. *Arch Otolaryngol Head Neck Surg* 1988; 114:661–663.
14. Tom MB, Rice DH: Presentation and management of neck abscess. *Laryngoscope* 1988; 98:877–880.
15. Guarisco JL, Grundfast KM: A technique for insertion and removal of an intraoral drain following treatment of a retropharyngeal abscess. *Laryngoscope* 1988; 98:242–243.
16. Osguthorpe JD, Hungerford GD: Transarterial carotid occlusion. *Arch Otolaryngol* 1984; 110:694–696.

Cervical Space Infections

Approach of

James N. Thompson, M.D.

Infections of the deep neck spaces comprise a group of inflammatory complications of primary infections of the upper aerodigestive tract. Abscesses of the deep neck spaces are potentially life threatening due to the anatomic approximation of those spaces to the airway and the great vessels of the neck. A clear understanding of the anatomy and pathophysiology of this group of complications is necessary for the appropriate treatment of patients who present with deep neck space abscesses. Prompt recognition of infection, along with early surgical drainage and appropriate antibiotic treatment, can be life saving.

The most common infection of the deep neck spaces is peritonsillar abscess, and it is described first in this chapter. Peritonsillar abscess not only occurs most commonly but also often precedes retropharyngeal or parapharyngeal abscess. One section of the chapter covers thrombophlebitis of the internal jugular vein, which can result from deep neck space infection and may require special radiographic studies for diagnosis. Prevertebral abscess is also described, although since the development of adequate tuberculosis treatment, this infection has been much less common.

PERITONSILLAR ABSCESS

Anatomy

The peritonsillar space is a potential space between the capsule of the pharyngeal tonsil and the surrounding superior constrictor muscle. The buccopharyngeal fascia is lateral to the constrictor muscle and forms the anterior limit of the peritonsillar space. The posterior boundary is formed by the posterior tonsillar pillar.[1]

Signs and Symptoms

Patients with peritonsillar infection will usually have pain and fever with a muffled voice. The pain can be quite intense and be associated with dysphagia and trismus. Physical findings include inflammation and medial displacement of the tonsil and uvula, as well as swelling of the anterior tonsillar pillar.

Diagnosis

The physician usually can make the diagnosis of peritonsillar abscess on the basis of history and physical examination. The findings in a febrile and toxic patient tend to be classic for this infection. Confirmation of the clinical diagnosis is by needle aspiration of the abscess. After injection of a small amount of local anesthetic (1% lidocaine), a 19-gauge needle is inserted just lateral to the superior pole of the tonsil, and aspiration is attempted. Since not all abscesses in the peritonsillar space are superior, aspiration should be attempted at the middle and inferior poles if the initial aspiration is unsuccessful. Aspirates are sent to the laboratory for culture and sensitivity. Radiographs are of minimal benefit in diagnosis.

Pathology

Peritonsillar abscess is a pathologic condition resulting from progression of a bacterial infection of the pharyngeal tonsils. It is perhaps the most common abscess of the deep neck spaces for which an otolaryngologist would be consulted. Peritonsillar abscess is more often found in adolescents and young adults, whereas peritonsillar cellulitis is more common in young children.[2]

Organisms most often responsible for this infection are the aerobic bacteria β-hemolytic streptococci, *Staphylococcus aureus,* and *Streptococcus pneumoniae.*[3] Increasingly, anaerobic organisms are being implicated as either primary or secondary pathogens.

Treatment

The treatment of peritonsillar abscess has been disputed for years. Suggested procedures include (1) immediate tonsillectomy; (2) incision, drainage, and antibiotics; and (3) needle aspiration and antibiotics. The latter two have been advocated with and without subsequent tonsillectomy, some otolaryngologists arguing that tonsillectomy should routinely follow antibiotic treatment, and others arguing that tonsillectomy should be reserved for patients who have recurrent peritonsillar abscesses.

In practice it is best to individualize treatment to each patient. For the severely ill patient who is having difficulty swallowing or who is dehydrated, hospitalization with IV rehydration and antibiotics is reasonable. In the small child who may require a general anesthetic for an adequate examination of the pharynx, immediate tonsillectomy is a suitable alternative and may shorten the patient's hospital stay without increasing the risk of intraoperative blood loss.[4] In the cooperative patient, however, I prefer the traditional incision and drainage procedure following the diagnostic aspiration.

I first make an incision in the mucosa over the site of pus aspiration with a no. 15 Bard Parker blade and insert a small curved hemostat, spreading it to increase the amount of drainage. I then hospitalize the patient until he or she has a normal temperature and can swallow comfortably. Penicillin G (1–2 million units every 4–6 hours for adults and 100,000 units/kg/day for children) is given intravenously. Clindamycin has excellent activity against the common aerobic and anaerobic organisms found in peritonsillar infections and is a reasonable alternative. The cephalosporins may also be used. During hospitalization, the patient is given analgesics and daily mouthwashes with half-strength hydrogen peroxide.

Postoperative laboratory tests should include a CBC count with a differential white blood cell (WBC) count, chest radiography, urinalysis, and the mononucleosis spot test. I reserve tonsillectomy for patients with recurrent abscesses unless there is a preexisting indication for surgery, such as multiple episodes of pharyngotonsillitis, or there are airway symptoms, such as obstructive breathing during sleep.

Complications

The peritonsillar space is in close proximity to the parapharyngeal and retropharyngeal spaces; consequently, a predictable complication of peritonsillar infection is spread of infection to these surrounding spaces with subsequent abscess formation. The spread of infection can be by direct extension, lymphatics, or venous thrombophlebitis. These infections of the deep neck space are discussed in detail later in the chapter.

Airway obstruction is a possible complication. It can occur from inflammatory swelling of the tonsillar region from spontaneous rupture of the abscess into the pharynx. Care must be taken in examining patients with peritonsillar abscess to avoid premature rupture of the abscess.

Necrotizing fasciitis has been described as a potentially lethal complication of peritonsillar abscess.[3] This complication, which fortunately is rare, seems to occur more often in the immunosuppressed patient, and gas-forming organisms have been implicated as the causative agents. Early recognition of necrotizing fasciitis and aggressive treatment with drainage of abscesses, IV antibiotic therapy, and major wound debridement are imperative.

PARAPHARYNGEAL SPACE INFECTIONS

Anatomy

The anatomy of the parapharyngeal space is of great interest to surgeons because of the high incidence of infection in this area following other head and neck infections. Infections of the parapharyngeal space commonly follow tonsillar and pharyngeal infections. The parapharyngeal space is also referred to as the peripharyngeal space, the lateral pharyngeal space, and the pharyngomaxillary space.

The parapharyngeal space is a cone-shaped potential space having its base at the base of the skull and its apex at the hyoid bone. It is bounded anteriorly by pterygoid and buccinator muscle fascia, the pterygoid mandibular raphe, and the submandibular gland. Its posterior limit is the fascia that covers the transverse process of the atlas, the rectus capitus, and the levator scapulae. The superior constrictor muscle forms the medial limit, and the medial pterygoid muscle, the parotid gland, and the ascending ramus of the mandible make up its lateral extent. The posterior extent of the parapharyngeal space is separated from the retropharyngeal space by a thin fascia, and spread of disease from one space to the other is not rare.[5] The great vessels of the neck (internal and external carotid arteries, the ascending pharyngeal artery, and the internal jugular vein), cranial nerves IX through XII, and the sympathetic trunk lie posteriorly in the parapharyngeal space; muscles, lymph nodes, and connective tissue lie anteriorly.[6]

One reason for the high incidence of infection in the parapharyngeal space is the close proximity of this space to other spaces in the head and neck. Infection can spread from the parotid, peritonsillar, masticator, and submandibular spaces. In addition, the mastoid bone can be a source when the bone near the digastric groove becomes eroded with infection, thereby allowing spread inferiorly and medially into the parapharyngeal space.[7] The most common mechanism is direct erosion from the peritonsillar space in a patient with tonsillitis.

Signs and Symptoms

The signs and symptoms of parapharyngeal space abscess can be somewhat variable, depending on the source of the infection and the anterior or posterior location of the abscess within the parapharyngeal space.

Anterior infection will present more often with trismus due to involvement of the internal pterygoid muscle. Induration of the lateral pharyngeal wall and swelling of the neck below the angle of the mandible are common findings. The patient will also usually have fever, neck pain, and tenderness.

Diagnosis

In most instances, parapharyngeal space abscess can be diagnosed by history and physical findings. Radiographic evaluation may help to confirm the diagnosis, and it may be particularly beneficial when the diagnosis is in doubt. However, plain radiographs are usually of little value. The greatest benefit is derived from CT, which not only is useful in identifying the abscess but also may help to rule out other disease within the neck. Ultrasonography is also useful and often can distinguish the separation between tissue planes and the accumulation of fluid in the parapharyngeal space, which are characteristic of these infections.

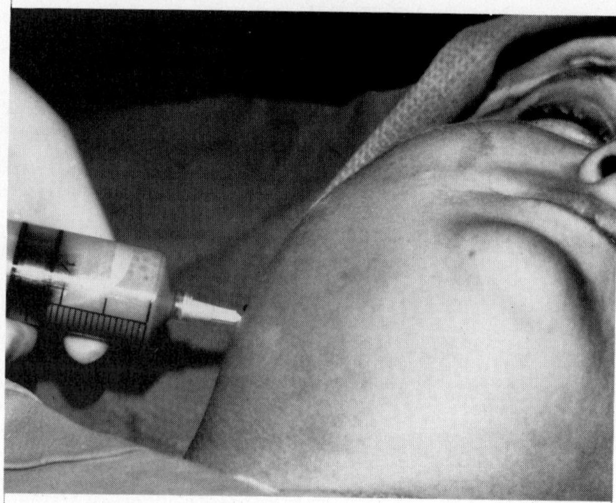

FIG 38–7.
Diagnostic aspiration of pus from adult patient with parapharyngeal space abscess.

Laboratory studies are of little benefit in establishing the diagnosis. An elevated WBC count and an elevated sedimentation rate would be expected and are usually present.

The diagnosis is made definitively by needle aspiration. After the skin overlying the abscess is prepared with alcohol or povidone-iodine, a 19- or 20-gauge needle attached to a syringe is introduced into the neck space. Aspiration of pus confirms the diagnosis (Fig 38–7).

Pathology

Since infections of the parapharyngeal space are most commonly caused by spread from tonsillitis or dental infection, the organisms that are cultured from the parapharyngeal space will most commonly be oropharyngeal pathogens, the majority of which are anaerobic. *Peptostreptococcus, Peptococcus, Bacteroides* species, and *Fusobacterium* are the anaerobic organisms most frequently cultured; group A *Streptococcus* is a common aerobic pathogen.

Treatment

The patient with an abscess of the parapharyngeal space has a potentially lethal disease and should be treated accordingly. Initially, the airway should be protected if it is compromised by pharyngeal swelling or possible rupture of the abscess into the oral cavity. If these possibilities are probable, a tracheotomy should be performed as soon as is feasible.

The patient should be admitted to the hospital for IV fluid replacement, antibiotic therapy, and surgical drainage. Initially, the choice of antibiotics should be based on the most likely infecting organisms—oral anaerobic bacteria and group A *Streptococcus.* Clindamycin is the first choice for antibiotic therapy. Its coverage includes the common aerobic organisms as well as the anaerobic organisms. Adults receive 300 to 900 mg intravenously or intramuscularly every 8 hours. Children receive

25 to 40 mg/kg/day intravenously in three divided doses. Penicillins and cephalosporins are universally effective in treating these organisms and are a reasonable alternative. Due to the possibility that β-lactamase-producing organisms are present, a cephalosporin such as cefoxitin (1–2 gm given every 4–8 hours intravenously) would be a good choice. In children the dosage should be 50 to 150 mg/kg/day in three or four divided doses. Ceftazidime would be another alternative. Antibiotic therapy should be continued for at least 10 days and should be adjusted according to sensitivities from wound cultures.

The hallmark of treating an abscess of the parapharyngeal space is surgical drainage. With the neck prepared as a sterile field and the patient under general anesthesia for safety and control of the airway, a transverse incision is made in a neck fold. The inferior landmark is the greater cornu of the hyoid bone. Dissection is performed anterior to the sternocleidomastoid muscle. After the cavity of the abscess is entered, purulent material is obtained for culture, and the wound is copiously irrigated with sterile saline. A Penrose drain is left in the wound, usually for 2 days. If drainage remains heavy at the end of that period, the drain may be left in place longer.

Posterior infection can involve the carotid sheath, which can lead to bleeding or sepsis. Septic erosion of the carotid artery can also occur if a peritonsillar infection spreads to the parapharyngeal space.[8] Thrombosis of the internal jugular vein, another potential complication of infection in the posterior area of the parapharyngeal space, is discussed in the following section.

SEPTIC THROMBOPHLEBITIS OF THE INTERNAL JUGULAR VEIN

Septic thrombophlebitis of the internal jugular vein is a potentially life-threatening complication of parapharyngeal space infection. A more common cause than parapharyngeal abscess is the introduction of needles or catheters into the neck for medical purposes or during the illegal use of drugs.

Three conditions can predispose to thrombosis within the internal jugular vein: (1) damaged vascular endothelium; (2) abnormal blood flow; and (3) altered blood composition, as in hypercoagulability states.

Clinical findings are often nonspecific. A vague fullness of the neck or a deep mass with tenderness may be present. Edema of the sternocleidomastoid has been reported. The symptoms are occasionally so vague that the delay between onset of symptoms and time when medical assistance is sought is considerable.

Diagnosis is established by CT scan or ultrasonographic imaging. The CT scan has the advantage of revealing any additional neck disease that is present. Computed tomography findings in the patient with thrombophlebitis of the internal jugular vein include an enlarged vein filled with material of low attenuation; the wall of the vein is often well defined (Fig 38–8). Venous collaterals can be seen on contrast studies.[9] Ultrasonography has the advantage of being less expensive than CT scanning; its equipment is often portable, and it does not expose

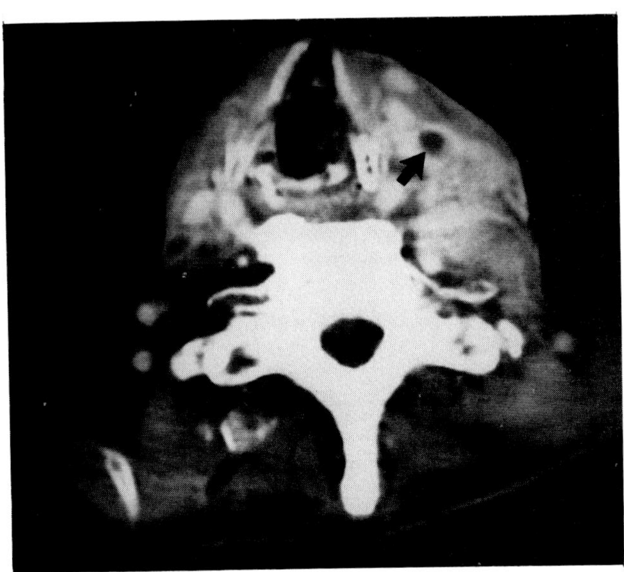

FIG 38–8.
Computed tomography scan showing thrombophlebitis of the internal jugular vein in a patient with metastatic cancer. Note well-defined wall of vein filled with material of low attenuation *(arrow)*.

the patient to ionizing radiation. When abnormal, it shows an echogenic area within a dilated internal jugular vein.

Causative organisms include anaerobic and aerobic *Streptococcus* species, *Staphylococcus* species, *Fusobacterium,* and *Bacteroides.* Initial antibiotic therapy should be adequate to cover those organisms and should include one of the following: (1) penicillin in combination with a penicillinase-resistant drug, (2) clindamycin, or (3) cefoxitin.

Treatment must address not only the underlying cause of the thrombosis but also the thrombosis itself. Anticoagulation should consist of 1 week of IV heparin therapy, followed by oral warfarin.[10] Anticoagulation should be monitored by regularly testing the prothrombin and partial thromboplastin times. If the underlying cause is a neck abscess, the abscess should be drained as discussed earlier.

Two other forms of treatment should be mentioned. Enzymatic thrombectomy remains controversial, but some suggest giving it if the thrombus is less than 72 hours old.[11] Surgical thrombectomy or ligation of the internal jugular vein is probably most beneficial when the patient has pulmonary embolism or septicemia in the presence of septic emboli. When a neck abscess must be drained surgically, it would seem reasonable to go ahead and ligate the internal jugular vein during the same anesthetic period.

RETROPHARYNGEAL ABSCESS

Anatomy

The retropharyngeal space is bordered by the deep and middle layers of the deep cervical fascia (Fig 38–9). Anteriorly, the visceral, or deep, layer of the middle cervical fascia extends

from the hyoid bone to the base of the skull behind the esophageal constrictors. It encloses the larynx, trachea, esophagus, and thyroid gland and sends a muscular component to enclose the strap muscles. The deep layer of the deep cervical fascia is divided into two layers, the more anterior being the alar fascia, which is the posterior border of the retropharyngeal space. The alar fascia extends inferiorly to the level of T1 or T2, where it fuses with the middle layer of the deep cervical fascia posterior to the esophagus. Consequently, the retropharyngeal space (bordered anteriorly by the visceral fascia and posteriorly by the alar fascia) extends from the skull base superiorly to the level of T1 or T2 inferiorly. Between the retropharyngeal space and the prevertebral space is the "danger space," which is bounded anteriorly by the alar fascia and posteriorly by the prevertebral fascia. The danger space extends from the skull base inferiorly to the level of the diaphragm and consequently represents a life-threatening route of spread of infection when retropharyngeal abscesses dissect posteriorly.

In childhood, the lymphatic drainage to the retropharyn-

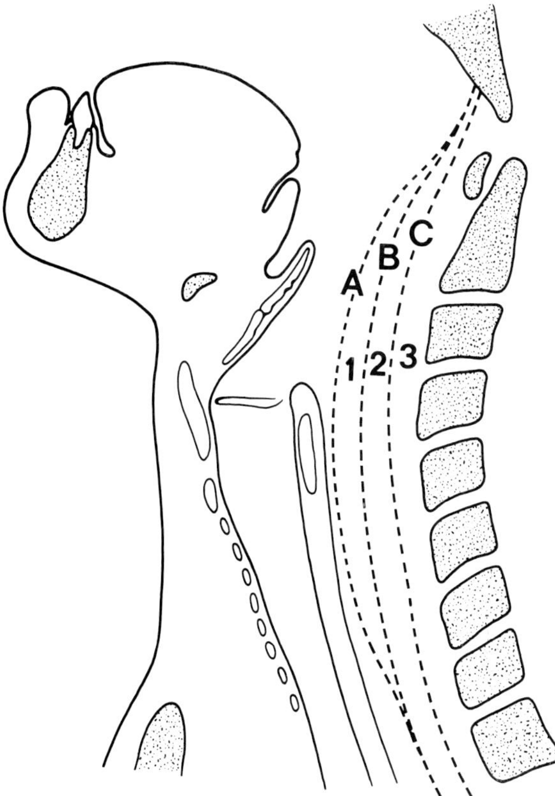

FIG 38–9.
Midline section through neck illustrating posterior pharyngeal fasciae (letters) and spaces (numbers). *A,* visceral fascia; *B,* alar fascia; *C,* prevertebral fascia; *1,* retropharyngeal space; *2,* danger space; *3,* prevertebral space. Inferior extent of retropharyngeal space is at the level of the first or second thoracic vertebra. The danger space extends to the level of the diaphragm, the prevertebral space to the coccyx.

geal space is extensive and probably accounts for the relatively high incidence of retropharyngeal infections in children compared with adults. Lymphatic drainage comes from the nasal cavities, the paranasal sinuses, the nasopharynx, the pharynx, the middle ears, and the eustachian tubes. The decreased incidence of retropharyngeal infection in adults is presumably related to atrophy of the lymphatics.[6]

Signs and Symptoms

Symptoms of retropharyngeal abscess in children are different from those in adults. Young children may exhibit only irritability, some neck stiffness and tenderness, and difficulty in feeding. Visudhiphan et al. described two children who presented with torticollis secondary to retropharyngeal abscess.[12] The voice may be muffled if there is swelling of the posterior pharyngeal wall, since the larynx of the child is relatively more superior than that of the adult. Airway compromise can occur and is possibly life-threatening if the abscess ruptures prematurely.

Physical findings in children include a soft tissue swelling of the posterior pharyngeal wall, which often stops at the midline, even though the retropharyngeal lymphatics are found on both sides of the midline. Cervical adenopathy may also be present. Great care must be taken when the pharynx of a child with a suspected retropharyngeal abscess is examined, since palpation of this area can cause rupture of the abscess and possibly death from aspiration.

In adults, the signs and symptoms more clearly point to the pharynx. Most commonly, patients will present with fever, sore throat, dysphagia, shortness of breath, stridor, neck tenderness and stiffness, and cervical lymphadenopathy. Extension of the disease into the mediastinum can cause chest pain, severe dyspnea, and radiographic evidence of a widened mediastinum. Although palpation of the retropharyngeal area is safer in the adult, one should still be aware of the potential for rupturing the abscess.

Diagnosis

A preliminary diagnosis of retropharyngeal abscess can be made with abnormal physical findings, including a soft, fluctuant mass behind the posterior pharyngeal wall. This part of the physical examination is not always easy, since children may be uncooperative and adults may have severe trismus, thus making it difficult to palpate the pharynx.

Radiographic evaluation of the neck may be the most helpful diagnostic test. A lateral roentgenogram will usually show widening of the prevertebral soft tissue of the retropharyngeal space (Fig 38–10). The retropharyngeal space is measured from the anteroinferior part of the second cervical vertebra to the posterior pharyngeal wall and is considered to be widened when this distance is greater than 7 mm.[13] In young children, however, this distance may vary some, since their soft tissues are quite pliable and may show radiographic variations with respiration and swallowing. The most reliable lateral view is that obtained during deep inspiration with the patient's neck extended. Findings other than thickening of the posterior pha-

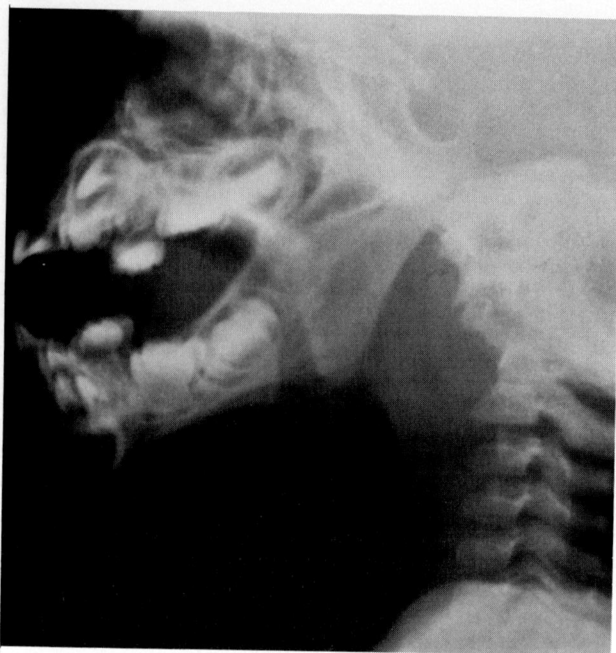

FIG 38–10.
Lateral radiograph showing widening of the prevertebral soft tissue of the retropharyngeal space.

ryngeal wall that suggest retropharyngeal abscess include air or air-fluid levels in the soft tissues, foreign bodies, and loss of the normal curvature of the cervical spine.

Computed tomographic imaging may be helpful in distinguishing abscess from cellulitis and in localizing the infection. However, if one is relatively certain of the diagnosis, a CT scan may unnecessarily delay emergency surgical intervention. Finally, a chest roentgenogram should be performed on all patients with suspected retropharyngeal abscesses to detect any evidence of spread to the mediastinum.

Pathology

Abscesses in the retropharyngeal space are usually acute. In children, they most often result from spread of infection in the ear, nose, and throat via the lymphatic system to the retropharyngeal lymph nodes. This type of spread typically occurs before age 3 or 4 years.

In adults, many retropharyngeal abscesses are caused by respiratory tract infections, but more often retropharyngeal abscess results from injury of the pharynx. Trauma from endotracheal intubation,[14] foreign body ingestion, endoscopic procedures, and blunt and penetrating neck trauma all can result in infection of the retropharyngeal space. The adult with a compromised immune system, such as a patient with diabetes mellitus or a cancer patient receiving chemotherapy, may also be predisposed to infections in this area.

The bacteria of retropharyngeal abscesses represent the entire spectrum of pathogens found in the oropharynx. Anaerobic organisms appear to predominate, but the disease is polymicrobial; it is fairly common for as many as ten bacterial isolates to be recovered from a single patient.[15] The common aerobic organisms include group A *Streptococcus, S. aureus,* and *Hemophilus influenzae.* The anaerobic organisms most commonly found are *Peptostreptococcus* species, *Fusobacterium,* and various species of *Bacteroides.*

Polymicrobial infections are probably more pathogenic than single-organism infections. There is a known synergism when aerobic organisms combine with anaerobic organisms, the presence of aerobic organisms creating an environmental milieu that facilitates anaerobic growth.

Treatment

The mainstay of treatment of retropharyngeal abscess is antibiotic therapy and surgical drainage. It is possible that early cellulitis of the retropharyngeal space can be treated successfully with antibiotics alone, but if there is any question of possible suppuration within the retropharyngeal space, surgery must be considered.

Any patient with a compromised airway demands immediate attention. As mentioned earlier, care must be taken not to rupture the abscess, since this can be fatal. Emergency tracheotomy may be necessary before the abscess is drained. Once an adequate airway is assured and antibiotic therapy has been started, surgical drainage can be performed.

The surgical approach depends on the clinical situation. In a child or adult who has an uncompromised airway and is otherwise healthy, I prefer general anesthesia with endotracheal intubation and an oral approach to the retropharyngeal space. With the patient in the Rose position, a stab incision is made into the mucosa overlying the abscess, and the purulent material is suctioned and cultured. If necessary, the wound is widened to provide continued drainage.

The traditional surgical approach to the retropharyngeal space in the patient whose airway is compromised is through a neck incision along the anterior border of the sternocleidomastoid muscle. With the carotid sheath retracted laterally and the thyroid gland, superior thyroid vessels, and superior laryngeal nerve retracted medially, the abscess is entered at the level of the hypopharynx. A Penrose drain is left in the incision until drainage from the wound becomes minimal.

Although retropharyngeal abscesses contain a high incidence of anaerobic organisms that are individually sensitive to penicillin, the prevalence of β-lactamase-producing bacteria necessitates alternative or supplemental treatment. Also, since *S. aureus* is a common aerobic pathogenic bacterium in retropharyngeal abscesses, a drug that is effective against penicillinase-producing strains of staphylococci may be helpful. Clindamycin given intravenously or intramuscularly every 8 hours (300–900 mg) is a good first-line choice (children receive 25–40 mg/kg/day intravenously in three divided doses). A cephalosporin is a good alternative (e.g., 1–2 gm of cefoxitin every 4–8 hours intravenously).

Complications

Most of the complications of retropharyngeal abscess are

life threatening. They include airway obstruction (from expansion of the posterior pharyngeal wall or from spontaneous or iatrogenic rupture of the abscess), hemorrhage, septicemia, spread of the abscess to other neck spaces or into the mediastinum with subsequent mediastinitis, thrombosis of the internal jugular vein, and erosion into the danger space through the alar fascia, with extension of infection to the level of the diaphragm. The gravity of these complications underscores the importance of prompt diagnosis and treatment of this disorder.

PREVERTEBRAL SPACE INFECTION

The prevertebral space is immediately anterior to the vertebral column and posterior to the prevertebral fascia. It extends from the skull base to the coccyx and is the route by which deep neck infections can extend as far inferiorly as the psoas muscle sheath.[13] However, since the prevertebral space is very compact, rapid extension of disease is rare.

The signs and symptoms of prevertebral space infection may be very subtle and include only neck stiffness and low-grade fever. Torticollis and neurologic deficits, such as extremity weakness, can occur when the disease has progressed to involvement of the cervical spinal cord.

Historically, before adequate chemotherapy was available, the principle source of infection in the prevertebral space was from spread of tuberculosis of the cervical spine. Today, acute infection of the prevertebral space should make one think of some nontuberculous chronic disease. Osteomyelitis is uncommon in the cervical spine, but when it is present, it can cause an abscess of the prevertebral space. Hematogenous spread of *S. aureus* is the most common mechanism by which cervical osteomyelitis results in prevertebral abscess.

Radiographic evaluation is more helpful with advanced disease of the cervical spine, and CT scans will demonstrate bone destruction. Bone scans may also be useful. Early disease may show no changes or only mild bony changes in the affected vertebral bodies.

Treatment of prevertebral space infection is directed at the underlying disease. Of course, if an abscess is present, adequate drainage is mandatory and may require exploratory laminectomy. If osteomyelitis is the underlying cause, long-term antibiotic therapy should be instituted. Clindamycin (300–900 mg every 8 hours intravenously or intramuscularly) is a good first-line drug, with penicillinase-resistant penicillins or cephalosporins being suitable alternatives.

REFERENCES

1. Blum DJ, McCaffrey TV: Septic necrosis of the internal carotid artery: A complication of peritonsillar abscess. *Otolaryngol Head Neck Surg* 1983; 91:114–118.
2. Shoemaker M, Lampe RM, Weir MR: Peritonsillitis: Abscess or cellulitis? *Pediatr Infect Dis* 1986; 5:435–439.
3. Wenig BL, Shikowitz MJ, Abramson AL: Necrotizing fasciitis as a lethal complication of peritonsillar abscess. *Laryngoscope* 1984; 94:1576–1579.

4. Harley EH: Quinsy tonsillectomy as the treatment of choice for peritonsillar abscess. *Ear Nose Throat J* 1988; 67:84–87.

5. Maran AGD, Mackenzie IJ, Murray JAM: The parapharyngeal space. *J Laryngol Otol* 1984; 98:371–380.

6. Paonessa DF, Goldstein JC: Anatomy and physiology of head and neck infections (with emphasis on the fascia of the face and neck). *Otolaryngol Clin North Am* 1976; 9:561–580.

7. Levitt GW: Cervical fascia and deep neck infections. *Otolaryngol Clin North Am* 1976; 9:703–716.

8. Garino JP, Ryan TJ: Carotid hemorrhage: A complication of peritonsillar abscess. *Am J Emerg Med* 1987; 5:220–223.

9. Rahn NH III, Rubin E, Koehler RE: Thrombophlebitis of the internal jugular vein: Noninvasive imaging. *South Med J* 1984; 77:1308–1310.

10. Cohen JP, Persky MS, Reede DL: Internal jugular vein thrombosis. *Laryngoscope* 1985; 95:1478–1482.

11. Anand VK, Morrison WV: Thrombophlebitis of the jugular vein. *Ear Nose Throat J* 1987; 66:64–69.

12. Visudhiphan P, Chiemchanya S, Somburanasin R, et al: Torticollis as the presenting sign in cervical spine infection and tumor. *Clin Pediatr* 1982; 21:71–76.

13. Barratt GE, Koopmann CF Jr, Coulthard SW: Retropharyngeal abscess—a ten-year experience. *Laryngoscope* 1984; 94:455–463.

14. Majumdar B, Stevens RW, Obara LG: Retropharyngeal abscess following tracheal intubation. *Anaesthesia* 1982; 37:67–70.

15. Brook I: Microbiology of retropharyngeal abscesses in children. *Am J Dis Child* 1987; 141:202–204.

CHAPTER 39

Neuro-otologic Infections

Approach of

Michael E. Glasscock III, M.D.

Dennis S. Poe, M.D.

and

Glen D. Johnson, M.D.

Complications from otitis media were frequent sources of major morbidity and mortality in the preantibiotic era. Temporal bone surgery was too often undertaken as a desperate life-saving effort. Today, with early recognition of otitis media and appropriate antibiotic therapy, such life-threatening advanced complications have become unusual. The management of several important temporal bone infections will be reviewed. Although these conditions are no longer common, their occurrence does present some challenging management problems. The evaluation and management of major otitis media complications will be presented.

Early recognition of otitis media complications is the single-most important aspect of their management. Early infections can usually be controlled entirely medically. A complication is said to have occurred when the inflammation has spread beyond the pneumatized temporal bone cells.[1–3] Bone destruction precedes the spread of disease to adjacent soft tissue spaces, and identification of bone destruction may be the earliest indication of an impending severe complication. Complications occur because an infection is trapped within a closed space, and therapy is going to require (1) establishment of drainage, (2) antibiotics, and (3) possible excision of infection tissues.

COMPLICATIONS OF ACUTE OTITIS MEDIA

Acute otitis media has been used to refer to acute suppurative infections of less than 3 weeks' duration. The treatment

of most acute suppurative infections is establishment of drainage and antibiotic therapy. The pneumatized space at the mastoid cavity has a volume of 15 to 20 mL and, when infected, it must drain through a middle ear space (having a volume of only 0.9 mL) and down a patent eustachian tube.[4] When blockage occurs, purulent material accumulates and builds pressure. Bone destruction develops from the combination of pressure and diffuse enzymatic absorption of broad areas adjacent to the inflammation. The resultant erosion in acute infections is broadly based as opposed to chronic ear disease, which more deeply penetrates adjacent bone. The severity of symptoms and rapidity of complication development determine what measures will be necessary to establish adequate drainage.

Minor complications can be handled with antibiotic therapy alone or with the possible addition of a decongestant to open the eustachian tube. More severe complications, such as evidence of bony destruction, will require a more rapid establishment of drainage via myringotomy if the tympanic membrane has not already perforated. Only when a true destructive abscess has occurred is a formal incision and drainage necessary. The bony destruction of acute coalescent mastoiditis necessitates a simple mastoidectomy. The situation may be likened to an abscess that requires incision and drainage for adequate resolution.

In summary, acute suppurative otitis media is usually adequately managed with antibiotics and establishment of drainage medically. Acute suppurative otitis media with any complication or bone destruction will usually require antibiotics with the addition of surgical drainage at least in the form of myringotomy. A mastoidectomy is necessary when bone destruction becomes extensive or coalescent.

COMPLICATIONS OF CHRONIC OTITIS MEDIA

Chronic otitis media is often defined arbitrarily as disease present in excess of 3 months, and clinical judgment is necessary to characterize an infection falling between 3 weeks and 3 months. Treatment of chronic infection requires establishment of drainage, antibiotic therapy, and usually excision of infected tissue. Complete removal of infected tissue may require a definitive middle ear and mastoid procedure that would be difficult in the face of acute inflammation. The first goal is to gain control of the acute suppurative process, ensuring the establishment of drainage and treatment with antibiotics. Local topical ear care is provided to reduce the acute inflammation that superinfects the underlying chronic process. Once the patient's medical condition is stabilized and the ear inflammation reduced, which may require several days, a definite mastoidectomy is indicated, and a systemic search for cholesteatoma, granulation tissue, bone destruction, and abscess formation is carried out at that time.

Bone destruction as a result of chronic inflammation is much deeper and more unpredictable than with acute infection. The erosive enzymes of cholesteatoma matrix or infected granulations can deeply penetrate bone, creating fistulae or extension of disease into the laryrinth, fallopian canal, or cranial cavity. The surgery for definitive removal of chronic disease requires a careful systematic exploration for foci of deeply penetrating infected tissue. Removal of erosive tissue is done carefully while constantly inspecting the bony margins at all time to assess the depth of penetration, always anticipating the exposure of underlying structures, for example, a semicircular canal, facial nerve, lateral sinus, or dura.

EARLY RECOGNITION OF OTITIS MEDIA COMPLICATIONS

Patients with acute otitis media who develop complications are generally young children. The onset of complications is usually quite rapid and obvious.

On the contrary, making the diagnosis of impending complications in patients with subacute or chronic otitis media is much more difficult. Frequently the patients have already been placed on antibiotics, which may mask some important symptoms, such as headache, fever, chills, and local pain that would suggest an impending complication. Otorrhea persisting more than 3 weeks despite reasonable antibiotic therapy should strongly suggest impending complications. Otitis media that recurs less than 2 weeks after antibiotic therapy implies persistent infected tissue within the temporal bone. A particularly foul-smelling drainage from the ear may also be indicative of bony erosion. Pulsatile serous drainage is common with acute and chronic suppurative infection; however, pulsatile purulent drainage may imply erosion of the posterior or middle fossa dural plates with an epidural collection.

In patients with potentially complicated otitis media, samples of the exudate and purulent material should be examined under a microscope and as much of this material debrided as possible for a thorough examination of the tympanic membrane. Any perforation is inspected, and the middle ear is examined, if possible, for obvious cholesteatoma or granulation tissue. In patients in whom systemic and topical treatment fails, specimens should be cultured for aerobes (e.g., *Mycobacterium tuberculosis*) and fungal organisms. A computed tomography (CT) scan has become the single most useful and most sensitive diagnostic examination. In the pre-CT era, evaluation of the mastoid bones and intracranial contents was challenging, often requiring some skillful sleuthing to arrive at a diagnosis. The current high-resolution CT scanners using bone settings and 1.5 mm cuts afford a remarkably accurate view of temporal bone detail. It is best to try to obtain both axial and coronal views to visualize small fistulas and tegmen defects. When complications of otitis media are suspected, a contrasted CT scan should follow the bone detail examination. The contrast material is readily taken up by any inflamed tissue within the cranial cavity causing marked enhancement. The thickened meninges in meningitis are enhanced, smaller abscess collections show a diffuse uptake, and larger abscesses present with a classic ringed lesion of enhancement surrounding hypodense center. Furthermore, the contrast material is taken into the venous sinuses and can demonstrate patency of the lateral sinus and internal jugular vein. Magnetic resonance imaging (MRI) has not proved to be as useful in the temporal bone because of its inability to visualize bone detail. Soft tissue detail is seen remarkably well, however. The MRI scanner is able to differentiate between fluid and soft tissue density within the mastoid cavity as opposed to a cholesteatoma or even a cholesterol granuloma. Tumors are extremely well demonstrated, and any brain abnormalities, such as a hernia, may be seen with exquisite detail that could be missed on a CT scan. When examination of soft tissue detail is important in making a diagnosis, and MRI scanner may prove to be invaluable. It is generally not as useful as the CT scanner in the evaluation of most otitis media complications, however.

The presence of any headache, fever, nausea, lethargy, alteration in level of consciousness, or any focal neurologic symptom should immediately raise the possibility of an intracranial complication that may become life threatening. A funduscopic examination is done to determine whether papilledema is present. A CT scan should be the next examination of choice to demonstrate any intracranial pathology. A brain abscess, subdural or epidural abscess, or lateral sinus thrombosis would demand emergent surgery in such a case. In the absence of any demonstrable mass lesion, a lumbar puncture (LP) is indicated to rule out meningitis. Performing the LP prior to obtaining the CT scan would run the risk of an uncal herniation if a mass lesion were, indeed, present. Finally, in the unusual circumstances of an ill patient with high spiking fever and in whom a CT scan with contrast has not shown any clear-cut pathology, an early lateral sinus thrombosis may be suspected. In such a case, a digital subtraction angiogram should be adequate to examine the lateral sinus suspected.

SUMMARY

Some general principles are applicable to the overall management of otitis media complications. Complications of acute suppurative otitis media without bony destruction will likely be adequately managed with the use of intravenous (IV) antibiotics and the possible addition of a myringotomy. Complications of acute suppurative otitis media associated with significant bony destruction require the addition of a mastoidectomy and an incision and drainage of any secondary soft tissue abscess.

Complications of chronic suppurative otitis media may present subtly when antibiotic use masks the true extent of pathology. A high index of suspicion may be necessary for the diagnosis. More severely ill patients require stabilization using high-dose antibiotics and examination debridement of the ear under a microscope. In both situations topical antibiotic drops and acetic acid irrigations are applied three times daily. Surgical establishment of drainage may be required in a critically ill patient, as well as incision and drainage of any secondary abscesses. Definitive mastoidectomy and tympanoplasty with a systematic search for residual disease are best delayed for several days to reduce the associated inflammation and to allow the patient's condition to stabilize. Patients presenting with intracranial complications are often desperately ill. Such patients are usually best managed with high-dose antibiotics to control the intracranial infection and prevent systemic sepsis. Once the patient's condition is stabilized, a mastoidectomy and drainage of the primary focus of infection can be carried out. The definitive tympanomastoidectomy should be staged to a later date.

It is also important to bear in mind that complications of otitis media are unusual, and unusual causes must be suspected. Tuberculosis, syphilis, connective tissue disorders, granulomatous disease, and malignancy all can present with a clinical picture resembling a chronic otitis media. Furthermore, patients who are immune compromised should raise a very high index of suspicion for the early development of otitis media complications. Such patients include infants, diabetics, elderly, and individuals on immunosuppressive therapy.

INTRATEMPORAL COMPLICATIONS OF OTITIS MEDIA

Acute Mastoiditis

The definition of mastoiditis requires clarification. The term, acute mastoiditis implies inflammation of the mastoid mucosa that would normally accompany any otitis media and would require only antibiotic therapy. Neely proposed the term "acute mastoiditis with bone destruction" as a more appropriate description for the bony necrosis and absorption of mastoid septae evolving as a complication of otitis media.[5] Synonymous terms for bone destruction are acute coalescent mastoiditis and acute mastoiditis with osteitis. Unchecked progression of such an infection may evolve into a subperiosteal abscess.

Subperiosteal abscesses occur by either direct extension of disease through cortical erosion or vascular extension through venous or lymphatic channels. An intact mastoid cortex was observed in 50% of the cases of subperiosteal abscess reviewed by Hawkins and Dru.[6] Subperiosteal abscesses most commonly occur over the area of Macewen's triangle. Less frequently, they can develop over the zygomatic root or erode through the digastric groove into the upper part of the neck, resulting in a Bezold abscess. A suppurative postauricular lymphadenitis can sometimes be confused with a true subperiosteal abscess.

Acute Mastoiditis With Bone Destruction

Acute otitis media is usually a disease of children and responds quickly to antibiotic therapy. It does not commonly progress to complications today. The natural history of an untreated acute suppurative otitis media is an initial presentation with a red, bulging tympanic membrane and acute pain. Relief of pain immediately follows rupture of the tympanic membrane. Bony destruction occurs in the case of acute purulent infection after 10 days to 2 weeks; therefore, a history of otorrhea for greater than 2 weeks should suggest the possibility of bony erosion.[7] There is often a recurrence of otaliga, particularly nocturnally. Periosteal edema and mastoid tenderness then develop, and a low-grade fever may be present. The skin of the posterosuperior external canal may appear to sag due to periosteal thickening overlying the antrum. With the widespread use of antibiotics today, the presentation of patients with acute coalescent mastoiditis are much more variable than the classic descriptions.

Despite antibiotic intervention, a small group of patients may still progress to this point due to blockage of drainage, inadequate blood levels of the drugs reaching the middle ear mucosa, a resistant bacterial strain, or immune compromise. Antibiotics occasionally serve only to mask the symptoms of fever, pain, and periosteal edema or tenderness until very late, despite the ongoing progressive bone destruction. The diagnosis may be suspected on the basis of persistent otorrhea alone.

A poorly responsive acute suppurative infection may be due to an underlying, previously unsuspected chronic otitis media. Superinfection of chronic ear disease is the most common cause of acute suppurative otitis media with complications. The chronic pathology has often already caused bony destruction, permitting rapid development of complications if early symptoms have gone unrecognized. Chronic otitis pathogens are usually gram-negative rods as opposed to the gram-positive cocci associated with acute otitis media.

Clinical Evaluation.—The patient with an acute coalescent mastoiditis is usually a young child or infant. Physical examination reveals either a bulging red tympanic membrane or, more likely, a profuse purulent otorrhea. Examination under the microscope may demonstrate a pulsatile thin purulent material draining from the perforation. A culture and sensitivity study of the drainage are obtained, if possible. There may be diffuse tender edema overlying the mastoid process or temporal area but without any focal fluctuant areas (Fig 39–1). Although needle aspiration can help determine whether a subperiosteal abscess is present, it is usually unnecessary and would be poorly tolerated in a young child. If the child is too young to undergo a CT scan without anesthesia, plain mastoid x-ray films can be obtained. A mastoid x-ray film should be adequate to demon-

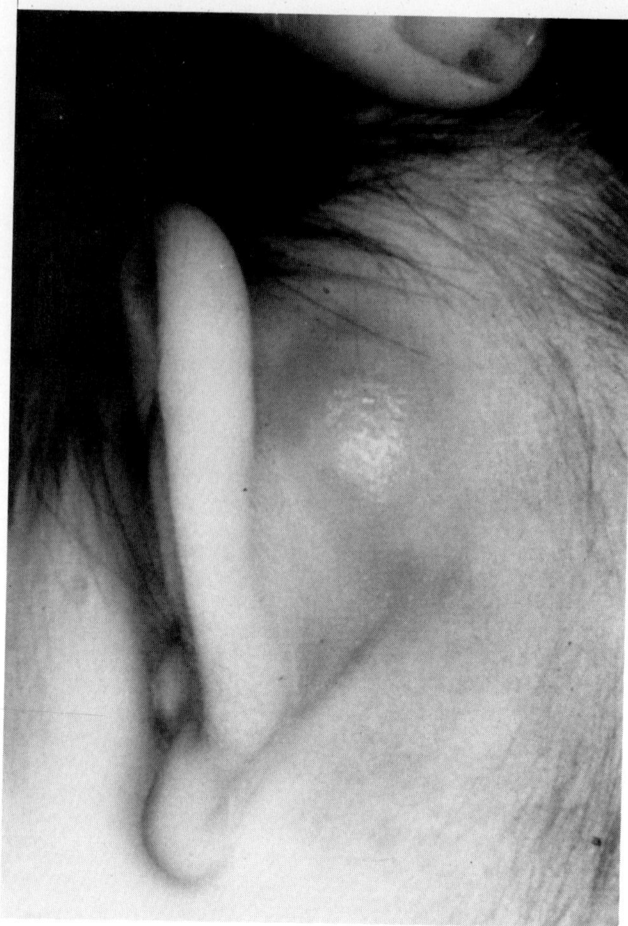

FIG 39–1.
Child with acute mastoiditis. (Courtesy of Eigi Yanagisawa, M.D.)

strate erosion and absorption of the bony septae as well as gross integrity of the posterior or middle fossa bony plates. In addition, a large labyrinthine fistula would be visible with a plain mastoid film. In an older child, a CT of the temporal bone is a preferable study. The temporal bone examination should include 1.5 mm high-resolution cuts rather than relying on coronal reconstructions. The study should be followed by a contrast-enhanced soft tissue scan. The CT is exceedingly accurate in demonstrating even small areas of bony erosion, fistula formation, and presence of intracranial inflammation or abscess, even at the earliest stages of development. It also affords examination of the subperiosteal tissues and helps distinguish between diffuse edema and true abscess.

Obtaining coronal views can be difficult in an uncooperative patient. The views are especially helpful in evaluating the descending seventh nerve and the integrity of the labyrinth and give an unparalleled picture of the middle fossa tegmen.

Children with acute coalescent mastoiditis are generally ill appearing with malaise, and therapy needs to be initiated quickly. Patients with a partially treated infection, as in the masked mastoiditis situation, are much less ill. Stable patients can be electively scheduled for a CT scan under anesthesia and then

transferred to the operating room under anesthesia to proceed with surgery.

The patient who appears to have an acute coalescent mastoiditis but appears desperately ill or toxic should be suspected of having a more serious intracranial process. A contrasted CT scan would be preferable in such a case, followed by an LP.

Management.—

Acute Mastoiditis Without Bony Erosion.—Acute mastoiditis without bony erosion on x-ray film is actually a severe, acute suppurative otitis media with an uncomplicated mastoiditis. Oral antibiotics are usually adequate therapy. A more severe case with significant overlying soft tissue edema in an ill patient may require IV antibiotics and a wide myringotomy if the tympanic membrane is still intact. The antibiotic therapy is guided by an infectious disease consultant and is based on intraoperative cultures and a Gram stain. We stress the use of an infectious disease consultant because it is impractical for the surgeon to keep fully abreast of all the uses of the third-generation cephalosporins and the evolving quinolones, as well as the regional resistant strains found in each particular hospital.

Acute Mastoiditis With Bone Destruction (coalescent mastoiditis).—The patient is most likely a young child or infant, ill appearing, with postauricular or temporal area diffuse edema possibly even rotating the auricle anteriorly and inferiorly but without any obvious subcutaneous fluctuance. Examination of the tympanic membrane would most likely show a thick, erythematous, bulging tympanic membrane with a perforation draining thin, purulent material, which is often pulsatile. If the tympanic membrane were intact, marked bulging of the drum would be seen. There would be no neurological changes to suggest an intracranial pathology. It is important to remember that these patients should not be desperately ill. If the patient does appear toxic, a more serious intracranial complication should be suspected. Antibiotics should be initiated intravenously as soon as possible on an empirical basis. Coverage should include gram-positive cocci and *Hemophilus influenzae.* An older patient would best be studied with a CT scan, if available, on an urgent basis.

Acute coalescent mastoiditis is a surgical condition. The patient can be stabilized on antibiotic therapy, but surgery should be undertaken as soon as possible for assuring resolution of the process. The situation closely resembles an abscess cavity necessitating incision and drainage, and a simple mastoidectomy with myringotomy is indicated. A definitive tympanomastoidectomy with facial recess approach would be extremely difficult in this situation of acute inflammation. It is also generally unnecessary, because providing drainage of the purulent material will result in a complete recovery. The discovery of underlying chronic disease may require a staged procedure.

Masked coalescent mastoiditis, a patient whose clinical symptoms and signs have been masked by antibiotics, will require a high index of suspicion to make the diagnosis of a slowly progressive bone destructive process. Such a patient should be

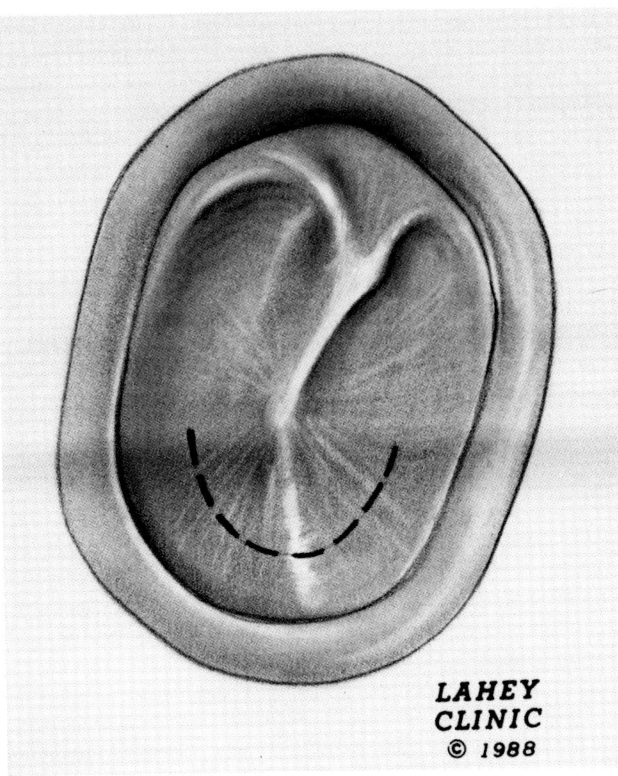

FIG 39–2.
Wide myringotomy.

best managed by a CT scan, under anesthesia if necessary, followed by a definitive mastoidectomy procedure.

In summary, all patients with mastoiditis and bony destruction will require IV antibiotics. Plain x-ray films are obtained in an infant, and a CT scan is obtained in older children and adults. If drainage has not already been established through a spontaneous perforation, a wide myringotomy is indicated on an emergent basis. In an infant, antibiotics alone may be sufficient therapy, even if coalescence has occurred, but the patient should be followed closely and a decision made after 24 hours to operate if the clinical picture has not improved. Except for infants, acute mastoiditis with coalescent bone destruction requires an urgent mastoidectomy. Antibiotics should then be continued for a minimum of 5 to 7 days before the patient is switched to oral antibiotics. In an older child or adult, a CT scan should be done at a later date once the acute disease process has resolved to ensure that no significant residual disease or underlying etiology exists.

Surgical Technique for Acute Mastoiditis with Bone Destruction.—

Wide Myringotomy (Fig 39–2).—A gravely ill patient can tolerate a myringotomy even without anesthesia at times. Cooperative patients may be given a local external meatus injection of 1% lidocaine with epinephrine 1:100,000. Topical anesthetic agents and iontophoresis techniques are not useful. An uncooperative patient will require a general anesthetic, and in such cases, mask anesthesia is usually adequate.

The tympanic membrane is markedly erythematous and bulging, and no landmarks may be visible. A semicircular incision paralleling the inferior tympanic ring can be safely made with a myringotomy knife. The incision is carried across the anterior and posterior inferior quadrants to produce a contraction of the superiorly based tympanic membrane flap and prevent rapid closure. Drainage of the purulent material should be immediate, and any hemorrhage should be self-limited. Cotton balls are then placed into the external meatus and changed frequently to monitor the degree of drainage.

Acute Mastoidectomy.—A simple mastoidectomy is sufficient for resolution of an acute mastoiditis with bone destruction. More detailed dissection within the mastoid cavity would be difficult because of the acutely infected tissues and significant hemorrhage. A masked mastoiditis with bone destruction is, however, a different situation. The patient would be less ill and the degree of inflammation suppressed, making it reasonable to open up the facial recess and improve drainage.

The simple mastoidectomy is begun with a postauricular incision. The incision must be modified in children less than 12 years of age because of variable stages of mastoid development, which may result in the seventh nerve exiting the skull base higher and more laterally than in an adult. The seventh nerve in children less than 2 years of age may lie within the line of the incision normally employed in adults. A smaller, more superior postauricular incision is necessary (Fig 39–3).

The skull base and mastoid tip are palpated at all times during the actual incision, because the marked mobility of the

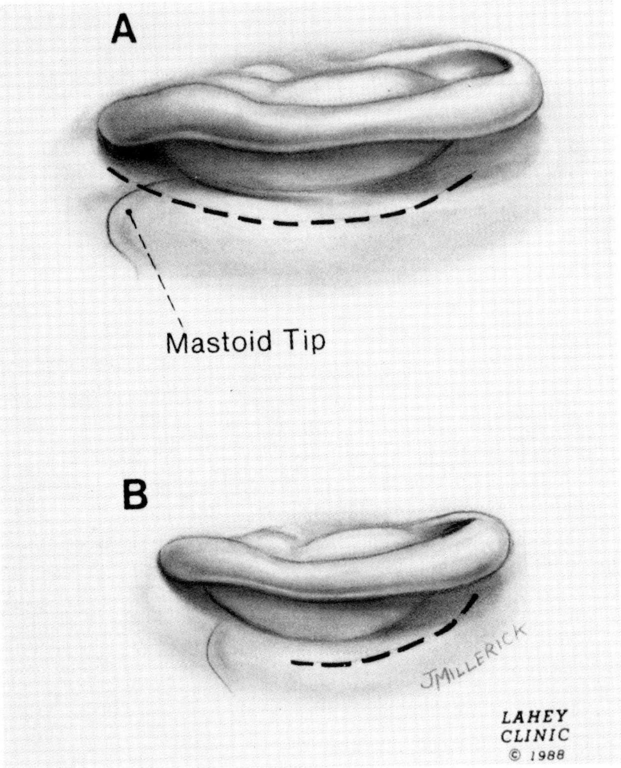

FIG 39–3.
Postauricular incision of adult (**A**) and child (**B**).

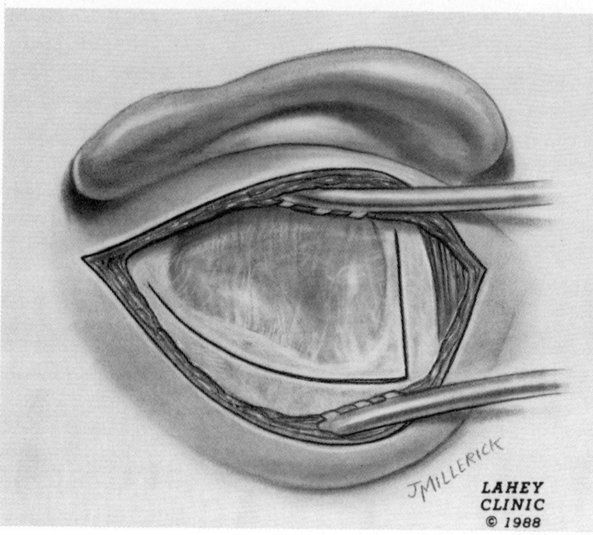

FIG 39–4.
Fascial and periosteal incisions with previous mastoidectomy.

skin in a young child may be disorienting. The smaller incision in children provides more than adequate exposure for complete mastoidectomy. In an adult, the incision is made similarly except that the inferior limb is carried down over the mastoid tip.

The incision is continued sharply to a level of the temporal fascia, pulling the auricle laterally to maximally expose the avascular plane overlying the fascia.

Ordinarily, bony cortex would next be exposed by a bold incision through the fascia, contacting bone with the knife along the temporal line. In the face of potential bony erosion, however, such an incision may plunge the knife into an exposed low-hanging temporal lobe or anterior sigmoid sinus. A T-shaped incision is made cautiously, with the horizontal limb following the temporal line. The vertical limb is made slightly more posteriorly than usual (lazy T) to place it behind the anticipated site of the sigmoid sinus in the event that cortical loss is encountered over the sinus (Fig 39–4). The incision should contract normal bone. The mastoid tip is again continually palpated during the actual incision.

The periosteal flaps are then elevated, constantly inspecting for subperiosteal collections or bony dehiscence. If a dehiscence were identified, the defect would be filled with infected soft tissue, and the flap would be sharply separated from the underlying soft tissue with the knife. Actual removal of the infected tissue can be delayed until exposure of the entire mastoid has been accomplished and the extent of bone destruction fully assessed. The flaps are elevated to expose the skin of the external meatus posterior wall, and it is not necessary to open into the external canal skin.

A complete mastoidectomy is then performed. Starting with a 6.0 mm cutting burr, the drilling is begun between Macewen's triangle and the temporal line. The middle fossa dura is visualized by thinning the tegmen, and any bony bleeding is usually controlled easily with a 5.0 or 6.0 mm diamond burr. Exposure of the dura in some areas will occur routinely and is no cause for concern. Bleeding from the dura itself must be controlled

using a bipolar cautery. Use of a monopolar Bovie on the dura can deeply injure the dura, even when it is turned down to minimal settings, and cerebrospinal fluid (CSF) leaks or delayed brain hernias often result.

The sigmoid sinus is identified secondly, then cortical bone removed anteriorly up to the posterior canal wall. Copious irrigation will be necessary to continually rinse away the purulent drainage and copious hemorrhage. The digastric ridge will be an important landmark for the stylomastoid foramen and is next identified. The sinodural angle can then be widely opened prior to proceeding toward the antrum. It may be necessary at times, because of bleeding, to stop working altogether, irrigate the wound copiously, and pack it with absorbable gelatin sponge (Gelfoam) strips soaked in epinephrine 1:1,000 for 3 to 5 minutes. Reducing the bleeding in such a fashion drastically reduces the dissection time wasted in fighting for visualization.

The antrum is then uncovered, staying high along the thinned tegmen. The posterior canal wall is thinned to remove all air cells, leaving a translucent bony plate. Now that maximal exposure of the antrum has been gained, the soft tissue within the antrum is carefully debulked, keeping in mind that bony erosion may have occurred deep to the soft tissue. Hemostasis is once again obtained.

The mastoid is completed using a diamond burr to thin the middle fossa tegmen and posterior fossa plates, inspecting the dura and sigmoid through the bone and ensuring that no extension of disease into the epidural or perisinus spaces has occurred. Residual infection into the perisinus cells is often overlooked and leads to recurrent infections. Other common sites to harbor residual infection are the mastoid tip cells and perilabyrinthine cells. Areas of soft infected bone should be drilled back to hard, good, viable bone at this time.

Once adequate removal of diseased cells and mucosa has been accomplished, the smooth rounded mastoid bowl should be relatively free of active oozing and pus other than that present from the middle ear. Copious irrigation with saline is done using at least 1 L.

The wound is closed in a standard fashion, approximating fascia and periosteum with 2-0 Vicryl interrupted sutures. The postauricular incision is closed over a single subcutaneous layer of 3-0 Vicryl sutures. A 1/4 in. Penrose drain is left in the inferior aspect of the wound and sutured to the skin edges. The drain is left in place generally 1 to 2 days, longer if the wound produces purulent material past that time. Intravenous antibiotics are continued for 5 to 7 days postoperatively, followed by 7 more days of oral antibiotics.

Mastoidectomy With Facial Recess Approach

In a patient with a masked mastoiditis and bone destruction, there will generally be less acute inflammation with reduction of the hyperemia and purulent material found in the acute mastoiditis situation. There is a higher chance for encountering greater bone destruction and complications of otitis media due to antibiotics masking the clinical picture. A facial recess approach may be added to further examine the middle ear, inspect for possible fistulae, and widen the drainage from the mastoid cavity.

A complete mastoidectomy is performed as previously described. Cholesteatoma and granulation tissue in the antrum area are debulked, leaving residual disease on the antral floor and fallopian canal until more anatomy can be identified. If the incus is present, an attempt to palpate it within the diseased mass can be made at this time. Cholesteatoma can be debulked, leaving matrix overlying the bony floor of the antrum, and it is often possible to inspect the integrity to the bony floor through the translucent matrix before any attempt is made to elevate the matrix. Following debridement of the diseased soft tissues, the ossicles are identified and palpated, if possible. If absent, the aditus ad antrum and lateral semicircular canal can usually be identified. The zygomatic root cells are then opened up, removing all the cells between the thinned superior wall of the bony canal and the middle fossa dura. Opening the zygomatic root cells gains access to the mastoid attic and epitympanum. Attempts to locate the malleus head and incus is again made at this point. The short process of the incus head, if intact, points to the bone that will be removed in the facial recess (Fig 39–5). The facial nerve second genu will be medial to the incus head, and it curves within the arc of the horizontal semicircular canal. The inside curve of the lateral canal and anterior aspect of the digastric ridge form the two endpoints of the descending facial nerve, which courses in a roughly straight line, occasionally deviating laterally at its midpoint. The descending facial nerve is identified using broad strokes with a 4.0 mm diamond burr and copious irrigation. Bleeding may be encountered in small air cells overlying the facial nerve, and can be controlled with Gelfoam and epinephrine (Adrenalin). The mucosa within these cells may be easily confused with hyperemic epineurium and can be differentiated by palpating the mucosa and cell. Small bleeders overlying the facial nerve may also be encountered and can be controlled with Gelfoam and epinephrine or by gently using the diamond burr. Persistent bleeders directly overlying the facial nerve may also be handled by using a Rosen needle to tuck the edges of the bleeder under some bone or by using a microbipolar set to the lowest possible setting to achieve cauterization. Once the operator is assured of the facial nerve course, the facial recess is opened using successively smaller diamond burrs. The facial nerve and the chorda tympani that form the boundaries of the facial recess are identified and even exposed, if necessary. As much bone as possible is removed with 1.0 and 2.0 mm diamond burrs within the confines of the triangular recess to maximize exposure and postoperative drainage. The middle ear is irrigated, packed with Gelfoam and epinephrine, and then reinspected for evidence of chronic disease. The ossicles are again inspected, and infected tissue is removed. Cholesteatoma matrix and granulations that were adherent to the floor of the antrum may now be elevated from either anteriorly or posteriorly. The cochleariform process is an excellent landmark to identify the facial nerve at its horizontal portion if difficulty is encountered locating landmarks. Granulations or cholesteatoma matrix are then gently teased away from the bone, starting preferably posteriorly and working anteriorly, looking for bony erosion that would suggest a fistula or exposed facial nerve. The management of these problems is discussed later in this section. The remaining infected tissue is removed. The last site to be carefully inspected is the epitym-panum, the anterior epitympanum in particular, which is the most common site for recurrence. The area can be difficult to evaluate, and it is important to fully open up the zygomatic root cells to properly visualize that area.

Once all of the chronically infected tissue has been removed and the lack of bony crevices and overhangs within the mastoid cavity is assured, wound closure is obtained as described for the complete simple mastoidectomy. A rubber band drain is substituted for the Penrose, which is used only in acute mastoiditis with coalescent bone destruction.

Incision and Drainage of a Subperiosteal Abscess

A standard postauricular incision is generally ideal for gaining access to the abscess, which is mostly commonly centered over Macewen's triangle. Great care is taken with the incision to avoid making the cut deeply over potentially exposed middle fossa dura or the lateral sinus. A finger is again maintained on the mastoid tip at all times to ensure proper orientation and to avoid any injury to the facial nerve. In a patient less than 12 years of age, the modified postauricular incision is used (see Fig 39–3). If the abscess has not been encountered superficial to the temporal fascia, the lazy T incision should be used to open the subperiosteal space. The abscess should be evacuated and irrigated copiously, and then the complete mastoidectomy should be performed.

The wound is closed, leaving a Penrose drain through the skin and fascia. The drain is withdrawn progressively when the purulent drainage begins to decrease. Antibiotics are given intravenously as described.

Facial Nerve Paralysis

Facial nerve paralysis occurs with four different types of temporal bone infection: (1) acute otitis media with mastoiditis, (2) chronic otitis media with cholesteatoma or granulation tissue, (3) malignant "otitis externa," and (4) herpes zoster oticus.

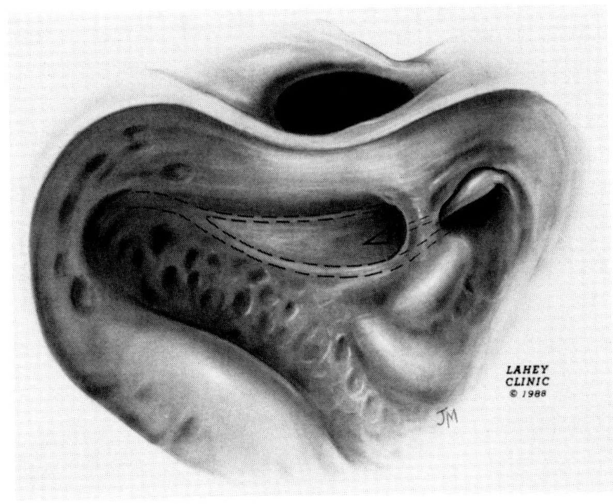

FIG 39–5.
Relationship of incus short process pointing toward facial recess.

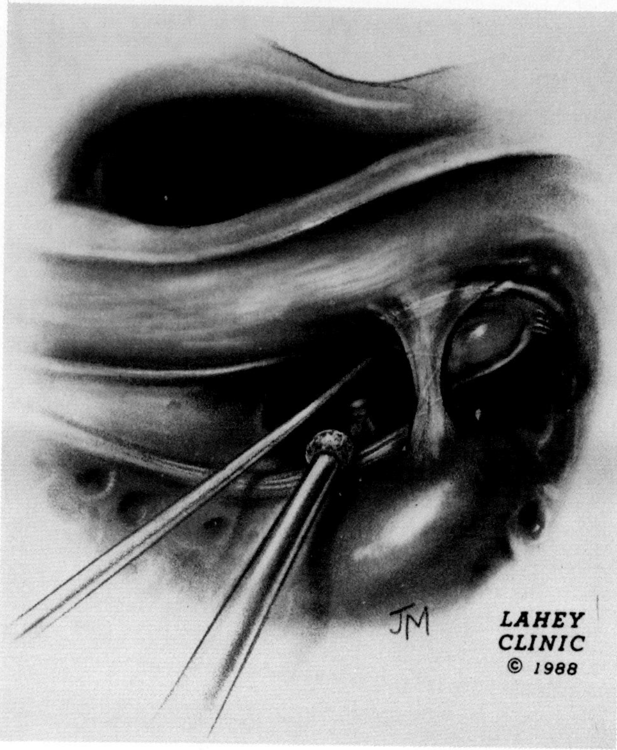

FIG 39–6.
Disarticulation and elevation of incus lenticular process to decompress seventh nerve through facial recess.

Facial paralysis in a child is most commonly due to acute otitis media with mastoiditis. On the contrary, paralysis in adults is due to a complication of chronic otitis media.

The most common site of injury is presumed to be the horizontal portion superior to the oval window, which is congenitally dehiscent in approximately 50% of individuals. However, dehiscence or exposure of the nerve is not a requirement for the development of paralysis.[1]

Chronic otitis media may induce paralysis by suppurative exacerbation of the chronic disease process, bony erosion with extrinsic pressure injury to the nerve, granulation tissue inciting an inflammatory reaction in the nerve, or actual invasion of the nerve.[2]

Sunderland stresses the importance of the perineurium as an effective physiologic barrier to the spread of infection as opposed to the epineurium, which is a poor barrier.[7] Therefore, diseased tissue involving the epineurium can be peeled off of the nerve. The tissue invading the perineurium should be left intact rather than risk further injury of adjacent perineurium with spread of disease.

The patient may present with either a paresis or a total paralysis. Site of lesion testing adds little to the evaluation.

Acute Suppurative Otitis Media With Facial Nerve Paralysis

Evaluation.—Facial nerve paralysis due to acute suppurative otitis media usually occurs in a child with symptoms of less

than 2 weeks' duration. The possibility of underlying chronic ear disease must always be remembered in older children or adults.

Acute inflammation is thought to cause nerve injury by local toxic effects, tissue edema, or venous congestion.[5]

Computed tomography scan of the temporal bone, with and without contrast, should be obtained to rule out any early associated intracranial pathology and any chronic erosive lesions impinging on the nerve.

Most commonly with acute suppurative processes, facial paresis is seen rather than complete paralysis. If complete paralysis does occur, however, excitability nerve testing is required. The facial nerve function is monitored using the Hilgar stimulator. Threshold testing will show a difference of more than 3.5 mamp between the two sides, and maximal stimulation testing will drop to less than 10% of the intact side when nerve degeneration is occurring. Electroneuronography (ENoG) may be used to objectively measure a 90% decrease in maximal stimulation testing. Should more than 90% nerve degeneration occur after 3 to 4 days, transmastoid nerve decompression would be indicated.

A wide myringotomy will usually provide adequate drainage and resolution of the inflammation with complete return of facial nerve function. The CT scan and wide myringotomy can be done under the same general anesthetic in a young child. Mastoidectomy and nerve compression are rarely necessary in acute suppurative otitis media situations.

Technique for Nerve Decompression in Acute Otitis Media.— A complete mastoidectomy with facial recess approach is performed. The recess is opened as widely as possible to maximize exposure. The most important landmark to identify is the cochleariform process as the site of the first genu of the nerve. All other landmarks may be initially obscured by the inflammatory disease, which may be overlying the horizontal portion of the nerve in particular. The bony shell of the skeletonized fallopian canal is then gently removed with small diamond burrs from the cochleariform to the stylomastoid process. If the sugreon works through the facial recess with 0.5 and 1.0 mm burrs and the newly available Skeeter drill, it is unusual to require removal of the incus to complete the full decompression. It is occasionally necessary to disarticulate the incus from the stapes to avoid noise transmission to the cochlea (Fig 39–6). The joint heals well when reapproximated and needs no further therapy.

When removal of the incus is necessary, the head of the malleus should also be nipped off and the recess widely opened to identify the tympanic annulus for maximum exposure. The incus is then sculpted and fitted from malleus handle to stapes at the termination of the case.

Decompression of the facial nerve is done with long strokes of the diamond burr made parallel to the course of the nerve and using copious irrigation. The stylomastoid artery branches, which frequently course along the lateral aspect of the descending nerve, will become apparent just prior to exposing the nerve itself.

Bleeding is controlled with long strokes of the diamond

burr, driving bone dust into the vessels, but occasionally bothersome bleeding ensues. The vessels should be further exposed with the drill, hemostasis obtained by tucking the loose bleeding ends of the vessel back under a small shelf of thin bone with a Rosen needle or by using a microbipolar cautery on a low setting and with irrigation during the cauterization. Extreme caution should be used with the cautery to ensure that the bipolar tips are not in contact with the facial nerve itself. A small pledget of Gelfoam soaked in epinephrine will also stop the oozing while the surgeon works on another site. The final decompression should ultimately expose the lateral surface of the nerve as close to 180 degrees around as possible.

The nerve sheath is not incised. The perineurium provides an important barrier to the spread of infection, and its integrity should be preserved. The epineurium is a much looser tissue layer and is a poor barrier for spread of infection.

Acute Suppurative Otitis Media With (Coalescent) Bone Destruction and Facial Paralysis

Acute and masked suppurative mastoiditis with bone destruction necessitates surgical management. The additional complication of facial nerve paralysis occurring due to bony invasion of the fallopian canal would require a minimum of a 2-week clinical history if the disease process is truly the result of acute suppuration. A CT scan should be obtained to document the bony erosion of air cell septae, but mastoid x-ray films are adequate in an uncooperative young child.

Management.—The patient should be immediately started on empirical antibiotics intravenously. A surgical drainage procedure would be indicated.

A wide myringotomy is made in all patients if spontaneous drainage has not already been established. A myringotomy is adequate in the very young patient or an older patient with acute suppurative otitis media and very early minimal evidence of bone destruction.

A complete mastoidectomy is indicated urgently in the patient with significant evidence of bone destruction and coalescence. If the nerve fails to return and begins to show evidence of degeneration within 3 days, a staged facial recess approach and nerve decompression can be done.

A complete mastoidectomy with facial recess approach for the primary operation can be done in the masked mastoiditis case. Such a patient can be managed with IV antibiotics for several days as long as there is no evidence of deterioration of the clinical picture or degeneration of the nerve excitability test. A complete paralysis followed by evidence of nerve degeneration would create a more urgent situation.

Technique of Facial Nerve Exploration With Acute Suppuration.—A complete mastoidectomy and facial recess approach is performed. The seventh nerve is identified within its intact fallopian canal from cochleariform to stylomastoid foramen. The fallopian canal is thinned to inspect the nerve through the bone, but the bone is preserved to prevent spread of infection to other portions of the nerve. Any sites of granulation tissue attached to the nerve are inspected to determine whether

the perineurium is invaded. Granulation tissue adherent only to the epineurium can be teased off of the nerve. Invasive granulations, however, should be trimmed to minimize their bulk without making an attempt to violate the perineurium. A full nerve decompression is not done at this time to prevent any spread of infection. Rather, if the nerve excitability tests continue to deteriorate postoperatively despite adequate drainage and antibiotics, a staged decompression is done.

Chronic Suppurative Otitis Media With Facial Paralysis.— A complete facial paralysis is more likely to develop because of chronic otitis media rather than with acute suppuration. In addition, the destructive cholesteatoma and granulation tissue may have created associated fistulae or erosion of the middle and posterior fossa bony plates. Patients are generally clinically stable, permitting the use of preoperative antibiotics for several days to reduce inflammation and allowing the meticulous dissection anticipated.

Routine cultures with sensitivities are obtained as well as fungal and tuberculin cultures. The ear is then debrided as much as possible under the microscope.

A CT scan with and without contrast is obtained to examine the extension of bony destruction and rule out intracranial pathology. If the seventh nerve paralysis seems inappropriate for what would be an otherwise mildly diseased ear and the CT scan does not demonstrate significant pathology, an MRI scan may be very helpful to actually visualize the nerve along its full length to inspect for an occult tumor.

Medical management is begun immediately with irrigations of the ear using 1.5% acetic acid solution warmed to near-body temperature, followed by topical antibiotic-steroid drops delivered three times daily. Intravenous antibiotics are initiated immediately.

A facial paresis is followed closely for any evidence of further degeneration. If a complete paralysis is present, nerve excitability testing should be done daily. If degeneration begins to develop, surgery is indicated much sooner.

Surgical Management of Chronic Suppurative Otitis Media With Facial Paralysis

A definitive mastoidectomy is performed. The decision to perform a facial recess intact canal wall procedure or to take the canal wall down is made based on the extent of disease present, and the presence of a facial nerve paralysis does not influence that decision. The canal wall is left intact for both procedures during the completion of the mastoidectomy until the extent of disease can be fully assessed.

Any cholesteatoma encountered in the antrum is debulked, leaving matrix on the floor of the antrum. The presence of bony destruction can then be best ascertained before elevation of the matrix is attempted. If a deep fistula is present, matrix can be left intact over the fistula to be removed at a second stage when the purulent infection has resolved. If an erosion is found to be present but is shallow, the matrix can be slowly elevated out of the depression, working from posteriorly to anteriorly, and constantly looking for any exposed endosteum. After the matrix has been elevated off of the bone overlying the lateral semicircular canal, the same technique is used to remove matrix from overlying the fallopian canal area. The canal is followed anteriorly to the cochleariform process, and constant palpation of the canal area is done to determine whether there is any bony dehiscence present. The most common site for bony dehiscence occurring congenitally is the inferior surface of the fallopian canal directly overlying the oval window area.

Granulation tissue may be encountered overlying the fallopian canal or even adherent to the facial nerve. Granulations are gently teased off of the nerve, again working posterior to anterior whenever possible, and any granulation tissues that appear to be deeply penetrating the nerve are left intact.

The facial nerve is inspected through thin bone or even exposed in areas for positive identification of the nerve along its full length from the cochleariform process to the stylomastoid foramen. It is not necessary to formally decompress the nerve; rather, examining the nerve for the site of injury and resolving the inflammation are sufficient to restore function to the nerve in most cases. A tympanic membrane may be grafted at this time regardless of whether the canal wall was left intact or taken down. With the intact canal wall procedure, a second-stage tympanoplasty to reinspect the mastoid cavity and reconstruct the ossicular chain should be planned for 6 months later.

INTRACRANIAL COMPLICATIONS OF OTITIS MEDIA

Intracranial complications of otitis media are frequently asymptomatic until the lesions become quite advanced. Any evidence of systemic symptoms, headache, particularly fever, or any early neurologic signs in a patient with chronic otitis media should immediately raise the suspicion of a developing intracranial complication.

Epidural Abscess With Temporal Bone Infections

An epidural abscess occurs by direct extension of disease through the thin middle or posterior fossa bony plates. There is usually erosion by cholesteatoma or granulation tissue, but at times bone can be grossly intact. Any purulent collection that has broken through the confines of the temporal bone to rest on the dura is, by definition, an epidural abscess. Frequently, small collections are located behind granulations, which may be quite indolent. With time they can progressively enlarge to either penetrate the dura producing subdural, intracerebral or intracerebellar abscesses, or extend to the lateral sinus, causing thrombosis or thrombophlebitis. Meningitis may follow either situation.

The clinical presentation may be quite variable. The majority of epidural abscesses are asymptomatic complications of long-standing chronic otitis media and are discovered only at the time of surgery. An epidural abscess may sometimes be suspected by the presence of profuse creamy purulent otorrhea that is pulsatile. The pulsatile otorrhea associated with acute otitis media is usually a thinner serous consistency. More symptomatic patients may complain of a headache or may have low-

grade fever. Even more serious infections may present with early, more advanced signs of meningitis. Finally, although more common with frontal epidural abscesses, a widespread otitic epidural abscess may present with signs of increased intracranial pressure: alterations of consciousness, nausea, vomiting, and papilledema. Advanced meningeal signs and hemiparesis may also occur.

Evaluation of Epidural Abscesses

The patient has a long-standing chronic ear with granulations and a very small, unsuspected collection on the surface of the middle or posterior fossa dura. A CT scan may be obtained in anticipation of a tympanomastoidectomy, and such a study would ordinarily be performed without contrast. The study would demonstrate the soft tissue disease within the middle ear and mastoid, but a small extradural collection with minimal bony destruction may be entirely missed. Such collections must, therefore, be diligently searched for during the mastoidectomy in a patient at risk.

A small epidural abscess may be suspected when chronic otitis media is associated with profuse, pulsatile, creamy, purulent otorrhea. The study of choice is CT scan with contrast, which would show irregular enhancement of thickened dura and may possibly demonstrate the actual collection (Fig 39–7).

A patient with any meningeal or neurologic signs must be treated as a medical emergency. A contrasted CT scan should be obtained, and emergent surgery is indicated. Lumbar puncture is contraindicated because of the possible elevated intracranial pressure. Consultation from a neurosurgeon is imperative, because a combined procedure may be required.

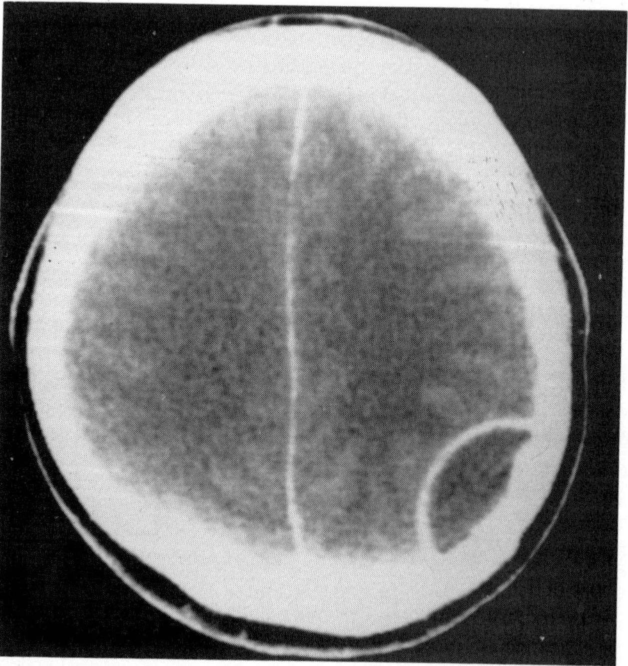

FIG 39–7.
Contrasted CT scan of epidural abscess. (Courtesy of G.E. Valvassori.)

Management of Epidural Abscesses Encountered Intraoperatively

Whenever exploration of a chronic mastoid reveals granulation tissue or pathologic bone erosion, a systematic search should be undertaken for possible presence of an epidural collection. The middle fossa tegmen should be thinned sufficiently to expose or provide visualization of the dura through the transparent bone. The dura is frequently uncovered in some areas, even in routine mastoid surgery. When chronic disease involves the perisinus cells, they must be fully opened up, skeletonizing the lateral sinus first and then the posterior fossa bony plate anterior and posterior to the sinus.

Epidural collections tend to involve the middle fossa when cholesteatoma is present. Involvement of the posterior fossa dura or lateral sinus more frequently accompanies acute suppurative disease or chronic otitis media with granulation tissue.[5]

Once an epidural collection is discovered, the bone is drilled away using a diamond burr and copious irrigation. Bipolar cautery of bleeding granulation is usually necessary. The drilling is continued to uncover the entire abscess and expose healthy dura. In the middle fossa area, it may be necessary to expose all the bone of the middle fossa tegmen, which does not risk a brain herniation unless an injury to the dura actually occurs. The zygomatic root cells are opened as anteriorly as possible, and the bone is removed laterally to the area of the junction of the tegmen with the vertical squamous portion of the temporal bone. Medially the bone is removed down to the level of the antral floor and posteriorly to the sinodural angle. Complete exposure of the posterior fossa dura at risk requires removal of bone 1.0 to 2.0 cm posterior to the lateral sinus and anterior to it the extending medially toward the posterior semicircular canal, which may also partially expose the endolymphatic sac.

Granulations are bluntly dissected off the dura if possible or, if adherent to the dura, can be trimmed down sharply or reduced with a bipolar, leaving some residual rather than risking penetration of the dura. Necrotic granulations are gently probed to ascertain whether a tract is present to the subdural space. Care must be exercised in this maneuver because it is easy to open up a walled-off tract into the CSF. An epidural collection that communicates into the subdural space is a neurosurgical problem, and intraoperative consultation is appropriate.

If subdural extension is in question, the procedure can be terminated, a CT with contrast, or preferably an MRI scan, obtained, and any neurosurgical exploration staged. Intraoperative ultrasound is available and is an ideal instrument to determine the presence and location of subdural or intraparenchymal collections.

Cerebrospinal fluid leaks will occasionally occur in the removal of dural granulations. The defect is plugged with temporalis muscle and fascia, and then a Gelfoam patch is placed over it and held against the defect with a cottonoid. A suction is applied to the cottonoid to dry up the Gelfoam against the defect and allow the patch to adhere to the dura. The patch will remain intact after 2 to 5 minutes of gentle pressure. If the leak cannot be controlled, it may be necessary to pack the cavity to maintain pressure against the Gelfoam and fascia. Gelfoam soaked in antibiotic solution or iodoform gauze may be used; however, the gauze would require a general anesthesia for removal.

Completion of the chronic ear procedure would then continue independently of the presence of the epidural abscess. The canal wall is left up or taken down as necessary for the complete removal of the chronic disease present, and tympanoplasty is performed. Ossicular reconstruction should be delayed for a planned second stage with the intact canal wall procedure.

Intravenous antibiotics are initiated intraoperatively empirically, and changes are made postoperatively at the recommendation of the infectious disease team.

Management of a Preoperatively Diagnosed Epidural Abscess

In a stable patient, IV antibiotics and local ear care should be given for several days preoperatively. The patient can then be taken to surgery for a possible combined neuro-otologic procedure, and the neurosurgeon is on standby. The complete mastoidectomy is performed and exposure of the abscess obtained and opened widely, exposing healthy bone and dura circumferentially. If necrotic granulations involve the dura, a neurosurgeon is called to evaluate a potential early subdural abscess. Development of a subdural empyema carries a very high mortality rate. All measures necessary for early recognition and management must be taken.

Management of Epidural Abscess With Neurologic Signs

Any neurologic changes associated with an epidural abscess implies complication of the abscess or a large collection with a mass effect. The situation is a surgical emergency requiring an immediate incision and drainage with empirical initiation of antibiotics in meningeal doses. A contrasted CT scan is obtained to determine the extent of disease. An abscess that has spread beyond the confines of the mastoid will require a craniectomy planned in conjunction with the neurosurgeon.

Middle Fossa Abscess (Fig 39–8).—A large extradural collection may require a formal middle fossa craniotomy to gain adequate exteriorization of the abscess. A linear incision is made vertically from the superior border of the zygomatic arch 1.0 cm anterior to the root of the helix and carried superiorly to approximately 4.0 cm from the vertex. The incision is carried down to the bone, and the temporal muscle, fascia, and periosteum are retracted to expose the squamous portion of the temporal bone. A rectangular bone flap is then outlined with a cutting 4.0 mm burr, and a diamond burr is used to complete the bone cut just overlying the dura. The bone flap is lifted out to expose the lateral middle fossa dura. The size of the bone flap is determined by the extent of disease where the inferior cut is made at the level of the root of zygoma. If the bone plate appears infected, it may be necessary to discard it and reconstruct the defect at a later stage. The abscess site is debrided and irrigated thoroughly. The incision is carried in continuity to the postauricular incision and a complete mastoidectomy

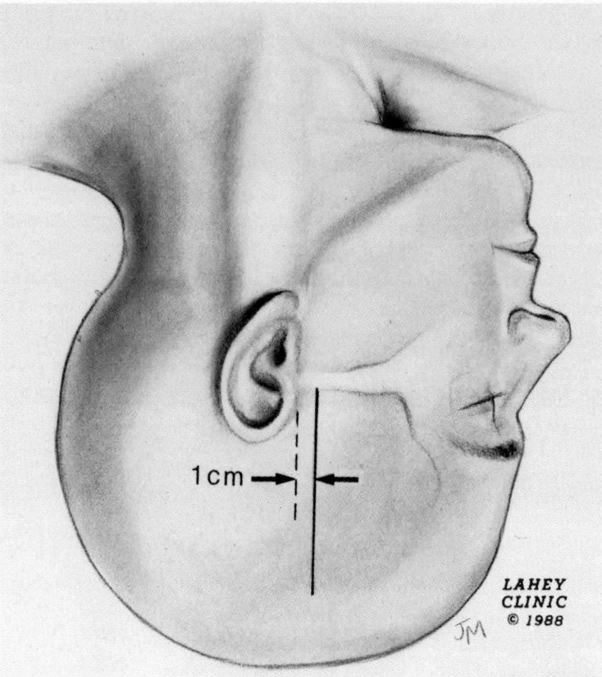

FIG 39–8.
Middle fossa incision.

performed. Facial recess and middle ear work are delayed for a later stage. Complete unroofing of the middle fossa tegmen is then accomplished, and the posterior fossa bone is thinned to ensure there are no other collections.

A catheter is sutured into the wound to permit frequent irrigation with antibiotic solution for several days postoperatively. A definitive mastoid procedure to completely eradicate any chronic disease from the ear will be done at a later date.

Posterior Fossa (Fig 39–9).—A postauricular incision is made over a 3.0 cm skin flap posterior to the auricle in the same fashion as done for a combined translabyrinthine-suboccipital acoustic tumor approach. A skin flap is elevated 2.0 cm anteriorly, allowing a staggered second incision to be made through fascia, temporal muscle, and periosteum 1.0 cm anterior to the skin incision. The full-thickness flap is elevated anteriorly up to the posterior external canal border. The musculature attached to the skull base is elevated with its periosteum and reflected inferiorly. A complete mastoidectomy is then done with a small craniectomy extending posterior to the sigmoid as far posteriorly as required to widely expose the abscess and uncover normal dura. The lateral side is completely exposed following it posteriorly to the transverse sinus and inferiorly to the sigmoid sinus. The transverse sinus would normally be the superior limit of the exposure, but further posterior and superior exposure of the transverse sinus may be necessary. The posterior fossa dura and sinus are totally uncovered, removing bone with 5.0 and 6.0 mm diamond burrs until leaving extremely thin flexible wafers of transparent bone overlying the soft tissue. Thinning the bone to that degree permits easy blunt

dissection from the dura and sinus by sliding a Penfield or freer elevator deep to the bone flecks and removing them carefully. The sinus must then be palpated to ensure that it is soft and uninvolved with disease and that there is no thrombophlebitis present. Further exposure of the posterior fossa dura is done by similarly lifting the bone. It is not always completely necessary to remove the bone over apparently healthy dura. The dura anterior to the sigmoid sinus extending toward the cerebellopontine angle is quite thin and easily disrupted if all the bone is removed from it. The wound is thoroughly irrigated with at least 1 L of saline and then closed over an irrigation catheter sewn in place. Antibiotic irrigation done at the bedside three times daily are initiated immediately, and the IV antibiotics started preoperatively are continued pending culture results. Definitive chronic ear surgery and tympanoplasty will be delayed until a later date.

Lateral Sinus Thrombosis

Lateral sinus thrombosis develops by thrombophlebitis of the small dural venules and emissary veins or by direct extension of posterior fossa extradural disease, which incites mural thrombosis and a propogation of infection. Although it rarely occurs today, its early recognition is critical, because the outcome can be rapidly fatal.

The classic description of lateral sinus thrombosis includes headache, malaise, "picket fence" high fever spikes, and possible increased intracranial pressure due to occlusion of the sinus. In addition, the mastoid may show signs of acute mastoiditis with Greisinger's sign (swelling over the posterior mastoid due to retrograde extension of thrombophlebitis into the emissary vein).

Antibiotic masking today complicates the clinical presentation of lateral sinus thrombosis, and a patient with early in-

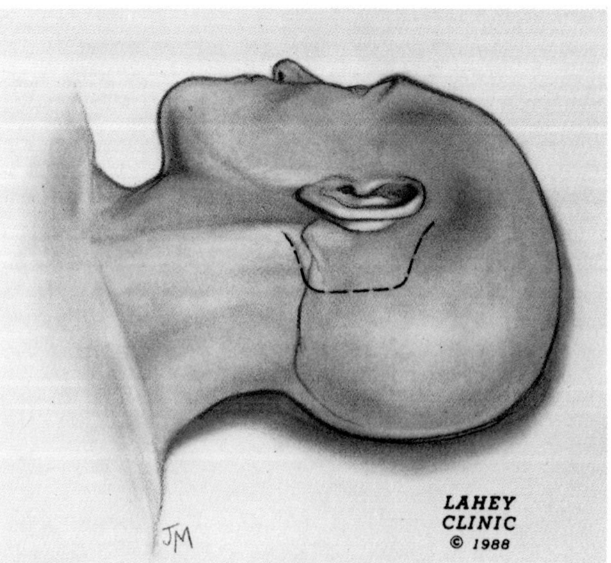

FIG 39–9.
Posterior fossa incision (combined approach flap).

volvement may have minimal symptoms of a possible headache and low-grade fever with malaise in a setting of either acute or chronic otitis media.

It must be stressed that any systemic symptoms associated with ear disease should always raise a concern over the possibility of intracranial complications.

A CT scan with contrast should be obtained, because it can readily demonstrate the dural and perisinus inflammation with bright enhancement of the sinus and surrounding dura. Sufficient contrast to adequately enhance the contralateral sinus is then given and its degree of enhancement compared with the ipsilateral potentially diseased sinus to estimate its patency. The right sinus is normally the dominant large vessel.

In a critically ill patient with a high fever and neurologic signs, the clinician would have a difficult time determining whether the etiology were a large epidural abscess, lateral sinus thrombosis, meningitis, subdural, or temporal lobe abscess or any combination. Rapid establishment of the diagnosis is essential. A CT scan with contrast would clearly demonstrate any abscess. A CT scan would also rule out the presence of cerebral edema, mass effects with shift, or hydrocephalus, which would then permit an LP in the absence of papilledema. Lateral sinus thrombophlebitis may be appreciated, but in a patent sinus with a mural thrombus, the CT scan could fail to elucidate the diagnosis.

The Queckenstedt and Tobey-Ayer tests are unreliable.[8] These tests involve observation of CSF pressure responses to internal jugular vein digital compression during the performance of an LP. The degree of sinus compromise necessary to evoke an abnormal test result, however, would most likely also require a sufficient elevation of intracranial pressure to make the LP potentially dangerous.

If the diagnosis of sinus thrombophlebitis is suspected on clinical grounds based on high-spiking daily or twice daily fever or signs of intracranial pressure elevation, and CT scan is unable to satisfactorily render a diagnosis, an angiogram can be performed. Digital subtraction angiography should be adequate to demonstrate any abnormalities of the sinus, including small mural thrombi.

Management

Unsuspected Lateral Sinus Thrombosis.—In an asymptomatic patient with chronic ear disease, a CT scan without contrast would most likely be obtained and the diagnosis missed until the time of surgery. During mastoidectomy, any extension of disease into the perisinus air cells suggests an aggressive process and requires examination of the whole posterior fossa dural surface, as well as the sinus, through thinned bone using large diamond burrs. Any granulations or infected cholesteatomas eroding through the bony plate are explored, and bone is widely removed surrounding the area to unroof any potential epidural collections. A lateral sinus thrombosis should be suspected in the presence of any posterior fossa epidural collection.

If such a collection is found, the sinus should be widely exposed, removing the overlying bone by drilling with the diamond until the thin eggshell covering remains. The freer elevator is then used to separate the sinus wall from the adherent

bone remnants. The sinus is palpated to ensure it is as soft and compressible as the internal jugular vein within the neck. Inflamed granulation tissue adherent to the wall is bluntly dissected off, if possible, and it may be necessary to sharply amputate granulations that are firmly adherent. In the absence of an actual thrombosis, nothing more need be done to the sinus.

If the vessel is indurated and thrombus is suspected, it must be incised and drained as in the treatment of any other abscess. Aspiration of the sinus through a 22-gauge needle is usually unnecessary but can be done if there is a question regarding the patency of the vessel. Proximal and distal control of the sinus is obtained using large sheets of oxidized cellulose (Surgicel), packing it extraluminally between the vessel wall and overlying bone at the limits of bony removal. Any thrombus extending more proximally will require further bony removal over the transverse sinus, because it can propogate as far back as the torcular Herophili. Distally it may be necessary to expose the jugular bulb to remove all visible clot. Surgicel packs are then partially removed to ensure good flow from both directions after the clot is removed.

Mokhtari has recently discussed the management of organized white thrombus occasionally found within the sinus.[8] In his series, no attempt was made to remove an organized clot, and such sinuses were packed with antibiotic-impregnated gauze, which was removed progressively over several days through the incision. If all of the clot can be removed, however, the vessel can be approximated with interrupted 6-0 Prolene suture. The Surgicel packs are then removed, and any leaks in the wall repair are controlled with a large wet Gelfoam pad placed on the sinus. A cottonoid is laid over the Gelfoam, and a suction tip is used to dry the cottonoid and Gelfoam while maintaining light pressure on the sinus. Even large tears in the sinus can usually be controlled by this very effective technique. Intraluminal and extraluminal packing of the sinus with Surgicel can be done in the event of uncontrolled hemorrhage but should be discouraged because of the infection in the site and the resultant cerebral edema and increased intracranial pressure.

Suspected Lateral Sinus Thrombosis.—The patient with preoperative evidence of a lateral sinus thrombosis showing neurologic changes or who is critically ill requires a lifesaving incision and drainage procedure rather than a definitive chronic ear operation. A complete mastoidectomy should be done, followed by examination of the middle posterior fossa dura through thin bony plates. Evacuation of the sinus thrombosis is accomplished. No facial recess dissection or tympanoplasty work is attempted at that time, and any definitive resection of chronic ear disease and hearing reconstruction should be staged.

The use of heparin to theoretically prevent propagation of thrombus is controversial and generally unnecessary with adequate surgical therapy. Heparin may be reserved for a patient with extensive clot beyond the limits of a reasonable surgical exposure (e.g., into the torcular Herophili or internal jugular vein).

Neck exploration and ligation of the internal jugular vein to prevent distant emboli were frequently necessary in the preantibiotic era. Currently, with earlier exploration of the thrombus site and effective antibiotic therapy, internal jugular vein ligation is unnecessary unless embolic phenomena actually develop.

Otitic Hydrocephalus

Otitic hydrocephalus is a delayed complication of otitis media characterized by an increased intracranial pressure. It has been classically described in the absence of any intracranial pathology and usually occurs several weeks after resolution of acute otitis media in children or adolescence. More commonly today, otitic hydrocephalus is a term applied to any elevation of intracranial pressure associated with temporal bone infection and has also been described and associated with chronic otitis media cases. There is disagreement as to the exact etiology of the elevated intracranial pressure, but it is generally believed to be due to sudden compromise of venous return. Shambaugh et al. pointed out that otitic hydrocephalus appears unrelated to the presence or absence of lateral sinus thrombosis, and, in fact, most cases of sinus thrombosis do not develop secondary elevation of intracranial pressure.[1] Otitic hydrocephalus is often associated with other intracranial complications of otitis media and requires a thorough evaluation to rule out the presence of mass lesions or intracranial infection.

Increased intracranial pressure presents clinically with headaches, vomiting, diplopia due to sixth nerve paralysis, decreasing levels of consciousness, possible focal neurologic signs if cerebral shift is occurring, and papilledema, which is the most consistent physical sign. An ophthalmologic consult should be obtained as soon as a diagnosis of papilledema is made, because the greatest danger from chronic hydrocephalus is persistent papilledema with visual loss. A decrease in the visual fields usually occurs before a loss of acuity.

A contrast CT scan is obtained because any brain or other intracranial abscess would be readily apparent. The scan is usually normal in the setting of otitic hydrocephalus. An LP can then be performed to confirm the diagnosis by demonstration of markedly elevated CSF pressure (>300 mm H_2O) with otherwise normal CSF levels. An LP should not be performed before a CT scan is obtained because of the risk of herniation should a mass lesion be present.

Management

Aggressive reduction of CSF pressure is important to prevent the optic nerve atrophy from progressive papilledema. The otitic hydrocephalus is self-limited but may require weeks to months for complete resolution. Control of the intracranial pressure can initially be obtained by repeated LP. More severe cases may require admission to an intensive care unit, insertion of a lumbar drain for about 1 week, and a regimen of 0.5 to 1.0 gm of mannitol/kg administered intravenously every 4 hours. A ventriculostomy may also occasionally be necessary. Definitive therapy of the underlying acute or chronic otitis media should be undertaken once the CSF pressure has been initially stabilized.

It is necessary to closely follow the patient for evidence of visual field or acuity changes and to repeat the LP as needed when papilledema recurs. Once the underlying disease is treated, the intracranial pressure will ultimately return spontaneously to normal levels.

Recurrent Meningitis

Recurrent meningitis can occur from numerous sources, including systemic foci with hematogenous dissemination, inherited immune deficiencies, extension of head and neck infections, and CSF fistulae. Identification of an occult source for the meningitis is a truly challenging problem that demands a careful systematic search for the site of infection or CSF leak. Having thoroughly eliminated the possibility of an infectious source, the otologist is challenged to locate the source of a likely CSF fistula.

The most common causes of CSF leak are trauma with skull base fracture or perilymph fistula, chronic otitis media with bone destruction, brain hernia due to surgical trauma or congenital dehiscence, postoperative fistula, congenital anomalous tracts, and transdural tumor resection. Identification of the true etiology is important, because recurrent meningitis is a potentially lethal problem; it must be dealt with by definitive surgery.

Evaluation

Differentiation between the anterior, middle, and posterior fossa source of leakage can be difficult. A careful history is extremely important. Rhinorrhea may present as a watery nasal drainage occurring when the patient is bending forward or may be subclinical and mistaken for persistent postnasal drip. Rhinorrhea does not differentiate between direct communication with the anterior fossa vs. otorrhea draining through the eustachian tube from a middle or posterior fossa source. The patient with otorrhea may have additional complaints of aural fullness, hearing loss, and vertigo. Physical examination may reveal a serous-appearing middle ear effusion, but it is often absent. A fistula test should be performed, but frequently the results are also unrevealing, even in patients with fistulae. Rhinorrhea can often be elicited by having the patient bend forward for a couple of minutes with gentle Valsalva's maneuvers. If clear otorrhea or rhinorrhea is produced, the fluid is collected for laboratory studies. If the drainage is insufficient to assay, dextrose sticks may be used to demonstrate the presence of glucose, which is normally absent in mucous secretions. Small amounts of glucose have been demonstrated in nasal secretions, causing false positive reactions. If sufficient fluid can be obtained, an assay for protein and glucose levels is usually sufficient to confirm the diagnosis. An immunofixation beta transferrin electrophoresis assay that is very specific for the identification of CSF is available.[9]

Differentiation between true rhinorrhea and otorrhea can be made with the use of CT scanning or radionucleotide injections. Injection of radioactive tracers into the basal cistern is useful for identifying the site of subtle leaks. Multiple intranasal pledgets are placed and maintained for several hours, and then the pledgets are withdrawn and individually counted for radioactive uptake. Computed tomography scans with water-soluble contrast injected into the cistern will show an active leak very

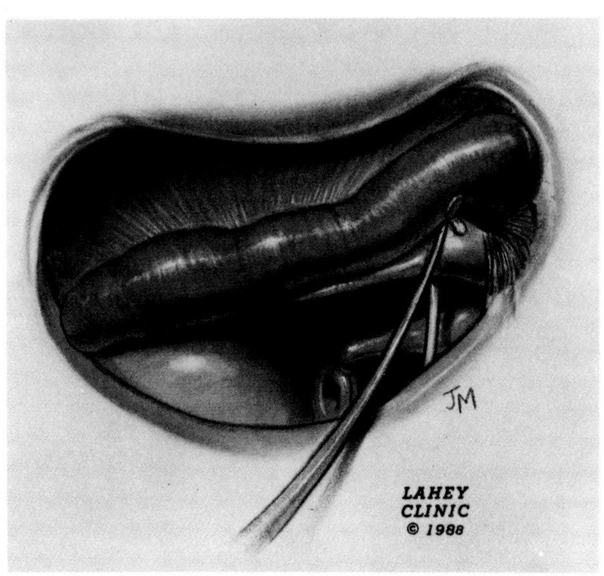

FIG 39–10.
Transcanal technique of elevating tympanic membrane off malleus and exposing anterior epitympanum.

nicely but may fail to show very small leaks. The management of anterior fossa CSF leaks is beyond the scope of this chapter.

Temporal Bone Trauma With Cerebrospinal Fluid Leak

The majority of CSF leaks following skull base trauma subside with conservative management. The patient who returns with meningitis, however, indicates there is a persistent leak requiring evaluation and surgical closure. Localization of the leak to the ear would require evidence of a middle ear effusion or demonstration of radionucletide uptake in pledgets packed at the eustachian tube orifice following injection of the basal cistern. A high-resolution CT scan with and without contrast should be done in axial and coronal planes using bone settings to look for evidence of bony trauma and examining the tegmen and labyrinthine integrity. Finally, a water-soluble contrast material can be injected into the cistern, followed by a CT scan if the diagnosis cannot be established.

The common sites of CSF communication would be a fracture running through the middle fossa tegmen over the epitympanum, subluxation or dislocation of the stapes footplate, or a round window fistula.

A middle ear exploration should be done if no definitive fracture or defect can be demonstrated on the CT scan. A transcanal tympanomeatal flap is elevated (Fig 39–10). If there is no serviceable hearing, the eustachian tube can be obliterated. The tympanic membrane is elevated off of the malleus starting from the short process and continuing inferiorly to release the tympanic membrane from the umbo. The whole tempanic membrane is then reflected anteriorly to reveal the eustachian tube orifice. Proplast implant is cut into small strips, soaked in gentamicin solution, and packed firmly into the eustachian tube, taking great care that no Proplast extrudes from the bony canal

into the middle ear space. Temporal muscle graft is then harvested from a small postauricular incision, cut into pieces, and packed to obliterate the whole middle ear space. The tympanic membrane is returned to its normal anatomic position, and Gelfoam is layered into the medial external canal to hold the drum in position. The remainder of the external canal is filled with polymyxin B sulfate (Polysporin) ointment.

If there is serviceable hearing, the round window and oval windows are examined for evidence of a perilymph fistula. Valsalva's maneuvers are performed. Stapes subluxation or dislocation is managed by a total stapedectomy, placing a House wire prosthesis on perichondrium overlying the oval window. A small oval window or round window fistula is sealed by elevating the mucosa from around the margins of the windows and packing ear lobule fat into the niches. Microfistulae may not be directly visualized. Multiple adhesions surrounding niches may be suggestive of an intermittent fistula. Even in the absence of a visualized fistula, fat is packed into both niches.

The epitympanum is carefully inspected for any small defects. Should a defect be revealed, a mastoidectomy exposing the area of the defect and leaving bone surrounding it can be performed. The dura is then elevated circumferentially around the bony defect with the freerer elevator and temporal fascia pushed through the hole to layer the tissue extradurally. Muscle graft is then placed on the under surface of the fascia, followed by Gelfoam to hold it in place and help seal the leak site. Tegmen defects are more commonly not clearly identifiable and require demonstration of an old fracture on CT scan to make the diagnosis. Extradural repair of presumed or confirmed tegmen defect can be performed through a middle fossa craniotomy approach. An extradural procedure is used, elevating the middle fossa dura off of the tegmen and holding it in place with a House urban retractor. A large graft of temporalis muscle fascia or fascia lata is then laid over the whole middle fossa floor and the dura returned to hold the fascia in place.

Cerebrospinal fluid leakage through the posterior fossa is much less common. A complete mastoidectomy is performed, with thinning of the posterior fossa bone to eliminate all adjacent air cells. Abdominal fat is then used to obliterate the mastoid cavity while preserving the middle ear space by packing it with Gelfoam.

Chronic Otitis Media With Bone Destruction and Cerebrospinal Fluid Leak

The presence of CSF otorrhea or rhinorrhea associated with chronic otitis media suggests bony destruction of the middle fossa tegmen by cholesteatoma or granulations with epidural invasion or brain herniation.

The most useful study is a high-resolution temporal bone CT scan taken in axial and, if possible, coronal planes focusing on the floor of the middle fossa for epidural collection and integrity of the tegmen. An unrevealing CT scan should be supplemented with high-resolution MRI to examine the floor of the temporal lobe on the coronal cuts for a brain hernia. Magnetic resonance imaging is much more sensitive in detecting very small hernias than CT.

Management.—A definitive tympanomastoidectomy is planned. The decision to use an intact canal wall procedure or a canal wall down operation will be determined by the type and extent of disease rather than the presence of a CSF leak. The complete mastoidectomy is performed, and exposure of the middle fossa dura for removal of granulations and drainage of epidural collections is done. Repeat tympanoplasty and middle ear work are then completed. Finally, the CSF leak is occluded using temporal fascia, muscle graft, and Gelfoam to repair the dural defect.

A brain hernia repair requires an additional middle fossa approach. A herniation unexpectantly encountered should not be repaired at that stage; rather, the tympanoplasty and mastoidectomy are completed removing all the disease surrounding the brain herniation as much as possible. It is important to leave the tegmen intact to provide bony support for the repair at the second stage. A broad Gelfoam pad can be laid over the hernia and the procedure terminated. The patient should then be restudied with MRI, CT, or both, and a combined transmastoid and middle fossa intracranial procedure will be planned.

Brain Herniation

Evaluation.—A middle fossa tegmen defect combined with a dural weakness or injury is necessary to allow the brain to herniate out of the cranial cavity. Extensive removal of bone can be done without any risk of herniation as long as the dura remains viable and intact. Herniations are most frequently due to previous surgical trauma to the dura, although congenital dehiscence can occur but is quite unusual. Ballance reported a 5.4% incidence of congenital tegmen defects in a large temporal bone study, but they rarely result in herniation.[10] The evaluation for true brain hernia requires a high-resolution CT scan in an attempt to demonstrate a tegmen defect with protrusion of brain substance into the middle ear or antral space and to rule out the presence of an abscess or soft tissue invasion of the epidural space. An MRI scan is very important, because the herniation is frequently too small to appreciate on CT. Coronal MRI cuts through the floor of the temporal lobe are exquisitively sensitive for even very small brain hernias.

Management.—There is considerable controversy as to the best type of approach for repair of brain hernias. There are advocates for the transmastoid approach, the middle fossa approach, or a combined approach. There is further discussion as to whether the fascia for repair should be placed intradurally or extradurally. The most effective technique to minimize the recurrence rate in our experience is a middle fossa intradural repair combined with a transmastoid extradural graft. Brain tissue within the hernia is nonviable, scarred, and infected. It is amputated at the base of its intracranial stalk, and the bony defect that transmitted the stalk is occluded.

A middle fossa incision is combined with a postauricular incision, and a complete mastoidectomy is done to preserve the tegmen. A neurosurgeon makes a vertical incision in the exposed dura and retracts the temporal lobe, inspecting the floor of the middle fossa until the hernia stalk can be identified. The brain hernia is then amputated and removed, thereby exposing

the tegmen defect. No attempt is made to dissect the dura from the tegmen. A large temporalis fascia or fascia lata patch is then laid over the defect and the brain allowed to reexpand, holding it in place. Temporalis muscle graft is placed in the bony defect from below and held in place with a plug of Surgicel. The extradural pack is then supported by layers of Gelfoam placed from below. The dura is closed to obtain a watertight seal, and the bone plate is sutured back into place using previously placed drill holes. A routine wound closure is performed and a pressure dressing applied (Fig 39–11).

Postoperative Fistula or Trauma

The most common postoperative source of otorrhea is a poststapes fistula. A polyethylene tube and Gelfoam wire prostheses were notorious for developing postoperative fistulae, but such complications are now infrequent with current techniques. A revision stapedectomy is required when a fistula is suspected, and the prosthesis and previous graft are left intact if at all possible. A large perichondral or fascial graft is wrapped around the base of the prosthesis and oval window graft.

Cerebrospinal fluid otorrhea can also follow an intraoperative trauma to the tegmen plate and dura with resultant brain herniation. Repair of such defect will usually require a combined intracranial middle fossa and transmastoid approach.

Congenital Anomalous Tracts

Evolution.—There are several sites of congenital communication between subarachnoid space and perilymph. The most common pathologic route of communication is along the perineural sheaths of the nerves within the internal auditory canal where the CSF gains access to the vestibule through the macula cribrosa. The second most important route is through an abnormally large cochlear aqueduct. Less important routes are along the endolymphatic duct, the subarcuate fossa, and Hyrtl's fissure.[9]

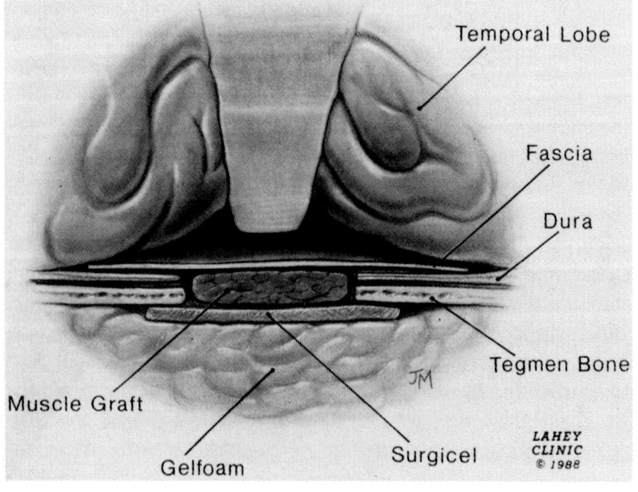

FIG 39–11.
Combined mastoid and middle fossa brain hernia repair.

Hyrtl's fissure is a communication between the subarachnoid space at the XIth nerve ganglion and enters the middle ear in the hypotympanum inferior and anterior to the round window. The tract usually closes in early infancy.

Cerebrospinal fluid gaining access to the vestibule may work its way up through congenital areas of weakness in the bony footplate, the anterior annular ligament, the round window, the fistula, ante fenestrum anterior to the oval window, and the fossula postfenestrum just posterior to the oval window. These fistulas are connective tissue-filled fissures within the otic capsule. The CSF fistulas are particularly common in patients with Mondini deformities of the cochlea and other cochlear malformations.

Management.—A middle ear exploration is performed in search of the site of leak, and the repair is effected. In the absence of useful hearing, the eustachian tube is packed with Proplast and the middle ear space obliterated. When useful hearing is present, careful search of the oval and round window niches, the areas anterior and posterior to the oval window, and areas inferior to the round window all must be inspected. Valsalva's maneuvers are sometimes useful but unreliable. Regardless of whether a fistula is seen or not, lobule fat is packed into both oval window and round niches after the mucosa is elevated out of the niches. A suspected leak from a congenital fissure may be repaired with perichondrium or fascia laid over the site. Mucosa is scraped off of the promontory prior to placement of the grafts as well. The fascia is then held in place with Gelfoam packing.

Refistulization in a hearing ear should prompt repeat exploration, but a postauricular approach should be considered. In a nonhearing, obliterated ear with a continued profuse leak, a transmastoid labyrinthectomy has been useful in closing the fistula. The macula cribrosa perforations are occluded with bone wax, and the mastoid is obliterated with abdominal fat.

SUMMARY

Complications of otitis media occur because of infection within a closed space with resultant bone destruction and spread to adjacent structures. Identification of the patient at risk for complications is important, because so many of the symptoms can be masked by the use of antibiotics. An area with otorrhea for greater than 2 weeks despite antibiotic therapy sets the stage for bone destruction in an acute suppurative infection. Any systemic symptom, such as headache or fever, in a patient with either acute or chronic otitis media is an immediate indicator of a possible complication. A particularly foul discharge usually suggests that bone destruction has occurred, and complications may be expected to follow. Any neurologic symptoms associated with otitis media require prompt evaluation, because the patient's condition may rapidly deteriorate into a life-threatening situation.

The time-proved, definitive management of otitis media complications is establishment of drainage by surgery. Conservative management is possible with the use of antibiotics, which permit the "medical" reestablishment of drainage through the natural middle ear pathways. Drainage may be further improved if more severe complications are present by performance of a wide myringotomy.

Complications of acute suppurative disease usually require only antibiotic therapy with possible addition of myringotomy for successful outcome. Advanced bone destruction, as with a coalescent mastoiditis or soft tissue abscess formation, demands a limited simple mastoidectomy and an incision and drainage type of procedure. A definitive tympanomastoidectomy is staged for a later date.

Intracranial complications must be treated aggressively. Contrast with CT aids greatly in establishing the diagnosis, and a drainage procedure is undertaken on an emergent basis from the discovery of any abscess formation or thrombophlebitis.

Surgical treatment of chronic otitis media complications is usually more technically difficult. For that reason, complications are first treated with antibiotics, and the patient's medical condition is stabilized. Topical local care is administered to the affected ear. After several days of therapy, a definitive mastoid procedure can be done with a tympanoplasty, if desired. Any hearing reconstruction is best delayed for a second stage.

REFERENCES

1. Shambaugh GE Jr, Glasscock ME III: *Surgery of the Ear,* ed 3. Philadelphia, WB Saunders Co, 1980.
2. Schuknecht JH: *Pathology of the Ear.* Cambridge, Mass, Harvard University Press, 1974.
3. Mawson SR: *Disease of the Ear,* ed 3. Baltimore, Williams & Wilkins Co, 1974.
4. Silbiger H: Uber das Ausmass der Mastoid Pneumatisction beim Menschen. *Acta Anat* 1950; 11:215.
5. Neely JG: Complications of temporal bone infection, in Cummings CW, Fredrickson JM, Harker LA, et al (ed): *Otolaryngology—Head and Neck Surgery.* St Louis, CV Mosby Co, 1986, pp 2988–3015.
6. Hawkins DB, Dru D: Mastoid subperiosteal abscess. *Arch Otolaryngol* 1983; 109:369.
7. Sunderland S: *Nerves and Nerve Injury.* New York, Churchill Livingston, 1972.
8. Mokhtari NA: Sigmoid sinus involvement in middle ear infection. *Laryngoscope* 1988; 98:310–312.
9. Hicks GW, Wright JW Jr, Wright JW II: Cerebrospinal fluid otorrhea. *Laryngoscope* 1980; 90(suppl 25):1–25.

Neuro-otologic Infections

Approach of

Herman A. Jenkins, M.D.

Neuro-otologic complications of chronic otitis media have greatly decreased since the advent of antibiotics and are now uncommonly seen by most otologists. However, these complications still occur, particularly in the indigent populations in which health care may not be readily accessible, and result in significant morbidity and mortality. The otolaryngologist must be aware of these entities and must be capable of making the correct diagnosis and implementing appropriate treatment.

LATERAL SINUS THROMBOPHLEBITIS

Etiology

Lateral sinus thrombophlebitis arises from direct extension of the infection from the mastoid onto the dura of the lateral sinus, inciting a perisinus abscess or a localized inflammatory response with formation of an intramural thrombus. The latter becomes infected and results in propagation of the clot and occlusion of the sinus. Thrombophlebitis of the small veins of the mastoid around the infected area or the surrounding soft tissues of the scalp may extend into the lateral sinus with resultant septic thrombosis and occlusion. β-Hemolytic streptococcal and pneumococcal infections have in the past been the most implicated organisms.[1]

Presentation and Diagnosis

Usual presenting symptoms in lateral sinus thrombophlebitis include postauricular edema, otorrhea, headaches, spiking temperatures (picket fence pattern), nausea, and vomiting.[2] Cervical tenderness, lymphadenopathy, and neck stiffness may be associated symptoms. Signs may include increased CSF pressure, with papilledema and altered sensorium, and evidence of septicemia. The presence of chronic ear disease and these symptoms should be a tip-off to the treating physician. In the past, diagnosis has been established by means of blood cultures documenting septicemia and the Queckenstedt test. This test demonstrates occlusion of the lateral sinus by elevation of the CSF pressure on manual occlusion of the normal venous drainage side, whereas no change in pressure occurs with pressure on the side of the sinus thrombosis. Today, with advances in imaging techniques, such tests with possible false readings have been abandoned. Computed tomographic scanning and MRI can be used to demonstrate the clot, particularly with the injection of new contrast materials to outline the vasculature. Arteriography may be necessary to finalize the diagnosis.

Treatment

Therapy for lateral sinus thrombosis requires a combination of medical and surgical management. Broad-spectrum antibiotics are required to control the septicemic portion of the disease, since chronic seeding of the bloodstream from the infected clot occurs. Primary management is surgery.

An extensive mastoidectomy unroofing the entire area of the dura around the lateral sinus should be performed. Any granulation tissue or perisinus abscess should be removed. A small needle may be inserted into the sinus to confirm occlusion by clot. The sinus is palpated to attempt to determine the limits of the thrombus. It should be easily compressible if blood is present and have a rubbery feel if a thrombus exists in the area of palpation. If blocked, the central portion of the sinus is opened to reveal the clot. It is evacuated as extensively as possible to obtain free flow of blood from both ends. If this is not possible due to central propagation, attempts should be abandoned. Control of bleeding can be obtained by occluding the lumen with ligatures, or the incision can be oversewn if the clot has been totally evacuated, and drainage can be reconstituted.

In the literature the role of anticoagulants is controversial, with authors fearing breakup of the clot, causing septic embolization.[2] However, this is the standard treatment of thrombophlebitis elsewhere in the body, and this fear has not been supported sufficiently. Certainly anticoagulants should be employed if free bleeding is not obtained from the intracranial end of the sinus, indicating persisting thrombus in the lateral and transverse sinus. Ligation of the internal jugular vein in the neck decreases the chances of septic embolization and permits use of anticoagulants to prevent more central propagation of the clot.

EPIDURAL ABSCESS

Temporal Bone

An epidural abscess is a collection of pus between the dura and the overlying bone. It represents direct extension of infection from the mastoid, and the dura serves often as an effective barrier to prevent further extension. The major hallmark of an epidural abscess is headaches, particularly in the presence of a chronic draining ear. Headaches may be relieved with ear drainage and recur when further drainage is prevented. Meningismus with stiff neck and pain on movement is common. Actual meningitis and intracranial abscess may be the final result.

Middle Fossa

An epidural abscess occurring in the middle fossa results from erosion of the tegmen tympani from the coalescent mastoiditis process. Extension in the middle fossa anteriorly may result in irritation of the cranial nerves, particularly the trigeminal and facial, both of which may be dehiscent for varying distances in the middle fossa. Diagnosis today is made primarily by CT scanning. This gives details of the temporal bone pathology, possible dehiscent areas of bone, and the extent of the abscess. Magnetic resonance imaging may fail to demonstrate the abscess if only small collections against the bone are present.

Middle fossa epidural abscess is managed with broad-spectrum antibiotic coverage and surgery. A complete mastoidectomy should be performed to evacuate any infected materials as completely as possible. If the collection of pus is small, an enlargement of the dehiscence can be made and the cavity drained into the mastoid. In larger abscesses with displacement of the dura, a middle fossa exploration is in order in combination with the mastoidectomy. The mastoid is first approached through a postauricular incision with exploration of the tegmen tympani in the mastoid and attic areas. The incision is then extended anteriorly and superiorly to expose the squamosal portion of the temporal bone. A small window of bone is removed, and the dura is elevated off the floor of the middle fossa. Care should be taken to prevent any tears in the dura and to prevent bleeding. The extent of the abscess should be fully exposed, any loculation broken down, and the cavity copiously irrigated with saline. An opening into the mastoid cavity through the tegmen is created if inadequate drainage sites are present.

Posterior Fossa

Posterior fossa epidural abscesses present with a similar hallmark of draining ear and headaches. Radiographically they can be depicted much like those in the middle fossa. A collection adjacent to the sinus, or perisinus, may lead to lateral sinus thrombosis. Once it is identified, treatment consists of mastoidectomy with removal of the infected material as well as unroofing of the posterior fossa dura to evacuate the abscess and promote drainage. A modified radical mastoidectomy may be necessary to control cholesteatoma; however, should this not be indicated, adequate treatment can be effected with evacuation and drainage into the mastoid. Extension along the sinus to the infralabyrinthine compartment may occur, and the surgeon must be ready to uncover the jugular bulb if needed. A mastoid-cutaneous drainage tube can be used for several days to ensure continued evacuation until the broad-spectrum antibiotic coverage has brought the infection under complete control.

OTITIC HYDROCEPHALUS

Otitic hydrocephalus results from both acute and chronic infections of the ear. The etiology of this condition is unknown, though a component of delayed venous drainage secondary to possible lateral sinus thrombosis has been proposed. Seen more commonly in children, it is characterized by the symptoms of headaches, vomiting, blurred vision, and other signs typically associated with increased intracranial pressure. Papilledema and cranial nerve weakness, particularly abducens nerve, are usual in this disease, with CSF pressures of 300 mm Hg or greater.[3] Otitic hydrocephalus is a diagnosis of exclusion and may mimic that of intracranial neoplasm and brain abscess. Computed tomographic scanning is normal, and arteriography shows changes in the late venous filling phases, indicative of the increased intracranial pressure.

Treatment of otitic hydrocephalus has varying degrees of success, and resolution may require several months. Acute management includes repeated LPs and dehydration. Acetazolamide, a carbonic anhydrase inhibitor, provides acute dehydration, and high-dose steroids may be beneficial. Eradication of the otologic disease induces resolution of the symptoms. The mastoid must be explored in its entirety with unroofing of the lateral sinus and removal of any granulation tissue or infected material. Evacuation of a possible thrombus from the lateral sinus is controversial since it is rarely septic and does not propagate.[4] Loss of vision must be monitored in patients with long-standing papilledema. Though unproved, long-term steroid treatment appears warranted.

RECURRENT MENINGITIS

Recurrent meningitis is one of the more common complications of chronic otitis media and chronically recurring acute otitis media. In contrast to lateral sinus thrombosis and associated meningitis, recurrent meningitis is most commonly due to direct connections between the CSF space and the extracranial cavity of the ear. These connections may be congenital in origin or related to traumatic injury of the temporal bone. The latter may result in retained epithelium in the fracture line with development of an infected cholesteatoma. Clinically, as well as subclinically, significant CSF leaks may be implicated in the recurrence. Documentation of CSF leaks is often difficult in the ear unless the flow is at a fairly vigorous level. Radiopaque dyes and radioactive tracers may help localize sites of leaks.

With or without the presence of a documented source of CSF leakage, the ear should be explored when CSF leakage is implicated in the etiology. If the site of leakage can be localized (e.g., a congenital dehiscence in the stapes footplate), local control with packing of fat or tissue around the leakage point may be effected. Fractures across the promontory with involvement of the tegmen tympani, however, require more extensive obliteration to control. In these cases, sealing the mastoid and middle ear cavity off from the outside will, in most instances, control the recurrent meningitis. An extensive mastoidectomy with removal of the canal wall, eardrum, and ossicles and closure of the external auditory canal in a blind sac is required to eradicate all the air cell tracts. The eustachian tube is then obliterated by drilling out the mucosa, and a combination of bone wax and bone pate is used to fill the residual orifice. The middle ear and mastoid cavity are obliterated with fat. By this procedure, the middle ear and mastoid connections to the CSF spaces are closed off, and the space is isolated from the outside world.

FACIAL NERVE PARALYSIS

The facial nerve may be involved in both acute and chronic ear infections. Management, however, of the paralysis in the two conditions differs.

Acute Otitis Media

Paralysis resulting from an acute otitis media represents extension of the infection along a dehiscence of the nerve with possible abscess collection in the fallopian canal. The prognosis for this condition is relatively good, and treatment is simply appropriate antibiotic therapy and a myringotomy to clear the acute infection. Should movement entirely cease, the electrical excitability of the nerve is followed similarly to that in Bell's palsy, and the paralysis is managed accordingly. Surgical decompression is used only if the electrical testing indicates that severe degeneration is impending, with the ultimate outcome for return of function expected to be poor. Criteria have been established in Bell's palsy and are adhered to in this condition as well. If results of the minimal excitability test are greater than 3.5 mamp difference between the paralyzed side and the normal, or electroneuronography shows greater than 90% degeneration of the involved nerve, a surgical decompression is undertaken.

Surgical decompression entails exploration of the vertical and tympanic segments up to the level of the cochleariform process. This should permit full exposure of the involved segment to reduce any pressure on the nerve. Decompression should be undertaken at the earliest signs of severe degeneration in an attempt to limit the degree of injury that will occur in the nerve. A middle fossa decompression with opening of the labyrinthine segment and internal auditory canal is contraindicated since meningitis is likely to ensue.

Chronic Otitis Media and Cholesteatoma

Facial nerve paralysis from chronic otitis media with cholesteatoma represents a different entity than that from acute infection. Here, involvement of the nerve results from pressure of the cholesteatoma and surrounding chronic inflammatory response. Facial paralysis in the presence of chronic infection represents a relative surgical emergency requiring prompt exploration. A complete mastoidectomy is performed, with exploration of the facial nerve throughout the tympanic and vertical segment. Great care must be exercised since the nerve may be encased in cholesteatoma and granulation tissue. Often dehiscences are present in the tympanic segment such that elevation of the infected material will also elevate the nerve out of its normal bed and produce additional stretch injury. Removal of the cholesteatoma matrix from the nerve should be done with gentle blunt dissection to prevent pressure injury. The matrix may be left on the nerve if too much damage would occur with removal. Incision of the sheath is controversial, but inadequate decompression of the nerve may occur if left intact. In incomplete paralysis, it is sufficient to remove the cholesteatoma and granulation tissue and not incise the nerve sheath.

ACUTE MASTOIDITIS

Though in previous years acute mastoiditis was a common presentation of acute infection of the ear, today it is unusual for an acute otitis media to reach this level. Symptoms typical of this disease are pain in the ear, fever, marked tenderness and swelling over the mastoid area, and signs of acute middle ear infection. In the later stages, the ear begins to profusely drain, and postauricular swelling increases, with the formation of a subperiosteal (Bezold's) abscess. Characteristically, the pinna moves downwardly and outwardly from its normal position. Acute mastoiditis occurs more frequently in children as a sequelae of acute otitis media, though occasionally it is seen in adults with cholesteatoma. Radiographic evaluation shows a well-pneumatized mastoid with clouding of the air cells and often coalescence or breakdown of the typical septa appearance.

If left untreated, the acute mastoiditis progresses to form a subperiosteal abscess and may extend intracranially to induce epidural abscesses and lateral sinus thrombosis. In the early phases, treatment consists of hospitalization and IV antibiotics. If otorrhea is not present, a myringotomy for culture and controlled drainage of the middle ear and mastoid are performed. If a subperiosteal abscess is evident on scanning or clinical examination, localized drainage is instituted. A postauricular incision is made and the tissues dissected down to the level of the periosteum. The periosteum is incised, and the abscess is evacuated. If the mastoid demonstrates evidence of coalescence on CT scanning, a simple mastoidectomy is performed. Postauricular Penrose drains are left in place and advanced slowly over 3 days to ensure adequate drainage. The abscess may extend up into the infratemporal space and require further dissection to assure adequate evacuation of the contents.

REFERENCES

1. Teichgraeber JF, Per-Lee JH, Turner JS: Lateral sinus thrombosis: A modern perspective. *Laryngoscope* 1982; 92:744–751.
2. Samuel J, Fernandes CMC: Lateral sinus thrombosis: A review of 45 cases. *J Laryngol Otol* 1987; 101:1227–1229.
3. Lenz RP, McDonald GA: Otitic hydrocephalus. *Laryngoscope* 1984; 94:1451–1454.
4. Wright I: The bacteriology of ear, nose and throat disease. *J Laryngol Otol* 1970; 84:283–308.

CHAPTER 40

Laryngotracheobronchial Infections

Approach of

Duncan S. Postma, M.D.

The evaluation and treatment of acute laryngotracheobronchial infections have contributed greatly to the number of gray hairs for the otolaryngologist-head and neck surgeon. The key, as in most aspects of medicine, is a previously carefully thought-out protocol. This works most smoothly when our medical colleagues and ancillary personnel share similar diagnostic and therapeutic approaches.

EPIGLOTTITIS

Epiglottitis, more appropriately called supraglottitis, is an acute infectious process that is most often caused by *Hemophilus influenzae* type b. It is a relatively unusual infection, occurring most often in infants, though adults occasionally are affected. It occurs especially in infants aged 2 to 4 years, with a relatively acute onset over 2 to 6 hours of high temperature with a drooling patient who sits upright with more inspiratory than expiratory stridor. In adults it often presents in a less fulminant manner. Since the management in children is different from that of adults, these age groups are discussed separately.

Initial Management in Children

There is controversy about examining children suspected of having epiglottitis because of reports of apparent precipitation of respiratory arrest. Respiratory obstruction is probably caused by at least two factors: a swollen epiglottis and aryepiglottic folds with supraglottic narrowing and excessive thick, tenacious oral and pharyngeal secretions, which accumulate because of odynophagia. Sudden respiratory arrest thus may be caused by mucous plugging of the narrowed supraglottic larynx during inspiratory efforts or laryngospasm, to which these infants may be particularly susceptible if examined aggressively.

In the child who is severely ill, presenting in a classic manner, the best course of action is to accompany the child to the operating room as soon as possible. Here, rigid bronchoscopy, foreign body forceps, and tracheotomy equipment should be set up and ready to be used. In the older and cooperative child, flexible laryngoscopy may be possible. Certainly, extreme caution should be exercised in all cases. In less severe cases, someone capable of handling the airway can accompany the child for radiographic examination of the soft tissues of the neck. This is not so much to make certain of the diagnosis of epiglottitis as to be certain that foreign bodies are not present. Although the x-ray film may be classic for epiglottitis, the clinician should be aware that recent studies have shown that radiographs can be very inaccurate in terms of making a diagnosis of epiglottitis.[1]

When skilled anesthesiologists and skilled nursing care are available, endotracheal intubation is the procedure of choice.[2, 3] The operating room should be completely set up for an emergency tracheotomy with the rigid bronchoscopy equipment available for immediate use. It is certainly comforting to know that, even with respiratory arrest in acute epiglottitis, most, if not all, of these patients can be resuscitated mouth to mouth or with bagging.[4] In most situations, safe induction with agents such as halothane and oxygen can be performed.

If these conditions cannot be met, a tracheotomy is a reasonable alternative.[5, 6] The advantages of endotracheal intubation are (1) 20 to 30 minutes of safety time if extubation occurs, because the endotracheal tube temporarily has decompressed the supraglottic edema; (2) earlier decannulation compared with tracheotomy and, therefore, shortened hospitalization; and (3) fewer complications after decannulation than with tracheotomy.[2,3]

The primary disadvantage in endotracheal intubation is the need for more skilled nursing care, but the problems of postoperative care of pediatric tracheotomy patients should not be underestimated. Although the tracheotomy thus enjoys only the single aforementioned advantage, its disadvantages are that (1) decannulation in the immediate postoperative period results in absolutely no airway since there has been no stenting of the supraglottic larynx; (2) the morbidity of the procedure, especially if done without a controlled airway, is significant; and (3) a longer hospital stay is necessary.

Observation without airway control in children with acute epiglottitis should be condemned. Reports of a 9% to 25% mortality with such expectant therapy contrasts with no mortality in the same studies when the airway is controlled at the time of initial diagnosis.[7,8] The duration of this necessary intubation ranges from 48 to 72 hours. With endotracheal intubation, direct or flexible laryngoscopy can be performed every 24 hours to determine the time of extubation. Decannulation after the tracheotomy usually can be accomplished in about 72 hours.

Initial Management in Adults

In adults, the most important aspect of epiglottitis is the diagnosis. One should be suspicious of the entity in a patient with a complaint of a "sore throat" out of proportion to the physical findings in the oropharynx. Indirect examination in adults is simple and affirms the diagnosis of acute epiglottitis. Thus, radiographic studies are usually superfluous and, in fact, can be very misleading.[1]

It is clear that *H. influenzae* type b infection is potentially as severe in adults as in children. However, most adults have epiglottitis from another cause, possibly viral, with a much less severe course.[9] The concept of supraglottitis, rather than epiglottitis, is especially appropriate in adults, because in some of these cases, it is clear that the epiglottis is less involved than the remainder of the supraglottic larynx. However, epiglottitis is so ingrained in literature that terminology will probably change slowly, if at all.

With adults, it is my practice to immediately start antibiotics, a single dose of corticosteroids (20 mg of dexamethasone), intensive humidification, and careful observation in the intensive care unit with oximetry monitoring. Nothing is given by mouth. Reevaluation at 2 to 4 hours, if the patient is stable, is helpful to predict the course of the illness. One should never be led into a sense of false security in the treatment of epiglottitis in adults, because deaths do occur.[10,11]

Once admitted to the intensive care unit, the patient is also placed on humidification, and is not allowed any oral intake. A tracheotomy tray and appropriate tracheotomy tube are placed at the bedside as well.

If intubation is required, it is done in a similar manner to that described for children. Use of a flexible bronchoscope to facilitate intubation can be especially useful in adults also.

Medical Treatment

Use of corticosteroids is controversial, and in children, they are clearly not needed unless there is some reason that airway control is not possible. In adults, I tend to use a single large dose (20 mg) of dexamethasone in addition to humidification. Racemic epinephrine is of no use in epiglottitis.

I use cefotaxime, ceftriaxone, or a combination of ampicillin and chloramphenicol until cultures and sensitivity results are available.[12,13] In the latter situation, if the organism is found to be sensitive to ampicillin, the chloramphenicol is discontinued. One should be aware that there have been rare reports of resistance to chloramphenicol and possibly to cephalosporins. All of these antibiotics cross the blood-brain barrier, which is important because of the propensity of *H. influenzae* to invade the central nervous system. I have tended to use ampicillin and chloramphenicol but vary from case to case. More data will probably give us reassurance about the cephalosporins. I explain to patients and their families the risk of aplastic anemia with chloramphenicol prior to using it. This changes the use of antibiotics on occasion.

Complications

Probably the most common major complication of epiglottitis is extubation or, in adults, airway compromise prior to intubation. Watchful waiting in adults should not be done without extremely careful follow-up as previously discussed. If patients are not responding appropriately to antibiotics, antibiotic resistance as well as other infections such as meningitis should be considered. Epiglottic abscesses can also occur as a complication of acute epiglottitis rather than a separate entity.[14,15] Diphtheria, *Streptococcus,* and *Staphylococcus* species have been implicated. The best treatment is wide drainage and the addition of oxacillin to the usual antibiotic coverage until sensitivities are available (Figs 40–1 and 40–2).

CROUP

Croup, or laryngotracheitis, can be defined as a subacute viral illness characterized by fever, barking cough, and stridor. Influenza viruses type 1 and 2 and *H. influenzae* type a are the most common causes.[16] It is much more common than epiglottitis; it occurs especially in infants aged 1 to 3 years, and it usually has a 3- to 7-day clinical course.

Diagnosis

Most cases of croup are handled by primary care physicians and respond to conservative management. When it is severe, further evaluation is necessary. Confirmatory data may be obtained from posteroanterior and lateral neck films, which may reveal subglottic narrowing with the classic "steeple" sign. However, neck films are not nearly as sensitive or specific as previously thought.[1,17] The possibility of a foreign body underscores the necessity of obtaining lateral films of the soft tissues in the neck in any child with stridor when the diagnosis is not oth-

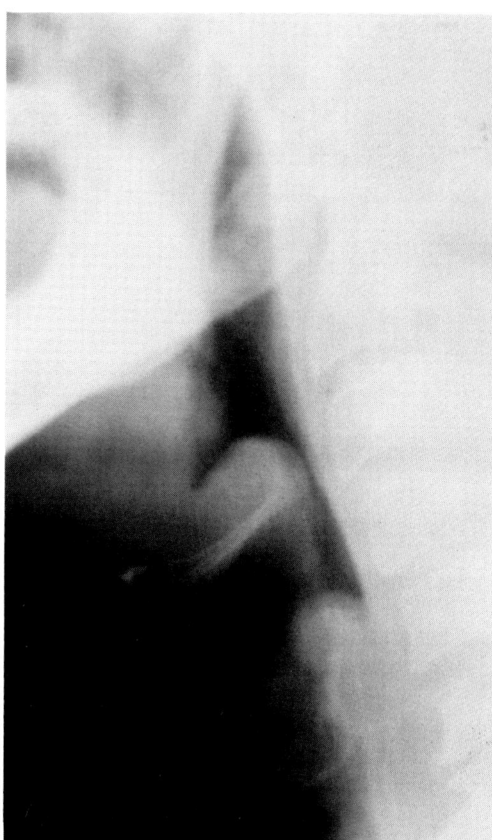

FIG 40–1.
Lateral view of middle-aged man with acute epiglottitis.

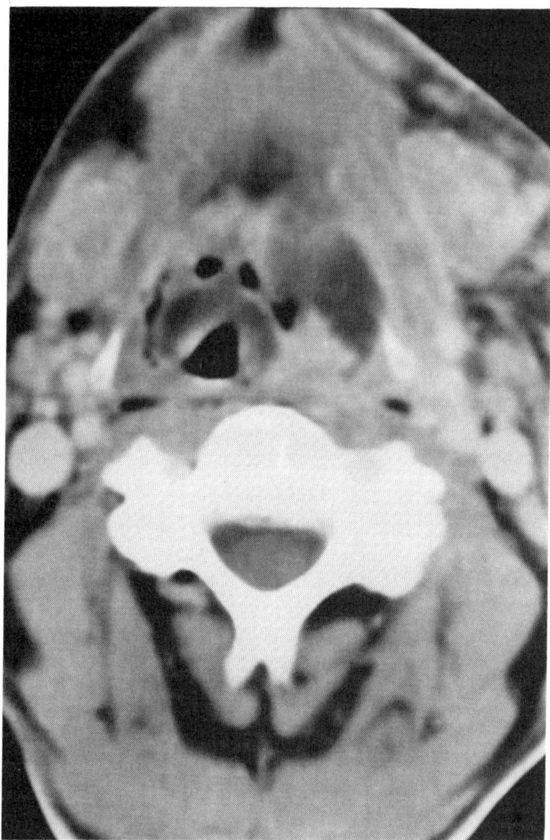

FIG 40–2.
Same patient as in Figure 40–1, who developed an epiglottic abscess, requiring drainage and temporary tracheotomy.

erwise obvious (Fig 40–3). White blood cell counts are usually elevated with croup.

The severity of the illness may be best judged by considering the infant's respiratory rate, degree of stridor and retraction, air movement, skin color, and general appearance. It should be emphasized that in the premoribund state, the respiratory rate and degree of stridor decrease as air movement decreases. Pulse oximetry monitoring has been very helpful in evaluating and following the course of these patients. Arterial blood gases are very upsetting and can often make patients much worse.

When epiglottitis is in the differential diagnosis, management should follow the same course as previously outlined. This will be further discussed in the next section. One should be aware of the "atypical" situations. Atypical croup can be defined as that occurring in infants less than 1 year old, lasting more than 7 days, or not responding to appropriate treatment (see Fig 40–3), as will be outlined. When the child is stable and in one of these atypical situations, flexible laryngoscopy can often be performed with very little chance of any morbidity. I have often done this in the intensive care unit when I believe the patient's situation has been stable over several days and when I am not worried about acute decompensation. Otherwise this should be done only in the operating room where the airway can be easily controlled.

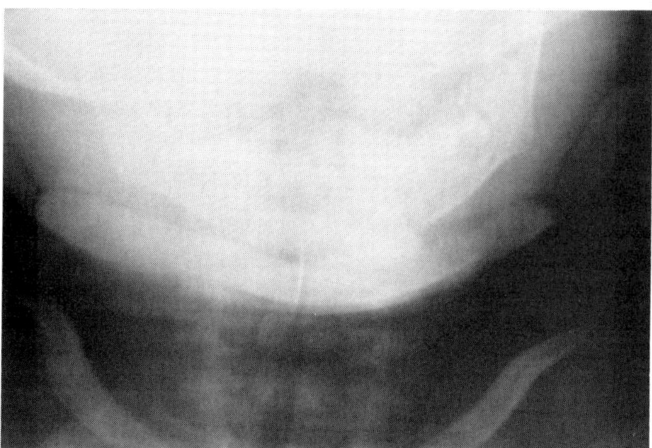

FIG 40–3.
A case of atypical croup. The curved white line seen in the glottic area represented glass seen en face. The photograph is from a fluoroscopic image. When I was first consulted, the subtle abnormality was believed to be present on all three chest radiographs performed during the previous week. This prompted the fluoroscopy on this moderately sick child. The glass could not be seen on lateral view. Dexamethasone decreased the edema in the subglottic area and improved the child's clinical status. Removal of the glass later that day was uneventful, as was the patient's postoperative course.

Management

When I am first consulted for a child with typical croup, after initial evaluation, my first step is to begin humidification and give at least 1.5 mg of dexamethasone/kg, as well as a treatment of racemic epinephrine as soon as possible. If the child is stable, an x-ray film can be obtained as long as someone who can handle the airway accompanies the child to the x-ray suite. Certainly the efficacy of racemic epinephrine is well established.[18–20] Furthermore, there is usually some beneficial effect within minutes. The racemic epinephrine may initially need to be repeated at frequent intervals, but this decreases as clinical improvement occurs. I believe that any child needing racemic epinephrine should be admitted to the hospital. Furthermore, any infant requiring racemic epinephrine should also receive a therapeutic dosage of dexamethasone or an equivalent corticosteroid. In edema caused from trauma, it is clear that corticosteroids work as quickly as 15 minutes and certainly by 1 hour.[21] Clinically, the beneficial effect of corticosteroids in croup is seen within 1 to 3 hours.

I think it is important to review and be familiar with evidence supporting the use of corticosteroids, because other health care personnel may not be as convinced as most otolaryngologists-head and neck surgeons.

A clear pattern is evident on reviewing and summarizing results of double-blind studies on the subject in the English language over the last 20 years[22–27] as well as an excellent double-blind study reported in the French literature.[28] There is clear evidence to support that less than 0.3 of dexamethasone/kg is an inadequate dose with which to treat croup.[29, 30] We have shown in animal studies of traumatic subglottic edema that less than 0.5 mg of dexamethasone/kg has significantly less effect than higher dosages.[21] Thus, it is not surprising that the two studies using a relatively small dose showed no effect.[22, 23] Five out of the six double-blind studies using more than 0.3 mg of dexamethasone/kg showed significant effects.[24–28] Of particular interest is that in these studies, six tracheotomies were performed in the placebo group, but none was performed in the steroid-treated groups. Further evidence for the tracheotomy-sparing effect of steroids is found in two random but not double-blind studies using low doses of steroids.[31, 32] In addition, a large retrospective report by Ross showed similar tracheotomy-sparing effects of steroids.[33]

As Haynes and Larner state, "A single dose of corticosteroid, even a large one, is virtually without harmful effects."[34] Thus, I believe the burden of proof is in the hands of those who doubt the value of corticosteroids. Because predicting which patients with severe croup will need later airway management is difficult, any patient with croup severe enough to warrant treatment with racemic epinephrine should receive at least one dose of 1.5 mg of dexamethasone/kg (maximum 20 mg) or its equivalent.[17] Since croup is usually of relatively short duration, one dose of a long-acting steroid such as dexamethasone is usually all that is required. However, occasionally a second smaller dose may be required.

Controversy surrounds the choice of airway support when it becomes necessary, as for a tiring infant. This may be manifested, for example, by rising carbon dioxide levels, a worsening neurologic status, or a decreasing respiratory rate in the face of poor gas exchange. The time-honored procedure is a controlled tracheotomy, preferably performed after an airway is established by endotracheal intubation or rigid bronchoscopy. A recent large series confirms the safety of tracheotomy under these circumstances, with no mortality in 24 patients with croup.[5] However, other large series successfully using endotracheal intubation have been reported.[35–37]

The clear potential disadvantage of endotracheal intubation is that it could cause further damage in an already edematous subglottic area, especially if the tube is particularly tight fitting. Certainly, the smallest size tube that allows ventilation should be used. Furthermore, younger infants with smaller subglottic spaces may be at increased risk for complication of endotracheal intubation. With this important reservation, strong support for both modalities of airway control exists, depending on local expertise. The duration of endotracheal intubation is usually 2 to 3 days. Most of these infants presumably will have received a dose of steroids before endotracheal intubation; I recommend that at least one additional dose be given 2 to 4 hours before extubation, with racemic epinephrine used as needed. Humidification should also be employed after extubation.

A tracheotomy tube in the uncomplicated cases can be removed at 5 to 7 days after appropriate evaluation. Despite some reports suggesting the contrary, not all cases are so straightforward; one inevitably will have patients who are difficult to decannulate.

BACTERIAL TRACHEITIS

Important in differential diagnosis of croup is bacterial tracheitis, or bacterial laryngotracheobronchitis. Although immunization against the toxin of *Corynebacterium diphtheriae* has dramatically reduced the incidence of this disease, cases still occur. Prompt recognition is important to facilitate treatment. If the disease is contracted despite immunization, the course is usually mild and uncomplicated.[38] Thus, a history of appropriate immunization is important.

The diagnosis must be made on clinical grounds alone, since treatment cannot be withheld until confirmation by culture.[39] Classically, a membrane appears on the tonsil with characteristic gray-green patches when necrosis has occurred. The membrane is several millimeters thick, may be difficult to dislodge, and often leaves a bleeding surface behind when it is removed. The membrane may spread medially to the palate and uvula and laterally to the pharynx. Laryngeal and tracheal involvement may be from direct extension or may be an isolated finding.

More recently, other bacteria have been implicated in causing bacterial tracheitis.[40, 41] Patients with bacterial tracheitis may have an otherwise typical croup, with fever, stridor, and barking cough. The illness is more severe, however, and does not respond to appropriate treatment. On bronchoscopy, in addition to findings consistent with croup, there is a thick mucopurulent material. Such material in an intubated patient with presumed croup should also help in making the diagnosis of bacterial tracheitis. The most common organism is *Staphylococcus aureus,* but group A *Streptococcus* and nontypable *H. influenzae* have also been reported.[40, 41] Whether this is a separate entity from bacterial tracheitis or a bacterial superinfection complicating bacterial tracheitis is unclear. Many cases can be handled with intubation. However, a tracheotomy may be indicated because of the thick secretions and possible higher mortality with endotracheal intubation for this disease.[41]

DIFFERENTIAL DIAGNOSIS

As noted earlier, one should always be aware of the atypical cases. Atypical croup (1) would be found in infants less than 1 year old, (2) would last more than 7 days, or (3) would be found in children who do not respond to appropriate treatment. One must think of such things as foreign bodies, subglottic stenosis, and subglottic hemangiomata. In many of these cases, flexible laryngoscopy can easily be performed, often in the intensive care unit, with adequate monitoring. In these situations, it is almost without risk. History of previous intubation would certainly point toward some degree of subglottic stenosis that may have been worsened by a viral illness. Subglottic tumors, especially hemangiomata, can present as croup. When epiglottitis is in the differential diagnosis in some of the atypical situations, I handle the child initially as if the diagnosis is epiglottitis. Thus, these children are taken to the operating room as soon as possible. If there is some delay, antibiotics, racemic epinephrine, and dexamethasone can be given, proceeding as soon as possible to the operating room. Remember that dexamethasone will decrease the edema around a foreign body, often improving the clinical status in this situation, which makes endoscopy safer. However, endoscopy is still important in these atypical cases. In children who are less seriously ill, one may give racemic epinephrine and dexamethasone in addition to appropriate x-ray studies as previously alluded to. In the more stable and older children, flexible laryngoscopy may often be performed with simple monitoring in the intensive care unit, obviating a trip to the operating room.

Spasmodic croup is an ill-defined entity characterized by the acute onset of a barking cough, dyspnea, and stridor. It may be recurrent and also may be associated with an upper respiratory tract infection but usually is without fever. Spasmodic croup almost always resolves with humidity and reassurance. The history, lack of fever, and radiographic findings help to distinguish it from croup.

Whooping cough, caused by *Bordetella pertussis,* has been reported with increasing frequency in this country.[42] Despite rates of immunization in high school greater than 95%, the rate has been reported to be as low as 70% in preschool children in some areas. The illness is less severe in immunized patients. After a 7- to 10-day catarrhal stage, the patient enters a paroxysmal stage with severe cough and posttussive cyanosis and vomiting.[43] In patients with these symptoms, whooping cough was reported in 41%, apnea was reported in 22%, and pneumonia was reported in 15%. Most patients were less than 1 year old. Treatment is supportive since antibiotics are not helpful.

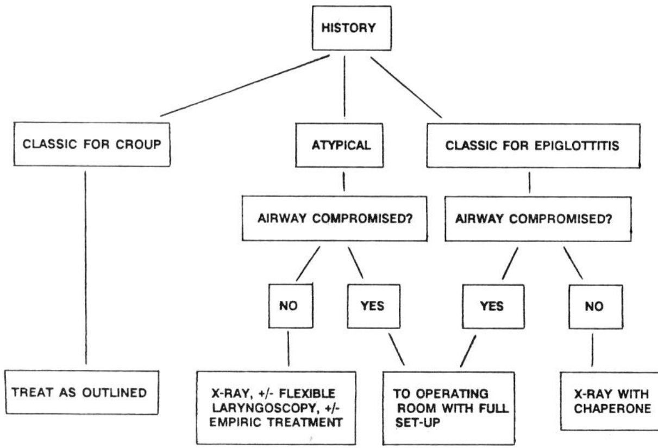

FIG 40–4.
Airway management in croup and epiglottitis.

In addition to epiglottitis, other causes of supraglottic swelling include cricoarytenoid arthritis, associated especially with rheumatoid arthritis but also with systemic lupus erythematosus.[44, 45] Treatment may include intra-articular injections of corticosteroids or an increase in systemic doses of corticosteroids or other immunosuppressive agents. The swelling may be severe enough to compromise the airway. Gout may also cause cricoarytenoid arthritis. The past medical history usually clarifies the situation.

CONCLUSION

An algorithm may be helpful to summarize the approaches to these different situations (Fig 40–4). One should not be rigid in following it, because it is meant only as a guide. In atypical cases, I err on the side of treatment with antibiotics and a single therapeutic dose of dexamethasone, proceeding with diagnostic workup as indicated by the clinical situation. Airway control is paramount, and it is always correct to proceed to the operating room, as for epiglottitis.

REFERENCES

1. Stankiewicz JA, Bowes, AK: Croup and epiglottitis: A radiologic study. *Laryngoscope* 1985; 95:1159.
2. Cantrell RW, Bell RA, Morioka WT: Acute epiglottitis: Intubation versus tracheostomy. *Laryngoscope* 1978; 88:994.
3. Schloss MD, Hannallah R, Baxter JD: Acute epiglottitis: Twenty-six years of experience at the Montreal Children's Hospital. *J Otolaryngol* 1979; 8:3.
4. Adair JC, Ring WH: Management of epiglottitis in children. *Anesth Analg* 1975; 54:622.
5. Carter P, Benjamin B: 10-year review of pediatric tracheotomy. *Ann Otol Rhinol Laryngol* 1983; 92:398.
6. Fearon B, Cinnamond M: Tracheotomy in acute supraglottitis (epiglottitis): The treatment of choice. *Laryngoscope* 1979; 87:879.
7. Margolis CZ, Ingram DL, Meyer JH: Routine tracheostomy in *Haemophilus influenzae* type B epiglottitis. *J Pediatr* 1972; 81:1150.

8. Rapkin RH: Tracheostomy in epiglottitis. *Pediatrics* 1973; 52:426.

9. Mustoe T, Strome M: Adult epiglottitis. *J Otolaryngol* 1983; 4:393.

10. Baker AS, Eavey RD: Adult supraglottitis (epiglottitis). *N Engl J Med* 1986; 314:1185–1186.

11. MayoSmith MF, Hirsh PJ, Wodzinski SF, et al: Acute epiglottitis in adults: An eight-year experience in the state of Rhode Island. *N Engl J Med* 1986; 314:1133.

12. Rhodes KH, Johnson CM: Antibiotic therapy for severe infections in infants and children. *Mayo Clin Proc* 1987; 62:1018

13. Abramowicz M et al (eds): The choice of antimicrobial drugs. *Med Letter,* March 1988, pp 33–39.

14. Hawkins DB, et al: Acute epiglottitis in adults. *Laryngoscope* 1973; 83:1211.

15. Heeneman H, Ward KM: Epiglottic abscess: Its occurrence and management. *J Otolaryngol* 1977; 6:31.

16. Cherry JD: The treatment of croup: Continued controversy due to failure of recognition of historic, etiologic, and clinical perspectives. *J Pediatr* 1979; 94:352.

17. Postma DS, Jones RO, Pillsbury HC: Severe hospitalized croup: Treatment trends and prognosis. *Laryngoscope* 1984; 94:1170–1175.

18. Adair JC, et al: Ten-year experience with IPPB in treatment of acute laryngotracheobronchitis. *Anesth Analg* 1971; 50:649.

19. Singer OP, Wilson WJ: Laryngotracheobronchitis: 2 years' experience with racemic epinephrine. *Can Med Assoc J* 1976; 115:132.

20. Westley CR, Cotton EK, Brooks JG: Nebulized racemic epinephrine by IPPB for treatment of croup. *Am J Dis Child* 1978; 132:484.

21. Postma DS, Prazma J, Woods CI, et al: Use of steroids and a long-acting vasoconstrictor in the treatment of postintubation croup: A ferret model. *Arch Otolaryngol Head Neck Surg* 1987; 113:844–849.

22. Eden AN, Larkin VD: Corticosteroid treatment of croup. *Pediatrics* 1964; 33:768.

23. Eden AN, Kaufman A, Yu R: Corticosteroids and croup: A controlled double-blind study. *JAMA* 1967; 200:403.

24. James J: Dexamethasone in croup: A controlled study. *Am J Dis Child* 1969; 117:511.

25. Koren G, et al: Corticosteroid treatment of laryngotracheitis v. spasmodic croup in children. *Am J Dis Child* 1983; 137:941.

26. Leipzig B, et al: A prospective randomized study to determine the efficacy of steroids in the treatment of croup. *J Pediatr* 1979; 94:194.

27. Skowton PN, Turner JA, McNaughton GA: The use of corticosteroid (dexamethasone) in the treatment of acute laryngotracheitis. *Can Med Assoc J* 1966; 94:528.

28. Massicotte P, Tetreault L: Evaluation de la methylprednisone dans le traitment des laryngites aigues de l'enfant. *Union Med Can* 1973; 102:2064.

29. Hawkins DB: Corticosteroids in the management of laryngotracheobronchitis. *Otolaryngol Head Neck Surg* 1980; 88:207.

30. Tunnessen WW, Feinstein AR: The steroid croup controversy: An analytic review of methodologic problems. *J Pediatr* 1980; 96:751.

31. Martennson B, Nilson G, Torbar JE: The effect of corticosteroids in the treatment of pseudocroup. *Acta Otolaryngol Suppl (Stockh)* 1960; 158:62.

32. Novik A: Corticosteroid treatment of non-diphtheric croup. *Acta Otolaryngol* 1960; 158:20.

33. Ross JA: Special problems in acute laryngotracheobronchitis. *Laryngoscope* 1969; 79:1218.

34. Haynes RC, Larner J: Adrenocorticotropic hormone; adrenocortical steroids and their synthetic analogs; inhibitors of adrenocortical steroid biosynthesis, in Goodman LS, Gilman A (eds): *The Pharmacological Basis of Therapeutics.* New York, Macmillan Publishing Co, 1974.

35. Allen TH, Steven IM: Prolonged nasotracheal intubation in infants and children. *Br J Anaesth* 1972; 44:835.

36. Mitchell DP, Thomas RL: Secondary airway support in the management of croup. *J Otolaryngol* 1980; 9:419.

37. Thompson PD, Olinsky A: Nasotracheal intubation in acute laryngotracheobronchitis. *S Afr Med J* 1975; 49:785.

38. Dobie RA, Tobey DN: Clinical features of diphtheria in the respiratory tract. *JAMA* 1979; 242:2197.

39. Branefors P: Epiglottitis and pseudocroup, in Braude AL (ed): *Microbiology and Infectious Diseases.* Philadelphia, WB Saunders Co, 1981.

40. Jones R, Santos JI, Overall JC: Bacterial tracheitis. *JAMA* 1979; 242:721.

41. Liston SL, et al: Bacterial tracheitis. *Am J Dis Child* 1983; 137:764.

42. Marks MI: Mumps, in Braude AL (ed): *Microbiology and Infectious Diseases.* Philadelphia, WB Saunders Co, 1981.

43. Schiff GM: Measles, in Braude AL (ed): *Medical Microbiology and Infectious Diseases.* Philadelphia, WB Saunders Co, 1981.

44. Connor JD: Pertussis, in Braude AL (ed): *Microbiology and Infectious Diseases.* Philadelphia, WB Saunders Co, 1981.

45. Editorial Leads From the MMWR: Pertussis—Maryland, 1982. *JAMA* 1983; 250:159.

Laryngotracheobronchial Infections

Approach of

Amelia F. Drake, M.D.

EPIGLOTTITIS

It is unfortunate that even in the 1980s there are known instances of childhood mortality due to epiglottitis (personal knowledge). The sudden onset and rapid clinical progression of the disease make consideration of the diagnosis critical in the development of effective and timely medical intervention. Although a more frequently considered diagnosis in the child, adults with supraglottitis may make multiple trips to the emergency room complaining of sore throat and air hunger before efforts are taken to alleviate a compromised airway. The medicolegal implications of dismissing a patient with possible epiglottitis should be considered by the examining physician.

Diagnosis

The appropriate clinical history is the key to making the diagnosis of epiglottitis, being marked by dramatic onset and rapid progression of symptoms, usually in the preschool-aged child. The classic presentation is one of high fever (temperature 38°C–40°C), lethargy, drooling, odynophagia, and muffled voice. After the history is obtained, the physical examination should consist primarily of an assessment of the degree of airway compromise. Physical signs may include stridor, intercostal retractions, extended neck, and circumoral cyanosis. Potentially stimulating or invasive procedures such as examination of the oropharynx with a tongue blade or blood work, if absolutely required, must be performed by medical personnel capable of and prepared to intervene if airway obstruction occurs. The same rationale can be applied to radiographic studies. If x-ray films are considered necessary in differentiating epiglottitis from croup, the child should be accompanied to the radiology suite by such personnel.

Lateral soft tissue radiograph of the neck classically shows the "thumbprint" of the edematous epiglottis, though this finding can be nonspecific and can also be seen in cases of laryngomalacia, when the clinical history is not appropriate (Fig 40–5). Epiglottitis may be distinguished from laryngomalacia by the presence of an air-filled hypopharynx on lateral soft tissue radiographs (Fig 40–6). Certainly resolution of the compromised airway precedes any laboratory or radiographic assessment.

The causative agent for epiglottitis is *Hemophilus influenzae* type b; in many cases, though, *Streptococcus pneumoniae* and *Staphylococcus* species have been associated with the disease. There is a bacteremia, with positive blood cultures for *H. influenzae* in 50% of the patients. Associated system involvement can include lungs, with pulmonary infiltrates seen on chest x-ray film.

Histopathologically, epiglottitis is characterized by edema of the lingual surface of the epiglottis with infiltration of polymorphonuclear leukocytes, causing progressive airway compromise. This sequence can proceed rapidly to total obstruction of the supraglottic airway. Laryngospasm is another proposed mechanism of airway obstruction.

Management

The initial management of suspected epiglottitis should follow a predetermined protocol. The operating room personnel and anesthesiologist should be alerted to the arrival of a patient with a compromised airway. When possible, this should be done even prior to the transfer of the patient to the institution. A rigid pediatric bronchoscope and tracheotomy tray should be available in the operating room for difficult intubations. A coordinated team approach should provide efficient and expeditious medical care with minimal potential complications.

Once the diagnosis is established, appropriate management of the disease requires that the airway be secure. If the patient is in distress, immediate efforts must be taken. Otherwise, the operating room is the safest site for intubation. The child should be left in the most comfortable position until intubation is to take place. The position assumed will be one of sitting, with the neck and jaw thrust forward to maintain an airway. Mask induction with first spontaneous, then assisted, ventilation is very effective. The intravenous line can be started once the child is under anesthesia. Blood cultures can be drawn simultaneously. Orotracheal or nasotracheal intubation can then be performed. Usually, orotracheal intubation is performed first. The tube may then be converted to the nasotracheal route. Laryngoscopy reveals a cherry-red, swollen epiglottis. After intubation, a nasogastric tube can be used to empty the stomach of

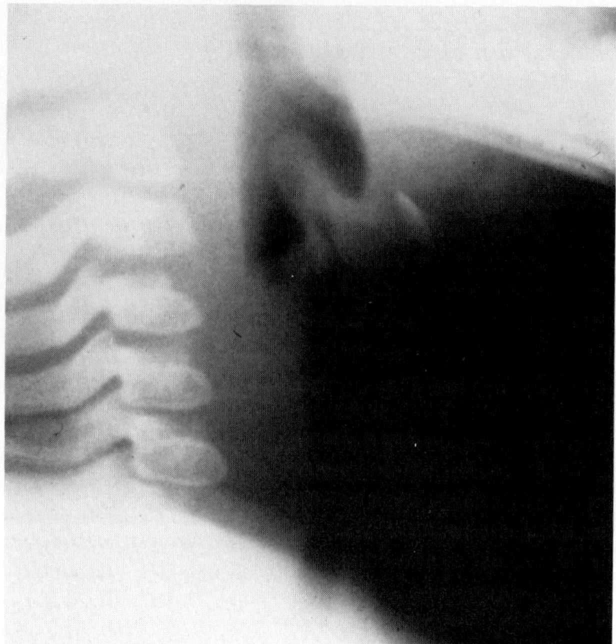

FIG 40–5.
Thickened epiglottis seen in laryngomalacia.

air caused by aerophagia. After the tube is firmly taped in place, a chest x-ray film should be taken to confirm the position of the tube.

The clinical course of epiglottitis usually follows rapid resolution (36–48 hours) once appropriate medical therapy is instituted. Extubation may be undertaken once the epiglottis is visualized and an adequate airway is confirmed. This can be performed at the bedside using either direct laryngoscopy or fiberoptic nasopharyngoscopy with sedation.

Medical management includes the safe establishment of the airway, hydration, and appropriate IV antibiotic coverage. The traditional medical approach employs ampicillin and chloramphenicol as the antibiotics of choice. The chloramphenicol is then discontinued once sensitivities show the organism to be sensitive to ampicillin.

Challenges

Controversies in the management of epiglottitis include selection of the means of airway support. Conservative management of the airway is disputed. The choice of antibiotic coverage has recently undergone a change with the advent of efficacious cephalosporins.

Means of airway support selects the safest method of support in a given situation. Formerly tracheotomies were performed as means of definitive intervention. In today's pediatric intensive care units, with improved methods of sedation and safe long-term positioning of the tube, nasotracheal intubation represents the standard of care.

It is well established that the course of supraglottitis in the adult is less severe than in the child. In certain cases, medical therapy including IV antibiotics and close airway observation

without intubation may be adequate. Frequently, however, the diagnosis is not considered in the adult patient, and the physical examination consists of examination of the oral cavity and oropharynx only. It is unknown how many adult patients with the disease are never diagnosed. Because of their larger airway, moderate edema of the supraglottic structures may be tolerated without obstruction occurring.

Conversely, conservative management of the airway has a more limited role in the treatment of the child with epiglottitis. Obstruction can occur at any time, for example, during transport of the patient, while obtaining radiographic studies, or in the emergency room. In such an event, if intubation cannot be accomplished, tracheotomy, cricothyroidotomy, or even transtracheal oxygenation via a large-bore angiocatheter must be considered before the child is allowed to die. Close observation of the airway in the intensive care setting is performed at some institutions but is not recommended. Antibiotics are initiated, and intubation can sometimes be avoided in these cases.

The traditional medical approach employing ampicillin and chloramphenicol as the IV antibiotics of choice was mentioned. Newer regimens employ cephalosporins such as cefuroxime or, more likely, ceftriaxone, whose efficacy is identical to chloramphenicol but without the rare, but potentially serious complication of aplastic anemia.

CROUP

Diagnosis

Laryngotracheobronchitis, also called laryngotracheitis or croup, may be contrasted with epiglottitis in terms of incidence,

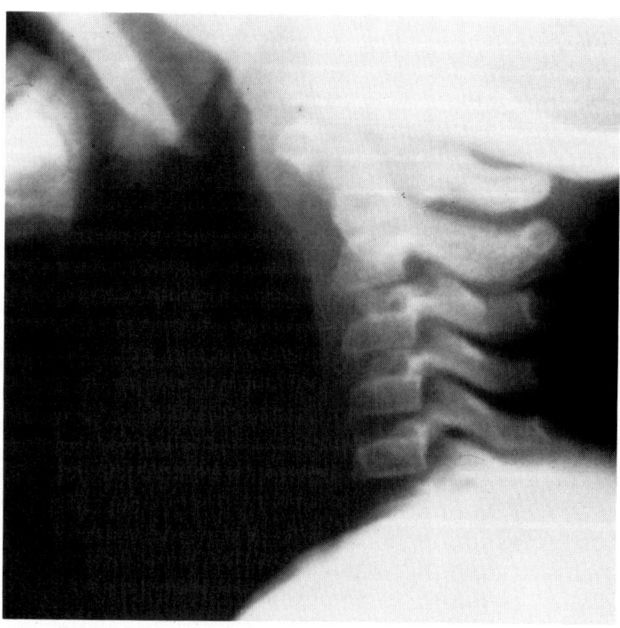

FIG 40–6.
Soft tissue radiograph of neck in epiglottitis.

age, history, severity of illness, and clincial course. The clinical progression follows that of a typical viral disease without the dramatic leukocytosis, rapidity of onset, or speedy progression of epiglottitis. The prodrome of an upper respiratory tract illness is generally present. The hoarse voice and coughing bark, likened to that of a seal, are the typical symptoms. Stridor, as well as intercostal retractions, may be present. The patient is frequently younger than the patient with epiglottitis, being an infant or toddler (in the 1- to 3-year age group). The disease has a seasonal predominance, occurring most often in the winter months.

Laboratory data demonstrate a mild leukocytosis on complete blood cell count, and blood cultures are negative. A radiographic feature typical of croup is the "steeple" sign on AP neck x-ray film, representing subglottic and tracheal narrowing by edema. Chest x-ray film may reveal pulmonary infiltrates.

Management

The disease of laryngotracheobronchitis is most often mild and can usually be treated at home with humidification and observation. The moderate case of croup may require the use of racemic epinephrine in the emergency room, and the patient should therefore be admitted to the hospital for continued treatment. Because of the rebound effect of racemic epinephrine (the symptoms recur or are worse after the drug wears off), no patient should be discharged from the emergency room after its use. Continued treatment on an inpatient basis with a mist tent, oxygen, racemic epinephrine, and possibly steroids should be employed. The severe case of croup may require support of the airway in addition to the other modalities, because the child tires despite medical management. The safest method available in the clinical setting should be used, which generally consists of nasotracheal intubation with a tube that is smaller than would normally be used for that size child.

Laryngoscopy at the time of intubation for severe croup reveals edema and hyperemia in the subglottic area. Because the disease is usually slower to resolve than is epiglottitis, intubation over 3 to 5 days or more may be necessary. When edema is present, an air leak developing around the endotracheal tube signals resolution of the edema and helps in timing extubation.

The causative organisms of laryngotracheobronchitis are the parainfluenza viruses (with parainfluenza type 1 being the most common), respiratory syncytial viruses and influenza A, as well as other less frequent agents.

Complications or possible sequelae of croup include recurrent croup and asthma. Of the children who require intubation for severe croup, some develop subglottic stenosis. It is unknown whether this is caused by intubation in the face of an already edematous subglottis or whether these patients represent undiagnosed congenital subglottic stenosis. The association of the later development of asthma provides evidence that croup may be a disease of the entire upper and lower airways.

Challenges

The role of antibiotics and steroids in what is usually a viral disease is still controversial. In severe cases, antibiotics may control secondary bacterial infection and should be used. Some experts have voiced the concern of using steroids in the setting of an acute infection. The potential immunosuppression and clinical masking of progressive disease are raised as objections. However, other studies have shown a benefit from very large doses of glucocorticoids (1–1.5 mg of dexamethasone/kg/day). This conflict has not been resolved in indication or in dosing. It would seem prudent at least to employ antibiotics in the patient receiving large doses of steroids.

The entity of recurrent croup represents a different diagnostic circumstance. In this case, an anatomic narrowing of the subglottic or tracheal airway may be the underlying cause of airway obstruction. The minimal edema resulting from a concurrent upper respiratory tract illness creates the critical difference in airway lumen, according to Poiseuille's law (diameter varies in inverse proportion to radius to the fourth power). Patients with recurrent symptoms or symptoms presenting at a very early age (<6 months) should undergo diagnostic laryngoscopy and bronchoscopy to evaluate them for congenital or acquired airway lesions. These can be accomplished with either rigid or flexible scopes but should include examination of the lower airway. Congenital airway lesions predisposed to recurrent croup as the presenting symptom include vascular rings, complete tracheal rings, and congenital subglottic stenosis. A history of previous intubation raises the concern of acquired subglottic stenosis.

BACTERIAL TRACHEITIS

Diagnosis

Bacterial tracheitis can be considered an uncommon complication of croup or a bacterial variant of croup, which presents as an acute illness of the upper airway. Bacterial tracheitis is intermediate in severity and incidence to croup and epiglottitis. The diagnosis of bacterial tracheitis should be suspected when a child with croup fails to improve or when the course of croup is refractory to medical treatment (cool mist, racemic epinephrine, steroids). Presenting symptoms are similar to those seen in viral laryngotracheobronchitis. The patient has a cough, a concomitant upper respiratory tract illness, and inspiratory stridor. Symptoms progress to include high fever and toxicity. The disease occurs more commonly in the winter months. *Staphylococcus aureus, Streptococcus pneumoniae,* or, occasionally, *H. influenzae* (which may not be typeable) are the causative organisms. Blood cultures are usually negative.

The pathology of bacterial tracheitis consists primarily of subglottic edema and purulent tracheal secretions. Radiographic features include a normal-sized epiglottis on lateral x-ray film of the neck and the characteristic subglottic narrowing seen also in croup on posterolateral views of the neck. Chest x-ray film reveals air trapping of the bronchi and pulmonary infiltrates.

Management

The mainstay of treatment is maintenance of a patent airway, which is accomplished with aggressive suctioning and antibiotic coverage. The thick tracheal secretions prevent racemic epinephrine from reaching the mucous membrane and, therefore, from being effective. Intubation, therapeutic bronchoscopy, or, occasionally, tracheotomy are required for removal of thick mucous plugs from the subglottic area and trachea and for ventilatory assistance. Cultures of the tracheal secretions can be performed at that time. Presumptive antistaphylococcal coverage is necessary until the culture results can be confirmed.

Challenges

The primary challenge in the care of bacterial tracheitis is timely diagnosis. As the clinical picture of the patient with presumed viral croup deteriorates, diagnostic laryngoscopy, bronchoscopy, and intubation must be considered before airway obstruction ensues.

SUGGESTED READINGS

Jones R, Santos JI, Overall JC: Bacterial tracheitis. *JAMA* 1979; 242:721.

Hawkins DB, Crockett DM, Shum TK: Corticosteroids in airway management. *Otolaryngol Head Neck Surg* 1984; 91:593.

Levison H, Tabachnik E, Newth CJ: Wheezing in infancy, croup and epiglottitis. *Curr Probl Pediatr* 1982; 12:1.

Lockhart CH, Battagli JD: Croup and epiglottitis. *Pediatr Ann* 1977; 6:262.

Mitchell DP, Thomas RL: Secondary airway management in the management of croup. *J Otolaryngol* 1980; 9:419.

Postma DS, Jones RO, Pillsbury HC: Severe hospitalized croup: Treatment trends and prognosis. *Laryngoscope* 1984; 94:1170.

Westley C, Cotton E, Brooks J: Nebulized racemic epinephrine by IPPB for the treatment of croup. *Am J Dis Child* 1978; 132:484.

Zach M, Erben A, Olinsky A: Croup, recurrent croup, allergy and airways hyper-reactivity. *Arch Dis Child* 1981; 56:336.

Bronchoesophagology

CHAPTER 41

Management of Laryngotracheobronchial Problems

Approach of

Sally R. Shott, M.D.

and

Robin T. Cotton, M.D.

AIRWAY BURNS

Approximately 2% to 3% of all patients who sustain thermal burns will also experience inhalation burns with damage to their airways. The majority of these patients have burns involving more than 80% of their total body area. Clinical criteria have been shown to be 96% accurate in predicting the presence of inhalation burns.[1] Thermal injury to the airway should be suspected in any patient who has a history of being burned in a closed space or where there is a history of fumes, choking, or loss of consciousness.

It should be assumed that facial burns involving the mouth and nose have concomitant airway injury until proved otherwise. Though 95% of patients with inhalation burns have associated burns in the head and neck regions, only a small percentage of patients with burns around the face actually will prove to have airway involvement. Singed nasal vibrissae is highly suggestive of potential airway involvement. Carbonaceous sputum has always been considered to be pathognomonic of inhalation injury, but this finding will disappear within 24 hours and may not always be present. A history of hypoxia or abnormal pulmonary findings with rales, rhonchi, or wheezes on auscultation can be suggestive of airway injury and require further evaluation.

The type of heat source can be important. Although hot fumes cause a reflex closure of the glottis, which provides protection to the trachea and lungs, steam injuries have 4,000 times the heat-carrying capacity and more easily cause distal injury.[2] In addition to direct thermal injury, toxic products associated with combustion must be considered. The chemical irritants given off can cause significant damage. When various noxious gases such as carbon dioxide, methane, helium, nitrogen, and nitrous oxide are released, chemical toxicity will also cause a severe inflammatory burn with sloughing and denuding of the respiratory tract mucosa.[2] Paralysis of respiratory cilia will occur, causing accumulation of secretions and debris in the smaller airways. Atelectasis, emphysema, and even complete lobar collapse can occur. From burning material, oxygen concentration can decrease, causing symptoms of asphyxia. Noxious substances, such as hydrogen cyanide and hydrogen sulfide, can also cause cardiovascular and central nervous system dysfunction.

Though the clinical history is important and suggestive of which patients may need further evaluation of their airways, it is highly nonspecific. For instance, hoarseness after a burn injury indicates injury down to the level of the glottis but tells nothing about the condition of the distal airways. Rales and wheezes are present in pulmonary parenchymal injury but tell nothing about the severity of the more proximal airway injury. Carbonaceous sputum may be considered pathognomonic of inhalation injury but tells nothing about the severity and exact location of the injury within the respiratory tract.

The two most helpful modalities of evaluation are direct visualization with bronchoscopy and indirect evaluation with lung scans. The xenon 133 lung scan is useful in identifying small airway and parenchymal damage and is most helpful if done within the first 3 to 4 days after the injury. A normal lung will completely clear the ^{133}Xe within 90 seconds. Prolonged clearance suggests bronchiolar spasm or edema.

Bronchoscopy allows direct visualization of the airway damage, but it should not be performed until the patient's cardiovascular status is stable. The normal physiologic response of tissue to heat injury is edema. This reaction is accentuated in the supraglottic structures, where the mucosal tissue is loosely attached to the underlying basal layer. Massive fluid resuscitation further accentuates the edema in this area. The exception to this is in a patient examined while in hypovolemic shock or prior to full fluid resuscitation. Though the examination may not seem too impressive at that time, the patient can develop significant airway edema and obstruction once fluid resuscitation is given.

Serial bronchoscopy allows evaluation of the healing process as well as examination for progression of disease. Supraglottic edema should resolve by the fourth or fifth day after injury. Laryngeal damage heals much more slowly, and the vocal cords may remain edematous and ulcerated for 3 to 4 weeks after injury. Examination of infraglottic lesions may show mucosal blisters, hemorrhage, and ulceration. Mucosal hemorrhage and ulceration are associated with more severe damage and may progress to purulent tracheitis and bronchopneumonia.[1]

Bronchoscopy on an intubated patient can be done by passing the bronchoscope through the endotracheal tube and then momentarily pulling the endotracheal tube above the vocal cords. Unfortunately, however, bronchoscopy on an intubated patient is not always accurate. The endotracheal tube can cause maceration of the tracheal mucosa, giving an unclear evaluation.[1] Once pulmonary sepsis sets in, the evaluation is even more difficult.

At present, the treatment for inhalation burns is only supportive. Though therapeutic measures such as systemic steroids, immediate tracheotomy, mechanical ventilation with positive end-expiratory pressure, nebulized antibiotics, and prophylactic antibiotics have been advocated, there are no current double-blind studies attesting to their effectiveness.[1]

The issue of tracheotomy in inhalation injuries continues to be controversial. There does, however, seem to be certain specific indications for a tracheotomy in airway burns[3]:

1. Acute onset of upper airway obstruction with the inability to intubate
2. Difficulty in handling secretions with recurrent aspiration
3. Severe facial burns with no safe airway access
4. Prolonged intubation with failure to extubate.

Though the need for prolonged intubation and ventilatory support has traditionally been an indication for tracheotomy, this indication is very controversial in inhalation injury. Many

believe that tracheotomy can increase the risk of pulmonary infection.[2–4] A direct causal relationship between length of intubation and development of subglottic stenosis was not found in the 100 children examined by Calhoun et al.[4] On the other hand, no direct relationship was found between tracheotomy and development of serious airway sequelae. Rather, it was the more seriously injured patients who required tracheotomy and therefore most likely had underlying damage to their airways prior to the tracheotomy. The Eckhauser et al.[5] study of tracheotomy in burn victims quotes a 100% mortality in trached patients vs. a 25% mortality in patients treated with intubation only.[3] However, the Calhoun et al. study shows that 24 of 54 patients treated with intubation died in the study, and only 5 of 22 who underwent tracheotomy died.[4] Sataloff and Sataloff point out the inconsistencies unfortunately present in most studies and emphasize that the two groups of patients in the Eckhauser et al.[5] article were quite dissimilar in degree of injury: "Most authors have either compared unlike groups or reported anecdotal observations and their conclusions are suspect."[2]

Theoretically, besides the specific indications for tracheotomy listed earlier, the reason for tracheotomy is to avoid mucosal disruption and scarring in the mobile portions of the larynx, especially in the subglottic area where the circumferential cartilage skeleton potentiates narrowing. If laryngoscopy and bronchoscopy show that the mucosa has been disrupted or that cartilage is exposed, a tracheotomy is indicated. If significant mucosal injury is present, early tracheotomy may be considered, though no specific studies are available.[2] If the patient is comatose or heavily sedated and does not have constant movement around the endotracheal tube, less damage is likely, and continued intubation is reasonable. Again, however, repeated examination with laryngoscopy and bronchoscopy are the most helpful way to determine the progression toward healing or stenosis.

Reconstruction of airway stenosis secondary to an inhalation injury should be delayed until the scar tissue is fully mature. Results appear to be more predictable and recurrences less common when surgery is delayed.[3]

TRACHEOTOMY

The technique of tracheotomy in an adult and in a child is different because of adherent anatomic differences between these two populations. The pediatric trachea has been described as being of a "soda straw" size.[6] Its high degree of malleability makes its identification difficult from the surrounding soft tissue. In view of this, subtle yet extremely important differences in the technique of tracheotomy in an adult and in a child are present.

In the adult tracheotomy, the procedures can be performed with either local or general anesthetic. In both instances, the patient is placed on the table with a rolled towel under the shoulder blades to facilitate hyperextension of the neck, bringing the trachea to a more anterior position. One percent lidocaine with epinephrine 1:100,000 is used to infiltrate the anterior neck skin at approximately a midway point between the cricoid cartilage and the suprasternal notch. If this procedure is performed under a general anesthetic, this local infiltration provides better hemostasis. If the patient is awake, this injection must also provide anesthesia. The patient is then prepped and draped. If this procedure is performed under local anesthesia, we find it best not to place a large number of drapes over the patient's face because this can be quite uncomfortable for the patient. A transverse incision midway between the cricoid cartilage and the suprasternal notch is used in our routine tracheotomy procedures and made with a knife blade through the skin, subcutaneous fat, and platysma muscle. Hemostasis is achieved as the procedure progresses, usually with electrocautery, though it is important to use ligatures rather than electrocautery when larger venous structures are encountered. When the strap muscles are reached, all dissection is performed in a vertical midline location. It is important for both the surgeon and assistant to work together, each picking up tissue with toothed forceps opposite each other and keeping the dissection in this midline plane. Dissection should be performed in a layer-by-layer fashion to cauterize or ligate vessels as needed. The strap muscles are retracted laterally, usually with Army-Navy retractors, which are frequently repositioned as the midline fascial layers are divided. When the thyroid cartilage is reached, several options exist depending on the level that the thyroid gland rests. If the majority of the gland overlies the thyroid cartilage, a simple superior retraction of the gland is adequate, possibly with minimal dissection freeing the inferior aspect of the gland from the trachea. However, if the gland rests in its more common position overlying the cricoid cartilage and the first several tracheal rings, it is important to divide and suture ligate the thyroid isthmus in the midline. In the adult, dependence on electrocautery division of the thyroid gland can lead to significant postoperative bleeding.

When the level of the trachea is reached, it is important to identify the cricoid cartilage as well as the most superior ring of the trachea. If the patient is awake, injection of an anesthetic solution into the tracheal lumen will minimize coughing and airway reaction once the trachea is opened. A tracheotomy hook is then placed just inferior to the cricoid cartilage, facilitating slight superior elevation of the trachea as well as providing immediate localization of the proper tracheal level should the patient strain and cough once the incisions are made.

In the adult, a tracheal window of cartilage is removed, usually removing the anterior wall of one or two tracheal rings, depending on their size. A horizontal incision is made between the tracheal rings, usually between the second and third rings, with a no. 11 scalpel blade. It is important to make this incision from a lateral to medial location only to the midline point. This protects from inadvertently incising too far laterally into important venous and neural structures should the patient move or cough during this part of the procedure. After the horizontal incisions both above and below the tracheal cartilage are made, the piece of cartilage is grasped with an Allis clamp and divided in a vertical direction using either a knife blade or heavy scissors, depending on the amount of calcification of the cartilage. It is important to have control of this piece of cartilage with the clamp so that it does not inadvertently fall into the airway. If the patient is intubated, the endotracheal tube is partially removed from the trachea, but only to a point just above the

tracheal opening. This provides constant airway control and access. Should there be difficulty in placing the tracheotomy tube at this point, the endotracheal tube can easily be placed distal to the tracheotomy opening and further ventilation achieved. Both the endotracheal tube and the cricoid hook remain in place until the tracheotomy tube has been placed, tested, and secured. We frequently find it advantageous to suction the trachea with a flexible suction catheter prior to placing the tube, because there is frequently some bleeding along the mucosal edges of the tracheal cartilages. Once the tracheotomy tube is placed and ventilation apparatus is attached, the tracheotomy tube is sutured into the skin of the neck using 0 Prolene sutures, one at each of the four corners. In addition, tracheotomy tape is applied, providing a second form of tube security.

A tracheotomy in the pediatric population is almost always performed under a general anesthetic. Because of the inherent soda straw size and malleability of the trachea in a child, it is often difficult to differentiate this structure from the surrounding soft tissues. It is therefore important that the procedure be performed over a bronchoscope or an endotracheal tube. The anesthesiologist can sit at the patient's head, holding both the bronchoscope and the patient's chin to provide better extension of the neck, because these patients frequently will have thicker and shorter necks than their adult counterparts. We have found it helpful in children with short, fat necks to remove some of the subcutaneous fat surrounding the horizontal skin incision. When the strap muscles are reached, the dissection is performed in a vertical direction just as in the adult. Because of the small size of the thyroid gland, we have found it safe to divide the isthmus, if necessary, using electrocautery. When the trachea is reached, the cricoid cartilage is once again identified and a vertical incision is made through the second and third tracheal rings. Before this vertical incision is made, 4-0 Prolene retraction sutures are placed just lateral to the proposed incision. These will provide airway access should the patient be accidentally decannulated in the first few postoperative days. After the incision is made, the endotracheal tube or bronchoscope is once again removed to a point just superior to the tracheal opening and the tracheotomy tube inserted. Because of the pliability and redundancy of the infant's skin, we have not found suturing the tracheotomy tube in place helpful. Tracheotomy ties, however, are secured. The 4-0 Prolene retraction sutures are labeled right and left and actually taped to the patient's anterior chest wall to protect them from being twisted. Only after the tracheotomy tube is in place and ventilation adequately confirmed is the endotracheal tube or bronchoscope removed.

There has been much discussion over the years concerning the proper incision into the trachea, especially in the pediatric population, where the morbidity and mortality related to a tracheotomy are approximately two times greater than that in the adult. One of the more common complications is collapse of the anterior tracheal wall in the suprastomal area. This is best visualized during bronchoscopy with the patient spontaneously ventilating. Due to deformity or pressure necrosis of the cartilagenous rings above the tracheotomy stoma either by long-term pressure from the tracheotomy tube or from weakening secondary to tracheitis, the anterior tracheal wall can be seen to actually collapse and cause obstruction during spontaneous ventilations. Fry et al. looked at several different types of tracheotomy incisions in a pediatric animal model to see if the type of tracheal incision affected the tendency to form either a stenosis at the tracheotomy site or suprastomal collapse.[6] Using three types of incisions (either an inferiorly based trapdoor, a vertical slit, or a horizontal H-type incision), they found a greater increase in resistance to airflow in both the inferiorly based trapdoor and horizontal H-type incisions. The vertical incision resulted in little appreciable increase in airway resistance. They also found that the inferiorly based trapdoor resulted in the most significant amount of tracheal stenosis. This animal model using ferrets suggested a statistical advantage in using the simple vertical slit tracheotomy incision.[6]

Removal of an actual button of tracheal cartilage in the pediatric population will lead to almost certain anterior tracheal wall collapse and fibrosis with tracheal stenosis.

In both the adult and pediatric tracheotomies, the tracheotomy ties are not changed until the third postoperative day. This eliminates any manipulation around the tracheotomy tube in those few critical postoperative days when the tracheotomy tract is still fresh and undeveloped. The first tracheotomy tube change is performed on the fifth postoperative day. In infants who cannot fully cooperate, this first tracheotomy change is performed in either the operating room or an area ajdacent to the operating room. If the patient becomes extremely uncooperative or an airway is dislodged and cannot be quickly replaced, it provides an environment where quick control of the airway can be facilitated.

In both the adult and pediatric population, a chest x-ray film is performed immediately following placement of the tracheotomy tube. This allows one to quickly identify a possible complication of pneumothorax. Closure of the surgical incision is not performed, because this can result in extensive subcutaneous and mediastinal emphysema. Kirschner has also noted in his review of avoiding problems in tracheotomy that it is important to confine one's dissection strictly to the midline once the skin incision has been made and to avoid raising tissue flaps, because this further predisposes to subcutaneous emphysema.[7]

A special condition arises in performing a tracheotomy in an obese adult where a significant layer of fat lies between the skin and the trachea. Frequently this increased distance to the trachea predisposes the patient to unplanned decannulation into the surrounding tissues. Use of a longer tracheotomy tube than the standard models can frequently protect the patient from this situation. A low tracheotomy performed with the patient's neck hyperextended may further place the patient at risk. Because of the long distance between the skin and the tracheal opening, once the patient's head is brought to its normal position, the tracheotomy tube may be pulled out of the trachea because of its short length in relation to the patient's neck thickness. In situations where tracheotomy is performed on an obese patient and there is greater potential for difficulty in localizing the tracheal opening, retraction sutures should be placed alongside the tracheal opening at the time of surgery to assist in locating the tracheal stoma.

CRICOTHYROIDOTOMY

The issue of tracheotomy vs. cricothyroidotomy has always been controversial. Before the 1900s, cricothyroidotomy and high placement of the tracheotomy tube were believed to be the best means to secure an airway, because this procedure was faster and less bloody than performing the procedure in a more inferior location. In the early 1920s, however, Jackson condemned these procedures because of the associated high incidence of laryngeal and subglottic stenosis.[8] Because of Jackson's influence, the trend then turned to performing the tracheotomy at approximately the third tracheal ring. Though this procedure soon became routine over the cricothyroidotomy, recent attention has been placed back to the previous technique.

Advocates of cricothyroidotomy stress that the cricothyroidotomy is especially useful in emergency situations, because hemorrhage is much less common. When the procedure is performed in the midline, usually the only structures traversed are the skin, the subcutaneous tissues, and the fascia between the strap muscles.[9] The minimal bleeding that does occur occurs when the cricothyroid membrane and the laryngeal mucosa are incised. Because the cricothyroid membrane does not calcify with age, entering the airway at this point is often easier than trying to divide calcified tracheal cartilages.[7] The higher placement of the airway is also of benefit in a patient undergoing a median sternotomy incision, because there is less risk of contamination.[9] Because the cricoid cartilage is so prominent in the neck, this procedure can be done with the patient either sitting or supine. The extreme hyperextension required in a lower tracheotomy is not required. It is advantageous in patients with cervical spine disease or injury and also more comfortable for those patients undergoing surgery under a local anesthetic.[7] It has also been suggested that a cricothyroidotomy is safer than the traditional tracheotomy because of the presence of a rigid cartilagenous posterior wall made up of the circumferentially formed cricoid cartilage at this level. In contrast to the tracheotomy when the posterior wall of the trachea at the incision site is made up of a posterior septum, the cricoid cartilage acts as a shield, making esophageal injury less likely during a cricothyroidotomy.[7]

There are several conditions, however, where a cricothyroidotomy is contraindicated. Because of the higher potential for subglottic stenosis occurring in a child at the level of the cricoid cartilage, cricothyroidotomies are contraindicated in this younger population. In addition, a cricothyroidotomy performed in a patient who has been intubated for an extended period may further exacerbate the subglottic and glottic erosion caused by the endotracheal tube.[9] If the patient fails extubation after a period of intubation, it is possible that this is due to subglottic edema or stenosis, and a cricothyroidotomy would then be performed through a diseased area.[10] These are situations where a tracheotomy would be more prudent. Critics of cricothyroidotomy also point to the potential of vocal cord damage, because the incision is just inferior to this site.[11] However, proponents note that the incision can be as far as 2 cm inferior to the vocal cords, and they do not believe that this is a justifiable objection.[12]

Most of the criticism and subsequent fear of subglottic stenosis developing at the level of the cricoid originated from Jackson's writings in 1921.[8] However, review of this patient population revealed a high incidence of concurrent tracheal infections in the patients who were undergoing cricothyroidotomy at that time, which most likely predisposed them to subglottic stenosis.[9] Proponents of cricothyroidotomy therefore stress that if this operation is performed in the absence of active tracheal or laryngeal damage, it is both a safe and easy procedure to perform with essentially the same risks and complications as a tracheotomy. It has been pointed out that both operations are usually performed in the face of serious disease and that because of these underlying conditions, both have intrinsically high risks of complications and death.

TRACHEOTOMY INDICATIONS FOLLOWING PROLONGED INTUBATION

The indications for tracheotomy following prolonged intubation continue to be controversial.[13, 14] It has been shown repeatedly that glottic and subglottic erosion develops within 72 hours of endotracheal intubation.[15, 16] Therefore, if it is obvious that a patient will require prolonged intubation, a tracheotomy should be performed as soon as possible. We continue to use the cutoff of approximately 2 weeks in less obvious cases and believe that a patient's prognosis for the need of continued intubation is usually determined by this time.

Much of this controversy rests in the premature infant population. As more premature infants survive, more cases needing prolonged ventilatory support exist. Critics of tracheotomy in this population point to the high overall morbidity and mortality rate associated with a tracheotomy.[14] Closer examination, however, reveals that the mortality rate related to the tracheotomy itself is low (3%), but the overall mortality related to the underlying pathology in this fragile group of patients is much higher (30%).[17] Arcand and Granger reviewed the incidence of subglottic stenosis in the 1970s and 1980s and found a significant increase in this last decade. A 2% rate of subglottic stenosis was noted in the 1970s, which, unfortunately, rose to as high as 23% in the 1980s. This reflects not only a larger population of premature infants with more severe pathology who go on to subsequently survive but also a higher reliance on endotracheal tubes.[17]

ENDOBRONCHIAL TUMOR MANAGEMENT

Laser technology in the past 20 years has allowed the surgeon to provide palliative treatment for malignant endobronchial tumors as well as definitive treatment for benign lesions. Currently, four lasers are available for surgical treatment: (1) the CO_2 laser, (2) the neodymium-yttrium aluminum garnet (Nd:YAG) laser, (3) the potassium titanyl phosphate (KTP) laser, and (4) the argon laser. Each laser is distinguished by the color of the laser light that it produces and the source of this light.

The CO_2 laser is characterized as a cutting and vaporizing laser. The CO_2 laser is highly absorbed by water, and since biologic tissue is 80% water, the CO_2 laser is believed to be ideal.[18] It is also noted for having a very minimal amount of scatter. Scatter is directly related to the amount of necrosis that occurs in tissue beyond the desired surgical site. A laser's precision in surgery is determined by a combination of the ability of the delivery optics to focus on a very small spot size and the amount of scatter produced in the surrounding tissue. Some scatter, however, is quite helpful, because it provides hemostasis to the surrounding tissues.

One of the main limitations of the CO_2 laser is its delivery system. Because it produces an infrared light that is invisible to the human eye, it requires a separate source of light, usually He, for the aiming beam. Because of the requirement of two separate beams, it is possible for malalignment to occur. The CO_2 laser light and helium neon are directed through a series of mirrors called the articulated arm to the tissue site.

The Nd-YAG laser is also produced using an infrared light that requires a separate light source for the aiming beam. It is known for producing the greatest amount of scatter in this group of four lasers and is best used as a coagulating laser. It is frequently used in treatment of gastrointestinal bleeding. Its use in the upper airway and pulmonary system has been minimal because of this high degree of scatter.

The KTP laser is within the visible spectrum. In general, visible laser lights can be focused to smaller spots than infrared lasers. It has been described as having an intermediate level of scatter, but the scatter is less so in hemorrhagic tissue due to its shorter extinction length in hemoglobin.

The argon laser is visible in the blue-green spectrum. It is preferentially absorbed by a red medium or tissue and is noted for its photocoagulation properties. Though its 90% extinction length is three times greater than the KTP laser, it is still believed to be minimal, with an extinction length between 0.154 and 0.219 mm. The visible laser beam allows for a smaller and more precise spot size than the infrared lasers.

Because treatment of endobronchial tumors occurs in a very confined area, control of the laser effect is of utmost importance. The CO_2 laser produces one half as much necrosis as the visible KTP laser, and the Nd-YAG produces twice as much necrosis. To better illustrate, if the CO_2 laser produces an effect in tissue of 1 mm, the KTP and argon lasers would produce 2 mm of tissue necrosis, and the Nd-YAG laser would produce 4 mm of necrosis. Therefore, use of the Nd-YAG laser in the tracheobronchial tree is not suggested at this time.

In general, laser removal of endobronchial lesions allows the surgeon much better accuracy than is provided by the traditional method of hand-held forceps removal. The CO_2 laser, passing through an operating microscope and micromanipulator, should provide surgical accuracy within 0.1 mm. The KTP laser, because it is transmitted through a visible light spectrum, should provide even better accuracy, because reliance on mirror transmission and a separate visible beam is not required. In addition, lasers provide coagulation of vessels up to 0.5 mm in diameter and even up to 2 mm in diameter in some instances.

This occurs through the scatter effect of the laser, which can be increased by defocusing the laser beam point.

In addition, less postoperative edema occurs through use of the laser. This may be due to the decrease in sensible fluid loss from sealing of the microcirculation and from the lack of physical contact with surrounding tissues as occurs with tissue manipulation with forceps or other surgical instruments. Postoperative pain is also believed to be less after lasers are used. It is hypothesized that this may be due to thermal sealing of nerve endings.

Delivery of the laser to endobronchial tumors is usually accomplished through a bronchoscope. The CO_2 laser can be coupled to a ventilating bronchoscope, allowing hands-off endoscopic surgery. The KTP laser, because it can be passed through a small coil, can be placed directly via this coil through the suctioning port of a ventilating bronchoscope. The lasers can be used for the management of recurrent respiratory papillomas as well as for resection of tracheal and proximal endobronchial adenomas. Tracheal webs have also been treated in this manner. Granulation tissue present in the trachea can also be excised. An airway can be established in patients with obstructing tracheal or proximal endobronchial malignant tumors.

In the pediatric population, use of lasers through the bronchoscope has been difficult because of the high degree of reflection of the CO_2 laser within the long thin bronchoscope. We have found that laryngeal and tracheal lesions are better approached using a variety of subglottiscopes. More distal and bronchial lesions are best reached using the KTP laser, which can easily be placed through the smaller pediatric bronchoscope.

Laser excision of endobronchial obstruction is not indicated when there is extraluminal compression of the trachea by an extrinsic tumor.

In the use of lasers, it is important to remove the char, or resultant necrotic tissue during the process of the procedure. It is possible to vaporize all of the water from the tissue and leave behind necrotic carbon or char. These carbon particles are able to absorb further energy and will vaporize only at temperatures greater than 2,000°C. The heat produced affects the surrounding tissue but is also in the surrounding air and can enter tissue further distal in the airway. It is therefore important that during the process of lasering, one stops and suctions away this char and lasers only fresh tissue.

The anesthesiologist and the surgeon must work closely when laser excision of endobronchial masses is performed. Only nonflammable anesthetic agents should be used, commonly a mixture of oxygen and nonflammable gas such as nitrous oxide, to oxygenate the patient at the lowest potential level for a fire.[19, 20] Because most of this surgery is performed through metal bronchoscopes, the danger of anesthetic and laser ignition of the endotracheal tube is usually not a problem.[21]

Unfortunately, multiple potential complications do exist when the lasers are used, and strict protocols are required in this type of surgery.[21] Both corneal burns and skin burns from misdirected laser beams or reflected energy are possible. Tracheal and bronchial perforation is perhaps the most feared complication. It is probably best to use the laser in a single or repeated pulsed mode to allow better differentiation of mucosa, perichondrium, and tracheal cartilage. The ability to determine one's exact location within the bronchus is more difficult in complete obstructing lesions where the exact site of the lumen is unknown. Caution is therefore always required. Delayed bleeding is possible if vessels greater than 1 mm in diameter are treated by laser cauterization. Delayed postoperative obstruction can also occur. It is rare but can occur within the first 18 to 24 hours after the procedure. This may be related to laryngeal and subglottic trauma associated with procedure.

Because of these well-known complications, it is important that every operating room using lasers have a laser safety committee and a laser safety officer. Protective eyeglasses should be used by the surgeon as well as by all personnel in the room. The patient's eyes should also be protected. All personnel, including the surgeons, should be certified in the use of the laser. Warning signs in the area where the laser is used should be posted. Adequate smoke evacuation is required and is especially necessary in the treatment of papillomas because recent data have suggested that papillomas can be transmitted through the laser vapors.[22] All drapes surrounding the patient and target area should be moistened to protect from fire in case of inadvertent firing or reflection of the laser beam.

Though laser excision of endobronchial tumors may be only palliative, it is helpful in reestablishing a patent airway or removing obstructive lesions that are causing postobstructive pneumonias and can therefore provide significant relief of the patient's symptoms.

REFERENCES

 1. Hunt JF, Agee RN, Pruitt BA: Fiberoptic bronchoscopy in acute inhalation injury. *J Trauma* 1975; 15:641–648.
 2. Sataloff OM, Sataloff RT: Tracheotomy and inhalation injury. *Head Neck Surg* 1984; 6:1024–1031.
 3. Miller RP, Gray SD, Cotton RT, et al: Airway reconstruction following laryngotracheal thermal trauma. *Laryngoscope* 1988; 98:1826–1829.
 4. Calhoun KH, Deskin RW, McCracken MM, et al: Long-term airway sequelae in a pediatric burn population. *Laryngoscope* 1988; 98:721–725.
 5. Eckhauser FE, Billote J, Burke JF, et al: Tracheotomy complicating massive burn injury. *Am J Surg* 1974; 127:418–423.
 6. Fry TL, Jones RD, Fischer ND, et al: Comparison of tracheotomy incisions in a pediatric model. *Ann Otol Rhinol Laryngol* 1985; 94:450–453.
 7. Kirchner JA: Avoiding problems in tracheotomy. *Laryngoscope* 1986; 96:55–57.
 8. Jackson C: High tracheotomy and other errors: The chief causes of chronic laryngeal stenosis. *Surg Gynecol Obstet* 1921; 32:392–398.
 9. McDowell DE: Cricothyroidotomy for airway access. *South Med J* 1982; 75:282–284.
10. Boyd AD, Conlan AA, Spencer FC: A clinical evaluation of cricothyroidotomy. *Surg Gynecol Obstet* 1979; 149:365–368.
11. Mitchell SA: Cricothyroidotomy revisited. *Ear Nose Throat J* 1980; 58:54–60.
12. Morain WD: Cricothyroidotomy in head and neck surgery. *Plast Reconstr Surg* 1980; 65:424–428.

13. Berlauk JF: Prolonged endotracheal intubation vs. tracheostomy. *Crit Care Med* 1986; 14:742–745.
14. Dankel SK, Schuller DE, McClead RE: Prolonged intubation in neonates. *Arch Otolaryngol* 1987; 113:841–843.
15. Whited RE: Posterior commissure stenosis from endotracheal intubation. *Laryngoscope* 1983; 93:1314–1318.
16. Dayal VS, El Masri W: Tracheotomy in intensive care setting. *Laryngoscope* 1986; 96:58–60.
17. Arcand P, Granger J: Pediatric tracheotomies: Changing trends. *J Otolaryngol* 1988; 17:121–124.
18. DiBartolomeo JR: The argon and CO_2 lasers in otolaryngology: Which one, when, and why? *Laryngoscope* 1981; vol 26 (suppl).
19. Ruder CB, Rapheal NL, Abramson AL, et al: Anesthesia for carbon dioxide laser microsurgery of the larynx. *Otolaryngol Head Neck Surg* 1981; 89:732–737.
20. Vourch G, Tannieres ML, Freeche G: Anesthesia for microsurgery of the larynx using a carbon dioxide laser. *Anesthesia* 1979; 34:53–57.
21. Meyers A: Complications of CO_2 laser surgery of the larynx. *Ann Otol Rhinol Laryngol* 1981; 90:132–134.
22. Garden JM: Papillomas in the vapor of carbon dioxide laser-treated verrucae. *JAMA* 1988; 259:1199–1202.

SUGGESTED READINGS

Brantigan CO, Grow JB: Cricothyroidotomy: Elective use in respiratory problems requiring tracheotomy. *J Thorac Cardiovas Surg* 1982; 71:282–284.

Council on Scientific Affairs: Lasers in medicine and surgery. *JAMA* 1986; 256:900–907.

DiVincenti FC, Pruitt BA, Reckler JM: Inhalation burns. *J Trauma* 1971; 11:109–117.

Moncreif JA: Tracheotomy in burns. *Arch Surg* 1959; 79:45–48.

Lund T, Goodwin CW, McManus WF: Upper airway sequelae in burn patients requiring endotracheal intubation or tracheostomy. *Ann Surg* 1985; 201:374–382.

Phillips AW, Tanner JT, Cope O: Burns therapy: Respiratory damage and the meaning of restlessness. *Ann Surg* 1963; 158:779–811.

Management of Laryngotracheobronchial Problems

Approach of

Bernard R. Marsh, M.D.

AIRWAY BURNS

Up to one third of all victims of major burns suffer a potentially lethal smoke-related inhalation injury.[1] The cause of injury may be (1) heat, (2) carbon monoxide toxicity, or (3) smoke inhalation.

Reflex closure of the larynx in conscious patients usually protects the lower airways, but thermal injury of the lung can occur with steam inhalation. Thermal injury of the respiratory tract affects primarily the larynx, especially the supraglottis. Such injuries occur from either inhalation of hot gases or the ingestion of hot or corrosive liquids. Upper airway edema, hemorrhage, and ulceration may compromise the airway, frequently within a few hours after injury. Airway obstruction occurs in 20% to 30% of burn victims with inhalation injury.[2]

The tongue and laryngeal surface of the epiglottis sustain thermal injury without appreciable swelling, but the lingual surface of the epiglottis, ventricular bands, aryepiglottic folds, and arytenoids may develop massive swelling following relatively brief exposure.

Carbon monoxide toxicity is a frequent, immediate cause of death, especially in fires occurring in closed spaces. This gas leads not only to tissue hypoxia, by shifting the oxyhemoglobin dissociation curve to the left, but also to a general toxic effect on oxidative metabolism. Early recognition is crucial to successful management.

Smoke can have any of a large number of toxic components. Water-soluble gases from burning plastics and rubber include ammonia, phosgene, sulfur dioxide, and chlorine. Other common products of combustion are cyanides, acroleins, aldehydes, and hydrocarbons. On contact with airway mucosa, various acids and alkalis are formed, causing a chemical laryngotracheobronchitis and resulting in epithelial damage. Within hours, the laryngeal mucosa may be denuded and ulcerated with sloughing epithelial debris. The severity of injury depends on the constituents of the smoke and other factors. Inhaled smoke may damage the alveolar membrane and capillary endothelium, increasing permeability and causing pulmonary edema. Smoke exposure also produces ciliary paralysis within minutes, and severe bronchospasm can occur almost immediately. Most deaths related to fires result from pulmonary damage caused by smoke inhalation.[3]

Diagnosis

Symptoms of dyspnea, cough, stridor, hoarseness, and pain may be present in varying degrees. Together with a history of exposure to a fire in a closed space, these symptoms suggest possible inhalation injury. Facial burns may or may not be present. Heat exposure is unnecessary to produce a chemical burn of the airway. Suspected inhalation burn injury to the respiratory tract requires prompt airway assessment. Fiberoptic examinations provide valuable information about the airway and should be repeated frequently since laryngeal edema can develop any time within the first 36 hours after smoke inhalation. The false cords may be red, swollen, and covered by a gray exudate over areas of second-degree burns. The true cords, if involved, are usually burned more in the anterior two thirds of the glottis.

Management

Intubation or tracheotomy may be necessary. There is some debate regarding the use of intubation in the presence of mucosal injury since there is a significant potential for glottic and subglottic stenosis. The majority of patients can be extubated within 3 to 5 days, making the risk acceptable. The major hazard of infection associated with tracheotomy makes endotracheal intubation the favored initial method of airway maintenance in spite of occasional late complications. A tracheotomy should be considered only if endotracheal intubation is impossible or a patient cannot be weaned from the ventilator after 1 to 3 weeks.

In addition to laryngoscopy and fiberoptic bronchoscopy, a chest radiograph and blood gas and electrolyte determinations should be obtained. In a study of 100 consecutive patients with serious burns examined with the fiberbronchoscope, one third had airway burns, and most of these had facial burns. The chest radiographs in these patients were initially quite unremarkable, but 73% of patients with airway burns eventually developed

pulmonary or airway complications.[4] Aggressive pulmonary toilet, fluid replacement, and adequate oxygenation contribute to effective management. Steroids should be avoided except for treatment of bronchospasm unresponsive to parenteral and inhaled bronchodilators. There is no proof that steroids are of any benefit, and their use increases the risk of pneumonia. Risk of superinfection militates against the use of prophylactic antibiotics, which are best reserved until there is clinical evidence of infection documented by Gram stain and culture.

Patients who are without symptoms but at risk for inhalation injury should undergo careful laryngoscopy; if edema or mucosal injury is evident, fiberoptic bronchoscopy should be performed. If there are no abnormal findings, observation is indicated.

TRACHEOTOMY

Technique

The technique used for tracheotomy depends to some extent on the circumstances necessitating the operation. This discussion assumes a relatively elective procedure performed in the operating room.

The patient should be positioned with a rolled sheet or towel under the shoulders to extend the neck. Adults properly sedated may tolerate the procedure under local anesthesia, but general endotracheal anesthesia is preferred. Patients in airway distress tolerate the extended neck position poorly under local anesthesia. Children should be intubated to secure the airway, provide satisfactory anesthesia, and improve identification of the trachea. I recommend that an esophageal stethoscope not be used in small children lest the esophagus rather than the trachea be opened.

In adults, after skin preparation with an antiseptic solution, the neck is completely isolated by sterile drapes and a half-screen to permit anesthesia access to the face. In the infant, the face is left undraped to allow full exposure for any necessary airway manipulation.

Local anesthesia and vasoconstriction can be obtained as needed by infiltrating lidocaine with epinephrine. The landmarks of the thyroid cartilage, cricoid cartilage, and suprasternal notch are easily identified in the adult, but in the infant the laryngeal cartilages are positioned higher in the neck and may be very difficult to identify.

In the adult the skin incision is usually performed in a horizontal skin fold over the cricoid cartilage except in an emergency airway obstruction, when a vertical incision should be used. In infants, I prefer a vertical incision in most cases. Any error in positioning a horizontal incision may cause the tip of the tracheotomy tube to ride against the anterior or posterior tracheal wall; erosion and granulation tissue are then likely, and tracheal obstruction or late stenosis may occur. The high position of the infant larynx and the poor definition of the cartilages make an inappropriately low incision a real possibility. A tube placed below the fourth tracheal ring may risk bronchial intubation in some patients. If the tube is shortened, one creates a risk of accidental decannulation.

A vertical incision permits the tube to be established in the most favorable position. My experience suggests that the cosmetic result of the short neck incision for an elective pediatric tracheotomy does not greatly depend on whether the incision is vertical or horizontal.

Skin and subcutaneous vessels can be controlled by electrocautery as required. The dissection should be kept strictly in the midline to avoid risk to the recurrent laryngeal nerves and major vessels. The assistant picks up the fascia opposite the surgeon as each layer in turn is incised, with care to avoid an anomalous carotid or innominate artery. Much of the procedure can be achieved by blunt dissection using either the scissors or a curved hemostat. These instruments should be spread slowly but to the maximum length of the incision at each level. The larynx should be palpated frequently to maintain a strictly midline position. The surgeon must be alert for anomalous vessels and the thyroid isthmus.

As the strap muscles are separated, retractors may be introduced to maintain adequate exposure. When the cricoid cartilage is identified, the pretracheal fascia should be entered to develop a plane beneath the thyroid isthmus, permitting its division and suture ligation. The first four or five tracheal rings should be identified and any remnants of fascia removed over the incision site. In infants, I pass a 3-0 silk suture longitudinally through the tracheal wall about 2 mm from either side of the intended incision. These sutures become the retractors to elevate the trachea into the incision. A tracheal hook is seldom needed. Each suture should be tied with a long loop, with the knot left outside the neck incision to facilitate removal after the first tube change. The electrocautery should then be adjusted to a very low level and any fine vessels along the incision site coagulated. The tracheotomy tube must be prepared and in hand as the anesthesiologist loosens the endotracheal tube tape.

Tubes in several sizes should be available in the operating room. I prefer plastic tracheotomy tubes in most cases. They are uncuffed for small children, but adults may require a cuffed tube. In children, I make a vertical midline incision through rings 2 through 4. Traction sutures evert the tracheal incision, allowing exposure of the endotracheal tube so that use of a tracheal dilator is seldom necessary. No cartilage is removed. The endotracheal tube should be withdrawn slowly, just enough to clear the tracheotomy site. The tracheotomy tube can then be inserted and adequate ventilation assured before the endotracheal tube is removed. One or two sutures may be used to close a portion of the skin incision, but a tight closure should be avoided.

The shoulder roll should be removed and the neck flexed before the tracheotomy tape is securely tied about the neck with a square knot to ensure that the tube cannot be inadvertently dislodged. I do not suture the tube to the skin. The tubes are soft enough to permit decannulation in spite of the sutures, and prompt restoration of the airway may be impaired by efforts to remove the sutures. A sterile dry dressing is fitted around the tube and underneath the ties. The traction sutures should be taped to either side of the chest and identified. In an emergency, such as a tube dislodgement, these sutures can be used to bring the tracheal fenestra into direct view for reestablishing the airway. The sutures may be removed after the first tube change about 1 week postoperatively. A chest radiograph and postoperative care should be provided in an intensive care unit until the airway is secure.

I do not use stay sutures in adults but remove a portion of tracheal wall corresponding to the size of the tracheotomy tube or create an inferiorly based U-shaped tracheal flap sutured to the skin. Such a flap may be used in children, but I am concerned that in small children a flap may nearly transect the trachea and increase the risk of stenosis.

Indications for Tracheotomy for Prolonged Intubation

The benefits of a tracheotomy in the patient requiring long-term ventilation include improved suctioning, greater patient comfort, less laryngeal complications, easier tube changes, and provision for oral intake.[5] However, it is generally agreed that an initial period of endotracheal intubation should precede tracheotomy. Optimal timing for conversion from endotracheal intubation to tracheotomy remains highly controversial. Optimism that extubation may eventually be achieved, combined with a desire to avoid possibly serious complications of tracheotomy, may lead to prolonged endotracheal intubation despite its potential for causing laryngotracheal stenosis.

A multitude of factors contribute to the relative risk of these two means for airway maintenance. I recently saw a patient with near total laryngeal stenosis after only 5 days of intubation. In the final analysis, there is no minimum period for endotracheal intubation during which it can be considered free from risk of significant laryngeal stenosis. In a prospective study of adult airway lesions evaluated by endoscopy, there was a 12% incidence of chronic laryngotracheal stenosis in patients intubated more than 10 days.[6] Patients in this study who were converted to tracheotomy had a higher incidence of tracheal stenosis, but in these patients the airways were already damaged from prior endotracheal intubation, suggesting that a long-term endotracheal tube increases the risk of tracheal injury from a subsequent tracheotomy. A study by Sasaki et al. suggests that tracheal contamination from the tracheotomy secondarily infects a larynx already injured by intubation.[7] This infection prolongs healing of injured tissue and predisposes to scar and stricture formation.

The determination of how long an endotracheal tube should remain in place also depends on factors such as the presence of diabetes mellitus, heart failure, pneumonia, agitation, and other systemic considerations that tend to increase the risk of laryngotracheal injury. No matter how carefully patients are selected or followed, the incidence of laryngotracheal sequelae increases with the length of intubation. In adult patients, intubation beyond 10 days should be subject to the most rigorous justification.

Premature infants may require prolonged ventilation and frequently develop complications with tracheotomy.[8] With advanced neonatal care, these patients can survive prolonged intubation, and conversion to tracheotomy is often deferred for some weeks. If the endotracheal tube size and care are optimal, these infants may tolerate intubation for 2 to 3 months. If there are multiple and traumatic intubations or a congenital subglottic stenosis, tracheotomy is advised as soon as development is sufficiently advanced to permit use of a standard tracheotomy tube.

In contrast to the premature infants, older children who

are intubated for an inflammatory edema of the larynx should be extubated as soon as possible. Efforts to determine just how long the tube may safely be left in place by evaluating the laryngeal reaction to it are usually unsatisfactory.

CRICOTHYROIDOTOMY

All forms of airway access are associated with damage to the airway. In recent years the relative merits and risks of cricothyroidotomy and tracheotomy have been considerably debated. Major complications of these two procedures can largely be avoided by proper patient selection, adherence to good surgical technique, and appropriate aftercare. Proper patient selection will strictly limit the population eligible for cricothyroidotomy and largely eliminate the most feared risk, which is chronic subglottic stenosis.

Indications

This procedure is an excellent emergency airway technique because of its simplicity and the speed with which it can be accomplished. Risks of pneumothorax and tracheoarterial fistula are virtually zero. On my service, cricothyroidotomy is used only in airway emergencies. It may be useful in cervical spine or maxillofacial injuries where endotracheal intubation is impossible or dangerous. Conversion to tracheotomy is recommended if there is a need for prolonged airway control.

It has also been used quite frequently in cardiac surgery for patients who require a median sternotomy and postoperative ventilatory assistance.[9] A low tracheotomy in this setting presents unacceptable risks of infection.

Occasionally, anatomic variations make this procedure an acceptable alternative to tracheotomy.

Cricothyroidotomy is contraindicated in any patient with laryngeal pathology, including preceding endotracheal intubation for more than 7 days. Such patients carry a significant risk of subglottic stenosis. It is not recommended for pediatric patients or for any inflammatory condition of the larynx.[10] For long-term tracheal access, it must be restricted to patients without laryngeal disease in whom a tracheotomy presents unacceptable risks. Even under these circumstances, there is a significant risk of voice impairment.[11]

TECHNIQUE FOR PERMANENT TRACHEOTOMY

Permanent epithelialization of a tracheotomy is facilitated by a skin-to-mucosa closure created at the initial surgery. A number of skin flap procedures have been described, none of which has received universal acceptance.[12, 13] The specific needs and the anatomic configuration of the individual patient must dictate the approach to be taken. The following procedure has proved useful for my patients in whom I expect a long-term need for tracheotomy.

A horizontal skin incision is placed over the intended site for the tracheal stoma. Upper and lower skin flaps are developed, and excess adipose tissue is excised. The strap muscles are separated in the midline and retracted. The thyroid isthmus should be divided between clamps and suture ligated and the stumps retracted laterally, exposing the first four tracheal rings. A U-shaped inferiorly based tracheal flap is then outlined with the cautery at a low setting. The flap width is tailored to the size of the anticipated tracheotomy tube and includes the second, third, and sometimes fourth ring. The tracheal flap is sutured to the inferior skin flap, which may be trimmed as necessary to provide an optimal stoma. The superiorly based skin flap may then be brought down and sutured to the superior aspect of the stoma. The lateral skin defects should not be closed.

This technique provides an easily accessible stoma, even though a tube or button is usually used.

Other forms of flap tracheotomy incorporating laterally based flaps have been reported and may be preferable in some circumstances.[14–16]

ENDOBRONCHIAL TUMOR MANAGEMENT

Tumors involving the tracheobronchial tree often result in cough, hemoptysis, dyspnea, and eventually postobstructive pneumonia, atelectasis, hypoxemia, and death. The availability of bronchoscopic lasers has given us a highly useful instrument for palliation in selected cases.

Indications

The patient must have respiratory symptoms resulting from a biopsy-proved malignancy that has failed all other reasonable therapy.

The lesion must be intraluminal within the trachea or main bronchi. Such lesions may be either primary or metastatic. Treatment of lesions within the lobar or segmental bronchi is seldom sufficiently beneficial to be worth the risk of bronchial penetration and fatal hemorrhage. Extrinsic compression of the airway is a contraindication to laser treatment.

The lesion must be situated such that there is a patent airway and functional lung distally. Tumors that arise in the distal segments and extend proximally should not be treated. Computed tomography and fiberoptic bronchoscopy each provide valuable information for determining suitability for laser therapy.

The patient's respiratory status and clinical condition should be such that successful treatment can be expected to make a meaningful improvement in quality of life. As a general rule, I do not treat patients who require a respirator for ventilation.

Operative Technique

Endoscopic laser treatment of obstructing airway tumors carries substantial risks. The bronchoscopist and the nursing and anesthesia staff must be well trained in working together efficiently to minimize the hazards of this procedure. Proper eye protection is mandatory for all persons in the area, and all personnel must have a clear understanding of all safety aspects of laser use. The patient must also be informed regarding the relevant risks and alternatives to this procedure.

Patient preparation should include a complete medical evaluation with special attention to the cardiovascular and pulmonary status, including values of blood.gases, chemistries, and hematology.

The CO_2 laser can be used for treatment of obstructing airway tumors, but its several disadvantages have led me to abandon its use in favor of the Nd-YAG laser in the treatment of friable endobronchial carcinomas.

These procedures should be performed in the operating room with full anesthesia support and monitoring, including a pulse oximeter. I investigate the tumor by first performing a fiberoptic bronchoscopy under local anesthesia and sedation. The nose should be anesthetized by application of 5% cocaine (or any other agent of choice) on a small cotton applicator. Supplemental oxygen is supplied by nasal prongs, which may be inserted between the lips to keep the nasal airway free of obstruction. The fiberscope is then passed gently along the floor of the nose into the pharynx, where 2% lidocaine is instilled through the bronchoscope into the larynx and trachea. The syringe should contain 2 mL of drug and about 2 cc of air so as to permit full discharge of the anesthetic into the airway. Usually several instillations are required to subdue the cough reflex, whereupon the fiberscope may be passed through the glottis into the lower airway. Additional lidocaine may be needed, especially in the left main bronchus and the upper lobes. In most instances the tumor will be immediately recognized and a decision made about the best approach.

There are two main options: (1) to continue under local anesthesia by using the laser fiber through the large channel (2.6 mm) fiberscope or (2) to use general anesthesia and the Nd-YAG rigid laser bronchoscope.

Option 1

This option may be considered for small lesions, especially in areas relatively inaccessible to the rigid bronchoscope. It can be used either under local anesthesia directly through the nose or through an endotracheal tube under general anesthesia. Disadvantages of this approach include greater risk of fire, much less facility for handling bleeding, accumulated secretions, laser smoke, and coagulated tumor as well as less efficiency for handling larger tumors and establishing an airway if problems develop. Great care must be exercised in patient selection and operative technique to minimize risks.

The laser power should be set to about 40 W and a pulse duration of 0.5 second. The patient and all personnel in the room must wear proper laser goggles. The fiberscope should be placed about 2 cm proximal to the tumor. The laser fiber can then be carefully inserted about 1 cm beyond the tip of the fiberscope, with care to avoid getting blood on the tip of the fiber. The laser fiber must be maintained in a position well distal to the end of the bronchoscope to lessen the risk of damage from laser backscatter as well as to prevent inadvertent laser activation within the scope (a sure prescription for a destroyed bronchoscope, at best, or a fire at worst). The laser fiber can then be activated directly onto the tumor and the effect observed. The bronchoscope may be advanced slightly to increase the effect, but great care should be exercised first to

obtain a blanching effect rather than vaporization. Bleeding may be minimized only by first fully coagulating the tumor in this way. The laser beam should be directed parallel to the bronchus wall; with perpendicular orientation there is risk of bronchial perforation. Fortunately, this is a rare complication and one I have never witnessed. It should usually be preventable, but it has been reported and can be associated with immediate fatal hemorrhage. The deep penetration of the Nd-YAG laser can also create sufficient damage to the bronchial wall and underlying structures that even without apparent penetration fatal complications may occur some time later when the tissue sloughs out. These patients are usually in marginal condition already, and almost any treatment is likely to fail. This emphasizes the importance not only of proper laser technique but also of proper patient selection and a full disclosure of potential risks.

After the tumor is fully coagulated, the lesion may be approached carefully to obtain greater power density and some tumor vaporization. At the conclusion of the procedure, the bronchus should be irrigated with saline to remove accessible debris.

This technique does not permit as effective removal of coagulated tumor as with the rigid instrument. Thus, if a large tumor is encountered, repeated laser treatments spaced some days apart may be required to accomplish what could be achieved in one sitting with the rigid system.

Approach through the large channel fiberscope may be performed under general endotracheal anesthesia. In this instance, a 9 mm endotracheal tube (clear plastic) is cut short to ensure that the distal end of the tube is several centimeters proximal to the tumor. A T adapter permits simultaneous ventilation and treatment. The fiberscope should be well lubricated to permit free passage through the endotracheal tube; I prefer silicone spray in addition to a small amount of water-soluble jelly. Some materials may be flammable, so care should be exercised in their use. The anesthesiologist should be reminded to place an oral airway between the teeth to protect the bronchoscope in the event of light anesthesia, to limit the forced inspiratory oxygen (FIO_2) to no greater than 30% during laser treatment, and preferably to use Heliox to reduce the risk of fire.

The fiberscope is then passed through the endotracheal tube to a point well beyond the tip of the endotracheal tube and approximately 2 cm proximal to the tumor. The laser fiber is inserted about 1 cm beyond the tip of the fiberscope and the procedure conducted as described earlier with similar laser settings.

This approach has the advantage of perfect cough control, making laser injury and fiber damage less likely. It also assures patient comfort through what may be a somewhat tedious procedure. If proper precautions are taken, the risk of fire and bleeding should be quite remote. Intraoperative bronchial tumor bleeding with a fiberscope in place can usually be managed by patience and judicious aspiration proximal to the bleeding site until control is obtained. The principal objective is airway maintenance with protection of the nonbleeding lung. Unfortunately, when bleeding is quite active, the bronchoscopic image may become lost from a blood smear over the distal lens just when critical decisions must be made. The view can usually be restored by quickly moving to the opposite lung to aspirate against clean mucosa and then immediately return to the bleeding bronchus. Expeditious action is needed to prevent clotting of the suction channel as well. The laser has no role in this setting as opposed to the same circumstance with the rigid bronchoscope in place when simultaneous suction and laser use may be quite helpful. Rarely is the bleeding severe enough to be life threatening and require more active measures. The patient should be positioned on his or her side with the bleeding side down and the table tilted head down. Use of Fogarty catheter with balloon inflation has been suggested as an option, though I have never found it necessary. A double lumen (Carlens) tube has also been used by some experienced in its placement. A rigid bronchoscope skillfully used may permit either intubating the nonbleeding lung, packing the bleeding site with ribbon gauze, or simultaneous using suction and the Nd-YAG laser. An intubated patient positioned as mentioned earlier can easily be suctioned with a large-bore catheter and may be adequately managed until spontaneous control occurs or other measures can be instituted. This condition demands the participation of the most skillful staff available but, even so, carries great risk. Emergency thoracotomy in these patients is usually not an option. Prevention is the key. Thorough coagulation with low power (35–40 W) before tumor manipulation will nearly always prevent such disasters. All tumors bleed, though some are much more bloody than others. Bronchial carcinoids, metastatic renal tumors, and thyroid tumors are notoriously bloody. Even so, these tumors can usually be managed with the Nd-YAG laser. If excessive bleeding does occur, the rigid laser bronchoscope permits much more effective control than can be achieved with the fiberscope. Simultaneous suction and laser use beginning around the bleeding vessel and gradually closing in on the bleeding site will usually suffice. Immediate postoperative bleeding of significant amount rarely occurs even when hemoptysis is the preoperative complaint. Recurrence of bleeding may occur some time later as the tumor extends, but it can usually be retreated in the same way.

All patients, whether under local or general anesthesia, should be monitored postoperatively in a recovery area staffed and equipped to treat potential hypoxia and ventilatory insufficiency.

Option 2

Use of a special rigid laser bronchoscope under general anesthesia provides several advantages over the fiberscope, as suggested earlier. Most important, the risk of fire is virtually eliminated, and second, one has greater control of the airway. Large tumors can be temporarily bypassed to establish an airway if necessary, and the instrument can be used to shave off coagulated tumor, making airway improvement more efficient. The view is unsurpassed through a large telescope, and laser and suction facilities are under continual simultaneous control. Somewhat greater laser power can be used, although I usually do not exceed 50 W and a 1-second pulse. The depth of penetration is much greater than is apparent, and greater power increases the risk of bronchial perforation and disaster. The FIO_2 is not so critical but should be limited to 50% or less, if

possible, since accumulated debris may ignite in the presence of laser heat and oxygen.

Use of this instrument requires a skilled bronchoscopist and an experienced anesthesia team. There will be some leakage around the bronchoscope during positive pressure ventilation; sometimes pharyngeal packing is required.

The instrument should be passed to about 1 cm from the tumor. The special suction catheter and laser fiber should be passed through their ports until they are just proximal to the distal end of the bronchoscope. The laser should be adjusted to no more than 40 W at first to obtain coagulation without bleeding. The laser fiber should be advanced to about the tip of the bronchoscope, leaving the telescope about 5 to 10 mm inside. This arrangement reduces the risk of smearing the lens and permits full view of the region. The instrument can then be advanced so as to position the laser fiber about 5 to 10 mm from the target. The entire surface of the tumor should be coagulated by rotation of the bronchoscope and movement of the laser fiber. If bleeding occurs, the suction catheter can be used for aspiration while the laser is simultaneously directed around the bleeding site, gradually closing in on the most active area. If there is concern about blood on the tip of the laser fiber, it should be removed immediately for cleaning before being used again.

When the tumor has been thoroughly coagulated, it can be shaved off with the lip of the bronchoscope and removed by suction or a foreign body forceps. There is always a degree of bleeding, but skillful use of this equipment makes the problem manageable, and the results are usually favorable. At the conclusion of the procedure, the bronchus should be irrigated with saline and debris aspirated.

Patients treated in this way should remain hospitalized overnight to ensure that the airway and ventilation remain satisfactory. They are usually in serious ventilatory jeopardy to begin with and will need close monitoring for several hours postoperatively.

Duration of the tracheobronchial airway after laser treatment depends on such factors as tumor growth rate, tumor bulk surrounding the bronchus, adequacy of tumor removal, length of the involved segment, diameter of the involved airway, and concomitant treatment. Results are more durable for short, squamous carcinomas of the main bronchi without extrabronchial extension. Several months of palliation can be expected; the treatment can be repeated, but as the tumor size increases, the period of benefit shortens. Little benefit is realized in treating most tumors of the segmental bronchi, and patients with large compressive tumors extending into the major airways may also experience benefit of only a few weeks' duration.

REFERENCES

1. Robinson L, Miller RH: Smoke inhalation injuries. *Am J Otolaryngol* 1986; 7:375–380.
2. Haponik EF, Summer WR: Respiratory complications in burned patients: Pathogenesis and spectrum of inhalation injury. *J Crit Care* 1987; 2:49–74.
3. Pecha BS, Raffin TA: Smoke inhalation: Averting long-term damage. *J Respir Dis* 1987; 8:87–93.

4. Moylan JA, Chin-Keung C: Inhalation injury—an increasing problem. *Ann Surg* 1978; 188:34–37.

5. Heffner JE, Miller DS, Sahn SA: Tracheostomy in the intensive care unit. *Chest* 1986; 90:269–274.

6. Whited RE: A prospective study of laryngotracheal sequelae in long-term intubation. *Laryngoscope* 1984; 94:367–377.

7. Sasaki CT, Horiuchi M, Koss N: Tracheostomy-related subglottic stenosis: Bacteriologic pathogenesis. *Laryngoscope* 1979; 89:857–865.

8. Kenna MA, Reilly JS, Stool SE: Tracheotomy in the preterm infant. *Ann Otol Rhinol Laryngol* 1987; 96:68–71.

9. O'Connor JV, Reddy K, Ergin MA, et al: Cricothyroidotomy for prolonged ventilatory support after cardiac operations. *Ann Thorac Surg* 1985; 39:353–354.

10. Cole RR, Aguilar EA: Cricothyroidotomy versus tracheotomy: An otolaryngologist's perspective. *Laryngoscope* 1988; 98:131–135.

11. Esses BA, Jafek BW: Cricoidthyroidotomy: A decade of experience in Denver. *Ann Otol Rhinol Laryngol* 1987; 96:519–524.

12. Cummings CW, Fredrickson JM, Harker LA, et al: *Otolaryngology—Head and Neck Surgery*. CV Mosby Co, 1986, vol 3, pp 2430–2431.

13. Ballenger JJ: *Diseases of the Nose, Throat and Ear*. Philadelphia, Lea & Febiger, 1969, pp 301–302.

14. Fee WE, Ward PH: Permanent tracheostomy, a new surgical technique. *Ann Otol Rhinol Laryngol* 1977; 86:635–638.

15. Sahni R, Blakley B, Maisel RH: Flap tracheostomy in sleep apnea patients. *Laryngoscope* 1985; 95:221–223.

16. Barnett MO, Chmiel SS, Windchy AM, et al: Customized stoma prosthesis for permanent tracheostomy patients with sleep apnea syndrome. *Ear Nose Throat J* 1987; 66:21–28.

CHAPTER 42

Issues in Laser Surgery

Approach of

Stanley M. Shapshay, M.D.

Since its introduction in 1972, endoscopic application of laser technology, especially in the larynx, trachea, and, to a lesser degree, bronchi has changed the practice of otolaryngology. The past 16 years of endoscopic laser surgery have been marked by initial enthusiasm, followed by scepticism, and more recently, general acceptance of the laser as a standard therapeutic modality. Endoscopic therapeutics became a buzzword in the 1980s because this treatment is effective and compatible with the important concepts of being less invasive and more cost effective.

The carbon dioxide laser (10.6 μm), with its precise soft tissue absorption, has proved to be the laser of choice for most applications in the larynx. When it is coupled to an operating microscope with a modern small-spot micromanipulator, precise delivery of laser energy is possible, with microscopic control and predictable excellent results.[1] Currently, small-spot micromanipulators are capable of delivering a 300 μm laser impact spot using a 400 mm lens on the operating microscope. This small laser spot with its increased power density reduces the power requirement for most laryngeal applications. For example, a power level of 1 to 3 W is sufficient for removing polyps and granulomas and for the incision and evacuation of Reinke's space edema (polypoid vocal cords).[2]

Recently, the neodymium-yttrium aluminum garnet (Nd-YAG) laser (1.06 μg) has gained popularity in endoscopic application because of its transmission through flexible quartz fibers. This laser is most useful when delivered through either flexible or rigid bronchoscopes but lacks the precise soft tissue interaction of the CO_2 laser. When hemostasis is important, deep tissue scatter and coagulation make this laser an excellent choice. A predictable depth of absorption is achieved through operator experience and a good understanding of laser soft tissue interaction and basic laser physics. What you see is not always what you get when you use the Nd-YAG laser. Because my clinical experience is limited to the CO_2 and Nd-YAG lasers, newer laser technologies, such as the potassium titanyl phosphate (KTP) laser (532 μm) will not be discussed in this chapter.

It is important to define clearly the best indications for the use of the laser and, equally important, when not to apply this technology. When is the laser clearly superior to more conventional, less expensive technology, such as electrocautery? Which ancillary techniques, delivery systems, and instruments are necessary for successful laser surgery? What is the best operative technique and approach to use to avoid complications?

The purpose of this chapter is to present a personal approach to the application of the laser in the upper airway. Selected operative situations, such as the endoscopic treatment of laryngeal carcinoma, will be discussed, stressing instrumentation, operative technique, and the prevention of complications.

APPLICATIONS IN THE LARYNX

In my 14 years of experience with laser technology, the most important and probably the most elegant application has been in microlaryngoscopy, using a micromanipulator attached to an operating microscope. With magnification powers $\times$ 16 and sometimes $\times$ 25 on the operating microscope, a precise depth of soft tissue absorption can be observed. When the laser power level is set just above the threshold for tissue vaporization (100°C) with pulsed or shuttered frequency to minimize adjacent soft tissue trauma, precise endoscopic surgery can be performed. When a microspot micromanipulator with a 0.3 mm spot size (400 mm lens on the microscope) is used, only 1 to 3 W of power are usually needed. Standard micromanipulators with 0.8 to 1.2 mm spot diameters (depending on the manufacturer) have a lower power density, requiring laser power around 10 W.

Special instruments in addition to standard microlaryn-

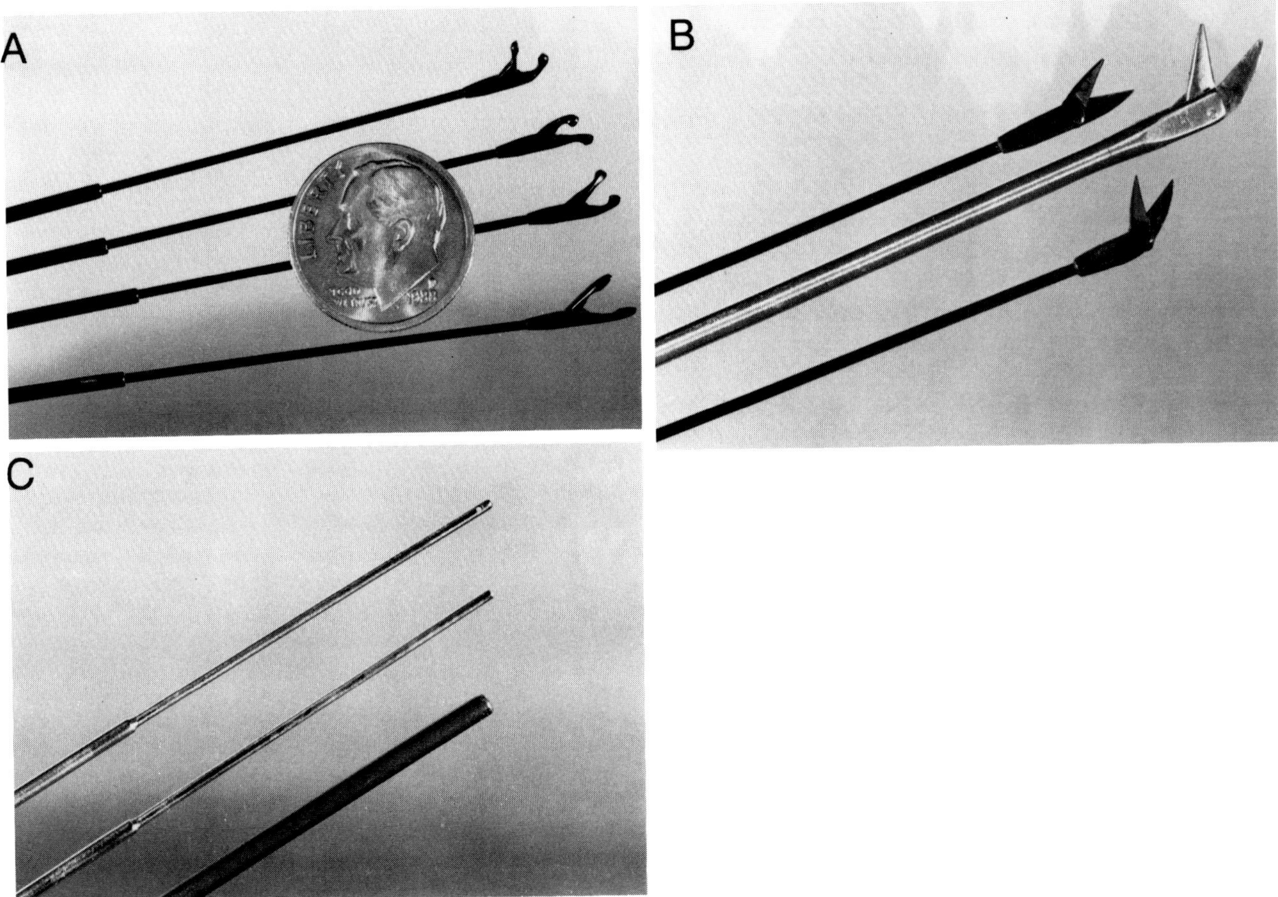

FIG 42–1.
A, microcupped forceps with straight, angled, and upbiting jaws with 1 mm grasping surface. **B,** straight and angled scissors, which are ebonized to avoid laser reflection, alongside standard *(silver)* scissors. **C,** microsuctions *(top)* have 1 mm lumen diameters compared with a standard 3 mm microlaryngeal suction.

goscopy fiberoptic wide-bore laryngoscopes are not absolutely necessary but are recommended. I prefer to use a Dedo-Jako laryngoscope (Pilling Company, Fort Washington, Pennsylvania) modified with built-in suction for smoke evacuation for the majority of adult patients. A dulled laryngoscope finish will prevent direct focused laser deflection; specially ebonized instruments can also be used. Approximately 60% of patients can be treated using the large-bore Dedo-Jako laryngoscope. The anterior commissure modification will expose most larynges, especially in female patients. A range of laryngoscopes of different sizes and lengths should be available for the treatment of children, adolescents, and adults.

Although the ideal laryngoscope suspension system has not yet been perfected, my current preference is for the Boston University suspension system (Pilling Co., Fort Washington, Pa.) attached to the side of the operating table. With the head of the table reversed so that the endoscopist can sit comfortably with the table's control mechanisms out of the way, the table may be tilted, raised, or lowered without changing the position of the laryngoscope. This is not possible when the more popular Lewy suspension (Pilling Co.) is used, which must be readjusted. In addition, this suspension device torques the laryngoscope, sometimes out of line with the laryngeal axis, and may also put considerable pressure on the patient's maxillary teeth.

A set of microlaryngeal instruments for application of the laser in the larynx is essential and should include vocal cord retractors and anterior commissure shields of different sizes. A set of microspot microlaryngeal instruments (Fig 42–1) has been developed by Karl Storz Endoscopy-America, Inc. (Culver City, Calif.) for precise laryngeal surgery for use with small-spot laser devices and pediatric microlaryngoscopy. This set of instruments includes 1 and 2 mm forceps and smaller suction lumen tubes for less tissue trauma.

BENIGN TUMORS AND LESIONS

Recurrent Respiratory Papillomas and Polyps

The first and probably the most common application of the laser in otolaryngology is the removal of benign lesions, such as recurrent respiratory papillomas and polyps. The laser has proved to be the instrument of choice for the treatment of patients with recurrent respiratory papillomas, which is a highly variable disease. The laser's precise removal of tumor with good hemostasis enables the surgeon to preserve laryngeal function and to avoid the problems associated with tracheotomy. Before the advent of laser endoscopic surgery, tracheotomies were more common, with subsequent recurrences of papillomas or polyps not only in the larynx but in the trachea and bronchi.

The goals of treatment vary with the age of the patient and the virulence of the disease process. Pediatric patients will often present with airway emergencies and sometimes require removal of lesions with the laser every 4 to 6 weeks. Older children will have varying rates of recurrence or tumor growth, requiring treatment every 3 to 4 months or yearly. Some adult patients may need treatments every 6 months or yearly, with vocal function a main concern.

Growth patterns of tumor vary between a sessile papillomatous growth, which tends to invade the submucosa, and a more frondlike exophytic pattern, which is easier to remove. Other considerations are the involvement of tumor with the anterior and posterior commissure, as well as with the subglottis. For an unknown reason, supraglottic growth is less common beyond the ventricle and false cords, with most of the disease located on the true vocal cords.

My treatment suggestions are based on the patient's age and on growth considerations. For pediatric patients, the main goal of treatment is airway preservation and the removal of all obstructing disease without causing scarring, especially at the anterior and posterior commissure. Because papillomatosis is mucosal, tissue removal should be limited to the mucosal and immediate submucosal area. Endoscopic laser surgery in the larynx is performed with the patient under general anesthesia, using nonflammable gases with oxygen concentration sufficient to maintain oxygen saturation in the mid-90% range. I prefer to use a red rubber endotracheal tube wrapped with a self-adherent metallic tape. These tubes generally range from 5 to 6 mm for the larynx of adult patients. A mixture of methylene blue dye and saline is put into the balloon, which acts like a self-contained sprinkler system if the balloon is perforated by the laser beam.

A biopsy is always performed to document the pathologic condition, because malignant change is a potential, albeit a rare occurrence. The laser should be equipped with an efficient smoke evacuation system, especially in the light of recent evidence showing the presence of DNA viral particles in the smoke of tissue vaporization.[3] The acute and long-term noxious effect of this smoke on the respiratory systems of the patient and operating room health care personnel is also a concern.

Laser power is set at 8 to 10 W (0.8 mm spot size); exposure time is set at continuous and shuttered by foot pedal control. Usually, laser exposure time is 1 to 2 seconds but varies with the extent of disease. All patients are given 4 (pediatric patients) to 10 mg of dexamethasone (Decadron) intravenously before manipulation of the larynx to minimize edema. The laser is employed in a sweeping fashion, removing papilloma layer by layer through vaporization; then, the resultant char is removed with a gentle application of the suction tube as a debriding instrument. Care is taken to avoid strong suctioning or unnecessary manipulation with probes and forceps to avoid postoperative swelling. Microlaryngeal suction is kept close to but not touching tissue while lasing to conduct heat away from the

surrounding tissue. Vocal cord retractors and anterior commissure protectors with built-in smoke evacuators are used to prevent heat trauma to the anterior commissure and the opposite vocal cord. The subglottic area can be exposed by advancement of the laryngoscope, by cord retractors, and from a special subglottic mirror reflecting the laser beam onto the diseased tissue on the undersurface of the vocal cords. New models of laryngoscopes have been specially designed to expose the subglottis as well.

It is important to realize that the larynx is a dynamic flexible organ, even when under suspension. The surgeon's or an assistant's hand placed on the neck skin over the thyroid cartilage can alter the position of the larynx, aiding endoscopic exposure. Frequent change of the position of the laryngoscope and resuspension are usually necessary when multiple areas (supraglottis, glottis, subglottis) are involved. Laser surgery should proceed efficiently, with a goal of 30 minutes or less of operating time. Longer procedures with excessive application of the laser dry tissues and increase postoperative morbidity, including pain, swelling, and inflammation. At the close of endoscopic laser surgery, the larynx is sprayed with a 2% lidocaine solution to diminish laryngospasm. Secretions, debris, and carbonaceous material are gently removed with suction and moist cottonoid applicators.

Postoperative care for the patient undergoing laser surgery of the larynx should include administration of humidified oxygen in the recovery room and during the first 12 to 24 hours after operation. When airway swelling is a concern, an additional dose of dexamethasone is given 6 to 8 hours after operation. Routine use of antibiotics is not indicated.

Vocal Cord Polyps

Vocal cord polyps vary from a single pedunculated lesion to bilateral polypoid changes, also known as Reinke's space edema. In both cases, the microspot CO_2 laser is used for precise treatment with minimal surrounding tissue damage and uncomplicated healing. Sessile polypoid change is bilateral in middle-aged women who are heavy smokers. An incision and suction removal technique described by Hirano[4] is employed for the treatment of patients with polypoid vocal cords filled with myxoid material in the submucosa, as opposed to the ablation or excision technique for patients with pedunculated well-formed polyps.

I have modified the incision and suction method by using a small-spot CO_2 laser to make a bloodless incision on the superior surface of the true vocal cords, well away from the vibrating free edges (Fig 42–2). Average laser power is 1 W at 0.5-second exposures. Care is taken not to approach the anterior commissure or vocal process during the incision. The incision is then opened into the submucosa, and the myxoid material is evacuated with microsuction instruments. A 2 mm microlaryngeal probe is used to break up thick loculations of gelatinous secretions, grasping one edge of the incision with side-biting 1 mm forceps to avoid traumatizing the epithelium (see Fig 42–1). It is important not to injure the underlying vocalis muscle, because scarring and subsequent loss of the mucosal wave during phonation would most likely occur. This complication is prevented by leaving a small amount of myxomatous material over the vocal muscle. After removal of the polypoid changes, excessive or redundant epithelium is obvious, and a portion is carefully removed for pathologic evaluation. A microwelding technique is employed for closure of the incision to "spot weld" the edges together. I believe this is superior to natural tissue adhesiveness, because postoperative coughing and throat clearing by the patient is likely to disturb the closure. After operation, 72 hours of almost complete voice rest are necessary for good healing. After this 72-hour period, patients are asked to use their voice sparingly and softly for 2 weeks.

The results of this technique in a series of 10 consecutive patients have been superior to those of my previous ablative technique with or without the laser (Fig 42–3). When the ablative technique was used, a granulating wound developed after the polyps were removed, increasing the chance of scarring and subsequent vocal dysfunction. Patients usually experienced 3 to 4 weeks of severe vocal dysfunction before improvement, which delayed their return to work and was a source of psychologic stress. With the incision, drainage, and welding technique, patients can speak satisfactorily 1 week to 10 days after operation and may return to work much earlier, depending on their employment requirements for vocal function.

Vocal Process Granuloma

Vocal process granuloma is, in my opinion, more a medical than a surgical problem. When a definite cause can be determined, such as reflux esophagitis, this condition must be corrected before the granuloma is treated. A history of trauma, such as previous intubation, is not uncommon in patients with granuloma and usually bodes well for ultimate resolution. Patients with idiopathic etiology are a concern because recurrence of the granuloma is more common. These patients usually have excessive laryngeal tension related to faulty vocal habits. A speech pathologist should be consulted for patients with idiopathic etiology, who are usually sales persons, auctioneers, teachers, or other professionals who require vigorous voice use.

Because granuloma is an inflammatory condition, operation is reserved for symptomatic patients who have vocal dysfunction, disturbing foreign body sensation, and, in rare instances, airway compromise. The goal of operation is atraumatic removal of granuloma without exposure of the vocal process. The granuloma is removed down to, but not through, the perichondrium of the vocal process. A biopsy is always performed rather than laser vaporization of the entire lesion. The granuloma has a rich blood supply, and the laser helps to control bleeding,

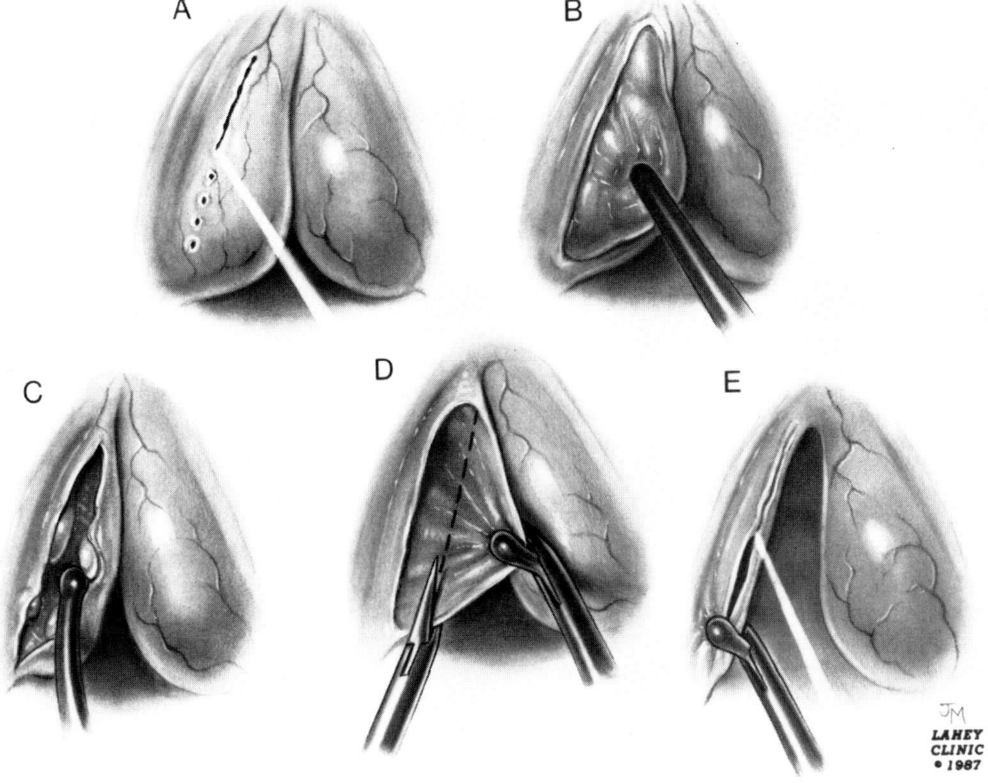

FIG 42–2.

A, laser incision with microspot micromanipulator using 1 W of power at 0.1-second exposures with a spot size of 0.3 mm. Note that incision is made on superior edge of vocal cord. **B**, microsuction removal of myxoid secretions from submucosa. **C**, a microprobe is used to break up loculations of myxoid material in submucosa. **D**, a microscissor is used to remove excessive lining after myxoid material is removed. **E**, free edges of vocalis mucosa are coated with microforceps and spot welded with CO_2 laser microspot using power levels of 750 mW at 0.1-second exposures.

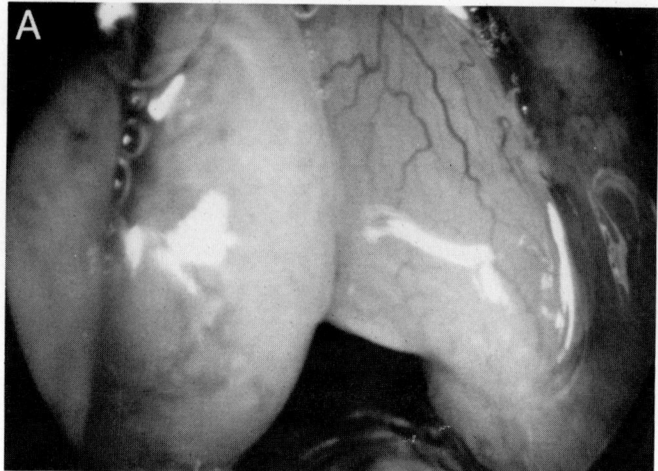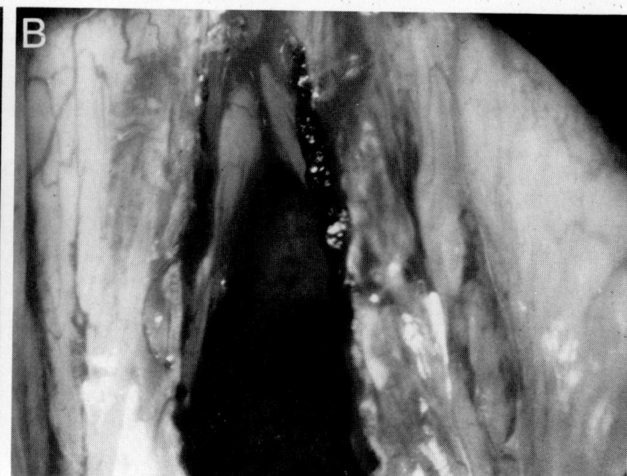

FIG 42–3.
A, endoscopic photograph shows polypoid changes of both vocal cords, also known as Reinke's space edema. **B,** endoscopic photograph after laser incision and evacuation of myxomatous polypoid changes. Vocal cords have been microwelded, closing incision after excessive lining has been removed as a pathologic specimen. (From Shapshay SM, Wallace RA, Kveton JF, et al: New microspot micromanipulator for carbon dioxide laser surgery: Early clinical results. *Arch Otolaryngol Head Neck Surg* [in press]. Used by permission.)

permitting precise removal of tissue. Hemostasis is difficult with forceps and scissors because of hemorrhage obscuring the operating field. The laser is used to excise most of the lesion, vaporizing the base with low power (0.8 mm spot size, 6 W power, 0.1-second exposures).

Endotracheal intubation and muscle relaxation anesthesia are preferred for patients with smaller granulomas, and Venturi jet ventilation by needle placement on the laryngoscope for patients with larger lesions. Intubation is with a small endotracheal tube (5–6 mm), displaced anteriorly by the laryngoscope. A posterior commissure laryngoscope with an anterior notch for the endotracheal tube is helpful. When Venturi jet ventilation is performed, it is important to remove the bulk of the lesion rapidly to prevent outflow obstruction and subsequent CO_2 retention. Acidosis and arrhythmias may occur when this is not corrected.

The postoperative management of patients undergoing laser surgery for granulomas is very important. I prescribe complete voice rest for 1 week to 10 days and then gradual soft voice use for the following 3 weeks. A broad-spectrum antibiotic, such as cephalosporin, is given for 1 month with systemic steroids (20 mg of prednisone/day). I have not found intralesional or inhalational steroids or zinc helpful. Despite these measures, approximately 40% of patients will have recurrences of granuloma. Fortunately, with time and treatment of underlying conditions, the majority of patients will be ultimately free of granulomas.

LARYNGEAL STENOSIS

Endoscopic treatment of glottic stenosis has been successful when patients are selected carefully. Anterior glottic webbing, usually from iatrogenic causes, such as overzealous surgery for vocal cord polyps with removal of the anterior commissure mucosa, can be managed easily with the CO_2 laser. I prefer

precise removal of scar tissue using the microspot micromanipulator (0.3 mm spot size) with power settings of 2 to 3 W and 0.1-second exposures. To prevent restenosis, which is more likely in patients with thicker more extensive stenosis, especially those patients with combined supraglottic and glottic webbs, an endoscopic 0.02 in. reinforced silicone rubber (Silastic) keel is inserted. This stent is fixed in place with a percutaneous 2-0 polypropylene (Prolene) suture and should stay in place for 4 to 6 weeks (Fig 42–4).[5]

The technique for placement of the stent is simple, consisting of two Prolene sutures threaded on a straight needle, one passing through the skin and cricothyroid and the other passing through the thyrohyoid membrane. The lower suture is grasped endoscopically and then passed through the anterior part of the stent in imbricating fashion. The upper percutaneous suture is passed through the thyrohyoid membrane in a straight needle with a double strand or complete loop. The eye of the needle is then broken off, permitting the upper percutaneous suture to be used as a pulling loop for the lower single strand suture. The free end of the single lower suture with its attached stent is pulled through the skin puncture as the stent is guided into place at the new anterior commissure. When satisfactory stent position is achieved, the suture, now a continuous loop through the stent, is fixed over a button.

Postoperative care includes administration of a broad-spectrum cephalosporin antibiotic until the stent is removed and meticulous wound care with hydrogen peroxide and antibiotic ointment three times daily. Systemic steroids are avoided because delayed epithelialization associated with their use is not desirable. The stent is removed endoscopically with the patient under general anesthesia, and any granulation tissue is removed carefully with the laser.

Posterior glottic stenosis is a more challenging problem than anterior scarring. The posterior commissure is harder to expose endoscopically, and the scar tissue tends to involve the

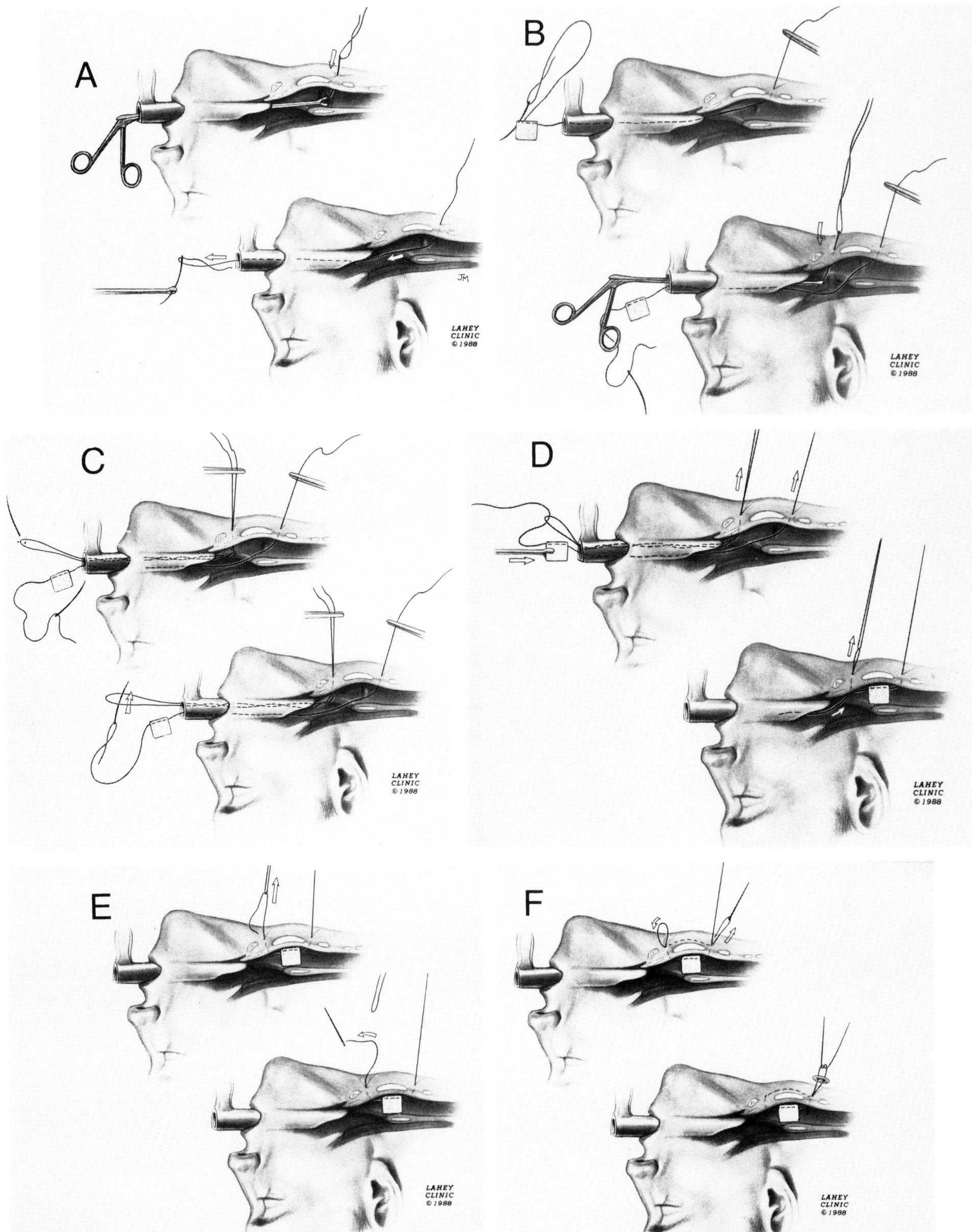

FIG 42–4.
A, endoscopic placement of anterior commissure reinforced Silastic stent with a percutaneous suture fixation technique. A Proline suture pierces the cricothyroid membrane and is brought out through the operating laryngoscope. **B**, lower (cricothyroid membrane) suture is placed through the leading edge of the Silastic stent in imbricating fashion. **C**, a double-stranded Proline suture is passed through the thyrohyoid membrane and brought out through the laryngoscope. The eye of the needle is broken, leaving a loop of double-stranded upper suture. The lower suture is then passed through this loop, which is used as a pull-out device. **D**, Silastic stent is guided into place into the anterior commissure as both sutures are gently pulled through the puncture sites. **E**, stent in place at the anterior commissure. The upper suture is passed through a straight needle. **F**, the upper suture is tunneled under the skin to exit with the lower suture. As tension is maintained on both sutures, fixation of the stent is accomplished by passing the sutures through a button and tying securely. A sterile dressing is placed under the button and changed daily.

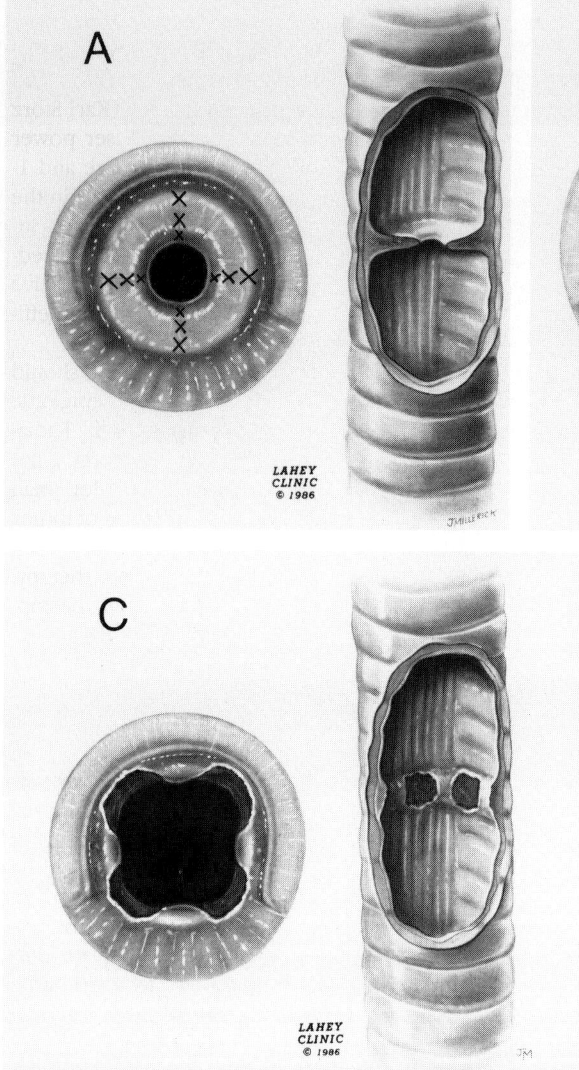

FIG 42–5.
Diagrammatic illustrations of tracheal lumen from endoscopic view and tracheal cross section. **A**, fibrous concentric tracheal stenosis with lumen size of 3 to 4 mm. Note radial laser incisions (*X*). **B**, lumen of airway is enlarged by radial incision and subsequent retraction *(arrows)* of scar tissue. **C**, tracheal size after radial laser incision and progressive dilation of lumen with 7.5 and 8.5 mm rigid bronchoscopes. Islands of epithelium are depicted between laser incisional areas.

interarytenoid muscle, fixating the arytenoids. Simple incision or excision of the scar tissue usually involves removal of epithelium, and some restenosis is common. The ideal treatment would be complete removal of scar tissue and epithelial resurfacing or grafting to prevent restenosis. This is a difficult task to perform endoscopically, because skin or mucosal grafts are not easily sutured into place. Endoscopic stents through the glottis are not easily tolerated by patients and can stimulate inflammatory changes in the form of granulation tissue. Scar tissue is usually the end process of inflammation.

With the advent of microflap techniques, especially those performed with small-spot laser devices and fine microlaryngeal instruments, an inferiorly based epithelial flap can be raised over the scar tissue underlying muscle.[6] The scar tissue is then ablated using a high-power setting (6 W at 0.5-second exposures). After the scarring is ablated, the arytenoids should be palpated to determine fixation. A fixed arytenoid will need to be lateralized by an external approach, preferably later. Additional endoscopic arytenoid scarring from the arytenoidectomy may lead to restenosis. Reepithelialization of the posterior glot-

tic wound occurs by spot welding the trapdoor flap back into place. A laser power setting of 500 to 750 mW at 0.5-second exposures is used for the welding process. Excessive laser energy will destroy the thin epithelial flap. Complete epithelial coverage is not possible because the flap will shrink slightly after elevation. The welding process is observed with the operating microscope set at magnification × 25. A slight blanching of the epithelial edges is seen at the desired endpoint. Additional blanching and heat coagulation will destroy the epithelium, mitigating against primary healing.

Supraglottic stenosis is less common but is treated by excision and dilation, usually without stenting. Subglottic stenosis is caused by a weblike concentric scar and is best treated by radial laser incisions using a high-power density of 4 to 6 W at 0.5-second exposures with a 0.3 mm spot size (Fig 42–5).[7] Dilation is best accomplished with ventilating bronchoscopes of gradually enlarging diameter, gently rotating and advancing the instrument after the lip of the bronchoscope is inserted into the stenotic area. When possible, tracheotomy is avoided to minimize infection after operation. However, most patients referred for treatment of subglottic stenosis have had tracheotomy. After operation, cephalosporin antibiotics are given for 3 weeks to prevent infection during this critical time of reepithelialization.

General anesthesia is used for patients undergoing operation for either subglottic or tracheal stenosis. Ventilation is delivered through a red rubber endotracheal tube wrapped with metallic reflecting tape. When the stenosis is accessible by laryngoscopic exposure, this method of delivery is preferable. Precise laser techniques can then be used under microscopic control. When the stenosis is more distal, requiring bronchoscopic exposure, a tracheoscope with laser fiber capability is used with the Nd-YAG laser-contact tip system. The contact tip (synthetic sapphire) has a high-power density, and its interaction with soft tissue is similar to that of the CO_2 laser.[8] Spontaneous ventilation with assist or Venturi jet ventilation with muscle paralysis is employed during operation.

VOCAL CORD PARALYSIS

Endoscopic laser arytenoidectomy for the treatment of bilateral vocal cord paralysis has been successful in the majority of patients. Advantages of laser surgery include no external wound healing, minimal postoperative morbidity, good voice, and minimal aspiration. The major disadvantages are imprecise unpredictable lateralization of the posterior commissure and marginal exercise tolerance. Endoscopic laser arytenoidectomy is ideal for the older patient with a more sedentary life-style than a younger active individual. My technique for laser arytenoidectomy is similar to that of Ossoff et al.,[9] who stress preservation of the posterior commissure mucosa to prevent scarring and poor cord lateralization. The posterior third of the vocal cord is ablated along with the arytenoid, care being taken not to heat coagulate the posterior commissure. When the medial aspect of the arytenoid ablated, intermittent application of the laser (10 W at 0.5-second exposures with a 0.8 mm spot size) is important. Superpulsed application of the laser is preferred for the body of the arytenoid. Most of the arytenoid is ablated down to the cricoid cartilage, except for the muscular process. A suction electrocoagulation device should be available, because hemorrhage is common when one is dissecting posterolateral to the vocal process; defocusing the laser is helpful to some extent. Laser ablation is preferred to excision of the body of the arytenoid because of superior hemostasis.

Antibiotics are administered for 3 weeks after operation, and steroids are given perioperatively to reduce edema. Usually, 6 to 8 weeks are required for lateralization and opening of the posterior commissure. Decannulation can occur between 2 to 3 months after operation when the final posterior glottic opening is at least 5 to 6 mm. Humidification is essential in the postoperative period.

LASER EPIGLOTTIDECTOMY

Endoscopic laser epiglottidectomy is not a common operation, requiring specific indication. Patients with chronic an-

gioneurotic edema of the epiglottis and early carcinoma have been treated in this fashion. Wide exposure of the epiglottis and vallecula is essential. I prefer to use a large Dedo-Jako laryngoscope or a distending Weerda laryngoscope (Karl Storz Endoscopy-America, Inc.) placed on suspension. Laser power settings are usually 8 to 10 W with a 0.8 mm spot size and 1- to 2-second exposures. Hemorrhage from blood vessels in the pharyngoepiglottic folds usually require electrocoagulation. Suprahyoid epiglottidectomy is usually performed because bleeding and exposure become problems when more extensive resections are attempted. As with laser arytenoidectomy, efficient smoke evacuation is essential.

In my opinion, larger T1 or T2 epiglottic carcinomas should not be treated in this fashion because spread to the preepiglottic space is common and not easily treated endoscopically. Radiation therapy or standard supraglottic partial laryngectomy is the treatment of choice for most of these lesions, except for small suprahyoid epiglottic tumors. However, laser ablation of tumor may be helpful in larger exophytic tumors to detect vocal cord invasion and to prevent tracheotomy before standard therapy. Perioperative steroids are given routinely to prevent postoperative airway edema.

VOCAL CORD CARCINOMA

My general approach for performing endoscopic laser surgery on the vocal cords is based on the concept of an excisional biopsy for patients with early carcinoma.[10] If an early T1 or in situ carcinoma is present on the middle to anterior third of the true vocal cord, excision with a 2 mm margin is performed. Involvement of tumor with the anterior commissure, vocal process, subglottis, or false cords is a contraindication to laser excision for curative intent. The excised specimen should be oriented so that the pathologist can prepare serial frozen sections.

The laser excisional biopsy concept is used as a diagnostic and staging procedure for all new cases of vocal cord cancer in the T1 and T2 categories. If tumor extends into the vocal muscle, this would indicate a "biologic" T3 tumor, although the TNM (primary tumor, regional nodes, metastasis) staging would be T2. Accurate assessment of tumor extension permits the surgeon to choose appropriate definitive therapy, such as radiation or vertical partial laryngectomy. Laser cordectomy is reserved for patients with superficial recurrence of tumor after radiation therapy or for patients who choose not to undergo an open operation after failure of radiation therapy. The 3-year control rate of laser surgery for accessible T1 vocal cord carcinoma is comparable with the control rate of radiation therapy (90%). I believe extension of laser surgery to lesions involving the anterior commissure or T2 tumors is dangerous, because histologic control becomes difficult. Patients with these tumors should be treated by radiotherapy or open partial laryngectomy.

The technique of endoscopic excisional biopsy demands good exposure through a large-bore laryngoscope and performance by an experienced laser endoscopist. The surgeon may become disoriented easily with a large specimen and unwittingly extend the resection into the subglottis. Resection of the vocal process is not catastrophic but undesirable; granulation tissue and poor vocal function are possible sequelae. Good tissue retraction while lasing without crushing the specimen is necessary for good pathologic evaluation. Excessive laser power with tissue coagulation renders the margins of frozen sections useless and creates postoperative edema. Uncomplicated wound healing without granuloma formation should be possible in most cases. The typical laser power setting is 8 to 10 W with a 0.8 mm spot size and 1- to 2-second exposures. The excised specimen is hand carried to the pathologist by the clinician for proper orientation during the preparation of frozen section margins.

Administration of humidified oxygen after operation and voice rest by the patient for approximately 3 days are important. Soft and infrequent phonation is prescribed for the next 2 to 3 weeks, depending on the extent of resection. Perioperative steroids are administered and continued for one to two doses (6–10 mg of dexamethazone intravenously) after operation every 6 hours.

The CO_2 laser is often used to treat patients with advanced or recurrent vocal cord carcinoma to preserve the airway (prevent tracheotomy) before definitive operation and in elderly patients who have failed radiation therapy as an alternative to total laryngectomy. Laser debulking of tumor before radiation therapy is attractive theoretically, but no randomized study proving its effectiveness has been reported. Prevention of tracheotomy in patients with partially obstructing larynx cancers by ablation of tumor with the laser is likewise appealing, but no evidence suggests that peristomal recurrence of tumor after total laryngectomy is decreased.

TRACHEAL MALIGNANCY

The Nd-YAG laser has clearly been established to be of value in the endoscopic management of patients with partially obstructing tracheobronchial tumors, the most common being squamous cell carcinoma, adenocarcinoma, and large cell carcinoma. Slower-growing less malignant tumors, such as carcinoid and adenoid cystic carcinoma, have a rich blood supply and also respond well to the deep coagulative effects of the Nd-YAG laser. It should be emphasized, however, that endoscopic Nd-YAG laser therapy for malignant disease is palliative only and is not intended to replace definitive potentially curable treatment, such as irradiation and operation. Carcinoid tumors, for example, are usually treated by sleeve resection, and laser bronchoscopy should be contemplated only when operation is not indicated.

The technique for Nd-YAG laser bronchoscopy, which is described succinctly in another report,[11] involves thorough photocoagulation of the tumor mass with a laser power of 40 to 45 W at 1-second exposures, keeping the fiber tip approximately 5 mm away from the tumor. After thorough blanching of the tumor is observed, the tumor is removed mechanically, shearing it free from the tracheal wall with the tip of the rigid ventilating bronchoscope, and the mass is grasped with bronchoscopic forceps. I prefer the laser fiber bronchoscope made by Karl

Storz-Endoscopy America, Inc. because it offers excellent telescopic optics as well as a choice of ventilation systems. I also prefer to use Venturi jet ventilation for patients with tumors around the carina, because the cough reflex is well controlled with muscle relaxants. For tumors partially obstructing the upper part of the trachea, topical anesthesia, mild intravenous sedation, and spontaneous ventilation with assist is a safer technique. More than 400 patients have been treated in this fashion at the Lahey Clinic Medical Center from 1980 to the present with low morbidity and only 1 intraoperative mortality.

LARYNGEAL HEMANGIOMAS

The hemangiomas most commonly involving the larynx are subglottic capillary hemangiomas in children and cavernous supraglottic hemangiomas in adults. The latter condition is usually an extension of a larger cavernous low-flow hemangioma of the oral cavity and hypopharynx. An isolated subglottic hemangioma is best treated by endoscopic ablation with the CO_2 laser, and the cavernous hemangioma responds best to low power (20–25 W) Nd-YAG laser photocoagulation. If the CO_2 laser is used to excise or ablate cavernous hemangiomas, serious hemorrhage is likely to occur. The Nd-YAG laser is well absorbed by the hemoglobin-rich cavernous hemangioma, stimulating thrombosis within the lesion. When low-power intermittent (0.5-second) exposures are used with an unfocused free fiber (no lens) approximately 2 cm away from the hemangioma, the laser penetrates and spares the overlying epithelium (Fig 42–6). Excessive laser power density will cause sloughing of tissue and possible delayed hemorrhage and infection.

SUMMARY

The CO_2 laser continues to have the wavelength of choice for most applications in the larynx and trachea. The deeper pentrating and scattering Nd-YAG laser is useful for photocoagulation of malignant tumors in the trachea and bronchi, especially because of readily available flexible fiberoptic delivery systems. Overall, however, with the exception of cavernous hemangiomas, the Nd-YAG laser has limited usefulness in otolaryngology. Wavelengths close to that of the argon laser, such as the KTP laser (532 μm) are clearly useful but do not challenge the precision of the CO_2 laser, especially for applications in the larynx.

Careful selection of patients cannot be overemphasized, because laser surgery has its limitations. Extending the application of the laser in the treatment of patients with early larynx cancer to applications in situations when the anterior commissure or false cord is involved may compromise the control of cancer by delaying definitive radiotherapy or open conservative surgery. With these limitations and precautions in mind, the CO_2 laser has changed the practice of laryngology, providing the clinician with an elegant tool for endoscopic surgery of the larynx and trachea.

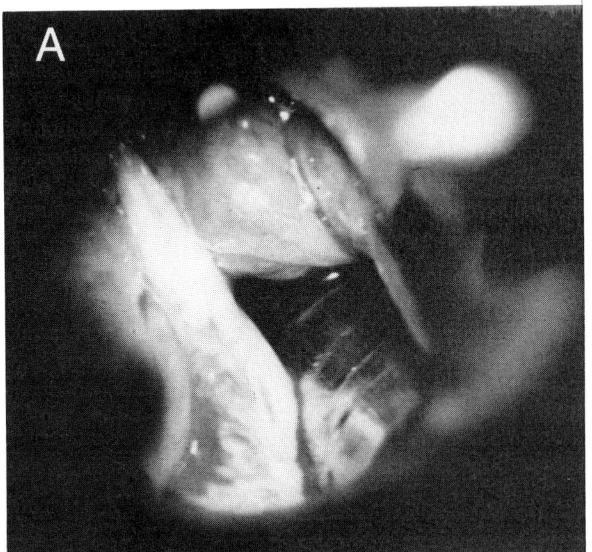
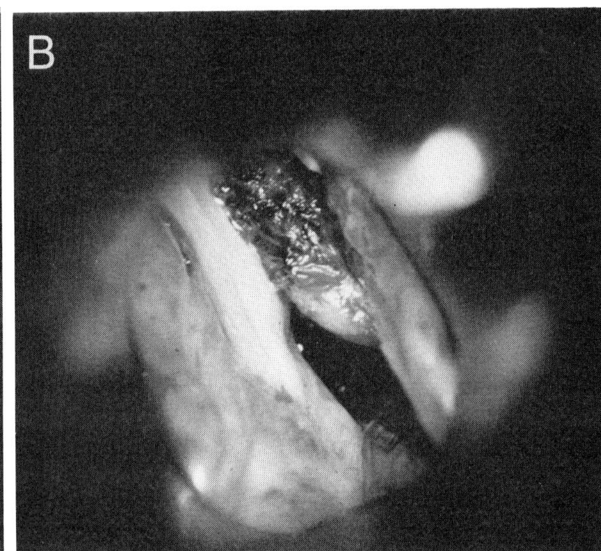
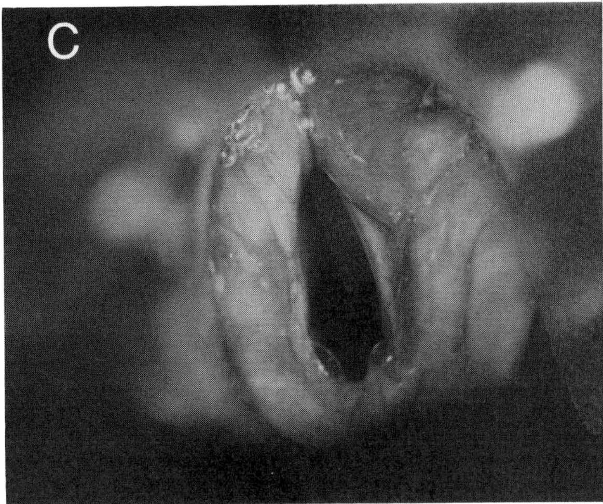

FIG 42–6.
A, endoscopic view of large cavernous hemangioma involving superior right vocal cord surface and ventricle. Occlusion of laryngeal airway is approximately 50%. **B,** immediately after Nd-YAG laser photocoagulation of right vocal cord, shrinkage of the mass with some carbonization of overlying epithelium is evident. No hemorrhage occurred intraoperatively or postoperatively. **C,** complete resolution of hemangioma 2 months after Nd-YAG laser photocoagulation. Small amount of fibrous tissue overlying the right anterior vocal cord remains. (From Shapshay SM: Application of the Nd-YAG laser in larynx and trachea, in Fried M [ed]: *The Larynx.* Boston, Little, Brown & Co [in press]. Used by permission.)

REFERENCES

1. Shapshay SM, Wallace RA, Kveton JF, et al: A new microspot micromanipulator for CO_2 laser application in otolaryngology. *Otolaryngol Head Neck Surg* 1988; 98:179–181.
2. Shapshay SM, Wallace RA, Kveton JF, et al: New microspot micromanipulator for carbon dioxide laser surgery in otolaryngology: Early clinical results. *Arch Otolaryngol Head Neck Surg* (in press).
3. Garden JM, O'Banion MK, Shelnitz LS, et al: Papillomavirus in the vapor of carbon dioxide laser-treated verrucae. *JAMA* 1988; 259:1199–1202.
4. Hirano M: Structure of the vocal folds in normal and disease states: Anatomical and physical studies, in Ludlow C, Hart M (eds): *Proceedings of the Conference on the Assessment of Vocal Pathology.* American Speech and Hearing Association Report. 1981, vol 11, pp 11–30.
5. Mouney DF, Lyons GD: Fixation of laryngeal stents. *Laryngoscope* 1985; 95:905–907.
6. Dedo HH, Sooy CD: Endoscopic laser repair of posterior glottic, subglottic and tracheal stenosis by division or micro-trapdoor flap. *Laryngoscope* 1984; 94:445–450.
7. Shapshay SM, Beamis JF Jr, Hybels RL, et al: Endoscopic treatment of subglottic and tracheal stenosis by radial laser incision and dilation. *Ann Otol Rhinol Laryngol* 1987; 96:661–664.
8. Shapshay SM: Laser applications in the trachea and bronchi: A comparative study of the soft tissue effects using contact and noncontact delivery systems. *Laryngoscope* 1987; 97 (suppl 41)2:1–26.
9. Ossoff RH, Sisson GA, Duncavage JA, et al: Endoscopic laser arytenoidectomy for the treatment of bilateral vocal cord paralysis. *Laryngoscope* 1984; 94:1293–1297.
10. Blakeslee D, Vaughan CW, Shapshay SM, et al: Excisional biopsy in the selective management of T1 glottic cancer: A three-year follow-up study. *Laryngoscope* 1984; 94:488–494.
11. Shapshay SM, Ossoff RH, Duncavage JA: Bronchoscopic laser surgery, in Johnson J (ed): *American Academy of Otolaryngology-Head and Neck Surgery: Instruction Course,* vol 1. St Louis, CV Mosby Co (in press).

Issues in Laser Surgery

Approach of

W. Paul Biggers, M.D., F.A.C.S.

The Outer Banks of North Carolina are unique in that many old, but powerful, lighthouses are strategically spaced along these barrier islands, warning ships of the dangerous shoals that have claimed many an unwary sailor over the past 400 years. Some of these beacons have beamed a powerful light out to sea for more than one hundred years. Although these lights are extremely powerful, they are not lasers, because the photons of light energy are not monochromatic, are not highly collimated, and are not coherent. These three factors endow laser light with its unique and medically useful properties. Our surgical colleagues in ophthalmology have pioneered the use of lasers in surgery, and we are indebted to them in leading the way for this exponentially expanding field of medicine. In this chapter, I will attempt to convey to the reader a few basic concepts in the use of lasers in otolaryngology. Basic understanding of laser physics is necessary before one can select the proper laser energy form for the surgical task at hand and to allow appropriate manipulation of laser energy with avoidance of potential intraoperative and postoperative complications.

BACKGROUND

Basic Laser Physics

Laser is an acronym for light amplification by the stimulated emission of radiation. It must be emphasized to ancillary personnel in the operating room that radiation in this sense does not mean ionizing radiation, affecting nuclear proteins with the threat of mutation, birth defect, and cancer production, but is radiation in the very broadest sense of the term, that is, the broad spectrum of electromagnetic radiation. Lasers commonly used in the operating room carry no risk of radiation injury via radioactive nuclear energy. Caution is required on the part of all personnel in regard to eye protection and skin protection while lasers are in use.

Since the dawn of time, basic elements and simple compounds formed by these elements have been endowed with the potential to produce photons of light energy at a specific wavelength, whether in the visible or invisible spectrum, when excited by various forms of energy. Laser theory was first postulated

by Albert Einstein early in this century. In 1958, the gas laser was first described by A. L. Schawlow and Charles Townes. Shortly thereafter, in 1960, T. H. Maiman built the first laser, a ruby laser, and in 1964 the first CO_2 laser was built by C. K. Patel. Later in the 1960s, G. J. Jako and T. G. Polanyi applied the laser to otorhinolaryngologic problems via the operating microscope, a major step forward. The contributions of these two individuals helped push otolaryngology ahead of most other specialties in application of laser technology.

Figure 42–7 is an oversimplification of one of the most common lasers in use in otolaryngologic surgery today, the CO_2 laser. In the laser chamber, CO_2 molecules are excited by high-voltage electrical current. The electrical energy imparted to the molecule of CO_2 forces electrons orbiting the nuclei of carbon and oxygen atoms into a higher orbit—the upper laser level (ULL). The electrons subsequently fall to the lower laser level (LLL) and, as a result of achieving this lower energy level, emit a photon of light energy. If within a very critical and short increment of time, (around 10^{-8} seconds) this photon of energy strikes another electron in the ULL, another photon of energy exactly the same wavelength and heading exactly the same direction is emitted. Thus, in this laser chamber, photons of light energy excite the emission of additional photons of light energy, which are reflected back and forth in the chamber. The photons strike a partially transmissive germanium mirror at one end and a highly polished gold mirror at the opposite end of the chamber. Control of release of the laser energy is accomplished by opening an aperture at the partially transmissive Ge mirror for a specified number of milliseconds, allowing a short burst of monochromatic, highly collimated, and tightly coherent light energy to be released.

The energy produced by this particular CO_2 laser has a relatively long wavelength and is invisible, being outside the visible spectrum of light in the far infrared zone of the electromagnetic spectrum. Since this is not visible light, it cannot be focused by the usual optical apparatus used to focus visible light. Selenide lenses have a configuration that allows for reflection and focusing of this particular light energy. The same basic principles apply to other commonly used medical lasers; however, the lasers producing energy in the visible spectrum

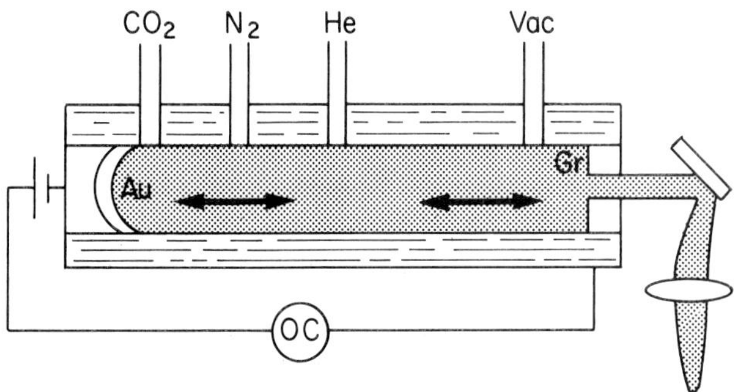

FIG 42–7.
Schematic drawing of the CO$_2$ laser chamber. Here the gas molecules are excited by electrical energy and caused to emit photons of light. In the CO$_2$ laser, the wavelength of the light is 10.6 μ near the infrared. The photons of energy are reflected between a gold mirror at one end of the chamber and a partially transmissive germanium mirror at the other end. The energy escapes the chamber through a variable aperture, which is precisely timed to be open for a set number of milliseconds. Monochromatic, tightly coherent, highly collimated bundles of photons can then be focused onto a target.

have an advantage in that this energy is much more easily manipulated, using standard, precisely ground glass lenses and flexible fiberoptic light conductors.

The amount of energy released from the laser is related to the input of electrical energy and to the number of milliseconds that the aperture at the Ge end of the chamber is open. Ordinarily, lasers are not very efficient machines. A great deal more energy must be put into the chamber compared with the amount of energy (in the form of light energy) that escapes from the chamber. The great advantage is that the light energy can be focused in a very precise way and accomplish tasks that electrical energy cannot accomplish as precisely, such as cutting, coagulation, and tissue vaporization. The effect of various forms of laser energy on tissues is both a function of the wave length of the laser energy and the inherent makeup of the target tissue in regard to water content, color, and thermal conductance.

TYPES OF LASERS

It is impossible to say that one type of laser is better than the other for surgical purposes. The choice of optimum laser energy depends on the task to be accomplished, the type of tissue involved, safety of utilization and inherent risks, and cost effectiveness of applications to common surgical procedures. Table 42–1 compares the two most common lasers used in ear, nose, and throat surgery, Ar and CO$_2$.

The sections that follow discuss the principal lasers used, or soon to be used, in otolaryngologic surgery in operating rooms across the country.

Carbon Dioxide Laser

Carbon dioxide produces laser energy at the far infrared end of the light spectrum, 10,600 nm. This energy is highly absorbed by intracellular water, which is 75% to 80% of the cells' contact. This water turns instantly into steam, causing cells to explode or vaporize.

Argon Laser

Argon gas produces blue-green laser light at 488 and 512 nm. This wavelength is very highly absorbed by the color red and is thus effective against highly vascular lesions, muscle, or darkly charred tissue. This energy is in the visible spectrum; therefore, it can be very precisely focused, allowing for very high-energy density at the point of focus (Fig 42–8).

Neodymium-Yttrium Aluminum Garnet Laser

Neodymium-yttrium aluminum garnet produces laser energy at the near infrared end of the light spectrum, approximately 1,064 nm. This is a very versatile wavelength, which possesses tissue vaporization properties as well as thermal conductance characteristics and excellent coagulation properties.

Potassium Titanyl Phosphate Laser

Potassium titanyl phosphate produces a green light at a wavelength of 532 nm by altering the output of the Nd-YAG laser with a KTP crystal. This light energy is more purely monochromatic than the Ar laser, but it otherwise is in a very similar light wavelength range. Champions of this newer laser believe that it can be focused to smaller spots, thus producing higher-powered densities for more precise cutting or photocoagulation.

TABLE 42–1.
Comparison of the Argon and Carbon Dioxide Lasers

Ar	CO$_2$
1. Argon can be carried through fiberglass rods and fibers, focused, and manipulated by glass lenses and glass mirrors.	1. CO$_2$ laser energy must be reflected off highly polished metal mirrors; it cannot be carried around corners with standard fiberglass instruments.
2. Precise optical focus is possible with intense power densities.	2. CO$_2$ laser must be focused with special selenide lenses; it will not penetrate glass. New micro focusing and manipulating devices allow for more precise small focal areas.
3. Wavelength of light energy produced by the Ar laser is highly absorbed by the color red; therefore it may be the best tool used against vascular lesions or dark lesions, especially when these lesions lurk under the skin.	3. CO$_2$ wavelength of energy is highly absorbed by intracellular water, making it the best tool for soft tissue destruction, regardless of the color of the tissue. Probably the best tissue vaporizer.

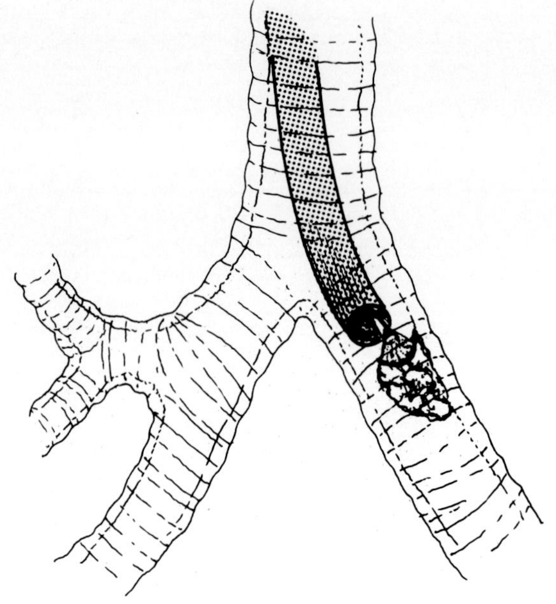

FIG 42–8.
Lasers that emit light in the visible spectrum have their light energy manipulated as we manipulate visible light; that is, it can be carried through glass lenses or down fiberoptic cables and delivered to a target around a corner. Here an endobronchial lesion is being vaporized by laser energy delivered through the flexible fiberoptic bronchoscope employing a flexible fiberoptic cable down the side arm to deliver Ar laser energy.

Free-Electron Laser

The free-electron laser allows for a variable wavelength output, including infrared, visible light, and ultraviolet light laser energy, as may be desired for various surgical tasks. This laser has the capacity for producing laser energy as a series of rapid superpulses consisting of megawatt levels of energy of very short duration. These high-energy superpluses are delivered in very short bursts to the tissue and are said to provide good surgical control and minimal thermal damage to tissue.

Sapphire Tip Laser

The sapphire tip affixed to the end of an Nd-YAG laser fiber allows it to cut precisely and sharply, producing less tissue coagulation and adjacent thermal injury. It also provides one with a tactile sense using laser energy that one does not get applying the energy from a distance. Many surgeons believe that this tactile sense is extremely important for certain types of surgery and less important for other types of surgery where sensing changes in tissue consistency and texture is not important. The major advantage of the sapphire-tipped Nd-YAG laser is for this tactile transfer of energy without diffuse spread producing surrounding coagulation. There is a major disadvantage; when these lasers are fired, and the tip is not in contact with tissue, these relatively expensive sapphire tips will melt and be ruined. There is no question that the sapphire tips allow the surgeon more precise control for incision purposes, but

they are less powerful and perform slower than some of the more powerful CO_2 lasers currently available.

Photodynamic Therapy-Pump Dye Laser

There is a growing interest in a new utilization of lasers that takes advantage of the fact that certain photosensitive drugs such as hematophorphin concentrate in tumor cells and may be activated by dye laser, producing a 632 nm wavelength of light energy. Ultimately, the interaction of the light energy and hematophorphin causes the liberation of singlet oxygen within the cell, which is toxic and destroys the cell rapidly. Other drugs that concentrate in cancer tissue are being tested. These drugs, when excited by certain wavelengths of laser light, become cytotoxic to various types of tumor. This exciting new aspect of laser technology is being pursued in various investigational centers.

ADVANTAGES AND DISADVANTAGES OF LASER USE

Some recent attempts have been made to produce flexible cables with certain chemicals that can bend CO_2 laser wavelengths (10.6 μm) around corners. These materials are not generally available at present. One important property of laser energy is that it can be used both in a focused or unfocused mode, depending on individual case requirement. When the laser is precisely focused, it becomes an excellent cutting tool. When it is unfocused and the power turned up, it becomes a more efficient tissue vaporizer and cautery or coagulator type of instrument. One of the major advantages is that of being able to apply the surgical cutting or vaporizing energy from a distance. Lasers are excellent for working in deep dark places, such as the larynx, gastrointestinal tract, female genital tract, nasopharynx, and even joint spaces, where the cutting or vaporizing tool can be employed but does not obstruct the operator's vision. Another useful quality of the laser's interaction with tissue is that the wound created is inherently sterile. The major attribution of lasers over more conventional surgical techniques lies in certain advantages that this form of energy has over "sharp steel" surgery or electrocoagulation. First, lasers can produce precise, nontraumatic and hemostatic removal of tissue. There is often less bleeding and usually less postoperative pain, especially in the first 24 to 48 hours. Then there is the quality of sterility. Laser wounds are inherently sterile. Perhaps the most important quality is that there is improved visibility when one is forced to operate in very limited spaces. There is minimal necrosis of adjacent normal tissue, less tugging and pulling on adjacent tissues, less tissue edema, and less scarring. Less tissue trauma often means less postoperative pain. Resection of muscle (e.g., tongue) with the laser results in a steady nonmoving target, in contrast to electrocautery.

Some of the major disadvantages of lasers include the initial expense of obtaining equipment and training personnel in its proper use. Perhaps the major hazard is that of combustion when the laser is used in the vicinity of oxygen-laden anesthetic gases. There have been a number of incidences where the flammable anesthetic tube has caught fire, and devastating injury of the trachea and larynx has ensued. It is the consensus that these problems are now preventable by using the noncombustible special endotracheal tubes made for laser surgery and available through several suppliers. For many years, I wrapped my endotracheal tubes with aluminum foil tape obtained from an electronic supply house as a sensing tape to automatically shut off cassette recorders at the end of the cassette. This was reasonably satisfactory when the tape was carefully wrapped, but was still combustible at high energy settings. Even with this technique and when the endotracheal balloon was protected with neurosurgical saline-soaked patties, the balloon cuff at times would suddenly deflate, with a backwash into the laser field of oxygen-laden gas that could be ignited. For some procedures in patients with adequate pulmonary reserve, room air can be used through the laser portion of the case, further reducing the risk of combustion.

It is the current consensus of those who have experience in laser surgery of the upper airway that should combustion of an endotracheal tube occur, the tube should be removed as quickly as possible, a new tube inserted, the airway lavaged with cool saline solution, and steroids administered.

Generally, CO_2 lasers have the advantage of mobility and can be rolled from operating room to operating room because they require no permanent plumbing and runoff of standard house current. Some argon lasers, older Nd-YAG lasers, and some of the other newer lasers require permanent installation with high-voltage connections and permanent plumbing for cooling. The questions of mobility and flexibility of use are important when small hospitals are making a decision regarding a laser that will be shared by different surgical specialties.

APPLICATIONS FOR LASERS IN OTOLARYNGOLOGY

The otolaryngologic surgeon has found the laser to be a uniquely advantageous tool in surgery on the upper airway and larynx. Laser laryngeal surgery of benign lesions is the most common widespread use of the CO_2 laser. In laryngeal surgery, the laser is an extremely valuable addition to our armamentarium. It is particularly useful for the following conditions in otolaryngology.

Laryngeal Surgery

The CO_2 laser is the most widely used laser in otolaryngology today, and its most common use is in laryngeal surgery. Laryngeal papillomatosis can be a particularly perplexing surgical problem in that most patients with this disorder require multiple excisions. Many of us have had patients who required operative intervention every 6 weeks to maintain an adequate airway. In any surgical procedure where numerous revisions are required, a technique that results in less scarring and distortion while producing the least amount of edema will be the technique chosen by most surgeons.

Having removed papillomas with both forceps, long-handled knives, and the CO_2 laser, I am convinced that employment of the laser has proved to be quite beneficial to these patients. Many of us who follow these patients for prolonged periods are convinced that the recurrence rate is slowed somewhat when the laser is used. Whether or not this is the result of less implantation of live virus at the time of surgery, sterilization of the field by heat at the time of surgery, or less seeding of tissue planes at the time of surgery remains as conjecture. Most of us find that with a very bulky papillomas, a combination of cupped forcep removal of the bulky external portion of the lesion, followed by refined vaporization of the deep invasive part of the lesion, seems to be the best and most expeditious technique. I believe also that use of the laser makes tracheostomy in children a less common occurrence. Most otolaryngologists believe that tracheostomies in the face of papilloma are to be avoided unless absolutely necessary to maintain adequate ventilation. Many adult patients who have had cupped forcep removal alone in the past now specifically request laser surgery because they have experienced less postoperative pain and swelling with better voice in the immediate postoperative period following laser surgery.

Laryngeal Webs

Laryngeal webs at the anterior commissure have been successfully managed using the laser on occasion without requiring stenting. I believe that the burn eschar that results as one burns through the web acts like a stent in many patients and prevents synnechial web formation during the early healing phase. Many webs require multiple procedures for satisfactory resolution and voice restoration. Fine incisions and less scarring follow use of the new microfocus micromanipulator attachments.

I use the continuous setting only for bulky lesions where a great deal of vaporization is required. Extreme care must be used when vacuuming away steam during the course of these procedures to protect the uninvolved vocal cord. In my opinion, the Pilling vocal cord retractor-protector with built-in suction in the adult and pediatric size for the right and left cord is particularly useful in laryngeal laser work. A small metal clip can be used to hold this steam suction instrument in a precise and steady position during the course of suspension laryngoscopy and laser ablation procedures. Often during the course of this type of surgery, pressure over the cricoid is required to bring the anterior larynx into better and more accessible view. It is particularly useful to have both hands free to operate the micromanipulator aiming device and to use another long narrow suction device to remove blood, eschar debris, and secretions. I recommend practice with the laser on laryngeal models or in the animal surgical suite to hone skills. This is particularly useful in learning to operate on the undersurface of vocal folds. I find it fascinating to use the highly polished metal mirrors, placing the aiming dot on the reflected image on the mirror and seeing the laser energy strike exactly where I placed the aiming dot. One feels like a wild West sharpshooter bouncing laser bursts off the mirror onto the target. This technique is quite useful and is very effective. It also makes distortion and tugging on the vocal cord unnecessary in many instances. The less pulling and tugging on the vocal cord during the course of surgery, the less the patient is troubled by lingering postoperative edema and intense hoarseness.

Other Laryngeal Lesions

I believe that healing following removal of a vocal cord nodule with laser is really no better than the healing process after removal with a no. 11 surgical blade on an extended knife handle. A very accurate line of resection is accomplished with the no. 11 blade, and a similarly accurate vibrating vocal cord edge can be produced with a laser in skilled hands. I do believe that lasers offer some advantage in the removal of polyps in that Reinke's space seems to be sealed much more adequately following laser surgery than sharp removal.

Leukoplakia of the vocal cords also lends itself quite well to laser removal. In my operating room, the vocal cord is initially freed of the hyperkeratotic lesion using conventional techniques, and the raw base is then subjected to laser coagulation. A specimen is thus obtained that is not denatured at its deep margin by heat, resulting in a better specimen for the pathologists to examine. Laser application to the resulting raw base discourages reformation of the keratotic lesion if the patient removes the exciting cause (e.g., exposure to tobacco smoke, vocal abuse, or other chemical irritants). I have become much more conservative lately, using the finely focused laser at much lower power settings, thus preventing tethering of the mucosa and preserving the normal mucosal wave.

I am less comfortable with removing malignant lesions using the laser. However, completely satisfactory cordectomy of verrucous-type carcinoma has been accomplished at my institution and at other centers with truly remarkable healing results and an absence of recurrence. The employment of the laser for cancer surgery requires consultation with an experienced laryngeal surgeon and should be reserved for only exophytic and relatively small lesions. The laser has also been used with mixed success to debride areas of infection in the larynx. I have found it particularly useful in the removal of pyogenic granulomas resulting from long-term intubation.

Other Less Common Otolaryngologic Applications

Other less common otolaryngologic conditions in which the laser may be useful include:

1. Rhinophyma
2. Tracheal granulomatosis
3. Subglottic stenosis
4. Partial glossectomy
5. Lesions of the buccal mucosa
6. Choanal atresia
7. Inferior nasal turbinate surgery
8. Capillary hemangiomas involving the respiratory tract

(The Nd-YAG laser may be a better choice than the CO_2 laser for this problem.)

Laser coagulation of bleeding ulcers has been pioneered by Dr. J. M. Brunetaud in France. He has successfully controlled massively bleeding gastric ulcers using laser coagulation. The photographic documentation of the healing lesions is truly remarkable. His work is also being continued at centers in this country.

I have had an occasion to use the laser to open up the distal airway on an emergency basis in the face of hypoxia secondary to near-total obstruction of the airway by tumor ingrowth. On one occasion, the CO_2 laser was turned up to its maximum power and was operated at 58 W on a continuous setting. This resulted in a great deal of steam, which escaped from the patient's mouth and nose despite vigorous use of suction aspiration. We were successful in opening up this airway and noted no particular ill effect despite the impressive escape of steam.

A number of individuals have delivered visible wavelength laser light and Nd-YAG laser light through flexible fiberoptic endoscopes to produce recannulization of obstructed secondary bronchi with good palliation of the patient and reversal, at least temporarily, of an ever-increasing hypoxia and its attendant symptoms. I have been favorably impressed with my initial laboratory experience with the Nd-YAG laser fine fiber with sapphire tip. It is rapidly becoming a useful tool for the head and neck surgeon and endoscopist.

Although not the subject of focus in this particular chapter, many otologists have become devotees of laser stapedotomy and are reporting excellent postoperative hearing results employing this technique for penetration of the stapes footplate. I have done this procedure elsewhere in the laboratory and believe it has promise in the right hands. The finely focused CO_2 laser (250 μm) may prove ideal for this purpose. Initial reports of other uses in otology are encouraging.

The Ar laser has been used with great success on hemangiomas involving the head and neck area, taking advantage of the fact that the laser energy in the visible spectrum passes through the relatively translucent epidermis, producing a second-degree burn but very little permanent scarring and destruction of the epidermis. The resultant healing after the vessels have been ablated through the skin is a remarkable achievement in the hands of a skilled and patient surgeon.

SUMMARY

All young otolaryngologic surgeons need to add laser techniques to their armamentarium, because with the continued refinement and improvement of laser energy sources, lasers will play an ever-expanding role in our surgery in the future. The skills developed now with our relatively crude instruments will certainly be transferable to the laser equipment of the future.

CHAPTER 43

Management of Esophageal Problems

Approach of

Mark C. Weissler, M.D.

ANATOMY

The esophagus is a muscular tube that connects the pharynx to the stomach. Ranging from 18 to 26 cm long, it is composed of an outer longitudinal and an inner circular muscle layer and lacks a true serosa. The normal esophageal mucosa is entirely nonkeratinizing squamous epithelium. Approximately the distal 54% of the longitudinal muscle and the distal 62% of the circular muscle are smooth muscle, whereas the more proximal portions are striated. The transition from striated to smooth muscle is not abrupt but is a transition zone of mixed striated and smooth muscle. This transition zone may account for more than one third of the esophageal length.

The esophagus has three areas of relative constriction that are the most frequently perforated areas at the time of esophagoscopy. These areas of constriction occur (1) at the upper esophageal sphincter (UES) at the level of the cricopharyngeal muscle (C-6) at the introitus to the esophagus, (2) at the level of the tracheal carina, and (3) at the lower esophageal sphincter (LES) at the junction of esophagus with stomach (T-10).

In the upper part of the chest, the esophagus lies in the midline. At the carina it passes slightly to the right of the midline and then turns leftward and posterior to pass beneath the left ventricle. It finally turns anteriorly and enters the stomach in a leftward direction.

PHYSIOLOGY

The act of swallowing is classically divided into three phases. The *oral phase* is under voluntary control and involves the passage of the food bolus from the mouth to the pharynx. The *pharyngeal phase* is largely reflexive and involves the passage of food through the pharynx and into the esophagus. The *esophageal phase* carries the food bolus, via peristalsis, into the stomach. A liquid bolus in an upright person may actually arrive in the stomach via gravitational forces ahead of the peristaltic wave.

Three forms of peristalsis are defined. Primary peristalsis consists of progressive esophageal contractions initiated by a swallow. Secondary peristalsis consists of progressive contractions of the body of the esophagus initiated by a bolus within the esophagus. Tertiary peristalsis consists of simultaneous contractions at different points within the esophagus.

With atmospheric pressure as the zero point, normal resting intraesophageal pressure is about -5 mm Hg secondary to negative intrapleural pressure. Gastric pressure is about $+5$ mm Hg, whereas the UES and LES have resting pressures of about $+100$ and $+20$ mm Hg, respectively.

CAUSTIC INJURY

Caustic injuries to the esophagus can be divided generally into alkali and acid injuries. Lye (alkaline) injuries tend to be more severe, since they cause a liquefaction necrosis in contradistinction to the somewhat self-limiting coagulative necrosis of acid injuries. Acid injuries tend to spare the esophagus and affect the gastric antrum most severely. Alkali injuries tend to affect the esophagus most severely, but the stomach and duodenum may also be affected. Solid alkalis tend to stick to the oral mucosa and are often spit out by children prior to swallowing. Liquid lye, however, is much more likely to be swallowed. Animal studies have shown that a 1-second exposure to 30% liquid sodium hydroxide will produce transmural necrosis of the cat esophagus. The critical pH appears to be 12.5, which is exceeded by an 0.4% NaOH solution. For comparison, Liquid Drano is a 9.5% NaOH solution.

Alkaline disc batteries can cause a particularly severe burn if they lodge in the esophagus and should be removed as soon as possible. If they pass into the stomach, they should be followed through the gastrointestinal (GI) tract with weekly radiographs or until the battery is found in the stool. Cathartics may shorten the transit time. If there is radiologic evidence that the battery has opened in the GI tract, signs of heavy metal poisoning should be checked for. The most commonly ingested batteries come from a child's own hearing aid.

Liquid bleach (sodium hypochlorite) ingestions rarely cause severe esophageal burns. Liquid detergents containing sodium tripolyphosphate (a common component of many denture cleansers) may cause mucosal ulcerations but rarely any stricture formation. Thermal injuries may be caused by a variety of hot foods. Among the more severe thermal injuries are those due to ingestion of Clinitest tablets (containing copper sulfate), which tend to lodge at the level of the carina and produce heat during hydration along with an alkali burn.

Diagnosis

In general, esophagoscopy to the first evidence of burn and no further has been the accepted diagnostic procedure. This should be done as early as possible after the injury. The presence of oral and pharyngeal burns does not correlate with the presence of esophageal burns. Direct laryngoscopy and bronchoscopy should be added to this procedure if the history or initial physical examination suggests injury to these structures. Recently, esophagogastroduodenoscopy with a flexible pediatric esophagoscope has been suggested[1,2] to better assess damage to the esophagus, stomach, and upper GI tract; however, this cannot be routinely recommended at this time. Routine radiologic studies are generally less helpful than endoscopy in the evaluation of the esophagus after caustic ingestion. Certainly, however, a chest x-ray film to look for evidence of aspiration of the caustic substance and an upright abdominal film to look for free air if there is any suspicion of peritonitis are indicated. Anteroposterior and lateral neck films may show evidence of laryngeal edema, though this will be better evaluated on the physical examination (possibly with the aid of fiberoptic laryngoscopy) and at the time of endoscopy. Acute esophogograms may be counterproductive, especially if performed with barium, since they make subsequent endoscopy more difficult. A carefully performed esophogogram with a water-soluble contrast medium may confirm a suspected perforation and serve to localize it. Barium esophogograms are indicated in follow-up to look for stricture formation.

Morbidity from caustic ingestion is due mainly to perforation leading to mediastinitis or peritonitis, stricture formation, and the delayed development of carcinoma. Treatment is aimed primarily at preventing stricture formation and perforation as well as treating their sequelae.

Treatment

The acute treatment of caustic ingestion includes a thorough physical examination to evaluate for evidence of oral and pharyngeal burns (which may not correlate with esophageal burns), laryngoscopy either with a mirror or fiberoptic scope passed transnasally, and evaluation of the chest and abdomen for evidence of aspiration or perforation. The value of neutralization is unclear but is probably not helpful and may only produce emesis with subsequent aspiration. Lye injuries occur almost immediately on contact, so that neutralization is unlikely to be beneficial. Acids tend to burn more slowly, and if a large quantity has been ingested, it may be helpful to pass a nasogastric tube into the stomach and aspirate any remaining material. Evidence of impending airway obstruction requires a tracheotomy. If there is evidence of perforation into the mediastinum or abdomen, immediate laparotomy and possible esophagogastrectomy may be lifesaving.

Prophylaxis against stricture formation becomes the next issue. Many techniques have been employed to prevent stricture formation, but definitive proof of efficacy is lacking. Many studies purporting to show good results use historical controls that may not be appropriate since strong alkalis and acids are not as readily available for home use as they once were, and most home-related caustic ingestions are now not as severe. Corticosteroids, antibiotics, prophylactic bougienage, passing of a nasogastric tube or stent, esophageal rest with total parenteral nutrition, and the use of substances such as colchicine, penicillamine, and β-aminoproprionitrile to block collagen synthesis all have been described, and there are experimental data to support the use of most of these methods.[3–7]

A reasonable approach is to base therapy on the results of esophagoscopy, the clinical examination, and the history of the type and amount of substance ingested. If the substance is one such as household bleach, which is rarely associated with stricture formation, and the esophagoscopy reveals minimal burns, the use of steroids and antibiotics on a prophylactic basis is probably not warranted. The patient can simply be observed for 48 hours, taking nothing by mouth, for fever or other evidence of perforation, and then advanced on an oral diet. A subsequent barium swallow should be obtained in about 1 month.

If, on the other hand, one suspects a more severe injury at the time of initial esophagoscopy, based on the findings of circumferential or deep burns or the type of caustic ingested, a more aggressive treatment is indicated. After the initial endoscopy (which should include bronchoscopy if there is a history, physical findings, or radiologic findings suggestive of aspiration), a nasogastric tube is passed as a lumen keeper.[8] Although several studies have shown that steroids can inhibit esophageal stricture formation if they are given within the first 48 hours of caustic ingestion,[9–11] this also resulted in an increased rate of septic complications. Antibiotics in and of themselves have not been shown to decrease stricture formation, but when they have been given with steroids in animals, they have decreased the risk of septic complications.[8] Clinical studies have both supported[12] and refuted[13] the effectiveness of steroids. In the most severe cases, the increased risk of septic complications would seem to negate any potential benefits, and in the least severe cases, they are probably not indicated, leaving only a select group of patients for whom they might be advantageous. Initially the patient is fed through the nasogastric tube unless a severe gastric burn is suspected, but oral feedings around the tube can begin in about 1 week. Barium swallows are obtained every 2 weeks for 6 weeks to look for stricture formation. If the patient otherwise does well for the first week after ingestion, and one suspects that the initial evaluation of the severity of the burn may have been overly pessimistic, gentle repeat endoscopy can confirm or refute one's initial impression. If findings are normal at this time, the nasogastric tube can be removed and the patient followed with serial barium swallows. Otherwise, repeat endoscopy is based on clinical symptoms and the findings on barium swallow. If a stricture is seen on follow-up barium swallows, early bougienage should be started. The clinical effectiveness of substances that interfere with collagen synthesis, such as colchicine, penicillamine, and β-aminopropionitrile, remains unproved.[14] Established strictures may be treated with repeated dilation or esophageal replacement with a gastric pull-up, colon interposition, or other procedure. In the most severe strictures retrograde dilation appears safest.[15]

OBSTRUCTIVE LESIONS

Postlaryngopharyngectomy Stenosis

Postlaryngopharyngectomy stenosis is a problem much better avoided than treated. A common cause of this problem is inadequate preoperative evaluation of a pyriform sinus carcinoma. For these lesions, thorough endoscopy prior to any operative procedure as a separate procedure is mandatory for adequate operative planning. Extension into the cervical esophagus or postcricoid hypopharynx will usually entail removing enough pharyngeal mucosa to make closure tight. Unless the surgeon has considered this possibility and spoken with the patient about it, he or she may be reluctant to perform some form of immediate reconstruction, thus performing an overly tight closure and condemning the patient to a liquid diet secondary to pharyngeal or esophageal stenosis. Worse, the surgeon may skimp on surgical margins to have enough mucosa for closure, thus performing an oncologically unsound procedure and increasing the likelihood of a primary recurrence as well as leaving the patient functionally deficient. The possible need for total laryngopharyngectomy must be foreseen and prepared for by preparing the patient for a free jejunal graft, gastric pull-up, or other form of reconstruction. For patients with a remaining strip of posterior pharyngeal mucosa, a pectoralis major myocutaneous flap cut with a fusiform end superiorly on the chest wall, which will be inserted inferiorly into a dart cut longitudinally in the anterior esophageal wall, gives consistently good results.

Once a stenosis has developed, the surgeon should first suspect a recurrent carcinoma and do a biopsy of the site. Repeated dilatations with a Maloney-type dilator may be effective but, as a rule, must be done frequently, usually with limited success, since the problem is one of actual tissue loss. Some patients can perform dilatation themselves at home, but this is the exception. Stenoses are most often best handled by reconstruction with a pectoralis major myocutaneous flap or other flap, preferably after waiting 1 to 2 years when the likelihood of recurrent cancer is lessened.

Esophageal Web

Esophageal webs and rings come in several varieties. The cervical esophageal web occurs most frequently in the postcricoid area on the anterior wall and has been associated with the Paterson-Brown-Kelly or Plummer-Vinson syndrome and an increased risk of postcricoid hypopharyngeal carcinoma. Lower esophageal rings (commonly known as Schatzki's rings) occur at or just above the gastroesophageal junction, are often covered by squamous epithelium above and gastric mucosa below, and are quite common. Their pathogenesis is unclear. Midesophageal webs may be secondary to caustic ingestion or other inflammatory disorders such as benign mucous membrane pemphigus or epidermolysis bullosa. Most esophageal webs are asymptomatic and require no treatment. Symptomatic webs are generally best treated initially with dilatation. Severe lower esophageal rings unresponsive to dilatation may require pneumatic dilatation or antireflux-type surgery with direct disruption of the ring.

Cervical Esophageal Tumors

Cervical esophageal squamous cell carcinomas often present as extensions of hypopharyngeal cancers. The risks of submucosal spread and skip lesions have led some authors to propose total esophagectomy for all of these patients.[16] Others have not found such a high risk and question the validity of requiring a 30 cm distal margin when no such equivalent margin can be obtained superiorly.[17] In general, most squamous cell cancers of the cervical esophagus, which present as extensions of hypopharyngeal cancers, can be managed by total laryngopharyngectomy and cervical esophagectomy with free jejunal, tubed pectoralis major, or other graft reconstruction. Total laryngopharyngoesophagectomy with gastric pull-up is an equally effective mode of therapy. Postoperative irradiation is used in all such cancers. When total thyroidectomy and parathyroidectomy are necessary, as is often the case in recurrent periostomal cancers, postoperative replacement of thyroid hormone and calcium, along with vitamin D, is required, and management may be difficult.

DISORDERS OF ESOPHAGEAL MOTILITY

Disorders of esophageal motility may be secondary to neurologic or muscular disorders or may be postsurgical or idiopathic. Most disorders of esophageal motility are best studied by manometric techniques with or without videofluoroscopy.

Cricopharyngeal Achalasia

Cricopharyngeal achalasia is a term that refers to incomplete relaxation of the UES during swallowing. It has been described as an isolated finding as well as in conjunction with thyrotoxic myopathy, poliomyelitis, after bilateral recurrent laryngeal nerve paralysis, after partial pharyngectomy, and in association with bulbar palsy.[18] Other disorders of the UES also exist. These consist of hypertensive or hypotensive resting pressure. Both have been associated with globus hystericus and reflux.[19] Reflux into the hypopharynx can sometimes present with complaints of dysphagia or hoarseness. A hypertensive UES has also been described in association with various neuromuscular disorders, after cricopharyngeal myotomy, and in association with certain connective tissue diseases. Premature closure of the UES has been associated with Zenker's diverticulum formation, and delayed relaxation has been associated with familial dysautonomia.

Some believe that a cricopharyngeal bar, which may be seen on barium swallow, represents a hyperactive cricopharyngeal muscle and evidence of cricopharyngeal achalasia; however, some manometric studies have failed to show definite evidence of this.[20]

Cricopharyngeal myotomy has been used to treat a variety of swallowing disorders. Its use in this setting must be based on good manometric evidence of cricopharyngeal hypertonicity or abnormal relaxation. The entire swallowing mechanism should be adequately studied to determine that the cricopharyngeal muscle is, indeed, the most likely source of the patient's difficulties. Cricopharyngeal myotomy is unlikely to help patients with a hypotonic cricopharyngeal muscle or with discoordination of the entire swallowing mechanism, including neuromuscular control of the tongue and the oral, voluntary phase of swallowing.

Zenker's Diverticulum

Though not universally accepted, pharyngoesophageal pulsion diverticulae (Zenker's diverticulae) seem to be associated with cricopharyngeal and UES dysfunction, specifically with premature contraction after swallowing. They tend to present to the left of the midline and emerge just above the level of the cricopharyngeal muscle through a weak area known as Killian's area, between the cricopharyngeal muscle and the remainder of the inferior pharyngeal constrictor muscle. They may also develop more laterally between the cricopharyngeal muscle and the upper esophagus through another weakened area known as the Killian-Jamieson area.

Symptoms include dysphagia, regurgitation of undigested food, and aspiration. Treatment consists of endoscopic opening of the mouth of the diverticulum with a special endoscope,[21] cricopharyngeal myotomy with superior pexy of the sac, or direct resection with cricopharyngeal myotomy. Resection and myotomy remain the most widely favored method of treatment. At the time of resection, it is helpful to have a nasogastric tube down the esophagus, as well as a separate structure, such as the tip of an endotracheal tube or packing, within the lumen of the diverticulum to make identification of these structures easier. This can be accomplished endoscopically immediately prior to resection.

Diffuse Esophageal Spasm

Diffuse esophageal spasm is an esophageal motility disorder characterized by simultaneous, painful, repetitive contractions of the smooth muscle portion of the esophagus, often associated with chest pain. There are few proved treatment regimens, though "long myotomy" and the calcium blocker nifedipine have been tried with some success.

Achalasia

Achalasia refers to an esophageal motility disorder characterized by incomplete relaxation of the LES and motor failure of the body of the esophagus. Radiologic studies reveal a classic bird's beak sign. Anatomic studies have shown loss of the myenteric plexus and vagal atrophy. Vigorous achalasia refers to a lack of LES relaxation combined with a picture similar to diffuse esophageal spasm. Some question whether all of these entities may simply represent a continuum of disease. Treatment includes pneumatic dilatation of the LES and, if this is unsuccessful, LES myotomy with or without a reflux procedure. The cause of achalasia remains unknown.

GASTROESOPHAGEAL REFLUX

Gastroesophageal reflux may present with symptoms of heartburn or even pharyngeal or laryngeal symptoms, but symptoms correlate poorly with its presence. Hiatal hernia may or may not be associated with reflux and vice versa. The diagnosis is best made by 24-hour esophageal pH monitoring or with various maneuvers after installation of 0.1N hydrochloric acid into the stomach while measuring lower esophageal pH; however, treatment usually begins on clinical grounds, and if a good clinical response is seen, further documentation is probably not necessary. Treatment includes avoidance of fats, tobacco, chocolate, alcohol, and any food for several hours before bedtime. Antacids may help and may raise LES pressure, as do some other cholinergic drugs such as bethanechol. The H_2 blockers may help symptoms by decreasing gastric acid secretion. For patients unresponsive to medical therapy, antireflux surgery may be necessary. Recently several authors have suggested a correlation between reflux and the development of laryngeal carcinoma.[22]

REFERENCES

1. Moore WR: Caustic ingestions: Pathophysiology, diagnosis, and treatment. *Clin Pediatr* 1986; 25:192–196.
2. Goldman LP, Weigert JM: Corrosive substance ingestion: A review. *Am J Gastroenterol* 1984; 79:85–90.
3. Knox WG, Scott JR, Zintel HA, et al: Bougienage and steroids used singly or in combination in experimental corrosive esophagitis. *Ann Surg* 1967; 166:930–941.
4. Krey H: On the treatment of corrosive lesions in the oesophagus. *Acta Otolaryngol (Suppl)* 1952; 102:1–49.

5. DiCostanzo J, Noirclerc M, Jouglard J, et al: New thera-peutic approach to corrosive burns of the upper gastroin-testinal tract. *Gut* 1980; 21:370–375.

6. Gehanno P, Guidon C: Prohibition of experimental esophageal lye strictures by penicillamine. *Arch Otolaryn-gol* 1981; 107:145–147.

7. Butler C, Madden JW, Davis WM, et al: Morphologic as-pects of experimental esophageal stricture. II: Effect of steroid hormones, bougienage, and lathyrism on acute lye burns. *Surgery* 1977; 81:431.

8. Wijburg FA, Beukers MM, Heymans HS, et al: Nasogastric intubation as sole treatment of caustic esophageal lesions. *Ann Otol Rhinol Laryngol* 1985; 94:337–341.

9. Haller JA, Bachman K: The comparative effect of current therapy on experimental caustic burns of the esophagus. *Pediatrics* 1964; 34:236–245.

10. Johnson EE: A study of corrosive esophagitis. *Laryngo-scope* 1963; 73:1651–1696.

11. McNeill RA, Welbourn RB: Prevention of corrosive stric-ture of the oesophagus in the rat. *J Laryngol Otol* 1966; 80:346–358.

12. Cardona JC, Daly JF: Current management of corrosive esophagitis: An evaluation of 239 cases. *Ann Otol Rhinol Laryngol* 1971; 80:521–527.

13. Kirsh MM, Ritter F: Caustic ingestion and subsequent damage to the oropharyngeal and digestive passages. *Ann Thorac Surg* 1976; 21:74–82.

14. Kikendall JW, Johnson LF: Esophageal injury: Caustics and pills, in Castell DO, Johnson LF (eds): Esophageal func-tion in health and disease. New York, Elsevier North-Holland 1983, pp 255–272.

15. Hawkins DB: Dilation of esophageal strictures: Compara-tive morbidity of antegrade and retrograde methods. *Ann Otol Rhinol Laryngol* 1988; 97:460–465.

16. Harrison DFN: Surgical management of cancer of the hypopharynx and cervical oesophagus. *Br J Surg* 1969; 56:95–103.

17. Gluckman JL, Weissler MC, McCafferty G, et al: Partial vs total esophagectomy for advanced carcinoma of the hypopharynx. *Arch Otolaryngol Head Neck Surg* 1987; 113:69–72.

18. Asherson N: Achalasia of the cricopharyngeal sphincter. *J Laryngol Otol* 1950; 64:747–758.

19. Gerhardt DC, Castell DO: Anatomy and physiology of the esophageal sphincters, in Castell DO, Johnson LF (eds): *Esophageal Function in Health and Disease.* New York, Elsevier North-Holland, 1983, pp 17–29.

20. Hellemans J, Pelemans W, VanTrappen G, et al: Manomet-ric studies in "achalasia" of the upper esophageal sphinc-ter. *Z Gastroenterol* 1981; 19:432–433.

21. Hollinger LD, Benjamin B: New endoscope for (laser) en-doscopic diverticulotomy. *Ann Otol Rhinol Laryngol* 1987; 96:658–660.

22. Ward PH, Hanson DG: Reflux as an etiological factor of carcinoma of the laryngopharynx. *Laryngoscope* 1988; 98:1195–1199.

23. Morrison MD: Is chronic gastroesophageal reflux a causa-tive factor in glottic carcinoma? *Otolaryngol Head Neck Surg* 1988; 99:370–373.

Management of Esophageal Problems

Approach of

Eugene M. Bozymski, M.D.

GASTROESOPHAGEAL REFLUX DISEASE

The reflux of gastric contents into the esophagus is common.[1] This can be documented in a normal population by use of a pH microelectrode. These episodes of reflux may be entirely asymptomatic or may be associated with the most frequently recognizable symptom, which is heartburn, or pyrosis.

When these episodes of reflux result in inflammatory changes in the esophageal mucosa, whether evident grossly or microscopically, the term reflux esophagitis is used. Gastroesophageal reflux disease includes not only the inflammatory changes that exist in the esophagus as a result of the reflux but also any other clinical condition that results from episodes of gastroesophageal reflux, such as airway disease, which may occur as a consequence of episodic gastroesophageal reflux.

Pathophysiology

Like peptic ulcer disease, gastroesophageal reflux disease is not caused by a single factor. Rather, there are a variety of mechanisms or combination of mechanisms whereby any one patient may develop symptomatic esophagitis. These various factors include (1) competency of the LES as well as other antireflux barriers, (2) the potency or composition and volume of the refluxate, (3) esophageal clearance mechanisms, (4) tissue resistance, and (5) gastric emptying.[2] It becomes apparent, then, that the final clinical syndrome resulting from gastroesophageal reflux may be quite variable depending on the interaction of these factors.

Lower Esophageal Sphincter

The LES remains one of the most important barriers to the development of reflux disease. This LES is comprised of smooth muscle, which is evident on esophageal manometric tracings as a high-pressure zone separating positive intragastric pressure from negative intrathoracic pressure. This resting pressure, or tone, is usually greater than 10 mm Hg above intragastric pressure and prevents reflux under ordinary conditions.[3] Anatomically smooth muscle from this high-pressure zone in the esophagus looks no different from the remainder of the esophagus but responds quite differently to a variety of neurohumoral substances. Gastroesophageal reflux occurs in several different ways, as pointed out by Dodds et al.[4] Spontaneous reflux can occur with transient relaxation of the LES unassociated with swallowing, or it may occur as spontaneous free reflux or in association with increased intra-abdominal pressure transients that exceed the LES pressure.[4]

It is of interest that gastroesophageal reflux most often occurs secondary to transient LES relaxations in normal individuals, and it is also the main mechanism wherein patients with esophagitis reflux also. As pointed out earlier, these patients are not a homogeneous group and the mechanisms by which any one patient refluxes may vary.

Basal LES pressure normally rests at levels greater than 10 mm Hg. Decreased basal LES pressure is noted in some patients with reflux esophagitis but there is not linear correlation between these two events. However, when LES pressure is less than 5 mm of mercury there is usually clinically evident esophagitis. The question remains as to whether the decreased LES pressure is a secondary phenomenon due to the reflux, as has been demonstrated in certain animal models,[5] or is a primary factor responsible for the gastroesophageal reflux in that it predates reflux symptoms and persists after resolution of esophagitis.[6, 7]

The relative contribution of other anatomic factors, such as the pinchcock action on the diaphragmatic hiatus, the acute angle at which the esophagus enters the stomach, creating a flap valve, the mucosal rosette, and the intra-abdominal segment of the esophagus, in preventing reflux is not entirely clear.

Potency and Volume of the Refluxate

It is not only acid that is problematic for the squamous epithelium of the esophagus but also other gastric content as well. Pepsin, a proteolytic enzyme produced by the chief cells of the stomach, can cause severe damage to esophageal epithelium.[8] In addition, other enzymes from the pancreas along with bile may make their way into the esophagus, particularly in patients who have had prior gastric surgery. Most certainly the constituents of bile can have a damaging effect on epithelial membranes and have been shown to increase the permeability of both esophageal and gastric mucosa to hydrogen ions.[9, 10] It is not entirely clear how important the role of bile is in the pathogenesis of reflux disease in the average patient.[11] That reflux injury is multifactorial is additionally pointed out by the report of esophagitis occurring in pernicious anemia.[12] The importance of volume of refluxate can be noted by the observation that patients with Zollinger-Ellison syndrome with marked hypersecretion of gastric acid may have very severe esophagitis.[13]

Gastric Emptying and Volume

The presence of reflux into the esophagus implies that there be a reservoir from which this refluxate originates. Increased gastric volume, whether due to increased gastric secretion, as seen in Zollinger-Ellison syndrome, or to delayed gastric emptying, which occurs as a consequence of a variety of diseases or medications, could act as a contributing factor in the development or progression of reflux disease. It has also been reported that in some patients with gastroesophageal reflux disease delayed gastric emptying is noted.[14]

Esophageal Clearance

The length of time that material refluxed from the stomach remains in the esophagus determines, in part, the adverse effects noted in the esophageal epithelium.[15] Esophageal clearance is dependent on esophageal peristaltic activity, which very effectively removes volume from the esophagus. The small amount of residual acid that is not swept back into the stomach by the peristaltic activity is neutralized by swallowed saliva.[16] The majority of the acid is returned to the stomach by the primary peristaltic wave, and the residual acid is buffered by swallowed saliva. The importance of the saliva is evident from studies that indicate that during times of increased salivation there is decreased acid clearance time, whereas if saliva is removed by suction there is a prolongation of esophageal clearance time.[16] It is thought that the saliva acts to provide bicarbonate ions that neutralize the residual hydrogen ions that remain in the unstirred layer that are not removed by primary peristaltic waves.[17] It should also be noted that it is the primary peristaltic wave that is important in clearing the esophagus after an episode of reflux rather than the secondary peristaltic waves, which are elicited by esophageal stretch receptors.[18]

Gravity also plays a role in clearing the esophagus, but unless there is some abnormality of peristaltic activity, this is not a predominant role. The clearance mechanisms certainly become more important when a patient is in the recumbent position and asleep because both peristaltic sequences and the production of saliva are diminished. This diminution allows refluxed material to remain in the esophagus for extended periods of time, placing those with nocturnal reflux at increased risk for epithelial damage.[19]

In addition to salivary secretion, there are submucosal glands, particularly in the cervical and distal part of the esophagus, that add their secretions to the esophageal lumen, and they may have some protective effect as well.[20]

Abnormal esophageal peristalsis can be demonstrated in some patients with reflux esophagitis, but it is not clear whether this is primary or secondary.[21]

Tissue Resistance

The constituents of tissue resistance as related to the squamous epithelium of the esophagus are not well defined or understood. The squamous epithelium is initially impermeable, but when it is damaged by agents such as pepsin, alcohol, or bile, backdiffusion of hydrogen ions is noted.[9] It appears that the unstirred mucous layer with its affinity for bicarbonate ions is a component of this function, as are the cell membranes and the intercellular junctions. The importance of blood flow to the epithelium as well as the ability of the epithelium to regenerate and repair itself obviously are very important, but the factors responsible for this are not well understood. The metabolites of the arachidonic acid cascade, particularly the prostaglandins and other mediators of inflammation, may well play a very important role in this area, but further studies are needed.

Clearly then, many factors or combinations of factors may be responsible for epithelial damage and inflammatory change in any given patient. Further questions as to the development of stricture in certain patients remain. Even more poorly understood is the replacement of the damaged squamous epithelium by columnar epithelium, as seen in Barrett's esophagus.

Hiatal Hernia

The relationship between gastroesophageal reflux disease and the presence of a hiatal hernia has come full circle. For a long period of time, it was believed that hernia and reflux were nearly synonymous. However, studies have shown that symptoms tend to correlate more closely with the presence of an incompetent LES mechanism than with the presence or absence of a hiatal hernia.[22] The present majority view, however, is that although many individuals have totally asymptomatic hiatal hernias, the majority of patients with problematic reflux disease have a coexistent hiatal hernia.[23] Part of the explanation may lie in the fact that patients with hiatal hernia have an increased acid clearance time.[24, 25]

Clinical History and Physical Examination

The classic symptom indicative of gastroesophageal reflux disease is heartburn, or pyrosis. If the physician can obtain the history of retrosternal burning pain aggravated by the recumbent position, with or without water brash, and prompt relief

by the ingestion of an antacid, the diagnosis appears to be evident. However, the extent of the damage to the esophageal epithelium varies considerably, and, in fact, no apparent damage may be evident at all. Chest pain other than heartburn can occur with reflux disease and is certainly responsible for some of the problems that we have in diagnosing the patient with "noncardiac chest pain." It is not entirely clear whether the chest pain is caused by stimulation of pain receptors by acid or secondary to localized spasm induced by reflux. Other symptoms related to reflux include regurgitation aggravated by positional change and frequently reported by the patient as hot liquid coming up into the back of the throat. This is to be distinguished from the symptom of water brash, which is a reflection of increased production of saliva as a consequence of reflux. Odynophagia, pain on swallowing, may occur when there is extensive erosive change in the esophagus. Dysphagia usually is indicative of some compromise of the lumen of the esophagus and heralds the onset of stricture formation.

Pulmonary symptoms may occur as a consequence of reflux and are related to the aspiration of refluxed material and include nocturnal cough and wheezing, asthma, bronchospasm, recurring pulmonary infections, laryngitis, hoarseness, and perhaps abnormalities of the gingiva and teeth.[23] Globus, a sensation of a lump in the throat, has been thought by some to be secondary to an increase in upper esophageal sphincter pressure secondary to acid reflux.[26] However, others have not demonstrated an increase in upper esophageal sphincter pressure.[27] This sensation of globus is frequently seen in patients in whom there is no relationship to gastroesophageal reflux and is often seen in younger people.

The physical examination in patients with gastroesophageal reflux disease is most often of no aid in arriving at a diagnosis. However, on occasion, physical findings secondary to complication, such as aspiration, may be present, or there may be indication of coexistent systemic disease that predisposes to reflux, such as diffuse systemic sclerosis.

Evaluation for Gastroesophageal Reflux and Reflux Esophagitis

Clearly the clinical setting in which symptomatic reflux occurs bears a great deal of importance relative to the evaluation that is undertaken. If one is dealing with the onset of heartburn in pregnancy or in a young patient with no other esophageal symptoms, a therapeutic trial can be undertaken, and if the patient does well, no further evaluation is warranted. Should the patient have associated symptoms, have an atypical history, or not respond to an antireflux program, further investigation is warranted. Likewise, if there is a suggestion that would indicate the presence of a complication such as nocturnal cough, dysphagia, or blood loss, for example, further evaluation would be mandatory.

Diagnostic Evaluation and Tests

Many tests are available to aid in the evaluation of the patient with reflux symptoms, including: (1) upper gastrointestinal (GI) x-ray studies; (2) intraesophageal, or upper esopha-

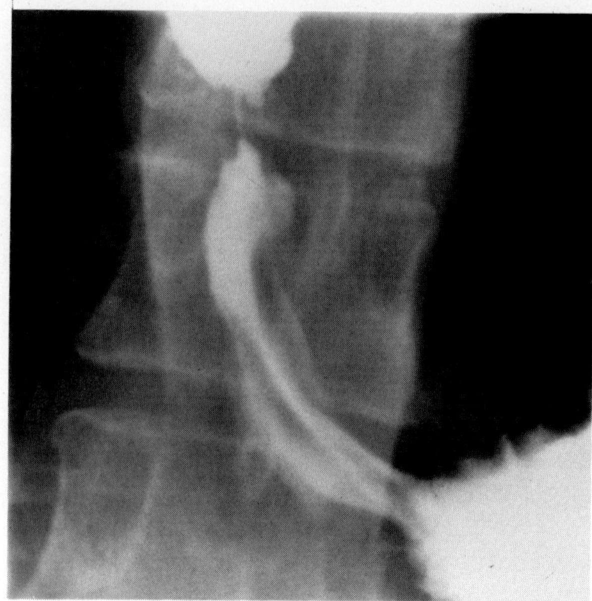

FIG 43–1.
Upper GI radiograph demonstrating a narrow stricture above a hiatal hernia.

geal, pH monitoring; (3) the acid infusion test of Bernstein; (4) esophageal manometry; (5) gastroesophageal scintiscan; (6) potential difference studies; (7) upper endoscopy; and (8) esophageal biopsy. Each has a different utility and allows us to answer slightly different questions relative to the patient's symptoms.

Upper Gastrointestinal X-Ray Examination

Radiography of the esophagus is clearly an excellent way to define any structural abnormality in the esophagus particularly related to the question of caliber or stricture (Fig 43–1). Double-contrast examinations allow one to define mucosal changes with more accuracy and may be particularly useful.[28] In addition, one can obtain good information relative to esophageal motility at the time of fluoroscopy of the esophagus and on occasion detect the presence of gross reflux as well.[29] The x-ray examination also allows one to note the presence of a hiatal hernia and provides an opportunity to examine the stomach and duodenum.

Intraesophageal pH Monitoring

Clearly, intraesophageal pH monitoring is a very useful way to document the presence of reflux in the esophagus. The development of small portable units that make ambulatory pH monitoring readily available have been essential for the development of this technique. Coupled with computer analysis of the data obtained by such monitoring, prolonged intraesophageal monitoring has now become the standard test by which other measures of gastroesophageal reflux are compared.[30] Although it is clear that this is an excellent method to detect reflux, we are still in the process of accumulating data to allow us to most wisely use this technique.[31] Prolonged pH monitoring provides a temporal profile of reflux events that can be correlated with the patient's symptoms. In addition, one can simultaneously record motor activity of the esophagus, which will, of course, have important research and clinical applications. The role of intraesophageal pH monitoring in the evaluation of patients with noncardiac chest pain continues to develop as well. pH monitoring also has the potential to assist us in monitoring the efficacy of our antireflux therapy.

Acid Clearance

Acid clearance can be assessed using intraesophageal pH monitoring and will aid in detecting the patient with abnormal esophageal motility and increased dwell time or delayed transit.

Bernstein Test

The acid infusion test, or the Bernstein test, is a simple test for detecting whether the patient's symptoms are indicative of an esophageal abnormality.[32] This test is performed by infusing 0.1N hydrochloric acid into the distal esophagus and attempting to reproduce the patient's pain pattern. A saline infusion serves as the control. This test is subjective and therefore should be performed carefully, with the patient being unaware of which solution is being infused, and, if possible, the technician should also be unaware of which agent is being infused. It must be remembered that false positive as well as false negative results occur with the Bernstein test, and a negative test result does not exclude the esophagus as being the source of the problem.

Generally the Bernstein test is done in conjunction with an esophageal manometric study or in conjunction with intraesophageal pH monitoring or other provocative testing.

Esophageal Manometry

Esophageal manometric studies allow us to assess the motility of the esophagus as well as the LES pressure. Measurement of LES pressure whether by station pull-through or rapid pull-through does not discriminate cleanly between patients with reflux disease and a control population. However, identifying those patients with decreased LES pressure (<10 mm Hg) may be useful; it appears that those patients having LES pressures less than 6 mm of Hg frequently do poorly on medical management (Fig 43–2).[33] It should be noted that some patients with decreased LES pressure do not have objective evidence of mucosal damage, and many times patients with normal LES pressure will have significant gastroesophageal reflux disease. This simply again serves to point out that there are many factors in addition to LES pressure that determine whether or not reflux disease occurs. It is, however, absolutely essential that any patient undergoing elective antireflux surgery have a preoperative esophageal manometric study to exclude the possibility of an unrecognized motor disorder as well as monitoring LES activity.

Gastroesophageal Scintiscan

Radioactive isotopes have also been used to evaluate the presence of reflux but have not gained wide clinical acceptance.[34] At present they are used mainly as a research tool.

Isotopic methodology can also be applied to test for the occurrence of pulmonary aspiration of refluxed gastric content.

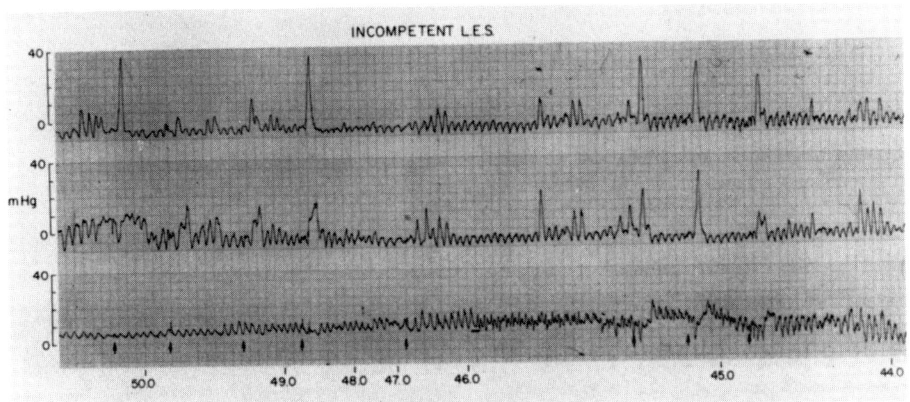

FIG 43–2.
Bottom channel shows the pressure profile of the LES in a patient with severe reflux esophagitis. Note the lack of any significant elevation above the baseline gastric pressure.

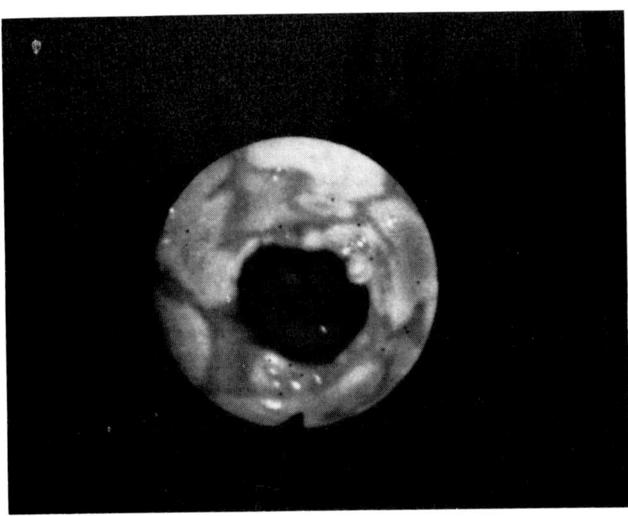

FIG 43–3.
Endoscopic appearance of erosive esophagitis. A small hiatal hernia appears below the esophagus.

Technetium 99m-sulfur colloid is placed in the stomach, and counts are then obtained over the lung fields the following morning in an effort to ascertain the occurrence of aspiration.[35]

Potential Difference Measurements

Potential difference measurements are dependent on the integrity of the epithelial membrane. Differing epithelia have different transport characteristics and therefore differ in their measured electrical potential difference. In the experimental animal when inflammation occurs, there is a rapid drop in potential difference indicative of increased permeability. This decrease in potential difference can also be seen in the clinical setting of esophagitis as well.[36] Like gastroesophageal scintiscan, however, it remains primarily a research tool.

Upper Endoscopy and Esophageal Biopsy

The endoscopic examination of the esophagus allows one to best determine whether or not gastroesophageal reflux has led to any adverse consequences relative to inducing inflammatory change in the esophagus (Fig 43–3). Clearly direct visual examination and biopsy of the esophagus are invaluable tools in assessing consequences of reflux. There are many instances in which symptoms are out of keeping with the endoscopic observation, and this becomes important information. Although it is clear that erosive esophagitis is easily detectable, on occasion esophagitis may escape detection, thus the need for biopsy and histologic confirmation in many clinical settings. It is exceedingly important in reflux disease to keep the possibility of columnar-lined lower esophagus (Barrett's esophagus) in mind. At times this epithelium is readily apparent by its more reddish appearance compared with the pink appearance of the esophagus, but on occasion, particularly when there is a very long segment of Barrett's epithelium, it may be difficult to detect. This affirms the need for biopsy and histologic confirmation.[37] The histologic hallmarks of esophagitis are erosions of the epithelium along the inflammatory infiltrate that may contain acute and chronic inflammatory cells. Intraepithelial inflammatory cells, including polymorphonuclear leukocytes and eosinophils, may be present. Histologic abnormalities that suggest reflux-associated changes consist of prominent papillae and basal cell hyperplasia, which may be related to increased cell turnover as a consequence of epithelial injury.[38, 39]

Summary

One can see from the description of these tests that many are available, and as always, the selection is highly dependent on the clinical setting and the severity of symptoms. Ancillary symptoms that might suggest complications of reflux disease also plays an important role. Clearly the clinical setting is the most important factor in suggesting which tests are most appropriate and deciding what specific question relative to the patient's presentation needs to be answered. The upper GI series allows one to critically examine the structural anatomy of the esophagus as well as exclude stricture. In addition, it imparts some information relative to motor activity and, on occasion, will show unsolicited gastroesophageal reflux. This, of course, is a very insensitive test to detect reflux, but if it is present without provocation, it is of note. The Bernstein acid infusion test allows us to determine whether the esophagus may be implicated in the genesis of the patient's symptoms. Ambulatory intraesophageal pH monitoring clearly is the standard to assess the presence or absence of gastroesophageal reflux and, along with the Bernstein test, is of value in determining whether the esophagus may be implicated in noncardiac chest pain. Esophageal manometric studies remain the par excellence method to determine whether or not motor disorders are present and is an absolutely mandatory test prior to elective antireflux surgery. Upper endoscopy and biopsy allow us to examine the esophagus for the consequences of reflux and to assess the impact of the disease on the mucosa as well as to look for certain complications and assess treatment modalities.

Complications

Gastroesophageal reflux is extremely common, and perhaps we are fortunate that more patients do not develop complications as a consequence. However, the problems that complications related to reflux create are sufficiently problematic to warrant a much more determined effort on our part to avoid them as best we can. It is very difficult to understand why some patients with reflux disease, for example, will develop columnar epithelium as a consequence of long-standing reflux, whereas others with reflux that appears clinically to be as problematic do not go on to develop Barrett's epithelium. A great deal of information is needed in these areas.

Esophageal Stricture

Peptic strictures generally occur in the distal esophagus and are a consequence of repeated prolonged exposure of the esophageal epithelium to the gastric refluxate (Fig 43–4). This continuing epithelial damage eventually leads to fibrosis and then stricture formation. Generally, strictures develop gradually over a period of time, but on occasion, their formation may be accentuated by placement of nasogastric tubes or ingestion of caustic materials, including some medications such as certain potassium chloride tablets, nonsteroidal antiinflammatory drugs, and many antibiotics. Epidermolysis bullosa, a genetic disorder, characterized by abnormalities in squamous epithelium and severe dystrophic changes of the skin, is occasionally associated with severe stricturing of the esophagus that may be multifactorial.[40] Finally, some patients presenting with peptic strictures have no history of heartburn or perhaps what appear to have been only minimal clinical symptoms.

The symptom that heralds the presence of a stricture is dysphagia. Dysphagia is an exceedingly "hard" symptom and one that demands immediate investigation. In the setting of a peptic stricture, the patient will first complain of solid food

sticking or slowing down in transit from mouth to stomach, and this may later progress to the point of soft foods as well. It is unusual for the patient to have trouble with liquids unless he or she has impacted a bolus of solid food in the distal esophagus. During such times, attempts to "wash the food down" will sometimes be helpful, and on occasion the ingestion of the liquid will induce regurgitation of the bolus and alleviation of the impaction in that manner.

Upper GI radiography is an excellent way to ascertain the status of the esophageal lumen and calibrate the stricture. On occasion because of the small size of the lumen, insufficient barium will enter the esophagus, making it difficult to adequately ascertain the exact length of the narrowing. Upper endoscopy may be necessary to evaluate the mucosa, exclude the possibility of neoplasm and columnar epithelium, and ascertain which method of dilatation would be most appropriate. It should be pointed out that using a small-caliber fibroscope may make it difficult to appreciate some moderate strictures, particularly if there is very little mucosal change. Prior to dilatation therapy, an attempt should be made to use an antireflux program to decrease the inflammatory change. In addition, if biopsies have been performed to exclude neoplasm or Barrett's epithelium, delaying the initial dilatation for approximately 1 week may be appropriate. If the patient is having considerable difficulty with nutrition, it may be advisable to initiate dilatation early on and obtain biopsies at a later date.

Therapy consists of a strict antireflux program, coupled with periodic sequential dilatations. A whole host of methods, including mercury-filled bougies such as the Hurst and Maloney dilators or fixed expansion balloons that can be passed either through the scope or over a fluoroscopically placed guide wire, are available. On occasion, passing a guide wire and then following with Puestow dilators or Savory-Guillard graded dilators and monitoring with fluoroscopic control will be most suitable. The exact method of dilatation will depend on a variety of factors, and it may be that initially dilatation with a "through

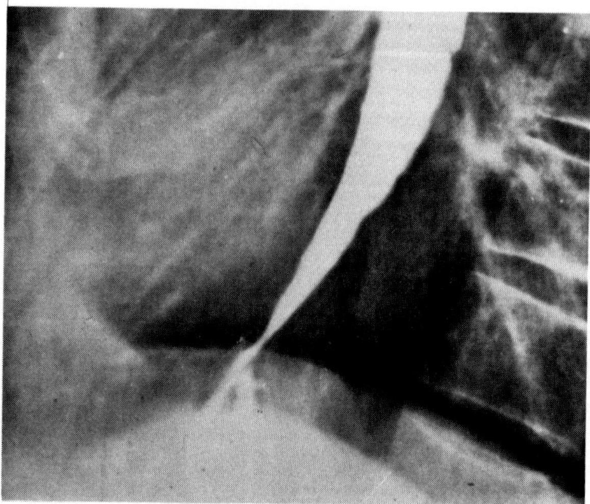

FIG 43–4.
Esophagogram demonstrating a smoothly tapered peptic stricture in a patient with long-standing reflux symptoms.

needed, to the posterior pharynx and larynx directly through the suction port of the fiberoptic bronchoscope. With practice, the endoscopist quickly learns to identify important anatomic landmarks while directing the scope into the trachea. An excellent text with realistic photography of the laryngeal and tracheal anatomy through a fiberoptic bronchoscope is available.[18] This book is a useful teaching aid in mastering fiberoptic bronchoscopy. Once the scope is in the trachea and the carina is visualized, the endotracheal tube is gently advanced over the fiberoptic bronchoscope into the trachea. The fiberoptic scope is removed, and the placement of the endotracheal tube is verified by auscultation, observation of symmetrical chest movement with positive pressure ventilation, and the presence of CO_2 by capnography. The patient is then expediently anesthetized with IV anesthetics. Fiberoptic bronchoscopy is safe, comfortable for the patient, atraumatic, easy to perform and, with practice, very reliable.

Other Options.—Although an awake fiberoptic intubation is my first choice, there are a number of other options and techniques in approaching the patient with an anticipated difficult airway. Each option certainly has its advantages and disadvantages as well as its appropriateness for a specific problem or a selected patient. The experience of the clinician is, of course, an important consideration in the selection of a particular method. The most important and primary goal is safety; a secondary goal is comfort for the patient. A discussion of some of the options follows.

Awake Oral Intubation.—An awake oral intubation is performed with a conventional retracting laryngoscope (MacIntosch or Miller) or a fiberoptic scope after application of topical anesthetics to the tongue and posterior pharynx and a careful IV titration of drugs to obtain appropriate analgesia and sedation. This approach is selected when access through the nose is limited. Such a technique requires a cooperative noncombative patient, since this method may be quite uncomfortable both physically and psychologically for the patient. Forceful manipulation may induce trauma of the airway. Bleeding, broken teeth, biting, wretching, gagging, laryngospasm, vagal reflex bradycardias, and vomiting all may occur.

Awake Blind Nasal Intubation.—An awake nasal intubation can be performed blindly after anesthetizing the nasal cavity and posterior pharynx with local anesthetics as previously described. A blind nasal intubation is performed surprisingly easily with practice. The patient's head is placed in a neutral position. An appropriately sized endotracheal tube is placed through the nose into the posterior pharynx. The tube is gently advanced a few centimeters with each inspiration as the patient is instructed to breath deeply. Covering the patient's other nostril and closing the mouth with a cupped hand enhances the movement of air through the advancing endotracheal tube. The clinician's ear is positioned near the proximal end of the tube as he or she continually listens for air movement through the endotracheal tube. As the tube is slowly advanced into the trachea with each

inspiration, the flow of air becomes louder and louder. During advancement, if suddenly no breath sounds are heard, the tube has either advanced into the esophagus or has impinged in the lateral recesses somewhere in the posterior pharynx or vallecula. The tube is slowly retracted until breath sounds are again heard, and the head is slightly repositioned. Repositioning of the head should follow a systematic approach. Attempts are made until finally the trachea is entered. Entrance into the trachea is clearly recognized because movement of air is excellent, the patient is unable to vocalize, and coughing usually occurs. Throughout the intubation process, the clinician's eye should continually, carefully observe the neck for any lateral bulging movements because of the tube becoming displaced from the midline and impinging in the lateral recesses of the posterior pharynx. Observations of such movements allow one to slightly twist and realign the tube into a midline position.

Nasal Insertion–Oral Visualization Intubation.—Another useful method is a combined nasal-oral approach to intubation. With this technique, after topical anesthesia to the tongue, pharynx, and nasal cavity, the tube is placed through the nose into the posterior pharynx, and orally under direct vision with a retracting laryngoscope, the tube is directed into the larynx with or without the aid of Magill forceps. Nasal intubations are selected when surgical access to the mouth is required or postoperative intubation is anticipated. The potential for bleeding in the nose or trauma to posterior pharyngeal tissue (adenoids, tonsils) is always a possibility.

Anticipated Anterior Larynx in the Uncooperative Patient

Inhalational Versus Intravenous Induction Technique.— Inhalational induction techniques are usually selected for the patient with a difficult airway who will not cooperate and will require an unconscious state under general anesthesia to facilitate endotracheal intubation. Patients who are mentally handicapped, children, or combative, uncooperative adults are examples. The important difference in an inhalational induction technique vs. an IV technique needs further explanation. The basic premise relates to the uptake and redistribution of IV anesthetics vs. inhalational anesthetics. Once an IV anesthetizing drug is injected, "bridges have been burned," and a considerable time is generally needed for recovery from anesthesia and return of reflex control of the airway. In contrast, for a patient to eventually become anesthetized with an inhalational technique requires that the airway be maintained and ventilation continued throughout the induction period. As induction proceeds, if the airway suddenly becomes obstructed as a result of the anesthetic state, ventilation ceases. However, the alveolar concentration of the anesthetic simultaneously decreases because the inflow of anesthetics into the lung has also ceased. The blood and brain concentrations of the anesthetic begin to immediately decline as the inhalational anesthetic continues to be rapidly redistributed to other tissue compartments throughout the body. The patient awakens and resumes control of the airway only a short time after airway obstruction is induced.

Advantages of an inhalational technique allow the airway to be tested as the patient becomes progressively anesthetized. Disadvantages are that if anesthetic-induced obstruction does occur, all of the hazards that accompany obstruction may still occur for a short period until the patient begins to awaken.

Finally, IV anesthesia with ketamine has been quite useful for short surgical procedures in the patient with a difficult airway. Ketamine works well as an anesthetic for somatic-type pain (skin and muscle) and has been useful in anesthetizing burn patients. A dissociative or catatonic state is produced. However, with intra-abdominal or intrathoracic type of surgical stimulation (visceral pain), ketamine alone is unsatisfactory. With ketamine anesthesia, airway tone and protective glottic reflexes usually remain remarkedly intact, and intubation is not required. In fact, pharyngeal stimulation often leads to laryngospasm. Thus, it is of limited use, since tracheal intubation may then subsequently be required under nonideal circumstances. However, ketamine has been extremely useful in many very difficult airway situations where tracheostomy would otherwise be necessary.

Laryngospasm

The definition of laryngospasm is a spasmatic closure of the larynx.[19] Phylogentically, laryngospasm is considered to be a protective reflex that prevents inspiration of noxious gases or aspiration of secretions and foreign bodies into the trachea. During anesthesia, laryngospasm is not uncommon, occurring in about 1% of a general population of patients and 2% of pediatric patients.[20] It may occur at any time, but typically it occurs during the induction and recovery from anesthesia in the twilight zones or periods of lighter anesthesia. Fink, in a classical article on laryngeal spasm, describes degrees of laryngeal spasm consisting of the three sphincteric levels of the larynx: the vocal cords, the false cords, and the aryepiglottic folds.[21] He describes varying degrees of spasm as related to "shutter" and "ball valve" mechanisms. The shutter mechanism consists of an active closure of the vocal cords via the adductor muscles of the larynx. The lateral cricoarytenoids and thyroarytenoids adduct the vocal cords by medially rotating the arytenoid cartilages. The ball valve mechanism occurs as the false cords and tissue between the hyoid bone and notch of the thyroid cartilage (preepiglottic body) are compressed. With contraction of the strap muscles, the hyoid and thyroid cartilages are drawn together, and the false cords and preepiglottic body become approximated to produce the ball valve mechanism.

Laryngeal spasm is a reflex autonomic reflex mediated by the vagus nerve through medullary control mechanisms. The reflex response occurs through sensory and motor innervation of the superior laryngeal nerve, which is a branch of the vagus nerve.[22, 23] Numerous reflexes such as spasm of the glottis, bronchospasm, apnea, bradycardia, cardiac dysrhythmias, and arterial hypotension can occur as a result of laryngovagal reflexes.[24] The afferent pathway for laryngospasm is induced by noxious stimuli, irritating gases, excessive secretions, or foreign bodies in the oropharynx. Extrinsic pain pathways from intense surgical stimulation of thoracic and abdominal viscera can also induce intense laryngospasm. Clinicians may sometimes use the term laryngospasm quite freely to describe either complete airway obstruction or partial airway obstruction with expiratory stridor and inspiratory stridor. Partial airway obstruction may result as decreased muscle tone is induced by the action of anesthetics or an active vocal resistance of the stuporous excited patient. Such obstruction is frequently accomplished by musical, high-pitched sounds, which may herald the onset of a complete obstruction mediated by an intense spasmotic closure of the larynx. Thus, from a clinical standpoint, laryngospasm is a process that occurs on a continuum from a partial to a complete emergency airway obstruction.

Clinically, laryngeal spasm is twice as common in children, perhaps as a result of a combination or heightened protective reflexes, smaller airway size, or a tendency to have more secretions throughout the airway. In addition, inhalational anesthetic induction techniques and barbiturates, which are quite advantageous in children, may be more likely to produce circumstances that precipitate laryngospasm.[25] The most dreaded complications that can occur from laryngospasm are hypoxia progressing to cardiac arrest and serious neurologic damage or death. Aspiration is a serious complication that can follow misadventures in airway management as a result of laryngospasm.

Prevention

Management of laryngospasm should be directed primarily at prevention. Laryngospasm can be induced by the accumulation of excessive secretions in the oropharynx and posterior pharynx, cough reflexes induced by the irritating effects of noxious anesthetic vapors, and excessive stimulation or manipulation of the upper airway in the lightly anesthetized patient. Preoperative medication with an antisialagogue drug such as atropine or glycopyrolate will decrease the potential for excessive secretions accumulating in the pharynx during the induction of anesthesia. In anticipation of potential aspiration, the histamine H_2 antagonists (cimetidine and ranitidine) can be used as a premedication to reduce the pH and volume of gastric secretions. Topical anesthesia sprayed over the oropharynx during the preinduction period or as induction proceeds is a useful adjunct to reduce the incidence of laryngospasm by blocking the afferent component of the reflex. Another advantage is that topical anesthesia allows oral manipulation such as the insertion of an oral airway at the critical time that the tongue relaxes and falls into the posterior pharynx to produce upper airway obstruction. Commonly in children, an inhalational induction technique is used. Such a technique requires patience, and a deliberate attempt is made to very slowly increase the concentration of the anesthetic vapor administered to the patient. During an inhalational induction of anesthesia, a sudden or rapid increase in the inhaled concentration of the anesthetic will invariably initiate coughing, breath holding, and laryngospasm. A similar analogy and response can be experienced if one suddenly inhales a very concentrated breath of an irritating vapor such as ammonia.

External rough manipulations of the head and neck, forceful ventilation, and premature stimulation of the tongue and pharynx during the induction period will incite laryngospasm in the lightly anesthetized patient. Airway management must be gentle, skillful, and executed with a soft touch at the right time.

Premature insertion of an oral airway in a lightly anesthetized patient can frequently precipitate coughing, bucking, breath holding, vomiting, and laryngospasm. There are conflicting reports that the prophylactic IV administration of 1.5 to 2 mg of lidocaine/kg will reduce the incidence of laryngospasm.[26, 27]

Management

Laryngospasm should not be confused with the most common cause of airway obstruction associated with the anesthetic state, which is loss of muscular tone and displacement of the tongue into the posterior pharynx. This is most successfully corrected with manual lifting of the jaw anteriorly and with the insertion of oral or nasal airways. Such a manual maneuver separates the hyoid and thyroid cartilage and thus removes the ball valve mechanism described earlier.[21] Partial obstruction caused by laryngospasm will generally improve as the depth of anesthesia is increased. Complete laryngospasm is initially treated with attempts to open the airway and insufflate oxygen under positive pressure past the obstruction. Some maintain that forceful positive pressure ventilation may be of no benefit and may worsen the situation by impelling anatomic obstruction and causing gastric distension.[21] This is important to realize, but in practice, controlled positive pressure ventilation, when coupled with anterior displacement of the mandible, may be quite effective and should be given a trial. If obstruction persists, 1.0 mg/kg IV succinylcholine is an emergency measure that should be initiated very early. If IV access is not available, 4 mg/kg of intramuscular succinylcholine is administered.[25] Direct laryngoscopy and intubation should rapidly be sequentially performed. Gastric distension should be avoided since it promotes or may initiate the process of vomiting, regurgitation, and aspiration. Following treatment of laryngospasm and successful intubation, any gastric distension should be relieved with a nasogastric tube.

Foreign Body

From an anesthetic standpoint, successful management of the patient with a foreign body in the airway again requires very careful planning, meticulous preparation for potential catastrophe, and a closely coordinated approach by the otolaryngologist and the anesthesiologist.[28, 29] A foreign body that acutely produces complete obstruction will require the Heimlich maneuver.[30] In infants, back blows and chest thrusts are recommended. Under less emergent circumstances, it is helpful, if possible, to know what the foreign body is and the present location. Is the foreign body above the vocal cords, in the trachea, in the esophagus, or in a bronchus? With radiopaque foreign bodies, a chest x-ray and lateral neck film are particularly useful, but in an acute life-threatening airway emergency, such diagnostic procedures waste valuable time.

In the cooperative patient, foreign bodies above the vocal cords usually can be removed atraumatically with topical anesthesia under direct visualization, but certain locations may require general anesthesia and endotracheal intubation to prevent dislodgment of the foreign body into the tracheobronchial tree. Such foreign bodies are usually immobile or have become fixed

since reflex and voluntary maneuvers by the patient have failed to free up or expell the object. Foreign bodies in the trachea, bronchi, or bronchioles may be impaled or may be quite mobile, depending on the length of time they have been in the tracheobronchial tree. These patients will always require a general anesthetic and direct bronchoscopy. Most commonly the patient is a young child who has aspirated a small foreign body, typically a bean, a peanut, or a small toy that has become lodged in a bronchus. Symptoms of foreign body in the airway are usually quite dramatic. Acutely, clinical symptomatology includes paroxysms of coughing, gagging, and bronchospasm. Eventually acute symptoms will abate, and inflammatory symptomatology will develop. In the lung, with time, pneumonia, atelectasis, or areas of hyperaeration usually accompany fever and leukocytosis.

Management

The anesthetic plan should include a careful preoperative assessment of the patient if at all possible. An excellent IV access is important to provide a lifeline for both anesthetic and any emergency drug administration. A unique competitive situation exists in that two or more individuals are working in the patient's airway. The anesthetist is maintaining ventilation; the endoscopist is searching for and removing the foreign body. A preoperative discussion and flexible plan should be developed and agreed on between the anesthetist and the endoscopist. Team work and mutual cooperation is mandatory. Routine and accessory airway equipment should be assembled and tested beforehand. The airway interface and connector links between the anesthetic equipment and the bronchoscopy equipment should be assured and tested for function. In addition, emergency equipment should include high-pressure jet ventilatory equipment, tracheostomy equipment, and an emergency resuscitation cart. A defibrillator should be readily available. Monitoring should include ECG, blood pressure, temperature, pulse oximetry, and capnography.

With foreign bodies in a bronchus, the patient is anesthetized using a rapid sequence technique. An anticholinergic drug (atropine or glycopyrolate) is administered to decrease secretions and prevent dangerous bradycardias from vagal stimulation. A precurarizing dose of a nondepolarizing muscle relaxant is administered intravenously to prevent fasciculation. This is followed by an appropriate dose of a short-acting barbiturate and succinylcholine. The Sellick maneuver (manual cricoid pressure) is applied by an assistant, and the trachea is rapidly intubated. The Sellick maneuver, via compressing the cricoid ring against the esophagus, reduces the potential for aspiration of gastric contents should regurgitation or vomiting occur during induction. Following intubation, the stomach is suctioned with a nasogastric tube. The endotracheal tube is replaced with a ventilating bronchoscope. Anesthesia is maintained with an inhalation anesthetic (halothane or isoflurane) and 100% oxygen administered through the bronchoscope. In most situations, muscle relaxation is continued with a succinylcholine drip (1 mg/mL) at a rate to maintain muscle paralysis. A neuromuscular monitor is used to access the intensity of paralysis. Ventilation is controlled and monitored by close observation, auscultation of the chest, pulse oximetry, and capnography. Ventilation performed by an educated hand is preferred over ventilation with a mechanical ventilator. Abrupt changes in airway compliance are immediately perceived with hand ventilation. Periods of partial ventilation and elective apnea are sometimes necessary as the endoscopist searches in a bronchus for the foreign body. These periods are carefully monitored and interrupted with periodic withdrawal of the bronchoscope back into the trachea to improve oxygenation and normalize CO_2. With removal of the foreign body, the bronchus is reexamined and alternately lavaged, suctioned, and the lung reexpanded. Tracheal aspirates should be sent for bacteriology analysis and culture. Once the foreign body and the bronchoscope are removed, the patient is reintubated and the succinylcholine drip is discontinued. With full return of muscle strength, the patient is awakened and then extubated. In the recovery area, a chest film is obtained to evaluate the lung fields and rule out pneumothorax. These patients are likely to have large areas of pneumonia and atelectasis that will require oxygen and aggressive physical therapy into the recovery period.

One particular problem that may be associated with the management of foreign bodies is an abscess in the airway. A postobstructive purulent asphyxiation syndrome can occur following spontaneous or elective drainage of an abscess in the upper airway or in the lung. With removal of a foreign body or incision and drainage of an abscess, purulent material can potentially enter the lung. With elective drainage of an abscess in the upper airway, the lung should be protected from aspiration by insertion of a cuffed endotracheal tube or tracheostomy tube. After insertion and inflation of a cuffed tube, the supraglottic area can be further protected with gauge packing and the head positioned down to provide conditions that will reduce the chance of aspiration once the abscess is electively drained. Another clinical situation where postobstructive purulent asphyxiation may occur is following the removal of a foreign body from a chronically obstructed bronchus. In this situation, purulent material is released to subsequently contaminate the contralateral or normal lung. In the management of adults with obstructed bronchi or lung abscess, the use of double-lumen endotracheal tubes can be highly effective in isolating the normal lung from areas of hemoptysis or purulent material released as a result of removing a foreign body or bronchial plug. Unfortunately, this problem is more common in children who have aspirated foreign material or organic matter such as a peanut or a bean, as has just been described. Double-lumen endotracheal tubes are not available and impractical for small children because of the very small airways. In children, it is important to aggressively suction the purulent material, which may be released in large quantities following removal of the foreign body. Positioning the child with the obstructed side and head down may facilitate gravity drainage and minimize aspiration into the normal lung.

Laryngeal Trauma

The anesthesiologist is frequently called on an emergent basis to treat a variety of airway emergencies in the trauma victim.[31–35] There are classic blunt traumatic syndromes that are important to immediately recognize if the patient is experiencing airway problems as a result of direct trauma to the chest, neck, and larynx. One classical example is the driver of an automobile who was wearing a seat belt and was involved in a high-speed deacceleration-type accident. Following sudden impact and deacceleration, the patient's upper half is thrown forward. The chest and neck make a forceful blunt impact on the steering wheel or steering column. This situation can result in multiple, serious intrathoracic, head and neck injuries. Frequently the patient is in shock and requires fluid resuscitation. Pneumothorax, hemothorax, cardiac tamponade, and myocardial contusion are emergency, life-threatening complications that should be suspected, promptly diagnosed, and treated.

It is not unusual for this type of injury to produce a fractured larynx. The patient with a fractured larynx presents in the emergency room with dysphonia, acute airway obstruction, pretracheal edema, hematemesis, echymosis, and subcutaneous emphysema of the neck and thorax. Fracture of the cervical spine must also be suspected and carefully evaluated. The preferred treatment of a fractured larynx is tracheostomy under local anesthesia.[31,34,35] This should certainly be expedited and performed by surgeons highly experienced with such an emergency surgical procedure. Cricothyrotomy may be a lifesaving procedure under emergency circumstances. Endotracheal intubation must be avoided in an effort to prevent further damage to the larynx. Following tracheostomy the patient should continue to be carefully evaluated for intrathoracic injuries. Surgical procedures of the larynx are performed electively once the patient has stabilized from other accompanying life-threatening injuries. An example of the disastrous consequences of endotracheal intubation in a patient with a fractured larynx is seen in Figure 44–6. The initial intubation resulted in insertion of the tube into the soft tissue of the neck, massive subcutaneous emphysema, and bilateral pneumothorax. A second endotracheal tube was inserted through an emergency tracheostomy and can be seen within the trachea. Pneumothorax was treated with bilateral chest tube insertion.

Atlanto-Occipital Subluxation in Rheumatoid Arthritis

Airway management in the patient with rheumatoid arthritis can be complicated by cervical neck deformities, temporal mandibular joint fixation, and arthritic involvement of the arytenoid cartilages.[36] The extent of these problems can usually be ascertained by a careful history and physical examination. A cautious inspection and range of motion examination should be performed for the mandible and the cervical spine. A past history of hoarseness and upper airway obstruction during an acute exacerbation of the rheumatoid disease is highly suggestive of arthritic involvement of the arytenoid cartilages. The inability to open the mouth occurs with advanced disease as fixation of the tempomandibular joint develops. The latter problem will necessitate an awake nasal intubation with the flexible fiberoptic bronchoscope and the potential for elective tracheotomy.

A particularly dangerous situation may exist in the patient with advanced rheumatoid arthritic cervical neck disease. Degeneration and involvement of the cervical vertebral bodies can

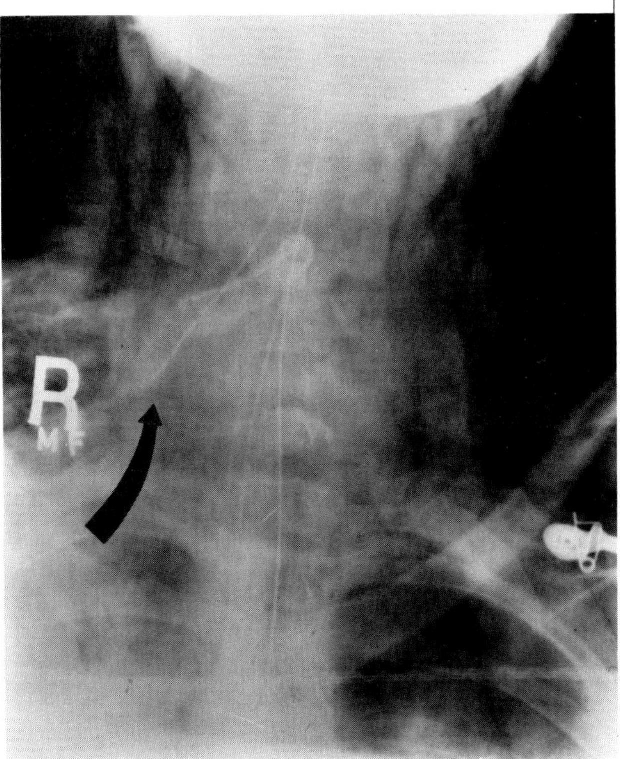

FIG 44–6.
This patient developed an unrecognized fractured larynx following an automobile accident. An initial endotracheal tube was inadvertently placed into the soft tissue of the neck (*arrow*). A second endotracheal tube, which was placed through an emergency tracheostomy, can also be visualized. Note the subcutaneous emphysema in the neck. Bilateral pneumothorax required chest tube placement.

produce an instability of the vertebral column, and the real possibility for fracture or subluxation of the atlanto-occipital joint exists during endotracheal intubation. Subluxation, or dislocation of the vertebrae, is a disastrous complication that has the potential to produce spinal cord transection and death. As the rheumatoid arthritic process progresses, synovial hypertrophy results in stretching or rupture of the transverse ligaments of the first cervical vertebra (C-1). This process allows subluxation of C-1 on C-2. It is therefore extremely important to obtain lateral radiographs of the cervical spine in both flexion and extension in patients with advanced cervical neck disease to evaluate any already existing subluxation (Fig 44–7). The use of muscle relaxants, combined with any forceful manipulations of the neck during intubation, has the grave potential to produce those conditions that will precipitate further subluxation and spinal cord damage.

Patients with advanced arthritic disease who cannot extend their necks or who have the potential for subluxation will require an awake fiberoptic intubation if a general anesthetic is indicated. Fiberoptic intubation is performed as previously described. Certainly if general anesthesia can be avoided, a regional technique is preferred. It is important to realize that other disease states such as osteoporosis, local or metastatic lytic lesions, and connective tissue disorders also have the potential

to produce cervical spine fracture or subluxation during intubation.

Complications

Pharyngeoesophageal Injury

Iatrogenic trauma and injury to the pharynx and esophagus is always a possibility whenever airways, endotracheal tubes, and nasogastric tubes are inserted into patients. Certainly in inexperienced hands or during emergency circumstances, such injuries can occur in patients with normal anatomy. However, the chance of injury is much more likely to patients who are difficult to intubate or who have pathologic inflammatory or neoplastic processes in the nose, mouth, posterior pharynx, esophagus, and larynx.

The process of intubation with a laryngoscope may sometimes require considerable force that may fracture teeth, injure nerves (lingual, hypogossal), and produce bleeding or tears anywhere along the airway or esophagus. The forceful insertion of an endotracheal tube blindly may dissect through the pharyngeoesophageal mucosa and may be directed into the soft tissue of the neck or into false passages of the mediastinum. A metal stylet protruding distal to the tip of an endotracheal tube is particularly dangerous in that it may tear the pharynx, larynx, trachea, or esophagus. Such false passages or tears produce catastrophic complications as positive pressure is applied into the tissue deadspace created by the injury. Mediastinal emphysema, pneumopericardium, and unilateral or bilateral tension pneumothorax rapidly lead to hypoxia, reduced cardiac output, hypotension, and cardiac arrest. In addition, such tears can produce acute hemorrhage and later inflammatory processes, which within the mediastinum carry a very high mortality. Rarely, blunt trauma or iatrogenic trauma during endoscopy procedures can produce tracheoesophageal fistula.[37]

Nasal tubes (endotracheal or nasogastric) should be inserted with extreme caution in patients with head and neck trauma. Tubes may be misdirected through fractures of the cribiform plate and into brain tissue. More commonly, posterior nosebleeds, adenoidectomy, and submucosal dissection into the pharyngeal sphincters can occur even in patients with normal anatomy. The latter problem is not uncommon with the insertion of nasogastric tubes where resistance is met and the tube cannot be visualized but can be palpated submucosally in the posterior pharynx.

Prevention.—Awareness and caution of such major complications should serve to alert one to pay particular attention to the earlier axion, "If it don't fit, don't force it!" Particular situations where serious supraglottic inflammatory lesions or large, vascular tumors prevent easy access to the larynx are best approached by elective tracheostomy.

Recurrent Nerve Palsy

Unilateral and bilateral vocal cord paralysis is an unusual complication of endotracheal intubation.[38,39] It occurs more commonly in adults than children, with a predilection for males.

EXTENSION

FLEXION

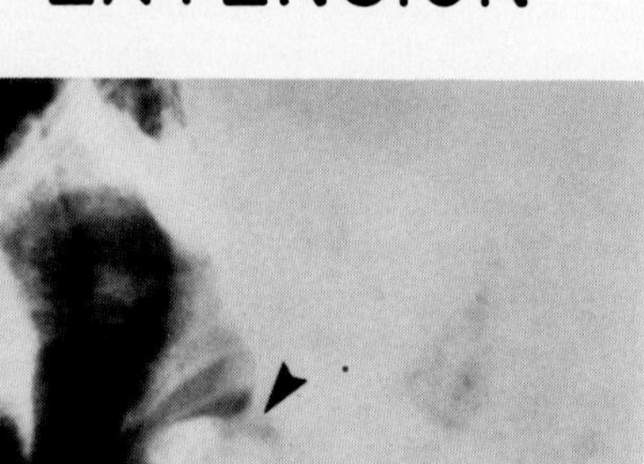

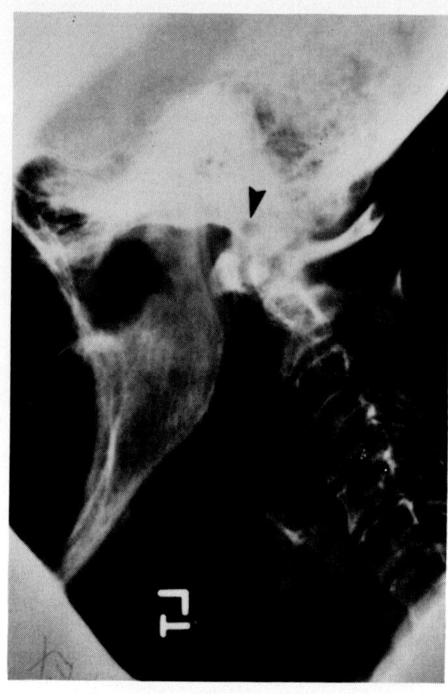

FIG 44–7.
Lateral flexion and extension radiographs of the cervical spine in a patient with rheumatoid arthritis. Note the area of subluxation of C = 1 on C = 2 (*arrows* point to opened space) with flexion of the neck.

Following endotracheal intubation and extubation, the patient will usually develop hoarseness and may sometimes experience aspiration of liquids with swallowing. The etiology of this complication is unclear. Ellis and Pallister have proposed that excessive cuff pressure exerted on the recurrent laryngeal nerve produces a traumatic neuropraxis.[38] In cadaver specimens, they have demonstrated that pressure can be exerted on the recurrent laryngeal nerve as it passes in the tracheoesophageal groove in close proximity to the inflated cuff of the endotracheal tube. Another explanation, proposed by Ellis, is that many patients may have an asymptomatic vocal cord paralysis prior to endotracheal intubation.[40] As a result of intubation, any local inflammation or edema of the cords would precipitate hoarseness, and on subsequent examination, the diagnosis of recurrent laryngeal nerve palsy would be made and intubation falsely incriminated as the cause. Prevention of this complication is best performed by gentle laryngoscopy, avoidance of oversized trachea tubes, and the use of high compliant, low-pressure endotracheal tube cuffs. During extubation, one should make sure that the cuff is fully deflated prior to extubation.

Recurrent laryngeal palsies may be temporary or permanent. Other important etiologies such as intrathoracic neoplasms and aneurysms of the aortic arch should be ruled out. Vocal cord paralysis may be associated with surgical procedures such as thyroidectomy or intrathoracic procedures involving the aortic arch. In the case of a bilateral nerve palsy, serious airway obstruction will necessitate reintubation or tracheostomy.

INTRAOPERATIVE PROBLEMS

Tracheal Fire

The word, "laser" is an abbreviation for *l*ight *a*mplification by *s*timulated *e*mission of *r*adiation. The laser beam has provided the surgeon with an exciting new tool—a microscalpel. One important medical application that continues to expand is microsurgery of the larynx and trachea. The microscalpelular laser beam can be precisely directed to meticulously excise localized pathologic lesions. Such a technique provides excellent conditions for the removal of small tumors such as laryngeal papillomas. The laser is particularly advantageous since microdissection can be performed in a relatively bloodless field and specifically focused to prevent damage to adjacent tissue. Numerous types of lasers have been applied to medicine, ruby, argon, neodymium–yttrium aluminum garnet (Nd-YAG), helium, neon, and CO_2.[41] The CO_2 laser has most commonly been used in otolaryngology. The beam produces an infrared light at 10,600 nm of wavelength that is invisible to the human eye.[41]

The potential for a fire requires three components: a spark, a combustible material, and oxygen. Historically, the use of flammable anesthetics and the introduction of electrocautery and sophisticated monitoring devices (ECG) into an anesthetizing location, produced the inevitable: fire and catastrophic explosion. After many explosive disasters involving serious injury to the patient and the operating team, flammable anesthetics such as ether, cyclopropane, and fluroxene were removed from the operating room environment. The incidence of operating room explosions and fires was greatly diminished. With the advent of modern laser surgery of the larynx, the problem of tracheal fires was rekindled. The high-energy laser beam produces the spark; the endotracheal tube, the combustible material and, of course, high flows of oxygen are in close proximity. The endotracheal or tracheostomy tube is at particular risk to ignite and burn.[41–44] Any other flammable objects such as airways, nasogastric tubes, or esophageal stethoscopes also have the potential to burn.

Prevention

Awareness of the problem, precautionary measures, and an emergency preconceived fire drill protocol are essential to both prevention and management of such a disaster. The surgeon can be particularly cautious and meticulous in attempting to avoid direct or prolonged bombardment of the endotracheal tube with the laser beam. No matter how cautious one is, because of the proximity and special confines of the surgical exposure, the tube is always at risk to be ignited. My approach, as well as others', is to protect the target areas of the endotracheal tube or tracheostomy tube with self-adherent aluminum tape, which is carefully applied to the tube beforehand. I use a type of tape that has been recommended and experimentally tested by others.[45] Realistic no. 100 metallic sensing tape no. 44-1155 can be obtained from the local Radio Shack Store (Radio Shack Corp., Fort Worth). Care must be taken in applying the tape to assure that the area to be exposed is covered. The metallic tape should be neatly and meticulously applied to the dry surface of the tube. The tape should be carefully trimmed to avoid any rough or sharp edges that could damage airway mucosa. In addition, inflammable endotracheal or tracheostomy tubes specially designed for laser surgery such as the Laser-Shield Endotracheal Tube (silicone elastomer; XOMED, Jacksonville, Fla.) and the Laser-Flex Tracheal Tube (metal; Mallinckrodt, Inc., Glenn Falls, N.Y.) are commercially available. Another recommended measure is to reduce the inspired oxygen concentration during the anesthetic.[45, 46] In the event a fire does occur, the intensity of the flame should be greatly reduced by this measure. Most recently, an He protocol for laryngotracheal operations with a CO_2 laser has been used.[46, 48] A 60% concentration of He with a forced inspiratory oxygen (Fio_2) concentration of 0.4 (40% oxygen) was used in more than 500 patients. A special polyvinylchloride tube without barium marking was used (Mallinckrodt, Inc.). Barium used to mark tubes increases the flammability. Only one instance of flash fire was reported, and this occurred in a patient in which the Fio_2 concentration was inadvertently increased to 0.70. The advantage of such a technique reportedly allows one to use ordinary polyvinylchloride endotracheal tubes. Another safety measure is to fill the endotracheal tube cuff with saline rather than air. If the cuff does become ruptured by the laser, an automatic fire extinguishing mechanism is activated as the saline escapes through the burning puncture site.

Management

In the case of the burning endotracheal tube, three immediate problems arise: (1) extinguishing the fire, (2) reestablishing the airway, and (3) treating the tissue burn. A preconceived stepwise fire drill protocol is useful:

1. Fire! Immediately and simultaneously the endoscopist should disconnect the tube from the anesthetic circuit and quickly remove the burning endotracheal or tracheostomy tube.
2. The tube is placed into a prepared bucket of water to extinguish the fire. (A portable fire extinguisher should also be in the immediate area.)
3. The patient is immediately reintubated with an endotracheal or tracheotomy tube, which should be held in readiness and made available by the anesthesiologist.
4. The tube is reconnected to the anesthesia circuit, and ventilation is resumed. The patient's airway will usually be easily visualized since a suspension laryngoscope is in place and the patient is paralyzed. However, since the patient is paralyzed, reintubation and resumption of ventilation must occur without delay to avoid hypoxia.

The third problem is the extent of burn damage to the posterior pharynx, larynx, and trachea. Minor localized burns, which are most commonly reported, are treated systemically by the IV administration of steroids to reduce inflammation (1 mg/kg dexamethazone) and antibiotics to prevent infection. Major airway burns may require tracheostomy and subsequent debridement.

Other Patient and Personnel Safety Precautions

Other dangerous complications can occur with the CO_2 laser. Damage to the eye is a particular hazard to both the patient and the medical personnel caring for the patient. The patient's eyes should have a soluble eye ointment applied, the lids taped, and protecting moisturized eye patches applied. All operating room personnel should wear protective eye goggles. Ordinary eye glasses are effective in blocking penetration of the laser beam into the eye. Entrances to an operating room area where the laser is being used should clearly caution circulating personnel of the potential for eye damage.

Inadvertent Extubation

Prevention of intraoperative extubation requires sophistication in initial placement, securement, and continual vigilance of the endotracheal tube. Inadvertent intubation is extremely uncommon in adult patients who have cuffed endotracheal tube since the inflated balloon itself tends to securely stabilize the tube. However, if the cuff is placed high and becomes situated within the larynx as the balloon is inflated, there is a natural tendency for extubation to occur. Because of the funnel-shaped anatomy of the larynx, with inflation of the cuff, the tube is self-extruded. This is a common cause of the leaking cuff in intensive care patients on ventilators where the tube and cuff may migrate to become situated between or above the cords. The distal end of the tube should be placed into the midtracheal area and taped securely. I prefer to place tape circumferentially around the upper part of the neck over the maxilli and securely around the tube. Benzoin applied to the skin is useful to enhance stability.

Children certainly have the highest risk of developing inadvertent extubation. In children, one can conveniently use the centimeter markings on the endotracheal tube to judge the distance that the tube is inserted. One useful technique to safely position the endotracheal tube in children has been recently described by Bloch et al.[49] The patient is intubated and the tube intentionally advanced into a mainstem bronchus, usually the right. This is determined by auscultation and observation of the chest. With the head in a neutral position, the tube is pulled back slowly just to the carina, where suddenly breath sounds are auscultated bilaterally. By observation of the centimeter markings on the tube at the teeth, the tube is then pulled back 2 cm from the carina. The tube is positioned in the midline and taped. The tape is placed around the tube and bilaterally over the buccal tissue under tension, which causes the lips to be folded in such a way to create a fish mouth appearance.[50] It is important to remember that extension and flexion of the neck can move the tube several centimeters, which in a child, if the tube is placed high in the neck, could lead to extubation; if the tube is placed too low, it could lead to endobronchial intubation.

Ripoll et al. reported an increased incidence of spontaneous dislocation of endotracheal tubes while experimenting with a new softer model polyvinylchloride tube.[51] One third of those intensive care patients orally intubated with the softer tube managed to extubate themselves spontaneously. The investigators attributed these extubations to the inspiratory pressures during mechanical ventilation forcing the tube cephalad as a result of unopposed rigidity of the softer tube. An analogy can be made to a cork popping out of a champagne bottle. Thus, endotracheal tubes made with softer plastic materials are more likely to result in spontaneous extubation.

My clinical impression is that nasal tracheal intubation improves stability and is far more comfortable for the patient. Particularly in children, I have found that the nasotracheal route is more stable and therefore decreases the incidence of spontaneous extubation in an intensive care environment. My colleagues and I have also used endotracheal stabilizing devices that incorporate rigid struts attached distally to the tube and secured to the forehead and maxilli with tape or Velcro material.[52, 53] Securing the tube to the fixed portion of the face (maxilli area) with tincture of benzoin and multiple strips of high-quality adherent tape is usually sufficient in the anesthetized patient.

During surgery, the most common times when a tube becomes accidentally dislodged is when the airway is covered up by drapes or when the tube is being moved to facilitate surgical exposure, such as during tonsillectomy. These situations can be prevented, recognized, and efficiently managed only by constant vigilance of the anesthesiologist and the otolaryngologist. Over the past decade, monitors of the airway interface such as capnography have become an invaluable aid in assisting anesthesiologists in their vigilance. Inadvertent extubation requires that

equipment be immediately available to manage the airway, particularly in the paralyzed patient. Face mask, ventilation bag, oral-nasal airways, and an extra styleted endotracheal tube should always be prepared and ready, both in the operating room and during transport.

Massive Subcutaneous Emphysema

Subcutaneous emphysema is the result of an air leak occurring somewhere within the respiratory tree. The source of the leak can occur from a surgical manipulation, a direct tear during endoscopy, or barotrauma to the respiratory tree. The communication from the leak to the subcutaneous tissue usually expands as air dissects along certain planes of connective tissue in the chest, in the neck, and into the subcutaneous tissue. The extent of spread is directly influenced by pressure within the airway. Pneumopericardium and pneumothorax may initiate the process or accompany it. Rupture of bronchioles within the lung parenchyma may initially present as pneumopericardium as air dissects from the ruptured bronchi retrograde up the sheath enclosing the bronchioles and vascular structures, back into the tissue planes of the mediastinum, and into the pericardium. Air may continue to dissect through the parietal pleura into the pleural cavity and produce a life-threatening tension pneumothorax, necessitating emergency chest tube insertion. This sequence of events is usually associated with adult or neonatal respiratory distress syndromes being treated with positive pressure ventilation and positive end-expiratory pressure (PEEP).

Trauma to the neck may produce a tear in the larynx or the tracheal rings and likewise produce subcutaneous emphysema into the neck and chest wall area. Air may dissect retrograde into the chest and produce a pneumothorax that again will require emergency chest tube insertion. An important principle in the spontaneously breathing patient is to minimize expiratory obstruction since any increase in obstruction above the leak will increase pressure and facilitate the volume of air escaping through the leak and into the tissue. Air leaks of the upper airway or trachea should be isolated by placing a cuffed tube distal to the leak. Tracheostomy will be required with damage to the larynx or upper trachea. A reinforced endotracheal tube placed at the carina through a tracheostomy can bypass midtracheal tears. During positive pressure ventilation, inspiratory pressures must be kept to a minimum, and one must be on guard for the development of a tension pneumothorax. Bilateral chest tube insertion may be necessary. Potential planes for dissection of air from tears along the airway are diagrammed in Figure 44–8.

Subcutaneous air may involve the head, neck, chest, and abdomen and may even dissect into the scrotum. Pneumopericardium is usually self-limiting and requires no treatment. The appearance of such massive infiltration of air may look quite frightening, but usually no harm is done if the airway is protected from the life-threatening complication of tension pneumothorax, which should be anticipated and aggressively treated with chest tubes. When anesthetizing these patients, one should avoid nitrous oxide; since any closed air spaces may enlarge as nitrous oxide diffuses into such spaces.

PROBLEMS FOLLOWING EXTUBATION

A number of acute airway problems may develop shortly after extubation of the trachea. Laryngospasm, postobstructive pulmonary edema, postintubation croup, and aspiration are complications that will require aggressive therapy once they develop. In the majority of situations, it is preferable to extubate the patient after important survival reflexes have returned. As consciousness returns, the ability to take a deep breath, to swallow, to cough, and to follow simple verbal commands may prevent such problems as laryngospasm or aspiration. If laryngospasm does develop after extubation, the therapy is identical to that described earlier.

Acute Problems

Postobstructive Pulmonary Edema

Postobstructive pulmonary edema is a rare syndrome that occurs in patients who have experienced airway obstruction and have developed high-inspiratory negative intrathoracic airway pressures as a result of the obstruction.[54] Upper airway obstruction may be a result of unconsciousness, laryngospasm, epiglottitis, or foreign body. Conditions that favor the formation of acute pulmonary edema are created as a result of high subatmospheric transpulmonary pressure gradients, associated changes in cardiovascular function, and hypoxia.[55] With the re-

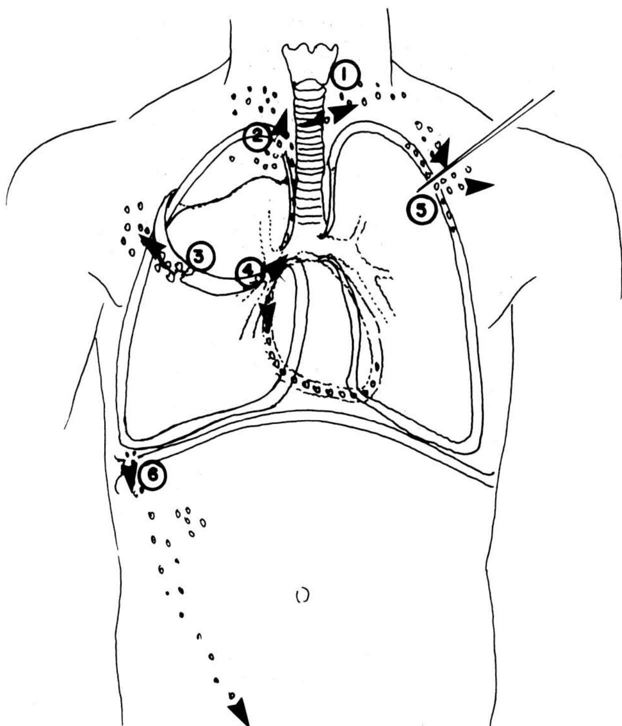

FIG 44–8.
Potential planes for dissection of air from tears along the airway: *1,* larynx and trachea; *2,* ruptured lung bulla; *3–5,* penetrating injuries or barotrauma to the lung; *6,* rupture of the diaphragm. Pneumothorax and pneumopericardium are common sequelae.

lief of the obstruction, pulmonary edema acutely develops. The treatment of postobstructive pulmonary edema includes reestablishing an airway and aggressive oxygen therapy.[56] Positive airway pressure may be necessary. Facial continuous positive airway pressure (CPAP), endotracheal CPAP, and controlled ventilation with PEEP are measures that will be selected depending on the severity of the patient's condition. Morphine (0.05 mg/kg) can be titrated for sedation; however, digoxin and steroids are usually not indicated in previously healthy patients.[56] The sitting position is helpful, and diuretics may be beneficial in selected patients.

Postintubation Croup

Postintubation croup is a syndrome that usually occurs in children 1 to 4 years of age following endotracheal intubation. In a large series of pediatric patients (7,875), the incidence of postintubation croup was 1%.[57] Postintubation croup is usually associated with an excessively large endotracheal tube and traumatic manipulations of the airway. Preventive measures include the use of a gentle atraumatic intubation technique and appropriately sized endotracheal tubes. The endotracheal tube should fit loosely enough in the larynx to allow a slight leak with positive pressure ventilation. A snugly fitting tube should be removed and replaced with a smaller-sized tube. Following intubation, excessive movement and manipulations of the tube should be avoided. The pathophysiology of croup is an edematous swelling of the larynx, which may involve the supraglottic, retroarytenoidal, and subglottic areas.[24] However, the subglottic area is the narrowest position of the airway and is most effected by an excessively large tube. Both viral and postintubation croup can be very effectively and dramatically treated with nebulized racemic epinephrine (Vaponephrin).[57–60] The dosage I use is 0.5 mL of a 2.25% solution of racemic epinephrine diluted in 4.5 mL of saline. Small amounts of the diluted racemic epinephrine are placed in a hand-held, acorn-type nebulizer with a 10-L oxygen flow and applied with a mask to the spontaneously breathing sitting child. Improvement usually occurs within 5 to 10 minutes of the inhalation therapy. The ECG should be carefully monitored. Racemic epinephrine has less beta effects when compared with epinephrine but is systemically absorbed and has the potential to produce cardiac dysrhythmias. Downs recommends that the total dosage of racemic (DL form) epinephrine nebulized not exceed the following over a 10-minute period: 2.5 mg for a 5 kg child, 5.0 mg for a 10 kg child, and 10.0 mg for a 20 kg child.[61] I also administer a single IV dose of 1 mg of dexamethasone (Decadron)/kg, which clinically has proved useful. Steroid therapy has been shown to be effective for croup in humans and in animal models of subglottic edema.[62–64] Failure to respond to racemic epinephrine and steroids is quite unusual; however, if the condition progresses, other measures such as reintubation may be necessary.

Aspiration Pneumonitis

Aspiration pneumonitis, or Mendelson's syndrome, is a most serious and life-threatening complication that must be treated very aggressively.[65] Aspiration of stomach contents produces a rapidly progressive diffuse chemical burn to the lung parenchyma. The extent of the chemical burn to the lung will be directly related to the pH and the volume of the aspirate.

Pathophysiology.—Damage to the lung parenchyma produces the acute onset of physiologic derangements that markedly interfere with respiratory gas exchange. Pulmonary edema, bronchospasm, atelectasis, and compliance changes rapidly progress as hypoxia, acidosis, and hypercarbia develop. The alveolar to arterial oxygen difference (A-aO$_2$ difference) is increased as physiologic shunting occurs in areas of the lung that are perfused but not ventilated. The deadspace to tidal volume (V_D/V_t) increases in areas that are ventilated but not perfused. These physiologic derangements produce extensive ventilation-perfusion abnormalities throughout the lung.

Prevention.—Preventive measures include making the patient take nothing by mouth and altering the stomach pH by the use of antacids and the prophylactic use of histamine H$_2$ antagonists drugs (e.g., cimetidine and ranitidine) that decrease the pH and volume of gastric secretions. A rapid sequence induction technique and the Sellick maneuver are useful measures to prevent aspiration during the induction of anesthesia. Trauma victims, comatose patients, obese patients, and patients with delayed gastric emptying or increased intra-abdominal pressure (e.g., pregnant patients in labor, those with bowel obstruction) have clinical conditions that predispose them to aspiration. In such high-risk patients, decompression of the stomach with nasogastric drainage is beneficial prior to the induction of general anesthesia.

Treatment.—Treatment of aspiration is extremely complicated and requires sophisticated oxygen therapy, endotracheal intubation, mechanical ventilation, and PEEP. Prevention of cardiac failure, meticulous fluid and electrolyte balance, and prevention of secondary infection of the lung are important elements in the management of aspiration. The pathophysiology and treatment of aspiration pneumonitis have recently been extensively reviewed by Roberts.[66]

Delayed Problems

Postintubation Granuloma

In 1932, Clausen described a patient who developed a granuloma of the larynx as a result of endotracheal intubation.[67] Since that early description, numerous series of cases involving postintubation granuloma as a complication of endotracheal intubation have been reported and recently reviewed.[68] The incidence of occurrence in adult surgical patients who have been intubated for a short period ranges from 1 in 800 to 1 in 20,000 patients.[69, 70] The incidence is higher in "awake," actively moving patients who are intubated for longer periods in an intensive care environment. Women comprise 75% to 90% of reported cases, and intubation granuloma is extremely rare in children.[68] Patients with debilitating disease, malnutrition, and infectious processes are more likely to develop granuloma.

Typically, the patient develops a persistent or progressive hoarseness and the sensation of fullness in the throat, which may develop within days or months following endotracheal intubation. Occasionally the lesion may enlarge to the extent to produce partial airway obstruction. Rarely, polypoid granulomatous lesions may spontaneously autoamputate to be aspirated or coughed up. The area of the larynx most affected is the vocal process of the arytenoid cartilage, which comprises the posterior one third of the vocal cords. The posterior area of tissue adjacent to the cricoid cartilage may also be affected. These posterior locations correspond to the areas of highest pressure exerted by tension forces of the endotracheal tube as it curves into the larynx.[71] Lesions are usually right sided, which is probably related to the common anesthetic practice of securing the tube on the right side of the mouth.[71, 72] Such a practice likely produces more pressure on the right cord as a result of torque.

Pathology.—The pathology of postintubation granuloma is a process of healing by secondary intention. Following trauma and pressure, the very thin layer of epithelium is denuded, and an ulcer crater is formed. The ulcer is accompanied by edema, localized hemorrhage, and fibrin pseudomembrane formation. Since the denuded epithelium leaves a space that cannot easily be bridged by reepithelization, granulation tissue begins to accumulate along the margins of the ulcer. The granulation tissue may resolve, become sessile, or progressively evolve into a polypoid lesion that may autoamputate or require surgical excision.

Prevention.—Multiple factors will influence the development of granuloma formation. Traumatic intubations associated with blind or rapid sequence techniques are more likely to produce injury than smooth, atraumatic techniques using appropriately sized endotracheal tubes under direct vision. Endotracheal tube size, malleability, and stability of the tube are important factors to control. Of historical interest, one important cause of granuloma formation was related to methods used to clean and sterilize endotracheal tubes. Caustic chemicals from disinfecting solutions and ethylene oxide residues on endotracheal tubes produced toxic necrotizing reactions following direct contact of the tube with epithelial tissue of the larynx or trachea. Modern endotracheal tubes are sterilely packaged, are not reused, and must confirm to regulated standards. These standards require that tubes are made of inert materials that do not cause localized tissue irritation.

Bolestrieri and Watson have made the following recommendations for minimizing the development of laryngotracheal complications following endotracheal intubation[68]:

1. Avoidance of traumatic intubation (using muscle relaxants if possible)
2. Use of direct vision techniques for placement of the endotracheal tube
3. Use of smaller endotracheal tubes with appropriate cuff placement and pressure control
4. Use of soft, conforming intubation tubes of anatomic design
5. Stabilization of the head and neck to minimize movement of the intubation tube

6. Use of nontoxic lubricants and tube materials
7. Use of disposable sterile tubes
8. Limitation of the duration of cannulation to the necessary minimum time
9. Frequent assessment of intubation tube position for inadvertent displacement
10. Reexamination of the larynx and trachea when intubation is prolonged with change to another tube or route if tissue damage occurs

I agree with their recommendations.

Subglottic Stenosis

Tracheal subglottic stenosis is an extremely serious late complication of trauma, tracheostomy, and intubation that, when symptomatic, will require surgical intervention.[73–75] Adult patients become symptomatic when the tracheal lumen is reduced to a diameter of 4 to 5 mm.[76] A congenital form of subglottic stenosis is uncommon but becomes symptomatic very early in infancy.[77] The greatest number of acquired cases of subglottic stenosis are in critically ill patients who have required long-term intubation, usually for greater than 1 week.

In the literature, the incidence of stenosis as a result of prolonged endotracheal intubation and tracheostomy is estimated to be around 10% but is quite varied. An incidence of 0.5% of tracheal stenosis was found in a Swedish study of 457 patients with prolonged endotracheal intubation.[71] In this same study, with secondary tracheostomy, 33% of patients developed tracheal stenosis. In a more recent study of 150 critically ill patients, a 19% incidence of stenosis after prolonged endotracheal intubation and a 65% incidence after tracheostomy were found.[78] Following tracheostomy, stenosis can develop at the tracheal incision, at the distal end of the tracheostomy tube, or adjacent to the balloon cuff. The higher reported incidence of stenosis with tracheostomy is expected since these are patients who cannot be weaned from endotracheal tubes and require longer-term airway management. The decision to perform tracheostomy is usually made after a patient has been intubated for a considerable period of time and has failed to make significant clinical improvement. The specific time that an endotracheal tube should remain in a patient before tracheostomy is performed continues to be controversial.

The prevention of tracheal stenosis from prolonged intubation of the trachea requires the same approach as just described for granulomas. Steward has listed numerous factors involved in producing subglottic stenosis: traumatic intubation, duration of intubation, size and composition of the tube, sterilization methods, and presence of upper airway infections.[79] Additional factors are movement of the tube, both relative to the patient (e.g., piston effect of the ventilator) and relative to the tube (e.g., coughing, bucking).[79] The general medical status of the patient is also certainly important. Debilitated patients and patients in shock are certainly at greater risk to develop subglottic stenosis.

Over the past 20 years, significant progress has occurred in respiratory therapy and the understanding of those factors important in producing tracheal stenosis. One particularly important area is attention to prevent undue pressure and movement of the endotracheal or tracheostomy tube cuff. Large-volume, high-compliant softer cuffs, which have undoubtedly decreased tracheal injury and the incidence of tracheal stenosis at the cuff site, have been developed. Older low-volume, low-compliant cuffs exerted very high pressures on the tracheal mucosa and tracheal rings. The tracheal rings were stretched, and submucosal blood supply was compromised as intraluminal pressures exceeded 25 mm Hg. Localized tissue edema, necrosis, chondritis, and the ingrowth of granulomatous tissue produced severe scarring that resulted in tracheal stenosis. The use of softer cuffs and monitoring of cuff pressure have certainly decreased the pressure trauma exerted by the cuff, but subglottic stenosis has not been eliminated. One simple preventive measure to reduce tracheal tube movement in patients with tracheostomies is the insertion of a corrugated rubber tubing between the tracheostomy tube and the rigid ventilator tubing. This "shock absorber" greatly reduces the to-and-fro motion produced by the ventilator.[80] Finally, the importance of proper humidification of the inspired gases during long-term respiratory care cannot be overemphasized.

Anesthesia for patients with tracheal stenosis is quite challenging. Recently at my institution, a 5 kg infant with congenital subglottic stenosis was successfully repaired using a high-frequency jet ventilation technique.[77] For the majority of symptomatic patients, an inhalation induction technique has been recommended by Donlon.[81] Such a technique avoids the use of muscle relaxants and allows the patient to breath spontaneously. The endotracheal tube is placed well above the stenotic lesion to avoid trauma, bleeding, and obstruction at the narrowed area. Following surgical dissection and resection of the stenotic area, the tube is advanced distally and the anastomosis completed. In some patients in whom ventilation is extremely precarious, immediately following sternotomy, a second sterile endotracheal tube can be quickly placed by the surgeon distally into the incised normal trachea to bypass the stenotic area. A second sterile ventilatory system is connected to the distal tube, and controlled ventilation is resumed. Surgical dissection of the stenotic area and proximal trachea can then be leisurely performed. Following dissection and resection of the stenotic area, the original proximal endotracheal tube is advanced into the distal trachea and the anastomosis completed. Intraoperative airway pressure should be kept to a minimum. In adults, to avoid positive pressure ventilation in the postoperative period, I have preferred to extubate the patient at the end of the procedure. Nasal or oral airways may be necessary to prevent upper airway obstruction since the patient's neck is fixed in a flexed position to prevent undue tension on the suture line.

REFERENCES

1. Berry FA: Anesthesia for the child with a difficult airway, in *Anesthetic Management of Difficult and Routine Pediatric Patients.* New York, Churchill Livingstone, 1986, pp 137–168.
2. Schuderi PE, McLeskey CH, Comer PB: Emergency percutaneous transtracheal ventilation during anesthesia using readily available equipment. *Anesth Analg* 1982; 61:867–870.

3. Smith RB: Transtracheal ventilation during anesthesia. *Anesth Analg* 1974; 53:225–228.

4. DeLisser EA, Muravchick S: Emergency transtracheal ventilation. *Anesthesiology* 1981; 55:606–607.

5. White A, Kander PL: Anatomical factors in difficult direct laryngoscopy. *Br J Anaesth* 1975; 47:468–473.

6. Bedger RC, Chang J: A jet-stylet endotracheal catheter for difficult airway management. *Anesthesiology* 1987; 66:221–223.

7. Aro L, Takki S, Aromaa U: Technique for difficult intubation. *Br J Anaesth* 1971; 43:1081–1083.

8. Finucane BT, Kupshik HL: A flexible stilette for replacing damaged tracheal tubes. *Can Anaesth Soc J* 1978; 25:153–154.

9. Berman RA: Lighted stylet. *Anesthesiology* 1959; 20:382–383.

10. Henderson JB, Bontrager E, Morse HT: An articulated stylet for endotracheal intubation. *Anesthesiology* 1970; 32:71–73.

11. Powell WF, Oxdil T: A translaryngeal guide for tracheal intubation. *Anesth Analg* 1967; 46:231–234.

12. Linscott MS, Horton WC: Management of upper airway obstruction. *Atolaryngol Clin North Am* 1979; 12:351–373.

13. Ovassapian A, Dykes MHM: The role of fiber-optic endoscopy in airway management. *Semin Anesth* 1987; 6:93–104.

14. Mulder DS, Wallace DH, Woolhouse FM: The use of the fiberoptic bronchoscope to facilitate endotracheal intubation following head and neck trauma. *J Trauma* 1975; 15:638–640.

15. Watson CB: Fiberoptic bronchoscopy for anesthesia. *Anesthesiol Rev* 1982; 9(9):17–26.

16. Gotta AW, Sullivan CA: Anaesthesia of the upper airway using topical anaesthetic and superior laryngeal nerve block. *Br J Anaesth* 1981; 53:1055–1058.

17. Dripps RD, Eckenhoff JE, Vandam LD: *Introduction to Anesthesia: The Principles of Safe Practice,* ed 6. Philadelphia, WB Saunders Co, 1982, p 255.

18. Patil VU, Stehling LC, Zauder HL: *Fiberoptic Endoscopy in Anesthesia.* Chicago, Year Book Medical Publishers, 1983.

19. Agnew LRC, Aviado DM, Brody JI, et al: *Dorland's Illustrated Medical Dictionary,* ed 24. Philadelphia, WB Saunders Co, 1965.

20. Olsson GL, Hallen B: Laryngospasm during anaesthesia. A computer-aided incidence study in 136, 929 patients. *Acta Anaesthesiol Scand* 1984; 28:567–575.

21. Fink BR: The etiology and treatment of laryngeal spasm. *Anesthesiology* 1956; 17:569–577.

22. Allen RJ, Towsley HA, Wilson JL: Neurogenic stridor in infancy. *Am J Dis Child* 1954; 87:179–191.

23. Suzuki M, Sasaki CT: Laryngeal spasm: A neurophysiologic redefinition. *Ann Otol* 1977; 86:150–157.

24. Blanc VF, Tremblay NAG: The complications of tracheal intubation: A new classification with a review of the literature. *Anesth Analg* 1974; 53:202–213.

25. Roy WL, Lerman J: Laryngospasm in paediatric anaesthesia. *Can J Anaesth* 1988; 35:93–98.

26. Gefke K, Andersen LW, Friesel E: Lidocaine given intravenously as a suppressant of cough and laryngospasm in connection with extubation after tonsillectomy. *Acta Anaesthesiol Scand* 1983; 27:111–112.

27. Leicht P, Wisborg T, Chraemmer-Jorgensen B: Does intravenous lidocaine prevent laryngospasm after extubation in children? *Anesth Analg* 1985; 64:1193–1196.

28. Chatterji S, Chatterji P: The management of foreign bodies in air passages. *Anaesthesia* 1972; 27:390–395.

29. Woods AM: Pediatric bronchoscopy, bronchography, and laryngoscopy, in Berry FA (ed): *Anesthetic Management of Difficult and Routine Pediatric Patients.* New York, Churchill Livingstone, 1986, pp 241–244.

30. Standards and guidelines for cardiopulmonary resuscitation (CPR) and emergency cardiac care (ECC). *JAMA* 1986; 255:2905–2992.

31. Seed RF: Traumatic injury to the larynx and trachea. *Anaesthesia* 1971; 26:55–65.

32. Brandenburg JH: Management of acute blunt laryngeal injuries. *Otolaryngol Clin North Am* 1979; 12:741–751.

33. Alonso WA: Surgical management and complications of acute laryngotracheal disruption. *Otolaryngol Clin North Am* 1979; 12:753–760.

34. Yarington CT: Trauma involving the air and food passages. *Otolaryngol Clin North Am* 1979; 12:321–327.

35. Snow JB: Diagnosis and therapy for acute laryngeal and tracheal trauma. *Otolaryngol Clin North Am* 1984; 17:101–106.

36. Edelist G: Principles of anesthetic management in rheumatoid arthritic patients. *Anesth Analg* 1964; 43:227–231.

37. Schmitz GL: Acquired tracheoesophageal fistula. *Otolaryngol Clin North Am* 1979; 12:823–827.

38. Ellis PD, Pallister WK: Recurrent laryngeal nerve palsy and endotracheal intubation. *J Laryngol Otol* 1975; 89:823–826.

39. Hahn FW, Martin JT, Lillie JC: Vocal-cord paralysis. *Arch Otolaryngol* 1970; 92:226–229.

40. Ellis PDM: Letter to editor. *Anesthesiology* 1977; 46:375.

41. Birch AA: Anesthetic considerations during laser surgery. *Anesth Analg* 1973; 52:53–58.

42. Snow JC, Norton ML, Saluja TS et al: Fire hazard during CO_2 laser microsurgery on the larynx and trachea. *Anesth Analg* 1976; 55:146–147.

43. Norton ML: Anesthesia for laser surgery in laryngobronchoesophagology. *Otolaryngol Clin North Am* 1983; 16:785–791.

44. Snow JC, Kripke BJ, Jako GJ, et al: Anesthesia for carbon dioxide laser microsurgery on the larynx and trachea. *Anesth Analg* 1974; 53:507–512.

45. Patel KF, Hicks JN: Prevention of fire hazards associated with use of carbon dioxide lasers. *Anesth Analg* 1981; 60:885–888.

46. Burgess GE, JeJeune FE: Endotracheal tube ignition during laser surgery. *Arch Otolaryngol* 1979; 105:561–562.

47. Pashayan AG, Gravenstein JS: Helium retards endotracheal tube fires from carbon dioxide lasers. *Anesthesiology* 1985; 62:274–277.

48. Pashayan AG, Gravenstein JS, Cassisi NJ, et al: The helium protocol for laryngotracheal operations with CO_2 laser: A retrospective review of 523 cases. *Anesthesiology* 1988; 68:801–804.

49. Bloch EC, Ossey K, Ginsberg B: Tracheal intubation in children: A new method for assuring correct depth of the tube placement. *Anesth Analg* 1988; 67:590–592.

50. Bloch EC: Personal communication, 1988.

51. Ripoll I, Lindholm CE, Carroll R, et al: Spontaneous dislocation of endotracheal tubes. *Anesthesiology* 1978; 49:50–52.

52. Valley RD, Norfleet EA: Pediatric endotracheal tube management: A new method of tube stabilization. *Crit Care Q* 1985; 8:31–34.

53. Steward DJ, Conn AW: A clip to retain and support nasotracheal tubes. *Can Anesth Soc J* 1968; 15:397–398

54. Oswalt CE, Gates GA, Homstrom FMG: Pulmonary edema

as a complication of acute airway obstruction. *JAMA* 1977; 238:1833–1835.

55. Lee KWT, Downes JJ: Pulmonary edema secondary to laryngospasm in children. *Anesthesiology* 1983; 59:347–349.

56. Brown RE: Negative pressure pulmonary edema, in Berry FA (ed): *Anesthetic Management of Difficult and Routine Pediatric Patients.* New York, Churchill Livingstone, 1986, pp 169–178.

57. Koka BV, Jeon IS, Andre JM, et al: Postintubation croup in children. *Anesth Analg* 1977; 56:501–505.

58. Adair JC, Ring WH, Jordon WS: Ten year experience with IPPB in the treatment of acute laryngotracheobronchitis. *Anesth Analg* 1971; 50:649.

59. Westley CR, Cotton EK, Brooks JG: Nebulized racemic epinephrine by IPPB for the treatment of croup. *Am J Dis Child* 1978; 132:484–487.

60. Diaz JH: Croup and epiglottitis in children: The anesthesiologist as diagnostician. *Anesth Analg* 1985; 64:621–633.

61. Downes JJ, Godinez RI: Acute upper-airway obstruction in the child. *American Society of Anesthesiologists Refresher Courses in Anesthesiology.* Philadelphia, Lippincott Co, 1980, vol 8, p 29.

62. Deming MV, Oech SR: Steroid and antihistaminic therapy for post intubation subglottic edema in infants and children. *Anesthesiology* 1961; 22:933–936.

63. Postma DS, Jones RO, Pillsbury HC: Severe hospitalized croup: Treatment trends and prognosis. *Laryngoscope* 1984; 94:1170–1175.

64. Postma DS, Prazma J, Woods CI, et al: Use of steroids and a long-acting vasoconstrictor in the treatment of postintubation croup. *Arch Otolaryngol Head Neck Surg* 1987; 113:844–849.

65. Mendelson CL: The aspiration of stomach contents into the lungs during obstetric anesthesia. *Am J Obstet Gynecol* 1946; 52:191.

66. Roberts RB (ed): Pulmonary aspiration. *Int Anesthesiol Clin* 1977; 15:1.

67. Clausen RJ: Unusual sequelae of tracheal intubation. *Proc R Soc Med* 1932; 25:1507.

68. Balestrieri F, Watson CB: Intubation granuloma. *Otolaryngol Clin North Am* 1982; 15:567–579.

69. Howland WS, Lewis JS: Postintubation granulomas of the larynx. *Cancer* 1956; 9:1244–1247.

70. Snow JC, Harano M, Balogh K: Postintubation granuloma of the larynx. *Anesth Analg* 1966; 45:425–429.

71. Lindholm CE: Prolonged endotracheal intubation. *Acta Anesthesiol Scand (Suppl)* 1969; 33:1–125.

72. Epstein SS, Winston P: Intubation granuloma. *J Laryngol* 1957; 71:37.

73. Maniglia AJ: Tracheal stenosis: Conservative surgery as a primary mode of management. *Otolaryngol Clin North Am* 1979; 12:877–891.

74. Strome M: Subglottic stenosis: Therapeutic considerations. *Otolaryngol Clin North Am* 1984; 17:63–68.

75. Fry TL, Fischer ND, Pillsbury HC: Tracheal reconstruction with pedicled thyroid cartilage. *Laryngoscope* 1985; 95:60–62.

76. Applebaum EL, Bruce DL: *Tracheal Intubation.* Philadelphia, WB Saunders Co, 1976, p 87.

77. Schur MS, Maccioli GA, Azizkhan RG: High-frequency jet ventilation in the management of congenital tracheal stenosis. *Anesthesiology* 1988; 69:952–955.

78. Stauffer JL, Olson DE, Petty TL: Complications and consequences of endotracheal intubation and tracheotomy. *Am J Med* 1981; 70:65–76.

79. Steward DJ: Congenital abnormalities as a possible factor in the aetiology of post-intubation subglottic stenosis. *Can Anaesth Soc J* 1970; 17:388–390.

80. Andrews MJ, Pearson FG: Incidence and pathogenesis of tracheal injury following cuffed tube tracheostomy with assisted ventilation: Analysis of a two-year prospective study. *Ann Surg* 1971; 173:249–263.

81. Donlon JV: Anesthesia for eye, ear, nose and throat, in Miller RD (ed): *Anesthesia,* ed 2. New York, Churchill Livingstone, 1986, vol 3, pp 1858–1879.

Management of the Airway in Anesthesia

Approach of

Kathryn E. McGoldrick, M.D.

Intubation clearly allows easier access to the surgical field during head and neck surgery and is intended to guarantee the integrity of the airway. Nonetheless, despite improved techniques and equipment, anesthesiologists are unable to honestly guarantee that intubation of the trachea will be an entirely benign procedure. To begin with, it is not always easy to insert an endotracheal tube. Then, once the tube is inserted, the mere presence of a tracheal tube may lead to edema, inflammation, desquamation, and ulceration of the airway. The first three processes are usually self-limited; ulceration is more ominous.

Safe practice is based on gentleness, careful observation and thorough preparation, knowledge of anatomy and physiology, common sense, and ever-present awareness and avoidance of potential mishaps.

I will now proceed to discuss in a systematic fashion the various complications related to the airway that may occur as a result of general endotracheal anesthesia. These complications may occur at the time of intubation, during intraoperative maintenance, with extubation, or as delayed problems presenting weeks to months after surgery.

INTUBATION-RELATED COMPLICATIONS

Anterior Larynx

The incidence of difficult intubations has been estimated to be approximately 1 in 750.[1] Cass et al. described prognostic signs of the difficult airway.[2] These included a short, muscular neck with a full set of teeth; micrognathia with obtuse mandibular angles; protruding maxillary incisors due to relative overgrowth of the premaxilla; poor mobility of the mandible due to temporomandibular arthritis or trismus; long, high-arched palate associated with a long, narrow mouth; and increased alveolomental distance. Others have mentioned the difficulties encountered with limited extension of the lower cervical vertebrae, increased posterior mandibular depth, and decreased (less than three finger-breadths) distance from the symphysis of the mandible to the thyroid notch with the head fully extended. Furthermore, Mallampati's signs describing the correlation between visibility of intraoral structures and ease of laryngoscopic exposure of the glottis may be helpful in predicting the difficult intubation.[3] For example, if the soft palate, fauces, uvula, and pillars are visible when the patient, in the sitting position, is asked to open the mouth and maximally protrude the tongue, an easy intubation should be expected. However, if both the hard and soft palate are not visible, extreme difficulty with intubation may be encountered. Moreover, the presence of stridor at rest can, of course, signal a challenging intubation.

Upper airway problems may be conveniently divided into three categories:

1. Patients with an unobstructed airway in whom the mask airway may be easily manageable. However, intubation is made difficult by physiognomic or pathologic anomalies.
2. Patients with an obviously obstructed airway.
3. Patients in whom impending obstruction of the airway is compensated or concealed on presentation but occurs on induction of anesthesia, administration of muscle relaxants, or extubation. Such situations may occur with certain supraglottic neoplasms, pedunculated intralaryngeal lesions, extremely large tonsils and adenoids, or various congenital deformities for which the patient ordinarily compensates by muscular effort.

Patients with a so-called anterior larynx clearly fall into category one. Certainly, all larynxes are anterior in the sense that they are anterior to the esophagus. Nonetheless, some conditions are characteristically associated with larynxes that are extremely anterior and difficult to visualize, and these include micrognathia, a hypoplastic mandible, or a very short neck. (These conditions, parenthetically, are not always characterized by a mask airway that is easily manageable.) A partial listing of syndromes associated with these problems includes arthrochalasis multiplex congenita, arthrogryposis, Cornelia de Lange's syndrome, cri du chat syndrome, DiGeorge syndrome, Goldenhar's, Klippel-Feil anomalad, Noonan's syndrome, Pierre Robin syndrome, Treacher Collins syndrome, and Turner's syndrome. Furthermore, a patient with no apparent stigmata may prove to have a larynx that is extremely difficult to visualize on laryngoscopy.

A variety of laryngoscope blades have been designed for use in patients with an anterior larynx, restricted mouth opening, or short, obese neck. These include the curved Bijarri-Griffrida and the Siker blades. The Siker has a mirrored surface, allowing visualization of the extremely anterior larynx, but has the disadvantage of reversing and inverting the image. In patients with an especially truncated thyroid cartilage to mandible distance, it may be helpful to attach Huffman prism clips directly onto the no. 3 MacIntosh blade. The Huffman prism clips do not invert or reverse the image, unlike the Siker blade. A stylet inserted into the endotracheal tube in such fashion as to impart an appropriate angle or curve to the tube may be helpful.

Not infrequently, an individual with a very anterior larynx that escapes visualization on laryngoscopy will do well with a blind nasotracheal intubation. First, the axes of the mouth, pharynx, and larynx are aligned by extending the head at the atlanto-occipital joint and flexing the neck at the cervical spine, achieving the so-called sniffing position. Intubation may then be performed under general anesthesia, with local anesthesia, or without anesthesia. However, for optimal results, spontaneous respiration should be preserved. Following application of a vasoconstrictor, such as cocaine, to the more patent naris, a nasotracheal tube is inserted into the chosen nostril and advanced gently into the oropharynx and then to the laryngeal entrance. Breath sounds are used to indicate the correct path through the larynx into the trachea. Skillful positioning of the head and neck may help guide the nasotracheal tube into the trachea. Head flexion tends to align the tube with the esophagus, whereas extension often aligns the axis of the tube with the trachea. In addition, tilting the head to the same side the tube enters the naris may help align the tip of the tube with the trachea.

Use of the pediatric flexible fiberoptic bronchoscope has gained popularity to accomplish difficult intubations in older children and adults. The fiberoptic scope is commonly introduced in an awake patient through a nostril previously treated with topical cocaine. Topical anesthetization of the larynx and trachea may be accomplished by superior laryngeal nerve block and by translaryngeal injection of 2 mL of 4% lidocaine through the cricothyroid membrane. An appropriately sized nasotracheal tube is inserted through the pretreated nostril into the pharynx. The flexible fiberoptic bronchoscope is then introduced through the nasotracheal tube into the oropharynx. After identification of the vocal cords, the scope is advanced into the trachea, and the tube is advanced over the scope into the trachea. Most skillful endoscopists emphasize that the successful use of the fiberoptic laryngoscope or bronchoscope in difficult situations requires considerable experience that should be acquired beforehand by using the instrument for elective, routine intubation in patients with normal anatomy. In addition, when fiberoptic equipment and expertise are available a strong case should be made for using this technique *before* attempting blind nasal intubation, lest inadvertent epistaxis obscure visualization.

In other instances where laryngoscopy proves unaccepta-
ble, retrograde passing of a catheter through the cricothyroid membrane into the pharynx and mouth and then passing of an endotracheal tube over the catheter into the trachea are possible.

Should the airway be lost during attempts to perform a difficult intubation, emergency measures such as cricothyrotomy or tracheostomy may prove lifesaving.

In summary, the key to accomplishing a challenging intubation is thorough preparation. This begins with careful preoperative examination of the mouth, pharynx, and neck, including assessment of range of motion. A variety of laryngoscope blades, different sized endotracheal tubes, stylets, and other equipment such as fiberoptic endoscopes and tracheostomy kits should be readily available, as well as an assistant to manipulate the position of the head and neck and to apply posterior laryngeal pressure as needed. Alternatives to routine intubation techniques are awake intubation, either oral or nasal, with topical anesthesia, and direct visualization; blind nasotracheal intubation with the patient either awake or asleep, breathing spontaneously; visualized, oral or nasal intubation under deep inhalation anesthesia; use of a fiberoptic laryngoscope or small-caliber fiberoptic bronchoscope; passage of a guide wire or catheter either anterograde or retrograde; and cricothyroidotomy or tracheostomy.

Above all, communication and cooperation among anesthesiologist, patient, and surgeon are essential to ensure optimal outcome in challenging cases of difficult intubation or difficult airway management.

Laryngospasm

The precise definition and mechanism of laryngospasm are still debated even today. In clinical practice, laryngospasm usually means that either the true vocal cords or both the true and false vocal cords have become apposed in the midline to close the glottis. The sensory portion of the superior laryngeal nerve probably carries the afferent limb of the reflex to the cervical vagal nuclei. Efferent potentials then travel along the vagus. Depending on the exact mechanism one chooses to believe, the intrinsic or extrinsic muscles (or both) of the larynx are stimulated, resulting in glottic closure.

Stimuli that may produce laryngospasm include the presence of blood, secretions, or vomitus in the airway; visceral pain; chemical irritation of laryngeal or pharyngeal mucosa; and an attempt to intubate the trachea with insufficient anesthesia. Prevention of laryngospasm includes ensuring adequate depth of anesthesia before instrumentation, using muscle relaxants, and using a full topical laryngeal block prior to intubation.

Treatment of a fully developed laryngospasm involves removing the stimulus, lifting the mandible up and out with the head in a sniffing position, and using a rapidly acting muscle relaxant. Gentle, intermittent positive pressure with 100% oxygen by mask has been used, but some think positive pressure causes the pyriform fossae to bulge and can occasionally worsen the laryngospasm by stimulating sensory areas supplied by the superior laryngeal nerve.

Foreign Body

Bronchoscopy for foreign body removal is extremely challenging. A plethora of potential problems arise from the anesthesiologist having to share the airway with the endoscopist while simultaneously providing adequate ventilation and unimpeded surgical access. Furthermore, most patients in this setting have some degree of compromise of the upper or lower airway. Without question, the removal of foreign bodies from the respiratory tract is one of the most exacting procedures known, and a successful outcome requires the optimum in expertise, communication, and teamwork of the endoscopist and anesthesiologist.

The nature of objects aspirated by children encompasses a wide spectrum, but most commonly one encounters food, such as peanuts, beans, seeds, or popcorn kernels. Plastic or metal pieces of toys are also aspirated with distressing frequency. Unfortunately, most aspirated objects are radiolucent. The peanut is especially perfidious if retained for any period of time, since it causes serious mucosal irritation, edema, and a greater incidence of pneumonitis distal to the bronchial obstruction than most other foreign bodies. Moreover, a single aspirated peanut or bean softens and expands from liquid absorption while it is lodged. This characteristic renders the peanut or bean especially vulnerable to fragmentation when grasped in the airway by the endoscopist's instrument. Fragmentation is notorious for causing death during the course of attempted removal if the divided pieces occlude both mainstem bronchi and totally prevent ventilation.

At this juncture, it is worth mentioning that not all aspirated foreign bodies exist or occur prior to induction. Iatrogenically induced foreign body aspiration may include such materials as teeth, blood, vomitus, adenoidal tissue, parts of the laryngoscope or the endotracheal tube, and soda lime dust!

Clinical findings with aspirated foreign bodies are most commonly those of partial bronchial obstruction. Hence, although air can enter around the foreign body on inspiration when the bronchus dilates, exhalation is obstructed because the foreign body functions as a unidirectional valve. Frequently radiographic findings will show unilateral hyperaeration, a lowered and flattened diaphragm, and mediastinal shift away from the affected side. However, not infrequently, chest films will be normal, particularly during the first 24 hours. Stridor, dyspnea, and wheezing are common. In cases of complete laryngeal obstruction, aphonia and cyanosis occur, and death will ensue within minutes unless the Heimlich maneuver or back slapping is successful. Not surprisingly, objects retained in the larynx or trachea cause much more distress and have a higher mortality than objects positioned more peripherally.

Fortunately, objects that are retained in the upper airway requiring urgent removal are relatively uncommon compared with foreign bodies that are located more distally. Ideally, the aspirated object should be removed within the first 24 hours to minimize the incidence of secondary pneumonia or other complications.

If urgent removal is mandated by the presence of cyanosis, 100% oxygen should be given while the child is taken immediately to the operating room under the care of an anesthesiologist and endoscopist. Awake laryngoscopy, rapid insertion of an endotracheal tube or bronchoscope, and positive pressure ventilation may dislodge a tracheal foreign body and push it more peripherally into a mainstem bronchus with relief of the immediate crisis. Intravenous atrophine is necessary to minimize secretions and reduce the incidence of bradycardia and other arrhythmias so common with airway manipulation and hypoxia. Nitrous oxide should be withheld because of its propensity to expand the trapped gas volume and pressure in the affected lung.

When bronchoscopy can be performed on a less urgent basis, atropine should still be given intravenously, and preoperative sedation should still be omitted. Following administration of thiopental or a mask induction, deep inhalation anesthesia with halothane and oxygen plus topical anesthetization of the larynx and trachea using 4% lidocaine ($\leq$5 mg/kg) allows vocal cord movement, appropriate jaw relaxation, and satisfactory anesthesia for airway endoscopy. It is essential to be patient and allow for the greatly increased time required for an inhalation induction in the presence of an obstructed bronchus. In addition, these patients should be assumed to have a full stomach; thus the necessity of extremely skillful airway management is critical.

Having briefly discussed management of induction, I will focus on maintenance of anesthesia for foreign body removal later in this chapter.

Laryngeal Trauma

The trauma of a difficult intubation frequently occurs not at the vocal cords but somewhat higher in the airway. For example, with nasal intubation, the difficulty usually is not in introducing the tube through the cords but in positioning the tube properly at the glottic opening. The more common lesions are localized abrasion, hemorrhage, ulceration, and, eventually, granuloma. Laceration of the larynx is an extremely rare event. The most serious complication is pseudomembranous laryngotracheitis, which, if not immediately treated, may cause sudden death. Indeed, pseudomembranous laryngotracheitis is not exclusively a result of trauma. The condition may occur after a completely uneventful anesthetic and in the absence of a history of upper respiratory tract infection.[4]

Long-term or delayed laryngeal complications are a function of the size, shape, and stiffness of the endotracheal tube; the pressure characteristics of the endotracheal tube cuff; the duration of intubation; the amount of movement of the head and neck about the tube; and, to a certain extent, the gentleness of the anesthesiologist.

Atlanto-Occipital Subluxation in Rheumatoid Arthritis

Ordinarily flexion of the cervical spine and extension at the atlanto-occipital joint achieves the sniffing position for laryngoscopy to facilitate visualization. However, this position may be difficult or impossible to obtain because of various conditions, including jaw or neck rigidity associated with trismus, rheumatoid arthritis, ankylosing spondylitis, burns, radiation therapy, and critically placed fractures. When one encounters a patient with any of these conditions, careful, gentle laryngoscopy is mandatory. The head should be maintained in neutral position, with the help of an assistant if necessary. Alternative intubation techniques that do not mandate neck manipulation or direct laryngoscopy, such as blind nasal intubation or fiberoptic techniques, should be considered.

It is essential to appreciate that in severe rheumatoid arthritis, there may be debilitating involvement of the cervical spine, the temporomandibular joints, and cricoarytenoid joints. Atlantoaxial subluxation is often present, particularly in those with severe hand deformities and subcutaneous nodules. Radiologic demonstration of a distance from the anterior arch of the atlas to the odontoid process in excess of 3 mm confirms the presence of atlantoaxial subluxation.[5] Its significance is that the displaced odontoid process can compress the cervical spinal cord or medulla, in addition to occluding the vertebral arteries. Even minimal trauma, as may be associated with movement of the neck during tracheal intubation, may cause further displacement of the odontoid process and damage to the underlying spinal cord. Furthermore, arthritic involvement of the cricoarytenoid joints is suggested by hoarseness or stridor. This involvement of the cricoarytenoids, limiting their movement, may result in narrowing of the glottic opening. Hence, a smaller than usual size endotracheal tube should be selected. Also, one must be aware of the potential for postextubation laryngeal obstruction to occur in this setting.

Other Intubation-Related Complications: Pharyngoesophageal Injury and Recurrent Nerve Palsy

Oral intubation can cause tissue trauma, damage to teeth (including dislodgement), mucosal lacerations, perforation of such anatomic structures as the esophagus or trachea, and bleeding with the risk of aspiration.

Other additional potential complications of nasal intubation include damage to septum and turbinates, nasal necrosis, epistaxis, sinusitis, and otitis media. Furthermore, a forced nasal intubation may take a false passage via the posterior pharyngeal wall from a retropharyngeal laceration. In cases of basilar skull fractures, nasotracheal intubation should not be attempted because of risk of intracranial penetration.

The complication of vocal cord palsy or paralysis can be unilateral or bilateral. With bilateral paralysis, symptoms of respiratory obstruction occur. However, usually hoarseness is the only symptom of unilateral damage. It is thought that pressure exerted by a distended endotracheal tube cuff on branches of the recurrent laryngeal nerve is the etiology of this complication, especially if the operation exceeds 2 hours. Fortunately, in most instances, the weakness or paralysis is transient. Nonetheless, with bilateral involvement a temporary tracheostomy is usually necessary.

Prevention of the rare complication of recurrent laryngeal nerve damage occurring in this setting includes (1) performing gentle intubation, followed by careful inflation of the high volume–low pressure cuff with a volume that allows a small, audible leak during inspiration; (2) abandoning the use of endotracheal tubes with cuffs that, on testing, inflate unevenly; (3) eliminating the practice of placing the cuff within the larynx

in a misguided attempt to avoid inadvertent endobronchial intubation (the cuff should be placed 1 or 2 cm below the larynx); and (4) filling the cuff with a sample of the inspired mixture of gases, regularly deflating the cuff, or using a simple pressure relief valve.[6]

INTRAOPERATIVE COMPLICATIONS

Tracheal Fire

To be certain, much has been written about tracheal fires during laser surgery, and this important topic will be reviewed in a few moments. However, it seems reasonable to begin by briefly mentioning that airway fires may occur in the absence of lasers and in the absence of such flammable or explosive agents as ether and cyclopropane.

The ingredients required for a fire include an ignition source, oxidizing agent or agents, and combustible material. These are provided by electrocautery, nitrous oxide and oxygen, and an endotracheal tube, respectively. A recent publication by Simpson and Wolf reported the hazard of using "spray" electrocautery during tonsillectomy and adenoidectomy in a 4-year-old boy.[7] Many techniques are available for reducing the risk of pharyngeal fire. These include reducing the concentration of oxidizing agents in the oral cavity by using a moist, occlusive pharyngeal pack, especially if an uncuffed endotracheal tube is in place, as well as by eliminating the use of nitrous oxide, and by minimizing the fraction of inspired oxygen concentration. Also, the risk of igniting the endotracheal tube with stray electrical current could be reduced by using bipolar rather than unipolar cautery since current density in the tissue surrounding the active electrode is much less with bipolar electrocautery. Hence, the risk of igniting a fire from heating nearby combustible material is appreciably reduced with the bipolar unit.

The laser is an intense heat source capable of igniting many materials. The ease with which this occurs depends on the material itself, the gas environment surrounding the material, and the focus of the laser beam. Indeed, Fried showed in a recent survey that endotracheal tube explosion was the most common serious complication of carbon dioxide laser laryngoscopic surgery.[8] Nonetheless, various maneuvers may be employed to reduce the incidence of this potential catastrophe, and these techniques begin by using either a metal endotracheal tube or a red rubber Rusch tube properly wrapped with reflective metallic tape. These rubber tubes are significantly more resistant to ignition at both higher energy exposures and greater durations of exposure than properly wrapped plastic Portex tubes.[9] Furthermore, it is imperative to appreciate that although nitrous oxide is nonflammable, it supports combustion. Hence, nitrous oxide is best avoided during laser surgery in the airway; rather, the minimum clinically acceptable concentration of oxygen should be used along with nitrogen and helium. Also, the cuff of the endotracheal tube can be inflated with normal saline instead of air to minimize the chance of ignition.

If a fire or explosion occurs, the anesthesiologist should be prepared to extinguish the fire immediately by occluding the endotracheal tube with a clamp, quickly disconnecting it from the breathing circuit, and then removing it from the patient. Another similar endotracheal tube and a bronchoscope should be readily available for reestablishing and examining the airway and performing pulmonary toilet. If necessary, a tracheostomy may be performed, preferably at the second tracheal ring.

Inadvertent Extubation

During major head and neck procedures, the anesthesiologist does not have direct visual and tactile access to the patient's airway. Hence, securement techniques appropriate to the nature of the surgery or accessibility of the endotracheal tube are essential to prevent accidental dislodgement. Careful application of adhesive tape, benzoin, and stainless steel wire to secure the tube to the teeth all are maneuvers that may be employed. More important, however, is the vivid realization that dislodgement is always a possibility. Thus, appropriate continuous monitoring with either a precordial or esophageal stethoscope to immediately detect tube displacement is critical, as is the preconsidered development of a plan to follow should dislodgement occur. In addition, capnography and pulse oximetry are extremely valuable. As in so many aspects of anesthetic care, meticulous attention to detail, careful and continuous observation, rapid diagnosis, and prompt institution of remedial measures are essential. Reintubation is not always easy in the middle of a bloody, complex dissection. Clearly, prevention is the best treatment.

Foreign Body

Airway management and other anesthetic considerations during induction in the presence of a foreign body were briefly discussed earlier. I will now focus on salient features of anesthetic maintenance in this challenging setting.

As the anesthesia is deepened with halothane (or another appropriate volatile agent) and oxygen, care should be taken to preserve spontaneous ventilation, at least until the location and nature of the foreign body have been ascertained by bronchoscopic examination. If the object is vegetable matter, with the potential for fragmentation during extraction, the possibility of placing the patient in the lateral position, affected side down, should be considered. If this is not possible, thoracotomy instruments and a thoracic surgeon should be immediately available since thoracotomy and bronchotomy may be instantly indicated if a fragmented object acutely occludes both mainstem bronchi. If the object occludes the trachea, it is often possible to succeed with less invasive steps merely by pushing the object into a mainstem bronchus. Also, a no. 3 Fogarty embolectomy balloon catheter may be helpful in dislodging impacted foreign bodies.

Sometimes, the size of the foreign body may exceed the internal diameter of the bronchoscope, necessitating the simultaneous removal of the aspirated object, the scope, and the forceps as a single unit through the vocal cords. This maneuver usually requires that the cords be rendered immediately, but briefly, immobile, and this can be nicely accomplished by giving 0.25 to 0.5 mg of succinylcholine/kg intravenously. If the object

is lost during attempted extraction, the pharynx should be inspected first. If the object is not found there, the bronchoscope should be reinserted and the foreign body sought in the larynx or trachea. The value of spontaneous respiration is readily apparent should tracheal occlusion be present, since breath sounds will be minimal or absent. As mentioned earlier, if the trachea is obstructed, the object must be pushed back to its initial position so that the patient can be ventilated. It is crucial to underscore that the foreign body must return to the affected side and not to the side of the only functioning lung, since then ventilation would be impossible in either lung. It is also important to realize that with the increased resistance inherent during bronchoscopy with the optical telescope in place, manual positive pressure ventilation is impaired, necessitating a higher inspiratory pressure and faster rate. Sporadically, the endoscopist should remove the telescope, occlude the orifice, and allow the anesthesiologist a brief interlude of unobstructed manual ventilation.

Following extraction of the foreign body, the endoscopist will need to check for additional pieces and to suction distal secretions. Since multiple bronchoscopic reinsertions may be necessary, mucosal edema with respiratory distress is not unusual following bronchoscopy. Measures to prevent or attenuate postoperation stridor and respiratory compromise include administration of steroids, humidified oxygen, and nebulized racemic epinephrine. Occasionally intubation for 1 or 2 days may be required until the edema resolves. Dexamethasone is given initially in doses of 0.5 to 1.5 mg/kg, with smaller doses repeated as needed at intervals determined by the individual situation. With ECG monitoring, racemic epinephrine (2.25%) is administered for 10 to 15 minutes through a nebulizer and face mask in a 1:6 dilution. This may be repeated, as indicated, every 2 hours.

Some aspirated objects may cause serious pneumonitis or other problems, including postobstructive purulent asphyxiation. Vegetable matter is likely to stimulate the proliferation of granulation tissue and attendant complications. The peanut, especially, is infamous for the variety of damage it can cause, including purulent asphyxiation. It seems that the peanut's rich content of arachidonic acid is especially likely to trigger inflammatory reactions, and eventually, copious purulence may result. It is possible for the purulence to block the airways and cause death. However, bronchoscopic suctioning is often helpful in ameliorating the obstruction. Fortunately, the complication of purulent asphyxiation is very rare.

Massive Subcutaneous Emphysema

Facial, cervical, and thoracic subcutaneous emphysema has been reported after both surgical and dental procedures, trauma to the upper airway and facial bones, and even after equipment failure.[10–12] Subcutaneous emphysema of the face, neck, or mediastinum often occurs unexpectedly and without a readily discernible cause. Frequently, it does not have important pathophysiologic consequences. However, subcutaneous emphysema may be progressive and can result in circulatory and respiratory embarrassment. Respiratory compromise may be due to airway obstruction from massive subcutaneous emphysema of the head and neck or reduced pulmonary compliance associated with tension pneumothorax. Dramatic circulatory consequences can develop as a result of increasing tension within the mediastinum, which may decrease cardiac output secondary to a tamponade effect.

It is essential to be mindful that airway perforation may occur secondary to mechanical trauma or airway pressure.[13] During orotracheal intubation, the airway may be perforated by pressure from the laryngoscope blade, the stylet, or even the endotracheal tube itself. Elevated airway pressure can cause rupture anywhere between the point of its application and the alveolus. Airway perforation from any cause may introduce air to unusual locations and trigger subcutaneous and mediastinal emphysema and pneumothorax.

Careful consideration of the risk/benefit ratio should precede certain procedures, such as subclavian or internal jugular venipuncture, especially prior to induction of anesthesia. Positive airway pressure and the use of high concentrations of nitrous oxide may escalate a small pneumothorax into a rapidly expanding tension pneumothorax. Indeed, tension pneumothorax should be included in the differential diagnosis of circulatory or respiratory instability following intubation, especially when there is a history of thoracic or upper abdominal trauma, inadvertent overinflation of the lungs, obstructive airway disease with emphysema, or when PEEP is being applied. Nitrous oxide should be immediately discontinued if surgical emphysema or pneumothorax is suspected, because this gas will diffuse into the trapped air and dramatically expand its volume in a concentration-related fashion.

Pneumothorax can occur via three mechanisms: Type 1 is intrapulmonary alveolar rupture, with retrograde perivascular dissection of air, producing mediastinal emphysema. Type 2 is injury to the visceral pleura, with escape of air into the pleural space. Type 3 is injury to the parietal pleura, with entry of air from adjoining structures, such as the thoracic wall or mediastinum. Type 1 may be associated with malfunctioning expiratory valve mechanisms on the anesthesia machine.[14, 15] Type 2 may be produced by subclavian and internal jugular venipuncture, tracheostomy, and mediastinoscopy. When there is visceral pleural discontinuity, regardless of etiology, airway pressures that ordinarily would be well tolerated can produce tension pneumothorax. Type 3 pneumothorax may be a complication of thyroidectomy, tracheostomy, or radical neck dissection, where exposure of the deep cervical fascia offers a route through which air may enter the mediastinum, since the deep cervical fascia surrounds the trachea and extends directly into the mediastinum.[16] Usually, paratracheal air dissection is associated with excessive negative airway pressure generated during labored or obstructed ventilation.

Signs of pneumothorax include hypotension, tachycardia, tachypnea, decreased pulmonary compliance, wheezing or distant breath sounds, and increased venous pressure. Treatment consists of insertion of a large-bore needle through the second intercostal space anteriorly, usually followed by tube thoracostomy.

To prevent barotrauma-related complications, one should exercise care to avoid excessive airway pressure during anesthesia. Intubation should be accomplished gently, and anesthesia equipment should be meticulously checked for valve integrity. Poorly compliant breathing bags should be discarded because of the potential for high-peak pressure to be produced during inadvertent overdistention. Furthermore, avoidance of airway obstruction or excessive negative airway pressure during neck surgery will prevent most cases of pneumothorax associated with air dissection along deep cervical fascia into the mediastinum.

Clearly, during the perioperative period of head and neck surgery, anesthesiologists should be alert for changes in pulmonary compliance, circulatory decompensation, or sudden swelling of tissues of the facial, cervical, or thoracic regions that may indicate undesirable air entry into the subcutaneous spaces.

EXTUBATION-ASSOCIATED COMPLICATIONS

Acute Problems

Laryngospasm

To diminish the likelihood of postextubation laryngospasm, the patient should be extubated while he or she is asleep but breathing adequately or when he or she is awake. Awake means that the patient opens his or her eyes spontaneously, moves all extremities well on command, and resumes a normal breathing pattern after a cough. When patients are extubated in the intermediate zone, somewhere between their being asleep and being fully awake, they are much more likely to develop postextubation laryngospasm. Furthermore, in unintubated patients who are inhaling anesthesia via a mask, it is wise to remove upper airway secretions while the patient remains fully anesthetized to avoid triggering laryngospasm as the airway reflexes return during awakening.

Applying positive airway pressure by mask may be briefly attempted to eradicate the laryngospasm, although some experts believe this maneuver actually exacerbates the condition. Certainly, laryngospasm that does not respond within 30 seconds to positive airway pressure and relief of soft tissue obstruction should be treated immediately with 1.5 to 2 mg of IV succinylcholine/kg to relax and open the vocal cords, controlled ventilation with high inspired concentration of oxygen, and reintubation, if necessary, to establish an adequate airway. It is often advisable to give 0.01 to 0.02 mg of atropine/kg intravenously prior to giving succinylcholine to avoid succinylcholine-associated, or hypoxia-associated, bradycardia.

Postobstructive Pulmonary Edema

Noncardiogenic pulmonary edema is uncommon and may arise from a variety of causes, including drugs, sepsis, head trauma, and high altitude. Although airway obstruction as a rare cause of acute pulmonary edema was recognized clinically in the 1960s, no case reports actually appeared until 1977.[17, 18]

Since many of the early series described pediatric patients with croup or epiglottitis, there was an initial perception that postobstructive pulmonary edema occurs mainly, if not exclusively, in children. However, in adults, a vast spectrum of conditions resulting in airway obstruction may also be linked with fulminating pulmonary edema, including laryngospasm,[19] epiglottitis,[20] sleep apnea,[21] goiter,[22] malignancy, and strangulation.[18]

The mechanisms underlying postobstructive pulmonary edema are obscure and probably multifactorial. However, forced inspiration against a closed glottis (modified Müller's maneuver), inducing large negative intrapleural and transpulmonary pressure gradients favoring the transudation of pulmonary edema fluid from the pulmonary capillaries into the interstitium, appears to be the predominant one. The amount of respiratory muscle force transformed to negative intrathoracic pressure is affected by chest wall compliance. Since children have more compliant chest walls than adults, this may explain the increased incidence of postobstructive pulmonary edema in children. Nonetheless, the possibility of prolonged hypoxia, or severe acidosis, being able to initiate pulmonary edema either by direct pulmonary effects or through cardiac depression cannot be cavalierly dismissed.

Certain patients, such as those with a forme fruste of sleep apnea or nasopharyngeal abnormalities, may be at increased risk for the development of postobstructive pulmonary edema.[23] This form of postobstructive pulmonary edema is characterized by rapid onset and, not uncommonly, resolution without the need for aggressive therapy or invasive monitoring, especially in children.

Those who need more aggressive therapy for this condition usually respond well to reintubation, ventilation with either continuous positive airway pressure or PEEP, judicious use of diuretics, and, arguably, steroids.

Given the potentially serious consequences, it seems reasonable to recommend that patients recently recovering from an acute episode of upper airway obstruction be observed closely for at least 12 hours for the appearance of this syndrome. If pulmonary edema develops, untoward sequelae can be averted by judicious management.

Postintubation Croup

Many irritant stimuli can initiate an inflammatory response with mucosal edema in the larynx or trachea. These stimuli include a traumatic intubation characterized by several attempts, the use of an endotracheal tube that is too large, a lengthy period of intubation, and surgery involving the head and neck with excessive movement around the tube. It is important to appreciate that movement of the tube in the airway occurs with each breath. Even though the tube is secured externally, the tracheobronchial tree moves with ventilation, especially with swallowing, coughing, and head movement.[24]

Certain ingredients in plastic tubes, such as antioxidants and plasticizers, are tissue irritants. Furthermore, when tubes are reused, residual cleaning agent may cause tissue injury. If inadequately aerated, gas-sterilized tubes may contain ethylene oxide that is liberated and then damages airway mucosa; ethylene oxide and water react to form ethylene glycol, a well-known irritant.

In the past, with the use of high-pressure, low-volume endotracheal tube cuffs, much damage was done to tracheal walls.

Modern cuffs, however, use larger inflation volumes requiring lower pressure more evenly distributed over a greater surface area. The net result is less mucosal and submucosal injury.

Children are those most frequently afflicted by the complication of glottic edema or postintubation croup. The edema may occur in the supraglottic, retroarytenoid, or subglottic regions. The complication of subglottic edema is most serious and requires immediate attention. Since edema encroaches on the airway lumen, resistance is greatly increased. This is especially true in infants in whom there is a disproportionate increase in resistance with a reduction in lumen radius since, from the Hagen-Poiseuille law, we know that flow in tubes varies as the fourth power of the radius. Recall also that expansion of edema outward is limited by the cricoid cartilage encircling the subglottic region. Moreover, the subglottic region has fragile respiratory epithelium with loose submucosal connective tissue that is easily traumatized and edema prone.

The peak incidence of croup occurs between 1 and 3 to 4 years of age.[25] Croup presents within minutes to hours of extubation with a barking cough and varying degrees of respiratory obstruction. There is associated dyspnea, stridor, suprasternal retraction, tachypnea, and tachycardia. Glottic edema persisting beyond 24 hours is often associated with more serious, permanent lesions. If resolution of the insult is followed by scar formation, subglottic stenosis may develop after several weeks or months.

Prevention of this complication starts with performing intubation as gently as possible and avoiding irritant stimuli, especially an oversized endotracheal tube. There should be a leak around the endotracheal tube, especially in pediatric practice, and this leak should be audible with 20 to 25 cm H_2O pressure applied. When feasible, the use of a face mask for pediatric patients should be encouraged. If postintubation subglottic edema occurs, humidification of inspired oxygen, cool mist, and 0.5 mL of 2.25% solution of racemic epinephrine diluted with 3 mL of saline, nebulized with intermittent positive pressure apparatus, are helpful therapeutic modalities.[25] Steroids, in some cases, have been said to be useful.

Aspiration

Since its description by Mendelson in 1946,[26] the acid aspiration syndrome has been a feared complication of anesthesia. Aspiration may be a sequel either to regurgitation or vomiting. Regurgitation is a passive phenomenon, depending on the pressure gradient between the stomach and oropharynx. Vomiting, however, is an active reflex and can occur at any time during anesthetic management. When protective reflexes are obtunded or abolished, as they are by reduced levels of consciousness, vomiting or regurgitation can result in liquids or solids being deposited in the tracheobronchial tree.

Morbidity and mortality associated with aspiration vary depending on the volume and chemical nature of the fluid aspirated. Patients at greatest risk are those with at least 25 mL (0.4 mL/kg) of gastric fluid of pH less than 2.5 in the stomach. The clinical picture produced by aspiration of gastric contents is a function of the type of material aspirated. Vomiting may produce aspiration of solid particulate matter capable of occluding the tracheobronchial tree. Physical signs are those of localized lung collapse distal to the blockage. The clinical course depends on the position of the occlusion and particulate size. Indeed, death may occur very quickly when the tracheal lumen is blocked. If liquid gastric contents are aspirated, the clinical effects depend on the acidity and volume of the aspirate. Generalized wheezing, rales, and expiratory rhonchi may be noted almost immediately, or these signs and symptoms can be quite delayed. Likewise, the chest x-ray film may be normal for some time after the injury, and the extent of the pneumonitis may not be radiologically obvious for many hours. Nonetheless, tachycardia, dyspnea, cyanosis, hypotension, and pulmonary edema may develop very quickly.

Solid matter aspirated into the airway requires prompt removal by bronchoscopy. When liquid is aspirated, suctioning should be performed to reduce pulmonary damage, although mucosal injury occurs within minutes. Small amounts (<10 mL) of saline may be used to facilitate airway suctioning. However, attempts to dilute and aspirate by lavage of the airways is not recommended, since it may only spread the damage.

The initial response to aspiration of liquid with a pH less than 2.5 is an irritative one of intense bronchospasm and transudation of large volumes of fluid from the respiratory epithelium, resulting in a profound hypoxemia. Tracheal intubation and mechanical ventilation with PEEP are often necessary to sustain an acceptable arterial oxygen tension. Aminophylline may be given as a 500 mg IV infusion to treat bronchospasm. Antibiotics are administered only if indicated (i.e., for treatment of the secondary infection that commonly develops following aspiration). Prophylactic antibiotics are indicated only in the setting of aspiration of obviously infected material, such as feces or pus from pharyngeal abscess. Steroids are not generally recommended.

Hiatus hernia, obesity, pregnancy, extreme nervousness, old age, diabetes, and conditions requiring upper abdominal surgery put patients at risk of aspiration. The most common factors that precipitate vomiting during anesthesia are partial respiratory obstruction and a level of anesthesia that is too light. Other factors include strong autonomic stimulation such as peritoneal traction or hypoxia and hypotension, administration of narcotics, and insertion of an oropharyngeal airway during light anesthesia. Regurgitation may be encouraged by the Trendelenberg position, prone position, palpation of the abdomen during light anesthesia, and conditions associated with delayed gastric emptying and, hence, increased intragastric pressure. The latter conditions include pain, anxiety, obstetric labor, pyloric or intestinal obstruction, metabolic derangements, increased intracranial pressure, and the administration of parasympathomimetic drugs and narcotics. In addition, succinylcholine-induced fasciculations are claimed by some to promote regurgitation. Since scleroderma and other collagen vascular diseases are associated with gastroesophageal valve incompetence, these patients are said to be at increased risk.

It is difficult to cite an exact figure denoting the incidence of aspiration under anesthesia. Several investigators have studied the problem of silent regurgitation and aspiration. Overall, an incidence of regurgitation between 14% and 26% was found.[27, 28] Silent aspiration was documented in 6% to 8%.[27, 29]

More recent studies in 1986 by Olsson et al. reported an incidence of aspiration pneumonitis confirmed by x-ray film after anesthesia of 2.2 per 10,000 anesthetics, with a mortality of 0.2 per 10,000.[30] Mortality rates had previously been thought to be more than 40% following confirmed aspiration.[31] However, Olsson et al. concluded that today the mortality due to anesthesia-associated aspiration is much lower.[30]

If we are to prevent aspiration, it is essential to appreciate that aspiration of vomitus or regurgitated material happens at the completion of surgery with nearly the same frequency as it does during induction. Moreover, aspiration pneumonitis is not confined to patients having general anesthesia but may occur even with regional techniques or in any patient whose level of consciousness is impaired by drugs or illness.

Much has been written about the prevention of aspiration during induction by recognizing those patients at greatest risk and performing either an awake intubation or a skillful rapid sequence induction with Sellick's maneuver (firm pressure on the cricoid cartilage, occluding the esophagus between the trachea and vertebral column). The insertion of a cuffed tracheal tube also affords protection against aspiration.

Proper airway management is the most important aspect of aspiration prophylaxis, but pharmacologic protection is another promising avenue. For example, antacids such as Bicitra (15 mL), given orally about 15 minutes prior to induction, reduce gastric acidity, although they do increase gastric volume. Rao et al. reported that a combination of 300 mg of cimetidine and 10 mg of metoclopramide taken orally more than 2 hours before induction markedly decreased gastric volume and increased pH.[32] Metoclopramide, a dopamine antagonist, increases lower esophageal sphincter tone and stimulates gastric motility. Cimetidine and other H_2 antagonists such as ranitidine reduce gastric acidity by blocking H_2 receptors and, thus, decreasing both basal and active acid secretion. Ranitidine has greater potency and duration of action than cimetidine and also a lower incidence of drug interactions. Both cimetidine and ranitidene, as well as metoclopramide, may also be parenterally administered.

The incidence of aspiration at the end of surgery can be reduced by passing a nasogastric tube and applying suction prior to extubation. Moreover, it is essential to extubate patients at risk only when they are fully awake and then to appreciate that depression of the glottic reflex lasts at least 2 hours and perhaps as long as 8 hours after extubation, even in patients who seem alert.[33] This, obviously, has implications for postoperative fluid ingestion.

In conclusion, it appears that if we are to reduce the incidence of aspiration pneumonitis, special emphasis should be placed on careful preoperative instructions as to the necessity of fasting for 8 hours prior to elective surgery and thorough questioning of patients about ingestion of food and liquids when they arrive for anesthetic induction. High-risk patients should be identified and treated accordingly in terms of anesthetic induction technique. Skillful airway management is essential. In addition, pharmacologic prophylaxis against acid aspiration seems reasonable. Finally, extubation should not be performed until the high-risk patient is wide awake, with reflexes intact.

Delayed Problems

Contact Granulomas of the Vocal Cords

The incidence of intubation granuloma is estimated to be about 1 in 1,000 endotracheal anesthesias,[34] but reports range from 1 in 800[35] to 1 in 20,000 tracheal intubations.[36]

It should be underscored that granuloma of the vocal fold is frequently unrelated to intubation. Moreover, even following intubation, the presence of granuloma is not per se evidence of inferior anesthetic technique. Many granulomas are caused by vocal fold trauma, ascribable to misuse of the voice.

Postintubation granulomata are thought to develop from tiny abrasions of the very delicate mucosa covering the vocal process of the arytenoid cartilage. The exposed surface becomes infected, an ulcer forms, and eventually a sessile granuloma develops. Through central proliferation, the lesion becomes an inflammatory polyp or pyrogenic granuloma. Laryngoscopy typically shows unilateral or bilateral involvement of the vocal fold at the vocal process of the arytenoid cartilage, near the junction of the middle, and posterior third of the fold. Women are afflicted five times as often as men, presumably because of their small larynx and thin mucoperichondrium.

Symptoms seem to vary with the size of the granuloma, and range from slight hoarseness and a foreign body sensation, to persistent cough and pain, and even to otodynia and respiratory obstruction. The first signs may occur as early as 4 days or as late as 7 months following intubation.

Factors associated with intubation granulomas include use of a large endotracheal tube, traumatic insertion of the tube, and intubation lasting more than $2^1/_2$ hours. Furthermore, friction of the tube against the larynx is probably related to development of granuloma. Significant friction is more likely to develop during neck surgery, especially thyroidectomy, and when lubricant for the tube is omitted. Overextension of the neck serves to press the tube against the arytenoid and increases the risk of contact pressure injury. Some cite contusion of the vocal folds produced by postextubation coughing as another contributory factor.

Prevention of intubation granuloma is predicated on etiologic considerations; hence, a sterile, smooth tube of appropriate diameter should be inserted as atraumatically as possible. Extension of the head after intubation should be discouraged, and surgical manipulation of the trachea should be gentle. Extubation should be timed so as to avoid vigorous coughing. If persistent hoarseness develops, early otolaryngologic evaluation is essential.

Treatment, depending on the severity of the lesion, ranges from voice rest to surgical excision of the granuloma.

Postoperative Vocal Cord Paralysis

Fortunately, vocal cord paralysis following intubation is uncommon. It usually follows head and neck surgery, especially thyroidectomy, where direct or indirect injury to the recurrent laryngeal nerves has transpired. As previously mentioned, the condition may also be attributed to neuropraxia from pressure on the recurrent laryngeal nerve by the cuff of the tracheal tube, and its incidence may be significantly reduced by eliminating the use of endotracheal tubes with cuffs that inflate unevenly and by placing the cuff sufficiently below the larynx.

Unilateral vocal cord paralysis is more benign, and its symptoms are generally limited to hoarseness that appears immediately postoperatively or soon after. Recovery is usually within a few weeks, although some slight degree of partial paralysis may persist.

Bilateral cord paralysis is much more serious and causes signs of increasing upper airway obstruction, which may follow immediately after extubation or be delayed for several hours. The patient will have difficulty vocalizing the latter E, and auscultation over the larynx discloses inspiratory and expiratory vibrations. As the respiratory obstruction worsens, stridor and paradoxical respiration develop, followed by complete obstruction. The usual methods of ameliorating respiratory obstruction, such as neck extension or oral airway insertion, do not help. Positive pressure ventilation through a face mask should be given, followed by reintubation. Most patients with bilateral vocal cord paralysis recover after 1 month or longer, but tracheostomy is often needed as a temporary measure.

Subglottic and Tracheal Injury Subglottic Stenosis

Subglottic stenosis may be a congenital condition but is usually associated with prolonged endotracheal intubation. This serious complication becomes apparent several months after intubation and is actually more common in adults than children. The stenotic lesion is usually situated where the cuff was positioned, or, less commonly, the site of damage may coincide with the tip of the endotracheal tube. Prevention consists of using appropriately sized endotracheal tubes with large volume–low pressure cuffs and of not allowing the tube to remain in place for weeks before resorting to a tracheostomy. Symptoms include coughing, dyspnea, and signs of respiratory obstruction. Treatment includes dilatation in the less serious cases or resection of the stenotic segment in more advanced cases.

Although tracheostomy protects the larynx from additional injury, trauma may still occur at the site of the inflated cuff and at the tip of the tracheostomy tube. In an attempt to prevent these injuries, standard tracheal tube cuffs have been replaced with large-volume, low-pressure cuffs, and many experts have advocated periodic deflation or inflation only during inspiration and various pressure-regulating devices. Moreover, tracheostomy is associated with tracheal erosion, especially into the innominate artery or esophagus, more often than laryngotracheal intubation, because tracheostomy tubes usually sit lower in the trachea and have a rigid, built-in curve that may exert undue pressure on tissues at the tube tip.

It is said that in adults, the inverted U flap incision in the anterior tracheal wall through the second and third tracheal rings circumvents damage to the first tracheal ring and may avoid the problem of tracheal stenosis following decannulation. In children, the tracheostomy site is deliberately placed lower than in adults, commonly ranging at a level from the fourth to seventh tracheal rings. This is to avoid complications associated with a high tracheostomy since tracheal stenosis can develop from an edematous and inflammatory reaction of the subglottic larynx or the cricoid cartilage.

REFERENCES

1. Edens ET, Sia RL: Flexible fiberoptic endoscopy in difficult intubations. *Ann Otol* 1981; 90:307–309.
2. Cass NM, James NR, Lines V: Difficult direct laryngoscopy complicating intubation for anaesthesia. *Br Med J (Clin Res)* 1956; 1:488–489.
3. Mallampati SR: Clinical signs to predict difficult tracheal intubation. *Can Anaesth Soc J* 1983; 30:316–317.
4. Komorn RM, Smith CP, Erwin JR: Acute laryngeal injury with short term endotracheal anesthesia. *Laryngoscope* 1973; 83:683.
5. Smith PH, Sharp J, Kellgren JH: Natural history of rheumatoid cervical subluxations. *Ann Rheum Dis* 1972; 31:222–223.
6. Stanley HT, Foote JL, Liu W: A simple pressure-relief valve to prevent increases in endotracheal tube cuff pressure and volume in intubated patients. *Anesthesiology* 1975; 43:478–481.
7. Simpson JI, Wolf GL: Endotracheal tube fire ignited by pharyngeal electrocautery. *Anesthesiology* 1986; 65:76–77.
8. Fried MP: A survey of the complications of laser laryngoscopy. *Arch Otolaryngol* 1984; 110:31–34.
9. Patel KF, Hicks JN: Prevention of fire hazards associated with use of carbon dioxide lasers. *Anesth Analg* 1981; 60:885–888.
10. Kirchner JA: Cervical mediastinal emphysema. *Arch Otolaryngol* 1980; 106:368–375.
11. Rosenberg MB, Wunderlich BK, Reynolds RN: Iatrogenic subcutaneous emphysema during dental anesthesia. *Anesthesiology* 1979; 50:80–81.
12. Jumper A, Sukumar D, Liu P, et al: Pulmonary barotrauma resulting from a faulty Hope II resuscitation bag. *Anesthesiology* 1983; 58:572–577.
13. Hawkins DB, House JW: Postoperative pneumothorax secondary to hypopharyngeal perforation during anesthetic intubation. *Ann Otol Rhinol Laryngol* 1974; 85:556.
14. Martin JT, Patrick RT: Pneumothorax: Its significance to the anesthesiologist. *Anesth Analg* 1960; 39:420.
15. Dean HN, Parsons DE, Raphaely RC: Bilateral tension pneumothorax from mechanical failure of anesthesia machine due to misplaced expiratory valve. *Anesth Analg* 1971; 50:195.
16. Schweizer O: Complications of anesthesia during radical surgery about the head and neck. *Anesthesiology* 1955; 16:927.
17. Travis KW, Todres ID, Shannon DC: Pulmonary edema associated with croup and epiglottitis. *Pediatrics* 1977; 59:695–698.
18. Oswalt CE, Gates GE, Holmstrom FM: Pulmonary edema as a complication of acute airway obstruction. *Rev Surg* 1977; 34:346–347.
19. Melnick BM: Postlaryngospasm pulmonary edema in adults. *Anesthesiology* 1984; 60:516–517.
20. Rivera M, Hadlock FP, O'Meara ME: Pulmonary edema secondary to acute epiglottitis. *AJR* 1979; 132:991–992.
21. Goldhill DR, Dalgleish JG, Lake RH: Respiratory problems and acromegaly. An acromegalic with hypersomia, acute upper airway obstruction, and pulmonary oedema. *Anaesthesia* 1982; 37:1200–1203.
22. Stradling JR, Bolton P: Upper airway obstruction as a cause of pulmonary oedema. *Lancet* 1982; 1:1353–1354.
23. Lorh DG, Sahn SA: Postextubation pulmonary edema following anesthesia induced by upper airway obstruction: Are certain patients at increased risk? *Chest* 1986; 90:802–805.
24. Blane VF, Tremblay NAG: Complications of tracheal intubation: A new classification with a review of the literature. *Anesth Analg* 1974; 53:202.
25. Jordan WS, Graves CL, Elwyn RA: New therapy for postintubation laryngeal edema and tracheitis in children. *JAMA* 1970; 212:585.
26. Mendelson CL: Aspiration of stomach contents into lungs during obstetric anesthesia. *Am J Obstet Gynecol* 1946; 30:191.
27. Berson W, Adriani J: "Silent" regurgitation and aspiration during anesthesia. *Anesthesiology* 1954; 15:644.
28. Turndorf H, Rodis ID, Clark TS: "Silent" regurgitation during general anesthesia. *Anesth Analg* 1974; 53:700.
29. Culver GA, Makel HP, Beecher HK: Frequency of aspiration of gastric contents by the lungs during anesthesia and surgery. *Ann Surg* 1951; 133:289.
30. Olsson GL, Hallen B, Hambraeus Jonzon K: Aspiration during anaesthesia: A computer aided study of 185,358 anaesthetics. *Acta Anaesth Scand* 1986; 30:84.
31. Dines DE, Titus JL, Sessler AD: Aspiration pneumonitis. *Mayo Clin Proc* 1970; 45:347.
32. Rao TLK, Suseeda M, El-Etv AA: Metoclopramide and cimetidine to reduce gastric pH and volume. *Anesth Analg* 1984; 63:264.
33. Tomlin PJ, Howarth FH, Robinson JS: Postoperative atelectasis and laryngeal incompetence. *Lancet* 1968; 1:1402.
34. Hefter E: Das intubations granulom. *Anesthetist* 1959; 8:194.
35. Howland WS, Lewis JS: Mechanisms in the development of postintubation granulomas of the larynx. *Ann Otol Rhinol Laryngol* 1956; 65:1006.
36. Snow JC, Harano M, Balough K: Postintubation granuloma of the larynx. *Anesth Analg* 1966; 45:425.

CHAPTER 45

Toxic Effects of Anesthetic

Approach of

Edward A. Norfleet, M.D.

The evolution and development of drugs that produce general or local anesthesia has been greatly influenced by both undesirable physical-chemical properties and the specific human toxicities of each drug. Unfortunately, all anesthetics have undesirable side effects that produce toxicity. The anesthetic state, in itself, can be considered a toxic reaction. It is well recognized that in addition to central nervous system (CNS) depression, marked depression of respiratory or cardiac function usually accompanies the anesthetic state. Anesthesiologists and biochemists continue to search for the perfect anesthetic to enhance the safety of the anesthetic state.

The important undesirable characteristics and toxic effects of some inhalational anesthetics are presented in Table 45–1. Inhalational anesthetics still in use today are nitrous oxide, halothane, ethrane, and isoflurane. Nitrous oxide for more than 100 years was thought to have no serious toxicity associated with it. It is noteworthy to recognize that the toxicity of nitrous oxide as it deactivates vitamin B_{12} has only recently been discovered and linked to numerous pathologies and occupational diseases associated with chronic human exposure.[1, 2] It has also been recently discovered that many of the toxicities associated with anesthetics are produced by toxic metabolites. The very interesting topic of the metabolism and toxicity of inhalational anesthetics has been extensively reviewed by Baden and Rice.[3]

In this chapter, I will discuss those topics of anesthetic toxicity that will be of great interest to the otolaryngologist. I have selected the malignant hyperthermia (MH) syndrome, cocaine overdosage, lidocaine toxicity, and the anesthetic-induced "sensitization" of the myocardium to catecholamines.

MALIGNANT HYPERTHERMIA

Malignant hyperthermia is a pharmacogenetic syndrome that is usually precipitated by a potent inhalational anesthetic drug in combination with depolarizing muscle relaxants. A generalized hypermetabolic state is activated in skeletal muscle, which, if not recognized and treated early, will rapidly advance to a progressive cascade of serious pathophysiologic derangements that may ultimately produce cardiovascular collapse and death. These derangements produce hyperthermia and extreme acidosis as a result of the accelerating hypermetabolic state. The basic biochemical defect resides in intracellular mechanisms that control and modulate intracellular calcium movements associated with the sarcoplasmic reticulium of skeletal muscle. The incidence of MH is reported to range between 1 in 15,000 and 1 in 50,000 anesthetic administrations.[4]

The first well-established case of MH syndrome associated with anesthesia occurred in 1960.[5] Britt and Kalow,[6] Gordon,[7] and Henschel and Locher[8] were early pioneers with this rare syndrome as they began to actively accumulate a worldwide registry of cases. Prior to recent therapeutic advances, the mortality was 70% once the syndrome was triggered. Over the past several decades, significant medical process has occurred with this rare but deadly syndrome. First, MH was recognized as a distinct syndrome. Second, a swine model of MH was discovered, which became a valuable tool to study the disease. Most recently, the drug dantrolene sodium (Dantrium) was found to be extremely therapeutic in preventing or interrupting the cycle of pathophysiologic events associated with the syndrome.[9]

Dantrolene sodium is a skeletal muscle relaxant, which initially was used to treat disorders of muscle spasticity. In the 1970s the drug was shown to be highly effective in reversing the biochemical events associated with the MH syndrome. Dantrolene inhibits the intracellular flux of calcium ions from the sarcoplasmic reticulum into the myoplasm and thus alters excitation-contraction coupling in skeletal muscle. With acute intravenous (IV) administration, there are minimal side effects in humans. However, with chronic oral usage, a small percentage of patients develop hepatotoxicity. The use of dantrolene to-

TABLE 45–1.
Undesirable Characteristics and Toxic Effects of Particular Inhalational Anesthetics

Name	Chemical Formula	Undesirable Physical-Chemical Properties and Toxicities
Nitrous oxide*	N_2O	Inactivation of vitamin B_{12} Diffusion into closed spaces Sympathomimetic
Ether	$C_2H_5OC_2H_5$	Flammability Nausea and vomiting
Chloroform	$CHCl_3$	Flammability Liver toxicity via centralobular necrosis
Cyclopropane	C_3H_6	Explosive Sympathomimetic Cardiac dysrhythmias
Trichlorothylene	C_2HCl_3	Production of phosgene with exposure to soda line Cardiac dysrhythmias
Halothane*	$CF_3CHClBr$	Respiratory and myocardial depression Cardiac dysrhythmias Hepatitis
Fluroxene	$CF_3CH_2OCH = CH_2$	Flammability Nausea and vomiting
Methoxyflurane	$CHCl_2CF_2OCH_3$	Renal damage secondary to fluoride ion
Enflurane*	CHF_2OCF_2CHClF	Respiratory and myocardial depression Seizure activity in EEG† with hypocarbia
Isoflurane*	$CHF_2OCHClCF_3$	Vasodilation ? Steal syndrome in coronary artery disease

*General anesthetics in common use today.
†EEG = electroencephalogram.

gether with verapamil to control the tachycardia associated with the MH syndrome should probably be avoided, because this combination produced hyperkalemia and cardiovascular collapse in swine.[10] In a multicenter study of the effects of dantrolene in treating MH, mortality was eradicated if the syndrome was recognized early and treated aggressively with 2.5 mg of dantrolene sodium/kg intravenously.[11]

All volatile anesthetic drugs and, in particular, the depolarizing muscle relaxant succinylcholine (Anectine) have, alone or in combination, triggered the development of the syndrome. Most commonly, the combination of halothane and succinylcholine have been implicated and associated with the development of hyperpyrexia in the majority of cases. This is predictable since over the past 30 years this specific combination of drugs has been the most popular general anesthetic technique available. Symptoms of MH include a hypermetabolic state characterized by extreme increases in oxygen consumption and carbon dioxide production. These hypermetabolic changes are accompanied by tachypnea, tachycardia, cyanosis, dysrhythmias, unstable blood pressure, hyperthermia, and muscle rigidity. Muscle rigidity frequently occurs as masseter muscle spasm, paradoxically in response to the administration of the muscle relaxant succinylcholine. Masseter spasm may be an important prodromal sign that should alert one to the great potential for the subsequent development of MH. Electrolyte disturbances (hyperkalemia), acidosis (mixed metabolic-respiratory acidosis), elevated creatine phosphokinase (CPK) enzyme levels, myoglobinemia, myoglobinuria, and an increase in arteriovenous oxygen difference are common laboratory findings associated with MH.

Management

The management of the patient with MH will be directed at either prevention in the susceptible patient or emergency treatment of a crisis in an unsuspected patient.

Prevention in the Susceptible Patient

The susceptible patient or a family member will by history have had an episode of hyperthermia during a previous anesthetic. The familial pattern of inheritance ranges from a dominant to recessive pattern, and thus a "genetic spectrum of susceptibility exists."[9] The patient or the family member may or may not have had an MH muscle biopsy test performed. In vitro, the patient's muscle is exposed to varying concentrations of halothane and caffeine to observe for the development of characteristic contracture patterns in susceptible muscle. Presently, there are controversies concerning the usefulness of such muscle biopsy tests. The test has not been universally rigidly standardized, is expensive, and is available at only a few medical centers. As with any laboratory test, false positives as well as false negatives may produce confusion concerning a particular patient. In the patient who has a positive history for unexplained hyperthermia during anesthesia, the results of the test will certainly not modify the anesthesiologist's approach.

Anesthetic Approach.—Fortunately, there are specific anesthetic techniques considered safe in the MH susceptible patient. The patient is heavily premedicated with benzodiazepines or barbiturates. If the surgical procedure can be performed under a regional anesthetic, this approach is preferred. Previously there was controversy concerning usage of ester (e.g., procaine) vs. the amide (e.g., lidocaine) local anesthetics. Formerly the amide group of local anesthetics was thought to be a trigger agent; however, presently all local anesthetics are considered safe.[12, 13] If the surgical procedure requires general anesthesia, a balanced technique must be used. A balanced anesthetic technique combines barbiturates, narcotics, nitrous oxide and oxygen, and a nondepolarizing muscle relaxant. This combination produces amnesia, analgesia, and muscle relaxation—the three essential components of a balanced anesthetic. One must avoid potent halogenated volatile anesthetics (e.g., halothane, ethrane, and isoflurane), succinylcholine, adrenergic agonists, and theophylline.[14]

I prefer to prophylactically treat the susceptible patient with dantrolene. Various methods of preoperative dantrolene prophylaxis have been advocated and continue to evolve. Currently it is my practice to administer 2 mg of dantrolene/kg intravenously just prior to the induction of anesthesia. Using the alternate technique of an oral loading dose over several days, my colleagues and I encountered the development of significant muscle weakness in a child with a muscular dystrophy.[15] Thus, the advantages of IV dantrolene given immediately preoperative avoids the potential for such adverse side effects, greatly shortens the patient's hospital stay, and assures an appropriate drug level of dantrolene at the most critical time of exposure. Flewellen also recommends IV dantrolene just prior to the induction of anesthesia.[13] Some consider the balanced technique in conjunction with close monitoring to be very safe and would administer dantrolene only if a crisis began to develop. The susceptible patient is monitored according to my routine standard, which includes blood pressure, ECG, pulse oximetry, capnography, and core temperature measurements. Following surgery, the patient is closely followed in the recovery room and for the first 24 hours postoperatively with close nursing surveillance, preferably in a critical care environment.

Management of Unsuspected Crisis

Efficient management of unsuspected crisis depends on a preconceived plan of therapy and organization of readily available equipment and drugs. I have found that the maintenance of a specialized cart for unexpected emergency treatment of malignant hyperthermia is invaluable at the time of crisis (Table 45–2).

Symptoms of crisis may include muscle rigidity during induction of succinylcholine or by increasing temperature, unexplained cyanosis, hypercarbia, or metabolic acidosis intraoperatively. The first clue may be the development of cardiac dysrhythmias. Any increase in temperature should be viewed with suspicion, because anesthetics and surgical exposure usually produce hypothermia. CAUTION: Hyperthermia may not always be the presenting symptom and may develop late in the syndrome. Once the suspicion or diagnosis of MH is made, the surgical team should be alerted and therapeutic modalities immediately started. I strongly advocate the therapy protocol as suggested by the medical authorities associated with the MHAUS, which is as follows:

1. Discontinue all inhalation anesthetics, and begin hyperventilation with 100% oxygen.
2. In the absence of blood gas analysis, administer 1 to 2 mEq of bicarbonate/kg.

TABLE 45–2.
Malignant Hyperpyrexia: Contents of Cart*

Top of Cart
  MHAUS† protocol for treatment of malignant hyperthermia
Top drawer
  Syringes
    1 mL for administration of insulin
    3 mL for drawing of blood for gas and electrolyte estimation
    Supply of heparin for heparinizing blood gas syringes
      IV cannulase and stopcocks for arterial line insertion
  Tubes
    For coagulation studies
    For serum thyroxine, CPK values
  Drugs
    Furosemide, three 20 mg vials, three 100 mg vials
    Procainamide, 3 g
    Dantrolene sodium, eight 20 mg vials
    Required sterile water for initial treatment in one adult
Second drawer
  Adult gastric lavage kit
  Four 50 mL syringes for dantrolene sodium
  Adult and pediatric peritoneal lavage catheters, fluid set and drainage bag
  Red rubber rectal tubes
  Disposable anesthetic circuit and bag (nonrebreathing type)
Refrigerator, left plugged in at all times
  Peritoneal dialysis fluid, 4,000 mL
  Regular insulin, 100 u/mL, 20 mL
  Dextrose 50%, 150 mL
  Potassium chloride, 160 mEq
  5% dextrose, 3 L
  Four glycerol freezer pouches for immediate surface cooling
On side of cart
  Collapsible plastic life raft and inflator

*From Mueller RA: *Probl Anesth* 1987; 2:242. Used by permission.
†MHAUS = Malignant Hyperthermia Association of the United States.

3. Obtain dantrolene, mix it with distilled water, and administer 1 mg/kg intravenously. At present, dantrolene is packaged as a lyophilized preparation that contains 20 mg of dantrolene per vial.
4. Simultaneously, begin cooling by all routes: surface, nasogastric lavage, IV cold solutions, wound, and rectally.
5. Change anesthetic tubing, and, if possible, soda lime.
6. Arrhythmias will usually respond to treatment of acidosis and hyperkalemia. If they persist or are life threatening, administer 200 mg of procainamide in repeated doses as required.
7. Administer further doses of dantrolene sodium as necessary, titrated to the heart rate, muscle rigidity, and temperature. Response to dantrolene should begin to occur in minutes; if not, administer more drug. Although the average successful dose of dantrolene is about 2 mg/kg, much higher doses may be needed ($\geq$10 mg/kg). Fortunately, dantrolene sodium does not produce significant myocardial depression at these doses.
8. Determine and monitor closely urine output, serum potassium level, calcium level, arterial blood gas values, and clotting studies. Hyperkalemia is common in the acute phase of MH; treat it with IV glucose and insulin.
9. Observe the patient in an intensive care setting for at least 24 hours since recrudescence of MH may occur, particularly following a case that was difficult to treat.
10. Follow CPK, calcium, and potassium values until such time as they return to normal.
11. Obtain and follow an ECG postoperatively.
12. Monitor body temperature closely, since overvigorous treatment of MH may lead to hypothermia. Temperature instability may persist for several days after the acute episode. Body temperatures of 41°C to 42°C are compatible with survival and normal brain function if treated promptly.
13. Ensure urine output of greater than 1 ml/kg/hour. Consider central venous pressure monitoring because of fluid shifts that may occur.
14. When the patient's condition has stabilized, convert from IV to oral dantrolene. Although data are not available regarding optimal doses and duration of treatment with dantrolene after an episode, the patient should probably receive a total dose of 4 mg/kg/day in divided doses for 48 hours postoperatively.

CAUTION: This protocol may not apply to every patient and must of necessity be altered according to specific patient needs.*

The most important objectives are removal of triggering agents, IV administration of dantrolene, and cooling of the patient to obtain normothermia. Dantrolene is dramatic in interrupting the crisis and should be available at the bedside during the recovery period. Prior to the development of dantrolene, surface and internal body cooling was the most effective treatment to abort the syndrome. Our emergency cart has equipment that allows us to quickly apply both external and internal hypothermia techniques. The entire patient can be packed in ice, or gastric lavage with cold saline can be quickly accomplished. One must use caution whenever aggressive hypothermia techniques are applied. Frostbite and ventricular fibrillation are complications caused by overly aggressive cooling. With early recognition and dantrolene administration, a previously rising temperature may begin to fall rapidly, and the need for aggressive hypothermic measures may not be necessary. The patient should be monitored very closely over the next 24 to 48 hours in an intensive care area. Appropriate laboratory data (arterial blood gas, electrolyte, and enzyme values) should be periodically followed until the patient has stabilized.

MHAUS* can provide extremely helpful information in understanding, recognizing, and treating the syndrome. In addition, they extend their efforts to the patient and the patient's family with up-to-date literature and continuing education programs. Referring my patients to MHAUS has greatly facilitated the extended care of the patient with MH. An excellent pamphlet entitled *Understanding Malignant Hyperthermia* is available to both physicians and their patients.

COCAINE TOXICITY

History

The history of our habitual abuse and therapeutic medical usage of cocaine from antiquity to the present time is extremely interesting. The ancient Inca civilization believed that cocaine was a divine plant provided as a gift of the Sun God. The Inca natives combined the coca leaf with lime (to release the alkaloid) and other ingredients to produce "cocada" paste, which was chewed for its powerful exhilarating effects. In other primitive cultures, there is evidence to suggest that cocaine was also used as a local anesthetic to facilitate trephining the skull to release evil spirits. Applications in medicine began to flourish in the 19th and 20th centuries as Koller, Freud, Halsted, Corning, Crile, and Cushing experimented with cocaine and applied the drug therapeutically as a local anesthetic[17]; unfortunately, both Freud and Halsted became habitually addicted to cocaine. Robert Lewis Stevenson is reported to have written the draft for Dr. Jekyll and Mr. Hyde while under the influence of cocaine as a prescribed remedy for tuberculosis. In 1888, the original Coca-Cola was introduced as a cocaine-containing cola, which was a stimulating tonic. These and other important historical events associated with the medical and illegal uses of cocaine have been summarized by Gay in a fascinating chronology.[17]

---

*From the Malignant Hyperthermia Association of the United States, Darien, Conn, 1986. Used by permission.

*Malignant Hyperthermia Association of the United States, Box 3231, Darien, CT 06820 (203-655-3007).

Among the street names for cocaine are nose candy, snow, happy trails, gold dust, Bernice, the star spangled power, the rich man's drug, Charlie, she, the Mercedes of drugs, goofy dust, lady, coke, happy powder, and dama blanca.

Cocaine Abuse

Cocaine abuse is perhaps the most serious, catastrophic social affliction invading our society today. Recent surveys indicate that one third of young American adults have tried cocaine at least once, and in the United States it is estimated that more than 22 million people are affected.[18, 19] It is not unusual to read about collegiate and professional athletes tragically developing "sudden death" following cocaine use.

The increasing severity of the medical problems associated with cocaine abuse requires that not only otolaryngologists but all physicians have a basic understanding of the pharmacology of cocaine, recognize the symptoms of toxicity, and be prepared to treat the life-threatening sequelae of an intentional or accidental overdosage. The majority of patients will be managed in an emergency room setting. Over the past decade, emergency room visits involving cocaine abuse have increased twofold.[20] Otolaryngologists are caring for a variety of nasal pathology, acute and chronic inflammatory disease, nose bleeds, ulcerations, and occasionally more serious complications such as nasal septal perforation, erosion of bony structures of the nasal cavity, and osteolytic sinusitis.[21–24] Ophthalmologists may see optic neuropathy associated with such osteolytic lesions.[25] The neurologist is consulted to manage clonic tonic seizures, unexplained periods of loss of consciousness, and cerebrovascular accidents.[36] The cardiologist is seeing with increasing frequency both young and elderly patients with sudden death or myocardial infarction induced as a result of cocaine abuse.[27, 28]

Pharmacology

Cocaine is extracted from the leaves of *Erythroxylon coca,* which is a tree indigenous to Peru, Bolivia, Mexico, and the West Indies.[29] Cocaine has the characteristic chemical structure relationships of other local anesthetics, where typically a hydrophilic amine is ester linked with a hydrophobic aromatic group. Cocaine is an ester of benzoic acid and ecgonine. Ecgonine is a parent compound of the important class of anticholinergic drugs atropine and scopolamine. Cocaine is an alkaloid and is chemically benzoylmethylecgonine $C_{17}H_{21}NO_4$.[29] Cocaine is rapidly absorbed through the mucous membranes of the respiratory tree and to a lesser extent through the membranes of the gastrointestinal (GI) tract. The serum concentration of cocaine peaks at 15 to 60 minutes after application to the nasal mucosa.[30] Following intranasal application of nasal pledgets soaked in 200 mg of 4% cocaine, the metabolic benzoylecgonine can be detected in the serum within 15 minutes, and a peak level occurs at 4.5 hours.[31] The serum half-life of cocaine is 1 hour.[32] In the serum, cocaine is quickly hydrolyzed by pseudocholinesterases into its major metabolites benzoylecgonine and ecgonine.[33] Cocaine is detoxified not only by serum pseudocholinesterase but also by enzyme hydrolysis in the liver.

Since the serum enzyme pseudocholinesterase is important in the hydrolysis of cocaine, any patient who has atypical pseudocholinesterase deficiency (frequency 1 in 3,200 patients) or who is taking drugs that enhance cholinergic actions, such as echothiophate, physostigmine, or prostigin, all of which inhibit ester hydrolysis, may be more likely to develop toxicity, since the metabolism of cocaine may be greatly delayed.[33] Following absorption of cocaine, 10% to 20% of unchanged drug and the inactive metabolite are subsequently excreted in the urine over the next 24 hours.

Physiologic Effects

Cocaine produces biphasic effects on the CNS and autonomic nervous system physiology. In the CNS, an initial generalized excitation is followed by profound depression. This is likely related to a depressive effect on central inhibitory centers. Smaller dosages of cocaine produce feelings of euphoria, self-confidence, and sexual excitement, whereas larger toxic dosages produce disorientation, clonic-tonic seizures, vomiting, incontinence, and ultimately respiratory failure as a result of depression of the medullary centers regulating respiration. Peripherally, cocaine produces many pathophysiologic effects on autonomic nervous system function.[19] The important effects are summarized and illustrated in Figure 45–1. A local anesthetic effect on neurons is produced as sodium channels are blocked by cocaine and propagation of neurotransmission is inhibited. Initially, cocaine stimulates the release of norepinephrine from presynaptic nerve terminals as a result of CNS activation. Subsequently, neuronal reuptake of epinephrine, norepinephrine, and dopamine is inhibited. This latter effect abolishes an important homeostatic mechanism responsible for regulating both endogenous and exogenous catecholamine metabolism and thus effects the blood levels of circulating catecholamines. As an additional effect within the neuron, cocaine can stimulate the synthesis of epinephrine, norepinephrine, and dopamine. All of these actions of cocaine on the brain, the spinal cord, and autonomic nervous tissue produce exaggerated sympathomimetic responses as circulatory levels of catecholamines are greatly increased.[19]

Dangerous cardiovascular complications such as tachydysrhythmias and malignant hypertension can result as systemic catecholamines are increased by the action of cocaine. Lethal complications as a result of these effects of cocaine are increasingly being reported in the medical literature.[24] Acute myocardial infarction in older patients is likely related to the sudden increase in myocardial oxygen demand induced by catecholamines. The increase in myocardial oxygen demand cannot be balanced with an increase in myocardial oxygen supply because of fixed atherosclerotic lesions of the coronary arteries. In younger patients, coronary artery spasm is a suggested mechanism responsible for acute myocardial infarction since in some patients selective coronary angiography fails to demonstrate specific atherosclerotic pathology.[27] Cerebrovascular accidents as a result of rupture of intracranial aneurysms and arteriovenous malformations occur following the hypertensive episodes associated with cocaine abuse. Spontaneous subarachnoid hemorrhage, transient ischemic episodes, and stroke are being re-

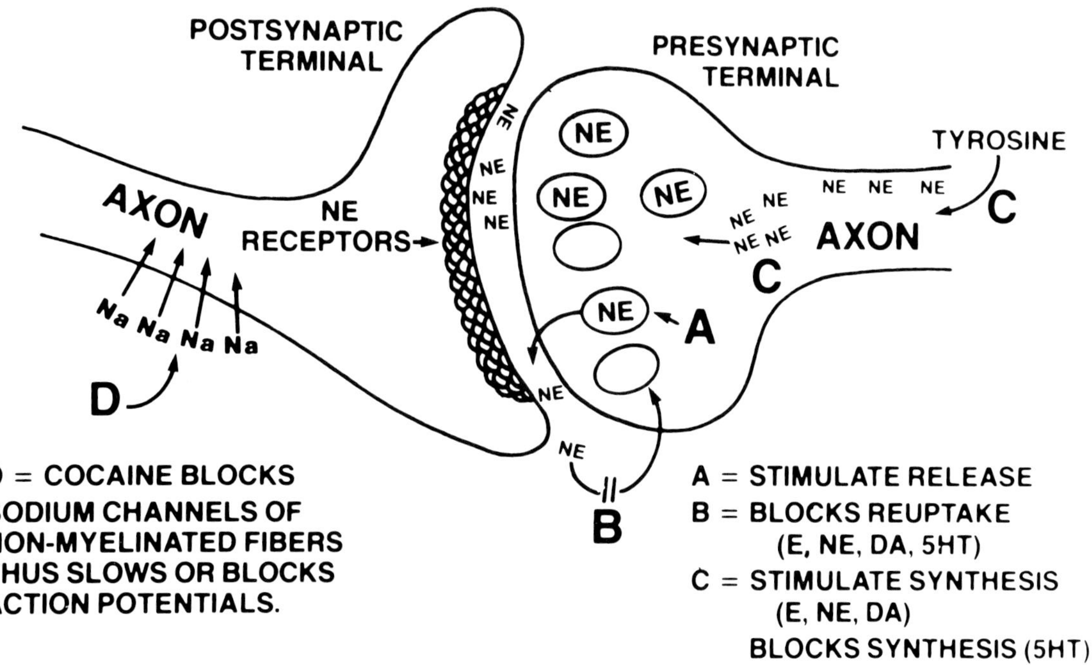

FIG 45–1.
Cocaine's local anesthetic and sympathomimetic effects. (From Gold MS, Dackis CA, Pottash ALC, et al: *Adv Alcohol Subst Abuse* 1986; 5(1–2):35–60. Used by permission.)

ported with alarming frequency in patients without accompanying congenital vascular abnormalities. The pathophysiologic mechanisms are unknown but are likely related to direct vasospasm or indirectly to the localized release and effect of the potent vasoconstrictor serotonin. Abnormalities in intravascular clotting mechanisms may follow because cocaine may indirectly induce increased platelet aggregation, prostaglandins are inhibited, and serum thromboxane levels rise.[26] Thromboxane is a potent vasoconstrictor and causes aggregation of platelets. The sudden death syndrome induced in healthy individuals may rarely result as a direct toxic effect on the myocardium but is more likely related to respiratory failure from profound central medullary depression. Cocaine abuse during pregnancy increases the incidence of stillbirth related to abruptio placenta and low birth weight of the infant.[34]

Clinical Usage

Cocaine has been an important and very useful drug as a local anesthetic to facilitate surgical procedures of the nose. Cocaine is an excellent local anesthetic, which, unlike other local anesthetics, also produces an intense vasoconstriction of the mucous membranes. These properties have made this drug ideal to induce profound local anesthesia and at the same time provide optimal operating conditions because the mucosa is decongested, bleeding is reduced, and, thus, surgical exposure is greatly enhanced. For anesthesiologists, these same properties have made the drug an excellent choice to facilitate awake nasal endotracheal intubation. In recent years, because of the problems associated with cocaine as a controlled substance, other local anesthetics combined with vasoconstricting drugs

have been used as a substitute to aid nasal tracheal intubation. Recently, Sessler et al. studied the efficacy of different solutions in nasal tracheal intubation.[35] They recommended the replacement of 5% cocaine solution with a 4% lidocaine and 0.5% phenylephrine solution to facilitate nasotracheal intubation.

In a hospital setting, whenever cocaine is used therapeutically, iatrogenic medical overdosage will rarely produce toxic symptomatology. Surprisingly, the toxic dosage of cocaine for each route of assimilation is not well established. Some of the dosages reported as lethal in an adult (70 kg) are 1.2 gm, with a median lethal dose being 500 mg from an oral ingestion.[17] Accidental absorption of large quantities of cocaine may sometimes occur in abusers known as "body packers," who conceal the drug in their GI tract for later use. They swallow large amounts of the drug, which has been packaged and tied securely in plastic bags or condoms. Accidental rupture of the packaged cocaine within the GI tract can suddenly release large quantities of the drug internally. Inhalational, IV, and subcutaneous dosages of 750 to 800 mg are considered lethal.[36] Of more importance to the otolaryngologist, Henderson and Johns, in a survey of practicing otolaryngologists, report that 47% of the physicians polled routinely use 200 mg of cocaine for nasal surgery without toxic effects.[37] However, caution should always be exercised since as little as 25 mg absorbed from mucosal surfaces have been reported to be lethal.[36] Cocaine is the most toxic local anesthetic drug available for medical use today. However, use of cocaine as a local anesthetic in an operating room or clinic environment is relatively safe, provided one is careful about dosage and aware of medical conditions that may enhance toxicity. One should be cautious when administering halothane or other halogenated anesthetics to patients in whom cocaine is concurrently being used. Potentially, dangerous cardiac dysrhythmias may result as halothane sensitizes the myocardium to the endogenously elevated catecholamine levels associated with cocaine.

Treatment

The treatment of an overdosage of cocaine is dictated by the severity of the respiratory, cardiovascular, and neurologic sequelae. Mild overdosage may not require any therapy whatsoever. Respiratory complications may include airway obstruction, hypoxia, and pulmonary edema, which are usually associated with tonic-clonic seizure activity. Management of respiratory failure will require oxygen therapy and establishment of a patent airway. Profound respiratory depression is treated aggressively with endotracheal intubation and assisted or controlled mechanical ventilation. Acid-base disorders may include both respiratory and metabolic components of acidosis, which are treated with ventilation and sodium bicarbonate as recommended by standard advanced life support protocols.

In an adult patient, extreme hypertension and tachydysrhythmias respond to 1 mg of IV propranolol injected slowly over 1 minute and repeated every 3 to 5 minutes until the desired cardiovascular effect is obtained.[38] Usually this will not require more than a total of 5 mg of propranolol. In the pediatric patient, a dosage of 0.01 to 0.1 mg of propranolol/kg has been recommended to control cardiovascular symptoms.[38] Following the excitement phase of cocaine toxicity, hypotension may occur. Hypotension is treated with the Trendleburg position and IV volume loading with lactated Ringer's solution. In the unresponsive hypotensive patient, 2 to 10 μg of dopamine/kg/minute may be needed if conservative measures fail. Recently, in patients with preexisting hypertensive cardiovascular disease, 0.25 mg of labetalol/kg has been advocated as a useful drug because of its combined alpha- and beta-blocking effects.[39] Because of its long half-life and hypotensive potential, labetalol is probably a poor choice for hypertensive management.

Seizures are treated with oxygen, establishment of an airway, and anticonvulsive drugs. Five to 10 mg of diazepam given intravenously is usually effective, but larger doses may be required. Small dosages of IV short-acting barbiturates (0.5–2 mg of pentobarbital/kg) are effective as well but may also require supportive airway management. At times, muscle paralysis combined with endotracheal intubation may be necessary if seizures cannot be controlled with conventional drug therapy.

Cocaine may occasionally produce hyperthermia as a result of the combined effects on the hypothalamus, peripheral vasoconstriction, and heat generated by muscular hyperactivity. Hyperthermic reactions are treated symptomatically by placing the patient in a cool environment. Chlorpromazine (Thorazine) produces a poikilothermic effect on the hypothalamus, which, in small dosages (25–50 mg intramuscularly), may be useful in normalizing temperature. In general, the toxic effects of cocaine are short lived because of the short half-life of the drug. In most crises of toxicity, symptoms should abate within a few hours. For the patient who presents in the emergency room with toxicity from cocaine abuse, a longer-range plan for psychologic help should be established following the management of the acute toxicity.

LIDOCAINE TOXICITY

Lidocaine (Xylocaine) is an extremely useful local anesthetic and antidysrhythmic drug of recent origin. The drug was first synthesized by Löfgren in 1943 and was introduced into medical practice as a local anesthetic in 1948.[40] In 1963, treatment of perioperative cardiac dysrhythmias in patients undergoing cardiac surgery was described by Harrison et al.[41] Today, lidocaine is the most popular and widely used local anesthetic and has certainly become the drug of choice for treating certain ventricular dysrhythmias, particularly those associated with myocardial ischemia and infarction. Intravenous lidocaine (1 mg/kg) is the drug of choice for the emergency treatment of premature ventricular contractions and ventricular tachycardia.

Pharmacology

Lidocaine is an amide local anesthetic. It produces local anesthesia by selectively blocking the permeability of the axon to sodium ions, which prevents depolarization of the neuron, and thus, conduction of the nerve impulse. As an antidysrhythmic drug, lidocaine is classified as a class Ib drug. Class I drugs are local anesthetics that act as membrane stabilizers of myocardial tissue. Electrophysiologically, lidocaine depresses phase IV depolarization in Purkinge's fibers and decreases the action potention duration (ADP) and the length of the effective refractory period (EFP) in cardiac conducting cells. The ADP is effected to a greater degree than ERP, so that the ERP/ADP ratio is increased.[42] The interesting electrophysiologic mechanisms responsible for producing local anesthesia and the dysrhythmic properties of lidocaine have been extensively reviewed elsewhere for the interested reader.[42, 43]

Metabolism

Lidocaine is metabolized in the liver, and small amounts are excreted unchanged in the kidneys. Metabolism occurs by *N*-dealkylation. The plasma half-life may vary from 30 minutes to 2 hours, with an average of 1.6 hours.[44] Therefore, a subsequent dose given 90 minutes after the initial dose should be halved.[44] Patients with reduced hepatic blood flow as a result of heart failure or shock and patients with hepatic dysfunction are much more likely to develop toxicity, and dosages should accordingly be reduced.

Clinical Usage

Lidocaine is a very versatile local anesthetic that is used for local infiltration, major nerve blocks, and a variety of conduction techniques (spinal, epidural, caudal). No matter which technique is used, the recommended total dosage in an adult should not exceed 300 mg, or 500 mg if epinephrine has been added to the solution. Infiltration anesthesia with 1% lidocaine will last approximately 2 hours but can be increased to 7 hours when it is combined with epinephrine 1:200,000.[44] The addition of epinephrine to a local anesthetic solution produces local vasoconstriction, which not only reduces bleeding locally but also greatly increases the duration of the block, reduces systemic absorption, and reduces toxicity of the drug. Thus, the addition of epinephrine increases the margin of safety as related to the total dosage of anesthetic. Lidocaine with epinephrine 1:200,000 is the most useful recommended dilution. When using lidocaine with epinephrine, one should consider not only the toxic dose of lidocaine but also the toxic dose of epinephrine. In an adult, no more than 200 μg of epinephrine should be injected at any one time (e.g., 40 mL of 1:200,000, 10 mL of 1:50,000).[45] Systemic absorption of small amounts of epinephrine generally produce sympathiomimetic effects, resulting in tachycardia and increased cardiac output (beta effects), whereas larger plasma concentrations of epinephrine produce hypertension and dysrhythmias (both alpha and beta effects).

The use of lidocaine to suppress ventricular dysrhythmias is a common practice in critical care units, particularly for patients being treated for recent myocardial infarction. A bolus loading IV dose of 1 mg/kg is followed by a constant infusion of 1 to 3 mg/minute. The plasma concentration at which cardiac dysrhythmias are suppressed is 2 to 5 μg/mL.

Cause

Xylocaine toxicity may occur following local anesthetic techniques for regional anesthesia or from accumulating toxic plasma levels when lidocaine is used in the management of cardiac dysrhythmia. Toxicity will be greatly influenced by the site of deposition of the drug. The most common cause of iatrogenic toxicity is accidental intravascular injection. Accidental intra-arterial or IV bolus injection can cause immediate toxicity with CNS symptoms or cardiac depression. Common symptoms of toxicity include tingling in the mouth and fingers, tinnitus, lethargy, and muscle twitching, which with higher dosages progresses to tonic-clonic seizure activity. Depression of cardiac contractility, reduced cardiac output, and heart block of varying degrees can occur particularly in patients with the "sick sinus syndrome."[46–49] The threshold when toxic symptoms begin to occur is at a blood concentration of 5 μg/mL, whereas seizures develop at 10 μg/mL.[44]

Perhaps the second most common intragenic cause of toxicity from local anesthetic administration is failure to closely monitor the specific amount and volume of drug actually being administered over a given time period. A basic principle that must be remembered and understood is the number of milligrams of drug in a standard percent solution. REMEMBER: 1 mL of a 1% solution contains 10 mg of the active substance. This follows, since to produce a 1% solution, 1 gm (or 1,000 mg) of the active substance is dissolved in 100 mL of the diluting solution. A 2% solution will contain 20 mg of the active substance in each milliliter of solution. Thus, in an adult patient, if a 1% solution of lidocaine is being used for local infiltration, the maximal volume should be 30 mL, since 300 mg is the limit (i.e., 300 mg total dose/10 mg/mL = 30 mL).

Prevention

Toxicity can best be prevented by avoiding intravascular injections and unintentional drug overdosage as a result of calculation errors. Intravascular injections are usually responsible for any immediate toxic symptoms. As the local anesthetic is injected, it is important to aspirate periodically to prevent inadvertent intravascular injections. Especially in the head and neck or posterior pharynx, accidental bolus injections of lidocaine into small branches of the carotid or vertebral arteries may retrogradely fill these vascular beds and thus cause extremely high brain concentrations, resulting in immediate seizures, coma, and respiratory depression. Dosage should be reduced in patients with low cardiac output syndromes and severe liver disease, since changes in regional blood flow to the brain and liver increase plasma concentrations and decrease the metabolism of lidocaine. Diazepam, because of its anticonvulsant properties, can be used to both prevent and treat seizures. Diazepam (0.15 mg/kg) is useful as a premedicant during regional anesthesia since the threshold for seizures can be increased by 50%.[50] Narcotic premedication, on the other hand, decreases the dose of lidocaine required to produce seizures because of the increased cerebral blood flow secondary to CO_2 retention.

Treatment

Prevention of hypoxia is the primary goal. As with cocaine toxicity, the principles of basic and advanced life support techniques should be immediately instituted. Oxygen administration, securement of an airway, and ventilation are directed at preventing hypoxia in patients who develop toxic CNS symptomatology. Seizures are most easily controlled by IV titration of diazepam or barbiturates. If seizures are not easily controlled, muscle relaxants may be required to facilitate endotracheal intubation.

Cardiovascular depression may consist of vasodilation, hypotension, low cardiac output, heart block, ventricular fibrillation, or cardiac arrest. Myocardial depression and hypotension may require 2 to 10 μg/kg of dopamine or other appropriate innotropic drug. Heart block may be transient but may require IV atropine, isoproterenol, or a transvenous pacemaker. Cardiac arrest and cardiovascular collapse is usually secondary to hypoxia and will require resuscitation with advanced cardiac life support protocols.[51]

CATECHOLAMINE-ANESTHETIC DYSRHYTHMIC INTERACTIONS

The catecholamines includes a group of structurally related sympathomimetic compounds that have a "catechol" aromatic moiety and an "amine" moiety, hence the chemical name catecholamines. The important biologic catecholamines includes dopamine, norepinephrine, and epinephrine. Endogenous catecholamines serve dual roles as important chemical transmitters to facilitate and modulate CNS and autonomic nervous system activity and to dynamically effect cardiovascular function. A steriospecific interaction occurs when these compounds are in proximity to alpha, beta, and dopimergic membrane receptors on specific end organs. In the periphery, alpha stimulation of vascular smooth muscle produces vasoconstriction. In the myocardium, once cellular beta receptors are activated, intracellular adenyl cyclase stimulates selected biochemical pathways to enhance inotropic, chromotropic, and dromotropic activities. All of these excitatory sympathomimetic events have the potential to induce or aggravate a wide variety of cardiac dysrhythmias. Dysrhythmias may occur as a result of release of endogenous catecholamines or from exogenous catecholamine administration. Excessive sympathetic stimulation is particularly dangerous in patients with advanced cardiovascular disease and may occasionally progress to life-threatening rhythm disturbances, such as ventricular tachycardia or ventricular fibrillation. The potential for the development of catecholamine induced dysrhythmias is greatly enhanced by a variety of other pathophysiologic conditions affecting the patient. These include hypoxia, hypercarbia, other acid-base disturbances, electrolyte imbalance, ischemia, certain tumors (pheochromocytomas), and the toxic effects of numerous cardiac drugs that modify the electrophysiologic properties of myocardial tissue.

Halogenated inhalational anesthetic drugs such as halothane, ethrane, and isoflurane produce potent reversible effects on myocardial automaticity, conduction, and contraction. Both conductive and contractile tissue throughout the heart are affected. Spontaneous excitation or synchronous depolarization of the sinoarterial node, the atrial muscle, the atrioventricular node, the Purkinge network, and ventricular tissue all are affected. Dysrhythmias during inhalational anesthesia and surgery are not uncommon, particularly during halothane anesthesia. Common dysrhythmias during halothane anesthesia include bradycardia, nodal rhythms, and premature ventricular contractions. All of the halogenated anesthetics sensitize the heart to the catecholamines; however, halothane certainly produces the most sensitivity. Sensitization is a term used to describe a phenomenon where an anesthetic drug such as halothane lowers the threshold for the development of ventricular dysrhythmias induced by elevations of either endogenous or exogenous catecholamines.

The infiltration of tissue with local anesthesia and epinephrine is a useful hemostatic adjunct to surgery. Although localized bleeding is significantly reduced as the epinephrine is systemically absorbed, the plasma concentration increases. Epinephrine produces dose-related cardiovascular effects as related to beta and alpha stimulation. Plasma concentrations of 1 to 2 µg produce beta stimulation, whereas larger concentrations (10–15 µg) produce alpha stimulation. The combined effects of drugs such as halothane and epinephrine produce unique dose-related interactions where inhomogenitics of automaticity, conduction, and refraction occur throughout the heart. Under such conditions, normal coordination of autonomic reflexes and synchronized regulation of excitation-contraction processes are perturbed. Premature ventricular contractions and dangerous ventricular tachycardias frequently develop. These rhythm disturbances may progress to ventricular fibrillation and cardiac arrest. These drug interactions are quite complex and not completely understood. The interesting subject of halothane-induced arrhythmias has been recently reviewed by Maze and Mason.[52] The use of epinephrine solutions should not be used indiscriminately and should be used with caution in patients with serious cardiovascular disease.

Prevention

During general anesthesia, whenever administration of an exogenous solution of epinephrine is anticipated, one should use the least sensitizing anesthetic technique. Narcotic techniques do not sensitize the heart to catecholamines; however, such techniques are not always the most desirable for certain surgical procedures. When an inhalational anesthetic is selected, enflurane and isoflurane produce less sensitization than halothane. Johnston et al. did an important comparative interaction study of epinephrine with enflurane, isoflurane, and halothane in humans.[53] These investigators determined how many micrograms of epinephrine per kilogram that could be injected submucosally to produce a dysrhythmia in 50% of patients (i.e., the median effective dose). The median effective dose was 2.1 µg/kg for halothane, 3.7 µg/kg for halothane-lidocaine, 10.9 µg/kg for enflurane, and 6.7 µg/kg for isoflurane (Fig 45–2). From this study, halothane produced the most sensitization that could be reduced by the addition of lidocaine to the epinephrine solution. The results of this study are presented in Figure 45–2. Katz and Epstein have recommended in an adult, no more than a total dose of 100 µg of epinephrine be subcutaneously injected in a 10-minute period or a total dose of 300 µg over 1 hour.[54]

One should avoid iatrogenic drug errors. Premixed dilutions of local anesthetic with epinephrine are safer than homemade dilutions since the potential for human error is greatly diminished. In my experience, the mathematical error of missing the decimal point when one is mixing epinephrine with a local anesthetic has been a major cause of overdosage progressing to dysrhythmia.

Another frequently confusing issue relates to the use of the pharmacologic designation of 1:100,000 or 1:200,000 when one is relating the concentration of epinephrine that has been added to a local anesthetic solution. An epinephrine solution labeled 1:1,000 (1 to 1,000) will contain 1 mg of epinephrine in 1 mL of solution. A 1:1,000 solution was made by adding 1 gm (or 1,000 mg) of epinephrine to 1,000 mL of solution. A useful method to quickly calculate how many micrograms per milliliter of epinephrine is contained in a specific anesthetic solution is as follows. Take the designated dilution, for example, 1:200,000, and mentally (or better still, with pen and paper!) set up the following equation to calculate how many micrograms are in 1 mL by dividing 1 million by the dilutional number (in this case, the dilutional number is 200,000, for 1:200,000):

$$X = \frac{1,000,000}{200,000 \text{ (dilution number)}}$$

$$X = 5 \ \mu g/mL$$

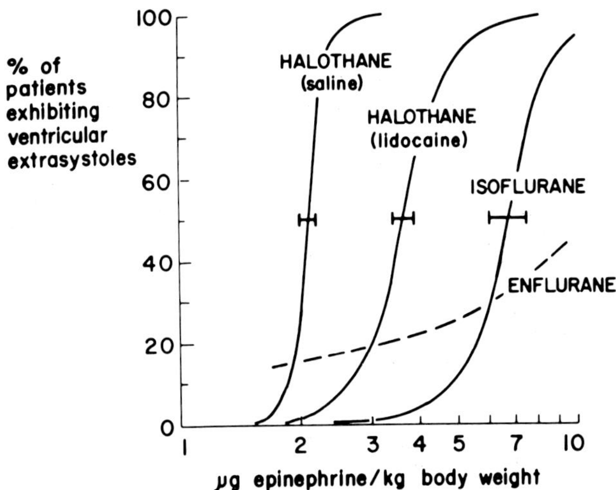

FIG 45–2.
The results of the statistical analysis suggest that the two halothane and the isoflurane curves (but not the enflurane curve) are parallel and that the median effective doses are significantly different from each other ($P < 0.01$). The bars indicate the standard deviation from the median effective dose. (From Johnston RR, Eger EI, Wilson C: *Anesth Analg* 1976; 55:709–712. Used by permission.)

Thus, 5 μg of epinephrine are in each milliliter of a 1:200,000 solution of epinephrine. For a 1:100,000 solution, it follows that there are 10 μg of epinephrine in each milliliter.

Treatment

The ECG should be monitored when epinephrine solutions are used. Following epinephrine-induced dysrhythmias, any inhalational anesthetic should be discontinued, and the patient should be given 100% oxygen. Premature ventricular contractions and ventricular tachycardia should be treated with 1 mg of IV lidocaine/kg, followed with an infusion of 1 to 3 mg of lidocaine/minute. Beta blockade with incremental dosages (1 mg) of propranolol are useful for tachydysrhythmias induced by catecholamines. The shorter-acting drug esmolol is a new beta blocker that is very useful in treating supraventricular tachycardia. A loading dose of 500 μg/kg/minute for 1 minute is followed by maintenance infusions of 50 μg/kg/minute. The titrating dosage can be increased until the desired heart rate is obtained. When very large dosages of epinephrine have been administered, both tachycardia (beta) and hypertension (alpha) occur. These effects usually disappear as the drug becomes metabolized. However, if both tachycardia and hypertension require therapy, labetalol is a useful new drug that blocks both the beta and alpha affects of epinephrine. Under anesthesia, in an adult, I give an initial IV dose of 5 mg (0.07 mg/kg) followed by 5 mg increments until the desired heart rate and blood pressure are obtained. During recovery, since the half-life of labetalol is much longer than that of epinephrine, labetalol can cause symptomatic postural hypotension after the epinephrine effect dissipates. All of the beta blocking drugs should be used with extreme caution in patients with asthma, cardiac failure, heart block, and severe bradycardia.

REFERENCES

1. Eger EI II: *Nitrous Oxide N₂O*. New York, Elsevier North-Holland, 1985.
2. Norfleet EA, Hackney RW, Waterson CK: Inhalational anesthetic toxicity: Controlling occupational exposure in the clinical environment, in Huisingh D (ed): *A Compendium of the Proper Management of Toxic and Hazardous Materials in Health Care Facilities*. Raleigh, NC, Board of Science and Technology, 1987, p 61.
3. Baden JM, Rice SA: Metabolism and toxicity of inhaled anesthetics in Miller RD (ed): *Anesthesia,* ed 2. New York, Churchill Livingstone, 1986, vol 1, pp 701–747.
4. Britt BA, Kalow W: Malignant hyperthermia: A statistical review. *Can Anaesth Soc J* 1970; 17:293.
5. Denborough MA, Lovell RRH: Anaesthetic deaths in a family. *Lancet* 1960; 2:45.
6. Britt BA, Kalow W: Malignant hyperthermia: Aetiology unknown. *Can Anaesth Soc J* 1970; 17:316–330.
7. Gordon RA: Malignant hyperpyrexia during general anesthesia. *Can Anaesth Soc J* 1966; 13:415–416.
8. Henschel EO, Locher WG: The Wausau story—malignant hyperthermia in Wisconsin, in Henschel EO (ed): *Malignant Hyperthermia: Current Concepts*. New York, Appleton-Century-Crofts, 1977, pp 3–7.
9. Gronert GA: Malignant hyperthermia. *Anesthesiology* 1980; 53:395–423.
10. Saltzman LS, Kates RA, Corke BC, et al: Hyperkalemia and cardiovascular collapse after verapamil and dantrolene administration in swine. *Anesth Analg* 1984; 63:473–478.
11. Kolb ME, Horne ML, Martz R: Dantrolene in human malignant hyperthermia. *Anesthesiology* 1982; 56:254–262.
12. Rosenberg H, Potter H, Gallamore R: *Understanding Malignant Hyperthermia*. Darien, CT, Malignant Hyperthermia Association of the United States, 1986.
13. Flewellen EH: Malignant hyperthermia and associated conditions: Dilemma, controversy, and unanswered questions, in *Review Course Lectures 1985*. Cleveland, International Anesthesia Research Society, pp 76–83.
14. Mueller RA: How to identify malignant hyperthermia. *Probl Anesth* 1987; 2:233–244.
15. Watson CB, Reierson N, Norfleet EA: Clinically significant muscle weakness induced by oral dantrolene sodium prophylaxis for malignant hyperthermia. *Anesthesiology* 1986; 65:312–314.
16. Malignant Hyperthermia Association of the United States: Darien, Conn.
17. Gay GR, Inaba DS, Rappolt RT, et al: "An ho, ho, baby, take a whiff on me." La dama blanca cocaine in current perspective. *Anes Analg* 1976; 55:582–587.
18. Johnston LD, Bachman JG, O'Malley PM: Student drug use, attitudes and beliefs: National Trends 1975–1982, publication (ADM) 83-1260. Washington, DC, Department of Health and Human Services, 1983.
19. Gold MS, Dackis CA, Pottash ALC, et al: Cocaine update: From bench to bedside. *Adv Alcohol Subst Abuse* 1986; 5(1–2): 35–60.
20. Grabowski J, Dworden S: Cocaine: An overview of current issues. *Int J Addic* 1985; 20:1065–1088.
21. Gossop M: Beware cocaine. *Br Med J Clin Res* 1987; 295:945.
22. Schweitzer VG: Osteolytic sinusitis and pneumomediastinum: Deceptive otolaryngologic complications of cocaine abuse. *Laryngoscope* 1985; 96:206–210.
23. Sawicka EH, Trosser A: Cerebrospinal fluid rhinorrhea

after cocaine snorting. *Br Med J (Clin Res)* 1983; 286:1476–1479.

24. Cregler LL, Mark H: Medical complications of cocaine abuse. *N Engl J Med* 1986; 315:1495–1500.

25. Newman NM, DiLoreto DA, Ho JT, et al: Bilateral optic neuropathy and osteolytic sinusitis. *JAMA* 1988; 259:72–74.

26. Levine SR, Jefferson MF, Kieran SN, et al: "Crack" cocaine–associated stroke. *Neurology* 1987; 37:1849–1853.

27. Cregler LL, Mark H: Cardiovascular dangers of cocaine abuse. *Am J Cardiol* 1986; 57:1185–1186.

28. Rollingher IM, Belzberg AS, Macdonald JL: Cocaine-induced myocardial infarction. *Can Med Assoc J* 1986; 135:45–46.

29. Gilman AG, Goodman LS, Gilman A: *The Pharmacological Basis of Therapeutics,* ed 6. New York, MacMillan Publishing Co, 1980.

30. Dyke CV, Barash PG, Jatlow P, et al: Cocaine: Plasma concentrations after intranasal application in man. *Science* 1976; 191:859–861.

31. Johns ME, Berman AR, Price JC, et al: Metabolism of intranasally applied cocaine. *Ann Otol* 1977; 86:342–347.

32. Van Dyke C, Jatlow P, Ungerer J, et al: Oral cocaine: Plasma concentrations and central effects. *Science* 1978; 200:211–213.

33. Verlander JM, Johns ME: The clinical use of cocaine. *Otolaryngol Clin North Am* 1981; 14:521–531.

34. Bingol N, Fuchs M, Diaz V, et al: Teratogenicity of cocaine in humans. *J Pediatr* 1987; 110:93–96.

35. Sessler CN, Vitaliti JC, Cooper KR, et al: Comparison of 4% lidocaine/0.5%/phenylephrine with 5% cocaine: Which dilates the nasal passages better? *Anesthesiology* 1986; 64:274–277.

36. Gay GR: Clinical management of acute and chronic cocaine poisoning. *Ann Emerg Med* 1982; 11:562–572.

37. Henderson RL, Johns ME: The clinical use of cocaine. *Drug Ther* Feb 7, 1977, pp 31–41.

38. Becker CE: *Cocaine Toxicity.* Poisindex, ed 55. Micromedex Inc, 1988.

39. Dusenberry SJ, Hicks MJ, Mariani PJ: Labetalol treatment of cocaine toxicity. *Ann Emerg Med* 1987; 16:235.

40. Fink BR: History of local anesthesia, in Cousins MJ (ed): *Neural Blockade in Clinical Anesthesia and Management of Pain.* Philadelphia, JB Lippincott Co, 1980, pp 3–18.

41. Harrison DC, Sprouse JG, Morrow AG: The antiarrhythmic properties of lidocaine and procaine amide. *Circulation* 1963; 28:486.

42. Covino BG: Perioperative management of arrhythmias, in Kaplan JA (ed): *Cardiac Anesthesia: Cardiovascular Pharmacology.* New York, Grune & Stratton, 1983, vol 2, pp 395–412.

43. De Jong RH: Clinical physiology of local anesthetic action, in Cousins MJ (ed): *Neural Blockade in Clinical Anesthesia and Management of Pain.* Philadelphia, JB Lippincott Co, 1980, pp 21–44.

44. Scott DB, Cousins MJ: Clinical pharmacology of local anesthetic agents, in Cousins MJ (ed): *Neural Blockade in Clinical Anesthesia and Management of Pain.* Philadelphia, JB Lippincott Co, 1980, pp 86–121.

45. Katz RL, Epstein RA: The interaction of anesthetic agents and adrenergic drugs to produce cardiac arrhythmias. *Anesthesiology* 1968; 29:763.

46. Dhingra RC, Deedwania PC, Cummings JM, et al: Electrophysiologic effects of lidocaine on sinus node and atrium in patients with and without sinoatrial dysfunction. *Circulation* 1978; 57:448–454.

47. Klein HO, Jutrin I, Kaplinsky E: Cerebral and cardiac toxicity of a small dose of lignocaine. *Br Heart J* 1975; 37:775–778.

48. Cheng TO, Wadhwa K: Sinus standstill following intravenous lidocaine administration. *JAMA* 1973; 223:790–792.

49. Lichstein E, Chadda KD, Gupta PK: Atrioventricular block with lidocaine therapy. *Am J Cardiol* 1973; 31:277–281.

50. Murphy TM: Nerve blocks, in Miller RD (ed): *Anesthesia* ed 2. New York, Churchill Livingstone, 1986, vol 2, pp 1015–1055.

51. Standards and guidelines for cardiopulmonary resuscitation (CPR) and emergency cardiac care (ECC). *JAMA* 1986; 255:2905–2992.

52. Maze M, Mason DM: Aetiology and treatment of halothane-induced arrhythmias. *Clin Anaesthesiol* 1983; 1:301–321.

53. Johnston RR, Eger EI, Wilson C: A comparative interaction of epinephrine with enflurane, isoflurane, and halothane in man. *Anes Analg* 1976; 55:709–712.

54. Katz RL, Epstein RA: The interaction of anesthetic agents and adrenergic drugs to produce cardiac arrhythmias. *Anesthesiology* 1968; 29:763–784.

Toxic Effects of Anesthetic

Approach of

Kathryn E. McGoldrick, M.D.

This chapter explores systemic complications, focusing on the metabolic complication of malignant hyperthermia (MH) as well as potential pharmacologic complications related to cocaine toxicity, lidocaine toxicity, and epinephrine-halothane interaction.

METABOLIC COMPLICATIONS

Malignant Hyperthermia

Initially described in 1960 by Denborough et al.,[1] MH represents one of the most dramatic complications of anesthesia and surgery. It may be defined as a fulminant hypermetabolic crisis triggered by anesthesia. Although mortality statistics initially hovered around 70%, with the advent of dantrolene sodium, the mortality rate has been greatly reduced and is now said to be approximately 10%. Nevertheless, MH is still one of the most common causes of anesthesia-induced death in North America. Infants, as well as septuagenarians, have been afflicted.

Perhaps the relative success we have achieved in coping with MH is due to the organized, aggressive approach adopted by several physicians involved with MH since the early days. Drs. Beverly Britt and W. Kalow, at the University of Toronto, established an international registry of reported cases that was very educational. Furthermore, assiduous attention has been devoted to rapid promulgation of current information regarding this still incompletely understood phenomenon via international symposia and frequent newsletters, such as those produced by the Malignant Hyperthermia Association of the United States (MHAUS) and the Malignant Hyperthermia Association of Canada (MHAC). Both MHAUS and its Canadian counterpart offer enthusiastic support to families and friends of MH patients.

Incidence

In the past, the incidence of MH was placed at 1 in 50,000 anesthetic episodes in adults and 1 in 15,000 children. However, new data collected in Denmark and published in 1985 disclosed fulminant MH approximately once in 260,000 general anesthetic episodes.[2] The number increased to 1 in 60,000 when succi-nylcholine was administered. If nonspecific signs of MH, such as masseter muscle rigidity, were included, the incidence rose to 1 in 12,000 anesthesia episodes. When additional nonspecific signs of MH, such as fever and unexplained tachycardia, were counted, this incidence increased further to 1 in 5,000 general anesthetics when an inhalation agent and succinylcholine were employed.

Presentation

Malignant hyperthermia has a plethora of symptoms. It is essential to appreciate that all forms may become fulminant and result in death. The so-called classic case is characterized by a rapid rise in body temperature that is associated with muscle rigidity, tachycardia and various other dysrhythmias, rhabdomyolysis, acidosis, hyperkalemia, and, eventually, disseminated intravascular coagulation (DIC). Most of these cases occur during anesthesia, although some may present in the postanesthetic period. There is often a family history of MH or of an unexplained perioperative death. In most instances, therapy for MH is successful if the correct diagnosis is promptly established. Unfortunately, the more fulminant forms are often associated with recrudescence. Hence, it is imperative to carefully monitor these patients' vital signs and certain laboratory parameters, as indicated, for at least 24 hours following the initial episode.

A common symptom of MH is masseter muscle rigidity following induction with succinylcholine. Approximately 50% of these individuals, if given muscle biopsy testing, are noted to be MH susceptible.[3] However, masseter rigidity following succinylcholine induction is not uncommon, especially in the pediatric population. Although the incidence in adults is 1 in 12,000,[2] in the pediatric population, at least one study reports the incidence approximates 1% when succinylcholine is used after halothane induction.[4]

Currently, it is popularly thought muscle rigidity after succinylcholine induction is a prodrome of MH and that the anesthetic should be immediately discontinued. Usually, if no other symptoms of MH, such as temperature elevation or generalized muscle rigidity, ensue, dantrolene treatment is not elected. However, the patient should be closely monitored in a recovery room or intensive care setting for a minimum of 8 hours. Urine myoglobin and blood CPK levels at 6, 12, 18, and 24 hours should be obtained. The CPK level usually peaks at 10 to 24 hours after trismus. Although preoperative CPK values are very unreliable predictors of MH susceptibility, in the setting of succinylcholine-induced masseter spasm, it has been noted that if the CPK level exceeds 15,000 IU, there is an 88% likelihood of MH susceptibility.[5] If the perioperative peak CPK value is 20,000 IU or more, the patient virtually invariably proves to be MH susceptible. Moreover, patients who develop masseter spasm following succinylcholine induction, even with nonimpressive peak CPK levels, should be tested with neurologic evaluation and muscle biopsy. Not uncommonly, a myotonic syndrome or other myopathy will be detected.

End-tidal CO_2 levels can be invaluable in detecting MH very early in its course, and these monitors have added many dimensions of safety to the anesthesiologist's armamentarium. Likewise, an apparently unexplained tachycardia may often be an early sign of MH. It is essential not to assume the latter is always due to light anesthesia or hypovolemia. Vigilance and a high index of suspicion are imperative if MH is to be detected while it is still reversible. It is vital to understand that temperature elevation may be a very late manifestation of MH, and generalized muscle rigidity may never be obvious.

Furthermore, since approximately one third of MH cases have occurred during induction of a second or subsequent anesthetic, a previously uneventful anesthetic experience does not imply impunity. However, a personal or family history of MH has great predictive value, and the importance of exploring these areas cannot be overemphasized.

The list of anesthetic agents that may trigger MH is extensive and includes depolarizing muscle relaxants and virtually all the potent inhalation anesthetics, such as halothane, ether, cyclopropane, methoxyflurane, enflurane, and isoflurane. Halothane has been the general anesthetic involved in approximately 60% of reported cases, and succinylcholine has been involved in 77%.

It had previously been thought that amide-type local anesthetics were capable of triggering MH. However, more recent wisdom holds that both amide and ester local anesthetics are safe.

Parenthetically, it should be mentioned that hyperthermia may be induced by nonanesthetic drugs such as certain psychotropic agents, and this condition is called the neuroleptic malignant syndrome (NMS). It is unknown whether there is a common etiology with anesthesia-induced MH.

Muscle Disorders and Malignant Hyperthermia

A variety of disorders have been associated with MH, and those with a strong association include Duchenne's muscular dystrophy and Becker's muscular dystrophy, as well as central core disease, myotonia congenita, the NMS, arthrogryposis, and the King syndrome, which is characterized by cryptorchidism, hypotonia, webbed neck, lordosis, and pectus deformity. In addition, there is some debate whether osteogenesis imperfecta has a strong link with MH. Nonetheless, most anesthesiologists would probably tend to avoid MH-triggering drugs in all of the aforementioned conditions.

It should also be noted that even mild and common muscle derangements may have a higher than usual risk of MH. These conditions include inguinal hernia, ptosis, strabismus, generalized muscle bulk, localized muscle weakness, and even simply a history of muscle cramps, especially if linked with caffeine ingestion.

Pathophysiology

Malignant hyperthermia is a disorder of skeletal muscle induced by exposure to certain pharmacologic agents. However, the specific site or sites of muscle abnormalities remain undetermined. It is postulated that the sarcoplasmic reticulum unloads calcium inappropriately, resulting in a rise in cellular calcium levels. Furthermore, it is thought that dantrolene reverses such an elevation. Nonetheless, the syndrome of MH may result from derangements at several sites. We simply do not know.

Inheritance

That more than one derangement in cellular physiology may result in MH may help to explain apparent vagaries in patterns of inheritance. McPherson and Taylor report a 50% frequency of autosomal dominant inheritance.[6] However, about 20% of families in their study seemed to have either recessive or multifactorial inheritance.

Intraoperative Diagnosis

Increased end-tidal CO_2 appears very early in the course of MH and should alert the anesthesiologist to rapidly and aggressively determine the etiology of the hypercarbia. Arterial blood gases will show hypoxemia, hypercarbia, and acidosis. In cases of MH, the degree of hypercarbia and acidosis may be quite dramatic. $Paco_2$ is often considerably more than 80 mm Hg, and pH is not infrequently in the 6.8 to 7.1 range.

Other laboratory concomitants include, eventually, hyperkalemia, hypermagnesemia, myoglobinemia with myoglobinuria, as well as elevated pyrurate, lactate, serum CPK, and aldolase values.

As previously stated, increases in body temperature may occur relatively late in the course of MH. However, it seems essential to carefully monitor continuously the body temperature of every patient receiving general anesthesia.

Screening Tests for Malignant Hyperthermia Susceptibility

Testing for MH is another controversial topic. Clearly, the most reliable and accurate test is the in vitro exposure of fresh biopsy muscle specimens to halothane and caffeine. An accentuated contracture response to halothane and caffeine is indicative of MH susceptibility. However, this test needs to be standardized since some laboratories test the response to caffeine only or halothane only, whereas others combine the two. Toward the goal of standardization, MHAUS in cooperation with the MHAC sponsored a workshop in November 1987, inviting investigators from the 17 North American laboratories currently performing the test to develop uniformity in the performance and reporting of the muscle biopsy test.

The calcium uptake test is currently viewed with disfavor, because it seemed to yield an inordinate number of false positive diagnoses and, hence, has not withstood scrutiny. Another method of ambiguous assistance in diagnosing MH susceptibility is the platelet adenosine triphosphate depletion test.

Serum CPK levels by themselves are nondiagnostic. About one third of MH-susceptible individuals have normal CPK values. Dramatic elevations of CPK levels may have some predictive value, but it is important to appreciate that exercise, stress, certain drugs, recent muscle injury, and other relatively benign conditions all may be associated with elevated CPK levels. However, abnormal serum CPK isoenzyme values may be helpful in establishing susceptibility since only the MM isoenzyme is normally found in adult serum. Hence, in adults, the presence of MB (cardiac) or BB (brain) isoenzyme is considered abnormal.

Recent work by Klip et al.[7] in *The Lancet* suggests that peripheral blood lymphocytes might provide a relatively noninvasive assay to determine susceptibility. The investigators suggested that halothane induces a significant increase in ionized calcium only in the blood of MH patients. If this test proves reliable in humans, it would be a valuable addition to our armamentarium, since certainly the best treatment for MH is prevention. However, at this time, there is no one single test that is completely devoid of false positives or false negatives.

Treatment of Acute Malignant Hyperthermia

Successful treatment of MH is inextricably linked to thorough preparedness, early detection, and aggressive therapy. Every anesthetizing area should have readily available a supply of iced IV fluids, dantrolene, cooling blankets, and a written protocol for counteracting MH.

Once the diagnosis of MH is made, inhalation anesthetics and succinylcholine should be immediately discontinued and the anesthetic tubing from the machine changed, lest any soluble volatile agent remain in the rubber tubing. The patient should be vigorously hyperventilated with 100% oxygen. An initial dose of 2.5 mg of dantrolene/kg is given intravenously as rapidly as possible, and 1 to 2 mEq of bicarbonate/kg is usually indicated. Additional doses of bicarbonate are titrated to arterial blood gases, and further doses of dantrolene are titrated to the patient's temperature elevation, degree of muscle rigidity, and cardiac status.

Arrhythmia control frequently follows dantrolene therapy and correction of acid-base and electrolyte status. However, procaine or procainamide may be necessary. Procainamide may be given over a 10-minute interval in a dose of 1 gm/70 kg, or 15 mg/kg, diluted in 500 ml of saline solution. Cardiovascular status must be carefully monitored for signs of myocardial depression.

Rapid correction of body temperature elevation is likewise critical, and appropriate methods include external ice packs, cooling blankets, and gastric, wound, and rectal lavage as well as rapid infusion of liberal amounts of iced saline. Other cooling methods have included peritoneal dialysis and cardiopulmonary bypass. Cooling should be discontinued once the body temperature falls to 38°C.

Urine output should be maintained by generous fluid administration and by the use of furosemide and mannitol. Insertion of a Foley catheter is essential to adequately monitor urine output. Prevention of renal failure secondary to myoglobin casts can usually be accomplished by keeping urinary output above 2 ml/kg every hour.

Temperature, ECG, urinary output, and central venous pressure should be continuously monitored. Arterial blood gas and serum electrolyte values should be frequently monitored. During and after the MH episode, hyperkalemia and then hypokalemia, hypercalcemia, and DIC can be observed. Over the next several hours, the MH patient will be very sensitive to iatrogenic potassium administration, even though previously hyperkalemic plasma levels fall precipitously once the temperature of the patient returns to normal. Plasma levels of 2 mEq/L are not unusual. Potassium replacement should rarely, if ever, be used because potassium may retrigger an MH episode.

In the early postepisode period, recrudescence may be a problem. Scrupulous monitoring of the patient over several hours is mandatory. There are no all-inclusive guidelines concerning the dose and duration of dantrolene therapy after apparent resolution of the acute MH episode. However, in fulminant cases, it seems advisable to continue 1 to 2 mg of dantrolene/kg every 4 to 6 hours for at least 24 hours.

Be aware that in addition to recrudescence, late complications of MH include renal failure, consumption coagulopathy, muscle necrosis, neurologic deficits, and inadvertent hypothermia.

An MH hot-line exists, and the number is 209-634-4917.

Management of the Malignant Hyperthermia–Susceptible Patient

Malignant hyperthermia–susceptible patients requiring anesthesia should be adequately reassured that the anesthetic implications of MH are known and that appropriate therapeutic modalities and monitoring will be employed. Dantrolene and iced saline must be available.

Some who believe that anxiety may predispose to MH susceptibility favor generous premedication. "Safe" agents include narcotics, benzodiazepines, barbiturates, and antihistamines. The phenothiazines, however, should be avoided since there are similarities between MH and the NMS.

Except for those patients scheduled for muscle biopsy for MH diagnosis, IV dantrolene pretreatment may be given in a dose of 2.5 mg/kg over a 15- to 30-minute interval immediately prior to surgery. Oral dantrolene prophylaxis is no longer thought to be efficacious.

An anesthetic machine devoid of vaporizers and with a disposable anesthetic circuit and freshly changed CO_2 absorbent is recommended, as is the use of capnography. Of course, continuous monitoring of body temperature is necessary. Arterial and central venous monitoring are employed as indicated by the nature of the surgical procedure.

Regional, local, or major conduction anesthesia is suggested due to their known safety. However, if general anesthesia is required, as is often the case in ear, nose, and throat surgery, a variety of agents may be safely used. These include barbiturates, narcotics, benzodiazepines, nitrous oxide, and most nondepolarizing muscle relaxants. (At worst, nitrous oxide may have some weak triggering properties.) Reversal of nondepolarizing relaxants has been a moot point, but it appears that use of neostigmine and atropine is appropriate.[8] Agents to be absolutely avoided are all of the potent inhalation agents, all depolarizing muscle relaxants, choline, and potassium.

In the absence of intraoperative signs of MH, most authorities do not advocate continuing dantrolene therapy into the postoperative period. However, at least 8 hours of close postoperative observation are mandatory.

Summary

Malignant hyperthermia, especially the abortive form, is probably more common than initially thought. Although much has been learned about MH since the first description of the syndrome more than 30 years ago, many questions still remain unanswered. Nonetheless, impressive strides have been made in reducing anesthetic mortality due to MH.

Vigilance is the sine qua non of safe anesthetic practice. It behooves the anesthesiologist to take a thorough personal and family anesthetic history and to monitor temperature continuously on all patients having general anesthesia. A written management protocol for MH as well as adequate supplies of dantrolene and iced IV infusions must be available in all anesthetizing areas. Furthermore, it is imperative to investigate promptly unexplained rises in temperature and changes in muscle tone, especially when they are linked to tachycardia and dysrhythmias.

PHARMACOLOGIC COMPLICATIONS

Lidocaine Toxicity

Systemic toxic reactions to lidocaine, or to any local anesthetic, occur when the anesthetic is administered in a fashion such that its rate of absorption exceeds its rate of destruction. This imbalance can be due to the injection of an excessive dose (either excessive concentration or volume or both). An accelerated rate of absorption may also result from the presence of lacerated veins or even from normally rich vascularity at the site of injection, from a very rapid rate of injection, or from application to mucous membranes or abraded skin. Of course, toxic reactions may also be due to unintentional intravascular injection, even of a therapeutic dose, because it is the sudden increase in systemic concentration that causes the reaction. Systemic toxic reactions may also be due to a decreased rate of detoxification of the local anesthetic. The detoxification rate is related to the chemical composition of the drug, and hence, its mode of metabolism, the functional status of the detoxifying organ, and the metabolic rate of the patient. Other factors that influence the development of a toxic reaction include the use of concurrent medications, the patient's general physical status

and acid-base balance (acidosis decreases the toxicity threshold), and variable and unpredictable individual sensitivity.

The signs and symptoms of CNS toxic reactions are manifested along a concentration-related spectrum. Drowsiness may be the first early subjective sign of local anesthetic toxicity, followed by light headedness, dizziness, tinnitus, a metallic taste, nausea, circumoral tingling or numbness, or blurred vision. Objectively, confusion, slurred speech, nystagmus, and muscle twitches or tremors can be noted.

Further along the spectrum of toxicity are gross convulsions. Drowsiness progresses to loss of consciousness, and muscle twitches progress to generalized tonic-clonic seizures. Cyanosis may appear if ventilation is impeded by seizure activity. Tachycardia and hypertension may occur as a sympathetic response to hypoxia and hypercarbia, but hypotension sometimes develops secondary to myocardial depressant effects of the local anesthetic.

There is an inverse relationship between the blood levels necessary to generate toxic symptoms and the relative potency of local anesthetic agents. For lidocaine, a level of 4 μg/mL is thought to be the threshold for early symptoms. However, with the more potent agent bupivacaine, toxicity begins to occur in the 2 μg/mL range. Wikinski et al.,[9] using lidocaine for psychiatric shock therapy, found a mean plasma level of 22 μg/mL at the time of convulsion.

Although local anesthetic agents can produce profound effects on the cardiovascular system, in general the cardiovascular system appears to be more resistant than the CNS. As the blood level of a local anesthetic approaches toxic concentrations, a decrease in blood pressure may be observed. This initial hypotension appears to be due to the negative inotropic action of local anesthetics more than to peripheral vasodilation. However, if it remains unchecked, ultimately decreased myocardial contractility and depressed heart rate and conductivity will combine with peripheral vasodilation to result in circulatory collapse and cardiac arrest.

As previously mentioned, alterations in acid-base status will influence the potential cardiovascular and CNS toxicity of local anesthetic agents. Hypercarbia and acidosis decrease the threshold for convulsive activity and augment the cardiodepressant effect of local anesthetics.

The best treatment for systemic toxic reactions is prevention. Hence, aspirate carefully prior to injecting at any site, inject slowly and cautiously, and use the optimum dose (i.e., minimum concentration and volume) for the desired effect. For lidocaine, the maximum suggested dose for infiltration is 4 mg/kg of plain solution and 7 mg/kg of epinephrine-containing solution.

Should the patient experience a mild reaction, observe him or her closely since the reaction may become more severe. Administer oxygen by face mask. If convulsions occur, assist ventilation by bag and mask with 100% oxygen, and administer an appropriate anticonvulsant. Diazepam (5–10 mg) or thiopental (50–100 mg) can be given intravenously. Convulsions are usually of brief duration, about 60 seconds or less. If they persist, succinylcholine administration and endotracheal intubation may be necessary to assure an adequate airway and proper oxygenation.

If cardiorespiratory collapse ensues, all of these measures may be necessary, as well as mechanical ventilation plus circulatory support with fluids and vasopressors. Closed-chest cardiac massage and resuscitative drugs should be given as indicated, with attention paid to acid-base status.

Since the possibility of this dramatic range of reactions is present every time local anesthesia is given, it is axiomatic that an IV line be established prior to administration of local anesthetics. Furthermore, lidocaine and other local agents should be given only in areas where adequate resuscitative equipment and properly trained personnel are readily available.

Cocaine Toxicity

Cocaine hydrochloride is the only local anesthetic that inherently produces vasoconstriction and shrinkage of mucous membranes. Hence, cocaine is extremely popular as a topical agent in nasal surgery. The drug is so well absorbed from mucosal surfaces that plasma concentrations comparable with those following direct IV injection are achieved. Since cocaine interferes with catecholamine uptake, it has a sympathetic potentiating effect.

An ester-linked benzoic acid, cocaine is rapidly hydrolyzed by plasma pseudocholinesterase to benzoyl escogonine. Such factors as echothiophate eye drops, liver dysfunction, and atypical pseudocholinesterase conditions will influence the metabolism of cocaine, but generally, with intranasal cocaine, a peak plasma concentration is reached within 1 hour and persists for 4 hours.[10]

Historically, epinephrine had often been mixed with cocaine in hope of enhancing the degree of vasoconstriction produced. This practice is both superfluous and deleterious since cocaine is a potent vasoconstrictor in its own right, and the combination of epinephrine with cocaine may trigger dangerous arrhythmias. It has been shown that cocaine used alone, without epinephrine, to shrink the nasal mucosa does not sensitize the heart to endogenous epinephrine during halothane or enflurane anesthesia.[11] However, animal studies have shown that following pretreatment with exogenous epinephrine, cocaine facilitates the development of epinephrine-induced arrhythmias during halothane.[12]

The usual maximum dose of cocaine employed in clinical practice is 200 mg for a 70 kg adult, or 3 mg/kg. However, 1.5 mg/kg is preferable if a volatile anesthetic agent is being used concomitantly since this lower dose has been shown not to exert any clinically significant sympathomimetic effect in combination with halothane.[13] Although 1 gm is considered to be the usual lethal dose for an adult, considerable variation occurs. Furthermore, systemic reactions may appear with as little as 20 mg.

Cocaine is commonly applied on pledgets or neurosurgical cottonoids as a 4% solution. Direct spraying may cause a greater amount to be absorbed. As a rule, similar doses can be applied more safely to the nasal mucosa than to the tracheobronchial mucosa, where uptake is especially rapid. It is obvious that meticulous attention must be paid to the volume used since there is a narrow range from safety, to toxicity, to death.

Meyers described two cases of cocaine toxicity during dacryocystorhinostomy, emphasizing that cocaine is contraindicated in hypertensives or in patients receiving alpha-modifying drugs such as guanethidine, reserpine, tricyclic antidepressants, or monoamine oxidase inhibitors.[14] In addition, sympathomimetics such as previously mentioned epinephrine hydrochloride or phenylephrine hydrochloride should not be given with cocaine.

Signs of cocaine toxicity are referable to the CNS, respiratory system, and cardiovascular system. The patient rapidly becomes excited, anxious, garrulous, and confused. Reflexes are augmented. Headache is common. The pulse becomes rapid and respiration erratic. A chill may herald the sudden onset of hyperthermia. The pupils become dilated, and exophthalmos occurs. Nausea, vomiting, and abdominal pain are common. The patient may complain of something crawling on his or her skin. Delirium, Cheyne-Stokes breathing, convulsions, and unconsciousness occur terminally. Indeed, death may be very rapid following acute cocaine overdosage, and therapeutic maneuvers must be performed with alacrity.

Before administering cocaine, the physician should carefully search out possible contraindications, including the use of certain concurrent medications. To avoid toxic levels, one should meticulously calculate and carefully administer doses of dilute solutions. Should serious cardiovascular effects occur, labetalol may be given.[15] Previously propranolol was widely used to control cocaine-induced hypertension.[16] However, a lethal hypertensive exacerbation has been attributed to unopposed alpha stimulation.[17] Labetalol thus offers the distinct advantage of both alpha and beta blockade. Intravenous barbiturates should be given to combat the CNS symptoms of cocaine toxicity. Cooling measures may be required for hyperthermia. These include use of a cooling blanket and ice water or alcohol sponging. In the unfortunate event of cardiovascular arrest, the usual resuscitative measures may be attempted.

Epinephrine-Halothane Interaction

Epinephrine is a commonly used vasoconstrictor in ear, nose, and throat surgery and is one of the most potent vasopressor drugs known. Epinephrine stimulates α_1-β_1-, and β_2-receptors and as such appears to interact with volatile anesthetic agents to induce cardiac arrhythmias. When the topic of epinephrine-induced cardiac arrhythmias is considered, it is important to realize that laboratory investigations have used primarily the dog as the animal model and that the canine myocardium is more resistant to the production of epinephrine-induced arrhythmias than is the human myocardium. Thus, arrhythmogenic doses in dogs are not applicable in humans at equivalent doses. However, comparisons between volatile anesthetic agent effects and relative changes are valid.

Sensitization of the myocardium has come to be defined clinically as a state in which the dose of epinephrine required to trigger an arrhythmia is less than the dose in the awake state. However, this is actually a misnomer since true pharmacologic sensitization involves inhibition of the adrenergic nerve membrane situated amine pump uptake mechanism, such as one sees with cocaine. Nonetheless, although the hydrocarbon anesthetics are not true sensitizers of receptors, the term myocardial sensitization endures.

The mechanism of so-called myocardial sensitization is incompletely understood. Nevertheless, the primary mechanism is probably related to an interaction on the myocardium that fosters favorable conditions for the generation of ectopic foci and reentrant arrhythmias.[18]

The worst offender of commonly employed clinical agents in terms of myocardial sensitization is halothane. Shortly after the introduction of halothane, guidelines were promulgated so that epinephrine could be safely used with halothane anesthesia, provided that precautions with regard to dose, concentration, and time course of administration were followed. The guidelines written by Katz and Katz[19] in 1966 proposed that:

1. Only solutions of epinephrine 1:100,000 or 1:200,000 be used. (In fact, more concentrated solutions do not necessarily afford increased vasoconstriction in the injected area.)
2. In any given 10-minute interval, an adult dose should not exceed 10 mL of 1:100,000 epinephrine.
3. In any given 1-hour interval, an adult dose should not exceed 30 mL of epinephrine 1:100,000.
4. Hypoxia and hypercarbia are to be avoided.

One should be aware there are many modifying factors that may alter the arrhythmogenic dose of epinephrine in a particular clinical setting. Factors such as the speed of injection, site of injection, and the presence of hypercarbia, hypocarbia, and hypoxia all may influence the epinephrine-halothane interaction. Concomitant use of adrenergic modifying drugs such as methyldopa, cocaine, tricyclic antidepressants, reserpine, monoamine oxidase inhibitors, and guanethidine is especially hazardous. Furthermore, aminophylline also lowers the arrhythmogenic dose of epinephrine under halothane anesthesia.

Fortunately, the pediatric population has been shown to be fairly resistant to the arrhythmogenic effects of epinephrine combined with halothane.[20] And other vasoconstrictors, such as ephedrine or phenylephrine, are much less likely to trigger arrhythmias under halothane anesthesia.[21]

Isoflurane has the widest margin of safety with respect to the arrhythmogenic dose of epinephrine. Indeed, other factors being equal, isoflurane should be the volatile agent of choice when injection of epinephrine is anticipated. Even with isoflurane, the dose of epinephrine should be limited to 5.4 μg/kg.

Risk of epinephrine-induced arrhythmias may be minimized by restricting the dose of submucosal epinephrine to 1.5 μg/kg during halothane anesthesia.[22] However, addition of 0.5% lidocaine as a vehicle for the epinephrine increases the dose of epinephrine, which triggers ventricular irritability by almost 50%.[22]

Management of epinephrine-induced arrhythmias under anesthesia is inextricably linked to prevention by using judicious doses of epinephrine and by adequately ventilating the patient. Furthermore, a thorough knowledge of the patient's drug history is essential. Should serious arrhythmias transpire, despite adherence to these guidelines, halothane should be discontin-

ued and another agent selected. The patient should be vigorously ventilated and the acid-base status determined. Lidocaine (1 mg/kg) should be given intravenously as indicated for ventricular irritability.

REFERENCES

1. Denborough MA, Forster JFA, Lovell RRH, et al: Anaesthetic deaths in a family. *Lancet* 1960; 2:45.
2. Ording H: Incidence of malignant hyperthermia in Denmark. *Anesth Analg* 1985; 64:700–704.
3. Rosenberg H, Reed S: *In vitro* contracture tests for susceptibility to malignant hyperthermia. *Anesth Analg* 1983; 62:415–420.
4. Schwartz L, Rockoff MA, Koka BV: Masseter spasm with anesthesia: Incidence and implications. *Anesthesiology* 1984; 61:772–775.
5. Rosenberg H, Fletcher JE: Masseter muscle rigidity and malignant hyperthermia susceptibility. *Anesth Analg* 1986; 65:161–164.
6. McPherson EW, Taylor CA: Genetics of malignant hyperthermia: Evidence for heterogeneity. *Am J Med Genet* 1982; 11:273–285.
7. Klip A, Elliott ME, Frodis W, et al: Anaesthetic induced increase in ionized calcium in blood mononuclear cells from malignant hyperthermia patients. *Lancet* 1987; 1:463.
8. Larach MG, Rosenberg H: Evaluation and management of pediatric patients for diagnostic muscle biopsy for malignant hyperthermia susceptibility. *Anesthesiology* 1983; 59:A228.
9. Wikinski JA, Usubiaga JE, Morales RL, et al: Mechanism of convulsions elicited by local anesthetics. *Anesth Analg* 1970; 49:504–510.
10. Johns ME, Berman A, Price JC, et al: Metabolism of intranasally applied cocaine. *Ann Otolaryngol* 1977; 86:342.
11. Chung B, Naraghi M, Adriani J: Sympathetic effects of cocaine and their influence on halothane and enflurane anesthesia. *Anesthesiol Rev* 1978; 5:16.
12. Koehntop DE, Liao J, Van Bergen FH: Effects of pharmacologic alterations of adrenergic mechanisms by cocaine, tropolone, aminophylline, and ketamine on epinephrine-induced arrhythmias during halothane-N_2O anesthesia. *Anesthesiology* 1977; 46:83.
13. Barash PG, Kopriva CJ, Langon R, et al: Is cocaine a sympathetic stimulant during general anesthesia? *JAMA* 1980; 243:1437.
14. Meyers EF: Cocaine toxicity during dacryocystorhinostomy. *Arch Ophthalmol* 1980; 98:842.
15. Gay GR, Loper KA: Control of cocaine-induced hypertension with labetalol. *Anesth Analg* 1988; 67:92.
16. Rappolt RT, Gay GR, Inaba DS: Propranolol: A specific antagonist to cocaine. *Clin Toxicol* 1977; 10:265.
17. Ramoska E, Sacchetti AD: Propranolol-induced hypertension in treatment of cocaine intoxication. *Ann Emerg Med* 1985; 14:1112–1113.
18. Reynod AK: On the mechanism of myocardial sensitization to catecholamines by hydrocarbon anesthetics. *Can J Physiol Pharmacol* 1984; 62:183.
19. Katz RL, Katz GJ: Surgical infiltration of pressor drugs and their interaction with volatile anaesthetics. *Br J Anaesth* 1966; 38:712.

20. Karl HW, et al: Epinephrine-halothane interactions in children. *Anesthesiology* 1983; 58:142.
21. Tucker WK, Packstein AD, Munson ES: Comparison of arrhythmogenic doses of adrenaline, metaraminol, ephedrine and phenylephrine during isoflurane and halothane anesthesia in dogs. *Br J Anaesth* 1974; 46:392.
22. Johnston RR, Eger EI, Wilson C: Comparative interaction of epinephrine with enflurane, isoflurane, and halothane in man. *Anesth Analg* 1976; 55:709.

Index